Seventh Edition

POLICY & POLITICS

in Nursing and Health Care

Diana J. Mason, PhD, RN, FAAN
Rudin Professor of Nursing
Co-Director of the Center for Health, Media, and Policy
School of Nursing
Hunter College
City University of New York
New York, New York

Deborah B. Gardner, PhD, RN, FAAN, FNAP
Health Policy and Leadership Consultant, LLC
Honolulu, Hawaii

Freida Hopkins Outlaw, PhD, RN, FAAN
Adjunct Professor
Peabody College of Education
Vanderbilt University
Nashville, Tennessee

Eileen T. O'Grady, PhD, NP, RN
Nurse Practitioner and Wellness Coach
McLean, Virginia

ELSEVIER

ELSEVIER

3251 Riverport Lane
St. Louis, Missouri 63043

POLICY & POLITICS IN NURSING AND HEALTH CARE   ISBN: 978-0-323-24144-1

Previous editions copyrighted 2014, 2012, 2007, 2002, 1998, 1993, and 1985.

Library of Congress Cataloging-in-Publication Data
Policy & politics in nursing and health care / [edited by] Diana J. Mason, Deborah B. Gardner, Freida Hopkins Outlaw, Eileen T. O'Grady.—Seventh edition.
     p.; cm.
  Policy and politics in nursing and health care
  Includes bibliographical references and index.
  ISBN 978-0-323-24144-1 (pbk. : alk. paper)
  I. Mason, Diana J., 1948-, editor. II. Gardner, Deborah B., editor. III. Outlaw, Freida Hopkins, editor. IV. O'Grady, Eileen T., 1963-, editor. V. Title: Policy and politics in nursing and health care.
  [DNLM: 1. Nursing–United States. 2. Delivery of Health Care–United States. 3. Politics–United States. 4. Public Policy–United States. WY 16 AA1]
  RT86.5
  362.17′3–dc23
                                                                2015008880

Senior Content Strategist: Sandra Clark
Content Development Manager: Laurie Gower
Senior Content Development Specialist: Karen Turner
Content Development Specialist: Jennifer Wade
Publishing Services Manager: Jeff Patterson
Senior Project Manager: Clay S. Broeker
Design Direction: Ashley Miner

Printed in the United States of America

Last digit is the print number: 9   8   7   6   5   4   3   2   1

Working together to grow libraries in developing countries

www.elsevier.com • www.bookaid.org

DIANA J. MASON, PhD, RN, FAAN, is the Rudin Professor of Nursing and Co-Founder and Co-Director of the Center for Health, Media, and Policy (CHMP) at Hunter College and Professor at the City University of New York. She served as President of the American Academy of Nursing (2013-2015) and as Strategic Adviser for the Campaign for Action, an initiative to implement the recommendations from the Institute of Medicine's *Future of Nursing* report, to which she contributed. From 2012 to 2015 she served as Co-President of the Hermann Biggs Society, an interdisciplinary health policy salon in New York City.

Dr. Mason was editor-in-chief of the *American Journal of Nursing* for over a decade. Under her leadership, the journal received numerous awards for editorial excellence and dissemination, culminating in the journal being selected by the Specialized Libraries Association in 2009 as one of the 100 most influential Journals of the Century in Biology and Medicine—the only nursing journal to be selected for this distinction.

As a journalist, she has produced and moderated a weekly radio program on health and health policy *(Healthstyles)* for 30 years. She blogs for *HealthCetera (www.centerforhealthmediapolicy.com)* and for the *JAMA News Forum*. In 2009, she was appointed to the National Advisory Committee for Kaiser Health News—the only nurse and health professional on the Committee.

She is the lead co-editor of *The Nursing Profession: Development, Challenges, and Opportunities,* part of the Robert Wood Johnson Foundation Health Policy Book Series. She has been the lead co-editor of all seven editions of *Policy & Politics in Nursing and Health Care.*

She is the recipient of numerous honors, including Honorary Doctorates from Long Island University and West Virginia University; fellowship in the New York Academy of Medicine; and the Pioneering Spirit Award from the American Association of Critical Care Nurses.

DEBORAH B. GARDNER, PhD, RN, FAAN, FNAP, is a health policy and leadership consultant. She has more than 35 years of health care experience as a clinician, manager, trainer, and consultant delivering care across diverse institutional and community settings. Dr. Gardner practiced as a psychiatric mental health clinical nurse specialist for 15 years. She received a PhD in Nursing Administration and Health Policy from George Mason University.

At the National Institutes of Health (NIH) Clinical Center she established and held the position as the Director of Organizational Planning and Workforce Development for 10 years. She served at the Bureau of Health Professionals, Health Resources and Services Administration (HRSA) as a senior consultant collaborating on the implementation of the Affordable Care Act (ACA) (2010-2012). As the Director of the Hawaii State Center for Nursing, she led the State's Campaign for Action Coalition, a Robert Wood Johnson Foundation Initiative to support the Institute of Medicine's *Future of Nursing* report.

In 2012 she served as a member of the Hawaii Governor's Healthcare Transformation Steering Committee to assess and refocus Hawaii's health care delivery system for alignment to the ACA goals.

A Fellow in the American Academy of Nursing and in the National Academy of Practice, she was instrumental in establishing the National Center for Interprofessional Practice and Education in Minneapolis, Minnesota. She has received numerous awards, including the HRSA Administrator's Special Citation for National Leadership in Interprofessional Education and Collaborative Practice, an International Coaching Federation Award for Excellence in the Establishment of an Outstanding Executive Coaching Program, the NIH Director's Award for Outstanding Mentoring and Innovation in Organizational Development Strategies, and the "Profiles in Excellence" alumni honors award from Oklahoma Baptist University.

Dr. Gardner has written numerous book chapters and articles. She serves on the Editorial Board for *Nursing Economic$* and writes the Policy and Politics column. She is a professional speaker on interprofessional practice and education teams, advanced practice nursing, and health policy issues.

FREIDA HOPKINS OUTLAW, PhD, RN, FAAN, is an adjunct professor in the Peabody College of Education, Vanderbilt University, Nashville, Tennessee. She served as the Assistant Commissioner, Division of Special Populations, Tennessee Department of Mental Health and Substance Abuse Services. In this role, she helped to develop policies and initiatives that improved treatment for children with mental health and substance abuse issues. She provided leadership in securing $32 million of federal funding to support transforming the mental health system for children and their families and was part of the leadership instrumental in passing legislation to create the Children's Mental Health Council, which developed a plan for a statewide system of care implementation, which continues today.

She participated in the American Nurses Association Minority Fellowship Legislative Internship Program. Her passion was further ignited when state and national policies impacted delivery of mental health services to children and their families to which she provided mental health services at the University of Pennsylvania nurse-managed health center. Dr. Outlaw received a Department of Health and Human Services Policy Academy Grant to lead a team of child-serving agencies, community stakeholders, families, and youth to work on transforming mental health care for children and families through planning, policy, and practice. Dr. Outlaw a member of the Robert Wood Johnson Foundation (RWJF) Collaborative National Advisory Committee, whose function is to advise the faculty of the RWJF Nursing and Health Policy Collaborative, University of New Mexico, College of Nursing. She is a Fellow in the American Academy of Nursing and is an active member of the Psychiatric Mental Health and Substance Abuse Expert Panel.

She has written frequently on the areas of depression, impact of racism, and stress on the health of African Americans; management of aggression; seclusion and restraint; religion, spirituality, and the meaning of prayer for people with cancer; and children's mental health. She has received recognition for her excellence in clinical practice and for her work to improve the mental health of children and their families.

EILEEN T. O'GRADY, PhD, NP, RN, is a certified Nurse Practitioner and Wellness Coach who uses an evidence-based approach with people to reverse or prevent disease. She believes deeply that more attention must be paid to getting us unstuck from lifestyles that do not support wellness.

She speaks professionally at universities, associations, corporations, schools, and communities on the importance of thoughtful self-care, patient engagement, and how to identify and remedy a life that is out of balance. She is currently adjunct faculty in the Graduate Schools of Nursing at Pace University, Georgetown University, Duke University, and George Washington University, where she was given an Outstanding Teacher Award.

She has held a number of leadership positions with professional nursing associations, most notably as a founder and vice chair of the American College of Nurse Practitioners (now the American Association of Nurse Practitioners). She was a 1999 Policy Fellow in the U.S. Public Health Service Primary Care Policy Fellowship and in 2003 was given the American College of Nurse Practitioners Legislative Advocacy Award for her leadership on nurse practitioner policy issues. She is the 2013 recipient of the Loretta Ford Lifetime Achievement Award and the Virginia Council of Nurse Practitioners Advocate of the Year Award.

She is a co-editor and author of *Advanced Practice Nursing: An Integrative Approach,* 5th edition (Elsevier, 2013) and has authored numerous articles and book chapters as well as a monthly column on advanced practice nursing and health policy for 10 years in *Nurse Practitioner World News.*

She has taught nurses and physicians both nationally and internationally with the U.S. Peace Corps. Dr. O'Grady has practiced as a primary care provider for 15 years and is now certified as a life coach through the International Coaching Federation and as an Adult Nurse Practitioner through the American Nurses Credentialing Center. Dr. O'Grady holds three graduate degrees: a Master of Public Health from George Washington University, a Master of Science in Nursing, and a Doctor of Philosophy in Nursing/Health Policy from George Mason University. She has dual citizenship in Ireland and the United States. *www.eileenogrady.net*

Contributors

Greg Abell
Principal
Sound Options Group, LLC
Bainbridge Island, Washington

Charles R. Alexandre, PhD, RN
Director
Quality and Regulation
Butler Hospital
Providence, Rhode Island

Carmen Alvarez, PhD, C-NP, CNM
Julio Bellber Post-Doctoral Fellow
Department of Health Policy
George Washington University
Washington, DC

Angela Frederick Amar, PhD, RN, FAAN
Assistant Dean for BSN Education and Associate
    Professor
Nell Hodgson Woodruff School of Nursing
Emory University
Atlanta, Georgia

Coral T. Andrews, MBA, RN, FACHE
Founding Executive Director
Hawaii Health Connector
Honolulu, Hawaii

Susan Apold, PhD, RN, ANP-BC, FAAN, FAANP
Robert Wood Johnson Foundation Executive
    Nurse Fellow
Clinical Professor of Nursing
New York University
New York, New York

Kenya V. Beard, EdD, GNP-BC, NP-C, ACNP-BC,
CNE
Associate Vice President for Curriculum and
    Instruction
Director
Center Multicultural Education and Health
    Disparities
Jersey College
Teterboro, New Jersey

Mary L. Behrens, MS, FNP-BC, FAANP
Family Nurse Practitioner
Westside Woman's Clinic
Casper, Wyoming

Susan I. Belanger, PhD, MA, RN, NEA-BC
Director
Education, Training, and Research
Sibley Memorial Hospital/Johns Hopkins
    Medicine
Assistant Professor
School of Nursing and Health Studies
Georgetown University
Washington, DC

Katherine N. Bent, RN, PhD, CNS
Assistant Commissioner, Compliance Policy
U.S. Food and Drug Administration
Silver Spring, Maryland

Jonathan Bentley, BS, RN
RN Care Coordinator
Harris Regional Hospital
Sylva, North Carolina

Carmina Bernardo, MA, MPH
Doctor of Public Health Student
Health Policy and Management Track
Graduate Center
City University of New York
New York, New York

Virginia Trotter Betts, MSN, JD, RN, FAAN
President and Chief Executive Officer
HealthFutures, Inc.
Nashville, Tennessee

Linda Burnes Bolton, DrPH, RN, FAAN
Vice President, Nursing and Chief Nursing Officer
Cedars-Sinai Medical Center
Los Angeles, California

Marilyn Waugh Bouldin, MSN, RN, PNP
Member
Board of Directors
Heart of the Rockies Regional Medical Center
Retired Director
Chaffee County Public Health
Salida, Colorado

Rebecca (Rice) Bowers-Lanier, EdD, MSN, MPH, RN
President
B2L Consulting
Richmond, Virginia

Patricia K. Bradley, PhD, RN, FAAN
Associate Professor
College of Nursing
Villanova University
Villanova, Pennsylvania

Edie Brous, MS, MPH, JD, RN
Nurse Attorney
New York, New York

Mary Lou Brunell, MSN, RN
Executive Director
Florida Center for Nursing
Co-Lead
Florida Action Coalition
Orlando, Florida

Kelly Buettner-Schmidt, PhD, RN
Associate Professor of Nursing
North Dakota State University
Fargo, North Dakota

Josepha E. Burnley, DNP, FNP-C
Nurse Consultant
Health Resources and Services Administration
Rockville, Maryland

Rachel Burton
Research Associate
Health Policy Center
Urban Institute
Washington, DC

Ann Campbell, MPH, MSN, AGPCNP-BC, RN
Primary and Palliative Care Nurse Practitioner
Mary Manning Walsh Home
Integrative Health Nurse Practitioner
The Original Bloom
New York, New York

Demetrius Chapman, PhD(c), MPH, MSN(R), APRN, PHCNS-BC
Associate Director
New Mexico Board of Nursing
Albuquerque, New Mexico

Peggy L. Chinn, PhD, RN, FAAN
Professor Emerita
University of Connecticut
Editor
Advances in Nursing Science
Oakland, California

Yoon Jeong Choi, MSN, MPhil, RN
PhD Candidate
School of Nursing
Columbia University
New York, New York

Glenda Christiaens, PhD, RN, AHN-BC
Former President
American Holistic Nurses Association
Salt Lake City, Utah

Mary Ann Christopher, MSN, RN, FAAN
Consultant
Avon, New Jersey

Angela K. Clark, MSN, PhD(c), RN
Graduate Student
College of Nursing
University of Cincinnati
Cincinnati, Ohio

Sean P. Clarke, PhD, RN, FAAN
Professor and Associate Dean
Undergraduate Programs
William F. Connell School of Nursing
Boston College
Chestnut Hill, Massachusetts

Sally S. Cohen, PhD, RN, FAAN
IOM/AAN/ANA/ANF Distinguished Nurse
   Scholar-in-Residence (2014-2015)
Virginia P. Crenshaw Endowed Chair
Director
Robert Wood Johnson Foundation Nursing and
   Health Policy Collaborative
College of Nursing
University of New Mexico
Albuquerque, New Mexico

Judith B. Collins, RNC, MS, WHNP, FAAN
Faculty Emerita
Schools of Nursing and Medicine
Founding Director
Health Policy Office and Women's Health Center
Virginia Commonwealth University
Richmond, Virginia

Karen S. Cox, PhD, FACHE, RN, FAAN
Executive Vice President and Co-Chief Operating
   Officer
Children's Mercy Kansas City
Kansas City, Missouri

Barbara I.H. Damron, PhD, RN, FAAN
Secretary
New Mexico Higher Education Department
Santa Fe, New Mexico

Patricia D'Antonio, PhD, RN, FAAN
Killebrew-Censtis Term Professor in
   Undergraduate Nursing Education
Senior Fellow
Leonard Davis Institute of Health Economics
School of Nursing
University of Pennsylvania
Philadelphia, Pennsylvania

C. Christine Delnat, MSN, RN
Assistant Professor
Department of Nursing
St. Mary-of-the-Woods College
Terre Haute, Indiana

Erin M. Denholm, MSN, RN, RWJENF
SVP Clinical Transformation
Centura Health
Denver, Colorado

Catherine M. Dentinger, FNP, MPH
Career Epidemiology Field Officer
New York City Department of Health and Mental
   Hygiene
Centers for Disease Control and Prevention
New York, New York

Betty R. Dickson, BS
Retired Contract Lobbyist
Barnardsville, North Carolina

Michele J. Eliason, PhD
Associate Professor
Department of Health Education
San Francisco State University
San Francisco, California

Jeanette Ives Erickson, RN, DNP, FAAN,
NEA-BC
Chief Nurse and Senior Vice President for Patient
   Care
Massachusetts General Hospital
Boston, Massachusetts

Carroll L. Estes, PhD
Professor of Sociology
Founding Director
Institute for Health and Aging
University of California, San Francisco
San Francisco, California

Robin Dawson Estrada, PhD, PNP-BC, RN
Assistant Professor
College of Nursing
University of South Carolina
Columbia, South Carolina

Sandra Evans, MAEd, RN
Executive Director
Idaho Board of Nursing
Boise, Idaho

Julie Fairman, PhD, RN, FAAN
Nightingale Professor in Nursing
Director
Barbara Bates Center for the Study of the History
    of Nursing
Co-Director
Robert Wood Johnson Foundation Future of
    Nursing Scholars Program
School of Nursing
University of Pennsylvania
Philadelphia, Pennsylvania

Lola M. Fehr, MS, CAE, PRP, RN, FAAN
President
Fehr Consulting Resources
Greeley, Colorado

Loretta C. Ford, PNP, EdD, RN, FAAN, FAANP
Professor and Dean Emerita
School of Nursing
University of Rochester, New York

Elizabeth B. Froh, PhD, RN
Clinical Supervisor
Lactation Team and Human Milk Management
    Center
Children's Hospital of Philadelphia
Philadelphia, Pennsylvania

Beth Gharrity Gardner, MA, PhD(c)
PhD Candidate
Department of Sociology
University of California, Irvine
Irvine, California

Catherine Alicia Georges, EdD, RN, FAAN
Professor and Chairperson
Department of Nursing
Lehman College
Bronx, New York

Rosemary Gibson, MSc
Senior Advisor
The Hastings Center
Garrison, New York

Greer Glazer, PhD, RN, CNP, FAAN
Dean
University of Cincinnati College of Nursing
Schmidlapp Professor of Nursing
Cincinnati, Ohio

Barbara Glickstein, MPH, MS, RN
Co-Director
Center for Health, Media and Policy
Hunter College
City University of New York
New York, New York

Bethany Hall-Long, PhD, RNC, FAAN
State Senator
State of Delaware 10th District
Professor of Nursing
University of Delaware
Newark, Delaware

Mary Mincer Hansen, PhD, RN
Adjunct Associate Professor
MPH Program and Global Health Department
Des Moines University
Des Moines, Iowa

Tine Hansen-Turton, MGA, JD, FCPP, FAAN
Chief Executive Officer
National Nursing Centers Consortium
Chief Strategy Officer
Public Health Management Corporation
Philadelphia, Pennsylvania

Charlene Harrington, PhD, RN
Professor Emeritus of Nursing and Sociology
School of Nursing
University of California
San Francisco, California

Mary Ann Hart, MSN, RN
Program Director
Graduate Program in Health Administration
Assistant Professor of Nursing and Health
    Administration
School of Nursing, Science, and Health
    Professions
Regis College
Weston, Massachusetts

Heidi Hartmann, PhD
President
Institute for Women's Policy Research
Research Professor
George Washington University
Washington, DC

Susan B. Hassmiller, PhD, RN, FAAN
Senior Adviser for Nursing
Director
Future of Nursing: Campaign for Action
Robert Wood Johnson Foundation
Princeton, New Jersey

Barbara Hatfield, RN
Former Delegate
West Virginia House
Charleston, West Virginia

Pamela J. Haylock, PhD, RN, FAAN
Oncology Care Consultant
Medina, Texas
Adjunct Instructor
Schreiner University
Kerrville, Texas

Margaret Wainwright Henbest, MSN, RN
Executive Director
Nurse Leaders of Idaho
Boise, Idaho

Karrie Cummings Hendrickson, PhD, MSN, RN
Finance Clinical Coordinator
Department of Analytic Strategy
Yale New Haven Health System
New Haven, Connecticut

Linda Hirota Hevenor, MPH, MS, RN
Director of Patient Safety
Department of Quality and Operational
  Excellence
Lifespan
Providence, Rhode Island

Sarah Hexem, JD
Law and Policy Program Manager
National Nursing Centers Consortium
Philadelphia, Pennsylvania

Anne Hudson, RN, C, BSN
Founder
Work Injured Nurses Group USA
Public Health Nurse
Coos County Public Health Department
Coos Bay, Oregon

Randall Steven Hudspeth, PhD, MS, APRN-CNP/CNS, FRE, FAANP
Executive Clinical Consultant
Hudspeth LLC
Boise, Idaho

Lauren Inouye, MPP, RN
Associate Director of Government Affairs
American Association of Colleges of Nursing
Washington, DC

Brenda Isaac, RN, BSN, MA, NCSN
Lead School Nurse
Kanawha County Schools
Charleston, West Virginia

Jean E. Johnson, PhD, RN, FAAN
Professor and Founding Dean (retired)
School of Nursing
George Washington University
Washington, DC

Jane Clare Joyner, RN, MSN, JD
Senior Policy Fellow
American Nurses Association
Silver Spring, Maryland

Louise Kahn, MSN, MA, RN, CPNP
Specialty Nurse
Center for Development and Disability
University of New Mexico
Albuquerque, New Mexico

David M. Keepnews, PhD, JD, RN, NEA-BC, FAAN
Professor and Director of Graduate Programs
Hunter-Bellevue School of Nursing
Hunter College, City University of New York
New York, New York

Karren Kowalski, PhD, RN, NEA-BC, ANEF, FAAN
President and Chief Executive Officer
Colorado Center for Nursing Excellence
Denver, Colorado
Professor
School of Nursing
Texas Tech University Health Sciences Center
Lubbock, Texas

Mary Jo Kreitzer, PhD, RN, FAAN
Director
Center for Spirituality and Healing
Professor
School of Nursing
University of Minnesota
Minneapolis, Minnesota

Bryan Krumm, MSN, CNP
Psychiatric Nurse Practitioner
Sage Neuroscience Center
Albuquerque, New Mexico

Ellen T. Kurtzman, MPH, RN, FAAN
Assistant Research Professor
School of Nursing
George Washington University
Washington, DC

Susan R. Lacey, RN, PhD, FAAN
Leadership, Research, and Empowerment
   Consultant
Huntsville, Alabama

Jean Larson, RN, MSN
Board Member
Canary Coalition
Leicester, North Carolina

Kathryn Laughon, PhD, RN, FAAN
Associate Professor
School of Nursing
University of Virginia
Charlottesville, Virginia

Roberta P. Lavin, PhD, APRN-BC
Associate Dean for Academic Programs and
   Professor
University of Missouri, St. Louis
St. Louis, Missouri

Judith K. Leavitt, RN, MEd, FAAN
Health Policy Consultant
Barnardsville, North Carolina

Sandra B. Lewenson, EdD, RN, FAAN
Professor
Lienhard School of Nursing
College of Health Professions
Pace University
Pleasantville, New York

Elena Lopez-Bowlan, APRN, MSN, FNP-BC
Examiner, Compensation and Pension
Veterans Administration Sierra Nevada Health
   Care System
Reno, Nevada

Robert J. Lucero, PhD, MPH, RN
Associate Professor of Nursing
College of Nursing
University of Florida
Research Health Scientist
HSR&D Center of Innovation on Disability and
   Rehabilitation Research
North Florida/South Georgia Veterans Health
   System
Gainesville, Florida

Beverly Malone, PhD, RN, FAAN
Chief Executive Officer
National League for Nursing
Washington, DC

Ruth E. Malone, PhD, RN, FAAN
Professor and Nursing Alumni/Mary Harms
   Endowed Chair
Department of Social and Behavioral Sciences
School of Nursing
University of California
San Francisco, California

Mary Lynn Mathre, RN, MSN, CARN
President and Co-Founder
Patients Out of Time
President and Founding Member
American Cannabis Nurses Association
Howardsville, Virginia

DeAnne K. Hilfinger Messias, PhD, RN, FAAN
Professor
College of Nursing and Women's and Gender
    Studies
University of South Carolina
Columbia, South Carolina

Gina Miranda-Diaz, DNP, MS/MPH, RN
New Jersey State Licensed Health Officer
Director
Health Department
West New York, New Jersey
Assistant Professor
Department of Nursing
Lehman College
Bronx, New York

Suzanne Miyamoto, PhD, RN
Senior Director of Government Affairs and Health
    Policy
American Association of Colleges of Nursing
Washington, DC

Wanda Montalvo, MSN, MPhil, RN
Montalvo Consulting
Staten Island, New York

Alan Morgan, MPA
Chief Executive Officer
National Rural Health Association
Washington, DC

Ellen S. Murray, MS
Colin Powell School for Civic and Global
    Leadership
City College of New York
City University of New York
New York, New York

Colonel (Retired) John S. Murray, PhD, RN, CPNP-PC, CS, FAAN
Pediatric Nurse Consultant and Graduate Student
Online Master of Science in Global Health
    Program
Feinberg School of Medicine and Professional
    Studies
Northwestern University
Boston, Massachusetts

Len M. Nichols, PhD
Professor of Health Policy
Director
Center for Health Policy Research and Ethics
George Mason University
Fairfax, Virginia

Karen O'Connor, PhD, JD
Jonathan N. Helfat Distinguished Professor of
    Political Science
American University
Washington, DC

Terry O'Neill, JD
President
National Organization of Women (NOW)
President
NOW Foundation
New York, New York

Douglas P. Olsen, PhD, RN
Associate Professor
College of Nursing
Michigan State University
East Lansing, Michigan

Katie Oppenheim, BSN, RN
Staff Nurse
Birth Center
Von Voigtlander Women's Hospital
University of Michigan Health System
Ann Arbor, Michigan

Judith A. Oulton, RN, BN, MEd, DSc (Hon)
Partner
Oulton, Oulton, and Associates
Tatamagouche, Nova Scotia, Canada

Sharon Pappas, PhD, RN, NEA-BC, FAAN
Chief Nursing Officer
Porter Adventist Hospital
Chief Nurse Executive
Centura Health
Denver, Colorado

Lynn Price, JD, MSN, MPH
Professor and Chair
Graduate Nursing
School of Nursing
Quinnipiac University
Hamden, Connecticut

Chad S. Priest, JD, MSN, RN
Assistant Dean for Operations and Community
   Partnerships
School of Nursing
Indiana University
Adjunct Assistant Professor of Emergency Medicine
Co-Director
Disaster Medicine Fellowship Program
School of Medicine
Indiana University
Indianapolis, Indiana

Joyce A. Pulcini, PhD, RN, PNP-BC, FAAN, FAANP
Professor
Director of Community and Global Initiatives
School of Nursing
George Washington University
Washington, DC

Frank Purcell, BS
Senior Director, Federal Government Affairs
American Association of Nurse Anesthetists
Washington, DC

Susan C. Reinhard, PhD, RN, FAAN
Senior Vice President
AARP Public Policy Institute
Chief Strategist
Center to Champion Nursing in America
Washington, DC

Victoria. L. Rich, PhD, RN, FAAN
Associate Professor
Nursing Administration
School of Nursing
University of Pennsylvania
Philadelphia, Pennsylvania

Nancy Ridenour, PhD, APRN, BC, FAAN
Dean and Professor
College of Nursing
University of New Mexico
Albuquerque, New Mexico

Karen M. Robinson, PhD, PMHCNS-BC, FAAN
Gerontology Professor
Executive Director
Caregivers Program of Research
School of Nursing
University of Louisville
Louisville, Kentucky

Beth L. Rodgers, PhD, RN, FAAN
Professor
College of Nursing
University of New Mexico
Albuquerque, New Mexico

Carol A. Romano, PhD, RN, FAAN
Rear Admiral (Retired)
USPHS
Dean and Professor
Graduate School of Nursing
Uniformed Services University
Bethesda, Maryland

Carol F. Roye, EdD, RN, CPNP, FAAN
Associate Dean for Faculty Scholarship
Professor
Lienhard School of Nursing
Pace University
New York, New York

Angie Ross, MEd
Consultant
Winter Park, Florida

Alice Sardell, PhD
Professor
Department of Urban Studies
Queens College
City University of New York
Faculty
Doctorate of Public Health Program
School of Public Health
City University of New York
Flushing, New York

Chelsea Savage, DNP, MSHA, BA, RN, CPHRM
Professional Liability Investigator
Virginia Commonwealth University Medical
  Center
Richmond, Virginia

Christine Ceccarelli Schrauf, PhD, RN, MBA
Associate Professor
School of Nursing
Elms College
Chicopee, Massachusetts

James Mark Simmerman, PhD, RN
Asia Pacific Regional Director of Epidemiology
Sanofi Pasteur Vaccines
Bangkok, Thailand

Arlene M. Smaldone, PhD, CPNP, CDE
Associate Professor of Nursing
Assistant Dean
Scholarship and Research
School of Nursing
Columbia University
New York, New York

Andréa Sonenberg, PhD, WHNP, CNM-BC
Associate Professor
Graduate Program
Lienhard School of Nursing
College of Health Professions
Pace University
Pleasantville, New York

Diane L. Spatz, PhD, RN-BC, FAAN
Professor of Perinatal Nursing
Helen M. Shearer Professor of Nutrition
School of Nursing
University of Pennsylvania
Nurse Researcher and Director of the Lactation
  Program
The Children's Hospital of Philadelphia
Philadelphia, Pennsylvania

Joanne Spetz, PhD, FAAN
Professor
Philip R. Lee Institute for Health Policy Studies
Associate Director for Research Strategy
Center for the Health Professions
University of California, San Francisco
San Francisco, California

Caroline Stephens, PhD, MSN, APRN, BC
Assistant Professor
Department of Community Health Systems
Associate Director
Hartford Center of Gerontological Nursing
  Excellence
School of Nursing
University of California, San Francisco
San Francisco, California

Elaine D. Stephens, MPH, FHHC, RN
Executive Vice President
National Association for Home Care and Hospice
Washington, DC

Patricia W. Stone, PhD, RN, FAAN
Centennial Professor in Health Policy
Director of the Center for Health Policy
School of Nursing
Columbia University
Visiting Professor for Faculty of Health
University of Technology, Sydney
Sydney, New South Wales, Australia

Lisa Summers, CNM, DrPH
Director of Policy and Advocacy
Centering Healthcare Institute
Boston, Massachusetts

Elaine Tagliareni, EdD, RN, CNE, FAAN
Chief Program Officer
National League for Nursing
Washington, DC

Carol R. Taylor, PhD, MSN, RN
Professor of Nursing, Senior Clinical Scholar
Kennedy Institute of Ethics
Georgetown University
Washington, DC

Clifton P. Thornton, MSN, BS, BSN, RN, CNMT
Pediatric Nurse Practitioner
Research Nurse
School of Nursing
John Hopkins University
Baltimore, Maryland

Cora Tomalinas, BSN, PHN, Retired RN
Commissioner
FIRST 5 Santa Clara County
Member
Governing Board Santa Clara County
Re-Entry Collaborative
Member
San Jose Mayor's Gang Prevention Task Force
   Policy and Technical Team
San Jose, California

Brian Valdez, JD
Policy and Development Specialist
National Nursing Centers Consortium
Philadelphia, Pennsylvania

Tener Goodwin Veenema, PhD, MPH, MS, RN, FAAN
Associate Professor
School of Nursing
John Hopkins University
Center for Refugee and Disaster Response
Johns Hopkins Bloomberg School of Public
   Health
Baltimore, Maryland

Antonia M. Villarruel, PhD, RN, FAAN
Professor and Margaret Bond Simon Dean of
   Nursing
School of Nursing
University of Pennsylvania
Philadelphia, Pennsylvania

Elizabeth Waetzig, JD
Founding Partner
Change Matrix, LLC
Granger, Indiana

Laura M. Wagner, PhD, RN, GNP, FAAN
Assistant Professor
School of Nursing
University of California, San Francisco
San Francisco, California

Jamie M. Ware, JD
Policy Director
National Nursing Centers Consortium
Manager of Strategic Policy Initiatives
Public Health Management Corporation
Philadelphia, Pennsylvania

Joanne R. Warner, PhD, RN
Dean and Professor
School of Nursing
University of Portland
Portland, Oregon

Catherine M. Waters, PhD, RN, FAAN
Professor
Department of Community Health Systems
School of Nursing
University of California, San Francisco
San Francisco, California

Ellen-Marie Whelan, PhD, CRNP, FAAN
Senior Advisor
Centers for Medicare and Medicaid Services
   Innovation Center
Washington, DC

Kathleen M. White, PhD, RN, NEA-BC, FAAN
Associate Professor and Track Coordinator
Health Systems Management and MSN/MBA
Director
Master's Entry into Nursing Program
Department of Acute and Chronic Care
School of Nursing
John Hopkins University
Baltimore, Maryland

Marie Davis Williams, MSW, LCSW
Deputy Commissioner
Tennessee Department of Mental Health and
    Substance Abuse Services
Nashville, Tennessee

Shanita D. Williams, PhD, MPH, APRN
Chief
Nursing Education and Practice Branch
Division of Nursing and Public Health
Bureau of Health Workforce
Health Resources and Services Administration
Rockville, Maryland

Rita Wray, BC, MBA, RN, FAAN
Founder and Chief Executive Officer
Wray Enterprises, Inc.
Jackson, Mississippi

Alixandra B. Yanus, PhD
Assistant Professor of Political Science
High Point University
High Point, North Carolina

Reviewers

Phyllis S. Brenner, PhD, RN, NEA-BC
Professor of Nursing and Nursing Administration
  Program Director
College of Nursing and Health
Madonna University
Livonia, Michigan

Dian Colette Davitt, PhD, RN
Associate Professor
Webster University
St. Louis, Missouri

Michelle L. Edmonds, PhD, FNP-BC, CNE
Professor of Nursing
School of Nursing
Jacksonville University
Jacksonville, Florida

Teresa Keller, PhD, RN
Associate Director for Undergraduate Studies
School of Nursing
New Mexico State University
Las Cruces, New Mexico

Karen Kelly, EdD, RN, NEA-BC
Director
Continuing Education
Associate Professor
School of Nursing
Primary Care and Health Systems Nursing
Southern Illinois University, Edwardsville
Edwardsville, Illinois

Carol A. Mannahan, EdD, RN, NEA-BC
Assistant Professor
Kramer School of Nursing
Oklahoma City University
Oklahoma City, Oklahoma

Brenda B. Rowe, MN, JD, RN
Associate Professor
Georgia Baptist College of Nursing of Mercer
  University
Atlanta, Georgia

Melissa V. Sirola, BSN, MSN, MBA, RN
Adjunct Instructor
Caldwell University
Caldwell, New Jersey

Annette Weiss, PhD, RN, CNE
Assistant Professor
Expressway RN Program Director
Misericordia University
Dallas, Pennsylvania

Contents

UNIT 2   Health Care Delivery and Financing

UNIT 3   Policy and Politics in the Government

UNIT 4   Policy and Politics in the Workplace and Workforce

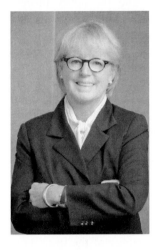

In 2010, the Institute of Medicine challenged the nation and the nursing profession to ensure that nurses are participating as leaders in decision making about health, health care, and health policy. The landmark report *The Future of Nursing: Leading Change, Advancing Health* is bringing attention to this most valuable resource for transforming health in the United States.

I've had the privilege of serving as Chairperson of the Strategic Advisory Committee for the *Future of Nursing:* Campaign for Action that is charged with overseeing the implementation of the report's recommendations. Specifically, the report recommends the expansion of "opportunities for nurses to lead and diffuse collaborative improvement efforts," including in health systems, and aims to "prepare and enable nurses to lead change to advance health." For this latter recommendation, the report specifically calls for "public, private, and governmental health care decision makers at every level [to] include representation from nursing on boards, on executive management teams, and in other key leadership positions."

Leading—as a clinical bedside leader, executive in a health care organization, member of a state or federal health advisory body, or a legislator at the local, state, or federal level—requires knowing how private and public policies are made, exquisite political skills, and the confidence and willingness to guide the decisions and actions of individuals and groups. These are not easy skills to learn but are essential for every nurse who wants to lead.

I know the importance of learning how to lead. For more than 10 years, I was Chief of Staff for former Senate Majority Leader and presidential candidate Bob Dole of Kansas, after working as a professional staff member for the Senate Committee on Finance and, later, as Deputy Staff Director of that committee. These superb opportunities gave me a deep understanding of policymaking and of the leadership and political skills that are required to shape policy. I never questioned that nurses should do this kind of work. It was my good fortune to "learn the ropes" as President of the California Student Nurses Association and later as Program Director for the National Student Nurses Association.

Society must recognize the important perspectives that nurses can bring to decision-making tables, but nurses must be ready to fully engage in the important health-related decisions of our day. *Policy & Politics in Nursing and Health Care* is an invaluable resource for nurses to learn the ropes of being leaders in local, state, national, and international organizations—from the bedside to the boardroom to the backrooms of policymaking. It provides guidelines and an important framework for developing leaders. For the more sophisticated nurse leaders, it offers in-depth analyses of important policy issues within a political context.

Policy & Politics in Nursing and Health Care has been in publication for 30 years. This essential resource continues to prepare the current and future generations of nurse leaders. We must use it wisely if we're to achieve the recommendations in *The Future of Nursing.* Our nation's health depends upon nurses being leaders in transforming health and health care in the United States and globally.

Sheila Burke, MPA, RN, FAAN
Faculty Research Fellow, Malcolm Weiner Center for Social Policy
Adjunct Lecturer, John. F. Kennedy School of Government at Harvard University
Chair, Government Relations and Public Policy, Baker, Donelson, Bearman, Caldwell & Berkowitz

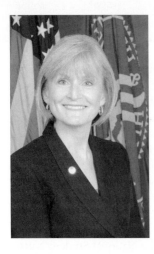

On the threshold of significant change, we find ourselves at a pivotal time for health care in the United States. For far too long, Americans have been served by a fragmented health care system and one that has heavily emphasized acute care, at the expense of keeping people well. It has come with a price tag of about $2.7 trillion a year. Costs have been ticking ever upward until recently. As a result, health care services have been unaffordable and largely inaccessible to millions of Americans. For all Americans, consistent care quality could not be guaranteed.

The Affordable Care Act has been instrumental in helping the nation reset this picture. Even in the midst of heated rhetoric and misinformation, the law is moving us forward on insurance coverage for previously uninsured Americans, access to care, improved care quality, and new payment mechanisms. Addressing these things is crucial to improving health care and the health of the nation.

Nurses are already central to this law and the change that it seeks to produce. The law includes opportunities to spread models of care that nurses were instrumental in developing, such as home visitation programs for high-risk mothers, programs for all-inclusive care of elders, nurse-managed health centers, and transitional care. The law uses provider-neutral language and improves the Medicare payment rate for nurse midwives. It also includes substantial funding to increase the primary care workforce, including nurses.

These and other elements of the law reflect engagement of various constituencies, including nursing. Policymaking is not for the timid. It requires mastery of knowledge and skills in the art and science of politics and the policy process. Though nursing organizations have long had influential leaders at national, state, and local levels, this set of competencies hasn't been universal across members of the profession.

I know well the growth in nursing's policymaking savvy. I have been a part of some of the important health policy discussions of our day and have watched as other nurses have sought to use their knowledge to inform laws and regulations that govern health care. Some years ago, as the director of a Center for Health Policy, Research and Ethics, I led an annual policy program on policy and political development for nurses. I also have had the privilege of serving as Chief of Staff to two U.S. Senators, serving as a member of the Institute of Medicine and the Medicare Payment Advisory Commission, and chairing the National Advisory Council for the Agency for Healthcare Research and Quality. In his first term, President Barack Obama appointed me to serve as the Administrator of the Health Resources and Services Administration, a division of the U.S. Department of Health and Human Services. In this capacity, my responsibilities included helping to lead the nation's efforts to ensure that we have a well-prepared nursing and health care workforce that can meet the vast and varied health needs of the nation. However, we need many more nurses at the multitude of policy tables at local, state, and federal levels. There may be as many opportunities for nurses to engage in this arena as there are nurses.

The health of the nation can directly benefit when nurses have sophisticated knowledge and skill in policymaking and its political context. We should expect no less of members of our profession—and deliver no less for our nation.

Mary Wakefield, PhD, RN, FAAN
Acting Deputy Secretary
U.S. Department of Health and Human Services

The Affordable Care Act (ACA) had just become the law of the land as the prior edition of *Policy & Politics in Nursing and Health Care* (sixth edition) was going to press. Now, its implementation is benefiting many of the previously uninsured, reducing health care costs, and moving our nation on the path toward the Triple Aim: improving people's experiences with care, improving health outcomes for the population, and reducing health care costs. And yet, it has illuminated the complexities and failures of a health care system that lags behind other nations in promoting health. Indeed, there is a growing recognition that health care's consumption of approximately 18% of the U.S. gross domestic product is undermining efforts to promote the health of families and communities rather than treating preventable illnesses—and at a very high price in humanistic and monetary terms.

This current edition of *Policy & Politics in Nursing and Health Care* focuses on the changes that the ACA has brought about, its deficiencies that mandate further reform in health care, and the importance of social determinants of health, or "upstream factors," that must be addressed if we are to have communities and a nation that thrive in terms of economic, social, and health dimensions. In concert with the Institute of Medicine's report *The Future of Nursing: Leading Health, Advancing Change,* this book highlights the role that nurses and other health professionals can play in leading the transformation of health care and creating healthy communities.

The book does this with the continuing aim of appealing to all nurses, from novice to expert, as well as other health professionals, although in this edition we have placed a stronger emphasis on the implications of the issues discussed for advanced practice nurses, including those pursuing or holding the doctorate of nursing practice (DNP). The DNP was designed to prepare nurses as clinical leaders who could develop evidence-based approaches to improving the health of specific populations. The book's emphasis on both reforming health care and addressing upstream factors that promote health is particularly suited to nurses with DNPs. However, we maintain that every nurse has a social responsibility to shape public and private policies to promote health. As such, this edition is designed to appeal to undergraduate, master's, DNP, and PhD students, as well as to practicing health professionals.

WHAT'S NEW IN THE SEVENTH EDITION?

This edition continues the almost 30-year approach of prior editions that have led others to describe the book as a "classic" in nursing literature. However, classics become stagnant if not refreshed. A new team of editors has brought a fresh perspective to this edition. The order of authorship on the cover does not reflect effort; rather, the editing of this book was truly a team effort. The new team is a result of transitions in the lives of former co-editors Judith Leavitt and Mary Chaffee. Certainly, their imprint, and that of the first-co-editor, Susan Talbott, continues to manifest throughout the book, but there is much that has changed.

Central to these changes are *updates on the Affordable Care Act* and its implementation, its impact on nursing and the health of people, the role of politics in our health care system, and the need for further policy reforms. As noted previously, the importance of improving the health of people while reducing health care spending by addressing *upstream factors or social determinants of health* is a major theme.

We have also further developed the *conceptual framework* for the book, as described in Chapter 1. This chapter also emphasizes the *competencies* that nurses are expected to demonstrate at the conclusion of undergraduate and graduate programs.

Evidence-based policy is another major theme that continues in this edition, but with more emphasis. Throughout the book, authors have provided more depth and breadth to the evidence that undergirds policy issues and potential responses, with the understanding that evidence is necessary, but often not sufficient, for policy change.

Indeed, it is the political context of policy change that must be addressed for success in many policy-related endeavors. As such, *individual and community activism* continue to be emphasized as ways for nurses and other health professionals to contribute to and lead policy change. New and updated vignettes (called Taking Action) provide real-life examples of such activism.

Some of the continuing chapters have new authors with fresh perspectives. *Other new content* includes:

- Using research to advance health and social policies
- Highlights of the ACA, with implications for nurses and other health professionals
- The politics of advanced practice nursing
- Ethical dimensions of policy and politics
- The new health insurance exchanges
- Patient engagement
- Overtreatment
- Social Security and women
- Women's reproductive health
- Public health
- Emergency preparedness
- Developing families
- Dual eligibles
- Nurses in boardrooms
- Quality and safety in health care
- Nurses' work environments
- The intersection of technology and health care
- Community-based organizations addressing health

USING THE SEVENTH EDITION

Using the book as a course text. Faculty will find content in this book that will enhance learning experiences in policy, leadership, community activism, administration, research, health disparities, and other key issues and trends of importance to courses at every educational level. Many of the chapters will help students in clinical courses understand the dynamics of the health system. Students will find chapters that assist them in developing new skills, building a broader understanding of nursing leadership and influence, and making sense of the complex business and financial forces that drive many actions in the health system. The book presents an in-depth view of the issues that impact nurses and suggests a variety of opportunities for nurses to engage in the policy issues about which they care deeply.

Using the book in government activities. The unit on policy and politics in the government includes content that will benefit nurses considering running for elective office, seeking a political appointment, and learning to lobby elective officials about health care issues.

Using the book in the workplace. Policy problems and political issues abound in nursing workplaces. This book offers critical insights into how to effectively resolve problems and influence workplace policy as well as how to develop politically astute approaches to making changes in the workplace.

Using the book in professional organizations. Organizations use the power of numbers. The unit on associations and interest groups will help groups determine strategies for success and how to capitalize on working with other groups through coalitions.

Using the book in community activism. With an expanded focus on community advocacy and activism, readers will find information they need to effectively influence remedies to policy problems in their local communities.

Acknowledgments

In every edition of this book, the co-editors have expressed their sincere gratitude to the many authors who have contributed their time and expertise to write a chapter out of a commitment to furthering the education of nurses and other health professionals on policy and politics. This edition is no exception. We are grateful for the thoughtful contributions of more than 100 authors and hope that readers will learn from them.

We are also grateful for the enduring contributions and imprint of the prior co-editors of this book that have made it the leading resource in its field. Susan Talbott was the co-editor on the first edition; Mary Chaffee on the fourth through sixth editions; and Judith Leavitt on the second through sixth editions. We hope that they are pleased with the continued development of the book.

We owe a huge debt of thanks to Beth Gardner, the book's editorial manager for this edition. She tracked and managed 92 manuscripts, kept the co-editors moving along, coordinated our communications, and was simply amazingly organized. In the midst of this, she married, pursued a doctoral dissertation, and remained in good humor. Beth, we are grateful for your superb work.

We also acknowledge the continuing support of Elsevier and the editorial team that worked with Sandy Clark, including Karen Turner. We are indebted to Clay Broeker, an extraordinary production manager who has worked on the last three editions of the book. Thank you, Clay, for your continued commitment to excellence in publishing.

Each of us has some special people to acknowledge.

Diana Mason

I want to acknowledge my husband, James Ware, for his continued support of my long days of work, including on this book.

My thanks, too, for the support I have received from Dean Gail McCain, Graduate Director David Keepnews, Barbara Glickstein, and my colleagues at Hunter College; the Center for Health, Media and Policy; and the City University of New York.

Deborah Gardner

Undertaking this editing experience would not have been possible without the consistent support of my husband, Dan. I also want to express my great joy in sharing this project with my daughter and colleague, Beth Gardner.

I also thank Mary Wakefield, who mentored me through my first experience in writing a policy chapter. As a co-author with her back in 1998, I learned from the best. Last but not least, Judith Leavitt, co-editor of four editions of this text, supported me as an author in other editions and believed I could take on this editing role.

Freida Outlaw

Special thanks to my husband, Lucius Outlaw, Jr., my greatest supporter; my delightful sons and the two lovely wives and one special woman in their lives; my mother, sister, and her family; my wonderful friends who have been with me from the beginning (BFF Lois Oliver); and my new friends. You are my village. I would like to express my gratitude to Martha Pride, PhD, RN, my psychiatric nursing professor at Berea College, and to Dr. Hattie Bessent and the Minority Fellowship Program for the support and guidance given to me.

Eileen O'Grady

A heartfelt thanks to Dr. Loretta Ford, founding mother of the nurse practitioner role. Writing a chapter with her is a privilege. We are so fortunate to see true leadership firsthand. She has shown us, with a sparkle in her eye, how to live courageously and be of maximal service. It is fortunate to know somebody so fearless and funny.

Thank you to all of those (including each author in this book) who stepped out of the safety of their clinical roles and took a risk to speak out on behalf of better health care in a larger venue.

CHAPTER 1

Frameworks for Action in Policy and Politics

Eileen T. O'Grady   Diana J. Mason   Freida Hopkins Outlaw   Deborah B. Gardner

"The most common way people give up their power is by thinking they don't have any."

Alice Walker

March 31, 2013 marked an important deadline in the implementation of landmark legislation, the Affordable Care Act (ACA)[1], also known as Obamacare. By that date those eligible to enroll for insurance coverage through the marketplace had to purchase a plan if they were to avoid a 2015 tax penalty of $95 or 1% of their annual income (whichever was higher). Amid a frenzy of media attention, an estimated 8 million people signed on for coverage during open enrollment—the period between October 2012 and the deadline—exceeding the revised target of 6.5 million (Kennedy, 2014). And the numbers kept increasing, as millions more enrolled in Medicaid or the Children's Health Insurance Program (known as CHIP) (Centers for Medicare and Medicaid Services [CMS], 2014).

Nurses were essential to these enrollments. For example, Adriana Perez, PhD, ANP, RN, an assistant professor at Arizona State University College of Nursing, used her role as president of the Phoenix Chapter of the National Association of Hispanic Nurses to organize town hall meetings with Spanish-speaking state residents to explain the ACA and encourage enrollment among those with a high rate of un- or under-insurance. She also developed a training model in partnership with AARP-Arizona and used it to empower Arizona nurses to educate multicultural communities on the basic provisions of the ACA. Through many such initiatives, the United States reduced the number of uninsured people by over 10 million in 2014; the number is projected to be 20 million by 2016 (Congressional Budget Office [CBO], 2014).

However, access to coverage does not necessarily mean access to care, nor does it ensure a healthy population. Health care access means having the ability to receive the right type of care when needed at an affordable price. The U.S. health care system is grounded in expensive, high-tech acute care that does not produce the desired outcomes we ought to have and too often damages instead of heals (National Research Council, 2013). Despite spending more per person on health care than any other nation, a comparative report on health indicators by the Organisation for Economic Co-operation and Development (2013) shows that the United States performs worse than other nations on life

---

[1]The Affordable Care Act (ACA) is the label used to refer to two laws passed by the House of Representatives and the Senate in 2010: the Patient Protection and Affordable Care Act and the Health Care and Education Affordability Reconciliation Act. We use the ACA terminology in this book.

expectancy at birth for both men and women, infant mortality rate, mortality rates for suicide and cardiovascular disease, the prevalence of diabetes and obesity in children, and other indicators.

In 1999, the Institute of Medicine (IOM) issued a report, *To Err is Human: Building a Safer Health System*, which estimated that health care errors in hospitals were the fifth leading cause of death in the U.S. (IOM, 1999). By 2011, preventable health care errors were estimated to be the third-leading cause of death (Allen, 2013; James, 2013). The ACA includes elements that can begin to create a high-performing health care system, one accountable for the provision of safe care, as well as improved clinical and financial outcomes. It aims to move the health care system in the direction of keeping people out of hospitals, in their own homes and communities, with an emphasis on wellness, health promotion, and better management of chronic illnesses.

For example, the ACA uses financial penalties to prod hospitals to reduce 30-day readmission rates. It also provides funding for demonstration projects that improve "transitional care," services that help patients and their family caregivers to make a smoother transition from hospital or nursing home to their own homes to help reduce preventable hospital readmissions. Based, in part, on research by Mary Naylor, PhD, RN, FAAN, professor of nursing at the University of Pennsylvania School of Nursing, these demonstrations are stimulating creative methods of accountability across health care settings, with most using nurses for care coordination and transitional care providers (CMS, n.d.; Coalition for Evidence-Based Policy, n.d.; Naylor et al., 2011).

UPSTREAM FACTORS

Promoting health requires more than a high-performing health care system. First and foremost, health is created where people live, work, and play. It is becoming clear that one's health status may be more dependent on one's zip code than on one's genetic code (Marks, 2009). Geographic analyses of race and ethnicity, income, and health status repeatedly show that financial, racial, and ethnic

disparities persist (Braveman et al., 2010). Individual health and family health are severely compromised in communities where good education, nutritious foods, safe places to exercise, and well-paying jobs are scarce (Halpin, Morales-Suárez-Varela, & Martin-Moreno, 2010). Creating a healthier nation requires that we address "upstream factors"; the broad range of issues, other than health care, that can undermine or promote health (also known as "social determinants of health" or "core determinants of health") (World Health Organization [WHO], n.d.). Upstream factors promoting health include safe environments, adequate housing, and economically thriving communities with employment opportunities, access to affordable and healthful foods, and models for addressing conflict through dialogue rather than violence. According to Williams and colleagues (2008), the key to reducing and eliminating health disparities, which disproportionately affect racial and ethnic minorities, is to provide effective interventions that address upstream factors both in and outside of health care systems. Upstream factors have a large influence on the development and progression of illnesses (Williams et al., 2008). The core determinants of health will be used to further elucidate and make concrete the wider, more comprehensive set of upstream factors that can improve the health of the nation by reducing disparities. Figure 1-1 depicts the core determinants of health developed by the Canadian Forces Health Services Group.

A focus on such factors is essential for economic and moral reasons. Even in the most affluent nations, those living in poverty have substantially shorter life expectancies and experience more illness than those who are wealthy, with high costs in human and financial terms (Wilkinson & Marmot, 2003). To date however, most of the focus on reducing disparities has been on health policy that addresses access, coverage, cost, and quality of care once the individual has entered the health care system–despite the fact that for more than a decade research has established that most health care problems begin long before people seek medical care (Williams et al., 2008). Thus, changing the paradigm requires knowledge about the political aspects of the social determinates of health and the broader

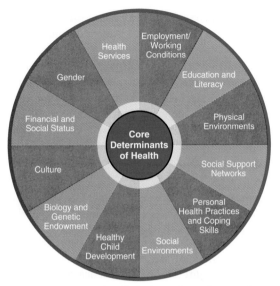

FIGURE 1-1 Surgeon General's Mental Health Strategy: Canadian Forces Health Services Group—An Evolution of Excellence. (From *www.forces.gc.ca/en/about-reports-pubs-health/surg-gen-mental-health-strategy-ch-2.page.*)

BOX 1-1 Political Aspects of the Social Determinants of Health

- The health of individuals and populations is determined significantly by social factors.
- The social determinants of health produce great inequities in health within and between societies.
- The poor and disadvantaged experience worse health than the rich, have less access to care, and die younger in all societies.
- The social determinants of health can be measured and described.
- The measurement of the social determinants provides evidence that can serve as the basis for political action.
- Evidence is generated and used in a continuous cycle of evidence production, policy development, implementation, and evaluation.
- Evidence of the effects of policies and programs on inequities can be measured and can provide data on the effectiveness of interventions.
- Evidence regarding the social determinants of health is insufficient to bring about change on its own; political will combined with evidence offers the most powerful strategy to address the negative effects of the social determinants.

Adapted from National Institute for Health and Clinical Excellence. (2007). The Social Determinants of Health: Developing an Evidence Base for Political Action. Final report to the World Health Organization Commission on the Social Determinants of Health. Lead authors: J. Mackenbach, M. Exworthy, J. Popay, P. Tugwell, V. Robinson, S. Simpson, T. Narayan, L. Myer, T. Houweling, L. Jadue, and F. Florenza.

---

core determinants. Political aspects of the social determinants of health appear in Box 1-1.

The ACA begins to carve out a role for the health care system in addressing upstream factors. For example, the law requires that nonprofit hospitals demonstrate a "community benefit" to receive federal tax breaks. Hospitals must conduct a community health assessment, develop a community health improvement plan, and partner with others to implement it. This aligns with a growing emphasis on population health: the health of a group, whether defined by a common disease or health problem or by geographic or demographic characteristics (Felt-Lisk & Higgins, 2011).

Consider the 11th Street Family Health Services. Located in an underserved neighborhood in North Philadelphia, this federally qualified, nurse-managed health center (NMHC) was the brainchild of public health nurse Patricia Gerrity, PhD, RN, FAAN, a faculty member at Drexel University School of Nursing. She recognized that the leading health problems in the community were diabetes, obesity, heart failure, and depression. Working with a community advisory group, Gerrity realized that

the health center had to address nutrition as an "upstream factor" that could improve the health of those living in the community. With no supermarket in the neighborhood until 2011, she invited area farmers to come to the neighborhood as part of a farmers' market. She also created a community vegetable garden maintained by the local youth. And area residents were invited to attend nutrition classes on culturally relevant, healthful cooking. 11th Street Family Health Services is one of over 200 NMHCs in the United States that have improved clinical and financial outcomes by addressing the needs of individuals, families, and communities

(American Academy of Nursing, n.d., b). The ACA authorizes continued support for these centers, although the law does not mandate they be funded. Congress would have to appropriate funding for NMHCs but has not done so. (See Chapter 34 for a more detailed discussion of NMHCs.)

The ACA may not go far enough in shifting attention to the health of communities and populations. One approach gaining notice is that of "health in all policies," the idea that policymakers consider the health implications of social and economic policies that focus on other sectors, such as education, community development, tax codes, and housing (Leppo et al., 2013; Rudolph et al., 2013). As health professionals who focus on the family and community context of the patients they serve, nurses can help to raise questions about the potential health impact of public policies.

NURSING AND HEALTH POLICY

Health policy affects every nurse's daily practice. Indeed, health policy determines who gets what type of health care, when, how, from whom, and at what cost. The study of health policy is an indispensable component of professional development in nursing, whether it is undertaken to advance a healthier society, promote a safer health care system, or support nursing's ability to care for people with equity and skill. Just as Florence Nightingale understood that health policy held the key to improving the health of poor Londoners and the British military, so are today's nurses needed to create compelling cases and actively influence better health policies at every level of governance. With national attention focused on how to transform health care in ways that produce better outcomes and reduce health care costs, nursing has an unprecedented opportunity to provide proactive and visionary leadership. Indeed, the Institute of Medicine's landmark report, *The Future of Nursing: Leading Change, Advancing Health* (2011), calls for nurses to be leaders in redesigning health care. But will nurses rise to this occasion?

Health care opinion leaders in a 2010 poll identified two reasons nurses would fall short of influencing health care reform: too many nurses do not want to lead, and with over 120 national organizations, nursing often fails to present a united front (Gallup, 2010). As the largest health care profession, nursing has great potential power. Yet, similar to many professions, it has struggled to collaborate within its ranks or with other groups on pressing issues of health policy. The IOM report has provided a rallying point for nursing organizations to work together and engage other stakeholders to advance its recommendations.

REFORMING HEALTH CARE

THE TRIPLE AIM

In 2008, Don Berwick, MD, and his colleagues at the Institute for Healthcare Improvement (IHI) first described the Triple Aim of a value-based health care system (Berwick, Nolan, & Whittington, 2008): (1) improving population health, (2) improving the patient experience of care, and (3) reducing per capita costs. This framework aligns with the aims of the Affordable Care Act.

The Triple Aim represents a balanced approach: by examining a health care delivery problem from all three dimensions, health care organizations and society can identify system problems and direct resources to activities that can have the greatest impact. Looking at each of these dimensions in isolation prevents organizations from discovering how a new objective, decreasing readmission rates to improve quality and reduce costs, for instance, could negatively impact the third goal of population health, as scarce community resources are directed to acute care transitions and unintentionally shifted away from prevention activities. Solutions must also be evaluated from these three interdependent dimensions. The Triple Aim compels delivery systems and payors to broaden their focus on acute and highly specialized care toward more integrated care, including primary and preventive care (McCarthy & Klein, 2010).

The IHI (n.d.) identified these components of any approach seeking to achieve the Triple Aim:
- A focus on individuals and families
- A redesign of primary care services
- Population health management

- A cost-control platform
- System integration and execution

Note that these possess the goal of creating a high-performing health care system but do not focus on geographic communities or social determinants per se. However, these two concepts can be incorporated into the Triple Aim of improving the health of populations and reducing health care costs.

The Triple Aim is easy to understand but challenging to implement because it requires all providers, including nurses, to broaden their focus from individuals to populations. The success of the nursing profession's continued evolution will hinge on its ability to take on new roles, more cogently and creatively engaging with patients and stepping into executive and leadership roles in every sector of heath care. But it must do so within an interprofessional context, leading efforts to break down health professions' silos and hierarchies and keeping the patient and family at the center of care.

THE ACA AND NURSING

The ACA is arguably the most significant piece of social legislation passed in the United States since the enactment of Medicare and Medicaid in 1965. Implementation continues to be a vexing process and a political flashpoint. It has defined the ideologies of U.S. political parties, and yet the public remains largely uninformed and misinformed about the legislation; 3 years after its passage, 4 out of 10 Americans were still unaware of many of its provisions and unsure that the ACA had become law (The Henry J. Kaiser Family Foundation, 2013). (Chapter 19 provides a thorough description of the ACA.) The ACA is over 2000 pages long, which reflects the complexity of creating a new health care infrastructure that addresses a wide array of issues including patient protections, health insurance industry reforms, and workforce development, to name a few. Newer systems of care are emphasized in the ACA that link patient outcomes to costs incurred in treatment and to high-value health systems. The legislation can be categorized into four main cornerstones (Figure 1-2).

The ACA was born out of national macroeconomic concerns. The United States spent $2.7 trillion in 2011, or $8680 per person, on health care; a

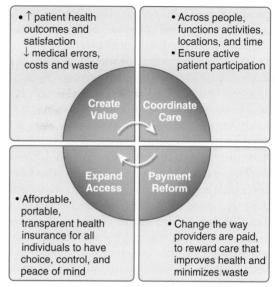

FIGURE 1-2 Four cornerstones of reform. (From O'Grady, E. T., & Johnson, J. [2013]. Health policy issues in changing environments. In A. Hamric, C. Hanson, D. Way, & E. O'Grady [Eds.], *Advanced practice nursing: An integrative approach* [5th ed.]. St. Louis, MO: Elsevier-Saunders.)

rate higher than inflation that is expected to consume nearly 20% of the gross domestic product by 2020 (CMS, 2013). With businesses having to spend such large amounts on health care for employees, the United States cannot compete in the global economy. Furthermore, such high health care expenses divert funds away from addressing the upstream factors that could prevent the need for costly acute care. Although previous presidents in the past 50 years tried unsuccessfully to pass health care reform legislation, President Obama was elected at a time when many Americans agreed that the United States could no longer afford to maintain a health care system that had neither spending controls nor accountability for improving clinical outcomes. The ACA was an outgrowth, in part, to "bend the cost curve," or reduce the rate of increase in health care spending (Cutler, 2010).

To improve the health of the public and reduce health care costs, health promotion and wellness, disease prevention, and chronic care management must be built into the foundation of the health care system (Katz, 2009; Wagner, 1998; Woolf, 2009). At the same time, acute care must use fewer resources, be made safer, and produce better outcomes (Conway, Mostashari, & Clancy, 2013).

Nurses are important players in shifting the focus of health care to one that prevents illnesses, promotes health, and coordinates care. Nurses have been performing in such roles without naming or measuring their activities for decades. But there are exceptions. The American Academy of Nursing's Raise the Voice Campaign (American Academy of Nursing, n.d., a) has identified nurses who have developed innovative models of care for which there are good clinical and financial outcome data. Known as "Edge Runners," these nurses have demonstrated that nursing's emphasis on care coordination, health promotion, patient- and family-centeredness, and the community context of care provides evidence-based models that can help to transform the health care system.

The ACA presents many opportunities for nurses to test new models of care that have already shown promise for improving health outcomes and the experience of health care, while lowering costs. The Center for Medicare and Medicaid Innovation (CMMI) was authorized to spend $10 billion over a decade to pilot-test programs that may improve the safety and quality of care. For example, under the *Bundled Payments for Care Improvement Initiative*, health systems will enter into payment arrangements that include financial and performance accountability for episodes of care. Currently being studied, an episode of care includes the inpatient stay and all related services during the episode up to 90 days after hospital discharge. These models may lead to higher quality, more coordinated care at a lower cost to Medicare. If the program is successful in achieving these outcomes, they are authorized to launch the program nation-wide.

If these can be shown to achieve the Triple Aim, the ACA authorizes the Secretary of the U.S. Department of Health and Human Services to put these programs in place permanently. The CMMI provides opportunities for nurse leaders and nurse researchers to demonstrate new methods of improving care in cost-effective ways. In addition, the ACA created the Patient-Centered Outcomes Research Institute (PCORI) with $3.5 billion to support comparative-effectiveness research that examines the outcomes that matter to consumers. Nurses serve on the governing board and review panels of PCORI. It provides nurses with opportunities to compare nursing interventions, head-to-head or with medications or other treatments that have sufficient evidence.

The following examples illustrate how nursing is embedded in the four cornerstones of reform. Some of these examples address only one cornerstone; others address all four.

1. **Create Value.** NMHCs are operated by advanced practice registered nurses (APRNs), primarily nurse practitioners (NPs). These clinics are often associated with a school, college, university, department of nursing, federally qualified health center, or an independent nonprofit health care agency. Managed by APRNs, NMHCs are staffed by an interprofessional team that may include physicians, social workers, public health nurses, psychiatric mental health nurses at the generic and advanced levels, and behavioral therapists. Barkauskas and colleagues (2011) found that quality measures for NMHCs compared positively with national benchmarks, particularly in chronic disease management. The founders of several NMHCs have been designated Edge Runners, including Patricia Gerrity of the 11th Street Family Health Service, as described earlier. NMHCs serve as critical access points for keeping patients out of the emergency room and hospitals, saving millions of dollars annually (Hansen-Turton et al., 2010).

2. **Coordinate Care.** The patient-centered "medical home" or "health home"[2] (PCMH) model was designed to satisfy patients' needs and to improve care access (e.g., through extended office hours and increased communication between providers and patients via e-mail and telephone),

---

[2]The ACA refers to refers to both "medical" and "health" homes. Reference to "health homes" is specific to Medicaid provisions in the law. In practice, facilities are designated as "medical homes" if they meet criteria set by the National Committee on Quality Assurance. This book will use that language, while recognizing that "health home" is more consistent with a health-promotion model.

increase care coordination, and enhance overall quality, while simultaneously reducing costs. The medical home relies on a one-stop-shopping approach by a team of providers, such as physicians, nurses, nutritionists, pharmacists, and social workers, to meet a patient's health care needs. Peikes and colleagues (2012) found that the PCMH model's attention to the whole person across care settings (such as from hospital to home) may improve physical and behavioral health, access to community-based social services, and management of chronic conditions. A number of NMHCs have achieved PCMH designation by the National Committee on Quality Assurance.

3. **Payment Reform.** Bundling payments and paying for care coordination, including through "accountable care organizations" (ACOs), are examples of payment reform. ACOs are similar to integrated delivery systems that combine services across health care settings and focus on ways to improve care delivery and outcomes under a bundled payment plan. Bundling payments allows for reimbursement of multiple services provided during an episode of care, rather than the traditional fee-for-service payments for each service or procedure for a single illness. ACOs differ from health maintenance organizations (HMOs) in that they are not incentivized to cut services but rather to keep people healthy. Indeed, one of the major differences between HMOs in the 1990s and ACOs today is that the latter are held to a higher standard of measuring, reporting, and making transparent the process and outcome indicators of quality. Each ACO has to have a minimum of 5000 Medicare patients (population health); if the ACO demonstrates that it keeps people healthy and saves Medicare money, those savings are "shared" with the ACO. Nurses are central to preventing complications in hospitalized patients, ensuring smooth transitions to home, and coaching the patient and family caregivers in self-care and health-promoting behavioral changes. As such, they are a vital component of ACO success.

But payment reform is proving to be challenging. The CMMI, authorized under the ACA, initially funded 31 "pioneer" ACOs. By mid-2014, only 22 remained, mostly because of difficulty in managing payment to the various entities in the ACO's network. Nonetheless, there is some consensus that the fee-for-service payment system encourages overtreatment (unnecessary and costly care) and must be replaced (Cutler, 2010; Gibson & Singh, 2012).

4. **Improve Access to Coverage.** The ACA does not guarantee health insurance coverage for all, including undocumented immigrants, but, by 2017, it will cover up to 30 million of the 45 million who were uninsured when the bill was signed in 2010 (89% of the total nonolder adult population; 92% of nonolder adult American citizens) (Congressional Budget Office [CBO], 2014). It makes it illegal for insurance companies to deny coverage to people with preexisting conditions, to drop people once they acquire a costly illness, or to apply annual and lifetime caps on coverage. As the demand for health care surges, it is expected that APRNs will be positioned to provide much of the needed primary care, creating the need for APRNs to practice to the full extent of their education and training. Barriers preventing such practice include mandated physician supervision or collaboration in two thirds of states, insurers refusing to credential or impanel APRNs, Medicare requirements for physicians—rather than NPs—to order referrals to home care and hospice, and other local, state, and national policies that limit APRN practice.

Access to coverage does not ensure that people will have access to care. There is a lack of primary care physicians (PCPs) serving the poor, in both rural and urban regions; approximately 210,000 PCPs currently practice, and it has been estimated that another 52,000 will be needed by 2025 (Petterson et al., 2012). This shortfall has led to the development of the APRN role. A workforce analysis center at the Health Resources and Services Administration reported that if primary care NPs and physician assistants (PAs) are fully integrated into a health care delivery system that emphasizes team-based care, the projected shortage of PCPs would be "somewhat alleviated" by 2020 (U.S. Department of Health and Human Services, 2013).

Community-based health care centers will be expanded in areas where there are health care provider shortages. Expansion of the National Health Service Corps is expected to ensure that providers, including registered nurses (RNs) and APRNs, will be available to staff these centers. An emphasis on primary care will increase the demand for NPs and RNs, and the ACA authorizes additional support for primary care workforce development (loans, scholarships, new educational program development, and expansion of existing programs). (See Chapter 60 for more on the nursing workforce.)

NURSES AS LEADERS IN HEALTH CARE REFORM

Coinciding with the passage of the ACA was the timely publication of *The Future of Nursing: Leading Change, Advancing Health* (IOM, 2011). It makes four recommendations, one of which is "Nurses should be full partners, with physicians and other health professionals, in redesigning health care in the United States" (Figure 1-3).

This presents a challenge to nurses: to identify opportunities to participate in policy decision making at all levels of society, the health care system, and health care organizations. Although nursing is well positioned to contribute to a reformed health care system, we cannot assume that those making the decisions about reform will automatically seek nurses' input. And, if invited to policy tables, will nurses show up and participate fully? The IOM report calls for the profession to develop its leadership capacity, while encouraging policymakers and others to appreciate nurses' perspectives on policy. Whether developing new models of care, sharing ideas for regulations with policymakers, developing demonstration projects that the new health care law seeks to test, or advocating new legislation to amend and improve upon the law (or preventing it from being dismantled), nurses must strengthen their social covenant with the public and more forcefully engage in shaping policy at all levels within government, workplaces, health-related organizations, and communities.

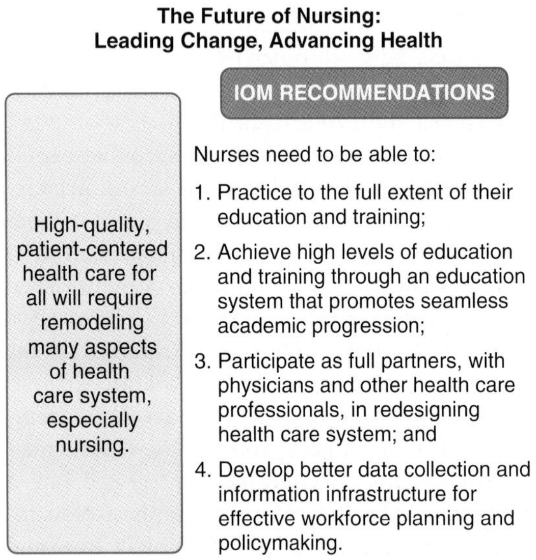

POLICY AND THE POLICY PROCESS

What do we mean by policy? *Policy* has been defined as the authoritative decisions made in the legislative, executive, or judicial branches of government intended to influence the actions, behaviors, or decisions of citizens (Longest, 2010). But that definition limits its application to sectors outside of government. For example, health care organizations set policy that affects employees, patients, and even surrounding communities (for example, by closing a neighborhood clinic or buying property for hospital expansion). Thus, a broader definition of *policy* is "a relatively stable, purposive course of action or inaction followed by an actor or set of actors in dealing with a problem or matter of concern" (Anderson, 2015, p. 6).

Public policy is policy crafted by governments. When the intent of a public policy is to influence health or health care, it is a *health policy*. *Social policies* identify courses of action to deal with social problems. All are made within a dynamic environment and a complex policymaking process. *Private policies* are those made by nongovernmental entities, whether health care organizations, insurers, or

The Future of Nursing: Leading Change, Advancing Health

IOM RECOMMENDATIONS

High-quality, patient-centered health care for all will require remodeling many aspects of health care system, especially nursing.

Nurses need to be able to:

1. Practice to the full extent of their education and training;

2. Achieve high levels of education and training through an education system that promotes seamless academic progression;

3. Participate as full partners, with physicians and other health care professionals, in redesigning health care system; and

4. Develop better data collection and information infrastructure for effective workforce planning and policymaking.

FIGURE 1-3 Four key messages: The IOM report. (From Institute of Medicine. [2011]. The future of nursing: Leading change, advancing health. Washington, DC: National Academies Press. Retrieved from *www.iom.edu/nursing.*)

others. Indeed, there is growing recognition that policies set by health care organizations and insurers, for example, can limit APRN practice even in states that have removed laws requiring physician supervision or collaboration. A hospital can limit what APRNs do as long as the organization does not call for APRNs to practice beyond the state's scope-of-practice policy.

Policies are crafted everywhere, from small towns to Capitol Hill. States use policies to specify requirements for health professions' licensure, to set criteria for Medicaid eligibility, and to require immunization for public university students, for example. Hospitals use policies to direct when visitors may visit patients, to manage staffing, and to respond to disasters. Public schools employ state policies to specify who may administer medications to schoolchildren and what may be sold from a school vending machine. Towns, cities, and other municipalities use policies to manage public water, to define who may run for office, and to decide if residents may keep exotic pets.

In a capitalist economy such as that of the United States, private markets can control the production and consumption of goods and services, including health care. The government often "intervenes" with policies when private markets have failed to achieve desired public objectives. But when is it necessary for the government to intercede? Broadly speaking, in the current U.S. political system, the divide between liberal and conservative political parties is a fundamental disagreement about the degree to which government can and should solve problems (Kelly, 2004) in education, national security, the environment, and nearly every other aspect of public life. The American political landscape is continuously shifting, as public mood shifts with new Representatives being elected and senior Representatives desiring to stay in office.

Longest (2010) describes two types of public policies the government develops:

- *Allocative policies* provide benefits to a distinct group of individuals or organizations, at the expense of others, to achieve a public objective (this is also referred to as the *redistribution of wealth*). The enactment of Medicare in 1965 was an allocative policy that provided health benefits to older adults using federal funds (largely from middle- and high-income taxpayers).
- *Regulatory policies* influence the actions, behavior, and decisions of individuals or groups to ensure that a public objective is met. The Health Insurance Portability and Accountability Act (HIPAA) of 1996 regulates how individually identifiable health information is managed by users, as well as other aspects of health records.

Policymaking is an often unpredictable dance that requires a high degree of political competence. Our system is based on continuous policy modification—incremental change is exceedingly more likely than revolutionary change. But there are exceptions; once in a generation a large social program is passed such as Medicare and Medicaid in the 1960s and the ACA in 2010.

FORCES THAT SHAPE HEALTH POLICY

Some of the most prominent forces that shape health policy appear in Figure 1-4.

VALUES

Values undergird proposed and adopted policies and influence all political and policymaking activities. Public policies reflect a society's values and also its conflicts in values. A policy reflects which values are given priority in a specific decision (Kraft & Furlong, 2010). Once framed, a policy reveals the underlying values that shaped it. Different people value different things, and when resources are finite, policy choices ultimately bring a disadvantage to some groups; some will gain something from the policy, and some will lose (Bankowski, 1996). To support or oppose a policy requires value judgments (Majone, 1989). Conflicts between values were apparent throughout the debates on the ACA; for example, despite a strong contingent of advocates for a government-run, nonprofit insurance option that would compete with private insurers, the insurance industry opposed it, as did others who saw it as an increase in government control, and it was not included in the law.

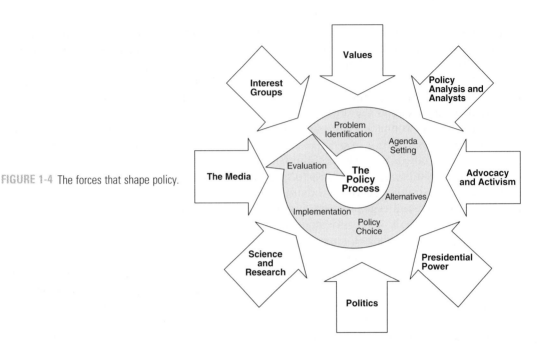

FIGURE 1-4 The forces that shape policy.

POLITICS

Politics is the use of relationships and power to gain ascendancy among competing stakeholders to influence policy and the allocation of scarce resources. Because inevitably there are competing interests for scarce resources, policymaking is done within a political context.

The definition of politics contains several important concepts. *Influencing* indicates that there are opportunities to shape the outcome of a process. *Allocation* means that decisions are being made about how to distribute resources. *Scarce* implies the limits to available resources and that all parties probably cannot have all they want. Finally, *resources* are usually considered to be financial but could also include human resources (personnel), time, or physical space such as offices (Mason, Leavitt, & Chaffee, 2012). Engaging in the political context of policymaking includes knowing the positions of key stakeholders and political parties, as well as the electoral process, public opinion, the influence of media coverage, and more (see Chapter 9 for an in-depth discussion of political analysis and strategies). Understanding politics is an invitation not to misuse power, people, or information but rather to align the health of the public with the interest of the policymaker. For example, a Congresswoman may have run her campaign focused on improving the economy. She may not have linked the rising obesity epidemic as a threat to the larger macroeconomy and American productivity. Nurses could link obesity to the economy by describing the catastrophic direct and indirect costs of the obesity epidemic and how it is making the United States less competitive in a global market. This is a way for nurses to use their power to create more urgency about the most pressing public health issues.

POLICY ANALYSIS AND ANALYSTS

Analysis is the examination of an object or a process to understand it better. Policy analysis uses various methods to assess a problem and determine possible solutions. This encourages deliberate critical thinking about the causes of problems, identifies the ways a government or other groups could respond, evaluates alternatives, and determines the most desirable policy choice. (See Chapter 7.) Policy analysts are individuals who, with professional training and experience, analyze problems and weigh potential solutions. Citizens can also use policy analysis to better understand a problem, alternatives, and potential implications of policy choices (Kraft & Furlong, 2010).

ADVOCACY AND ACTIVISM

Advocacy of one patient at a time has long been a central role for nurses. But nurses can be advocates on a larger scale by working in policy and politics, which is endorsed in "nursing's social policy statement" (American Nurses Association [ANA], 2003), a document that defines nursing and its social context. Political activism may be associated with protests but has grown to include additional diverse and effective strategies such as blogging, using evidence to support policy choices, and garnering media attention in sophisticated ways.

INTEREST GROUPS AND LOBBYISTS

Interest groups advocate for policies that are advantageous to their membership. Groups often employ lobbyists to advocate on their behalf and their power cannot be underestimated. In 2009, 1814 U.S. businesses and organizations spent $554,566,269 on lobbying and employed 3527 lobbyists to advocate for their interests in the health care reform debate and other issues (Center for Responsive Politics, n.d., a). This was a peak year that coincided with interest groups' attempts to influence the ACA. In 2013, 1299 organizations spent $483,078,712 on lobbying and used 2918 lobbyists to advance their interests, including over $1.6 million by the ANA and $940,000 by the American Association of Nurse Anesthetists (Center for Responsive Politics, n.d., b).

THE MEDIA

The power of media is demonstrated in political and issue campaigns, whether through paid political advertisements or the "talking heads" on "news" programs that present polarized views. The aim is to deliver messages that resonate with the values and emotions of a target audience to support or oppose a candidate or proposed policy. The strategic use of media is imperative in today's cacophony of information. Gaining the attention of a target audience is power. Persuading that audience to behave the way you want is ultimate power.

In this information age, nurses must proactively use media to influence policy and make themselves available to speak with journalists about policy matters. However, nurses have not always been eager to enter the media spotlight (see Chapter 14 on using media as a policy and political tool), particularly when it comes to talking with journalists. Social media is a tool for influencing policymakers (Grande et al., 2014) and provides nurses with an opportunity to control their message. Nurse bloggers such as Barbara Glickstein are getting visibility as "media makers." Theresa Brown writes for the *Opinionator* column for *The New York Times*. Both are bringing nursing perspectives on policy matters to the public's attention.

SCIENCE AND RESEARCH

The information age has created an emphasis on evidence-based practice and policies. Scientific findings play a powerful role in the first step of the policy process: getting attention to particular problems and moving them to the policy agenda. Research can also be valuable in defining the size and scope of a problem and substantiating policy recommendations. This can help to obtain support for a proposed policy and in lobbying for support of it. Evidence should be used to inform policy debates and shape policy choices to help ensure that the solution will be effective. That said, evidence is essential but may not be sufficient to advance policies. Values and politics can trump evidence, as has been apparent in recent debates over two issues: climate change and decreasing rates of vaccinations. Despite the evidence showing that humans are contributing to potentially devastating changes in the earth's climate or that childhood vaccinations do not cause autism, debates about these issues continue and affect whether policies are or are not adopted to address the problems.

THE POWER OF PRESIDENTS AND OTHER LEADERS

The president embodies the power of the executive branch of government and is the only person elected to represent the entire nation. As the most visible government official, the president is able to propel issues to the top of the nation's policy agenda. Although the president cannot introduce legislation, he or she can provide draft legislation and legislative guidance. The president can also issue executive orders when he or she cannot get support for policy change from Congress. President Obama has done so in the face of a paralyzed Congress, as did his Republican and Democratic predecessors. This force also applies to the leaders of many public and private entities. Never underestimate the power of the official leader or of those who seek to remove or thwart the leader.

THE FRAMEWORK FOR ACTION

Nursing has a covenant with the public. The profession's practice laws, standards, and ethics have roots in its history of activism for social justice. A social contract with society demands professional responsibility. Thus, every nurse must continuously consider the policy context of daily practice in any setting. The solutions to today's most intractable health care problems, including perverse payment mechanisms, deeply disturbing social injustice, and shocking ethnic and racial disparities, are not simple to solve. But, according to the annual Gallup poll (Gallup, 2013), the public regards nurses'

"honesty and ethical standards" more highly than those of any other profession. This public trust places a moral imperative on nurses to vigorously engage in influencing policy. Nurses see close up how policies get played out in patient care and can report on unintended consequences. This imperative requires nurses to expand their involvement in policy decisions at the institutional, community, state, federal, or international realm and need not be restricted to any one setting.

The Framework for Action (Figure 1-5) illustrates that nurses operate in four spheres: government, workplace, interest groups (including professional organizations), and community to influence policies that affect health and health care and core/social determinants of health.

SPHERES OF INFLUENCE

The four spheres of influence provide a visual medium for understanding the policy arena. These spheres are not discrete silos. Policy can be shaped in more than one sphere at a time, and action in one sphere can influence others. To achieve greater

FIGURE 1-5 A framework: Spheres of influence for action. Nurses need to work in multiple spheres of influence to shape health and social policy. Policies are designed to remedy problems in the health system and to address social determinants of health; both of which aim to improve health.

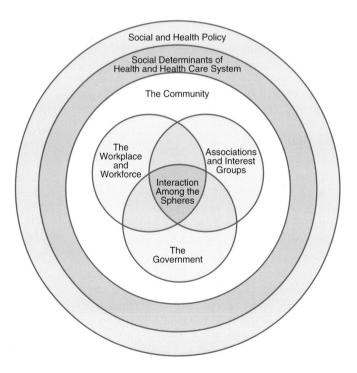

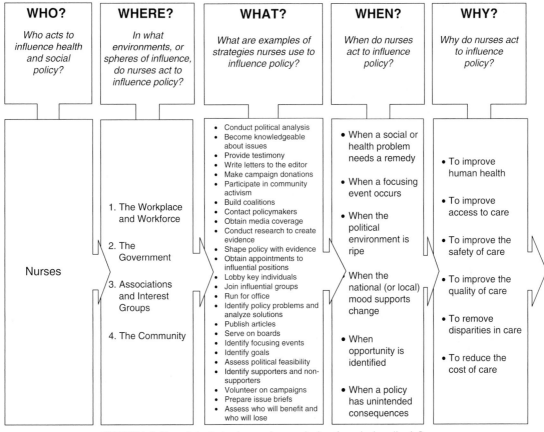

FIGURE 1-6 The who, what, where, when, and why of nursing's policy influence.

access to care for the uninsured, for example, nurses may work in their own organization to alter policy to increase access to services. They may also use political strategies in the media, such as blogging or being interviewed on television, to express their support for better access to care. They may work with a professional association or an interest group to communicate their views to policymakers. Additional context (the who, what, where, when, and why of nursing's policy influence) is provided in Figure 1-6.

THE GOVERNMENT

Government action and policy affect lives from birth until death. It funds prenatal care, inspects food, controls the safety of toys and cars, operates schools, builds highways, and regulates what is transmitted on airwaves. It provides for the common defense; supplies fire and police protection; and gives financial assistance to the poor, aged, and others who cannot maintain a minimal standard of living. The government responds to disaster, subsidizes agriculture, and licenses funeral homes.

Although most U.S. health care is provided in the private sector, much is paid for and regulated by the government. So, how the government crafts health policy is extremely important (Weissert & Weissert, 2012). Government plays a significant role in influencing nursing and nursing practice. States determine the scope of professional activities considered to be nursing, with notable exceptions of the military, veterans' administration, and Indian health service. Federal and state governments determine who is eligible for care under specific benefit programs and who can be reimbursed for providing care. Sometimes government provides leadership in defining problems for both the public and private sectors to address. There are more than a dozen House and Senate committees and subcommittees that shape policy on health, and many more committees address social problems that affect health. In the House of Representatives, the Congressional Nursing Caucus, an informal, bipartisan group of legislators who have declared their interest in helping nurses, lobbies for federal funding for nursing education (Walker, 2009).

Abraham Lincoln's description of a "government of the people, by the people, for the people" (Lincoln, 1863) captures the intricate nature of the relationship of government and its people. There are many ways nurses can influence policymaking in the government sphere, at local, state, and federal levels of government. Examples include:

- Obtaining appointment to influential government positions
- Serving in federal, state, and local agencies
- Serving as elected officials
- Working as paid lobbyists
- Communicating positions to policymakers
- Providing testimony at government hearings
- Participating in grassroots efforts, such as rallies, to draw attention to problems

THE WORKFORCE AND WORKPLACE

Nurses work in a variety of settings: hospitals, clinics, schools, private sector firms, government agencies, military services, research centers, nursing homes, and home health agencies. All of these environments are political ones; resources are finite, and nurses must work in each to influence the allocation of organizational resources. Policies guide many activities in the health care workplaces where nurses are employed. Many that affect nursing and patient care are internal organizational policies such as staffing policies, clinical procedures, and patient care guidelines. External policies are operative in the health care workplace also; for example, state laws regulating nursing licensure. Federal laws and regulations are evident in the nursing workplace such as Occupational Health and Safety Administration regulations

regarding worker protection from bloodborne pathogens.

Policy influences the size and composition of the nursing workforce. The ACA authorizes increased funding for scholarships and loans for nursing education, potentially augmenting existing workforce programs funded under Title VII and Title VIII of the Public Health Service Act. The nongovernmental Commission on Graduates of Foreign Nursing Schools is authorized by the federal government to protect the public by ensuring that nurses and other health care professionals educated outside the United States are eligible and qualified to meet U.S. licensure, immigration, and other practice requirements (Commission on Graduates of Foreign Nursing Schools, 2009). The National Council of State Boards of Nursing is a not-for-profit organization that brings together state boards of nursing to act on matters of common interest affecting the public's health, safety, and welfare, including the development of licensing examinations in nursing (National Council of State Boards of Nursing, 2009). These are just a few examples of the external forces that shape workforce and workplace policy.

ASSOCIATIONS AND INTEREST GROUPS

Professional nursing associations have played a significant role in influencing practice. Many associations have legislative or policy committees that advocate policies supporting their members' practice and advance the interests of their patient populations. Working with a group increases the effectiveness of advocacy, provides for the sharing of resources, and enhances networking and learning. In fact, these associations can be excellent training grounds for novice nurses to learn about policy and political action (see Chapter 4). Nurses can be effective in association policy activities by serving on public policy or legislative work groups, providing testimony, and preparing position statements.

When nursing organizations join forces through coalitions, their influence can be multiplied. For example, The Nursing Community (*www.thenursingcommunity.org*) is an informal coalition of national nursing organizations that formed to speak with one voice on matters important to national policy and political appointments (see

Chapter 75). The Coalition for Patients' Rights (*www.patientsrightscoalition.org*) is a group of more than 35 national organizations representing health care professionals that is working to fight the American Medical Association's attempts to limit patients' access to nonphysician providers. Twenty members are nursing organizations.

Nurses can be influential, not just in nursing associations, but by working with other interest groups such as the American Public Health Association or the Sierra Club. Some interest groups have a broad portfolio of policy interests, whereas others focus on one disease (e.g., National Breast Cancer Coalition) or one issue (e.g., driving while intoxicated, the primary focus of Mothers Against Drunk Driving). Interest groups have become powerful players in policy debates; those with large funding streams are able to shape public opinion with media advertisements.

THE COMMUNITY

A limited number of nurses will have the opportunity to influence policy at the highest levels of government, but extensive opportunities exist for nurses to influence health and social policy in communities. Nursing has a rich history of community activism with remarkable examples provided by leaders such as Lillian Wald, Harriet Tubman, and Ruth Lubic. This legacy continues today with the community advocacy efforts of nurses such as Cora Tomalinas, Mary Behrens, Ellie Lopez-Bowlan, the Nightingales who took on Big Tobacco, and the nurses who are a part of the Canary Coalition for Clean Air (their stories appear in this book).

A community is a group of people who share something in common and interact with one another, who may exhibit a commitment to one another or share a geographic boundary (Lundy & Janes, 2001). A community may be a neighborhood, a city, an online group with a common interest, or a faith-based network. Nurses can be influential in communities by identifying problems, strategizing with others, mobilizing support, and advocating change. In residential communities (such as towns, villages, and urban districts), there are opportunities to serve in positions that influence policy. Many groups, such as planning boards, civic organizations, and parent-teacher associations, offer opportunities for involvement.

HEALTH

The Framework for Action includes health as an element of the model to represent that optimal health is viewed as the goal of nursing's policy efforts. Optimal health (whether for the individual patient, family, a population, or community) is the central focus of the political and policy activity described in this book. This focus makes it clear that the ultimate goal for advancing nursing's interests must be to promote the public's health.

Nursing embraces a broad definition of health that aligns with the World Health Organization (1948): "Health is a state of complete physical, mental and social well-being and not merely the absence of disease or infirmity." It incorporates the concept of positive health, not just ill health (Greene et al., 2014). This definition requires a focus on creating communities that thrive economically, have safe environments, and use resources to ensure that their members have access to good nutrition and other elements that can promote health.

HEALTH AND SOCIAL POLICY

This definition of health leads to the focus on health and social policy as key elements in the Framework for Action. Many factors that affect health are social ones, such as income, education, and housing. Although nurses involved in policy often focus on health policies, the emphasis on upstream factors requires a broader focus on the socioeconomic factors that affect health, including labor policy, laws that can stimulate job creation, or local ordinances on smoking bans.

HEALTH SYSTEMS AND SOCIAL DETERMINANTS OF HEALTH

The health care system is the focus of most discussions of health policy to date. Much of this book focuses on understanding the complex and sometimes chaotic U.S. health care system, the ACA's role in augmenting the system's performance, and other policies needed to achieve the Triple Aim. It also addresses the powerful impact that upstream factors have on the health of populations. A singular focus on the health care system is limited in the extent to which it can lead to higher levels of health for individuals, families, and communities.

NURSING ESSENTIALS

Nursing has also developed a competency-based educational curriculum supporting future nurses' involvement in policy. The American Association of Colleges of Nursing (AACN) publishes the necessary curriculum content and expected competencies of all nursing school graduates from baccalaureate, master's, doctor of nursing practice, and research doctorate (PhD) programs. These documents serve as a framework for twenty-first-century nursing and ground the profession in the direct and indirect care of individuals, families, communities, and populations. The content builds on nursing knowledge, theory, and research and derives knowledge from a wide array of fields and professions.

A study by Byrd and colleagues (2012) found that undergraduate nursing students for the most part are largely unaware of the importance of political activity for nurses. After participating in a robust and active public policy learning activity, students measured high on a political astuteness scale. This study suggests that political skills can be learned when presented with relevance to nursing and used to hone skills such as inquiry, critical thinking, and complex problem solving. These results highlight the importance of increasing students' awareness of how to participate in the political process, as well as encouraging their participation in student and professional organizations.

For each level of nursing education—BSN, MSN, DNP, and PhD—there is a clear expectation that graduates will have policy competency, with increasing emphasis on policy leadership as nursing students progress academically, although this is less well defined for PhD graduates (AACN, 2006; AACN Task Force, n.d.). These essentials make it clear that health policy directly influences nursing practice and every aspect of the health care system.

It is understood that patient safety and quality cannot be addressed outside of the context of policy. The broader policy context is emphasized throughout nursing degree programs. It is expected that DNP graduates are able to design, implement, and advocate health policies that improve the health of populations. The powerful practice experiences of nurses can become potent influencers in policy formation. Additionally, a DNP graduate integrates these practice experiences with two additional skill sets: the ability to analyze the policy process and the ability to engage in politically competent action (AACN, 2006). See Table 1-1 for a summary of the policy competencies in successive nursing education programs.

POLICY AND POLITICAL COMPETENCE

Competence is being adequately prepared or qualified to perform a specific role. It encompasses a combination of knowledge, skills, and behaviors that improve performance. Nurses are often reluctant to become involved in policy because of the "politics." Political skill has a bad reputation; for some, it conjures up thoughts of manipulation, self-interested behavior, and favoritism (Ferris, Davidson, & Perrewe, 2005). "She plays politics" is not generally considered to be a compliment, but true political skill is critical in health care leadership, advocating for others, and shaping policy. It is simply not possible to succeed in any decision-making arena by ignoring the political realm. Ferris, Davidson, and Perrewe (2005) consider political skill to be the ability to understand others and to use that knowledge to influence others to act in a way that supports one's objectives. They identify political skill in four components:

1. *Social astuteness:* Skill at being attuned to others and social situations; ability to interpret one's own behaviors and the behavior of others.
2. *Interpersonal influence:* Convincing personal style that influences others featuring the ability to adapt behavior to situations and be pleasant and productive to work with.
3. *Networking ability:* The ability to develop and use diverse networks of people, and the ability

TABLE 1-1 AACN's Nursing Essentials Series: Policy Competencies for Nurses

Nursing Program	Policy Essential: All Nurses at This Level Must Have Expertise in:	Description
BSN Policy Essential VI[1] (2008)	Health care policy, finance, and regulatory environments	Health care policies, including financial and regulatory, directly and indirectly influence the nature and functioning of the health care system and thereby are important considerations in professional nursing practice.
MSN Policy Essential VI[1] (1996)	Health policy and advocacy	Recognizes that the master's-prepared nurse is able to intervene at the system level through the policy development process and to employ advocacy strategies to influence health and health care.
DNP Policy Essential V[1] (2011)	Health care policy for advocacy in health care	The DNP graduate has the capacity to engage proactively in the development and implementation of health policy at all levels, including institutional, local, state, regional, federal, and international levels.
		DNP graduates, as leaders in the practice arena, provide a critical interface among practice, research, and policy.
		Preparing graduates with the essential competencies to assume a leadership role in the development of health policy requires that students have opportunities to contrast the major contextual factors and policy triggers that influence health policymaking at various levels.
Research-Focused Doctorate in Nursing (PhD)[2] (2010)	*Curricular elements include:* Communicate research findings to lay and professional audiences and identify implications for policy, nursing practice, and the profession	Strategies to influence health policy. Leadership related to health policy and professional issues.

Sources:

[1]The American Association of Colleges of Nursing. Essentials Series. Baccalaureate (2008); Masters (1996); DNP (2011). Retrieved from *www.aacn.nche.edu/education-resources/essential-series.*

[2]The American Association of Colleges of Nursing. (2010). The Research-Focused Doctoral Program in Nursing: Pathways to excellence. Report from the AACN Task Force on the Research-Focused Doctorate in Nursing. Retrieved from *www.aacn.nche.edu/education-resources/phdposition.pdf.*

to position oneself to create and take advantage of opportunities.

4. *Apparent sincerity:* The display of high levels of integrity, authenticity, sincerity, and genuineness (pp. 9-12).

In most cases, policymakers are generalists who make decisions on a broad range of issues. Nurses can have a profound impact on policymaking by using their knowledge to frame and define health policy alternatives. Influencing policy at all levels requires a strong set of interpersonal skills, integrity, and knowledge. According to O'Grady and Johnson (2013), political competency, at either the individual or the organizational level, can be defined by three main elements: deep knowledge, political antennae, and power (Figure 1-7).

DEEP KNOWLEDGE

Deep knowledge requires freely sharing expertise and gaining the knowledge you need from others. Subject-matter expertise without knowledge of policy and its processes is a doomed strategy. Deep knowledge involves knowing the viewpoints of others, including the opposition, and having a clear message and data at the ready to support your position and neutralize opposition. For example, many physicians' organizations oppose expansion of practice for APRNs, citing patient safety as a primary concern. Politically competent nurses can arm themselves with a summary of decades of evidence citing no such concerns (Newhouse et al., 2011; O'Grady, 2008).

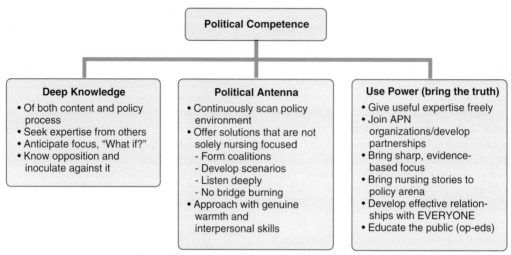

FIGURE 1-7 Political competencies. (From O'Grady, E. T., & Johnson, J. [2013]. Health policy issues in changing environments. In A. Hamric, C. Hanson, D. Way, & E. O'Grady [Eds.], *Advanced practice nursing: An integrative approach* [5th ed.]. St. Louis, MO: Elsevier-Saunders.)

POLITICAL ANTENNAE

Developing political competence requires a continuous scanning of the environment, and it is critical that nurses offer solutions to policy problems that are not solely nursing focused but also address the Triple Aim. Agendas cannot be advanced without the formation of coalitions and networks. Influencers of policy must consider alternative scenario development to use if opposition develops. For example, the 2008 recession had an impact on the nursing shortage: many nurses chose not to retire during that uncertain economic period. The nursing community was able to maintain nursing education funding despite the lessening of the nursing shortage using scenario development. For example, during the economic downturn and slashing of many federal programs, nurses were able to create a scenario in which the aging population explodes, the nursing workforce nears retirement age, and there is a dire nursing faculty shortage. Projections were made predicting catastrophic hospital vacancy rates and unmet health care needs. This scenario was highly effective in preventing cuts in federal funding to nursing education.

Having political antennae requires active listening with policymakers to understand their motives and to develop strategies that fit their political objectives. So if policymakers promised constituents they would not raise taxes, the politically competent nurse would work in a coalition to help find a budget-neutral solution.

Finally, having political antennae requires the avoidance of bridge-burning. Ruptured relationships can cause lasting damage, not only to the nurse involved but also to the profession. Many wounds can develop during policymaking, and it may be crucial that one exercises restraint. Political and policy disagreements require a response of genuine warmth, a quality that can go a long way in building trust. Learning how to navigate differences and agreeing to disagree without being disagreeable are important political skills.

USE OF POWER

Power is the ability to act so as to achieve a goal. In the policy process, power is knowing who has it, who is on what committee, and who are the thought leaders in the community. A coalition is one important way nurses can augment their policymaking power. But an individual nurse can claim it by being articulate and having an elevator speech that can spark interest.

Application of power requires raising one's awareness about what is true and what is false. Being grounded in truth, such as knowing the value of human caring and the role that nursing can have on individuals and populations, is a form of personal integrity that leads to power. Using power is a choice that requires a noncondemnatory and helpful attitude. By freely giving expertise away and approaching "difficult" people with a benign attitude (they are doing the best they can), we hold onto our integrity, build trust, and keep emotions in check. To be effective in the policy arena, nurses must have a sharp focus on the evidence, not emotion. Advancing nursing's policy agenda through such a use of power demands that we drop narcissism and nursing parochialism and focus on problem solving. Nursing *narcissism* is when a nurse shows an inordinate fascination with oneself, self-centeredness, and a high degree of smugness. This can include taking sole responsibility for some action or project in which a team was responsible. Nursing *parochialism* is when a nurse is in a problem-solving context (policy meeting) and only offers up the solution of "nurses" as the remedy to every problem. Parochialism is an approach that narrows options and interests and appears self-serving. Both of these destructive approaches do not deploy the cost-quality-access triad framework to problem solving and therefore severely constricts nursing power. They are to be avoided at all costs and nurses exhibiting these attitudes must be removed from decision-making tables. Effective use of power avoids polarization, egotism, and self-serving postures at all costs. Bringing nurses' stories to the policy arena is, however, a powerful way to pair the human story to the scientific evidence.

Corralling the political power of the 3.1 million registered nurses in the U.S. can only occur if individual nurses join, support, and fully engage with professional nursing organizations. More than any other effort to date, *The Future of Nursing: Leading Change, Advancing Health* (IOM, 2011) has brought disparate nurses together to engage across associations and educational institutions, and with new community partners, to change policy. Many of the recommendations direct policy changes resonant with nurses. This effort is increasing nursing's political competence, but more could be done: printed op-eds, blog posts, and interviews with nurses in major media outlets could capitalize on the high regard the public has for nursing.

Nurses who effectively use power are a sought-after and a valued asset. They get invited to the table, but they are asked back and often invited to more tables with ever-expanding influence. This requires a great degree of knowledge, along with humility, a problem-solving attitude, and a patient-centered lens. Such activities and attitudes strengthen an individual's interpersonal power and integrity, which can inspire others.

DISCUSSION QUESTIONS

1. What are the most pressing health care problems you see in your community? How can you frame that issue in a health policy context?
2. Can you identify areas in your own political competence that requires growth? What do you need to learn to be more effective?
3. Why has nursing made policy and political competence such a strong part of the nursing curriculum and role development?

REFERENCES

Allen, M. (2013). How many die from medical mistakes in U.S. hospitals? *Scientific American*. Retrieved from *www.scientificamerican.com/article/how-many-die-from-medical-mistakes-in-us-hospitals/*.

American Academy of Nursing. (n.d., a). Raise the voice. Retrieved from *www.aannet.org/raisethevoice*.

American Academy of Nursing. (n.d., b). Edge Runners: The Eleventh Street Family Health Service, Drexel University. Retrieved from *www.aannet.org/edge-runners–eleventh-street-family-health-services*.

American Association of Colleges of Nursing. (2006). The essentials of doctoral education for advanced nursing practice. Retrieved from *www.aacn.nche.edu/publications/position/DNPEssentials.pdf*.

American Association of Colleges of Nursing [AACN] Task Force on the Research-Focused Doctorate in Nursing. (n.d.). The research-focused doctorate in nursing: Pathway to excellence. Retrieved from *www.aacn.nche.edu/education-resources/phdposition.pdf*.

American Nurses Association. (2003). *Nursing's social policy statement: The essence of the profession*. Washington, DC: American Nurses Association.

Anderson, J. E. (2015). *Public policymaking* (8th ed.). Farmington Hills, MI: Cengage Learning.

Bankowski, Z. (1996). Ethics and human values in health policy. *World Health Forum*, *17*(2), 146–149.

Barkauskas, V. H., Pohl, J. M., Tanner, C., Onifade, T. J., & Pilon, B. (2011). Quality of care in nurse-managed health centers. *Nursing Administration Quarterly*, *35*(1), 34–43.

Berwick, D., Nolan, T., & Whittington, J. (2008). The Triple Aim: Care, health, and cost. *Health Affairs*, *27*(3), 759–769. Retrieved from *content.healthaffairs.org/content/27/3/759.full*.

Braveman, P., Cubbin, C., Egerter, S., Williams, D., & Pamuk, E. (2010). Socioeconomic disparities in health in the United States: What the patterns tell us. *American Journal of Public Health*, *100*(Suppl. 1), S186–S196.

Byrd, M. E., Costello, J., Gremel, K., Schwager, J., Blanchette, L., & Malloy, T. E. (2012). Political astuteness of baccalaureate nursing students following an active learning experience in health policy. *Public Health Nursing*, *29*(5), 433–443.

Centers for Medicare and Medicaid Services (CMS). (2013). National health expenditures 2012 highlights. Retrieved from *www.cms.gov/Research-Statistics-Data-and-Systems/Statistics-Trends-and-Reports/NationalHealthExpendData/Downloads/highlights.pdf*.

Centers for Medicare and Medicaid Services (CMS). (2014). Medicaid & CHIP: February 2014 monthly applications, eligibility determinations, and enrollment report, April 4, 2014. Retrieved from *www.medicaid.gov/AffordableCareAct/Medicaid-Moving-Forward-2014/Downloads/March-2014-Enrollment-Report.pdf*.

Centers for Medicare and Medicaid Services (CMS). (n.d.). Community-based care transitions programs. Retrieved from *innovation.cms.gov/initiatives/CCTP/*.

Center for Responsive Politics. (n.d., a). Influence and lobbying: health. Retrieved from *www.opensecrets.org/lobby/indus.php?id=H&year=2009#clients*.

Center for Responsive Politics. (n.d., b). Health professionals: lobbying, 2013. Retrieved from *www.opensecrets.org/industries/lobbying.php?cycle=2014&ind=H01*.

Coalition for Evidence-Based Policy. (n.d.). Social programs that work: Transitional care model—Top tier. Retrieved from *evidencebasedprograms.org/1366-2/transitional-care-model-top-tier*.

Commission on Graduates of Foreign Nursing Schools. (2009). Commission on graduates of foreign nursing schools: Mission and history. Retrieved from *www.cgfns.org*.

Congressional Budget Office [CBO]. (2014). Insurance Coverage Provisions of the Affordable Care Act—CBO's April 2014 Baseline. Retrieved from *www.cbo.gov/sites/default/files/cbofiles/attachments/43900-2014-04-ACAtables2.pdf*.

Conway, P. H., Mostashari, F., & Clancy, C. (2013). The future of quality measurement for improvement and accountability. *JAMA*, *309*(21), 2215–2216.

Cutler, D. (2010). How health care reform must bend the cost curve. *Health Affairs*, *29*(6), 1131–1135.

Felt-Lisk, S., & Higgins, T. (2011). Exploring the promise of population health management programs to improve health. Mathematica Policy Research Issue Brief. Retrieved from *www.mathematica-mpr.com/publications/PDFs/health/PHM_brief.pdf*.

Ferris, G., Davidson, S., & Perrewe, P. (2005). *Political skill at work: Impact on work effectiveness*. Mountain View, CA: Davies-Black Publishing.

Gallup. (2010). Nursing leadership from bedside to boardroom: Opinion leaders' perception. Retrieved from *newcareersinnursing.org/sites/default/files/file-attachments/Top%20Line%20Report.pdf*.

Gallup. (2013). Honesty and ethics in professions. Retrieved from *www.gallup.com/poll/1654/honesty-ethics-professions.aspx*.

Gibson, R., & Singh, J. P. (2012). *Medicare meltdown: How Wall Street and Washington are ruining Medicare and how to fix it*. New York: Rowman & Littlefield Publishers.

Grande, D., Gollust, S., Pany, M., Seymour, J., Goss, A., Kilaru, A., et al. (2014). Translating research for health policy: Researchers' perceptions and use of social media. *Health Affairs*, *33*(7), 1278–1285. Retrieved from *content.healthaffairs.org/content/33/7/1278.abstract?sid=aa8bb4ab-5fcd-490d-abc0-1069d3d18819*.

Greene, R., Dasso, E., Ho, S., & Genaidy, A. (2014). A person-focused model of care for the twenty-first century: a system-of-systems perspective. *Population Health Management*, *17*(3), 166–171. doi:10.1089/pop.2013/0040.

Halpin, H. A., Morales-Suárez-Varela, M. M., & Martin-Moreno, J. M. (2010). Chronic disease prevention and the New Public Health. *Public Health Reviews*, *32*, 120–154.

Hansen-Turton, T., Bailey, D. N., Torres, N., & Ritter, A. (2010). Nurse-managed health centers. *American Journal of Nursing*, *110*(9), 23–26.

The Henry J. Kaiser Family Foundation [KFF]. (2013). Kaiser health tracking poll: August 2013. Retrieved from *kff.org/health-reform/poll-finding/kaiser-health-tracking-poll-august-2013*.

Institute for Healthcare Improvement. (n.d.). The Triple Aim: IHI Triple Aim Initiative. Retrieved from *www.ihi.org/Engage/Initiatives/TripleAim/Pages/default.aspx*.

Institute of Medicine. (1999). *To err is human: Building a safer health system*. Washington, DC: National Academies Press.

Institute of Medicine. (2011). *The future of nursing: Leading change, advancing health*. Washington, DC: National Academies Press. Retrieved from *www.iom.edu/nursing*.

James, J. (2013). A new, evidence-based estimate of patient harms associated with hospital care. *Journal of Patient Safety*, *9*(3), 122–128. Retrieved from *journals.lww.com/journalpatientsafety/Fulltext/2013/09000/A_New,_Evidence_based_Estimate_of_Patient_Harms.2.aspx*.

Katz, M. H. (2009). Structural interventions for addressing chronic health problems. *JAMA*, *302*(6), 683–685.

Kelly, N. (2004). Does politics really matter? Policy and government's equalizing influence in the United States. *American Politics Research*, *32*(3), 264–284.

Kennedy, K. (2014). Health exchange enrollment reaches 7.5 million. *USA Today*. Retrieved from *www.usatoday.com/story/news/nation/2014/04/10/health-exchange-enrollment-reaches-75-million/7545495/*.

Kraft, M., & Furlong, S. (2010). *Public policy: Politics, analysis, and alternatives* (3rd ed.). Washington, DC: CQ Press.

Leppo, K., Ollila, E., Peña, S., Wismar, M., & Cook, S. (Eds.) (2013). *Health in all policies: Seizing opportunities, implementing policies*. Helsinki, Finland: Ministry of Social Affairs and Health. Retrieved from *www.euro.who.int/__data/assets/pdf_file/0007/188809/Health-in-All-Policies-final.pdf*.

Lincoln, A. (1863). Gettysburg Address. Retrieved from *www.ourdocuments.gov/doc.php?flash=old&doc=36*.

Longest, B. (2010). *Health policymaking in the United States* (5th ed.). Chicago, IL: Health Administration Press.

Lundy, K., & Janes, S. (2001). *Community health nursing: Caring for the public's health*. Sudbury, MA: Jones and Bartlett.

Majone, G. (1989). *Evidence, argument, and persuasion in the policy process*. New Haven, CT: Yale University Press.

Marks, J. (2009). Why your zip code may be more important than your genetic code. Robert Wood Johnson Foundation. Retrieved from *www.rwjf.org/en/research-publications/find-rwjf-research/2009/04/why-your-zip-code-may-be-more-important-to-your-health-than-your.html*.

Mason, D., Leavitt, J., & Chaffee, M. (2012). Policy and politics: A framework for action. In D. J. Mason, J. Leavitt, & M. Chaffee (Eds.), *Policy and politics in nursing and health care* (6th ed.). St. Louis, MO: Elsevier.

McCarthy, D., & Klein, S. (2010). *The Triple Aim journey: Improving population health and patients' experience of care, while reducing costs*. The Commonwealth Fund. Retrieved from *www.commonwealthfund.org/*

Publications/Case-Studies/2010/Jul/Triple-Aim-Improving-Population -Health.aspx.

National Council of State Boards of Nursing. (2009). National Council of State Boards of Nursing—About NCSBN. Retrieved from www.ncsbn.org/about.htm.

National Research Council. (2013). U.S. health in international perspective: Shorter lives, poorer health. Washington, DC: The National Academies Press. Retrieved from www.nap.edu/catalog.php?record_id=13497.

Naylor, M., Aiken, L., Kurtzman, E., Olds, D., & Hirschman, K. (2011). The care span: The importance of transitional care in achieving health reform. Health Affairs, 30(4), 4746–4754.

Newhouse, R. P., Stanik-Hutt, J., White, K. M., Johantgen, M., Bass, E. B., Zangaro, G., et al. (2011). Advanced practice nursing outcomes, 1990-2008: A systematic review. Nursing Economics, 29(5), 1–21. Retrieved from www.nursingeconomics.net/ce/2013/article3001021.pdf.

O'Grady, E. T. (2008). Advanced practice registered nurses: The impact on patient safety and quality. In R. G. Hughes (Ed.), Patient safety and quality: An evidence-based handbook for nurses. AHRQ Publication no. 08-0043. Rockville, MD: Agency for Healthcare Research and Quality.

O'Grady, E. T., & Johnson, J. (2013). Health policy issues in changing environments. In A. Hamric, C. Hanson, D. Way, & E. O'Grady (Eds.), Advanced practice nursing: An integrative approach (5th ed.). St. Louis, MO: Elsevier Saunders.

Organization of Economic Co-operation and Development (OECD). (2013). Health at a glance 2013: OECD indicators. OECD Publishing. Retrieved from dx.doi.org/10.1787/health_glance-2013-en.

Peikes, D., Zutshi, A., Genevro, J., Parchman, M., & Meyers, D. (2012). Early evaluations of the medical home: Building on a promising start. The American Journal of Managed Care, Retrieved from www.ajmc.com/publications/issue/2012/2012-2-vol18-n2/early-evaluations-of-the-medical-home-building-on-a-promising-start/1#sthash.7GyzblEQ.dpuf.

Petterson, S. M., Liaw, W., Phillips, R. L., Rabin, D. L., Meyers, D. S., & Bazemore, A. W. (2012). Projecting the U.S. primary care physician workforce needs: 2010-2025. Annals of Family Medicine, 10(6), 503–509. Retrieved from www.annfammed.org/content/10/6/503.full.

Rudolph, L., Caplan, J., Ben-Moshe, K., & Dillon, L. (2013). Health in all policies: a guide for state and local governments. Washington, DC and Oakland, CA: American Public Health Association and Public Health Institute. Retrieved from www.phi.org/uploads/files/Health_in_All_Policies-A_Guide_for_State_and_Local_Governments.pdf.

U.S. Department of Health and Human Services, Health Resources and Services Administration, National Center for Health Workforce Analysis. (2013). Projecting the supply and demand for primary care practitioners through 2020. Rockville, MD: U.S. Department of Health and Human Services. Retrieved from bhpr.hrsa.gov/healthworkforce/supplydemand/usworkforce/primarycare/projectingprimarycare.pdf.

Wagner, E. H. (1998). Chronic disease management: What will it take to improve care for chronic illness? Effective Clinical Practice, 1(1), 2–4.

Walker, I. (2009). Caucusing for a cause. The American Journal of Nursing, 109(9), 26–27.

Weissert, C., & Weissert, W. (2012). Governing health—The politics of health policy (4th ed.). Baltimore, MD: The Johns Hopkins University Press.

Wilkinson, R., & Marmot, M. (Eds.) (2003). Social determinants of health: The solid facts. Geneva: World Health Organization. Retrieved from www.euro.who.int/__data/assets/pdf_file/0005/98438/e81384.pdf.

Williams, D. R., Costa, M. V., Odunlami, A. O., & Mohammed, S. A. (2008). Moving upstream: How interventions that address the social determinants of health can improve health and reduce disparities. Journal of Public Health Management and Practice, 14(Suppl.), S8–S17. doi:10.1097/01.PHH.0000338382.36695.42.

Woolf, S. H. (2009). A closer look at the economic argument for disease prevention. JAMA, 301(5), 536–538.

World Health Organization. (1948). Preamble to the Constitution of the World Health Organization. Retrieved from www.who.int/about/definition/en/print.html.

World Health Organization. (n.d.). Social determinants of health. Retrieved from www.who.int/social_determinants/en/.

ONLINE RESOURCES

Institute of Medicine: The Future of Nursing: Leading Change, Advancing Health
www.iom.edu/nursing
The Future of Nursing: Campaign for Action (current efforts to implement the IOM recommendations)
www.campaignforaction.org
The Affordable Care Act
www.hhs.gov/healthcare/rights/law

CHAPTER 2

An Historical Perspective on Policy, Politics, and Nursing

Patricia D'Antonio   Julie Fairman   Sandra B. Lewenson

"Reform can be accomplished only when attitudes are changed."

Lillian Wald

In 1893, Lillian Wald, then a young medical student, visits the sick mother of a poor and vulnerable New York City family. What she sees—a young mother struggling to recover in a ramshackle tenement, with little access to fresh air and healthy food—and what she does—leaving medical school and returning to nursing because she believed nurses could have a greater impact—changes her life (Wald, 1915). She and her nursing school colleague, Mary Brewster, establish the Henry Street Settlement House in New York City's lower east side. Like many reformers in the late nineteenth century, Wald and Brewster believed that only by living in impoverished, immigrant communities could they effect meaningful change in the city's housing, sanitation, nutrition, and educational policies. But Wald takes her vision one step further. She establishes the Visiting Nurse Service at the Henry Street Settlement (D'Antonio, 2010). At a time when the best in health care centered on the home, she decides that those most vulnerable would have the best in nursing care when ill at home and they would also have the best in health promotion and disease prevention; these families would learn from visiting nurses how to keep themselves healthy in the face of the infectious diseases rampant at the time. And, these visiting nurses would respond to calls from the families in the community just as she would respond to the calls from physicians. Turing her vision into a reality took hard work and strategic partnerships with insurance companies, donors,

schools, and the New York City's Department of Health. However, she prevails—and changes the structure of the U.S. health care system. What come to be known as public health nurses remain central to developing programs addressing public health efforts to promote health and prevent disease. Wald's skill lay in her ability to harness the support of those in power.

Recognizing the strength of coalitions to enact change Wald, along with her colleagues at the settlement house and other nurse leaders, participated in the establishment of the National Organization of Public Health Nursing in 1912, creating an organization to control the standards and practice of public health nurses. She created coalitions, such as that with the American Red Cross, when concerned about the need for access of care in rural communities (Lewenson, 2015), and she knew how to procure the financial resources from private foundations and donors to support many of her public health initiatives. Her success lay in creating coalitions that first identified problems, then found the right resources, and effected successful solutions by making the issues ones that the public "owns."

Why should anyone care about one story about one famous nurse? Because the issues that Wald and her colleagues set out to address remain central to the current debates about how to get the best in health care to vulnerable and dispossessed individuals, families, communities, and populations. Rates of infectious diseases are again climbing in the U.S. and across the globe, adding to the increasingly recognized and growing burden of noninfectious diseases. Certainly, major policy initiatives such as the Affordable Care Act (ACA) promise to increase access to health care, improve quality, and contain costs by shifting the focus from acute care hospitals to homes, communities, and primary care sites. The ACA privileges health promotion and disease prevention in ways unprecedented since the early 1920s. Remembering Wald's story is a reminder that nurses have been, and will continue to be, active participants in health policy debates from the home to the national level and in turning ideas into reality.

Stories create the foundation upon which policies move forward or fail, but the reason for exploring the intersections of history and health policy transcends simply knowing stories. Examining points at these intersections allows for a richer understanding of the possibilities as well as the problems that resonate in health policy deliberations. The distance of time as one studies change over time, the core of historical methods, allows a different view of the tensions existing between public and private spheres of influence, community needs and professional prerogatives, best evidence, and political power. This chapter uses historical case studies, looking to the past to find themes, ideas, and actions that can provide tools for considering future policy deliberations and actions.

"NOT ENOUGH TO BE A MESSENGER"

Buoyed by the success of public health initiatives like Wald's, public health officials returned from rebuilding post–World War I Europe to implement a bold new vision in the United States. The turn toward health care, in addition to illness care, was one of the hallmark characteristics of the "new public health" of the 1920s. If the prewar public health agenda of reformers like Wald focused on the ill individual and environment then the postwar agenda would focus on the individual alone and how that individual could experience even greater health through the practices of personal hygiene, mental hygiene, and social hygiene. Its centerpiece was the "periodic medical examination"—now being urged for women as well as children. Public health leadership were well aware that cancer and degenerative heart disease were emerging as leading causes of death and they urged nurses to preach to patients to demand, and physicians to provide,

examinations that would detect susceptibility to these diseases or identify them when there were still treatment options. They also recognized that routine prenatal examinations that identified and treated medical problems offered the best hope of decreasing appallingly high rates of maternal mortality and launched campaigns that urged mothers and fathers to see pregnancy as akin to a disease and not as a normal phenomenon (D'Antonio, 2014). The problem lay in convincing the public.

In New York City, the focus of this section and the epicenter of both the public health and nursing worlds, public health leadership in the city turned to nurses to deliver this message. This decision seemed self-evident. Public health nurses had long considered themselves and had been considered by others as the "connecting link" between patients and physicians, between and among institutions, and between scientific knowledge and its implementation in the homes they visited. They became the centerpiece of the city's "demonstration projects," an envisioned mix of different types of public and private partnerships that would test ways of delivering this message that were carefully coordinated for efficiencies, cost-effectiveness, and high quality.

Public health nursing leaders in New York City believed that the turn toward health, particularly that of mothers and young children, would define their professional identity and disciplinary independence to a broader community. Health work with mothers and young children had been part of their traditional practices; and, as men were more likely to have periodic medical examinations associated with the purchase of life insurance policies and employment, women and young children seemed particularly vulnerable. In 1921, with funds from an anonymous donor, a small group of white New York City public health nurses, some also involved in the demonstration projects, launched The Citizen's Health Protective Society in the middle-class Manhattanville section of the city. This would be a self-sustaining insurance program that promised prenatal care for mothers; attendance at a medically supervised childbirth if delivered at home, and nine visits for all mothers in the postpartum period. It also promised health supervision of babies and preschool children and bedside nursing if sick at home. Do you want, it queried in handouts to families in Manhattanville, a carefully selected white, middle-class community, a self-supporting nursing and health service for $6 per year for an individual and $16 per year for families of three or more? Manhattanville did not. The Society moved to a more promising location at 134 Street and Amsterdam Avenue. This community remained uninterested as well. The Society closed in 1924. Families appreciated health work but they would only pay for illness care. They would not pay for nursing health care (Maternity Center Association, 1924).

Public health nurses in the city's demonstration projects had more success. These nurses, similar to progressive urban colleagues throughout the country, went one step farther than their health education mandate. They used their experiences in the demonstration projects to move to identifying families as their practice domain. They built knowledge that bridged the biological sciences that supported their public health practices with the new social sciences that buttressed their work with families. This practice, however, brought them out of bounded disciplinary interests and into a place at the center of not only their own but also others' agendas. Foundations, families, physicians, and other public health workers all had particular ideas about what nurses should and could do as they delivered their messages of health.

This placed the demonstration project nurses squarely in the middle of escalating tensions among New York City's Department of Health, the private agencies who delivered home health care, and the Rockefeller Foundation and Milbank Memorial Fund who provided the financing, over who controlled the public health agenda. The private or (as they referred to themselves) voluntary agencies and philanthropies publically ceded control to the official agency that the Departments of Health represented. But privately they constantly sought ways to turn the Department of Health toward their priorities. In New York City, both the private agencies and Rockefeller Foundation and the Milbank Memorial Fund believed public health nurses were key to this process. Indeed, the involvement of the city's public health nurses in the demonstration projects operating in the East Harlem section of

the city had been a central element in the Rockefeller Foundation's support. It could not be a true demonstration of care control, the Foundation believed, unless it involved the city's own public health nurses who ran clean milk and infant welfare stations; and who implemented programs of case finding, case holding, and case control of tuberculosis and other infectious diseases. And it could not be a true maternal-child nursing service without the support of the city's school nurses who worked with those over 6 years of age. The Foundation's policy, in the United States and abroad, was one of only working through governmental public health authorities to ensure the sustainability of its initiatives. It hoped to use a consolidated private and public health nursing system in East Harlem to ultimately do the same in New York City (D'Antonio, 2014).

But the public health nursing leaders of the city's demonstration projects never persuaded the various heads of the New York City's Department of Health to let its nurses join any of their projects. The Department of Health maintained that its nurses were official agents of the city with real police power that it hoped they would rarely use; it needed to maintain control of their practices. The Department of Health had its own agenda for its nurses. It wanted to position them as representatives of a new public health message clothed in tact and sympathy rather than, as in the past, the bearer of quarantine placards and sanitary citations.

More importantly, the nurses involved in the health demonstration projects had shared no investment with their supporting philanthropies in involving the city's own public health nurses. Because, in the end, they won what they themselves wanted. By the end of the formal demonstration period in 1928, both private and public health nurses in New York City—not the physicians who had done so in the past—supervised the independent practices of other public health nurses. This was a substantive achievement. Public health nurses employed by New York City finally gained control of their own nursing practices.

At the same time, nurses in the demonstration projects thrived in their missions of service to mothers and young children and of research on the most pressing issues in public health nursing. It launched a program that continued a long-standing nursing mission to provide bedside nursing to sick residents in their own homes. It also strengthened its outreach to pregnant women, encouraging medically supervised births preferably in hospitals, and providing both prenatal and postpartum care in homes. It started new health education services for preschool children. It also began sustained research projects about the organization of public health nursing work, particularly that situating generalized nursing as the standard for urban public health nursing. And, in 1928, in response to the needs of the discipline for more advanced clinical education, it recast itself as a postgraduate training site for public health nursing students in New York, from around the nation and from international sites of Rockefeller Foundation philanthropy (D'Antonio, 2013).

New York City's health demonstration projects eventually established what are now the norms for primary, pregnancy, dental, and pediatric care. However, this change came almost painfully slowly through the day-to-day work of public health nurses going door to door, street to street, school to school, and neighborhood to neighborhood preaching the gospel of good health to those without access to the resources that class, race, ethnicity, and financial stability provided to others. As importantly, however, it came through the efforts of families to first incorporate and then to normalize these messages of health by removing them from stigmatizing sites of health and social welfare (in which the public health nurses were located) and placing them within the schools that the community embraced. The nurses in New York City's health demonstration projects slowly moved from understanding their role as bringing "medicine and a message" of middle-class values to immigrant families they wished to assimilate, to conceiving it as one of being "more than just a messenger" as they sought to serve as embodiments of a new emphasis on sound mental as well as physical health. Support for public health nursing did decline in the 1930s as nurses painfully realized that it was "not enough to be a messenger." But the decline was less about no longer serving families who needed to assimilate, as other historians have suggested. The decline was as much about families taking responsibility for their health (D'Antonio, 2014).

New York City's public health nurses were also working in a context increasingly dominated by the rise in hospitals and their outpatient clinics where families increasingly sought health care. But the nurses in New York City's demonstration projects paid little attention to warnings about the implications of these new clinical sites for public health practice. They steadfastly maintained the site of their practices to that place where it could be most effectively and independently exercised: with cooperative families in their own homes, in the clinics the nurses controlled, and in the classrooms they created. Despite their commitment to maternal-child health initiatives, this narrow focus allowed them to professionally ignore one of the most pressing public health issues in the city—and indeed the United States—in the early 1930s: the newly rising rates of maternal mortality attributed by both the New York Academy of Medicine and the Maternity Center Association to poor obstetric practices in hospitals that women were increasingly choosing as sites of their infants' births. These nurses could not see or take responsibility for solving problems that lay inside public health policies but outside their defined disciplinary purviews and sites of practice (D'Antonio, 2014).

BRINGING TOGETHER THE PAST FOR THE PRESENT: WHAT WE LEARNED FROM HISTORY

Generations later, a different group of constituents gathered to consider a new agenda for nursing in the twenty-first century that would situate patient care, rather than professional self-interest, at the forefront. In 2009, the Robert Wood Johnson Foundation (RWJF) in collaboration with the Institute of Medicine (IOM) commissioned a new study charged with developing recommendations for reconceptualizing nursing practice and education within a reformed health care system. The Committee appointed by the IOM was indicative of the changing health care political landscape and reflected the multiple stakeholders and thought leaders who were or would be partners with nurses to improve patient care. The Committee was very diverse in age, profession, political leanings, and race/ethnicity, and included consumer representation. The 6 nurses on the 18-member committee all came from diverse backgrounds and served as a contrast to the dominance of white women in the profession seen in the demonstration projects and public health leadership of the 1920s and 1930s. The pivotal role of foundations had changed: they now shared influence with multiple stakeholders such as the federal government, pharmaceutical corporations, consumer groups, and the insurance industry. These groups were now critical players in shaping the scope of nursing practice. In ways unthinkable in the 1920s and 1930s, consumers of nursing care played pivotal roles.

The final report, *The Future of Nursing: Leading Change, Advancing Health*, and its recommendations, reflected the diversity of the committee and the stakeholders as well as the political landscape of health reform being debated as the committee deliberated (IOM, 2011). The first recommendation that nurses should practice to the fullest extent of their knowledge and skills links the story of the New York public health nurses to the nurses of the present. The conceptualization of the role of the public health nurses with families and communities as well as their aims and efforts to fully incorporate their skills and knowledge into their practice reflects historic continuities of nursing practice over the past century. This continuity resonated strongly with the public, professional organizations, and federal and state governments. Since the IOM report was issued seven states have removed practice barriers to allow nurse practitioners to practice independently and numerous other states are expanding their practice acts. At the national level, retail clinics, health care service sites in drug stores, and big box stores typically staffed with nurse practitioners are growing in number and popularity, and nurse-managed health centers are recognized by the ACA as a practice model that can provide access to high-value care for people with limited resources (Fairman et al., 2011). In general, policymakers and the public still see nurses—but now nurse practitioners rather than, as in the past, public health nurses—as a viable and valuable policy solution to the current primary care provider shortage and misdistribution.

Health policy researcher Debra Stone notes there is no strict dichotomy between reason and power, and between policy and politics (Stone, 2001, p. 377). The IOM *Future of Nursing* report placed nurses at the center of a perfect storm of these forces and reflected the political, economic, and social context that propelled both professional and public interests (IOM, 2011). The report recommendations were also strategically shaped to position the patient as the focus of care within a reformed health system and the history of both public health nurses and nurse practitioners is a reminder of the importance of public need when public disciplinary interests are articulated. History is also a reminder that sometimes small, piecemeal changes or events can be the springboard for larger policy issues at the right time and place.

When thinking about the policy levers that drive our health care system, we can look to history as a way of providing perspective and for pulling apart the power dynamics that drive policymaking. Our examples demonstrate how the IOM report placed nurse practitioners, just as the Public Health Department and the Rockefeller Foundation situated the earlier public health nurses, as policy solutions for improving the health care of the nation at a particular time and place. Our histories show that polcymaking is untidy; we want it to be rational but "reasoned analysis is necessarily political. It always involves choices to include things and exclude others and to view the world in a particular way when other visions are possible" (Stone, 2001, p. 378). The public health nurses of the 1920s and 1930s were perhaps not as facile at understanding this reality or not as skilled at thriving within an environment when the political alliances were flexible and shifting. But they did adjust. These are important lessons to learn and remember. Today, as we try to reformulate our health care system to be more accessible, efficient, and inclusive, policymakers are making choices about providers and services. Nurse practitioners are part of policy solutions as seen through the ACA support of retail clinics and nurse-managed health centers. However, they need to remember that strategic alliances shift, that new stakeholders emerge, and that future policy decisions may not always be rational, but they will always be political.

There are both historical continuities and differences in the stories of public health nurses of the 1920s and 1930s and the growing appeal of nurse practitioners today to policymakers and stakeholders. The ability to build coalitions and partnerships is as critical today as it was in the 1920s and 1930s. In the early 1960s, when nurse Loretta Ford and physician Henry Silver serendipitously found they shared common interests of providing better care to rural poor families, they knew physician manpower was unavailable and that the nurse with additional skills and knowledge could provide the needed level of care. The United States was suffering from a primary care shortage similar to the current shortage. Although they published their model early, they were not alone in coming to these conclusions. Nurse Barbara Resnick and physician Charles Lewis in Kansas City in the mid-1960s were also situating nurses as the solution to patient dissatisfaction with the lack of continuity of care in their university outpatient clinics. Although models like these were part of larger changes occurring where physicians were in short supply or nurses initiated their own practices, individual and sporadic efforts such as these were not enough to drive changes in policy even when analytic reasoning indicated their effectiveness. Nurse practitioners lacked a unified coalition to move their interest forward—for example, to change restrictive state practice regulations and payment structures—and they lacked interested groups and partners outside of nursing to help broaden their appeal. Although individual physicians were supportive, organized medicine was not.

Having data is important, as the public health nurses understood, but, as Stone (2001) also argued, politics may trump data. Data supporting the value and quality of nurse practitioner services began appearing in the early 1970s. A meta-analysis of 1970s-era studies of nurse practitioner effectiveness done by the Congressional Office of Technology Assessment documented their effectiveness in 1984. Although powerful in its scope and innovation, this study did not stimulate the interests of lawmakers at the state and federal level, who could have used the data to develop a reasoned policy analysis. Although professional nursing did have lobbyists working on professional issues, the organizations

were more focused on workplace issues than broader policies, and not mature or flexible enough to work together as a larger, powerful group until the late 1970s. Organized medicine was indeed "organized" and had powerful lobbies and leadership that kept its message simple and consistent, and one that would be replayed for decades. The message was that physicians were the only safe providers because of their longer and more intensive education; yet, their position actually lacked data.

Another lesson learned from the public health nurse narrative that resonates today is the importance of the creation of bridges between the community and the health system. In the late 1970s, professional nursing organizations such as the American Nurses Association (ANA) seized a strategic opportunity to reformulate their policy agenda. Building on the growing body of studies that indicated high patient satisfaction and clinical effectiveness of nurse practitioners as providers, and a growing strategic and political movement that situated the patient as the focus of professional legitimacy, the ANA built policy positions that situated nurse practitioners as normative providers for groups of patients such as older adults, children, and healthy adults. A deceptively strong and influential patient movement was also beginning to support nurse practitioner-provided care. Although patient support was unorganized and lacked a single leader, patients across the country showed their appreciation by returning for follow-up and bringing in their family and neighbors. The ANA effectively built upon the momentum patients provided to begin to form coalitions and work more effectively with the nascent nurse practitioner organizations to generate more powerful policy positions and partnerships.

We also learn from history that sometimes coalitions are not enough to move the policy levers. Even as nurses built coalitions and patients became their advocates through the 1980s and 1990s, there were pieces missing. For example, medical organizations influential in the policy arena did not offer nurses large-scale support. Physician organizations were not interested in partnerships and still held strong political capital at the state and national level. Individual physicians certainly supported nurse practitioners in their own practices, but organized medicine did not see them as independent providers or partners.

Organized medicine could situate nurses in this way because it still had enormous political power and resources. But physicians' cultural authority has now been challenged. Fraud and payment scandals and exposes of physicians' relationships with pharmaceutical companies generated public skepticism during a time of patient empowerment movements and civil and women's rights movements. As historians Beatrix Hoffman and Nancy Tomes (2011) noted, patients reinvented "new terms for themselves—consumers, clients, citizens, and survivors—in their search to be heard in the health care arena" (p. 2) and exercised greater control over their care. In their search, patients found nurse practitioners qualified and value-based providers, educated and willing to see the patient as the "source of control" as the IOM report *Crossing the Quality Chasm* posited (IOM, 2001).

The stories of nurse practitioners and public health nurses are also connected by the ability to thrive and continue negotiations within a slow and subtle policy process. Incremental change occurred in health policy at the turn of the twenty-first century, although this was not a naturally rational or progressive movement. One of the ways this transformation can be illustrated is by the shift in the language defining who could provide care and receive payment. Many stakeholders worked over decades to bring about these changes. These categories are politically constructed worldviews, bestowing advantages and disadvantages. The change in language signified the slowly occurring power shift and the power of professional nursing and its allies to renegotiate the boundaries of patient care. Federal legislation began to include the term "provider" instead of "physician," or the more inclusive phrase "physicians and nurses." Medicare recognized nurse practitioners as primary care providers, although the states still maintain their regulatory authority to allow or not allow full scope of practice.

Another lesson learned is that coalitions must be flexible and ready to change. As the power dynamics in health care started to shift, nurse practitioners gained new partners and support. Since

the 1980s, the Federal Trade Commission produced advocacy letters declaring restrictive practice acts anticompetitive and against the interests of consumers. Their activity in this area accelerated in the first decade of the twenty-first century. The American Association of Retired Persons (AARP), the largest consumer group in the world, had nurses in key leadership positions to steer the organization, which developed policy positions that supported nurse practitioners. As medicine was becoming more corporatized and less patient-centric, the public began rating nurses as the most trusted health professional in Gallup polls, with the exception of 2001 when firefighters topped the list (Gallup, n.d.). Even so, nurse practitioners were not always part of the policy solutions to the primary care shortage. Building more capacity in medical education, even when it became harder and harder to attract physicians into primary care, continued to be the traditional policy strategy although its sustainability as policy is weakening. Policymaker recognition of the high cost of physician education and the viability of nurse practitioners as a reasonable and faster option to provider supply growth was supported by reports by the Rand Health Foundation and the National Governors Association.

By the time the IOM's *Future of Nursing* report was published in 2011, patient support, coalition building, and new partnerships had positioned nurse practitioners to be a consistent part of the policy process. Although the IOM report might have served as the spark, it was nested in both the policies and politics of the past century as well as the context surrounding health reform debates occurring in Congress. A litany of factors including rising health care costs, a shifting focus from specialty to primary care, and a shortage of primary care providers created a demand for new and more efficient models of care. Nurses gained willing and energetic partners in the public media and with the patients they served. A large private foundation, RWJF, leveraged its long-term interest in nursing to support the IOM report. Other new partners came forward; in particular, the Association of American Medical Colleges showed courage and strength by supporting nurse practitioners in press releases and policy statements. The nursing profession as a driver of policy change had come of age. It developed coalitions across nursing professional organizations that were focused on policy, and it developed new partnerships with powerful organizations outside of nursing that saw nursing's value while creating new opportunities and connections with nursing to both influence policymakers and drive policy change.

CONCLUSION

The two stories—about public health nurses shaping health outcomes of immigrant populations during the early twentieth century and about the evolving policy support (via the IOM report) for nurse practitioners—show how health care policies and politics, perhaps even more than nurses' work, shape the delivery of care and the outcomes sought. For the public health nurses, the day-to-day politics between and among professionals, the various private and public enterprises that offer health care options, especially to vulnerable populations, have typically looked to more traditional methods of providing care rather than seeking nursing as part of the solution to the delivery of primary health care. Yet, the value public health nurses brought to community and population health argue for nurses to participate in policymaking and to advocate their inclusion in health care solutions. For nurse practitioners, history is a reminder of how they gained policy momentum amid the shifting weights of reasoning and power, and with the growing power of consumer movements. Both stories illustrate how messy policymaking can be, how alliances can be tenuous while understanding the value of coalitions and partnerships as stabilizing agents in uncertain policy environments. History provides rich data that can help nurses advocate the role this profession can make as part of a larger solution to improve health care in the United States.

DISCUSSION QUESTIONS

1. What types of alliances exist and what types need to be cultivated to affect change in your own areas of nursing practice?

2. What are the problems and/or the possibilities in developing cross-disciplinary as well as public and private alliances to affect change?

3. What type of historical evidence can be used to support nursing's political advocacy in providing primary health care?

4. Explore the advocacy efforts Lillian Wald, public health nurses in urban and rural settings, and nurse practitioners used to affect change in health care.

REFERENCES

D'Antonio, P. (2010). *American nursing: A history of knowledge, authority and the meaning of work.* Baltimore, MD: Johns Hopkins University Press.

D'Antonio, P. (2013). Cultivating constituencies: The story of the East Harlem Nursing and Health Service, 1928–1941. *American Journal of Public Health, 103*(6), 988–996.

D'Antonio, P. (2014). Lessons learned: Nursing and health demonstration projects in New York City, 1920-1935. *Policy, Politics and Nursing Practice, 14*(3–4), 133–141. doi:10.1177/1527154413520389.

Fairman, J., Rowe, J., Hassmiller, S., & Shalala, D. (2011). Broadening the scope of nursing practice. *New England Journal of Medicine, 364*(3), 193–196.

Gallup. (n.d.). Honesty/ethics in professions. Retrieved from *www.gallup.com/poll/1654/Honesty-Ethics-Professions.aspx.*

Institute of Medicine. (2001). *Crossing the quality chasm: A new health system for the 21st century.* Washington, DC: National Academy Press.

Institute of Medicine. (2011). *The future of nursing: Leading change, advancing health.* Washington, DC: The National Academies Press.

Lewenson, S. B. (2015). Town and country nursing: Community participation and nurse recruitment. In J. Kirchgessner & A. Keeling (Eds.), *Nursing rural America* (pp. 1–19). New York: Springer.

Maternity Center Association, Columbia University Health Sciences Center, Box 52, Folder 2, 1924.

Stone, D. (2001). *Policy paradox: The art of political decision making* (revised ed.). New York: Norton.

Tomes, N., & Hoffman, B. (2011). Introduction: Patients as policy actors. In B. Hoffman, N. Tomes, R. Grob, & M. Schlesinger (Eds.), *Patients as policy actors.* New Brunswick, NJ: Rutgers.

Wald, L. D. (1915). *The house on Henry Street.* New York: Henry Holt and Company.

ONLINE RESOURCES

American Association for the History of Nursing
www.aahn.org
Learning Historical Research
www.williamcronon.net/researching/
Nursing History and Health Care
www.nursing.upenn.edu/nhhc/Pages/Welcome.aspx

CHAPTER 3

Advocacy in Nursing and Health Care

Chad S. Priest

"I come to present the strong claims of suffering humanity. I come to place before the Legislature of Massachusetts the condition of the miserable, the desolate, the outcast. I come as the advocate of helpless, forgotten, insane men and women; of beings sunk to a condition from which the unconcerned world would start with real horror."

Dorothea Dix

Nurses have a long history of advocating on behalf of and alongside patients, families, and communities to promote health, equality, and justice. Nursing is widely respected for effective professional advocacy that has expanded the professional role of the registered nurse and created safer working conditions for nurses. Florence Nightingale's revolutionary advocacy around the environment of care and Margaret Sanger's pursuit of reproductive freedom for women exemplify nursing advocacy.

Despite a history rooted in speaking for and working on behalf of the most vulnerable in the United States, nursing's relationship with advocacy is complicated. Perhaps this is because the profession was for many years defined by loyalty to others—namely to physicians and hospitals—and not to patients. Echoes of this tension reverberate today, as nurses are routinely challenged as they navigate between loyalty to physicians and hospitals and advocacy on behalf of patients, families, and communities. Complicating matters, nursing schools and institutions do not necessarily prepare students to serve as advocates. Many nurses find the idea of advocacy on behalf of patients (and even themselves) to be daunting. The nursing profession has also sent mixed signals about the value of advocacy, and there has been

scant research into what exactly nursing advocacy looks like.

This chapter is about advocacy at the individual, community, and system levels—and the relationship between advocacy and policy. Because this chapter is about advocacy, this chapter is also about nursing. Although the relationship between nursing and advocacy deserves refinement, nursing practice is rooted in advocacy on behalf of and alongside those who are sick, vulnerable, and in need of care.

THE DEFINITION OF ADVOCACY

The word *advocacy* is derived from the Latin word *advocatus*, meaning to plead the cause of another (Advocate, n.d.). Although the word *advocacy* is most frequently associated with legal and political settings, the definition has expanded to encompass a wide range of activities undertaken in support of individuals, families, systems, communities, and issues. Nurses are widely viewed as advocates for patients and their families. Some have suggested that patient advocacy is an integral part of nursing practice (Hanks, 2010a, 2010b; Vaartio et al., 2009; Vaartio et al., 2006). In modern nursing practice, nurses serve as advocates when they ensure that patients understand the treatments they are receiving while in the hospital, or serve as a translator between the patient and members of the health care team. Many nurses work to coordinate care and help patients navigate the complexities of the health system.

In the community setting, nurses frequently work with residents and community leaders to advocate for healthier neighborhoods. Working alongside members of the community, community health nurses seek to mitigate the social determinants of illness through advocacy at the individual, system, and policy levels. As experts in the delivery of health care and the promotion of health, nurses are also frequently engaged in issue advocacy, addressing such issues as access to care and disease prevention.

Through professional organizations such as the American Nurses Association (ANA) and the American Association of Nurse Anesthetists (AANA) (see Chapter 74), nurses serve as advocates for the nursing profession itself by educating and appealing to state and federal legislators and policymakers to promote safe workspaces for nurses and to safeguard the nursing scope of practice.

THE NURSE AS PATIENT ADVOCATE

Patient advocacy is a frequently described, but poorly understood, concept in nursing. It is viewed as a central tenet of nursing practice, both in the United States and around the world (Allcock, 1989; Altun & Ersoy, 2003; Bu & Jezewski, 2007; Foley, Minick, & Kee, 2000; Gale, 1989; Hanks, 2005; Jugessur & Iles, 2009; Kohnke, 1978; Mathes, 2005; McSteen & Peden-McAlpine, 2006; Morra, 2000; Vaartio et al., 2006). Despite widespread acceptance of the role of patient advocate by nurses in the published literature, there is only an emerging understanding of what nursing advocacy is, how (and whether or not) it is performed by nurses, and what results from nursing advocacy (Baldwin, 2003; Grace, 2001; Mallik, 1998). Advocacy has traditionally been associated with legal and political activity. As advocacy has evolved in nursing, it has taken on a number of meanings—from advocating for social justice (Paquin, 2011) to simply performing nursing functions adequately and safely.

Winslow (1984) identified two major metaphors —loyalty and advocacy—espoused by nursing leaders and educators from the profession's birth through the mid-1980s. Loyalty as a metaphor for practice was rooted in the "battle against disease" and featured rigid hierarchies that were prevalent in military practice settings through the 1940s (Winslow, 1984). Instructional books from the early period of the profession characterized the nurse as a warrior in the battle against disease and

illness, glamorizing a life of "toil and discipline" in which nurses pledged loyalty to their physician leaders (Winslow, 1984). The primary goal of loyalty by nurses was to project and reinforce confidence in the health care enterprise. Nurses were explicitly taught that loyalty to the physician equated with faithfulness to the patient (Winslow, 1984).

The primacy of loyalty as a nursing ethic came under attack in 1929 in a most unusual place. In a hospital in Manila, The Philippines, a physician ordered a new graduate nurse, Lorenza Somera, to administer cocaine injections, instead of *procaine* injections, to a tonsillectomy patient (Winslow, 1984). Somera loyally carried out the physician's order, resulting in the death of the patient. Although it was clear that the physician had erred in ordering the incorrect medication, he was acquitted of all charges while Somera was found guilty of manslaughter for failing to question the orders of the physician (Winslow, 1984). The Somera case sparked worldwide protests from nurses and served to push nursing toward independent practice and accountability. It was also one of many events that led to a reconceptualization of the dominant nursing metaphor from loyalty to physicians to advocacy for patients (Winslow, 1984).

CONSUMERISM, FEMINISM, AND PROFESSIONALIZATION OF NURSING: THE EMERGENCE OF PATIENTS' RIGHTS ADVOCACY

During the 1960s and 1970s, influenced by feminist and consumer-rights ideologies, nursing advocacy became the dominant metaphor for nursing (Hewitt, 2002; Mallik, 1998; Winslow, 1984). The concept of "nurse as advocate for the patient" recognized the inherently oppressive nature of patienthood, wherein the patient is vulnerable as a result of his or her illness and unable to care for himself or herself (Bu & Jezewski, 2007). Advocacy for the patient was thus framed as rejection of loyalty to the physician, freeing nurses to develop their own professional identity. Indeed, adoption of the patient advocate role occurred simultaneously with the professionalization of nursing (Porter, 1992;

Shirley, 2007). As a construct for nursing practice, advocacy had the advantage of being seen as morally good for patients, as well as providing an opportunity for nursing to promote professional autonomy (Kosik, 1972; Winslow, 1984).

Early forms of nursing advocacy borrowed heavily from legal models of advocacy and centered on consumerism and patients' rights. Through this lens, the nurse acted as a guardian and intervened when these rights were threatened by the medical establishment (Bramlett, Gueldner, & Sowell, 1990; Mallik, 1997a; Mallik & Rafferty, 2000; Winslow, 1984). This form of advocacy was eventually codified in the ANA Code of Ethics in 1978, which proclaimed that:

[I]n the role of client advocate, the nurse must be alert to and take appropriate action regarding any instances of incompetent, unethical, or illegal practice(s) by any member of the health care team or the health care system itself, or any action on the part of others that is prejudicial to the client's best interests. (Bernal, 1992, p. 18.)

Some U.S. state boards of nursing have codified, and thus mandated, nursing advocacy by including language in nurse practice acts that either explicitly or implicitly defines an advocacy role. For example, the Indiana Nursing Practice Act defines Registered Nursing to include "advocating the provision of health care services through collaboration with or referral to other health professionals" (Indiana Nursing Practice Act, 2008).

PHILOSOPHICAL MODELS OF NURSING ADVOCACY

GADOW

Although patients' rights advocacy formed the basis of nursing advocacy and remains the dominant conception of nursing advocacy, nursing theorists have advanced competing conceptualizations of advocacy that seek to define a unique nursing advocacy. Sally Gadow advanced an "existential advocacy" whereby the nurse's role is to help patients clarify their values and the illness experience, and exercise their right to self-determination (Gadow, 1983). The premise underlying existential advocacy was that nurses are uniquely situated to advocate for patients, because they frequently spend the most time with patients and have an intimate connection with patients and their families. She also viewed advocacy as a moral imperative, with the ultimate goal being to increase patient autonomy (Hanks, 2005).

CURTIN

Writing during the same period as Gadow, Curtin (1979) sought to situate nursing advocacy as "human advocacy." Curtin invited nurses to help patients identify meaning and purpose in their illnesses with the ultimate goal of enhancing patient autonomy (Curtin, 1979; Mallik, 1997a).

KOHNKE

Occupying something of a middle ground between patients' rights advocacy and the philosophical advocacies of Gadow and Curtin, Kohnke developed a model of functional advocacy that called nurses to serve as brokers of information and supporters of patient decision making (Kohnke, 1978, 1980). More than any other theorist of the time, Kohnke expressly suggested that physicians persecuted patients (whom she calls victims) through their "we know best" attitude (Kohnke, 1980). An illustration appearing with her work in the *American Journal of Nursing* depicts the physician as a puppet-master manipulating a helpless patient, with the nurse as a "rescuer," attacking the physician with the banner of health (Kohnke, 1980).

Although nursing advocacy has been widely internalized as a core professional value by many nurses, critics have questioned the utility of nursing advocacy as a framework for practice and have argued that few nurses are actually engaged in advocacy activities. Several critics have questioned whether or not nurses have the capacity to serve as advocates, noting that many nurses lack the institutional and personal power required to advocate for patients' rights (Bernal, 1992; Grace, 2001; Hanks, 2007; Hewitt, 2002; Mackereth, 1995; Martin, 1998). Hewitt (2002) points out that "for the nurse to be in a position to empower patients, it is necessary for the nurse to be first empowered" (Hewitt, 2002, p. 444).

Although it is well understood that the oppressive nature of the medical establishment impairs patient autonomy, it is less clear why nurses view themselves as well suited to act as patient advocates (Mallik, 1997b; Martin, 1998; Negarandeh et al., 2008; O'Connor & Kelly, 2005). One central theme in the nursing advocacy literature is that nurses are uniquely situated to serve as patient advocates because they spend the most time with patients and have the most influence over the patient's experience while the patient is hospitalized or ill (Bu & Jezewski, 2007; Curtin, 1979; Hanks, 2007; Martin, 1998; Schroeter, 2002, 2007). The intimacy of nursing care has been suggested as the mechanism by which nurses are able to engage in existential advocacy behaviors (i.e., empowerment advocacy) (Curtin, 1979). In a study of nursing elite in the United Kingdom, Mallik (1998) found that nursing leaders viewed the intimate nursing relationship with suspicion. One subject in her study stated:

[T]his complete "under the skin oneness" is a piece of impertinence really. I mean somebody who has 55 years of history behind them walks through the door and suddenly you are their best friend and you know everything there is to know about them, it's a bit beyond the pale. (Mallik, 1998, p. 1005.)

Others have argued that when nurses assume the role of advocate, they unfairly and inappropriately stake an exclusive claim to the role, alienating other health care team members that arguably engage in advocacy behaviors in the course of their professional duties (Hewitt, 2002; Mallik, 1997a).

Perhaps the most devastating critique of nursing advocacy, especially considering the high value nurses place on evidence-based practice, is that the phenomenon is poorly understood (Hewitt, 2002). Despite substantial attention to nursing advocacy since the early 1970s, there is a dearth of scientific research exploring the phenomenon. Only a handful of researchers have undertaken any scientific exploration of nursing advocacy. Most of these are qualitative researchers who have focused on understanding

the concept of nursing advocacy and how nurses internalize and enact the nursing advocacy role. Despite their inability to fully explain nursing advocacy, these studies have resulted in remarkable consistency with respect to identifying advocacy functions and personal traits and characteristics of nurses that appear to promote or inhibit advocacy behaviors.

ADVOCACY OUTSIDE THE CLINICAL SETTING

Nursing advocacy is not limited to clinical settings. Nurses are expert health care providers who are well positioned to advocate for policies and practices that promote and encourage health. Three types of nursing advocacy influence policy, population health, and the profession of nursing: issue advocacy, community and public health advocacy, and professional advocacy.

ISSUE ADVOCACY

The nursing care of patients necessarily extends beyond the hospital or clinic. Consider that symptom management for many patients requires interventions that are not purely medical. For example, mental health nurses frequently set goals with their patients to integrate patients into the community. The reality is that patients with mental illness cannot be expected to integrate into the community without the existence of health care services and programs that support such integration. Mental health nurses are frequent advocates for these programs and services. This issue advocacy directly promotes improved patient outcomes, although it does not involve advocacy on behalf of any one individual.

Importantly, issue advocacy is almost always best accomplished through the formation of coalitions. Nurses are excellent coalition partners, bringing evidence-based expertise and professional credibility to any debate. For example, Muckian (2007) describes a successful grassroots coalition of nurses, patients, families, and other advocates that organized to reverse budget cuts to a Wisconsin in-home Medicaid program for children with autism.

COMMUNITY AND PUBLIC HEALTH ADVOCACY

Although reforming the health care system is important, and nurses' input into reform is critical, advocacy in support of health extends beyond issue advocacy. There is wide agreement among researchers, policymakers, and providers that social structures and behaviors have a significant impact on health. The quality of the environment, the nature of human relationships, the durability of the social infrastructure, and the justice inherent in the social order are all, in isolation and in combination, powerful determinants of health status. These social determinants of health and illness are complex, multifactorial, and almost entirely unresponsive to the biomedical interventions that are the core of the current health system.

Nurses, however, are well positioned to work with communities to mitigate social determinants of illness and promote health. Oftentimes this involves explicitly advocating for social justice (Paquin, 2011). Community health nurses routinely interact with community leaders to improve community conditions that impact health. For example, Longo and colleagues (2010) described a nursing-led indoor air quality assessment for persons exposed to volcanic air pollution from the ongoing eruption of the Kilauea volcano in Hawaii.

PROFESSIONAL ADVOCACY

Nursing, and nurses, matter. Consider the following:

- Nurses compose the largest segment of the health care workforce.
- Patients are in frequent contact with nurses who deliver almost all of the care to patients in the hospital setting (Needleman, 2008).
- Research has demonstrated that the amount and quality of nursing care that patients receive is directly related to a number of health outcomes (Needleman, 2008).

Because nurses have a direct relationship to the health of patients, advocacy on behalf of the nursing profession is a powerful form of patient advocacy. Advocacy on behalf of the profession frequently involves examining issues such as workplace safety, nurse/patient ratios, expanded scope of practice, and limitations on malpractice liability. At the national level, organizations such as the ANA attempt to provide broad representation of nursing interests to members of congress, policymakers, and thought leaders. Advanced practice nurses (APRNs) and their representative organizations are known to be highly effective advocates at the state and federal levels. Through advocacy of advanced practice nursing, these nurses also advocate for improved access to care and the reduction of health disparities in communities.

BARRIERS TO SUCCESSFUL ADVOCACY

Similar to any political activity, advocacy is time-consuming and requires a significant commitment on the part of the nurse. Whether it is direct patient advocacy requiring the nurse to stay late after a shift to work with a family, or issue advocacy involving research around an issue and meetings with members of the legislature, some nurses are unwilling or unable to devote the time needed for successful advocacy.

For those who make the commitment of time and energy to become advocates, other barriers may exist, including lack of education and training about advocacy skills or outright fear of retribution from employers or governmental organizations as a result of advocacy activities (Galer-Unti, Tappe, & Lachenmayr, 2004). Each of these barriers is discussed in the following sections.

EDUCATION AND TRAINING

One of the major barriers to successful nursing advocacy is a lack of education and training in advocacy during formal nursing education. Although some schools of nursing offer programs or units to expose students to political processes, typically limited to visits to state board of nursing meetings or legislative committees, few educational programs are designed to promote advocacy skills in nurses. Additionally, faculty may not model effective advocacy behaviors.

In one of the few examples of research into how nurses learn and engage in advocacy, Foley, Minick, and Kee (2002) discovered that some nurses reported feeling as though advocacy was "deeply rooted in who they were" so that advocacy skills were essentially ingrained in their personhood (Foley, Minick, & Kee, 2002, p. 184). Other nurses reported learning advocacy skills by watching their colleagues or mentors engage in advocacy behaviors (Foley, Minick, & Kee, 2002). Still others reported that it wasn't until they gained confidence as a nurse that they felt comfortable engaging in advocacy (Foley, Minick, & Kee, 2002). These findings are problematic for those interested in teaching advocacy skills, as they suggest that advocacy skills are primarily a part of individual personalities or are learned in practice, and not during formal education.

Zauderer and colleagues (2008) outlined a political-organizing educational program for nursing students that focused on empowering students to be aware of, and to participate in, the political process. This program focused on political activism and included a trip to the state capital to lobby legislators (Zauderer et al., 2008). Although this training approach is likely to be useful to build skills in advance of a specific legislative encounter and is certainly valuable, it is not clear if a political-organizing framework is sufficient to prepare students to act as advocates in their practice upon graduation.

McDermott-Levy (2009) described a unique opportunity to train students in advocacy for environmental health. During a clinical experience, one of McDermott-Levy's students cared for a patient with laryngeal cancer (McDermott-Levy, 2009). In the course of caring for the patient, the student discovered a history of laryngeal cancer in the patient's immediate family. Further investigation revealed that the family may have been exposed to carcinogens while living in a coal-mining community (the patient's father worked in a coal mine as well). McDermott-Levy suggests that nurses trained in environmental health would be well positioned to advocate for patients and communities in these situations. Considering the work of Foley and colleagues (2002) described earlier in this chapter, organic clinical encounters are likely to be extraordinary opportunities to introduce students to advocacy skills. Consider that these students could have engaged in any number of advocacy activities related to the environmental exposure—all from an encounter with one patient. In their groundbreaking study of nursing education, Benner and colleagues (2010) call for greater attention to nursing advocacy in the schooling, learning, and teaching process. They accurately point out that "[e]nthusiasm for nursing as a social good is a motivation for both students and teachers, and a 'moral source' against frustration and fatigue" (p. 206).

INSTITUTIONAL BARRIERS AND FEAR OF RETRIBUTION

Advocacy, whether on behalf of patients or in support or opposition to issues, is typically associated with some degree of "rocking the boat." After all, if the status quo were effective, there would be no need for advocacy (unless, of course, you were advocating for the preservation of the status quo). Speaking up for what you believe can be a risky endeavor. Consider that many nurses avoid advocating for better workplace conditions, or for patient safety, for fear that their employers will retaliate against them. Although many health care institutions respect the contribution of nursing and promote nursing autonomy, nurses who fear retaliation for doing the right thing have plenty of examples to substantiate their concerns. And it is not just health care organizations that have retaliated against nurses who were strong advocates: governmental organizations such as state boards of nursing also send mixed signals about nursing advocacy.

Consider the interesting, and perhaps troubling, case of Ellen Finnerty, a Registered Nurse from California who was terminated from her job and had her Registered Nursing license revoked by the California Board of Registered Nursing based on her advocacy for a patient under her care. Finnerty had worked as a Registered Nurse for 20 years and was serving as a charge nurse on a medical-surgical floor when one of her patients developed respiratory problems (Finnerty v. Board of Registered Nursing, 2008). According to the court records, the patient was exhibiting labored breathing, but had stable vital signs. The treating physician ordered that the patient be intubated immediately while on the medical-surgical unit. Finnerty disagreed with the physician's order, claiming that the patient should be taken to the intensive care unit (ICU) for the intubation because the medical-surgical unit lacked the appropriate equipment to perform the procedure and nurses were distracted handling many patients during the change of shift. Despite Finnerty's objection, the physician reaffirmed the order for the intubation. Finnerty then countermanded the order directly, unplugged the patient's bed, and transferred the patient directly to the ICU where the patient arrived in stable condition and was successfully intubated.

Unfortunately, the patient experienced respiratory arrest a few minutes later and died. Although the patient's demise was not related to any delay in intubation that may have taken place caused by the transfer to the ICU, Finnerty's employer terminated her employment (although the termination was later changed to a resignation) as a result of her "gross negligence—failure to follow direction from [the] treating physician." Shortly thereafter, the California Board of Registered Nursing filed a complaint against Finnerty alleging unprofessional conduct and gross negligence and incompetence and seeking the revocation or suspension of her license (Finnerty v. Board of Registered Nursing, 2008). The Board determined that Finnerty had inappropriately substituted her clinical judgment for the physician's and that her actions violated the nurse practice act, and they issued a revocation of her license.

Finnerty appealed the decision up to the California Court of Appeals, claiming that "she was required by the Board's standards of competent performance to act as Mr. C.'s advocate by taking him to the ICU for intubation, rather than permitting intubation to take place in an environment that was not equipped for intubation." The case of Ellen Finnerty calls into question whether and how nurses can act as advocates for patients in the face of questionable decision making by other members of the health care team. What would happen if the nurse did not question the intubation in the medical-surgical environment and the patient had an adverse outcome?

SUMMARY

Advocacy is widely viewed as a fundamental nursing role, whether on behalf of patients, communities, or the profession, and in crafting policy solutions. Although many nurses are engaged in advocacy behaviors, there are significant barriers to advocacy by nurses. First, whereas some boards of nursing require that nurses engage in advocacy, others appear to punish nurses who stand up for what is right. Second, there is tension between nurses' loyalty to patients (or communities, the profession, or policies) and nurses' obligations to institutions (e.g., hospitals). Finally, advocacy education and training is not a routine component of most formal nursing education programs, leaving nurses to rely on their colleagues to learn effective advocacy behaviors. Despite these barriers, advocacy on behalf of health can be extremely rewarding, and nurses are in a unique position to advance the cause of patients' interests in the complex health care system.

DISCUSSION QUESTIONS

1. What examples of advocacy do you see in your own nursing practice, or the nursing practice of others?
2. What are the barriers you have experienced to effective nursing advocacy? What are ways to mitigate those barriers?
3. How can schools of nursing more effectively prepare nurses to serve as advocates?

REFERENCES

Advocate (n.d.). Dictionary.com unabridged. Retrieved from *dictionary .reference.com/browse/advocate*.

Allcock, D. (1989). The psychiatric nurse as advocate. *Nursing Standard, 3*(37), 29–30.

Altun, I., & Ersoy, N. (2003). Undertaking the role of patient advocate: A longitudinal study of nursing students. *Nursing Ethics, 10*(5), 462–471.

Baldwin, M. A. (2003). Patient advocacy: A concept analysis. *Nursing Standard, 17*(21), 33–39.

Benner, P., Sutphen, M., Leonard, V., & Day, L. (2010). *Educating nurses: A call for radical transformation.* San Francisco, CA: Jossey-Bass.

Bernal, E. W. (1992). The nurse as patient advocate. *Hastings Center Report, 22*(4), 18–23.

Bramlett, M. H., Gueldner, S. H., & Sowell, R. L. (1990). Consumer-centric advocacy: Its connection to nursing frameworks. *Nursing Science Quarterly, 3*(4), 156–161.

Bu, X., & Jezewski, M. A. (2007). Developing a mid-range theory of patient advocacy through concept analysis. *Journal of Advanced Nursing, 57*(1), 101–110.

Curtin, L. L. (1979). The nurse as advocate: A philosophical foundation for nursing. *Advances in Nursing Science, 1*(3), 1–10.

Finnerty v. Board of Registered Nursing (2008). Cal. App. 4th 219.

Foley, B. J., Minick, P., & Kee, C. (2000). Nursing advocacy during a military operation. *Western Journal of Nursing Research, 22*(4), 492–507.

Foley, B. J., Minick, P., & Kee, C. (2002). How nurses learn advocacy. *Journal of Nursing Scholarship, 34*(2), 181–186.

Gadow, S. (1983). Existential advocacy: Philosophical foundations of nursing. In C. P. Murphy & H. Hunter (Eds.), *Ethical problems in the nurse-patient relationship.* Boston, MA: Allyn and Bacon.

Gale, B. J. (1989). Advocacy for elderly autonomy: A challenge for community health nurses. *Journal of Community Health Nursing, 6*(4), 191–197.

Galer-Unti, R. A., Tappe, M. K., & Lachenmayr, S. (2004). Advocacy 101: Getting started in health education advocacy. *Health Promotion Practice, 5*(3), 280–288.

Grace, P. J. (2001). Professional advocacy: Widening the scope of accountability. *Nursing Philosophy: An International Journal for Healthcare Professionals, 2*(2), 151–162.

Hanks, R. G. (2005). Sphere of nursing advocacy model. *Nursing Forum, 40*(3), 75–78.

Hanks, R. G. (2007). Barriers to nursing advocacy: A concept analysis. *Nursing Forum, 42*(4), 171–177.

Hanks, R. G. (2010a). The medical-surgical nurse perspective of advocate role. *Nursing Forum, 45*(2), 97–107.

Hanks, R. G. (2010b). Development and testing of an instrument to measure protective advocacy. *Nursing Ethics, 17*(2), 255–267.

Hewitt, J. (2002). A critical review of the arguments debating the role of the nurse advocate. *Journal of Advanced Nursing, 37*(5), 439–445.

Indiana Nursing Practice Act (2008). Ind. Code §23-25-1-1.1(b)(4).

Jugessur, T., & Iles, I. K. (2009). Advocacy in mental health nursing: an integrative review of the literature. *Journal of Psychiatric and Mental Health Nursing, 16*(2), 187–195.

Kohnke, M. F. (1978). The nurse's responsibility to the consumer. *American Journal of Nursing, 78*(3), 440–442.

Kohnke, M. F. (1980). The nurse as advocate. *American Journal of Nursing, 80*(11), 2038–2040.

Kosik, S. H. (1972). Patient advocacy or fighting the system. *American Journal of Nursing, 72*(4), 694–698.

Longo, B. M., Yang, W., Green, J. B., Longo, A. A., Harris, M., & Bibilone, R. (2010). An indoor air quality assessment for vulnerable populations exposed to volcanic vog from Kilauea Volcano. *Family & Community Health, 33*(1), 21–31.

Mackereth, P. A. (1995). HIV and homophobia: Nurses as advocates. *Journal of Advanced Nursing, 22*(4), 670–676.

Mallik, M. (1997a). Advocacy in nursing—A review of the literature. *Journal of Advanced Nursing, 25*(1), 130–138.

Mallik, M. (1997b). Advocacy in nursing—Perceptions of practising nurses. *Journal of Clinical Nursing, 6*(4), 303–313.

Mallik, M. (1998). Advocacy in nursing: Perceptions and attitudes of the nursing elite in the United Kingdom. *Journal of Advanced Nursing, 28*(5), 1001–1011.

Mallik, M., & Rafferty, A. M. (2000). Diffusion of the concept of patient advocacy. *Journal of Nursing Scholarship, 32*(4), 399–404.

Martin, G. W. (1998). Communication breakdown or ideal speech situation: The problem of nurse advocacy. *Nursing Ethics, 5*(2), 147–157.

Mathes, M. (2005). On nursing, moral autonomy, and moral responsibility. *Medsurg Nursing, 14*(6), 395–398.

McDermott-Levy, R. (2009). Education: Nurses' tool for advocacy in environmental health. *The Pennsylvania Nurse, 64*(2), 10–13.

McSteen, K., & Peden-McAlpine, C. (2006). The role of the nurse as advocate in ethically difficult care situations with dying patients. *Journal of Hospice and Palliative Nursing, 8*(5), 259–269.

Morra, M. E. (2000). New opportunities for nurses as patient advocates. *Seminars in Oncology Nursing, 16*(1), 57–64.

Muckian, J. (2007). Influencing policy development: The whirling dervish of the autism in-home program. *Journal of Pediatric Nursing, 22*(3), 223–230.

Needleman, J. (2008). Is what's good for the patient good for the hospital? Aligning incentives and the business case for nursing. *Policy, Politics & Nursing Practice, 9*(2), 80–87.

Negarandeh, R., Oskouie, F., Ahmadi, F., & Nikravesh, M. (2008). The meaning of patient advocacy for Iranian nurses. *Nursing Ethics, 15*(4), 457–467.

O'Connor, T., & Kelly, B. (2005). Bridging the gap: A study of general nurses' perceptions of patient advocacy in Ireland. *Nursing Ethics, 12*(5), 453–467.

Paquin, S. (2011). Social justice advocacy in nursing: What is it? How do we get there? *Creative Nursing, 17*(2), 63–67.

Porter, S. (1992). The poverty of professionalization: A critical analysis of strategies for the occupational advancement of nursing. *Journal of Advanced Nursing, 17*(6), 720–726.

Schroeter, K. (2002). Ethics in perioperative practice—Patient advocacy. *AORN Journal, 75*(5), 941–944, 949.

Schroeter, K. (2007). Advocacy: The tool of a hero. *Journal of Trauma Nursing, 14*(1), 5–6.

Shirley, J. L. (2007). Limits of autonomy in nursing's moral discourse. *Advances in Nursing Science, 30*(1), 14–25.

Vaartio, H., Leino-Kilpi, H., Salantera, S., & Suominen, T. (2006). Nursing advocacy: How is it defined by patients and nurses, what does it involve and how is it experienced? *Scandinavian Journal of Caring Sciences, 20*(3), 282–292.

Vaartio, H., Leino-Kilpi, H., Suominen, T., & Puukka, P. (2009). Nursing advocacy in procedural pain care. *Nursing Ethics, 16*(3), 340–362.

Winslow, G. R. (1984). From loyalty to advocacy: A new metaphor for nursing. *Hastings Center Report, 14*(3), 32–40.

Zauderer, C. R., Ballestas, H. C., Cardoza, M. P., Hood, P., & Neville, S. M. (2008). United we stand: Preparing nursing students for political activism. *The Journal of the New York State Nurses' Association, 39*(2), 4–7.

ONLINE RESOURCES

American Nurses Association
www.nursingworld.org
The American Association of Nurse Attorneys
www.taana.org

CHAPTER 4

Learning the Ropes of Policy and Politics

Andréa Sonenberg   Judith K. Leavitt   Wanda Montalvo[1]

"Were there none who were discontented with what they have, the world would never reach anything better."

Florence Nightingale

Every politically active person, from U.S. Presidents to chief executive officers, *learned* the political and policy skills that catapulted them into positions of power and responsibility. Nurses arrive in those positions in a similar fashion. Although one can learn about the policy process and political analysis through formal education, it is only through experience and practice that one can apply what has been learned to become effective in the position. A most important catalyst in becoming involved is to find mentors—colleagues and friends who are politically savvy—to teach us, to believe in and support us, and to celebrate our successes and help us learn from our failures.

This chapter explores how to become involved through mentoring, education, and experience. Students new to politics, as well as experienced nurses, have unlimited ways to expand their knowledge and involvement. Whatever one's experience, engaging in the process serves to improve one's skills. There are infinite causes and issues in health care to stimulate one's interest if one wants to become engaged. The first step is to decide how much energy and time one is willing to devote. Success in the world of policy and politics demands the strengths and skills that nurses possess. Working in the policy arena will open doors to opportunities where nurses can become significant participants and leaders. This book includes many of their inspirational and motivational stories.

POLITICAL CONSCIOUSNESS-RAISING AND AWARENESS: THE "AHA" MOMENT

How does one get started? Many find that there is a defining moment when the old ways of reacting to issues of injustice, inequality, or powerlessness no longer work. It is the moment when a person realizes that an issue or problem is caused by failures in the system. For instance, lack of support staff on an acute care unit may be related to decreased reimbursement rates rather than an uncaring hospital administration. Denial of care for a patient eligible to receive Medicaid or Medicare could be related to cuts in federal funding, rather than the patient's need for care. Ultimately, disparity in health outcomes may be due, in part, to health care policies. Realizing that a problem may be caused by a policy failure is a critical first step toward becoming part of the policy solution. This is political consciousness-raising and an "aha" moment. It is the adrenaline rush that urges, "Something must be done—and I need to become involved."

Until that defining moment, nurses may feel frustrated, angry, or hopeless. When the "aha" moment hits, they begin to understand that they can and must influence those who make the laws

[1]We'd like to acknowledge Janet Y. Harris, DNP, RN, NEA-BC; Mary W. Chaffee, RN, PhD, FAAN; and Connie Vance, RN, EdD, FAAN for their work on the previous editions of this chapter.

and regulations that create the inequities. Nurses then recognize the personal nature of policy issues ("the political is personal"). Advancing a solution requires skills that can be learned. When nurses accept they are not at fault for the inadequacies of the health care system and believe that nursing can shape solutions, the profession becomes political. Nurses become proactive rather than reactive. The result is individual nurses and the profession become empowered to act. Feeling empowered is essential to true advocacy (Sessler Branden, 2012).

Being politically active as a nurse is grounded in the role of *advocacy*, which many nurses equate with patient advocacy. In the professional realm of nursing, advocacy should be approached from a broader definition. Florence Nightingale saw nursing in all of its forms as advocacy; a "calling" that required nurses to look for, and act in, ways to be world citizens for the sake of human health (Dossey et al., 2005). Through her grounded theory research, Sessler Branden (2012) identified the following far-reaching conceptual definition of advocacy that emerged: "a dynamic process through which the nurse engages in a set of actions with broadly stated goals ultimately affecting a desired change at any level of patient care, health care systems and/or health policy." A more extensive discussion of advocacy can be found in this text (see Chapter 3).

GETTING STARTED

Through interviews with 27 American nurses involved in health policy at the national, state, and local levels, Gebbie, Wakefield, and Kerfoot (2000) set out to discover how and why these activist nurses became involved. Their results corroborated what we knew anecdotally:

- The majority of respondents had parents, most often fathers, who were active in policy and politics and who created a mentoring, supportive environment.
- Many were raised to be independent and to believe in their capacity to accomplish what they wanted.
- High school provided a training ground in political socialization.

- Nursing education provided role modeling and mentoring by faculty, deans, and alumni as well as the opportunity to increase political awareness through courses in policy, political science, and economics.
- Clinical practice often provided strong role models and experiences in public health and community health provided opportunities for political insights.
- Graduate education opened doors for many, through such avenues as the study of law, health economics, and health policy.
- Some had their consciousness raised gradually through work experiences that exposed them to public policy and the need to understand how to influence the process.

Nurses who were interviewed confirmed that there are multiple points of entry into the policy arena. Whether this book, a course in policy and politics, or a conversation with a colleague is your first exposure, you have already started.

Political skills can be learned. Nurses bring many skills to the political arena that are learned through education and refined in clinical practice. Politics requires the kind of communication skills that nurses use to persuade an unwilling patient to get out of bed after abdominal surgery or a child to swallow an unpleasant-tasting medication. Nurses are health care experts. We speak knowledgeably about what patients and communities need because we experience it firsthand.

THE ROLE OF MENTORING

THE MENTOR ADVANTAGE

Emerging nurse leaders seeking to advance their careers and develop political skills should secure a mentoring relationship. Stewart (1996) defines mentoring in nursing as a teaching–learning process acquired through personal experience within a one-to-one, reciprocal relationship between two individuals diverse in age, personality, life cycle, professional status, and/or credentials. It is a developmental relationship where the mentor provides the protégé with career and psychosocial supports, such as counseling, friendship, acceptance, role modeling, challenging assignments, and sponsorship (Fagenson, 1989; Kram, 1983; Zey, 1984). Mentoring occurs at many levels and should be continuous, goal directed, and under the aegis of a capable person to serve the protégé as a trusted teacher and counselor (Vance & Olson, 1998). The characteristics of successful mentors include being trustworthy, an active listener, accessible, and able to support the protégé's professional development (Cho, Ramanan, & Feldman, 2011). Good mentors are able to identify strengths and limitations in their protégé and provide critical feedback to support career and political skill development. Compared to nonmentored individuals, productive mentoring relationships result in the protégé gaining increased visibility, self-efficacy, access to new social networks, and greater career mobility (Allen et al., 2004; Fagenson, 1989; Scandura, 1992).

As a way of learning "the ropes," mentoring is a vehicle for developing political skill and contextual knowledge, part of a critical set of competencies used throughout a protégé's career. The mentor-protégé transfer of knowledge occurs through observation of role-modeling, encompassing mentor behavior that can be observed and imitated by the protégé (Chopin, 2012). Political skill is composed of four underlying dimensions and requires a degree of personal learning, discernible mainly through application and not easily taught or learned (Blass, 2007). The question for the protégé is "what are the components of political skill and how do I go about developing them?" Ferris (2007) defined four distinct factors of political skill:

- *Social astuteness:* Individuals possessing political skill are astute observers of others and are keenly attuned to diverse social situations. They comprehend social interactions and accurately interpret their behavior; they are able to discern the situation and are self-aware.
- *Interpersonal influence:* Politically skilled individuals have a subtle and convincing personal style that exerts a powerful influence to persuade those around them. They are able to strategically modify their behavior to different persons in different settings.
- *Networking ability:* Individuals with strong political skill are adept at developing and

building partnerships with diverse networks of people for beneficial alliances and coalitions.
- *Apparent sincerity:* Politically skilled individuals appear to others as possessing high levels of integrity, authenticity, sincerity, and genuineness. This dimension of political skill strikes at the very heart of whether or not influence attempts will be successful because it focuses on the perceived intentions. If actions are not interpreted as manipulative or coercive, individuals high in apparent sincerity inspire trust and confidence from those around them.

The protégé learns through observation of the mentor, modeling the new skill with repeated practice (May & Kahnweiler, 2000). This happens most effectively when seeing the mentor in real situations as they influence others; through body posture, use of language, and listening to their messaging. More importantly, the mentor allocates time to debrief about the observed interaction to help the protégé understand how and why the mentor acted in such a manner. The development of these skills occurs over time. The protégé must be mindful and respectful of the mentor's time, proactively prepare and schedule meetings with the mentor, and be open to mentor feedback (Straus, 2013). Informal mentor–protégé relationships tend to gain better results as compared to formal mentoring systems because "assigned" relationships may remain superficial (Armstrong, Allinson, & Hayes, 2002). Mentors should be on the lookout for emerging nurse leaders to identify a protégé with a similar cognitive styles; this will help to facilitate a mutual understanding and effective communication and supports a positive attitude about the mentoring relationship (Armstrong, Allinson, & Hayes, 2002; Chao, 1997).

Participating in lobby days and observing skilled lobbyists negotiate with policymakers is a great way to sharpen one's skills. At these events, nurse lobbyists and activists serve as mentor-guides and role models to nurses and students. They provide information and strategies and they model effective behaviors while lobbying policymakers on specific legislation. These activists also provide the inspiration and vision for what can be done if nurses work together toward shared goals. This is real-life

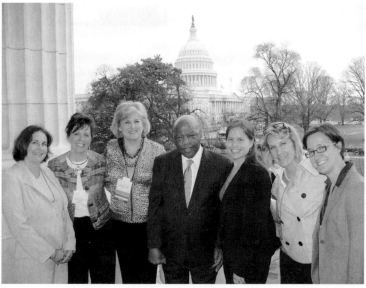

FIGURE 4-1 Dr. Linda Streit *(second from left)*, Dr. Lisa Eichelberger *(third from left)*, and Congressman John Lewis (D), Georgia *(center)*; the rest are nursing students attending the American Association of Colleges of Nursing Annual Student Health Policy Summit in Washington, DC.

learning and it is a highly effective and practical way of developing political awareness and know-how.

FINDING A MENTOR

To find a mentor, it is important to determine what you would like to learn or in what area of politics and policy you would like to be involved. Start with self-reflection and write down your areas of strength along with areas of self-improvement. Consider the types of political skill you want to develop at either an organizational level or health policy level. Answering these questions helps you to begin thinking of the type of qualities you are searching for in a mentor. Then identify people whom you have noticed, heard, or read about who are activists in your area of interest. Leverage your networks. Good sources for finding mentors are nursing associations, schools of nursing, professional organizations, local governmental departments or offices, and local political organizations and campaigns. You may contact the person directly, via e-mail, by phone, or with a note, or ask a colleague to help with an introduction. Make clear why you think the person would be a good mentor. Tell them what you want to learn

and why you would like them to assist you. Consider connecting with someone outside of nursing. For instance, nurses can get involved in local political campaigns where they are warmly welcomed, particularly if they identify themselves as nurses. The important criteria for a mentor are knowledge and an interest in you. Remember to give the relationship time to develop and be honest about expectations and time available. Sometimes the mentor need only get you started; in other situations a mentor can become a lifelong friend and role model.

COLLECTIVE MENTORING

Learning politics is not a solitary activity. This means that nurses should be on the lookout for mentors who can serve as their teachers and guides as they hone political and policy skills. Every nurse should assume responsibility for actively mentoring others as they refine their repertoire of skills and deepen their involvement. Reciprocal collective mentoring is extremely effective in expanding the political power of the profession and its members. Collective mentoring can occur in schools, clinical agencies, and professional associations.

Inherent in this form of mentoring is the development of networks of persons who are active in policy and who take responsibility for expanding these networks. Nurses in these networks should develop strategies for mentoring political neophytes and for "claiming" nurses who may not be in traditional careers (Gebbie, Wakefield, & Kerfoot, 2000). For example, politically active faculty members can network with political leaders in professional associations to provide undergraduate and graduate students with lobbying and leadership opportunities. Many state nursing associations are successfully reaching out to collectively mentor hundreds of nursing students through lobby days in national and state capitols. Nursing students and practicing nurses have many opportunities to experience collective mentoring in learning the political ropes through relationships with leaders and peers in organizations such as the National Student Nurses Association, American Nurses Association (ANA), specialty and state nursing associations, and volunteer health-related organizations. Also, local political parties, community organizations, and the offices of elected officials offer nurses opportunities to learn through mentored experiences. These organizations offer mentoring opportunities for involvement in lobbying, policy development, media contacts, fund-raising, and the political process in various venues.

Mentoring in policy development also requires connections to knowledgeable leaders. In the workplace, one can learn from health professionals who serve as leaders on influential committees. For example, if you want to work on improving staffing systems, you would need to learn about the cost of staffing, the cost of bringing in temporary staff, and the budget allocation for staffing on the unit. A clinical unit manager should have that information and can help guide your learning. In addition, one would need to know how much Medicare and Medicaid allocate to particular types of patients (outside the control of the institution) and the acuity level of patients. By working with knowledgeable staff, one can learn how to put this information together, how to influence colleagues to support a proposed policy, and how to gain access to and support from organizational leaders.

EDUCATIONAL OPPORTUNITIES

There are many ways to learn how to influence health policy; some will depend on your own learning style, where you live, and your interests. Whatever your educational and political goals, there is something for everyone; from continuing education programs to graduate programs in political science and policy, from workshops run by campaign organizations to fellowships and conferences.

PROGRAMS IN SCHOOLS OF NURSING

Health policy is one of the "essentials" of nursing education at the baccalaureate, master's, PhD, and DNP levels. (American Association of Colleges of Nursing, 2006, 2008, 2010, 2011). Nursing programs offer courses, either as core requirements or electives, related to health policy or with health policy content embedded. Many of these can be taken as continuing education credits even if you are not enrolled as a part-time or full-time student. Additionally, several schools of nursing have established graduate degree programs in policy. Schools of nursing offering health policy concentrations on the graduate level can be found on the American Association of Colleges of Nursing (AACN) website.

DEGREE PROGRAMS AND COURSES IN PUBLIC HEALTH, PUBLIC ADMINISTRATION, AND PUBLIC POLICY

College and university departments of public health, political science, policy science, political administration, and others are a rich source of policy content in academic programs. Programs leading to degrees that include health policy content are widely available at the baccalaureate, master's, and doctoral levels. These are easily accessible through online catalogs.

CONTINUING EDUCATION

Annual conferences on health policy topics are conducted by academic institutions and professional associations. Specialty nursing associations and state nursing associations often offer legislative workshops. Health policy organizations are also sources of continuing education through webinars and conferences. Check websites for the most current offerings, and monitor your state nursing association's meeting announcements. Search the Internet using *health policy meeting, health policy conference*, or *health care meeting* as search terms.

WORKSHOPS

A quick, intensive, and participatory approach to learning is to take a one- or two-day workshop in politics, campaigning, or policy from political or educational institutions. Political parties hold campaign workshops at state and national level as do other nonpartisan groups. Do a websearch for *political training* and you will find options for learning.

LEARNING BY DOING

There are many ways to obtain valuable practical experience in health policy and politics, from volunteerism to internships to self-study programs.

Internships and Fellowships. Internships and fellowships provide great learning experiences. In addition to teaching nurses the ropes, these practical placements offer valuable mentoring and networking opportunities and may lead to employment options. Internships may be arranged for credit in academic programs. Summer or year-long internships are available at local, state, and federal legislative bodies and in government agencies. Professional associations can be a good resource for finding such opportunities. The ANA offers a year-long mentored experience called American Nurses Advocacy Institute *(www.nursingworld.org)*. The Nurse in Washington Internship (NIWI) sponsored by The Nursing Organizations Alliance (The Alliance) is a two and a half day experience *(www.nursing -alliance.org/content.cfm/id/niwi)*.

Volunteer Service. A great way to learn politics is to volunteer to work on a political campaign (Figure 4-2). Volunteer time and energy are welcomed by candidates for elective office at all levels of government, local, state, and federal. First-time candidates with tight budgets are especially appreciative of volunteers. Building relationships through volunteer service is a critical part of learning the ropes and of networking. Also consider contacting

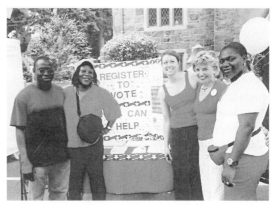

FIGURE 4-2 Nursing students with faculty member Dr. Connie Vance *(second from right)* participating in voter registration.

political party headquarters for training and information about volunteer activities.

Professional Association Activities. Many professional nursing associations offer opportunities for volunteer service that lead to rich educational, mentoring, and networking experiences. In addition to the ANA, many other nursing organizations offer opportunities. The American Association of Critical Care Nurses (AACN) and the Oncology Nursing Society (ONS), along with many specialty organizations, offer tool kits, training materials, legislative briefs, and mentoring around policy issues of concern to their practice. Other health professional associations, such as the American Public Health Association, the American Cancer Society, and the American Heart Association, have strong advocacy and legislative programs. Check their websites for volunteer opportunities.

Internet Discussion Boards and Other Resources. There are numerous sites where one can become involved in discussions on various policy topics. Not only is this a learning experience, but it is also a valuable networking opportunity. One strategy to find discussions is to join a professional networking site, such as LinkedIn, and find various relevant groups through it. Be broadminded about what groups discuss health policy; they range from policy and nursing to public and global health groups. Individual professional organizations are also creating their own professional networks with discussion boards. Professional organization webpages may also link to political action or government affairs webpages. Current legislative agendas are often listed, with user-friendly links to generate letters to one's legislators by simply inputting one's zip code. Although the letters can be sent as written, it is always beneficial to include personal anecdotes related to the issue being addressed.

SELF-STUDY

The value of reading and self-directed learning cannot be underestimated in learning about policy and politics. Many types of literature exist covering diverse interests:

Professional Journals. Many professional nursing, health care, and social sciences journals include updates on current political issues. Some are wholly focused on policy and politics (e.g., *Policy, Politics, & Nursing Practice; Health Affairs*); others publish regular political and policy content (e.g. *American Journal of Nursing, Nursing Outlook, Nursing Economics, Journal of the American Medical Association* [*JAMA*]).

Organizational Newsletters. Some organizational newsletters, both professional and interest group, feature health policy related columns. One that is particularly committed to disseminating health policy information to its members is the American Association of Retired Persons (AARP).

Books. Browse through the political science, government, or current events sections of your favorite bookstore and you are likely to find a goldmine. You can also browse online booksellers. Search for the words *politics*, *policy*, or *health policy*, and see what piques your interest.

Newspapers. Major metropolitan newspapers offer political analysis of national, regional, and local politics. Those recognized for in-depth political reporting on health issues include the *Washington Post (www.washingtonpost.com)*, the *New York Times (www.nytimes.com)*, the *Los Angeles Times (www.latimes.com)*, and the *Wall Street Journal (www.wsj.com)*.

Television. Network and cable news programs and television news-magazines address political issues and government activities. The ultimate viewing experience for politicos is C-SPAN. This channel is available as a public service created by the U.S. cable television industry to provide access to the live gavel-to-gavel proceedings of the U.S. House of Representatives and the U.S. Senate and to other forums in which public policy is discussed, debated, and decided. C-SPAN provides a wealth of information about the democratic process, without editing, commentary, or analysis. Television programs have become interactive by integrating social media, such as Twitter, so viewers can participate in televised stories and discussions.

Radio. Radio continues to be a rich source of political information and debate on AM, FM, and satellite radio stations. Policy-focused stations include the following:
- National Public Radio (NPR) via public radio stations and the Internet *(www.npr.org)*. NPR provides carefully researched in-depth reporting.
- C-SPAN Radio offers public affairs commercial-free programming 24 hours a day, accessed through the radio or the Internet. The broadcast schedule is available at *www.c-span.org*.
- Liberal and conservative political talkfests. Many political "talking heads" have radio programs that serve as forums to debate hot political topics. Check your local radio program website for air time and station.

Internet. An all-you-can-eat political buffet exists on the Internet. All major news organizations, activism groups, political parties, issue advocates, and many others have a presence on the Internet. A diverse universe of political discussion exists, from well-substantiated journalism to blogs with absolutely no quality control. Through social networking sites, both personal and professional, one can participate in discussions, become informed, and have the added benefit of networking.

APPLYING YOUR POLITICAL, POLICY, ADVOCACY, AND ACTIVISM SKILLS

The purpose of learning the ropes of policy, politics, and advocacy is to influence health policy. The only way to become an effective political leader, advocate, or activist is through experience and practice, so that one can apply strategies and skills learned to influencing decisions made by governments, communities, organizations, institutions, and associations. Much political activity occurs in the sphere of government. The U.S. government is a complicated system that determines the direction of a complex nation. Activism has made a difference in many communities and has been recognized as a powerful force in promoting equity in access to quality, culturally competent, preventive health and mental health services, and community resources (Buresh & Gordon, 2013; Jansson, 2011). For example, in May 2012 New York City passed the "Soda Ban," which limited the public sale of sugary drinks to 16 oz. Mayor Bloomberg had introduced the legislation as a public health initiative to mitigate one of the risk factors of obesity, a national epidemic (Peltz, 2013; Weissner, 2013). There was a public and corporate outcry about government involvement in personal decision making and purchasing power. A grassroots effort by concerned soda-loving citizens, local and national businesses, and corporations, such as Pepsi, Coca-Cola, and Snapple, successfully fought to overturn the ruling by filing a lawsuit against the city (Peltz, 2013). In March 2013, on the eve of the implementation of the ban, a State Court ruled the ban to be illegal and the law was overturned. Mayor Bloomberg continues in his efforts by filing an appeal with the state's highest court, the New York State Court of Appeals, which has agreed to hear the case (Weissner, 2013). Advocates of the law hold that the public health campaign is not over. Dr Ludwig, professor of pediatrics and nutrition at Boston Children's Hospital, points out that "the individual liberty argument would have more weight if the health effects weren't spilling over into society in the form of higher insurance premiums and a greater share of public dollars going to Medicare and Medicaid"

(Tavernise, 2013). This case is an example of how political efforts on both sides of an initiative can be effective, and that arguments must be based on both the evidence and the precedence.

POLITICAL COMPETENCIES

The Spectrum of Political Competencies (Figure 4-3) portrays the range of activities from which nurses can draw to influence health and health care. It demonstrates the breadth and variety of competencies ranging from novice to more sophisticated levels, including running for elective office. These skills can be learned and applied in a wide variety of activities aimed at improving health and health care. Some nurses have their initial experience of activism and advocacy in school. For example, students in the RN-to-BSN program at Valdosta State University in Georgia learned to address community health problems through political strategies aimed at fluoridating a community water system (Wold et al., 2008). Senior nursing students at New York Institute of Technology attended New York State Nurses Association's Lobby Day to develop skills in civic engagement (Zauderer et al., 2008–2009). In the community, nurses can participate in a variety of activities aimed at influencing decisions, including writing letters to the editors of newspapers, writing letters to legislators, calling in to radio talk-shows, commenting on health policy blogs, participating in professional social-network group discussions, working on campaigns, serving in volunteer positions, speaking at hearings, and participating in rallies (Figure 4-4).

More sophisticated political skills are required for effective organizational leadership, obtaining political appointments, and seeking elective office. Many skills that nurses develop in clinical roles are directly transferrable to influential policy roles and paid political positions. Ohio State Senator Sue Morano, RN, identified skills that nurses can bring to elective office that help them become effective advocates. These include setting priorities, leadership, conflict resolution, collaboration, communication, and having conversations about difficult issues (Iacono, 2008). There are limitless

LEARNING THE ROPES	PARTICIPATING IN DEMOCRACY	INFLUENCING AND ADVOCATING	USING ADVANCED POLITICAL SKILLS
• Get a mentor • Educate self about policy and politics • Read and consider health care and social issues • Get an internship • Read, listen to, and discuss the news and current issues • Network with other nurses • Participate in nursing legislative events • Learn about advocacy and activism • Study policy • Strengthen communication skills (written and verbal) • Attend educational programs or camps • Learn the structure of governments • Identify your elected representatives • Learn the scope of influence of groups with authority (e.g., local board of health, organizational groups, congressional committees) • Join policy and advocacy groups on professional social networking sites	• Volunteer on a political campaign • Vote • Explain political views to others • Learn about political candidates and their views • Participate in voter registration activities • Sign petitions • Post candidates' signs on your property or vehicle • Weigh pros and cons of political positions • Join a political party • Research the status of a bill • Serve as a volunteer poll worker on election day	• Post opinions on blogs • Participate in professional organization's legislative activities • Write op-eds and letters to editors of newspapers and other media • Express opinions via social media (e.g., Twitter) • Speak at public hearings • Cultivate a relationship with elected representatives • Respond to "action alerts" sent out by professional organizations • Participate in rallies and protests • Network with opinion leaders (local organizers, business owners, and others) • Support a political candidate (go door-to-door, attend meetings, make calls) • Express opinions to elected officials via letter, e-mail, call or visit • Make financial contributions to political action committees • Hold a house party fundraiser for a candidate • Participate in community meetings	• Run for elective office • Obtain a political appointment • Serve as a paid political staff member • Provide expert testimony • Hold a media event • Host television, radio or other media broadcasts • Write a newspaper column • Serve as a policy analyst • Obtain an appointment to a board or committee • Serve as a speechwriter • Participate in political surveys and polling • Manage a political campaign • Become a lobbyist • Publish articles on health care issues and solutions • Provide an interview with the media

FIGURE 4-3 The spectrum of political competencies and examples of activities.

opportunities for nurses from all educational levels and experience to learn new skills and use them to improve health for individuals and populations.

CHANGING POLICY AT THE WORKPLACE THROUGH SHARED GOVERNANCE

JANET HARRIS, RN, DNS

Infrastructures and processes within institutions offer great opportunities for nurses to get involved in policy change as well as learn internal political processes. One such example is actions by a group of nurses from a Bone Marrow Transplant Unit at a medical center in Mississippi that had rolled out Relationship-Based Care as a practice model. This model was one vehicle used in the implementation of a shared governance model.

In this model the front line staff members were engaged and empowered through Unit-Based Practice Councils. This particular council was concerned that outpatients coming to their area for chemotherapy were sitting in the admissions office for 4 to 6 hours awaiting registration and lab results. Often, not feeling well and after a long wait, patients were sent home because their counts were too low for chemotherapy administration on that day. The council decided to work to improve the process. Their initial collaborative discussions with physicians were disheartening, but the council persisted and proposed a pilot project.

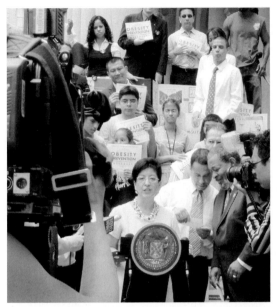

FIGURE 4-4 Wanda Montalvo, RN, leads a press conference asking the NYC Council to support the Childhood Obesity Initiative.

Imitating the example of communication savvy demonstrated by their manager, the practice council representatives worked with various multidisciplinary groups across the organization to garner support for the project. The pilot included process redesign of laboratory specimen collection at the local doctor's office or clinic prior to the patient's travel to the infusion center. Blood counts were assessed locally and unnecessary trips to the center were avoided. Upon arrival at the center, a streamlined admissions process expedited the patient transfer to the chemotherapy infusion area. The resultant patient waiting time was less than 30 minutes. Not only were the patients delighted with the change, the nursing staff members were proud of their ability to successfully navigate the complex academic system, and to develop a new policy that provided better quality care for patients.

This front line group used several "learning the ropes" strategies. First, elected council members all attended training workshops on effective teamwork within the council as well as teamwork across the organization. Crucial conversation content was offered through "Lunch and Learn" activities; staff

learned how to communicate when stakes were high and opinions varied. They discussed their plans at length by evaluating the pros and cons of each step in the proposed process. The unit manager, who was one of the most senior and experienced staff members in the organization, served as a mentor to the group; a unit practice council advisor also assisted in the mentorship and advocacy role. Lastly the council learned by doing. They researched their topic using the Internet and an online reference center. They combined the evidence with the skills used in continuous quality improvement throughout the organization. The results demonstrated the organization's front line nurses' influence and political savvy to drive improved care for a specific patient population.

DISCUSSION QUESTIONS

1. Create a one-page plan for your own learning about policy and politics.
2. Give examples of four opportunities for learning-by-doing.
3. List three places you can look for a mentor.

REFERENCES

Allen, T. D., Eby, L. T., Poteet, M. L., Lentz, E., & Lima, L. (2004). Career benefits associated with mentoring for protégés: A meta-analysis. *Journal of Applied Psychology, 89*(1), 127–136.

American Association of Colleges of Nursing. (2006). The essentials of doctoral education for advanced nursing practice. Washington, DC: AACN. Retrieved from *www.aacn.nche.edu/publications/position/DNPEssentials.pdf.*

American Association of Colleges of Nursing. (2008). The essentials of baccalaureate education for professional nursing practice. Washington, DC: AACN. Retrieved from *www.aacn.nche.edu/education-resources/BaccEssentials08.pdf.*

American Association of Colleges of Nursing. (2010). The research-focused doctoral program in nursing pathways to excellence. Washington, DC: AACN. Retrieved from *www.aacn.nche.edu/education-resources/PhD Position.pdf.*

American Association of Colleges of Nursing. (2011). The essentials of master's education for advanced practice nursing. Washington, DC: AACN. Retrieved from *www.aacn.nche.edu/education-resources/MastersEssentials11.pdf.*

Armstrong, S. J., Allinson, C. W., & Hayes, J. (2002). Formal mentoring systems: An examination of the effects of mentor/protégé cognitive styles on the mentoring process. *Journal of Management Studies, 39*(8), 1111–1137.

Blass, F. R. (2007). Leader reputation, the role of mentoring, political skill, contextual learning, and adaptation. *Human Resource Management, 46*(1), 5–19.

Buresh, B., & Gordon, S. (2013). *From silence to voice: what nurses know and must communicate to the public* (3rd ed.). Ithaca, NY: ILR Press.

Chao, G. T. (1997). Mentoring phases and outcomes. *Journal of Vocational Behavior, 51*(1), 15–28.

Cho, C. S., Ramanan, R. A., & Feldman, M. D. (2011). Defining the ideal qualities of mentorship: a qualitative analysis of the characteristics of outstanding mentors. *The American Journal of Medicine, 124*(5), 453–458. doi: dx.doi.org/10.1016/j.amjmed.2010.12.007.

Chopin, S. M. (2012). Effects of mentoring on the development of leadership self-efficacy and political skill. *Journal of Leadership Studies, 6*(3), 17–32.

Dossey, B., Slanders, L., Beck, D. M., & Attewell, A. (2005). *Florence Nightingale today: Healing, leadership, global action.* Silver Spring, MD: ANA.

Fagenson, E. A. (1989). The mentor advantage: Perceived career/job experiences of proteges versus non-proteges. *Journal of Organizational Behavior, 10*(4), 309–320.

Ferris, G. R. (2007). Political skill in organizations. *Journal of Management, 33*(3), 290–320.

Gebbie, K. M., Wakefield, M., & Kerfoot, K. (2000). Nursing and health policy. *Journal of Nursing Scholarship, 32*(3), 307–315.

Iacono, M. (2008). Senator Sue Morano, RN: Nursing advocacy in the Ohio Senate. *Journal of Perianesthesia Nursing, 23*(3), 204–206.

Jansson, B. S. (2011). *Improving healthcare through advocacy: A guide for the health and helping professions.* Hoboken, N.J.: John Wiley & Sons, Inc.

Kram, K. E. (1983). Phases of the mentoring relationship. *Academy of Management Journal, 26*, 608–625.

May, G. L., & Kahnweiler, W. M. (2000). The effect of a mastery practice design on learning and transfer in behavior modeling training. *Personnel Psychology, 53*(2), 353–373.

Peltz, J. (2013, March 11). Soda ban halted by judge; NYC large sugary beverage restriction rejected day before scheduled enforcement. *The Huffington Post.* Retrieved from *www.huffingtonpost.com/2013/03/11/soda-ban-halted-by-judge-large-sugary-beverage_n_2854807.html.*

Scandura, T. A. (1992). Mentorship and career mobility: An empirical investigation. *Journal of Organizational Behavior, 13*(2), 169–174. doi:10.1002/job.4030130206.

Sessler Branden, P. (2012). *The nurse as advocate: A grounded theory perspective.* (Doctoral dissertation: Vanderbilt University).

Stewart, B. M. (1996). An evolutionary concept analysis of mentoring in nursing. *Journal of Professional Nursing, 12*(5), 311–321.

Straus, S. E. (2013). Characteristics of successful and failed mentoring relationships: A qualitative study across two academic health centers. *Academic Medicine, 88*(1), 82–89.

Tavernise, S. (2013, March 12). A bumpy road to a soda ban. *The New York Times.* Retrieved from *well.blogs.nytimes.com/2013/03/12/a-bumpy-road-to-a-soda-ban/?_r=0.*

Vance, C., & Olson, R. K. (1998). *The mentor connection in nursing.* New York: Springer Publishing Company.

Weissner, D. (2013, October 17). New York court to hear Bloomberg's appeal to restore soda ban. *Reuters.* Retrieved from *www.reuters.com/article/2013/10/17/us-nycsodaban-appeal-idUSBRE99G0T620131017.*

Wold, S., Brown, C., Chastain, C., Griffis, M., & Wingate, J. (2008). Going the extra mile: Beyond health teaching to political involvement. *Nursing Forum, 43*(4), 171–176.

Zauderer, C., Ballesas, H., Cardoza, M., Hood, P., & Neville, S. (2008-2009). United we stand: Preparing nursing students for political activism. *Journal of the New York State Nurses Association,* Fall/Winter, 4-7.

Zey, M. (1984). *The mentor connection.* Homewood, IL: Dow Jones Irwin.

ONLINE RESOURCES

American Association of Colleges of Nursing Grassroots Network
capwiz.com/aacn/home
American Nurses Association Policy and Advocacy
nursingworld.org/MainMenuCategories/ANAPoliticalPower.aspx
C-SPAN
www.c-span.org
Henry Kaiser Family Foundation
kff.org
Robert Wood Johnson Foundation Policy
www.rwjf.org/en/topics/rwjf-topic-areas/health-policy.html

CHAPTER 5

TAKING ACTION:
How I Learned the Ropes of Policy and Politics

Chelsea Savage

"This is the true joy in life, the being used for a purpose recognized by yourself as a mighty one; the being thoroughly worn out before you are thrown on the scrap heap; the being a force of Nature instead of a feverish selfish little clod of ailments and grievances complaining that the world will not devote itself to making you happy."

George Bernard Shaw

I began my career at the bedside. But being at the bedside wasn't enough to stoke my commitment to social justice and making change in the world. This story of "Taking Action" describes my journey so far, including the successes and challenges along the way, and my own assessment of how passion, combined with mentoring, can produce change in policy. I began my commitment to social justice in 2007 as a Fellow in Richmond, Virginia, for "Hope in the Cities," a program sponsored by Initiatives of Change, USA, that focuses on building trust through honest conversations on race, reconciliation, and responsibility *(www.us.iofc.org)*. From the rich discussions I had with diverse individuals and groups, I developed an ability to look for and understand the story of the "other" and to use this in conversations to facilitate peace and understanding. This has served me well in the political arena where differences can collide or lead to more creative policy solutions to today's problems.

I was able to connect that commitment to social justice with my passion for nursing and health care advocacy as Chair of the Legislative Committee for the Virginia Organization of Nurse Executives in

2007. That chairmanship led to a 2-year term as Chair of the Legislative Coalition of Virginia Nurses. In 2009, I became a Fellow of the American Nurses Advocacy Institute, an initiative of the American Nurses Association to develop and mentor nurses into political leaders. A year later, I was selected to participate in the University of Virginia (UVA) Sorensen Institute Political Leaders Program. This program is designed for Virginians who want to learn the political ropes and become more active in public service. I am active in the Virginia Nurses Association (VNA), serving as Secretary and Assistant Commissioner of Government Affairs. However, I had no clue that I ever was going to do any of those things; they weren't even in my realm of possibilities. So how did all of this happen?

MENTORS, PASSION, AND CURIOSITY

Three things created these opportunities. The first was my passion for social justice, the second was my mentors, and the third was an insatiable curiosity that propelled me to venture into uncharted territories. I was finishing a fellowship in Health Law when Shirley Gibson, a mentor and president of the Virginia Organization of Nurse Executives at that time, asked "Chelsea, will you chair the Legislative Committee for the Virginia Organization of Nurse Executives?" I said yes and within a couple of weeks I was networking with leaders in the state, leading advocacy on health care and nursing issues. I was one of the representatives of several diverse nursing organizations that comprised the

49

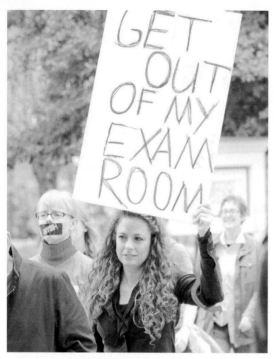

FIGURE 5-1 Author Chelsea Savage participated in a protest against state legislation that would have mandated transvaginal ultrasounds prior to abortions in Virginia.

Legislative Coalition of Virginia Nurses (LCVN), founded in part by one of my mentors, Becky Bowers-Lanier. Becky, a well-regarded nursing leader in health policy, and Sallie Eissler, a pediatric nurse practitioner, decided nursing needed a succession plan and I was supposed to help with that. So I was elected Chair of LCVN. Highlights of my time included meeting with policymakers and campaign managers for the governor's race, creating legislative platforms that outlined succinctly our legislative priorities, and assisting with the passage of the Virginia Indoor Clean Air Act that banned smoking in restaurants and certain other public places.

Sallie Eissler was also head of the Political Action Committee for the VNA and a political junkie. She suggested that I learn about politics in Virginia by applying to the Sorensen Institute Political Leaders Program (PLP) through the UVA. PLP had nothing to do with nursing and everything to do with building political networks and learning to function in the system. Because of my connections though PLP, I was tapped to be Co-Chair for Nurses for Obama in Virginia. Our mission was to educate the public on the Affordable Care Act (ACA). Radio interviews and newspaper articles followed.

I was aware that, if you are not careful, working publicly on behalf of candidates in an election year can create problems with your employer and non-partisan nursing professional organizations. A colleague advised me that nurses are certainly able to wear more than one hat. I could be a supporter of the ACA and even President Obama as an individual nurse, but it was up to me to make it clear I was not representing the views of my employer or my professional association.

I am lucky to have several mentors in my life, such as Becky and Sallie. I didn't choose them, but for some reason they chose me, perhaps because I was an enthusiastic, "can do," productive individual with a passion for creating a healthy society. Through their example, I look for opportunities to mentor. I look for passion in nurses. If a tree falls in the woods and no one is around to hear it, does it make a sound? Replace tree with "nurse" and falls in the woods with "has a passion for the health of their patients and profession" and ask: "Does quiet passion really count for anything?"

Let's go back to professional organizations because this is how "it makes a sound." Strength is in numbers and in nurses wanting to be heard. Bring this back to the bedside. I was a nurse manager of a 27-bed medical-telemetry unit when I started on my journey in health policy and politics. We had a significant number of full-time employment (FTE) positions that were unfilled; there just weren't any applicants. The nursing shortage had reduced me to spending half of my time calling overworked nurses to ask them to do overtime. I was working with three professional nursing organizations at the time, and the consensus was that the shortage was linked to a shortage of nursing faculty, resulting in hundreds of qualified applicants to Virginia's schools of nursing being turned away. Testifying before Virginia state legislators on behalf of those nursing professional associations, I verified the need to raise nursing faculty salaries. Two things happened that made that a success. The first was that my passion found a voice; the second was that the voice was backed by numbers of constituents who vote. There are over 100,000 nurses in the Commonwealth of Virginia. Together with our numbers and the respect the public has for our profession, we create a voice that gets attention and that is successful in creating change.

Where does passion and a commitment to become an agent for change in our society come from? Different places, but for me a good part of it came from adversity. I grew up in a strict religious sect and was not allowed to go to school after the 6th grade. I was supplied with books, and my passion led me to teach myself and obtain my GED when I was 15 years old. Education became my passion, and what I experienced created in me a commitment to social justice, advocacy for nursing, and better health care for Virginians.

Consider another example. I have a dynamic friend who was diagnosed with ovarian cancer; she immediately founded CancerDancer *(www .ocancerdancer.org)*, an organization with almost 10,000 members, to spread the word on ovarian cancer signs and symptoms. A special characteristic of us humans is that what should discourage us often makes us a powerful catalyst for change. We are so resilient. Find your passion, then find your voice; and go out and change the world.

CHAPTER 6

A Primer on Political Philosophy

Sally S. Cohen   Beth L. Rodgers

"If I were to attempt to put my political philosophy tonight into a single phrase, it would be this: Trust the people."

Adlai Stevenson

In this chapter, we present major concepts from political philosophy so that nurses will be mindful of the ideological, philosophical, and political themes that structure contemporary health policy debates. Such knowledge can enhance the ability of nurses to develop strategies that take into account political and ideological perspectives, many of which are not always evident, but nonetheless often drive political deliberations and outcomes. After an introduction to political philosophy, we present an overview of the role of the state, present major political ideologies and their evolution, summarize how political philosophy relates to contemporary gender and race issues, and discuss the "welfare state." We conclude with a discussion of the implications of political philosophy for nurses involved in health politics and policy.

POLITICAL PHILOSOPHY

Political philosophy examines, analyzes, and searches for answers to fundamental questions about the state and its moral and ethical responsibilities. It asks questions such as, "What constitutes the state?," "What rights and privileges should the state protect?," "What laws and regulations should be implemented?," and "To what extent should government control people's lives?" Political philosophy encompasses the goals, rules, or behaviors that citizens, states, and societies ought to pursue. It provides generalizations about proper conduct in political life and the legitimate uses of power

(Hacker, 1960). Today's political philosophers build on the classic works of the past and apply them to contemporary issues, including health policy. From another perspective, political philosophy addresses two issues. The first is about the distribution of material goods, rights, and liberties. The second issue pertains to the possession and determination of political power. It includes such questions as, "Why do others have rights over me?," "Why do I have to obey laws that other people developed and with which I disagree?," and "Why do the wealthy often have more power than the majority?" (Wolff, 1996).

Political philosophy is a normative discipline, meaning that it tries to establish how people ought to be, as expressed through rules or laws. It involves making judgments about the world, rather than simply describing or observing people and society. Political philosophers attempt to explain what is right, just, or morally correct. It is a constantly evolving discipline, prompting us to think about how the concerns and questions just described, although as ancient as society, still affect us today.

For nurses, political philosophy offers ways of analyzing and handling situations that arise in practice, policy, organizational, and community settings. For example, it helps determine how far government authorities may go in regulating nursing practice. It offers ways of understanding complex ethical situations—such as end-of-life care, the use of technology in clinical settings, and reproductive health—when there is no clear answer regarding what constitutes the rights of individuals, clinicians, government officials, or society at large. Political philosophy offers normative ways of addressing such situations by focusing on the relationships among individuals, government, and society. Finally, political philosophy enables nurses to think about their roles as members of society, organizations, and health care delivery settings in attempting to attain important health policy goals, such as reducing the number of people without health care coverage and eliminating disparities among ethnic groups.

THE STATE

The "state" in political philosophy (and political science) does not pertain to the 50 states of the United States. Rather, it is a "particular kind of social group" (Shively, 2005, p. 13). The state arose from the notion that people cannot rule at their will. As Andrew Levine (2002) explained, "Few, if any, human groupings have persisted for very long without authority relations of some kind" (p. 6). Today's modern state is a highly organized government entity that influences many aspects of everyday lives (Shively, 2005). It typically refers to the "governing apparatus that makes and enforces rules" (Shively, 2005, p. 56). Therefore the terms *state* and *government* may be interchangeable. It is the role of the state (or government) in health policy issues—such as licensure of health professionals and institutions, financing care, ensuring adequate environmental quality, protecting against bioterrorist attacks, and subsiding care—that affects nurses in their professional practice and personal lives. Usually people think of national governments as the modern state. However, local and state governments also assume important roles in protecting individuals, regulating trade, and ensuring individual rights and well-being. In distinguishing between a nation and a state, note that a state is a political entity "with sovereignty," meaning it has responsibility for the conduct of its own affairs. In contrast, a nation is "a large group of people who are bound together, and recognize a similarity among themselves, because of a common culture" (Shively, 2005, p. 51).

Despite these distinctions, the terms *state* and *nation* may overlap in common parlance because government leaders often appeal to the "emotional attachment of people in their nation" in building support for the more legal entity, a state (Shively, 2005, p. 52). Furthermore, the cultural diversity of most countries makes claims of common cultural

ties as the distinguishing feature of any nation increasingly difficult to uphold. That said, few would dispute that the political culture of the United States is different from that of other countries. We pride ourselves on individualism, a laissez-faire approach to government and economics, and a strong belief in the rights of individuals. Policy analysts often point to the unique political culture as an explanation for why U.S. social policy deviates from that of other countries. An example is the difficulty in establishing any type of national health insurance program. The Affordable Care Act (ACA) can be considered progress in this regard but it still relies on a combination of private and public initiatives, while most other developed countries have strong state-sponsored health care insurance (Canada) or delivery systems (United Kingdom).

INDIVIDUALS AND THE STATE

Thomas Hobbes (1588-1679). Hobbes was one of the major political philosophers to describe the relationship between individuals and the state. Hobbes developed the concept of the "social contract," which basically claims "individuals in a hypothetical state of nature would choose to organize their political affairs" (Levine, 2002, p. 18). As Shively succinctly explained, "Of their free will, by a cooperative decision, the people set up a power to dominate them for the common good" (Shively, 2005, p. 38). Hobbes's theory was important in establishing governance and authority, without which people would live in a natural state of chaos. To avoid such situations, according to Hobbes, people living in communities voluntarily establish rules by which they abide.

Nurses can view the social contract as a rationale for government intervention in aspects of practice, public health, and delivery of care. We turn to government to protect us from situations such as unregulated care and unlicensed practice, which might cause harm to patients if professionals and administrators were left to their own devices. We voluntarily adhere to these rules to prevent danger and minimize the consequences of unmonitored care.

John Locke (1632-1704). Locke was a British political philosopher who greatly influenced liberal thinkers, including the writers of the U.S. Constitution, by emphasizing the importance of individual rights in relationship to the state. His defense of individual rights was fundamental to liberalism (discussed later) and the development of democracies around the world. For Locke, individual rights were more important than state power. States exist to protect the "inalienable" rights afforded mankind. One of the premises of Locke's theories is that people should be free from coercive state institutions. Moreover, the rights inherent in such freedom are different from the legal rights established by governmental authority under a Hobbesian contract. They are basic to the nature of humanity.

Jeremy Bentham (1748-1832). Bentham, heralded as the father of classic utilitarianism, rejected the natural law tradition. His utilitarianism theory basically asserted that individuals and governments strive to attain pleasure over pain. When applying this "happiness principle" to governments, "it requires us to maximize the greatest happiness of the greatest number in the community" (Shapiro, 2003, p. 19). Instead of relying on natural law, Bentham favored the establishment of legal systems "enforced by the sovereign" (Shapiro, 2003, p. 19). Bentham's utilitarianism has become foundational to many contemporary theories in economics, political science, bioethics, and other disciplines.

The tension between individual rights and the role of the state is inherent in many health policy discussions. Consider, for example, substance abuse. On one hand, individuals have the right to smoke tobacco and drink alcohol. One might even argue that the state should protect individuals' rights to do so. On the other hand, such freedoms may interfere with others' rights to fresh air and freedom from harm (e.g., from second-hand smoke inhalation or from incidents related to alcohol use). In such cases, the state has a legitimate role to intervene and protect the rights of others; the greater good. The challenge lies in finding the right balance between the rights of individuals on both sides of the issue and balancing them with the rights of the state.

POLITICAL IDEOLOGIES

A political ideology is a "set of ideas about politics, all of which are related to one another and that

modify and support each other" (Shively, 2005, p. 19). Political ideologies are characterized by distinctive views on the organization and functioning of the state. Ideologies give people a way of analyzing and making decisions about complex issues on the political agenda. They also provide a way for policymakers to convince others that their position on an issue will advance the public good. Three major political ideologies, liberalism, socialism, and conservatism, originated with 18th- and 19th-century European philosophers and are the basis of political deliberations and policies throughout the world (Shively, 2005). The terms and definitions of *liberalism* and *conservatism* as they have evolved over time are not necessarily consistent with these two ideologies as they exist today. Nevertheless, without appreciating their origins, the nuances in their rhetoric and their role in health policy cannot be fully understood.

LIBERALISM

American political thought was greatly influenced by 18th-century European liberalism and the political thinking of Hobbes, Locke, and others. This 18th-century liberalism meshed well with political, economic, scientific, and cultural trends of the time, all of which sought to free people from confining and parochial values. Liberalism relies on the notion that members of a society should be able to "develop their individual capacities to the fullest extent" (Shively, 2005, p. 24). People also must be responsible for their actions and must not be dependent on others.

John Stuart Mill (1806-1873). Mill, a British political philosopher, is considered a major force behind contemporary liberalism. His essay "On Liberty" (1859) is foundational to modern liberal thinking. Mill was committed to individual rights and freedom of thought and expression, but not unconditionally. He based his work on Locke's philosophies, tempered by Bentham's utilitarian philosophy.

Mill contended that individuals were sovereign over their own bodies and minds but could not exert such sovereignty if it harmed others. He provides a way of reconciling Locke's emphasis on individual rights with Hobbes's focus on the importance of an authoritarian state. A leading contemporary political philosopher and political scientist, Ian Shapiro, applied Mill's balancing of individual rights with his "harm principle" as follows:

… although sanitary regulations, workplace safety rules, and the prevention of fraud coerce people and interfere with their liberty, such policies are acceptable because the legitimacy of the ends they serve is "undeniable." (Shapiro, 2003, p. 60)

The best form of government under liberal ideology is a democracy, in which individuals participate in political decision making and express their views freely. The right to vote confers an important privilege to members of a democracy in that it is a form of political expression free from domination by others.

In sum, liberal ideology is based on the importance of democracy; intellectual freedom (e.g., freedom of speech and religion); limited government involvement in economic activities and personal life; government protections against abuse of power by one person or group; and placing as many choices as possible in the private realm (Shively, 2005). In many ways, liberalism lies at the center of American political thought.

CONSERVATISM

In response to liberals' calls for changing the existing social and political order, conservatives countered with a preference for stability and structure. They preferred patterns of domination and power that had the benefit of being predictable and gave people familiar political terrain. Under conservative thought, those in power had the "awesome responsibility" to "help the weak." In contrast, liberals preferred to give such individuals "responsibility for their own affairs" (Shively, 2005, p. 26). Liberals wanted people to be free of government intrusion in their lives; conservatives favored a strong government role in helping those in need of assistance.

Guided by the notion that government had a responsibility to provide structured assistance to others, 19th-century European conservatives, especially in Great Britain and Germany, developed many programs that featured government support to the disadvantaged (e.g., unemployment assistance and income subsidies). They accepted welfare policies (discussed later) that were foundational to the revival of Europe after World War II. They have been major players in contemporary European politics, especially in Great Britain, offering a synergy with American conservatism.

SOCIALISM

Socialism grew out of dissatisfaction with liberalism from many in the working class. Unable to prosper under liberalism, which relied on individual capacities, socialists looked to the state for policies to protect workers from sickness, unemployment, unsafe working conditions, and other situations.

Karl Marx (1818-1883). Marx, a German philosopher, is widely considered the father of socialism. For Marx, individuals could improve their situation only by identifying with their economic class. The 19th-century Industrial Revolution had created the working class, which, according to Marx, was oppressed by capitalists who used workers for their profits. According to Marx, only revolution could relieve workers of their oppression.

As a political ideology, socialism encompasses many ideas. Among them are equality, regardless of professional or private roles; the importance of a classless society; an economy that contributes equally to the welfare of a majority of citizens; the concept of a common good; lack of individual ownership; and lack of any type of privatization. Therefore socialism is also an economic concept under which "the production and distribution of goods is owned collectively or by a centralized government that often plans and controls the economy" (Socialism, 2005). The collective nature of socialism is in contrast to the primacy of private property that characterizes capitalism.

Socialism originated and proliferated in Europe toward the end of the 19th and into the early 20th centuries. Then it split into two ideologies, communist and democratic socialist. In 1917, communists, under the leadership of V. I. Lenin, took over the Russian Empire and formed a socialist state, the Union of Soviet Socialist Republics (USSR). Lenin and his communist followers believed in revolution as the only way to advance socialism and achieve total improvement in workers' conditions. Democratic socialists, in contrast, were more willing to work with government institutions, participate in democracies, and "settle for partial improvements for workers, rather than holding out for total change" (Shively, 2005, p. 33). Between 1989 and 1991, communist regimes in Eastern Germany, the USSR, and throughout Eastern Europe collapsed. In their quest for economic and political change, the new Eastern European governments have turned to democracy, democratic socialism, capitalism, and other economic and political models.

Today, only a handful of countries (e.g., Cuba, China, North Korea, Vietnam) are under communist rule. Socialists, especially democratic socialists, have prevailed in Scandinavia and Western Europe. They have been instrumental in advancing the modern welfare state in those countries and elsewhere around the world (Shively, 2005).

CONTEMPORARY CONSERVATISM AND LIBERALISM

Contemporary political conservatism, which grew in popularity in the late 20th century, is similar to classic conservatism (described previously) but differs from it in several ways. In particular, conservatives oppose a strong government role in assisting the disadvantaged. Recall that the conservative political philosophers of the 18th and 19th centuries supported the state's role in helping individuals through social policies. Now, liberals are the ones who generally favor a strong government role in social policies, such as health, welfare, education, and labor, whereas conservatives prefer minimal government intervention and reliance on privatization and individual choice.

Contemporary conservatives oppose rapid and fundamental change, as did proponents of earlier models of conservatism. They call for devolution of federal responsibility for health and other social issues to state governments, a diminished presence of government in all aspects of policy, a reduced tax burden, and the importance of traditional social values. Many political observers point to the 1980 election of President Ronald Reagan as a turning point for the rise of American conservatism.

In contrast to conservatives' calls for a decreased federal presence in health care policy, liberals today support an expanded government role to help people who need income support, health care coverage, child care assistance, vocational guidance, tuition, and other aspects of social policy. The Great Society programs of President John F. Kennedy and Lyndon B. Johnson in the 1960s and early 1970s boosted American liberal policies. Among the highlights of the Great Society initiatives were the enactment of Medicare, Medicaid, and Head Start. These federal government initiatives are founded on the importance of the state helping the disadvantaged through government-sponsored programs. They are in line with traditional liberal philosophies, described previously, which support the notion that individuals should be given equal opportunities to pursue their inalienable rights. Such rights include their health and welfare, broadly defined, even though the right to health care is not a legal one under the U.S. Constitution.

Since the mid-1990s, conservatives and liberals have found themselves in a somewhat ironic situation. Conservatives have deviated from their preference for the status quo by favoring rampant changes in certain aspects of social policy, among which are privatizing Social Security and inserting the federal government into the public education domain under the No Child Left Behind (NCLB) law. Liberals, on the other hand, often find themselves as the defenders of the status quo as they fight to sustain public programs, such as Medicaid. Each of these stances also reflects ideologies of their respective camps.

George Lakoff, a well-known linguist and political scientist, has developed an interesting way of explaining the differences between contemporary liberals and conservatives by designating each as a particular type of parent. For Lakoff, conservatism revolves around the so-called "Strict Father" model, an authoritative structure that emphasizes the traditional nuclear family (Lakoff, 2002).

According to Lakoff, liberalism favors an entirely different approach to family life, the so-called "Nurturant Parent." In this approach, "children become responsible and self-reliant through being cared for, respected, and caring for others, both in their family and in their community" (Lakoff, 2002, p. 34). Liberals focus on investing in social programs as a form of social support. Conservatives oppose this approach because they think it fails to sustain self-discipline and reinforces moral weakness.

Lakoff's typology places liberals and conservatives at two extremes of an ideological continuum. Most people's views, however, lie between these two extremes. Moreover, many organizations take policy positions on health care and other issues that are in concert with a certain ideological perspective (Table 6-1). However, similar to elected officials, they may deviate from these positions on any given issue. Nursing organizations welcome members of all political persuasions and strive to foster tolerance among different ideological and partisan points of view.

GENDER AND RACE IN POLITICAL PHILOSOPHY

In the postmodern era in philosophy, which started in the mid-20th century, scholars noted that the traditional philosophy failed to represent the voices of numerous groups. Two perspectives that were particularly absent were those based on gender and race.

Critical to feminist political philosophy is the idea of politics as a social contract and rejection of the contract as being necessarily male centered. Pateman (1988) notes that the social contract fails to recognize the unique needs of women and, instead, tends to subjugate them to the concerns of the males who formulated the earlier ideas of political philosophy.

Several other positions linked with feminist philosophy include, first, the idea that the views most widely espoused with regard to philosophy and politics are those of men, resulting in a patriarchal and androcentric bias reflected in social and cultural traditions. Second, there is the notion that a woman-centered view can counter this androcentric bias and provide a balanced perspective. A third viewpoint argues specifically for philosophy to advance the status of women.

Feminism, as a political philosophy, ranges from a call for consideration of women's perspectives to radical feminism and may be extended to rejection of the heterosexual norm (MacKinnon, 1989). Democratic feminism, a variant of democratic theory, argues for an egalitarian foundation in which there are "norms of equality and symmetry" and "open debate" is possible (Benhabib, 1996, p. 70). This theory in political philosophy is related to "deliberative democratic theory," which focuses on deliberation in the process of decision making. Democratic feminists would argue that deliberation must include diverse perspectives, including those of women, to be effective.

One drawback to feminist political philosophy is that it can divide people based on gender. Someone's identity is not merely female or male, but is likely connected with ethnicity, socioeconomic status, work role, and other influences. Consequently, a focus on gender as a key point in political philosophy may fail to recognize the intricate interplay of the various facets that constitute identity.

In the 1990s, and building on Carol Pateman's *Sexual contract*, Charles W. Mills identified the "Racial Contract" as another example of how

TABLE 6-1 Organizations and Think Tanks That Are Aligned with a Political Ideology on Health Policy Issues

Organization	Website
Conservative	
American Enterprise Institute	www.aei.org
Concerned Women for America	www.cwfa.org/main.asp
Family Research Council	www.frc.org
Heritage Foundation	www.heritage.org
National Center for Public Policy Research	www.nationalcenter.org
Liberal	
Americans for Democratic Action	www.adaction.org
Center for Law and Social Policy	www.clasp.org
Center for American Progress	www.americanprogress.org
Families USA	www.familiesusa.org
People for the American Way	www.pfaw.org/pfaw/general

traditional approaches to political philosophy overlooked the realities of most of the world's population; nonwhites or people of color, which includes Black people, Native Americans, people of Asian origin, and millions of others who are nonwhite in ancestry.

Mills (1997) explained that the "social contract tradition," which is essential for much of "Western political theory," did not extend to all people. Instead, it was a contract that white men wrote and intended only to apply to themselves (p. 3). Nonwhite people did not have the same relationship with the state or government as white people. They were considered objects of government or property. Because the traditional social contract is only among the people of one race, Mills refers to it as a Racial Contract.

Mills (1997) claimed that the narrow scope of contracts that were based on mainstream political philosophy was not intentional. It reflected the reality of the "the power structure of formal or informal rule, socioeconomic privilege, and norms for the differential distribution of material wealth and opportunities, benefits and burdens, rights and duties" (p. 3).

Mills (1997) provided examples of how racial oppression existed globally and was not limited to whites over nonwhites, even though that's the scenario with which those of us in the western world are most familiar. He also discussed how the Racial Contract and "the reality of systematic racial exclusion, are obfuscated in seemingly abstract and general categories that originally were restricted to whites" (p. 118). For example, Mills pointed to the Japanese occupation of China in the 1930s as a different version of a Racial Contract, in this case a "Yellow Racial Contract," which referred to longstanding disputes over power and supremacy between different people of Asian origin (p. 128).

In contrast to ideal contracts embedded in mainstream political philosophy, which one might use as guides for living a good or moral life, Mills (1997) contended that "nonideal contracts" are to be "demystified and condemned" for overlooking race and racial oppression by whites all over the world (p. 5). Analyzing the "nonideal contract" enables one to understand how its "values and concepts have functioned to rationalize oppression, so as to reform them" (p. 6). Thus, the "Racial Contract," with all its flaws, can provide a path to reform by identifying normative aspects of a revised contract that might "establish…what a just 'basic structure' would be, with a schedule of rights, duties and liberties that shapes citizens' moral psychology, conceptions of the right, notions of self-respect, etc." (p. 10).

THE WELFARE STATE

The welfare state refers to the "share of the economy devoted to government social expenditures" (Hacker, 2002, pp. 12-13). Health policy analysts often compare aspects of the welfare state among developed countries. In such comparisons, the United States typically ranks lowest for public social expenditure as a percentage of the gross domestic product (GDP). However, if one adjusts for tax burdens, such as income taxes, and other public subsidies, then the United States ranks closer to the middle (Hacker, 2002). A unique aspect of the American welfare state is that most health care spending comes from the private sector.

The origins for much of the modern welfare state in Europe and the United States can be traced to the post-World War II period, when government leaders wanted to provide health and other social services to rebuild their national economies after the war's devastation. One of the best examples of such activities was the establishment of the British National Health Service (NHS), a government-administered and government-financed health insurance and delivery system to which all United Kingdom residents are entitled. The cornerstone of the U.S. welfare system is the 1935 U.S. Social Security Act, which established the Social Security program, welfare, federal maternal and child health programs, and other important initiatives to ameliorate the devastation of the Great Depression.

Since the 1980s, the welfare state has been in a state of flux in the United States and across Europe. One response to the constraints on the welfare state in countries such as the United States and Canada, the United Kingdom, and Germany has been the infusion of competition, accountability, and requirements for increasing private sector responsibility in the provision of health care. The growth of managed care in the United States, the increased accountability of physicians, the infusion of market-oriented practices in the United Kingdom, and tightening of rules regarding physician income in Canada exemplifies this. Shifts in political mood, as with the 2008 election of President Barack Obama, demonstrate how the ideological pendulum can swing from one side to another in a relatively short time.

TYPES OF WELFARE STATES

There are many different types of welfare states, based on the division of responsibilities for social services between public and private sectors and the role of a central government authority. The most well known categorization is Esping-Andersen's (1990) description of three types of welfare state: social-democratic, corporatist, and liberal. Remember that this categorization encompasses all aspects of social policy.

Social-democratic welfare states refer to the Scandinavian countries, where most social programs are publicly administered and relatively few privately sponsored social benefits are offered. These countries have "pursued a welfare state that would promote an equality of the highest standards" (Esping-Andersen, 1990, p. 27).

Corporatist welfare states are typically the Western European nations (e.g., France, Italy, and Germany), where social rights and status differentials have endured and affected social policies. These countries grant social rights to many, but primarily provide state interventions when family capacities fail.

Liberal welfare states include the United States, Canada, and Australia, where privately sponsored benefits dominate. Among liberal welfare states, the United States is distinctive for its large percentage of social spending in the form of privately sponsored benefits (Hacker, 2002). In liberal welfare states, welfare and other social benefits are highly stigmatized, and the state encourages market

involvement as much as possible (Esping-Andersen, 1990).

POLITICAL PHILOSOPHY AND THE WELFARE STATE: IMPLICATIONS FOR NURSES

How might nurses apply these concepts of political philosophy to their involvement in health politics and policy? Rather than sitting on the sidelines, nurses, regardless of partisan preference, can participate in the ideological and political debates that shape health policies. Each of us has perspectives on the role of government and the rights of individuals with regard to certain health policies. They form our own ideology and political positions. Determine where you stand on an issue and the underlying ideology that informs your views. Then use that knowledge as the basis for advocating for policies that have the potential to improve health policy and patient outcomes. In so doing, be mindful of the philosophical traditions that shape your views.

When engaging in political deliberations, listen to the rhetoric that others use and identify the underlying political and philosophical threads. Use similar language, as long as it is based on sound knowledge, when you meet with policymakers, or use written texts to advance your positions. The following two cases, covering the uninsured and motorcycle helmet use, clarify these points.

First, consider the issue of reducing the number of uninsured Americans. If one believes that the government's role should be minimal and individuals should largely be accountable for health care purchasing and costs, then tax credits and other types of individual health care accounts would be the policy of choice. If, on the other hand, one believes that the state is largely responsible for ensuring a basic minimum level of health care, then one would prefer the expansion of government-sponsored programs, such as Medicare, Medicaid, and CHIP, to cover those presently lacking insurance.

Similar issues arise when considering issues of public health, such as motorcyclists' use of helmets. For example, one view, taken predominantly by traditional liberals, might be that motorcyclists have the right to decide for themselves whether or not they wear helmets. Others, using a Hobbesian or social contract framework, might argue that it is in the best interest of society at large for riders to wear helmets and abide by laws requiring them to do so. This is partly because of the cost to society, but mostly because the state has a responsibility to protect individuals, which in turn promotes a peaceful and orderly society. Individuals, in turn, have a responsibility to yield to the state in its attempts to maintain order. There are some cases in which the state may need to limit individual freedoms to protect the state at large. Variations among the American states in helmet laws depict the different approaches to the balance of power among individuals, the state, and the community at large.

The relationship between nursing and the state has yet to be carefully explored. Connolly (2004) states, "Undertaking political history requires an understanding of how government works, in both theory and practice" (p. 16). Yet, there are many aspects of nursing's political history that remain untapped and that warrant a close examination of how the profession has interacted with state structures in the policy process.

Whether working with public officials, strategizing to create links between policy and practice, or studying the role of the state in public policies that pertain to nursing, political philosophy is the foundation of thought and action. It can be a lively aspect of nurses' strategic thinking in linking policy, politics, and practice.

DISCUSSION QUESTIONS

1. If you were meeting a delegation of nurses from ten different countries, how might you use political philosophy to explain the U.S. health care system (access, quality, and financing), the role of the U.S. welfare state, and the position of certain national nursing organizations on related issues?

2. In thinking about certain groups that have been excluded from mainstream political philosophy, what do you see as nursing's role (individually and collectively) in ensuring that they receive the same benefits and privileges as people from other groups?

REFERENCES

Benhabib, S. (1996). *Democracy and difference: Contesting the boundaries of the political.* Princeton, NJ: Princeton University Press.

Connolly, C. A. (2004). Beyond social history: New approaches to understanding the state of and the state in nursing history. *Nursing History Review, 12,* 5–24.

Esping-Andersen, G. (1990). *The three worlds of welfare capitalism.* Princeton, N.J.: Princeton University Press.

Hacker, A. (1960). *Political theory: Philosophy, ideology, science.* New York: MacMillan.

Hacker, J. S. (2002). *The divided welfare state: The battle over public and private social benefits in the United States.* New York: Cambridge University Press.

Lakoff, G. (2002). *Moral politics: How liberals and conservatives think.* Chicago: University of Chicago Press.

Levine, A. (2002). *Engaging political philosophy from Hobbes to Rawls.* Malden, Mass.: Blackwell Publishers.

MacKinnon, C. A. (1989). *Toward a feminist theory of the state.* Cambridge, Mass.: Harvard University Press.

Mills, C. W. (1997). *The racial contract.* Ithaca, NY: Cornell University Press.

Pateman, C. (1988). *The sexual contract.* Stanford, CA: Stanford University Press.

Shapiro, I. (2003). *The moral foundations of politics.* New Haven: Yale University Press.

Shively, W. P. (2005). *Power and choice: An introduction to political science* (9th ed.). Boston: McGraw-Hill.

Socialism. (2005). Answers.com. Retrieved from *www.answers.com/topic/socialism.*

Wolff, J. (1996). *An introduction to political philosophy.* Oxford, UK: Oxford University Press.

ONLINE RESOURCES

Open courses on political philosophy, such as this one offered by Professor Stephen B. Smith at Yale University, including short lectures on YouTube *oyc.yale.edu/political-science/plsc-114*
Internet Encyclopedia of Philosophy
www.iep.utm.edu

CHAPTER 7

The Policy Process

Eileen T. O'Grady

"A problem clearly stated is a problem half solved."
Dorothea Brande (1893-1948)

The purpose of this chapter is to provide a conceptual framework for understanding policymaking. When provided with a clear understanding of the policymaking process, nurses can more strategically and effectively influence policy. By using conceptual models, complex ideas may be depicted in a simplified form to help organize and interpret information, and to this end, political scientists have established a number of conceptual models to explain the highly dynamic process of policymaking (Dye, 1992). This chapter reviews two of these conceptual models.

HEALTH POLICY AND POLITICS

Health policy is significantly broader than nursing care policy alone. Health policy encompasses the political, economic, social, cultural and social determinants of individuals and populations and attempts to address the broader issues in health care (see Box 7-1 for policy definitions). This distinction is important because nurses need to be aware of the relevancy and significance of health policy in any position they hold. To influence the process, a clear understanding of the points of influence is essential and this includes correct framing of the health care problem itself. For example, if a nurse working in a nurse managed clinic is troubled by the staff shortages or long patient waits, they may be inclined to see themselves as the solution by working longer hours and seeing more patients. Defining and framing the problem in a broader policy context involves assessing the history, patterns of impact,

resource allocation, and community needs as a first step in the policy process. Broadening and framing the problem to influence or educate stakeholders at the community, city, state, or federal level could include advocating for better access or funding for nursing workforce development. The next step is to bring the problem to the attention of those who have the power to implement a solution. Other key factors to consider include the generation of public interest, availability of viable policy solutions, the likelihood that the policy will serve most of the people at risk in a fair and equitable fashion, and consideration of the organizational, community, societal, and political viability of the policy solution.

Public interest is a fascinating dynamic relevant to the development of public policy and is particularly important to influencing policy agendas at the community and broader policy levels. Taft and Nana (2008) have classified the sources of health policy within three domains. The first is professional, such as the need for standards and guidelines for practice. The second is organizational, which should be consistent with the needs of health care purchasers (employers), payers (insurers), and suppliers (health systems and providers). The third relates to the community stakeholders (patients and consumers) and public sources, including special interest groups and government entities.

Whatever the source, public awareness is often necessary for political action to take place and for the policy process to be initiated. For example, trends associated with health behaviors, such as the increased rates of childhood obesity, drunk driving, smoking, or gun violence, either gradual or resulting from a crisis situation, can all shift public perception and open the policy debate. Research

---

BOX 7-1 Policy Definitions

Policy is authoritative decision making (Stimpson & Hanley, 1991) related to choices about goals and priorities of the policymaking body. Generally, policies are constructed as a set of regulations (public policy), practice standards (workplace), governance mandates (organizations), ethical behavior (research), and ordinances (communities) that direct individuals, groups, organizations, and systems toward the desired behaviors and goals.

Health Policy is the authoritative decisions made in the legislative, judicial, or executive branches of government that are intended to direct or influence the actions, behaviors, and decisions of others (Longest, 2010, p.5).

Health Determinants include the physical environment in which people live and work, people's behaviors, people's biology, social factors, and health services (Longest, 2010 p. 2).

Policy analysis is the investigation of an issue including the background, purpose, content, and effects of various options within a policy context and their relevant social, economic, and political factors (Dye, 1992).

Stakeholders are those directly impacted by specific policy decisions and who may be involved in the policymaking process.

Advocacy is a role, often performed by nurses, that works to promote or protect rights, values, access, interests, and equality in health care. Much of the policy process involves advocating for policy on behalf of patients and public health.

---

consistently shows that a wide range of social and economic factors affect health although this broader causality is not well understood by the public. An opinion survey probing public opinion determined that most respondents think access to care and behaviors are most important. Far fewer respondents considered broader social determinants such as income, safe housing, race, and ethnicity to be important factors impacting a person's health status (Robert & Booske, 2011). This gap in public understanding adds to the confusion and politicization of health policy in developing solutions that fundamentally impact a person's health status. As public knowledge increases, however, trends

become increasingly objectionable to some members of society, which propels them to seek solutions. The rate of deaths caused by drunk driving, for example, resulted in strict nationwide drunk driving laws, and research on the impact of secondhand smoking led to the near universal ban on smoking in shared open spaces.

When people have a strong sense that the status quo is unacceptable, they begin to organize in a predicable fashion, leading to actions such as coalition forming or the establishment of a nonprofit organization. To move policy agendas forward, organizations must mature and build the resources needed to be effective in the policy realm.

Interest groups can stimulate a shift from interest in a policy solution to action wherein people work collectively to find solutions. Unions, trade associations, and political action committees are such examples. Professional nursing organizations serve as an interest group for nurses, not only to explore issues about the advancement of nursing but also to focus on societal issues such as the need for health reform, informing the public of emerging diseases and health threats, and the consequences of health disparities

Identifying and framing a problem is the first step, but it is also necessary to identify potential solutions. For example, concerns were raised in Washington state about the ability of insured workers to access health care in rural areas. This resulted in a delay in workers returning to work as well as insufficient reporting of injuries. Because nurse practitioners had been restricted in performing some of the functions related to certifying worker disability compensation, worker access to these providers was underused. As a result, the Washington State legislature enacted a pilot program to allow nurse practitioners (NPs) to expand their scope of practice to include serving as attending providers for injured workers. Despite some stakeholder concerns, the evidence concerning NP competency in undertaking this service was positive and subsequent analysis of the pilot program established that it was not only effective, it was also efficient in terms of use of resources (Sears & Hogg-Johnson, 2009). A policy intervention that will solve the problem is dependent on a thorough understanding of the problem itself as well as viable, evidence-based policy options.

Fairness and equity is a primary value driver that inspires nurses to participate in the policy process. Fawcett and Russell (2001) consider the equity of a policy as the extent to which it allows the benefits and burdens of nursing practice to be equally distributed to all; in particular, equal access to health services. For many nurses, advocating for fairness and equity is an application of patient advocacy, especially when human rights and health disparities are at stake. As noted in Chapter 1, social determinants of health illustrate that, in addition to individual choices, there are important environmental factors beyond the control of the individual that require collective action if health and health care are to be accessible for all (Dorfman, Wallack, & Woodruff, 2005).

Political viability is a further issue that must be considered. Policy that is considered desirable to both politicians and stakeholders will have the best chance of passage by a policymaking body. For example, public concerns about health effects from exposure to second-hand smoke have been communicated to policymakers many times. Although policymakers may want to take action to protect the public from tobacco smoke in public places, the pressure from tobacco companies for policymakers not to act has been equally powerful. As a result, public policy related to second-hand smoking languished for years in many states. However, when local communities in these states changed their ordinances to restrict smoking in public, there was increased pressure on state legislators to take action.

UNIQUE ASPECTS OF U.S. POLICYMAKING

Cost, quality, access, patient safety, and racial disparity problems persist across U.S. health delivery systems. Although the causes of these problems are multiple, the U.S. stands out from its peers across the globe for having one of the most complicated health care delivery and health care finance systems in the world. It has a highly decentralized system of

government with a health care finance system that includes a mix of public and private payers. What is most unique about the United States is that no single entity, authority, or government agency is ultimately responsible for health care. All of these facts lead to a complex patchwork of decision making, causing health care policy in the United States to be a highly complex and politically polarizing process. The current health care structure reflects policy decisions from the values of current society, together with residual policies from the colonial era. The U.S. Constitution does not specifically mention health care but the preamble indicates that the federal government should "promote the general welfare." This lies at the heart of the current political debate between the Democrat and Republican Parties regarding the role of the federal government in health care.

Federalism is the system of government in which power is divided between a central authority (federal) and constituent political units (state governments).This division of power and authority, while purposely designed by the founding fathers, is the source of much tension, acrimony, and complexity in U.S. policymaking. The locus of tension between the states and federal government is very relevant to health care policy. Medicare, Medicaid, and CHIP are examples of federally driven policies that create a partnership with states to administer health care under federal guidance. Meanwhile, regulation of health professionals, private health insurance coverage and long-term care policies have long been the domain of the individual states. This complexity between the state and federal spheres illuminates the fragmented and seemingly chaotic approach to solving health care problems in the United States.

Many aspects of the Affordable Care Act (ACA) protect states' rights to choose the degree to which they carry out some of its most important provisions, such as creating health exchanges to expand access to care. This built-in flexibility allows states to experiment with local solutions because, for example, what works in Minnesota may not work in Manhattan. The ACA escalated tensions between federal mandates and states' rights as evidenced by the United States Supreme Court's role in settling the dispute resulting from the multistate lawsuit challenging the constitutionality of the ACA's mandate that every citizen purchase health insurance. Although the Supreme Court upheld the individual mandate as a federal law that states must accept, the court also ruled expansion of the Medicaid program constitutional, but protected the right of states by ruling that states cannot be penalized if they choose not to participate in the expansion (O'Connor & Jackson, 2012).

The trend to allow states increased flexibility in recent decades adds complexity to health policymaking and amplifies the need for nurses to understand the policymaking process. Nurses must be knowledgeable regarding the appropriate authorities so that decision-making bodies are targeted appropriately. For example, there have been incidences of nurses who have approached federal legislators to persuade them to increase funding for school nursing, unaware that the issue was a state issue and funded at the state level.

The U.S. Constitution gives the federal government the power to block state laws when it chooses to do so. As noted earlier, state governments have authority to regulate health professionals as part of their charge to protect the public; although this is not in the Constitution, it has been the case since the formation of the United States (Safriet, 1992). This status quo is no longer appropriate as new forms of remote care delivery can render geographic boundaries irrelevant. Federalism is intended to create and sustain a highly decentralized locus of authority and is one of the most important dynamics in U.S. policymaking. This dynamic also, however, makes health care delivery systems complicated and difficult to reform.

Just as the federalist power structure creates tension between state and federal government policymaking, another outcome has been incremental policymaking. Historically, the most politically viable model, incrementalism, is used to describe policymaking which proceeds slowly by degrees. It represents a conservative approach to decision making and is viewed as a way to improve current policy. Within the U.S. Constitution, the three branches of government are designed deliberately to prevent one person or group from obtaining dictatorial powers. The disadvantage of this checks and balances structure is that it is very difficult for far-reaching policy reforms to succeed.

Once in a generation there is a major reform in U.S. health policy. The 1930s saw the implementation of Social Security, and 1965 saw the passage of Medicare and Medicaid. CHIP in the 1990s and the 2010 passage of the ACA are also examples. However, most health policy reform in the United States has been incremental. Fukuyama (2013) has described the U.S. system as a vetocracy which empowers political players who represent a minority viewpoint to block the actions of the majority resulting in paralysis. This vetocracy was illustrated in 2013, 3 years after the ACA was signed into law, when members of the House of Representatives shut down the government for 16 days (at an estimated cost of $24 billion) in an attempt to defund some of the provisions in the ACA.

Policies in the United States are far easier to stop and obstruct than pass and implement. Policymaking is largely a process of continuous fine-tuning of what already exists. A good example of incrementalism is the policy toward gays in the military. In the early 1990s it was highly controversial to implement the don't ask, don't tell mandate that allowed gays to serve. By the early 2000s, public opinion on homosexuality shifted dramatically and the military now accepts individuals with this sexual orientation.

Lindblom (1979) first described the concept of incrementalism in the early 1950s. When policymakers face a highly complex, theoretical, or resource-intensive decision and lack the time, capacity, or understanding to analyze all of the various policy options, they may limit themselves to a set of particular strategies instead of tackling the problem holistically. Policy solutions may be restricted to a set of familiar policy options that align with the status quo and lack a thorough evidence base (Lindblom, 1979). Therefore, incrementalism, although effective in limiting the power of any one person, group, or branch of government, also creates a process that is neither proactive, goal-oriented, nor ambitious; it ossifies timely policy, and limits innovation (Weiss & Woodhouse, 1992).

CONCEPTUAL BASIS FOR POLICYMAKING

The policy process consists of a series of actions, each critical to resolving a problem through analysis and formulation of solutions and can involve many organizations and individuals as well as requiring multiple steps. Two models from political scientists are relevant to nurses' understanding of the policy process. The purpose of reviewing these models is to provide two different yet complementary approaches for readers to see how the seemingly chaotic policymaking process has a form, rhythm, and predictability.

LONGEST'S POLICY CYCLE MODEL

Health policy is a cyclical process. Longest (2010) mapped out an interrelated model to capture how U.S. policymaking works. It is a continuous, highly dynamic cycle that captures the incrementalism inherent in U.S. governmental decision making (Figure 7-1). In its simplest form, there are three phases to the policy process: a policy formulation phase, an implementation phase, and a policy modification phase. Each phase contains a set of actions and activities that produce outcomes or products that influence the next stage. Although simple in design, this model is deceptively complex. Defining the policy problem with adequate clarity so that it gains the attention of policymakers and stakeholders is challenging; each policy problem has many solutions and competitors seeking a place on the policy agenda. Although policymaking is dependent on good data and evidence about what works, data and evidence may not be enough to outweigh the influence of the political environment.

Policy formulation includes all of the activities that are involved in policy design, including those activities which inform the legislators. It is in this phase that nurses can serve as a knowledge source to legislators in helping frame the problem and bringing nursing stories and patient narratives to illustrate how health problems play out with individual constituents/populations. The most effective

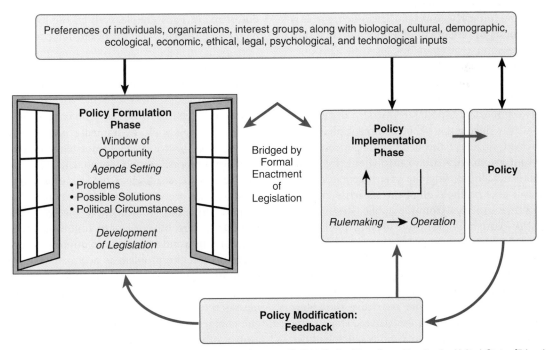

FIGURE 7-1 Longest's Policy Framework. (Redrawn from Longest, B. [2010]. *Health policymaking in the United States* [5th ed.]. Chicago: Health Administration Press.)

time to influence legislation is before it is drafted, so that nurses can help frame the issues to align with their desire for policy outcomes that are patient-centered.

Policy implementation comprises the rule-making phase of policy development. The legislative branch passes the law to the executive branch which is charged with implementation. This includes adding specificity to the law and may also include, for example, defining the provider to include advanced practice nurses. The writing of rules after legislation is passed is a crucial and often overlooked aspect of policymaking. At this juncture, nurses with appropriate expertise can monitor and influence how the rules are written. Once written, federal regulations are published in the daily Federal Register for 60 days to receive public comment. States also have regulation processes that provide designated times for public input.

Stakeholder groups can exert enormous influence during the implementation phase (Regulations .gov, 2013). When strong letter-writing campaigns are employed, the rulemaking agency may be forced to publish those comments and make adjustments according to their volume and scientific rigor. It is not unusual for the intent of a policy to get lost in the translation to program development. This rule-making phase is an important leverage point for nurses to closely monitor and respond to regulations through grassroots campaigns.

Two important aspects of American democracy are at play during the public comment phase: (1) informed citizenry: the democratic process only works if its citizenry is informed; and (2) government is not all-knowing: the government acknowledges it does not hold all of the expertise, it must solicit that expertise from the public (Regulations. gov, 2013). An example of rule making that limited nursing occurred when the Georgia legislature revised its scope of practice law for nurses. The law had many benefits for APNs, but the executive branch of the Georgia state government made the rules and regulations more restrictive than they were before the legislation was passed. The restrictions caused many APNs to avoid practicing under the new scope of practice but to continue to work under the old scope of practice that is still in effect

as it is less restrictive (Center to Champion Nursing in America, 2010).

Policy modification allows all previous decisions to be revisited and modified. Polices that are wholly pertinent at one time may, over time, become inappropriate. Almost all policies have unintended consequences which is why many stakeholders seek to modify policies continuously.

KINGDON'S POLICY STREAMS MODEL

Kingdon (1995) proposed a policy streams model to reflect the issue of policy looking for a problem. He described three streams of policy activity: the problem stream, the policy stream, and the political stream. These three conditions must stream through the open policy window at the same time (also referred to as the Garbage Can Model because the three streams must make their way through a minefield of debris). The problem must come to the attention of the policymaker, it must have a menu of viable policy solution options, and it must occur in the right political circumstances.

The problem stream describes the complexities in focusing policymakers on one specific problem out of many. For example, early in the process of developing the language for health reform legislation, policymakers engaged in a long process to define exactly which problems associated with the U.S health care system should be included in a legislative package (addressed by the government vs. private markets). Driving the problem stream are values, so access could be framed as a free market versus social justice issue. Values tend to have a stronger emotional component attached to them so that part of the challenge is the lack of agreement about which problems are the most urgent and require legislation. Some believe that cost is the biggest problem, others want to limit health reform to tort reform, and some want to improve access or quality. Until the problem is adequately defined, appropriate policy solutions cannot be identified.

The policy stream describes policy goals and the ideas of those in policy subsystems, such as researchers, congressional committee members and staff, agency officials, and interest groups. Ideas in the policy stream disseminate through policy circles in search of problems. The third stream, the political stream, describes factors in the political environment that influence the policy agenda, such as an economic recession, special interest media, or pivotal political power shifts.

The political circumstances that push problems to the top of the policy agenda need a high degree of public importance and a low degree of stakeholder conflict around the proposed solutions. A great deal of stakeholder conflict weakens the possibility that the policy window will open. If these three conditions occur at the same time, a policy window opens and progress can be made on the issue. Kingdon (1995) sees these streams as moving constantly and waiting for a window of opportunity to open through couplings of any two streams (particularly the political stream), creating new opportunities for policy change. However, such opportunities are time-limited: if change does not occur while the window is open, the problems and options will not be addressed.

For example, although health reform was a high priority for newly elected President Obama in 2009, the economic crisis and recession became a powerful political stream bringing to bear a major debate about how escalating health care costs were making the United States less competitive in the global marketplace. The movement of U.S. jobs overseas and the recession were linked to out-of-control health care costs and the need to reform health care, thus, a policy window was opened.

BRINGING NURSING COMPETENCE INTO THE POLICYMAKING PROCESS

There are many ways to think about stakeholders and interest groups. For example, some interests may be considered public interest rather than self-interest. All people affected by health policy want to know how it will affect the people and things they care about and how they can influence those policies. To effectively influence the policymaking process, nurses must successfully analyze the process and influence it with a high degree of political competence. Policy development that is dominated by public interest generally follows a course of action that is based on

data, information, and community values and addresses a solution to an actual or potential problem. It tends to be practical decision making. Policy generated by self-interest often follows a course of action with a predominantly special interest focus connected to the concerns of individuals or group interests over public interest.

Organizations that are provider-focused tend to focus on access, cost, and revenue. There is a focus on the structure of the health delivery system and points of access to their services. Stakeholder organizations that are not solely of a single provider type tend to have a broader agenda, including educational programs that develop the health workforce, insurers, pharmaceutical industry, hospitals, and medical supply companies. Although these other stakeholder organizations each have agendas of their own, it is easy to see where coalitions or policy networks can form around issues (Longest, 2010). For example, hospitals and educational programs can form coalitions around health workforce development. These stakeholder coalitions exert enormous influence in shaping health policy.

An example of a provider interest group is the National Association of Pediatric Nurse Practitioners (NAPNAP) which identified childhood obesity as a organizational priority and, as a result, created a childhood obesity special interest group which participated in a wide range of governmental committees, interviews on news media, and development of clinical practice guidelines, as well as creating culturally appropriate resources for parents. Pediatric NPs have effectively participated in a range of policy and clinical endeavors to address the alarming childhood obesity epidemic (NAPNAP, 2013) (See Box 7-2).

According to Longest (2010) there are best practices that leaders of advocacy organizations undertake to promote their health-related mission. Once the organization makes policy influence a priority, a governmental relations (or affairs) team is formed (or a firm is contracted) to do the work. If these teams are competent, they can transform the effectiveness of the organizations by giving the CEO (and/or board of directors) anticipatory guidance and lead-time. The ability of organizations to anticipate lead time and direct resources

---

BOX 7-2 **Think Like a Policymaker: Nurse Staffing Ratios**

Staffing ratios have been mandated in some states through legislative action as a solution to inadequate nurse staffing and concerns about the quality and safety of patient care. Opinions vary widely about whether the implementation of mandatory staff ratios in hospitals will have the desired effect. Some say that these mandatory ratios will remove the ability of hospitals to effectively manage their costs, resulting in higher costs for taxpayers and patients. Others argue that voluntary methods to improve safe staffing have not worked and nurses are placed in high-risk care environments. Buerhaus (2009) has proposed several nonregulatory solutions to safe staffing including improving hospital work environments, incentives to hospitals for high quality care, and focused efforts on reducing the nursing shortage. Do you think this health related issue is amenable to a public policy solution, or could safe staffing standards be managed as a policy within the workplace? As a policymaker, what information would you need to decide whether this problem would benefit from a public policy solution?

Recommended reading: Buerhaus, P. (2009) Avoiding mandatory hospital nurse staffing ratios: An economic commentary. *Nursing Outlook, 57*(2), 107-112. (Also see Chapters 53 and 61.)

---

appropriately is the key function of a strong public policy team. This anticipatory approach moves maturing organizations away from reacting to policy changes and toward strategic leadership (Longest, 2010). Effective advocacy organizations are continuously analyzing the environment. This requires that politically competent organizations primarily look out (not in) at the ever-changing political landscape.

Professional nursing organizations (e.g., the American Academy of Nursing, the American Nurses Association, and many nursing specialty groups) are concerned not only with public policy that impacts the health of all people, but also with policy that impacts nurses and the practice of nursing. These organizations, individually and collectively, support policies that are in the best interest of their members.

ENGAGING IN POLICY ANALYSIS

Issue analysis is similar to the nursing process: it is necessary to clearly identify the problem (including the context of the problem, alternatives for resolution and the consequences of each, along with specific criteria for evaluating the alternatives) and recommend the optimal solution. Issue papers provide the mechanism to do this. This is a process that identifies the underlying issue, identifies the stakeholders, and specifies alternatives along with their positive and negative consequences. Issue papers help to clarify arguments in support of a cause, to recognize the arguments of the opposition, to lay out the evidence or lack thereof to an issue, and to develop strategies to inform policy analysts and advance the issue through the policy cycle (Box 7-3).

It is helpful to compare alternatives by creating a scorecard. This is a two-dimensional grid with the evaluation criteria on the vertical axis and the different alternative policies on the horizontal axis with a notation for each alternative facilitating comparison of their strengths and weaknesses.

Another mechanism for helping people to understand an issue is a policy decision brief often referred to as a one page leave-behind. This provides a summary for the policymaker to read and to gain a grasp of the issue quickly. A standard format for a policy brief includes: summary of the issue, background information, analysis of alternatives, a recommendation for action, references, and personal contact information (Box 7-4).

INFUSING THE EVIDENCE BASE INTO HEALTH POLICY

The role of data and research is highly valuable in understanding a health policy issue and in developing a solution to the problem. It assumes that health policy driven by an evidence base will link the evidence, policy solution, and the significance of the situation. However, evidence may support opposing views of a policy solution. For example, will expanding access to care for the poor increase or decrease costs? There is evidence that supports both sides of this policy debate and the cost shifting currently in place for most delivery systems makes it difficult to ascertain which view is correct.

BOX 7-3 Example of a Policy Decision Brief

Re: Health Care Fraud in the Military Health System
Issue Summary: Health care fraud burdens the Department of Defense (DOD) with enormous financial losses while threatening the quality of health care. Assuming that between 10% and 20% of paid claims are fraudulent, the annual loss to DOD is $600 million to $1.2 billion.

Background

- The U.S. Attorney General has identified health care fraud as the second priority for law enforcement, following only violent crime.
- Because health care fraud perpetrators target DOD, Medicare, Medicaid, and private health insurers simultaneously, the Defense Criminal Investigative Service (DCIS) cooperates extensively with many federal agencies in joint health care fraud investigations.
- Federal agencies fighting health care fraud, except DOD, have received additional resources to enhance their efforts.
- The TRICARE Program Integrity Office currently has a staff of 10, and a caseload of 1000 active cases.
- The 1996 Kennedy-Kassebaum legislation provided for 80 additional U.S. attorneys to be hired specifically to prosecute health care fraud and abuse.

Alternatives

1. **Enhance prosecution.** Provide state attorneys general with an incentive to participate in the prosecution of DOD health care fraud by offering a portion of recovered funds from successfully prosecuted cases.
   Advantages: Could increase the total number and speed with which DOD health care fraud cases are prosecuted.
   Disadvantages: Does not address the problem of inadequate resources dedicated to detecting and investigating DOD health care fraud cases.
2. **Enhance detection and investigation.** Provide a portion of recovered funds (5% to a maximum of $15 million annually) to the federal agencies charged with detection and investigation of DOD health care fraud to enhance their efforts.
   Advantages: The bottleneck in government efforts to control military health care fraud occurs within the first two steps: detection and investigation. Returning a portion of recovered funds would serve as an incentive for superior performance, as well as allow for increased efforts in the fight against fraud. Current budget restrictions have precluded significant deterrent efforts; additional resources would be used to develop computer applications that detect and deter health care fraud more effectively.
   Disadvantages: Funds previously recovered and returned to the DOD would be returned to detection/investigation agencies.
3. **Continue current efforts.** No change in current detection, investigation, and prosecution efforts.
   Advantages: Current efforts will uncover a certain level of health care fraud and will continue to recover a portion of fraudulent claims to the government.
   Disadvantages: Fraud perpetrators will become increasingly sophisticated in their activities and will be able to stay one step ahead of overburdened government investigators.
4. **Develop additional data about the problem.** Direct the Government Accountability Office to conduct a study on the feasibility of the alternatives.
   Recommendation: Direct the Controller General of the U.S. to undertake a study and provide a report to Senator Smith on the feasibility of the above alternatives. Because of the magnitude of federal expenditures on health care, and the loss from health care fraud, it is essential to determine the best alternative based on empirical data.

Another barrier to crafting policy is that there can be a lack of clarity about the evidence that is needed. Nurses generally understand that evidence-based practice is based on science. However, there is a hierarchy of what constitutes evidence from scientific inquiry that ranges from systematic review, randomized controlled trials, cohort studies, case control studies, cross-sectional surveys, case reports, expert opinion, and anecdotal information (Glasby & Beresford, 2006). This hierarchy can make it difficult to reach an agreement among stakeholders, policymakers, and the public about what evidence is appropriate for health policy. As noted by Hewison (2008), practitioners and consumers may be at odds over which type of evidence is the more valuable. New evidence may need to be

---

BOX 7-4 Example of a One-Page "Leave-Behind" Summary of a Nursing Policy Issue

Remove Barriers to Nurse Practitioners' Ability to Practice

ACTION NEEDED: Enable NPs to practice to the full extent of their license

By amending current statutes or directing the Centers for Medicare and Medicaid Services to revise outdated rules and manuals, Congress should take action to remove obsolete limitations in federal laws and regulations that do not recognize nurse practitioners' advanced education and clinical education to furnish the full range of services.

Background: The landmark Institute of Medicine 2011 report, *The Future of Nursing: Leading Change, Advancing Health,* includes recommendations for Congress and the Department of Health and Human Services to remove barriers limiting the ability of nurse practitioners and other advanced practice nurses to practice at the full extent of their license. These recommendations are supported by extensive evidence of the high quality, safety, and effectiveness of care provided by nurse practitioners. To ensure increased access to better care at lower cost in the U.S., federal health care programs must eliminate policies that prevent nurse practitioners from providing patient care at the fullest extent of their license.

In spite of their recognized scope of practice, Medicare does not permit nurse practitioners to conduct assessments to admit the patients to skilled nursing facilities even though it authorizes them to order skilled nursing care. Similarly, Medicare does not allow NPs to provide the initial certification for hospice care, although they are authorized to serve as attending providers and to recertify patients' eligibility. The need to revise these and other Medicare policies are discussed in separate fact sheets. In addition, Congress should address the following barriers to NP practice:

- Provide coverage of nurse practitioners' services as physician services are covered.
- Several outdated regulatory barriers to NP practice could be removed simply by correcting the interpretation of the term physician to be consistent with current Medicare payment policies that authorize Part B payment to NPs for services within their scope of practice. This simple change would enable nurse practitioners to certify Medicare beneficiaries for home health and hospice services and to conduct examinations to admit patients to skilled nursing facilities.
- Recognize NPs as primary care providers in all health care plans and programs.
- The Institute of Medicine's definition of primary care should serve as a benchmark for any legislation to expand access to primary care services.

Request: Congress and CMS should update and revise statutes and regulations to ensure patient access to nurse practitioner services.

For additional information, please contact the AANP Federal Health Policy Office at (703) 740-2529 or *federalpolicy@ aanp.org.*

---

developed before one can move ahead with a policy recommendation that may include evidence informed by input from community stakeholders.

POLICY-RELEVANT RESEARCH

Despite the debate over what constitutes evidence and which evidence is relevant for health policy, health services research (HSR) can be very effective in developing policy options. HSR is a far broader form of research than clinical research in that it is a multidisciplinary field of scientific inquiry that looks at how people gain access to health care, how much care costs, and what happens to patients as a result of this care. The main goals of HSR are to identify the most effective ways to deliver high quality cost effective safe care across systems (Agency for Healthcare Research and Quality

[AHRQ], 2013a). These include issues such as the restructuring of health services, human resource use in health care settings, primary care design, patient safety and quality, and patient outcomes. For example, Linda Aiken's work on safe staffing (Aiken, 2007; Aiken et al., 2002), Mary Naylor's work on transitions in care for older adults (Naylor et al., 2004), and Mary Mundinger's work on the use of nurse practitioners (Mundinger et al., 2000) are widely cited in policy literature. There has been an increase in comparative effectiveness research, which uses a design to inform decisions about Medicare. It uses a range of data sources to compare the costs and harms of various treatment decisions and is commonly used to study the cost effectiveness of drugs, medical devices, and surgical procedures (AHRQ, 2013b).

INFLUENCING THE POLICY PROCESS AS NURSING PRACTICE

Many opportunities exist for nurses to become involved in the policy process. Involvement in health policy is a natural extension of the role as advocate. Nurses who seek elective office have chosen to take on the role of policymaker as their primary practice. In this case, nurses in elected office are practicing the highest form of civil service that a professional nurse can engage in to advance the public's health. If running for elected office is not feasible or desired, the less difficult form of civic engagement is to participate in the electoral process. This includes a large menu of activities including, at the least, being informed of candidates' positions regarding health care, but also potentially supporting financially candidates who advocate sound health policy reforms as well as working on campaigns, hosting fundraisers, and/or serving as policy advisors to candidates.

In addition to elective office, nurses serve in policy research roles; as policy analysts within professional nursing or patient advocacy organizations and health care institutions and within state or federal agencies; and as staff to policymakers. Nursing leaders have had considerable impact on policy from their leadership positions in organizations such as the AARP, the Institute of Medicine (IOM), the Health Services and Resources Administration (HRSA), and the Centers for Disease Control and Prevention (CDC).

professional nursing associations ought to extend the reach of nurses to include significant input into the debate regarding the widespread access issues for the disenfranchised. This includes nurses getting elected to Congress, becoming involved in policy-making, and serving on influential advisory and corporate boards.

The health care policy environment is rapidly changing and incremental reforms will be undertaken continuously. All nurses must see how the policy process is core to their role as nurses, advocating for patients on an increasingly broad level. The very first step in engaging effectively in the policy process is for nurses to understand how that process works. Nurses must also be knowledgeable of the current and emerging issues that are relevant to nursing practice and must develop the political competence to effectively shape health policy.

DISCUSSION QUESTIONS

1. Identify a problem you face regularly in your clinical setting. Next, identify how this problem could be framed as a policy issue.
2. The Longest and the Kingdon models help us interpret how policy works. Select one model and apply it to a policy issue you care about.
3. What do you think yourself and your peers can do to strengthen nursing's influence in the policy process?

CONCLUSION

Atul Gawande (2009) has emphasized that it is the leaders within health care who will implement policies on health reform. Nurses should be active in all policy arenas to assure that solutions improve the health of people. Mahlin (2010) asserts that nursing organizations must do more than advocate for patients, for there are many in the United States who require care yet have inadequate or nonexistent access. This author suggests it is a worthwhile goal for nurses to engage and participate more fully in the wider health policy realm because those who are outside the system cannot adequately address systematic problems and also asserts that

REFERENCES

Agency for Healthcare Research and Quality [AHRQ]. (2013a). An organizational guide to building research capacity. Retrieved from *www.ahrq.gov/funding/training-grants/hsrguide/hsrguide.html.*

Agency for Healthcare Research and Quality [AHRQ]. (2013b). Effective Health Care Program: What is comparative effectiveness research? Retrieved from *effectivehealthcare.ahrq.gov/index.cfm/what-is-comparative-effectiveness-research1/.*

Aiken, L. (2007). Supplemental nurse staffing in hospitals and quality of care. *Journal of Nursing Administration, 37,* 335–342.

Aiken, L., Clarke, S., Sloane, D., Sochalski, J., & Silber, J. (2002). Hospital nurse staffing and patient mortality, nurse burnout, and job dissatisfaction. *JAMA, 288*(16), 1987–1993.

Buerhaus, P. (2009). Avoiding mandatory hospital nurse staffing ratios: An economic commentary. *Nursing Outlook, 57*(2), 107–112.

Center to Champion Nursing in America. (2010). Access to care and advanced practice nurses: A review of Southern U.S. practice laws. AARP Public Policy Institute. Retrieved from *www.achi.net/hcr%20docs/2011hcrworkforceresources/access%20to%20care%20apns.pdf.*

Dorfman, L., Wallack, L., & Woodruff, K. (2005). More than a message: Framing public health advocacy to change corporate practices. *Health Education & Behavior, 32*(3), 320–336. Retrieved from *www.bmsg.org/node/369.*

Dye, R. (1992). *Understanding public policy* (7th ed.). Englewood Cliffs, NJ: Prentice Hall.

Fawcett, J., & Russell, G. (2001). A conceptual model of nursing and health policy. *Policy, Politics, & Nursing Practice, 2*(2), 108–116.

Fukuyama, F. (2013, October 6). Why are we still fighting over Obamacare? Because America was designed for a stalemate. *The Washington Post.* Retrieved from *washingtonpost.com/2013-10-04/opinions/42696476_1_affordable-care-act-majority-obamacare.*

Gawande, A. (2009). The cost conundrum. *The New Yorker*, June 1, 2009, 36–44.

Glasby, J., & Beresford, P. (2006). Who knows best? Evidence-based practice and the service user contribution. *Critical Social Policy, 26*(1), 268–284.

Hewison, A. (2008). Evidence-based policy: Implications for nursing and policy involvement. *Policy, Politics & Nursing Practice, 9*(4), 288–298.

Kingdon, J. W. (1995). *Agendas, alternatives, and public policies.* Boston: Little, Brown.

Lindblom, C. (1979). Still muddling, not yet through. *Public Administration Review, 39*(6), 517–526.

Longest, B. (2010). *Health policymaking in the United States* (5th ed.). Chicago: Health Administration Press.

Mahlin, M. (2010). Individual patient advocacy, collective responsibility and activism within professional nursing associations. *Nursing Ethics, 17*(2), 247–254.

Mundinger, M., Kane, R., Lenz, E., Totten, A., Tsai, W., Cleary, P., et al. (2000). Primary care outcomes in patients treated by nurse practitioners or physicians: A randomized trial. *JAMA, 283,* 59–68.

National Association of Pediatric Nurse Practitioners [NAPNAP]. (2013). Childhood obesity special interest group. Retrieved from *www.napnap.org/Files/CO%20SIG%20Newsletter%20Winter%202011.pdf.*

Naylor, M., Brooten, D., Campbell, R., Maislin, G., McCauley, K., & Schwartz, J. (2004). Transitional care of older adults hospitalized with heart failure: A randomized, controlled trial. *Journal of the American Geriatric Society, 52*(7), 675–684.

O'Connor, M., & Jackson, W. (2012). Analysis: U.S. Supreme Court upholds the affordable care act: Roberts rules? *The National Law Review.* Retrieved from *www.natlawreview.com/article/analysis-us-supreme-court-upholds-affordable-care-act-roberts-rules.*

Regulations.gov. (2013). eRulemaking Program [website to enable citizens to search, view and comment on regulations issued by the US Government]. Retrieved from *www.regulations.gov/#!aboutProgram.*

Robert, S., & Booske, B. (2011). U.S. opinions on health determinants and social policy and health policy. *American Journal of Public Health, 101*(9), 1655–2663.

Safriet, B. (1992). Health care dollars and regulatory sense: The role of advanced practice nursing. *Yale Journal on Regulations, 417,* 442–445.

Sears, J., & Hogg-Johnson, S. (2009). Enhancing the policy impact of evaluation research: A case study of nurse practitioner role expansion in a state workers' compensation system. *Nursing Outlook, 57*(2), 99–106.

Stimpson, M., & Hanley, B. (1991). Nurse policy analyst. Advanced practice role. *Nursing and Health Care, 12*(1), 10–15.

Taft, S. H., & Nanna, K. M. (2008). What are the sources of health policy that influence nursing practice? *Policy, Politics, & Nursing Practice, 9*(4), 274–287.

Weiss, A., & Woodhouse, E. (1992). Reframing incrementalism: A constructive response to the critics. *Policy Sciences, 25,* 255–273.

ONLINE RESOURCES

American Association of State Colleges and Universities: The American Democracy Project
www.aascu.org/programs/ADP
Campaign to Promote Civic Education
new.civiced.org/programs/promote-civics
The Commonwealth Fund
www.commonwealthfund.org
Health Affairs
www.healthaffairs.org
Kaiser Family Foundation
kff.org

CHAPTER 8

Health Policy Brief: Improving Care Transitions

Rachel Burton

An example of a well-written policy brief is presented here. It was developed by Health Affairs and the Robert Wood Johnson Foundation. Website resource: *www.healthaffairs.org/health policybriefs/ brief.php?brief_id=76.*

> ## IMPROVING CARE TRANSITIONS: BETTER COORDINATION OF PATIENT TRANSFERS AMONG CARE SITES AND THE COMMUNITY COULD SAVE MONEY AND IMPROVE THE QUALITY OF CARE[1]

WHAT'S THE ISSUE?

The term *care transition* describes a continuous process in which a patient's care shifts from being provided in one setting of care to another, such as from a hospital to a patient's home or to a skilled nursing facility and sometimes back to the hospital. Poorly managed transitions can diminish health and increase costs. Researchers have estimated that inadequate care coordination, including inadequate

management of care transitions, was responsible for $25 to $45 billion in wasteful spending in 2011 through avoidable complications and unnecessary hospital readmissions.

Several new federal initiatives aim to encourage more effective care transitions. In addition, debate continues over how to restructure fee-for-service payments to motivate providers across care settings to work as a team to make transitions smoother.

This brief examines the factors contributing to poor care transitions, describes the elements of effective approaches to improving patient and family experience with transitions, and explores policy issues surrounding payment reforms designed to address the problem.

WHAT IS THE BACKGROUND?

For years, health policy experts have identified poor care transitions as a major contributor to poor quality and waste. The 2001 Institute of Medicine (IOM) report, *Crossing the Quality Chasm,* described the U.S. system as decentralized, complicated, and poorly organized, specifically noting "layers of processes and handoffs that patients and families find bewildering and clinicians view as wasteful."

The IOM noted that, upon leaving one setting for another, patients receive little information on how to care for themselves, when to resume activities, what medication side effects to look out for, and how to get answers to questions. As a result, the conditions of many patients worsen and they may end up being readmitted to the hospital. For example, nearly one fifth of fee-for-service Medicare beneficiaries discharged from the hospital are readmitted within 30 days; three quarters of these

---

[1]Health Policy Brief: Care Transitions, Health Affairs, September 13, 2012. Written by Rachel Burton, Research Associate, Urban Institute. Editorial review by Eric Coleman, Division Head Health Care Policy and Research, University of Colorado Medical Campus; Debra J. Lipson, Senior Researcher, Mathematica Policy Research; Ted Agres, Senior Editor for Special Content, Health Affairs; Anne Schwartz, Deputy Editor, Health Affairs; and Susan Dentzer, Editor-in-Chief, Health Affairs. Health Policy Briefs are produced under a partnership of Health Affairs and the Robert Wood Johnson Foundation. Reprinted with permission.

readmissions, costing an estimated $12 billion a year, are considered potentially preventable, especially with improved care transitions.

Root Causes. There are several root causes of poor care coordination. Differences in computer systems often make it difficult to transmit medical records between hospitals and physician practices. In addition, hospitals face few consequences for failing to send medical records to patients' outpatient physicians upon discharge. As a result, physicians often do not know when their patients have been released and need follow-up care. Finally, current payment policies create disincentives for hospitals to invest in smoother care transitions. For example, although Medicare does not allow hospitals to bill for readmissions that occur within 24 hours of discharge, it does pay full price for most readmissions that occur after that time. This means that the prevailing financial incentive for hospitals is to not expend resources on improving care transitions because a poor transition often leads to readmission, which generates additional revenue.

Moreover, some analysts believe that Medicare and Medicaid payment policies have unintentionally created incentives to unnecessarily transfer patients back and forth between hospitals and nursing homes. Their suspicion is that nursing homes, which are primarily paid by Medicaid with generally low payment rates, unnecessarily transfer patients to hospitals to qualify for more generous Medicare payment rates when their patients return to them after discharge.

Lending credence to this claim, researchers have found that states with lower rates of Medicaid spending on dual-eligible patients under age 65 (people who are eligible for both Medicaid and Medicare) have higher rates of Medicare spending on these patients, and vice versa, suggesting that providers are gaming the system.

Transition to Primary Care. As mentioned, one of the biggest barriers to smoother care transitions is the fact that primary care physicians often have little or no information about their patients' hospitalizations. A review of the literature published in the *Journal of the American Medical Association* in

2007 found that physicians had received a hospital discharge summary about their patients, and had it on hand, in only 12% to 34% of first postdischarge visits. Even when discharge summaries are received, they often lack key information, such as test results, treatment course, discharge medications, and follow-up plans. The situation is even worse for those patients who have no usual source of care.

Patients often do not consistently receive follow-up care after leaving the hospital. Among Medicare beneficiaries readmitted to the hospital within 30 days of a discharge, half have no contact with a physician between their first hospitalization and their readmission. (Figure 8-1 shows 30-day hospital readmissions under Medicare as a percentage of admissions, by state.)

This problem may be worsening because of an ongoing shift in practice patterns. Increasingly, outpatient primary care physicians are no longer visiting their patients when hospitalized, and hospitalized patients' care is now being managed by hospitalists, physicians who only treat patients in the hospital. Although hospitalists are generally believed to have improved the quality and coordination of patients' in-hospital care, their presence, and the removal of patients' outpatient primary care physicians from the hospital, has led to an increased need for care coordination among providers that doesn't always occur.

Care Transition Models. Several models for improving transitions after hospitalization have been developed and rigorously tested. One of the most widely disseminated is the Care Transitions Intervention developed by Eric Coleman at the University of Colorado. This approach involves transitions coaches, primarily nurses, and social workers, who first meet patients in the hospital and then follow up through home visits and phone calls over a 4-week period.

The coaches promote development of patients' skills in four key self-care areas: managing medications; scheduling and preparing for follow-up care; recognizing and responding to red flags that could indicate a worsening condition, such as the onset of a fever or worsening breathing problems; and taking ownership of a core set of personal health

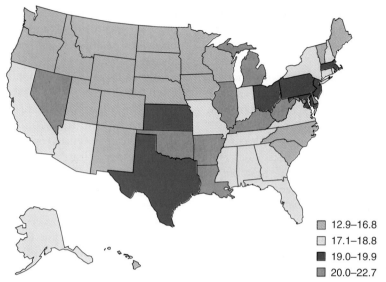

FIGURE 8-1 Medicare 30-day hospital readmissions as a percentage of admissions, 2009. (From Commonwealth Fund [2009, October]. *Medicare 30-day hospital readmissions as a percent of admissions: National metrics.* Washington, DC: Commonwealth Fund.)

Legend:
- 12.9–16.8
- 17.1–18.8
- 19.0–19.9
- 20.0–22.7

information by having patients brainstorm and ask their providers questions about their conditions or self-care routine. In a large integrated delivery system in Colorado, the Care Transitions Intervention reduced 30-day hospital readmissions by 30%, reduced 180-day hospital readmissions by 17%, and cut average costs per patient by nearly 20%. The intervention has been adopted by more than 700 organizations nationwide.

Another rigorously tested transitional care model, developed by Mary Naylor and her colleagues at the University of Pennsylvania, involves a longer period of intervention targeted at a high-risk, high-cost subset of older adult patients, such as those hospitalized for heart failure. In six academic and community hospitals in Philadelphia, this approach reduced readmissions by 36% and costs by 39% per patient (nearly $5000) during the 12 months following hospitalization. Under the Naylor model, an advanced practice nurse not only coaches patients and their caregivers to better manage their care but also coordinates a follow-up care plan with patients' physicians and provides regular home visits with 7-day-a-week telephone availability.

WHAT IS IN THE LAW?

The Affordable Care Act contains several provisions that could improve care transitions. These include both carrots (financial incentives) and sticks (financial penalties).

Among the carrot approaches, starting October 1, 2012, hospitals can receive increases to their Medicare payments if they achieve or exceed performance targets for certain quality measures, including whether they told patients about symptoms or problems to look out for postdischarge; whether they asked patients if they would have the help they needed at home; and whether they provided heart failure patients with discharge instructions. (See the Health Policy Brief published on April 15, 2011, for more information on improving quality and safety: *healthaffairs.org/healthpolicy briefs/brief_pdfs/healthpolicybrief_45.pdf.*)

Among the stick approaches, also beginning October 1, 2012, the Centers for Medicare and Medicaid Services (CMS) can reduce payments by 1% to hospitals whose readmission rates for patients with heart failure, acute myocardial infarction, or pneumonia exceed a particular target. According to a recent analysis by the Kaiser Family Foundation, more than 2200 hospitals will forfeit about $280 million in Medicare payments over the next year because of these readmissions penalties.

Medical Homes. The law also authorizes paying providers for care transition services as part of payments to primary care practices that operate as medical homes, practices that closely manage and coordinate the care of patients with chronic conditions. One demonstration project, which pre-dates the Affordable Care Act, is the Multi-Payer Advanced Primary Care Practice Demonstration in which Medicare offers practices that have been for-mally recognized as medical homes in eight states up to $10 per beneficiary per month to cover the cost of medical home services, which include care transition planning.

Another demonstration, the Comprehensive Primary Care Initiative, offers monthly payments to practices that average $20 per beneficiary in the first 2 years and then transitions to $15 plus the opportunity to earn shared savings in the last 2 years. Again, a portion of these programs are intended to compensate practices for the costs of care coordination and care transitions planning.

In addition, the Federally Qualified Health Center Advanced Primary Care Practice Demon-stration will pay $6 per beneficiary per month to health centers that adopt the medical home model and apply for Level 3 medical home recog-nition, having the most stringent requirements, from the National Committee for Quality Assur-ance (NCQA) by the end of the 3-year demon-stration. NCQA's medical home standards ask practices to establish processes to identify patients admitted to the hospital, share clinical informa-tion with the admitting hospital, obtain patient discharge summaries from the hospital, and contact patients for follow-up care, among many other expectations.

Medicaid and Medicare. State Medicaid agen-cies can now offer providers enhanced reimburse-ment, such as through monthly care management payments, to cover the cost of "comprehensive transitional care" and other services if the practice qualifies as a "health home"; a practice that cares not only for Medicaid patients' physical conditions but also helps them obtain such other services as behavioral health care and long-term care services and supports.

Also, a 5-year, $500 million Community-Based Care Transitions Program pays organizations that partner with hospitals with high readmission rates to provide care transition services for high-risk Medicare beneficiaries. All-inclusive payments cover the cost of care transition services provided to individual beneficiaries in the 180 days following an eligible discharge plus the cost of systemic changes made by partner hospitals to improve care transitions. So far 47 awardees have been announced, and applications continue to be accepted. Partici-pating organizations initially enter into 2-year agreements, which can be extended annually through the end of 2015.

Incentives in New Payment Models. The Medicare Shared Savings Program for accountable care organizations (ACOs) will give groups of pro-viders an incentive to coordinate care more closely to keep patients healthy and out of the hospital because they will be eligible to share in the savings they are able to generate relative to a spending benchmark. The quality metrics that must be met by ACOs to benefit financially under the program include six that pertain to care coordination, including preventing unnecessary hospital read-missions. (See Health Policy Brief published on January 31, 2012, for more information on ACOs: *healthaffairs.org/healthpolicybriefs/brief_pdfs/health policybrief_61.pdf.*)

The Affordable Care Act also authorizes 5-year bundled payment pilots in Medicare and Medicaid to test whether making a single payment to one entity for services provided by several providers for an episode of care, such as a knee replacement, will give providers an incentive to work together to ensure that patients receive all the services they need, including hospital and follow-up care, in a more efficient manner. Managing care transitions to prevent costly hospital readmissions will be par-ticularly important because, in the Medicare pilot, at least, the bundled payment will cover services beginning 3 days before a hospital admission for an eligible condition and extending 30 days after hospital discharge.

Signaling the importance of care transitions to the success of these efforts, the Medicare pilot requires bundled payments to cover the cost of transitional care services. CMS's new Innovation Center has begun accepting applications from providers interested in piloting four bundled payment models through a separate Bundled Payments for Care Improvement initiative. The Medicaid pilot, meanwhile, requires participating hospitals to have "robust discharge planning programs."

In addition, a new Medicare-Medicaid Coordination Office in CMS is charged with better integrating benefits for dual-eligible beneficiaries. It also works to ensure "safe and effective care transitions," among other goals. This office has awarded contracts of up to $1 million each to 15 states to design models to coordinate primary, acute, behavioral, and long-term care for Medicare-Medicaid enrollees. CMS has also invited proposals from states to test two new payment models to better integrate care for this population and allow states to share in savings from these improvements. Twenty-six states, including the 15 states awarded demonstration design contracts, have developed proposals for this demonstration. The new payment and delivery system models are likely to focus on improving care transitions, among other strategies. (See the Health Policy Brief published on June 13, 2012, for more information on dual eligibles: *healthaffairs.org/healthpolicybriefs/brief_pdfs/health policybrief_70.pdf.*)

Physicians and Nurses. The Affordable Care Act also requires the Department of Health and Human Services to develop and implement a plan by 2013 that would lead to reporting physician-level quality measure data on the new Physician Compare website (*www.medicare.gov/physician compare/search.html?AspxAutoDetectCookieSupport =1*), including measures of the quality of care transitions. CMS has until 2019 to decide whether to conduct a demonstration giving Medicare beneficiaries financial incentives to seek care from physicians who score highly on these measures.

The law also creates a $200 million, 4-year workforce development demonstration aimed at increasing the number of advanced practice registered nurses trained in care transition services, chronic care management, preventive care, primary care, and other services appropriate for Medicare beneficiaries.

Mixed Messages. Taken as a whole, the inclusion in the Affordable Care Act of these carrots and sticks aimed at different types of providers suggests a tension over whom to pay and how to pay them to improve care transitions. On the one hand, the payment cuts that high-readmission hospitals nationwide will soon face create an expectation that hospitals take responsibility for improving care transitions using existing resources. But the fact that another program will provide new care transitions payments to hospitals and community-based organizations suggests that they may require additional resources to provide these services.

And although physicians' performance on care transitions quality measures will be reported on Physician Compare, no provision in the Affordable Care Act requires hospitals to alert physicians when their patients are discharged, typically the needed first step before a physician can become involved in a care transition.

OTHER POLICY OPTIONS

If these Affordable Care Act provisions fail to improve care transitions or if CMS decides to pursue other policies, the agency's statutory authority gives it some additional options, as follows:

- **Pay physicians for care transition services.** Under the Medicare physician fee schedule, CMS could create a new billing code that would enable physicians to bill for delivery of care transition services. In a proposed rule issued in July 2012, CMS would create a code to bill for care transition services delivered to Medicare beneficiaries in the 30 days following a discharge from a hospital, skilled nursing facility, or community mental health center. The code would apply to Medicare patients whose medical or psychosocial problems, or both, require moderate or high complexity medical decision making.

To qualify for the new payment, physicians would have to obtain and review a patient's hospital discharge summary, update the patient's medical records to reflect changes in health conditions and ongoing treatments, and establish or adjust a patient's care plan. Physicians would be required to communicate with a beneficiary or their caregiver within 2 business days of discharge to resolve medication discrepancies and inform them about possible complications. Whether physicians will consider the payment level assigned to this billing code adequate for the effort required, however, remains unclear.

- **Track whether hospitals transmit records to physicians.** Another policy option would be to add a care transitions measure to Medicare's Hospital Inpatient Quality Reporting program, a pay-for-reporting program. Adding such a measure would create a modest incentive for hospitals to better communicate with physicians about patients' hospitalizations, especially if CMS chose to include that measure in the subset that is displayed on the Hospital Compare website (*www.medicare.gov/physiciancompare/search.html?AspxAutoDetectCookieSupport=1*).

If CMS wanted to further elevate hospitals' focus on this measure, it could include it in the subset of measures it uses in the Hospital Value-Based Purchasing Program, the new pay-for-performance program for hospitals created in the Affordable Care Act and scheduled to go into effect in October 2012.

A hospital-related care transitions measure has been developed by a group of physician specialty societies and endorsed by the National Quality Forum, a nonprofit organization that works with providers, consumer groups, and governments to establish and build consensus for specific health care quality and efficiency measures. This indicator, called Timely Transmission of Transition Record (measure no. 0648), measures how often a hospital sends a transition record to a patient's physician within 24 hours of discharge. Having this information would allow primary care physicians to identify which patients needed follow-up care.

However, hospitals may not welcome this additional reporting burden because transmittal of such records to outpatient physicians is not a billable hospital service, which means claims data cannot be used to easily calculate how often such transmittals occur. Instead, for hospitals that don't have good electronic health record systems, labor-intensive chart reviews would be required to calculate such a measure.

If CMS were to pay hospitals to develop discharge plans, discuss them with patients, and transmit them to outpatient physicians for follow-up care, the hospitals would have a greater incentive to perform these crucial activities. CMS could also then use the hospitals' billing records for these services to calculate quality measures assessing how often the hospitals performed these important services.

However, in the current strained federal fiscal environment, offering a new carrot to hospitals may have little appeal for policymakers. Indeed, because Medicare already gives hospitals lump-sum payments to cover all the costs associated with a hospitalization and because Medicare's conditions of participation require hospitals to have a discharge planning process in place, policymakers may feel hospitals are already being paid for care transition services but are simply not performing them as routinely as they should be.

- **Strengthen hospital do-not-pay policies.** Another policy stick would be to further limit payment for hospital readmissions. For example, CMS could extend its current policy of not paying for Medicare readmissions that occur within 24 hours of a hospital discharge for the same condition to 72 hours, or even 15 or 30 days, postdischarge. Doing so would require carefully defining which readmissions would be ineligible for payments and how to account for co-occurring conditions. Already, hospitals as a group are upset about CMS's decision to penalize them for certain planned readmissions because they do not think it adequately distinguishes between readmissions that are truly necessary compared to readmissions that are truly preventable.

WHAT'S NEXT?

Given the current budgetary environment and the fact that Medicare is estimated to spend $12 billion per year on potentially preventable hospital readmissions, interest in improving care transitions to reduce Medicare spending is likely only to grow.

Although some care transitions interventions have generated cost savings, uncertainty remains over how best to encourage providers to use these approaches. Evaluation of the changes brought about by the Affordable Care Act will begin filling gaps in our knowledge. And if the health care law's approaches fail to make a strong enough case for providers to pay attention to care transitions, policymakers may want to explore bigger carrots and sticks.

REFERENCES

Bubolz, T., Emerson, C., & Skinner, J. (2012). State spending on dual eligibles under age 65 shows variations, evidence of cost shifting from Medicaid to Medicare. *Health Affairs*, *31*(5), 939–947.

Coleman, E. A. (2003). Falling through the cracks: Challenges and opportunities for improving transitional care for persons with continuous complex care needs. *Journal of the American Geriatrics Society*, *51*(4), 549–555.

Hackbarth, G. (2007, June). *Report to the Congress: Promoting greater efficiency in Medicare*. Washington, DC: Medicare Payment Advisory Commission.

Kripalani, S., LeFevre, F., Phillips, C. O., Williams, M. V., Basaviah, P., & Baker, D. W. (2007). Deficits in communication and information transfer between hospital-based and primary care physicians. *JAMA*, *297*(8), 831–841.

Kronick, R., & Gilmer, T. P. (2012). Medicare and Medicaid spending variations are strongly linked within hospital regions but not at overall state level. *Health Affairs*, *31*(5), 948–955.

Naylor, M. D., Aiken, L. H., Kurtzman, E., Olds, D. M., & Hirschman, K. B. (2011). The importance of transitional care in achieving health reform. *Health Affairs*, *30*(4), 746–754.

Pham, H. H., Grossman, J. M., Cohen, G., & Bodenheimer, T. (2008). Hospitalists and care transitions: The divorce of inpatient and outpatient care. *Health Affairs*, *27*(5), 1315–1327.

Tilson, S., & Hoffman, G. J. (2012). *Addressing Medicare hospital readmissions*. Washington, DC: Congressional Research Service.

ONLINE RESOURCES

The Women's and Children's Health Policy Center
www.jhsph.edu/research/centers-and-institutes/womens-and-childrens-health-policy-center/de/policy_brief/index.html

CHAPTER 9

Political Analysis and Strategies

Kathleen M. White[1]

"The difficult can be done immediately, the impossible takes a little longer."
Unknown author, Army Corps of Engineers motto, World War II

The knowledge and expertise of nurses regarding health and health care are critical to the political process and the development of health policy. However, the word *politics* often evokes negative emotions and many nurses may not feel inclined to get involved. Nonetheless, nurses have the skills to be active participants in the political arena for a number of reasons. First, nurses are skilled at assessment, and being engaged in the political process involves analysis of the relevant issues and their background and importance. Second, nurses understand people and, in order to understand an issue, it is critical to know who is affected and who is involved in trying to solve the problem. Finally, nurses are relationship builders and the political process involves the development of partnerships and networks to solve problems. As skilled communicators, nurses have the ability to work with other professionals, patients, families, and their communities to solve health care problems that affect their patients and the health care system. Nurses have much to offer in the political process and need to develop skills in political analysis and strategy to truly make a difference.

WHAT IS POLITICAL ANALYSIS?

Political analysis is the process of examining an issue and understanding the key factors and people that might potentially influence a policy goal. It involves the analysis of government and organizations, both public and private; people and their behavior; and the social, political, historical, and economic factors surrounding the policy. It also includes the identification and development of strategies to attain or defeat a policy goal. Political analysis involves nine components.

IDENTIFICATION OF THE ISSUE

The first step in conducting a political analysis is to identify and describe the issue or problem. Identifying and framing the issue involves asking who, what, when, where, and how questions to gather sufficient information to lay the groundwork for developing an appropriate response to the issue. Start with what you know about the issue:

- What is the issue?
- Is it my issue and can I solve it?
- When did the issue first occur, is it a new or old problem?
- Is this the real issue, or merely a symptom of a larger one?
- Does it need an immediate solution, or can it wait?
- Is it likely to go away by itself?
- Can I risk ignoring it?

Beware of issue rhetoric (Bardach, 2012) that is either too narrowly defining an issue in a technical way, or defining the issue too broadly in a societal way. Decide what is missing from what you know about the issue and gather additional information:

- Why does the problem exist?
- Who is causing the problem?
- Who is affected by the issue?
- How significant is the issue?

---

[1]This chapter is an updated adaptation of the chapter developed in prior editions by Susan Talbott, Diana Mason, Judy Leavitt, Sally Cohen, and Ellen-Marie Whelan.

- What additional information is needed?
- What are the gaps in existing data?

Don't cut corners or overlook the importance of this step in the political analysis, as a well-defined issue is important to the whole process, as is identifying and defining the right issue. The way a problem is defined has considerable impact on the number and type of proposed solutions (Fairclough, 2013). The challenge for those seeking to get policymakers to address particular issues (e.g., poverty, the underinsured, or unacceptable working conditions) is to define the issue in ways that will prompt decision makers to take action. This requires careful crafting of messages so that calls for solutions are clearly justified. This is known as framing the issue. In the workplace, framing may entail linking the problem to one of the institution's priorities or to a potential threat to its reputation, public safety, or financial standing. For example, inadequate nurse staffing could be linked to increases in rates of morbidity and mortality, outcomes that can increase costs and jeopardize an institution's reputation and future business.

It is important not to confuse symptoms, causes, or solutions with issues. Sometimes what appears to be an issue is not. For example, proposed mandatory continuing-education for nurses is not an issue; rather, it is a possible solution to the challenge of ensuring the competency of nurses. After an analysis of the issue of clinician competence, one might establish a goal that includes legislating mandatory continuing-education. The danger of framing issues as solutions is that it can limit creative thinking about the underlying issue and leave the best solutions uncovered.

CONTEXT OF THE ISSUE

The second part in the political analysis process is to do a situational analysis by examining the context of the problem. This analysis should include, at a minimum, an examination of the social, cultural, ethical, political, historical, and economic contexts of the problem. Several questions can guide you in analyzing the background of the issue:

- What are the social, cultural, ethical, political, historical, and economic factors that are creating or contributing to this problem?

- What are the background and root causes of each of these factors?
- Are these factors constraining or facilitating a solution to the problem?
- Are there other environmental obstacles affecting this issue?

It is important to be as thorough as possible at this stage and to consider whether the source of the information is verifiable and impartial. It is also important to understand any opposing views.

When assessing the political context, nurses need to clarify which level of government (federal, state, or local) or organization is responsible for a particular issue. Scope of practice is a good example. Although typically defined by the states, there are examples where the federal government has superseded the state's authority, such as in the Veteran's Administration and the Indian Health Service. Nurses also need to know which branch of government (legislative, executive, or judicial) has primary jurisdiction over the issue at a given time. Although there is often overlap among these branches, nurses will find that a particular issue falls predominantly within one branch.

Knowledge of past history of an issue can provide insight into the positions of key public officials so that communications with those individuals and strategies for advancing an issue can be developed accordingly. For example, if it is known that a particular legislator has always questioned the ability of advanced practice registered nurses (APRNs) to practice independently, then that individual may need stronger emphasis on the evidence about the quality and value of APRNs to support legislation allowing direct billing of APRNs under Medicare.

This type of context analysis is also applicable to the workplace or community organization. Regardless of the setting, assessing the history of the issue would include identifying who has responsibility for decision making for a particular issue; which committees, boards, or panels have addressed the issue in the past; the organizational structure; and the chain of command.

At an institutional level, once the relevant political forces in play have been identified, the formal and informal structures and the functioning of those structures need to be analyzed. The formal dimensions of the entity can often be assessed through documents related to the organization's mission, goals, objectives, organizational structure, bylaws, annual reports (including financial statement), long-range plans, governing body, committees, and individuals with jurisdiction. The informal dimensions of the organization, such as personal relationships and personal communication networks that could be positive or negative, are more difficult to analyze but need to be understood to get a full picture of the context of the issue.

One final example in the analysis of the context of the issue is worth mentioning. Does the entity use parliamentary procedure? Parliamentary procedure provides a democratic process that carefully balances the rights of individuals, subgroups within an organization, and the membership of an assembly. The basic rules are outlined in Robert's Rules of Order *(www.rulesonline.com)*. Whether in a legislative session or the policymaking body of large organizations, one must know parliamentary procedure to develop a political strategy to get an issue passed or rejected. There have been many issues that have failed or passed because of insufficient knowledge of rule-making.

POLITICAL FEASIBILITY

The third part of a political analysis is to analyze the political feasibility of solving an issue. There are several ways to conduct a political feasibility analysis. A simple analysis is conducting a force field analysis (Lewin, 1951) to identify the barriers and facilitators to making change to solve the issue. The force field analysis asks you to think critically about the issue and the forces affecting it by creating a two-column chart. One column lists the restraining forces, or all of the reasons that preserve the status quo and any reasons why the issue should stay the same. The second column lists the driving forces, or forces that are pushing the issue to change. This exercise requires that the whole picture is considered and provides a list of the important factors that surround the issue.

A second option is to use John Kingdon's (2010) model of public policymaking (see Chapter 7). Kingdon proposes three streams or processes that affect whether an issue gets on the political agenda;

the problem stream is where people agree on an issue or problem, collect data about the issue, and share the definition of problem; the policy stream is characterized by discussion and proposal of policy solutions for the issue; and the political stream is when public mood and political will exists to want to address the issue. Kingdon's model explains that an issue gets on the political agenda only when the three streams couple or converge and a window of opportunity is thereby created. This analysis provides consideration of what needs to happen for the issue to advance to the public policy agenda, including an analysis of the policy and political factors.

THE STAKEHOLDERS

Stakeholders are those parties who have influence over the issue, are directly influenced by it, or could be mobilized to care about it. In some cases, the stakeholders are obvious. For example, nurses are stakeholders on issues such as staffing ratios. In other situations, one can develop potential stakeholders by helping them to see the connections between the issue and their interests. Other individuals and organizations can be stakeholders when it comes to staffing ratios. Among them are employers (i.e., hospitals, nursing homes), payers (i.e., insurance companies), legislators, other health care professionals, and consumers.

The role of consumers cannot be underestimated. In the political arena, these are the constituents and therefore the voters, and they can wield tremendous power over an issue and its solution. In many cases, nurses are advocates and work on behalf of stakeholders such as the patients who are affected by the care they receive. Nursing has increasingly realized the potential of consumer power in moving forward nursing and health care issues. For example, a consumer advocacy organization such as AARP possesses significant lobbying power. When nurses wanted to advance the idea of a Medicare Graduate Nursing Education (GNE) benefit, similar to the Medicare Graduate Medical Education funding to hospitals for the clinical training of interns and residents, AARP championed the proposal because it views the nursing shortage as a threat to its members' ability to access health care. GNE was included in the ACA as a pilot project.

In commencing a stakeholder analysis it is important to evaluate the relationships you, or others in your group, have with key stakeholders. Look at the connections with possible stakeholders throughout your organization, community, places of worship, or businesses. Consider the following when doing a stakeholder analysis:

- Who are the stakeholders on this issue?
- Which of these stakeholders are potential supporters or opponents?
- Can any of the opponents be converted to supporters?
- What are the values, priorities, and concerns of the stakeholders?
- How can these be tapped in planning political strategy?
- Do the supportive stakeholders reflect the constituency that will be affected by the issue?

For example, as states expand coverage of health services through the state's Medicaid program, it is vital to have those who now qualify let their policymakers know how important the issue is for them and to share their personal stories of how this insurance coverage has made a difference. Yet stakeholders who are recipients of the services are too often not identified as vital for moving an issue forward. Nurses, as direct caregivers, have an important role in ensuring that recipients of services are included as stakeholders; especially when bringing issues to elected officials.

ECONOMICS AND RESOURCES

An effective political strategy must take into account the resources that will be needed to address an issue successfully. Resources include money, time, connections, and intangible resources, such as creative solutions. The most obvious resource is money, which must be considered when defining the issue and getting it recognized or on the public agenda. Thus, before launching an initiative to champion an issue, it is necessary to determine the resources that will be necessary, how much it will cost, who will bear those costs, the source of the money, and what value will be achieved from the outlay of the resources. It is critical to fully examine, despite the initial financial outlay, the potential for cost savings it may produce. It could be helpful to know how

budgets are formulated for a given organization, professional group, or government agency. What is the budget process? How much money is allocated to a particular cost center or budget line? Who decides how the funds will be used? How is the use of funds evaluated? How might an individual or group influence the budget process?

Money is not the only resource to evaluate. Sharing available resources, such as space, people, expertise, and in-kind services, may be best accomplished through a coalition. It may require a mechanism for each entity to contribute a specific amount or to tally their in-kind contributions such as office space for meetings; use of a photocopier, telephone or other equipment; and use of staff to assist with production of brochures and other communications. Other cost considerations include publicity efforts such as printing materials, paying for postage, and accessing electronic communications.

VALUES ASSESSMENT

Every political issue should prompt discussions about values. Values underlie the responsibility of public policymakers to be involved in the regulation of health care. In particular, calls for extending the reach of government in the regulation of health care facilities imply that one accepts this as a proper role for public officials, rather than as a role of market forces and the private sector. Thus, electoral politics affect the policies that may be implemented. An analysis that acknowledges how congruent nurses' values are with those of individuals in power can affect the success of advancing an issue. There are issues that would be considered morality issues—those that primarily revolve around ideology and values, rather than costs and distribution of resources. Among well-publicized morality issues are abortion, stem cell research, and immigration. However, most issues that are not classified as morality issues still require an assessment of the values of supporters and their opponents.

Any call for government support of health care programs implies a certain prioritization of values: Is health more important than education, or jobs, or military action in the Middle East? Elected officials must always make choices among competing demands. And their choices reflect their values, the needs and interests of their constituents, and their financial supporters such as large corporations. Similarly, nurses' choice of issues on the political agenda reflects the profession's values, political priorities, and ways to improve health care.

Although nurses may value a range of health and social programs, legislators review issues within the context of demands from all of their constituencies. When an issue is discussed, it is critical to link the issue to the problem it may solve. It is also important to make sure issues are framed to show how they will help the public at large and not just the nursing profession. For example, when a request for increased funding for nursing education is made, linking this request to the need to alleviate the nursing shortage or to increase the number of nurses necessary for successful implementation of health care reform would be important.

NETWORKS AND/OR COALITIONS

Although individuals develop political skill and expertise, it is the influence of networks and coalitions, or like-minded groups that wield power most effectively. It is critical to the political analysis process to evaluate what networks or coalitions exist that are involved with the issue.

Too often nurses become concerned about a particular issue and try to change it without help from others. In the public arena particularly, an individual is rarely able to exert adequate influence to create long-term policy change. For instance, many advanced practice registered nurses (APRNs) have tried to change state Nurse Practice Acts to expand their authority. As well intentioned as the policy solutions may be, they will likely fail unless nurses can garner the support of other powerful stakeholders such as members of the state board of nursing, the state nurses association, physicians, and consumer advocacy groups. Such stakeholders often hold the power to either support or oppose the policy change. (See Chapter 75 for a discussion of building coalitions.)

POWER

Effective political strategy requires an analysis of the power of proponents and opponents of a particular solution. Power is one of the most complex political and sociological concepts to define and measure. It is critical to be aware of the sources of power, regardless of setting or issue, to understand how influence happens and to build your own sources of power for leadership in the political process.

Power can be a means to an end, or an end in itself. Power also can be actual or potential. Many in political circles depict the nursing profession as a potential political force considering the millions of nurses in this country and the power they could wield if more nurses participated in politics and policy formation. Any discussion of power and nursing must acknowledge the inherent issues of hierarchy and power imbalance that arise from the long-standing relationships between nurses and physicians. Some of nurses' discomfort with the concept of power may also arise from the inherent nature of "gender politics" within the profession. Male or female, gender affects every political scenario that involves nurses. Working in a predominantly female profession means that nurses are accustomed to certain norms of social interactions (Tanner, 2001). In contrast to nursing, the power and politics of public policymaking typically are male dominated, although women are steadily increasing their ranks as elected and appointed government officials. Moreover, many male and female public officials have stereotypic images of nurses as women who lack political savvy. This may limit officials' ability to view nurses as potential political partners. Therefore nurses need to be sensitive to gender issues that may affect, but certainly not prevent, their political success.

Any power analysis must include reflection on one's own power base. Power can be obtained through a variety of sources such as those listed in Box 9-1(French & Raven, 1959; Benner, 1984). An analysis of the extent of one's power using these sources can provide direction on how to enhance that power. Although the individual may hold expert power, it will be limited if one attempts to go it alone. An individual nurse may not have sufficient power to champion an issue through the legislative or regulatory process, but a network, coalition, or alliance of nurses or nursing organizations can wield significant power to move an issue to the public agenda and to successfully solve it.

Consider the nursing organization that is seeking to secure legislative support for a key piece of legislation. It can develop a strategy to enhance its power by finding a highly regarded, high-profile individual to be its spokesperson with the media (referent power), by making it known to legislators that their vote on this issue will be a major consideration in the next election's endorsement decisions (reward or coercive power), or by having nurses tell the media stories that highlight the problem the legislation addresses (expert power). A longer-range power-building strategy would be for the nursing organizations to extend their connections with other organizations by signing onto coalitions

---

BOX 9-1 Sources of Power

1. **Legitimate (or positional) power** is derived from a belief that one has the right to power, to make decisions and to expect others to follow them. It is power obtained by virtue of an organizational position rather than personal qualities, whether from a person's role as the chief nurse officer or the state's governor.
2. **Reward power** is based on the ability to compensate another and is the perception of the potential for rewards or favors as a result of honoring the wishes of a powerful person. A clear example is the supervisor who has the power to determine promotions and pay increases.
3. **Expert power** is based on knowledge, skills, or special abilities, in contrast to positional power. Benner (1984) argues that nurses can tap this power source as they move from novice to expert practitioner. It is a power source that nurses must recognize is available to them. Policymakers are seldom experts in health care; nurses are.
4. **Referent power** is based in identification or association with a leader or someone in a position of power who is able to influence others and commands a high level of respect and admiration. Referent power is used when a nurse selects a mentor who is a powerful person, such as the chief nurse officer of the organization or the head of the state's dominant political party. It can also emerge when a nursing organization enlists a highly regarded public personality as an advocate for an issue it is championing.
5. **Coercive power** is based on the ability to punish others and is rooted in real or perceived fear of one person by another. For example, the supervisor who threatens to fire those nurses who speak out is relying on coercive power, as is a state commissioner of health who threatens to develop regulations requiring physician supervision of nurse practitioners.
6. **Information power** results when one individual has (or is perceived to have) special information that another

individual needs or desires. For example, this source of power can come from having access to data or other information that would be necessary to push a political agenda forward. This power source underscores the need for nurses to stay abreast of information on a variety of levels: in one's personal and professional networks, immediate work situation, community, and the public sector, as well as in society. Use of information power requires strategic consideration of how and with whom to share the information.
7. **Connection power** is granted to those perceived to have important and sometimes extensive connections with individuals or organizations that can be mobilized. For example, the nurse who attends the same church or synagogue as the president of the home health care agency, knows the appointments secretary for the mayor, or is a member of the hospital credentialing committee will be accorded power by those who want access to these individuals or groups.
8. **Persuasion power** is based in the ability to influence or convince others to agree with your opinion or agenda. It involves leading others to your viewpoint with data, facts, and presentation skills. For example, a nurse is able to persuade the nursing organization to sponsor legislation or regulation that would benefit the health care needs of her specialty population. It may be the right thing to do, but the nurse uses her skills of persuasion for her own personal or professional agenda.
9. **Empowerment** arises from any or all of these types of power, shared among the group. Nurses need to share power and recognize that they can build the power of colleagues or others by sharing authority and decision making. Empowerment can happen when the nurse manager on a unit uses consensus building when possible instead of issuing authoritative directives to staff, or when a coalition is formed and adopts consensus building and shared decision making to guide its process.

that address broader health care issues and expanding connections with policymakers by attending fundraisers for key legislators (connection power); getting nurses into policymaking positions (legitimate power); hiring a government affairs director to help inform the group about the nuances of the legislature (information power); using consensus building within the organization to enhance nurses' participation and activities (empowerment), or, finally, by identifying a legislative champion for the issue who could garner the use of several power bases at once.

GOALS AND PROPOSED SOLUTIONS

Typically, there is more than one solution to an issue and each option differs with regard to cost, practicality, and duration. These are the policy options. The political analysis of the issue involves the context of the issue, stakeholders, values, power, and what is politically feasible. By identifying the goal, and developing and analyzing possible solutions, nurses will acquire further understanding of the issue and what is possible for an organization, workplace, government agency, or professional organization to undertake. There needs to be a full understanding of the big picture and where the issue fits into that vision. For example, if nurses want the federal government to provide substantial support for nursing education, they need to understand the constraints of federal budgets and the demands to invest in other programs, including programs that benefit nurses and other health care professionals. Moreover, support for nursing education can take the form of scholarships, loans, tax credits, aid to nursing schools, or incentives for building partnerships between nursing schools and health care delivery systems. Each option presents different types of support, and nurses would need to understand the implications of the alternatives before asking for federal intervention.

The amount of money and time needed to address a particular issue also needs to be taken into account. Are there short-term and long-term alternatives that nurses want to pursue simultaneously? Is there a way to start off with a pilot or demonstration program with clear paths to expansion? How might one prioritize various solutions? What are

the tradeoffs that nurses are willing to make to obtain the stated political goals?

Such questions need to be considered in developing a political strategy.

POLITICAL STRATEGIES

Once a political analysis is completed, it is necessary to develop a plan that identifies activities and strategies to achieve the policy goals. The development and implementation of a political strategy to solve an issue requires that there is a tightly framed message, an aligned common purpose or goal, and a well-defined target audience. Messaging is critical to the development of a political strategy. Nurses need to be able to communicate with policymakers, other health care leaders, and the public, and may sometimes use social media for messaging to advise on institutional and public policy.

LOOK AT THE BIG PICTURE

It is human nature to view the world from a personal standpoint, focusing on the people and events that influence one's daily life. However, developing a political strategy requires looking at the larger environment. This can provide a more objective perspective and increase nurses' credibility as broad-minded visionaries, looking beyond personal needs.

In the heat of legislative battles and negotiations, it is easy to get distracted. However, the successful advocate is the one who does not lose sight of the big picture and is willing to compromise for the larger goal. It is critical for nurses to frame their policy work in terms of improving the health of patients and the broader health delivery system, rather than a singular focus on the profession.

DO YOUR HOMEWORK

We can never have all the information about an issue, but we need to be sufficiently prepared before we advocate. Usually it is unlikely to know beforehand when a particular policy will be acted on; nonetheless, it is not sufficient to claim ignorance when confronted with questions that should be answered. However, if one has done everything possible to prepare and is asked to supply information that is not anticipated, it is reasonable and preferable to indicate that one does not know the answer. The information should then be obtained as soon as possible and distributed to the policymaker who requested it. Remember not to let perfection be the enemy of good; gather the requested information, and present it as clearly and simply as possible.

Some of the ways to be adequately prepared are provided in Box 9-2.

READ BETWEEN THE LINES

It is as important to be aware of the way one conveys information as it is to provide the facts. When legislators say they think your issue is important, it does not necessarily mean that they will vote to support it. A direct question such as, Will you vote in support of our bill? needs to be asked of policymakers to know their position. Communication theory notes that the overt message is not always the real message (Gerston, 2010). Some people say a lot by what they choose not to disclose. What is not being said? Are there hidden agendas that the stakeholders are concerned about? When framing the issue, know the hidden agendas and covert messages. Be careful to make the issue as clear as possible and test it on others to be certain that reading between the lines conveys the same message as the overt rhetoric.

BOX 9-2 Being Prepared for Political Advocacy

Here are some ways to ensure that you're prepared for advocacy around a specific issue. Conducting a full political analysis will inform your preparation strategy.

- Clarify your position on the problem, your goal in pursuing the issue, and possible solutions.
- Gather information and data, and search the clinical and policy literature.
- Prepare documents to describe and support the issue.
- Assess the power dynamics of the stakeholders.
- Assess your own power base and ability to maneuver in the political arena.
- Plan a strategy, and assess its strengths and weaknesses.
- Prepare for the opposition.
- Line up support.

IN GOD WE TRUST, ALL OTHERS BRING DATA

This quote is attributed to W. Edwards Deming (Hastie, Tibshirani, & Friedman, 2011) who developed principles for managers to transform business effectiveness through the application of statistical methods. He suggested that by presenting data to workers, they can see the outcomes or intended results of their work and make improvements to meet goals. This quote resonates in today's current heath care environment in that it requires measurement and data reporting by most health care organizations, by many health care professionals, and at all levels of practice, including the institutional, local, state and national. Data are important to the political analysis process and again during strategy development to move an issue through the policy process. Decision makers are often dissatisfied with their ability to get or understand the data needed to make good policy decisions. They need an interpretation of the data in a form that is understandable and useable for their purposes. Nurses are skilled are interpreting and reporting data in the clinical setting and as researchers and consumers of clinical research. A nurse can make himself or herself valuable to a policymaker by preparing a report of the important points on an issue under consideration that translates data into concise information.

MONEY TALKS

Follow the money and understand the flow of funds within a private health care organization/system or the public sector. Money is important in both the public and private sectors, and the more money you have, the more powerful you appear to others, whether the money is revenue, profits, or donations. In the political arena, special interest groups, such as professional organizations (for example, the American Nurses Association), solicit money from their members and spend it to maintain a presence in Washington, DC, and 50 state capitals through political action committees (PACs). Other organizations, such as labor unions, trade associations, and some large corporations, also make donations to influence the agenda in Washington and the state capitals. One other type of influential group is the

"527 committees" that get their name from the IRS code section that governs their existence. These 527 committees are advocacy issue groups that are outside the mainstream of special interest groups and corporate America. They may have ties to some of the other groups, but they have less stringent rules to follow on the use of money and how it influences the political process.

These advocacy groups hire professional advocates or lobbyists to monitor the policy and political environments and influence elected and appointed officials on issues of importance to their special interest group. Even though money is important to have and can be very influential, the problem with money in politics is who is spending the money, what they are asking for in return, and how that affects the allocation of public resources.

COMMUNICATION IS 20% *WHAT* YOU SAY AND 80% *HOW* YOU SAY IT AND TO WHOM

Using the power that results from personal connections can be an important strategy in moving a critical issue forward. In the example of APRN reimbursement, the original legislation that gave some APRNs Medicare reimbursement was greatly facilitated by the fact that the chief of staff for the Senate Majority Leader was a nurse. Or consider the nurse who is the neighbor and friend of the secretary to the chief executive officer (CEO) in the medical center. This nurse is more likely to gain access to the CEO than will someone who is unknown to either the secretary or the CEO. Building relationships and partnerships and networking are important long-term strategies for increasing influence but can also be short-term strategies.

Equally important is the way the message is framed and conveyed to stakeholders. We have often been told, it's not what you say but how you say it. When delivering the message, learn to use strong, affirmative language to describe nursing practice. Use the rhetoric that incorporates lawmakers' lingo and the buzz words of key proponents. This requires having a sense of the values of the target audiences, whether they are legislators, regulators, hospital administrators, community leaders, or the consumer public. Stakeholders

appreciate a succinct and framed message that is responsive to the values and concerns of your supporters or opponents. For example, during health reform discussions, APRNs framed their issue in terms of quality of care and cost savings. Since the nation continues to be concerned about the amount of money spent on health care, the message of reducing costs without compromising quality resonated with the Administration, Members of Congress, insurers, employers, and the public alike. How you convey your message involves developing rhetoric or catchy phrases that the media might pick up on and perpetuate. Nurses need to develop their effectiveness in accessing and using the media, an essential component of getting the issue on the public's agenda.

Learn and use good communication techniques; in particular, the use of a persuasive and assertive communication style that focuses on the facts and the data, and limits any emotional appeals to stories that illustrate the human impact of the problem. As discussed above, it is important to develop a message that is important to your target audience.

And finally, don't be afraid to toot your own horn. Don't assume that your good work will be recognized or valued by others. If nursing is leading an initiative or has generated the research evidence to support the issue, present the evidence to the policymakers and let them know what has been studied or found to be effective and inform them that nurses led the work.

YOU SCRATCH MY BACK AND I'LL SCRATCH YOURS

Developing networks involves keeping track of what you have done for others and not being afraid to ask a favor in return. Often known as quid pro quo (literally, something for something), it is the way political arenas work in both public and private sectors. Leaders expect to be asked for help and know the favor will be returned. Because nurses interface with the public all the time, they are in excellent positions to assist, facilitate, or otherwise do favors for people. Too often, nurses forget to ask for help from those whom they have helped and who would be more than willing to return a favor.

Consider the lobbyist for a state nurses' association who knew that the chair of the Senate public health and welfare committee had a grandson who was critically injured in a car accident. She visited the child several times in the hospital, spoke with the nurses on the unit, and kept the legislator informed about his grandson's progress and assured him that the boy was well cared for. When the boy recovered, the legislator was grateful and asked the lobbyist what he could do to move her issue. Interchanges like this occur every day and create the basis for quid pro quo.

STRIKE WHILE THE IRON IS HOT

The timing of an issue will often make a difference in terms of a successful outcome. A well-planned strategy may fail because the timing is not good. An issue may languish for some period because of a mismatch in values, concerns, or resources but then something may change to make an issue ripe for consideration. The passage of the ACA is a good example. President Obama knew from studying the history of legislation in this country that the best chance of passing sweeping legislation was in the early years of a presidential term. Once elected, with both the U.S. House of Representatives and the U.S. Senate under the control of the Democratic Party, the President knew that the only hope of passing comprehensive health care reform would be if it became his priority within his first year.

UNITED WE STAND, DIVIDED WE FALL

The achievement of policy goals can be accomplished only if supporters demonstrate a united front. Collective action is almost always more effective than individual action. Collaboration through networking, alliances, and coalition building can demonstrate broad support for an issue.

A 2010 Gallup poll of health care leaders found that the lack of a united front by national nursing organizations was viewed as a major reason why nursing's influence on health care reform would not be significant. To maximize nursing's political potential, we must look for opportunities to reach consensus or remain silent in the public arena on an issue that is not of paramount concern.

Sometimes diverse groups can work together on an issue of mutual interest, even though they are opponents on other issues. Public and private interest groups that identify with nursing's issues can be invaluable resources for nurses. They often have influential supporters or may have research information that can help nurses move an issue forward.

THE BEST DEFENSE IS A GOOD OFFENSE

A successful political strategy is one that tries to accommodate the concerns of the opposition. It requires disassociating from the emotional context of working with opponents and is the first step in principled negotiating. A person who is skillful at managing conflict will be successful in politics. The saying that politics makes strange bedfellows arose out of the recognition that long-standing opponents can sometimes come together around issues of mutual concern, but it often requires creative thinking and a commitment to fairness to develop an acceptable approach to resolving an issue.

It is also important to anticipate problems and areas for disagreement and be prepared to counter them. When the opposition is gaining momentum and support, it can be helpful to develop a strategy that can distract attention from the opposition's issue or that can delay action. For example, one state nurses' association continually battles the state medical society's efforts to amend the Nurse Practice Act in ways that would restrict nurses' practice and provide for physician supervision. Nurses have become concerned about the possibility of passage during a year when the medical society's influence with the legislature was high. A key strategy to deal with this specific example is to develop coalitions and alliances to work with other health provider organizations engaged in similar battles with the physicians (e.g., optometrists, pharmacists) to monitor the current environment and be vigilant if changes arise. With this type of strategy in place, the physician groups will know that there would be a large coalition to deal with if any changes are proposed.

In developing a good defense, arm yourself with data and information about the issue. Be sure to understand how the issue fits in to either the organization's current priorities or other important public agenda items. Know the supporters and opponents of the issue. Many groups maintain voting records of legislators on their key legislative agenda priorities. Finally, learning as much as you can about current public agenda items and organizational priorities is critical to being an informed health care professional. Visit your professional organization websites, including NursingWorld.org, the online home of the American Nurses Association. Also, the websites of specialty nursing organizations can provide valuable up-to-date information on the key issues facing the profession and health care in general.

DON'T MAKE ENEMIES AND DON'T BURN BRIDGES

To burn one's bridges is to cut off any potential future support or collaboration with a person or organization. Because nursing or even health care is such a small world, it is critically important not to burn bridges, no matter how tempted you might be! Building bridges rather than burning them is a much smarter option for the future. It is critical to handle tricky political maneuvers with care and finesse. Everyone has experienced a sound defeat at some stage and the person who can congratulate the winner and move on to learn from the experience will thrive.

ROME WAS NOT BUILT IN A DAY

It is important to remember that it takes a long time to do important work, to create something long lasting and sustainable. This is very true when referring to influence in the political process, whether it is governmental or organizational. It is often reported that it feels like the arguments have been going on for years, but policy successes will not happen immediately. It will take the involvement of many workers or volunteers and countless meetings, going through the political analysis of an issue and pursuing a political strategy to find a policy solution. It is critical not to overestimate the importance of that building process nor underestimate the importance of adding another brick.

DISCUSSION QUESTIONS

1. When you are attempting to undertake a political analysis of an issue, one of the key questions to continually ask during the process is: "In this political [or social or economic] climate, can we get this done?" How would you evaluate the barriers that arise from climate or context or timing on a specific issue of interest?
2. For the same issue, who are the stakeholders and how could they be used in a political analysis that might be different from their use in political advocacy?
3. What are the political strategies that could leverage facilitators and constraints into political momentum to move the issue forward?

REFERENCES

Bardach, E. (2012). *A practical guide for policy analysis* (4th ed.). Washington, DC: CQ Press.

Benner, P. (1984). *From novice to expert.* Menlo Park, CA: Addison-Wesley.

Fairclough, N. (2013). *Critical discourse analysis: The critical study of language.* New York: Routledge Press.

French, J., & Raven, B. (1959). The basis of social power. In D. Cartwright (Ed.), *Studies in social power* (pp. 150–167). Ann Arbor, MI: University of Michigan Press.

Gallup (2010). Nursing leadership from bedside to boardroom: Opinion leaders' perception. Retrieved from *newcareersinnursing.org/sites/default/files/file-attachments/Top%20Line%20Report.pdf.*

Gerston, L. N. (2010). *Public policy making: Process and principles.* Armonk, NY: M.E. Sharpe.

Hastie, T., Tibshirani, R., & Friedman, J. (2011). *The elements of statistical learning* (2nd ed.). New York: Springer.

Kingdon, J. (2010). *Agendas, alternatives and public policies* (2nd ed.). (Longman Classics in Political Science). New York: Pearson.

Lewin, K. (1951). *Field theory in social science.* New York: Harper and Row.

Tanner, D. (2001). *Talking from 9 to 5: Women and men at work* (reprint ed.). New York: William Morrow Paperbacks.

ONLINE RESOURCES

American Nurses Association's Take Action
www.rnaction.org/site/PageServer?pagename=nstat_take_action_home
American Association of Colleges of Nursing
www.aacn.nche.edu/government-affairs/AACNPolicyHandbook_2010.pdf
National League for Nursing
www.nln.org/publicpolicy
American Organization of Nurse Executives
advocacy.aone.org

CHAPTER 10

Communication and Conflict Management in Health Policy

Elizabeth Waetzig   Greg Abell

"In great teams, conflict becomes productive. The free flow of conflicting ideas is critical for creative thinking, for discovering new solutions no one individual would have come to on his own."

Peter Senge

Nurses engage in conflict every day. They are trained to listen to, and advocate for, their patients and are, at times, called to resolve conflict among family members, providers, and others. Participating in health policymaking requires using these familiar skills, but also requires some very specific communication and conflict engagement skills. As Phyllis Kritek (1994), a nurse leader and educator, suggested in *Negotiating at an Uneven Table*, the frustration over having been excluded from the decision-making table for years sometimes has led nurses to a stubbornness of an intensity that might be a barrier to effective participation. To increase the capacity of nurses to engage effectively in politics and policymaking aimed at influencing health reform, and to be thought leaders in many other policy and political venues, this chapter will explore the following: (1) a definition of conflict; (2) a process to engage in complex and challenging conversations; (3) skills to preserve opportunities available in these conversations; and (4) methods for effective engagement of conflict.

UNDERSTANDING CONFLICT

Senge (1990) in the opening quote identifies conflict as a place of possibility where we will find opportunities for creativity and innovation. If this is true, then, why do many people demonstrate a significant aversion to conflict? The answer may lie in some key characteristics of conflict:

- The issues are considered significant to at least one of the parties.
- Around these issues there is a perception of an incompatible difference or threat.
- When experiencing threat, we move to defend ideas, perspectives, and plans of action.
- We believe "the best defense is a good offense" and attacking the other person and their ideas increases the level of threat.

What might this look like in real time:

- When we are experiencing strongly held differences of opinion, we believe there is obviously a right and a wrong answer.
- From our perspective, it is obvious that we are right.
- Given that we cannot both be right, then the other person is obviously wrong.
- Therefore it is my job to fix this by convincing you that "I am right and you are wrong."

This paradigm compromises effectiveness in engaging conflict. People pursue polarized positions and thinking, and behavior becomes focused on defending these positions. Little effort is directed to understanding the other person's thinking because they are now often seen as an adversary. Effective strategies for conflict engagement must challenge this paradigm. The value in conflict is not found in fixing it but in acknowledging and understanding differences. While we say we respect diversity of opinion, this respect is often absent from our most challenging conversations.

TYPES OF CONFLICT AND RAMIFICATIONS TO CHALLENGE

Conflict is experienced daily that is quickly resolved or effectively ignored. Conflict can also cause us to lose sleep and dominate our waking thoughts. Bernard Mayer (2009) describes the six faces of conflict as follows:

- *Low impact:* A decision needs to be made and although there is a potential for differences of opinion, the issue is not particularly significant or critical. Where do you want to have lunch? On what color of paper should we print the agenda for the meeting?
- *Latent:* There are issues about which we know there is potential for conflict. We know strongly held differences of opinion exist. The conflict remains latent until something exposes it. Topics of religion and politics at social gatherings can expose latent conflict.
- *Transient:* Some conflicts occur within a time frame. For example, filing a workplace grievance or labor dispute often places the conflict into a context in which there are rules defining a time frame for engagement and resolution of the dispute.
- *Representative:* Almost all conflict is, to some extent, representative and not about what we think it is about. For example, the filing of a contract grievance is often representative of a deeper breakdown in a relationship between a supervisor and a direct report.
- *Stubborn:* Conflict has become complex, challenging, and resistant to resolution. The stakes feel high and there may be significant emotion attached to the issues and to the ways they are being addressed. However, when handled well, resolution may be reached.
- *Enduring:* Enduring conflict is deeply rooted in structures, systems, identity, and values. Ongoing engagement is required, and there may not be a final resolution. Engagement is to reach agreements that allow for forward movement. One way to engage enduring conflict and stay with it even when it is not resolvable is to agree to policies and procedures that clarify individual and organizational expectations and that increase the ability to function effectively together.

THE PROCESS OF CONVERSATIONS

Complex conversations require a process that provides time for thought, reflection, and structure that is inclusive, productive, and innovative. The four stages include:

1. Preparing to participate
2. Entering or initiating the conversation
3. Increasing mutual understanding
4. Moving from inquiry and advocacy to action (This is a process that the authors developed while teaching *Leading Through Conflict,* an original work.)

PHASE I: PREPARING TO PARTICIPATE

Who do you choose to be? To effectively prepare for a complex conversation, there are three objectives to consider:

1. Decide who you are committed to *being* in this process.
2. Align what you are *doing* with who you are committed to *being.*
3. Support others to prepare to engage effectively.

Preparation must be comprehensive, built on a lifelong process of reflection and a desire to stay grounded in the midst of surprise, disappointment, conflict, and change. We suggest the following questions in support of this level of preparation.

Who is the conversation calling me to be? Know what motivates you to participate and influences your choices at the table. Motivations for advocacy may include exposing problems, revenge, or assuaging ego. More positive motivators are beliefs that the thing advocated for would benefit the profession, the organization, and/or the entire population.

Why am I being invited to participate? You may bring experience and/or expertise that is essential. You may represent a group whose buy-in is necessary for implementation of a new policy. There may be a need for a person of a certain gender, ethnicity, or profession to increase the credibility of the process. If you know the reason, is it one that aligns with your values? Can you participate with authenticity and support the outcome?

Who am I representing? Are you representing the interests of a larger group? It could be the organization or agency that employs you, the nursing profession, the health of the population served, or all of the above. Be clear about your representation and ensure that you can authentically represent those voices. This may sometimes require you to represent perspectives with which you do not entirely agree.

What are my own personal positions, philosophies, aims, intents, limits, and interests related to the issues? There are times when the values and interests of those who invited you or those you represent are such that remaining in the conversation would not serve you, those you represent, or the individuals in the conversation.

What biases, blind spots, or vulnerabilities might get in the way? How have diverse experiences, ideas, knowledge, and strengths shaped your current thinking?

Can you commit to self-reflection, awareness, and honesty even if it means potential isolation? It takes courage to stand alone when something does not feel right.

What is the situation calling you to do? When promoting change, you may agitate. When creating new policy, you are called to collaborate. You may also need to be the voice of dissent.

Are you comfortable with the role you are taking? Discomfort can show up as defensiveness and limit your ability to listen and contribute productively.

What will be most challenging? Anticipating challenges such as the issue(s), a person, or process will allow you to recognize them when they arise and to address them appropriately.

What kind of conversation do you want to have? If the group is shifting from one conversational structure to another, stop, evaluate the reason for the shift, and decide to continue as is or make a mid-course correction. Examples of conversational structures include:

- A persuasive conversation is used to influence in a way that is honest and compelling.
- A distributive conversation is used to divide up a fixed resource.
- A dialectic conversation is a discussion used to investigate the truth of a theory or opinion.
- An integrative conversation is used to put the parts together into a whole.
- A generative conversation is used to create entirely new possibilities. (Isaacs, 1999, p. 38)

After preparing psychologically, focus on preparing substantively. The following questions are useful in preparing for a conversation around policy.

What is prompting this conversation? Why are we engaging at this time? Who is asking for this conversation? Is this one in a series of conversations, the subsequent ones contingent on the outcome of this one? Some reasons may be undisclosed.

What is/are the issue(s)? Does the group share a definition of the issues?

What information needs to be gathered, shared, or reviewed before and during this conversation? What data, process, and political information may be valuable?

How likely is conflict to arise in the conversation? If you can anticipate conflict, the better able you are to identify and effectively engage it when it surfaces.

What options do I have for engaging in and resolving conflict? Options include disengaging, asking for facilitative help, and identifying shared interests that may keep others at the table.

Our third focus is on procedural preparation. If the process feels fair and inclusive, then the outcome is more acceptable. The interpretation of a fair process is dependent on a number of factors:

- *What is your relationship to this issue?* How important is the topic or issue to you, your organization, your patients, your profession, or your community?
- *What authority do you bring?* Can you commit the organization you represent? To what extent is it important to clarify your authority?
- *What is your level of responsibility and/or accountability?* Colleagues, peers, and leaders will want to hear about the progress or outcome. Knowing your level of responsibility and to whom you are accountable gives clarity to emotional elements of a conversation.
- *How will you organize to complete the work?* If people are not given information about the time, location, participants, or premeeting information, the conversation may feel unorganized and trust is compromised.
- *What is the structure of your work?* Having everyone engage all issues at all times may be inefficient and frustrating. Instead, convene a conceptual meeting where the principles of the

work are agreed upon and then a design team can provide details for the whole group to react to. Phase I prepares participants to think through psychological, substantive, and procedural issues and clarify what they mean for their participation. Participants in this phase have prepared those being represented and those with whom they are meeting by building shared expectations.

PHASE II: ENTERING INTO THE CONVERSATION

In Phase II, a foundation is laid for the group as they begin to engage. The objectives include:
1. Creating a safe space
2. Increasing trust in the process and the people
3. Including all of the voices

As you prepare, think about your needs regarding safety, trust, and your role. You must consider your relationships to those in the conversation and those external to it, the issues, and your own capacity to remain honest and compassionate in the face of diversity. As you convene the conversation, be intentional about the environment and the process.

Determine whether the process is confidential. If the conversation or process is to be confidential, what does that mean to the group? If it is not to be kept confidential, who will be informed and how will they be informed? Will the group create a unified message?

Identify and clarify potential parameters such as time and expected outcome. In most complex conversations, there are external factors that should be named and acknowledged by the group. Who convened the process and why? What is the sense of urgency? Is there a deadline? Is it firm? Is there funding attached to the process?

Define the principles to guide the conversation. Sometimes called ground rules or group norms, these are the shared expectations about participation (attendance and level of engagement), behaviors (checking e-mail/text/Facebook and taking phone calls), logistics (how often you meet and where), and communication (disclosing helpful information).

Clarify the purpose of the conversation. Are you gathering information to better understand the problem, various points of view, and possible direction? Making decisions? Debating alternatives? Creating something new? Do you have the authority and ability to innovate?

Manage your tone. You can model the conversational structure. If you enter the conversation to tell rather than learn, others will probably do the same. If you engage in dialogue that leads to innovation rather than persuade others to take your path, you promote that conversational structure. If you work to include all of the voices with respect, others are likely to follow.

How will decisions be made? Most individuals have their own assumptions about how decisions will be made in a group. They do not prepare for the situation where a decision is needed and the group is not in agreement. Have this conversation before disagreements arise.

If you choose how to have a conversation thoughtfully, you set patterns and group norms that will serve the group well when challenging topics are addressed and divergence occurs. Knowing what to expect creates safety, increases trust, and promotes participation by everyone.

PHASE III: INCREASING MUTUAL UNDERSTANDING

Even when advocating or persuading, it is important to increase mutual understanding. Everyone has to be willing to share their information, ideas, knowledge, and narrative, as well as understand the same from others. The objectives of increasing mutual understanding are to:
1. Support group dialogue to create deeper shared understanding of the challenge.
2. Create a shared understanding of issues and desired outcomes.
3. Clarify outcomes with sufficient detail to prepare for implementation.

To increase mutual understanding the following is suggested:
- *Balance inquiry and advocacy.* To inquire is to keep an open mind and a willingness to explore other perspectives. To advocate is to promote a point of view or position. When you think that you have less power in the conversation, you are likely to advocate. Inquiry is a way to gain and build trust. To create mutual understanding, you must find a balance of exploring what is

important to others as well as explaining what is important to you and those you represent.

- *Be familiar with typical decision-making patterns and possibilities.* Individuals tend to believe (or hope) that they move in similar directions at the same pace as they move to decisions. However, people do not think in straight lines, but tend to go off on tangents and lose track of central themes. Usually individuals start in a familiar place and, if allowed, stray to a point where they find the unfamiliar, feel uncomfortable, and stall. Can you stay with uncertainty and discomfort or do you retreat to safe and obvious solutions (or remain stuck in conflict)? Sometimes people choose to stay stuck in conflict because the adversarial relationship is frequently a most familiar place for many people. If you can consider a broader range of possibilities in the unfamiliar, creative and more innovative options may emerge.
- *Build trust and increase mutual understanding.* The questions we ask and the way in which we ask them either invite or discourage responses. Good questions are intentional and purposeful, come from curiosity, and cause the inquirer and the respondent to ponder.

When you gain mutual understanding through inquiry, advocacy, persistence, and compassion, you increase opportunities to create, innovate, decide, and move forward in an informed and productive way. And if divergence shows up, you are ready to explore it rather than let it shut you down. At some point, though, the conversation must lead to action.

PHASE IV: FROM INQUIRY TO ACTION; MOVING FORWARD

It is difficult to know when to stop talking and start doing. The shift can be intentional and structured to provide a measure of safety and consensus while implementing and evaluating an action. Here are some guiding questions for moving to action:

- *To what extent are we on the same page?* Have you reached mutual understanding and are you ready to move toward action? If you think that action is possible, test it out. Summarize the learning and assess the level of consensus. If you have reached agreement in principle, move to identifying and clarifying the details for action and implementation.
- *Are you stuck?* If you are stuck, there are still decisions to make about how to move forward. Is it okay to remain stuck? Remaining stuck for a defined amount of time may allow for creative solutions to emerge. If you remain stuck, decide when to reconvene and create expectations for what should happen in the short term.
- *Has the proposed solution been reality tested?* Talk about the impact and possible reactions to a proposed course of action or decision, especially if the action will require change.
- *What are the details?* Provide details about who will do what, by when. Leaving these details undefined can lead to unmet expectations, conflict, and distrust.
- *Is there a plan for accountability?* How will we know if our action is having the desired effect? Indicators of success help in making decisions to stay the course or to make corrections.
- *When do you opt out?* In *Getting to Yes*, Fisher and Ury (1983) describe a concept called your Best Alternative to a Negotiated Agreement (BATNA). If what you could accomplish on your own is better than the proposed outcome of the conversation, then you are better off proceeding with your BATNA. If not, then stay with the process. Be aware that there are consequences for relationships when you opt to proceed with your BATNA (Fisher and Ury, 1983).

Complex and challenging conversations often lead to creative and innovative policies that are often accompanied by political relationships and structures. It is helpful to know and be able to apply a process that includes preparing for the conversation, establishing safety, trust, and space for multiple voices, increasing mutual understanding, and moving to action and implementation.

LISTENING, ASSERTING, AND INQUIRING SKILLS

Complex and challenging conversations including ones that generate some conflict will require interpersonal interaction. Effective engagement is dependent on critical communication skills. While the topics we choose to talk about are critical, how we talk about them is equally important. We will unpack the skills of listening, asserting, and inquiring as they relate to the challenge of conflict.

LISTENING FOR SHARED UNDERSTANDING

Many in the helping professions have undergone training on effective listening. Effective listening is built on the ability to recognize and balance two critical elements: It is about both doing AND being when listening.

When introducing the skill of active listening, a participant will occasionally raise their hand and state something like, "Oh yeah I know what that is. I hate it when people do that to me." When asked to explain, they describe someone who has learned to do active listening while not really understanding what it means to be an active listener. They are experiencing someone as disingenuous in the conversation. The impact words have shift when delivered by one who is truly engaged in being an active listener. This level of listening and responding is driven by a deep commitment to understanding and learning. They are listening from a place of mutual respect, curiosity, and a desire to learn. It is this shift in orientation that is essential to move from simply doing active listening to truly being an active listener.

The way we listen must be in integrity with our commitment to collaboration, mutual purpose, and shared learning. In fact, many identify respect for diversity of opinion as a core shared value for collaboration. However, basic civility too often disappears with the arrival of diverse opinions about high stakes, complex, and often emotional issues.

In a conversation committed to mutual purpose, some fundamental things you need to do are:
- Understand the perspective by understanding objectives, needs, and interests around the issue held by the other person(s).
- Share your perspective by understanding objectives, needs, and interests around the issue.
- Jointly clarify and understand where everyone shares interests and separate interests, not necessarily opposed to each other.
- Create options that, to the greatest extent possible, will meet both your shared and individual interests.

There are a number of reasons that listening is critical:
- Listening to the other person and sharing your understanding of what has been shared lets them know if they have been heard. People will often repeat themselves and advocate their perspective until they know they have been heard.
- Listening and responding helps to clarify if what you heard is, in fact, what was intended.
- As you listen to others and provide feedback, it facilitates the others' ability to share what is most important to them. For example, upon hearing your feedback they might say, "Yeah, that is what I said, and it is not really what I meant. Let me try it again."
- Effective listening can defuse emotion. People have often escalated their anger and hostility because no one is listening to them.
- Listening encourages the group to slow the conversation down. For many who struggle with a lack of time, this may seem counterproductive. However, groups spend a lot of time generating solutions to challenges that they have not taken sufficient time to fully understand. They then wonder why their plan does not meet their objectives.

These are not simply behaviors to make it look like we are really listening. These behaviors are in service of both the speaker and listener. In service of the speaker, they convey that what is being shared is important and that you are putting all of your attention into understanding what the speaker wants to have understood. In service of the listener, these behaviors position you to be receiving and processing all that is being shared. The ideas that people share are not only conveyed by their choice of words but equally by their body language, tone of voice, facial expression, and vocal inflections.

ASSERTING FOR SHARED UNDERSTANDING

Many who are uncomfortable with conflict are also uncomfortable requesting what they need or sharing what they think. It is assumed that by initiating a request or sharing a divergent opinion, there is a risk of upsetting others. Depending on the nature of the request it might be perceived as critical of that person and upset the relationship. The request may also be denied, the opinion ignored, thinking and ideas demeaned and berated, and subsequent conflict that may develop.

The question we often face is this: "Is this context safe, and is this a safe person with whom to share my needs, thoughts, and ideas?" We engage in a cost-benefit analysis, calculating the risks of sharing and the potential benefits of putting forth ideas. Although this may be valid, our analysis of the situation does not always provide a complete or accurate understanding of the situation. We too often focus on the risks and lose sight of the benefits. Asking the question, "Should you share?" may be appropriate. However, a more complete question is, "How do you share in a way that will make it easy for the others to hear, understand, and respond?"

There are some basic and very effective strategies that support success in this aspect of engaging in challenging and complex conversations and navigating conflict. First is to consider shifting your overall orientation when engaging a potentially challenging conversation. Move from either/or thinking to both/and thinking. When engaged in either/or thinking you can become polarized around the notion that one of you is right and one is wrong. A defensive or adversarial posture is adopted and little time spent in joint exploration. Shifting to both/and thinking is inclusive in that it seeks to hear from and explore the multiple perspectives around what is typically a complex issue. You are sharing your perspective, not as a rebuttal to another point of view, but in service of your shared learning and understanding. It communicates a commitment to mutual purpose.

While this commitment sets the stage, it does not make the conversation easy. Significant issues and often emotions that are strong still exist. It is essential to maintain civility and respect in the conversation. A key question introduced previously asks, "How do you share in a way that will make it easy for others to hear and respond?" Both what you say and how you say it are critical. At this point you want to share your perspective in a way that it neither negates nor disrespects the other person or the ideas. You are looking to maintain a conversation that is safe and supports a full exploration of the issues.

DIFFERENTIATING FACT AND INTERPRETATION

How often when sharing your perspective are you sharing it as fact? How often are your "facts" your interpretation and understanding of a situation? How often do you become committed to your interpretation, unwilling to acknowledge and explore the perspective of others? Be clear to yourself and with those to whom you are sharing, when you are describing facts and when you are sharing your interpretation of these facts.

When preparing to share your perspective it may be useful to reflect on the following questions:
1. What is the current situation? What can you state with certainty? (Facts)
2. What does the situation mean to you? Individually? Collectively? (Interpretation)
3. What are you working to accomplish in this situation? Individually? Collectively? (Individual and collective purpose)

You may understand the distinction and now need to determine what to share of your perspective. The answer is all of it. The critical consideration is in the how of sharing. When sharing in the context of facts and interpretation of the facts, it is essential to share both if others are truly going to understand your perspective. Start by sharing the data and/or facts that are informing your perspective. Describe specific events or behaviors that you have observed. Delineate that which you can observe from your interpretation of it without judgment.

Next, add your interpretation of what these events or behaviors mean to you. It is at this point that the how becomes most critical as you are sharing your interpretation as a hunch. As a hunch, it has not become fixed as fact and remains open to alternate interpretations. You are open to the possibility that you may have misinterpreted a situation or that a radically different interpretation might make more sense. You remain open to learning.

INQUIRING FOR SHARED UNDERSTANDING

An essential skill for achieving deeper, shared understanding of an issue is the ability to ask good questions. Our questions are often focused on identifying the flaw in the other person's thinking or looking to find an easy solution to the problem. It is not possible to generate appropriate responses to a challenge that we do not fully understand and full understanding is achieved when we can articulate both our shared *and* individual perspectives.

There is a decision to be made at this point in a conversation. Will we ask questions in service of divergent thinking or convergent thinking? Will the questions expand shared understanding of the issue(s) or will we look for a quick and readily accessible solution? The conversation ultimately will be determined by the questions we ask. In general, questions focused on divergent thinking are intended to increase the depth and breadth of understanding of an issue. These are questions that push the conversation beyond the known into the unknown. Questions intended to support divergent thinking focus on increasing awareness of alternatives, encourage open discussion, are designed to gather diverse viewpoints, and facilitate unpacking the logic of a problem.

For some, this may increase discomfort and frustration. For problem solvers, the goal is to make a decision and find a plan of action as quickly as possible. As such, our questions are too often oriented to convergent thinking. The focus becomes evaluating alternatives, summarizing key points, sorting ideas into categories, and arriving as quickly as possible at a general conclusion or decision.

In many situations, this is the appropriate response. As health care professionals, nurses are educated and are prepared to respond quickly and decisively during critical incidents. The ability to individually and collectively assess the needs within a situation and quickly draw on experience and technical expertise is critical to the role.

This same strategy for responding to challenges can compromise the ability to achieve one of the key values in jointly engaging complex conversations around policy: leveraging individual thinking into shared thinking to generate new and innovative thinking in the group. Some challenges are complex and will not be solved with existing solutions; they require the adaptive work of shared learning.

INTENTIONAL INQUIRY: ASKING QUESTIONS IN SERVICE OF A CONVERSATION OF SHARED LEARNING

Author Marilee Adams (2004), in a book entitled *Change Your Questions Change Your Life*, introduces a strategy she calls Question Thinking. She refers to it as a "system of tools using questions for vastly better results in almost anything you do" (Adams, 2004, p. 18). Questions make up a significant part of both your internal and external dialogue and therefore have significant impact on the way(s) in which you engage your world and others. Adams (2004) states "questions drive results" (p. 18). They virtually program how we behave and what types of outcomes are available.

Adams distinguished between two paths of engagement, referred to as the Learner Path and the Judger Path. Different types of questions characterize the paths. For example, when choosing the Judger Path, you are inclined to ask:
- What is wrong with them?
- What is wrong with me?
- Why are they so stupid?
- How do I fix this?

In contrast, when choosing the Learner Path, you are more likely to ask questions such as:
- What happened?
- What is useful?
- What do I want?
- What can I learn?
- What is the other person thinking, feeling, needing, and/or wanting?

The options of Judgers Path and Learners Path are a choice. Who are you committed to being in the conversation? What is the nature of the challenge? Is quick decisive action called for? Would it be wise to slow down and explore the challenge more completely? What choice is most in line with your intentions? Learner questions are born out of thoughtful choices, a commitment to mutual purpose and mutual benefit.

Intentional Inquiry is a method of asking questions with purpose in mind and does not mean manipulating the conversation or to coercing a specific outcome. These questions inspire reflection and new thinking. The term "intentional" is significant. Questions in this context become tools by which you intentionally seek greater understanding of the issue. Below are some examples:

- Broadening questions are nonthreatening and provide a range of response options. Tell me more about that? What might that look like?
- Clarifying questions clarify what is unclear or potentially misunderstood. What do you mean when you say the situation is unsafe? What would better communication look like?
- Explaining questions invite a person to share their line of reasoning or thought process. What leads you to that perspective? How did you reach that conclusion?
- Exploring questions are designed to get at what is most important about an issue. What do you most need us to understand that you do not think we currently understand? What is most important to you about this issue?
- Challenging questions explore apparent inconsistencies in what is being said. Please help me understand, on the one hand you say the policy should be flexible and yet on the other hand you want to significantly limit the response options.
- Brainstorming questions generate ideas or options. What options have you considered? Given the situation, what might we consider?
- Consequential questions focus attention on the ramifications of a potential course of action. How will this decision impact the patients? How might the night staff be affected by this policy?

Questions can move us outside our comfort zone, yet possibilities worth exploring are outside our comfort zone. It is where we will find creative and innovative responses to our biggest challenges.

CONCLUSION

Engaging in politics and policymaking require complex and challenging conversations that often include conflict. To be effective in these conversations requires an understanding of conflict, identifying it when it emerges. Prepare by reflecting and choosing who you want to be, so that you can choose how you want to act while engaged. Enter into the conversation with confidence so that you can create a safe and trustworthy environment in which all can participate. Create mutual understanding using the communication skills of listening, asserting, and inquiring. This is the most thorough and intentional way to move forward effectively in advancing health policy and being influential in politics related to health care delivery.

DISCUSSION QUESTIONS

1. How would you describe your current relationship to conflict? Describe a time when you were significantly challenged when confronting conflict as a health care professional at an uneven table. Describe a time you successfully engaged conflict as a health care professional.
2. What challenges related to communication and conflict are you currently experiencing as a health care professional?
3. How will you apply what you have learned in this chapter to your challenges?

REFERENCES

Adams, M. (2004). *Change your questions change your life.* San Francisco, CA: Berrett Kohler Press.
Fisher, R., & Ury, W. (1983). *Getting to yes: Negotiating agreement without giving in.* New York, NY: Penguin Press.
Isaacs, W. (1999). *Dialogue: The art of thinking together.* New York, NY: Currency.
Kritek, P. (1994). *Negotiating at an uneven table.* San Francisco, CA: Jossey-Bass.
Mayer, B. (2009). *Staying with conflict.* San Francisco, CA: Jossey-Bass.
Senge, P. (1990). *The fifth discipline: The art and practice of the learning organization.* New York, NY: Currency.

ONLINE RESOURCES

Harvard Program for Health Care Negotiation and Conflict Resolution
www.hsph.harvard.edu/hcncr
Mediate.com (although the website is focused on mediation, it includes many books and articles on national and international collaboration and conflict engagement)
www.mediate.com
Negotiation Skills for Minority Nurses
www.minoritynurse.com/article/negotiation-skills-minority-nurses

CHAPTER 11

Research as a Political and Policy Tool

Lynn Price

"If politics is the art of the possible, research is surely the art of the soluble."

Sir Peter Medawar

That research has any nexus to politics or policy may strike one as curious, if not an outright oxymoron. Research, using any methodology, is carefully considered, designed, implemented, and interpreted. Politics is, well, messy. Policy is birthed from political process, and is therefore often complex and messy in its own right. Yet, research is a powerful lever in the world of politics and policymaking. In the past few decades, research has come to play an increasingly influential role in the crafting of both political messages and policy declarations in nursing and health generally.

SO WHAT *IS* POLICY?

Policy is usually thought of as formal rules, set by Congress, state legislatures, or agencies at city, county, state, or federal levels. But it is also made by private entities. Clinics and hospitals have infection-control policies, visitation policies, and other rules pertaining to the work. Nursing schools have policies about student conduct and grading. Insurance companies create policies about how much of the physician's rate for services will be paid to advanced practice registered nurses (APRNs). Increasingly, policymakers in both private and public venues look to evidence to inform decisions.

In both venues, research alone is not responsible for producing policy. The rules for the use of data are the same, but as policy and political players change, so do considerations about research, how best to use findings, or even what research question

to ask. One can think of this as the political ecology of policymaking; that is, the many subtle and sometimes overt influences that surround the making of any policy.

WHAT IS RESEARCH WHEN IT COMES TO POLICY?

Research in policymaking venues involves the usual suspects in quantitative methodology, including the randomized controlled trial, although the opportunities for using this gold standard are fewer than in bench science. In recent years, systematic reviews and meta-analyses have become popular in advancing policy positions. These reviews sift, distill, and analyze quantitative data from the existing literature on a topic. The end product is a solid summary of evidence in one package; efficient for both advocates and policymakers.

Several recent systematic reviews examined the plethora of studies on nurse practitioner (NP) care, concluding that NP health outcomes compare favorably to those of physicians across a wide variety of measures (Newhouse et al., 2011; Stanik-Hutt et al., 2013). Research into NP practice, care, and outcomes is hardly novel; Walter Spitzer and colleagues published the first such study in 1973 (Spitzer et al., 1973). In the 40 years since, NPs have been extensively studied. Thus, systematic reviews of this literature, which summarize the best evidence, provide a useful reference for NPs in advocating for expanded scope of practice.

Data mining, the use of data collected from large data sets residing in large health systems and governments, offers a window into the discovery of problems and crafting of policy solutions; this marriage of data and health care policymaking also has a long history (Almasalha et al., 2013; Cheung, Moody, & Cockram, 2002; Diers, 2007; Duffield et al., 2009; Eriksen et al., 1997; Heslop et al., 2004). Using secondary data is challenging but rewarding given its immense scope in time and data points, compared with what most researchers can accomplish in traditional data collection (Smith et al., 2011).

Other sources of data also provide grist for the policymaking process. Policymakers are asked to make decisions in many different areas, and to do so most likely without personal expertise in any given area. Reports from expert panels, foundations, and government research agencies can all carry great weight, if introduced in the context of moving an issue forward. Op-ed pieces by experts and position papers generated by legislative staff or others can also be powerful. The point is that one must be wide open to sources when looking for evidence to support or oppose a policy position (Béland, 2010).

In presenting data to policymakers, it behooves the advocate to be short and to the point. Policymakers deal with a tremendous number of issues across economic, health, and social terrains. Keeping the focus on one's issue requires policy briefs that are short and specific to the problem and the policy solution (Food & Agriculture Organization of the United Nations, 2011).

Narrative, that is, the telling of a pertinent story to bring the issue to life, also has its place in the process (Epstein, Heidt, & Farina, 2012). Deborah Stone, a prominent observer of policymaking, refers to what she calls causal stories as necessary to the very genesis of a policy initiative. She notes that people have to view any particular trend, experience, or event as problematic and capable of solution (Stone, 2006); narrative data provide an effective mechanism for crafting this view.

THE CHEMISTRY BETWEEN RESEARCH AND POLICYMAKING

Research can be extremely useful in casting light on a problem and nudging policymakers to action. Nursing has a distinguished lineage of nurses affecting policy through the use of data, from Nightingale's Crimean data to American midwives who accomplished great things for their practice by persistent and consistent collection of ordinary practice data (Diers & Burst, 1983). Today, health care research examines how intricately intertwined in practice are the pieces of the health care puzzle: delivery, providers, procedures, patients, families, cultures, reimbursement, and so on. One consequence is a growing acknowledgement by non-nurse researchers of the role of nursing, and particularly advanced practice nursing in contemporary health care (Kuo et al., 2013).

USING RESEARCH TO CREATE, INFORM, AND SHAPE POLICY

Research rarely exists in a vacuum, particularly health services research which ideally knits the worlds of research and policy together. Béland (2010) and Béland and Waddan (2012) argue that research design and dissemination should be used strategically and tactically. The 2011 Institute of Medicine (IOM) seminal report, *The Future of Nursing: Leading Change, Advancing Health*, exemplifies strategic thinking. This evidence-based report summarizes the position of nursing in the United States health system and focuses on the barriers nursing faces in implementing the full effect of the profession's capacity to positively affect American health care. Savvy health services researchers seek to amplify that message, with studies tactically aimed at answering questions policymakers might have about the qualifications of APRNs to step into full leadership within the health care system as it evolves. In 2011, Newhouse and colleagues presented a systematic review of literature comparing APRN and physician health patient outcomes, with positive findings. In 2012, Newhouse published an article explaining the policy implications of the 2011 review. In 2013, Stanik-Hutt and colleagues published a systematic review, *The Quality and Effectiveness of Care Provided by Nurse Practitioners*, which provides a concise source of data on NP practice (Stanik-Hutt et al., 2013). Since the release of *The Future of Nursing* in 2011, other researchers have published on NPs in the wider venue of health services research (Carruth & Carruth, 2011; Dill et al., 2013; Kuo et al., 2013; Morgan et al., 2012; Pittman & Williams, 2012; Traczynski & Udalova,

2013). Each of these articles seeks to inform the greater conversation about advancing APRN practice within the context of promoting full practice authority as recommended by the 2011 IOM report.

RESEARCH AND POLITICAL WILL

The key to moving any issue into the public or institutional eye is transforming it into a political issue; that is, casting the issue as problematic enough to make public or private policymakers want to fix it. Effective research casts the problems it exposes as bad, even immoral, situations that must be addressed (Stone, 2006). But how will any particular issue be perceived among the numerous issues competing for attention? Sometimes political leaders themselves offer the issue as important, as has been the case with health care reform under the Obama administration. Other times, the issue comes to the fore because of particular news events, as with the increasing emphasis on human trafficking as a social and health problem. Framing the policy question at hand is essential, because it is fundamental to setting up the argument. Thus, the strategic use of research will anticipate the viewpoints of other stakeholders and seek to place the issue at hand at the top of the policy agenda.

Highlighting a problem and getting it on the agenda is not enough to advance policy in most instances. There must be enough political will to devote attention, time, and effort to solve the problem, particularly when the problem is pervasive or long-standing. Complex problems are challenging because it is difficult to capture a single framing perspective, leading to many differing opinions about what the real problem is and a subsequent dilution of political will about the issue. Health disparities have been extremely well documented, for example, and embraced by several presidential administrations as an issue that needs fixing. The ultimate measure of eliminating disparities is improved health status, but figuring out exactly what leads to good health is enormously complex. So it is difficult to propose a straightforward solution to ending disparities and thus difficult to capture sustained political will to undertake the work of eliminating this form of discrimination (Stone, 2006).

It is this interplay of research, political will, and policymaking that frequently frustrates action-oriented people such as nurses, who want to see change happen in a timely manner. Forty years of outcomes research documenting that APRNs are safe, competent providers is now coupled with a policy environment that is trying to solve the primary care provider shortage. It seems pretty straightforward, right? Several factors intervene that make the progress to full autonomous practice nationwide slow, sometimes agonizingly so. Nursing and, in particular, advanced practice nursing is not well understood outside of the outdated (and questionable) paradigm of working under physician orders. It is surprising how many legislators, even those whose personal provider *is* a nurse practitioner, have no idea that nurses are diagnosing and prescribing on their own, and very safely.

There is a second reason policymakers often do not jump readily toward removing barriers to practice. Often a very powerful stakeholder (e.g., organized medicine in one form or another) sits at the table, opposing any further entry into its world by nursing or other professionals. And like it or not, this is a potent disincentive for policymakers to move off the dime on an issue. So there must be a compelling story to engage legislators in advancing full autonomous nursing practice. In the past, the theme has been access to health care in rural areas. A quick look at the states who first achieved APRN practice independent of physician involvement (e.g., Alaska, Maine, and New Mexico) reveals that they have large rural populations in need of competent providers. Lately, the theme is turning to the decreased number of physicians entering or staying in primary care practice; something known from research into health care workforce distribution.

A number of recent studies illustrate that states with full practice for APRNs appear to provide the optimal environment to maximize use of APRN providers.[1] States with nurse practice acts or regulations

---

[1] Full practice means there is no mandate for physician presence such as supervision or collaborative agreement before an APRN can practice; it is not accurate to call this independent practice, as practice itself for any discipline is collaborative within the discipline and beyond.

that allow full APRN practice experience higher levels of APRN providers and thus higher levels of patients who have an APRN primary care provider (Kuo et al., 2013). APRNs enjoy consumer confidence, particularly among those most likely to have APRNs as the only choice of primary care provider (Dill et al., 2013). Full APRN practice does not negatively affect physician wages (Pittman & Williams, 2012). Examination of practice patterns in the federal Veterans Affairs health care settings confirms that there is no significant difference in the patient populations served by APRNs, physicians, or physician assistants (Morgan et al., 2012).

So in addition to setting the scene for policy intervention by illuminating a problem, research has a vital role in creating an atmosphere conducive for policymakers to step up to the plate, especially when the issue is likely to be controversial. Ginsburg (2008) offers some valuable insights about nursing in the hospital setting and the research necessary to capture policymakers' interest in nursing intensity and hospital payment; for instance. Moodie (2009) suggests that researchers interested in moving policy forward pay attention to what policymakers need answered, as well as the constituencies to which they have to answer, a theme also echoed by the September 2009 *Briefing Paper* from the Overseas Development Institute (Overseas Development Institute [ODI], 2009).

Moodie and the ODI are looking at research from a marketing viewpoint: the researcher is using data to persuade a policymaker that a certain policy answer is the one called for, based on the evidence. Moodie (2009) describes the various ecologic factors that a researcher should assess before designing any particular research with an eye toward influencing policy. The ODI paper (2009) also emphasizes Moodie's point that research needs to be mindfully performed *and* presented. "Simply presenting information to policymakers and expecting them to act upon it is very unlikely to work" (ODI, 2009, p. 1). The ODI sets forth five other lessons for policy entrepreneurs who want to involve policymakers in evidence-based decisions. This advice from non-nurse policy researchers recognizes that, in addition to highlighting a problem, research can enhance, perhaps even shape, the political climate in which change can occur; this is valuable advice to nursing as it continues its political and policy evolution. And along these lines, there is one other way research is influencing the policy context, through artful dissemination in documentaries seen on television and in movie theaters.

RESEARCH: NOT JUST FOR JOURNALS

In 2005, David Satcher (former Surgeon General in the Clinton Administration), with a host of public health and academic colleagues, published a study entitled, *What if we were equal? A comparison of the black-white mortality gap in 1960 and 2000* (Satcher et al., 2005). The study concluded that annually more than 83,000 excess deaths in the African-American community could be prevented if health disparities and their consequent gulag effect on access to care for minority populations were addressed.

This research, and other health disparity documentation, was picked up and studied again, journalistically, by Larry Adelman in 2008. He produced a 7-hour series called *Unnatural Causes*, which aired on PBS (Adelman, Stange, & Rutenbeck, 2008). During the segment entitled *In Sickness and in Wealth*, Dr. Adewale Troutman, Director of the Louisville, Kentucky, Metro Health Department, offers a compelling visual tour of both the physical and sociological realities of his city, vividly illustrating the interplay of poverty, social class, and health outcomes in what could be a new frontier of compelling qualitative research, which seeks to engage the public (and policymakers) directly through visual and narrative data. It is worth noting how effective such documentaries can be at getting an issue out into public discourse while bypassing special interests.

Nursing's future rests on the clear and convincing record of research on nursing work. Moving the future forward requires that nurses and others understand nursing's role in the complex and dynamic world of health and health care. As nursing is increasingly recognized as a vital pillar in the temple of health care, nurses must continue to document and broadcast who they are, what they do, and why it matters to patients, to policymakers, to budgets, and to the delivery of meaningful health care to all.

DISCUSSION QUESTIONS

1. What contexts inform the crafting of policy?
2. When and how does research connect with policymaking?
3. You and your research team have concluded that the consistent use of high-energy drinks by adolescents negatively impacts memory retention. Describe your strategy for bringing this to the attention of policymakers, such as your local school board or state legislators.

REFERENCES

Adelman, L., (Producer), Stange, E., (Director), & Rutenbeck, J., (Director) (2008). *Unnatural causes: Is inequality making us sick?* San Francisco, CA: California Newsreel with Vital Pictures. Retrieved from *www .unnaturalcauses.org*.

Almasalha, F., Xu, D., Kennan, G. M., Khokhar, A., Yao, Y., Chen, Y. C., et al. (2013). Data mining nursing care plans of end-of-life patients: A study to improve healthcare decision making. *International Journal of Nursing Knowledge, 24*(1), 15–24.

Béland, D. (2010). Policy change and health care research. *The Journal of Health Care Politics, Policy and Law, 35*(4), 615–641.

Béland, D., & Waddan, A. (2012). *The politics of policy change: Welfare, Medicare, and social security reform in the United States.* Washington, DC: Georgetown University Press.

Carruth, P. L., & Carruth, A. K. (2011). The financial and cost accounting implications of the increased role of advanced nurse practitioners in U.S. healthcare. *American Journal of Health Sciences, Fall*, 1–8.

Cheung, R. B., Moody, L. E., & Cockram, C. (2002). Data mining strategies for shaping nursing and health policy agendas. *Policy, Politics, & Nursing Practice, 3*(3), 248–260.

Diers, D. (2007). Finding midwifery in administrative data systems. *Journal of Midwifery and Women's Health, 52*(2), 98–105.

Diers, D., & Burst, H. V. (1983). Effectiveness of policy-related research: Nurse-midwifery as a case study. *Image–the Journal of Nursing Scholarship, 15*(3), 68–74.

Dill, M. J., Pankow, S., Erikson, C., & Shipman, S. (2013). Survey shows consumers open to greater role for physician assistants and nurse practitioners. *Health Affairs, 32*(6), 1135–1142.

Duffield, C., Diers, D., Aisbett, C., & Roche, M. (2009). Churn: Patient turnover and case mix. *Nursing Economics, 27*(3), 185–191.

Epstein, D., Heidt, J. B., & Farina, C. R. (2012). *The value of words: Narrative as evidence in policymaking.* Ithaca, New York: Cornell eRulemaking Initiative, Cornell Law School. Retrieved from *www.lawschool.cornell .edu/ceri/upload/2012-06-23-SitautedKnowldge-IPA-Final.pdf*.

Eriksen, L. R., Turley, J. P., Denton, D., & Manning, S. (1997). Data mining: a strategy for knowledge development and structure in nursing practice. *Studies in Health Technology and Informatics, 46*, 383–388.

Food & Agriculture Organization of the United Nations. (2011). *Food security communications toolkit.* Rome: Food & Agriculture Organization of the United Nations.

Ginsburg, P. B. (2008). Paying hospitals on the basis of nursing intensity. *Policy, Politics, & Nursing Practice, 9*(2), 118–120.

Heslop, L., Gardner, B., Diers, D., & Poh, B. C. (2004). Using clinical data for nursing research and management in health services. *Contemporary Nurse, 17*(1–2), 8–18.

Institute of Medicine. (2011). *The future of nursing: Leading change, advancing health.* Washington, DC: National Academies Press.

Kuo, Y. F., Loresto, F. L., Rounds, L. R., & Goodwin, J. S. (2013). States with the least restrictive regulations experienced the largest increase in patients seen by nurse practitioners. *Health Affairs, 32*(7), 1236–1243.

Moodie, R. (2009). Where different worlds collide: Expanding the influence of research and researchers on policy. *Journal of Public Health Policy, 30*(S1), S33–S37.

Morgan, P. A., Abbott, D. H., McNeil, R. B., & Fisher, D. A. (2012). Characteristics of primary care office visits to nurse practitioners, physician assistants and physicians in United States Veterans Health Administration facilities, 2005-2010: A retrospective cross-sectional analysis. *Human Resources for Health, 10*, 1–8.

Newhouse, R. P., Stanik-Hutt, J., White, K. M., Johantgen, M., Bas, E. B., Zangaro, G., et al. (2011). Advanced practice nurse outcomes 1990-2008: A systematic review. *Nursing Economics, 29*(5), 1–21.

Overseas Development Institute [ODI]. (2009). *Briefing paper 53: Helping researchers become policy entrepreneurs.* London: Overseas Development Institute.

Pittman, P., & Williams, B. (2012). Physician wages in states with expanded APRN scope of practice. *Nursing Research and Practice, 2012*, 671974.

Satcher, S., Fryer, G. E., McCann, J., Troutman, A., Woolf, S. H., & Rust, G. (2005). What if we were equal? A comparison of the black-white mortality gap in 1960 and 2000. *Health Affairs, 24*(2), 459–464.

Smith, A. K., Ayanian, J. Z., Covinsky, K. E., Landon, B. E., McCarthy, E. P., Wee, C. C., et al. (2011). Conducting high-value secondary dataset analysis: An introductory guide and resources. *Journal of General Internal Medicine, 26*(8), 920–929.

Spitzer, W., Kergin, D., Yoshida, M., Russell, W., Hackett, B., & Goldsmith, C. (1973). Nurse practitioners in primary care III: The southern Ontario randomized trial. *Canadian Medical Journal, 108*, 1005–1016.

Stanik-Hutt, J., Newhouse, R. P., White, K. M., Johantgen, M., Bass, E. B., Zangaro, G., et al. (2013). The quality and effectiveness of care provided by nurse practitioners. *The Journal for Nurse Practitioners, 9*(8), 492–500.

Stone, D. (2006). Reframing the racial disparities issue for state governments. *Journal of Health Politics, Policy and Law, 31*(1), 127–152.

Traczynski, J., & Udalova, V. (2013). Nurse practitioner independence, health care utilization, and health outcomes. Retrieved from *www .lafollette.wisc.edu/research/health_economics/Traczynski.pdf*.

ONLINE RESOURCES

Kaiser Family Foundation. This site has a wealth of current information about American health care and reform efforts in the states and at the federal level.
kff.org

World Health Organization. This site is the leading voice for global health data and public health initiatives across the world.
www.who.int/en/

State Nursing and/or Advanced Practice Nursing Organization's websites. These sites are often the best source for information and initiatives affecting the current and future practice in nursing.

CHAPTER 12

Health Services Research: Translating Research into Policy

Patricia W. Stone   Arlene M. Smaldone   Robert J. Lucero   Yoon Jeong Choi

"Research is formalized curiosity. It is poking and prying with a purpose."

Zora Neale Hurston

The high cost of health care, large numbers of uninsured Americans, uncontrolled health care spending, and an unstable economy have led to the most recent efforts to reform health care in the United States. Most health policy experts agree that the nation must control health care costs, improve efficiency, increase access to health care, and improve the quality of care. However, it is often unclear how best to make these improvements. A strong evidence base is needed to inform decision makers on what does and does not work to improve the health care system. Research that attempts to provide this evidence is often called health services research (HSR).

DEFINING HEALTH SERVICES RESEARCH

AcademyHealth, the preeminent professional society for health services researchers, defines HSR as "the multidisciplinary field of scientific investigation that studies how social factors, financing systems, organizational structures and processes, health technologies, and personal behaviors affect access to health care, the quality and cost of health care, and ultimately our health and well-being. Its research domains are individuals, families, organizations, institutions, communities, and populations" (AcademyHealth, 2008). The Agency for Healthcare Research and Quality (AHRQ) states

that HSR "examines how people get access to health care, how much care costs, and what happens to patients as a result of this care. Health services research aims to identify the most effective ways to organize, manage, finance, and deliver high-quality care; reduce medical errors; and improve patient safety" (Helping the Nation with Health Services Research, 2002).

A recent focus of HSR, based on the Comparative Effectiveness Research Act of 2008, is the conduct and synthesis of research comparing the benefits and harms of various interventions. HSR also studies strategies for preventing, diagnosing, treating, and monitoring health conditions in real-world settings (Conway & Clancy, 2009). The purpose of comparative effectiveness research (CER) is to improve health outcomes by developing and disseminating evidence-based information to patients, clinicians, and other decision makers about interventions that are most effective for patients under specific circumstances (Iglehart, 2009; Volpp & Das, 2009). The U.S. Department of Health and Human Services (HHS), as part of the American Recovery and Reinvestment Act of 2009, provided $400 million of financial support for CER. In June 2009, the Institute of Medicine recommended 100 national priorities for CER (Committee on Comparative Effectiveness Research Prioritization, Institute of Medicine, 2009). Of the top 25 priorities, the following may be of particular interest to nurses: (1) Compare the effectiveness of various primary care treatment strategies and (2) compare the effectiveness of literacy-sensitive disease management programs and usual care in reducing disparities in children and adults with low literacy and chronic disease. The Affordable Care

Act (ACA) authorizes CER and a number of demonstration projects that will use HSR methods.

The Patient-Centered Outcomes Research Institute (PCORI) is the United States–based nongovernmental institute created as part of the ACA. The mission of the PCORI is to examine and evaluate relative health outcomes, clinical effectiveness, and appropriateness of different medical treatments through existing studies and conducting its own. Its board includes patients, nurses, physicians, hospitals, drug makers, device manufacturers, insurers, payers, government officials, and health experts. The PCORI is different from other international bodies such as the United Kingdom's National Institute for Health and Clinical Excellence, which determines cost-effectiveness directly, based on quality-adjusted life year valuations. The PCORI does not have power to mandate or even endorse coverage rules or reimbursement for any particular treatment. However, the HHS may take research findings funded by the PCORI into account when deciding what procedures it will cover.

A long-standing challenge has been the capacity of the U.S. health care system to translate innovation from research into practice at a faster pace. Dougherty and Conway (2008) developed a model intended to accelerate implementation of innovations in clinical settings to address the how of health care delivery (Figure 12-1). This transformational model suggests that basic science and its translation into clinical practice is only the first step to achieve effective and safe delivery of high-quality care (translation 1 or T1). Translation 2 (T2) processes focus on the translation of clinical efficacy knowledge into clinical effectiveness, and the policy changes needed to improve outcomes is addressed in translation 3 (T3) activities. HSR and CER are the necessary population-based research activities at the T2 level and serve as the foundation for effective health policy.

HSR METHODS

HSR researchers use both quantitative and qualitative research methods, and these methods are not unique to the field. However, it is the use of these methods to generate knowledge to inform health policy development and changes that is the hallmark of HSR. Edwardson (2007) reported on the theories and conceptual frameworks used by HSR nurse researchers in studies funded by the AHRQ between 2000 and early 2005. A total of 28 different frameworks were identified in the 49 studies reviewed. The frameworks most often used were Donabedian's Quality Paradigm (Donabedian, 1966) (i.e., structure-process-outcome), Rogers' Diffusion of Innovation Theory (Rogers, 2003), Reason's Theory of Human Error (Reason, 1990), and Aday and Andersen's Model of Health Care Access (Aday & Andersen, 1974). The common

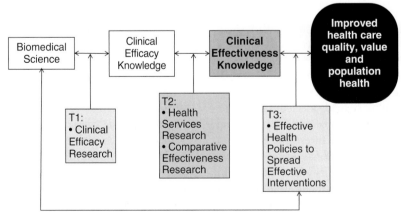

FIGURE 12-1 Transforming health care across the research spectrum. (Adapted from Dougherty, D., & Conway, P. H. [2008]. The "3T's" road map to transform US health care: The "how" of high-quality care. *Journal of the American Medical Association, 299*[19], 2319-2321.)

theoretical underpinning among these frameworks is their conceptualization of variables at the system level rather than the individual level.

QUANTITATIVE METHODS AND DATA SETS

Using quantitative multivariate methods, HSR researchers often analyze data from administrative data sets, such as hospital discharge data, and national survey data to examine health care access and quality, regional differences in care delivery patterns, health behavior patterns, and health outcomes from a population perspective. Various types of data are available to HSR researchers through the federal agencies in the HHS including the Centers for Disease Control and Prevention's National Center for Health Statistics (NCHS) and AHRQ. Additionally, population census and employment data are available through the U.S. Census Bureau and the Bureau of Labor Statistics.

Often researchers must combine data from multiple sources or over multiple years. The researcher must become familiar with the data set methodology report and list of variables with their respective definitions to ascertain how variables are categorized, the sampling methodology employed, and how missing data were handled. National surveys often use complex sampling frames and employ sampling weights enabling generalizability of survey findings to the population at large. To effectively use data sets that employ weighted sampling requires expertise in the use of statistical analysis software such as SAS (SAS Institute Inc., Cary, NC, USA) that allows for incorporation of sampling weights into the data analysis process. Table 12-1 provides descriptions of several publically available data sets that are available to health services researchers. What follows are examples of how these data have been used to inform policy.

Using data from the Hospital Consumer Assessment of Healthcare Providers and Systems, Kutney-Lee and colleagues (2009) designed a cross-sectional study using multivariate regression modeling techniques to examine the relationship between nurse staffing levels and patient perceptions of their nursing care across 430 hospitals in 4 states

(California, New Jersey, Pennsylvania, and Florida). Higher nurse-patient ratios and better work environments were associated with greater patient satisfaction. These findings demonstrate that appropriate staffing levels are important to patient satisfaction and support ongoing efforts to improve hospital performance.

The National Health and Nutrition Examination Survey (NHANES) data (n.d.) have been instrumental in tracking the prevalence of health problems such as obesity and diabetes over time, and examining factors that may be associated with changes in prevalence. Using 24-hour dietary recall data from two cross-sectional NHANES surveys (NHANES III 1988-1994 and NHANES 1999-2004), researchers examined national trends in sugar-sweetened beverage consumption among adults 20 years of age or older (Bleich et al., 2009). During this study period, both the percentage of adults who consumed sugar-sweetened beverages (58% vs. 63%) and daily caloric intake from these beverages (239 vs. 294 calories) increased and accounted for a significant proportion of daily caloric intake. Based on these and other findings, the taxation of sugar-sweetened beverages has received increasing interest as a policy option to decrease obesity (Brownell & Frieden, 2009).

Another group of researchers (Mark et al., 2004) used longitudinal National Inpatient Sample data (1990-1995) combined with other national data sets to examine the effects of changes in registered nurse (RN) staffing on quality of care in a sample of 422 hospitals from 11 states. The quality of care was based on measures of inpatient mortality and three nurse-sensitive outcomes: hospital-acquired pneumonia, urinary tract infection, and pressure sores. Hospitals were stratified by level of RN staffing. The magnitude of effect of a one-unit increase in RN staffing on inpatient mortality was greater for hospitals at the 25th percentile of staffing compared with the 75th percentile of staffing, suggesting a nonlinear relationship between RN staffing and inpatient mortality. There may be a staffing threshold that dictates an optimal level of staffing to improve patient outcomes. The evidence supports administrators to develop nurse staffing

TABLE 12-1 Examples of Publicly Available Data for Use in Health Services Research

Data	Description	Fees
U.S. Department of Health and Human Services (HHS)		
Hospital Consumer Assessment of Healthcare Providers and Systems (HCAHPS) *www.medicare.gov/ hospitalcompare*	• National patient survey of hospital care quality • 32 items • 9 key areas: communication with doctors, communication with nurses, responsiveness of hospital staff, pain management, communication about medicines, discharge information, cleanliness of the hospital environment, quietness of the hospital environment, and transition of care	Free
Area Health Resource File (AHRF) *www.arf.hrsa.gov*	• National county-level health resource information database • >6000 county-level variables on health care professionals, hospitals and health care facilities, population characteristics, health care use, and socioeconomic and environmental characteristics	Free
Centers for Disease Control and Prevention (CDC)		
Behavioral Risk Factor Surveillance System (BRFSS) *www.cdc.gov/brfss*	• State-level national estimates of health risk behaviors among U.S. adult populations • Largest telephone health survey system in the world • Cell phone survey added in 2008 for more representative sample • Contains survey questions on smoking, alcohol use, physical inactivity, diet, hypertension, and seatbelt use • Asthma call-back survey piloted in three states in 2005 and conducted each year • Data available from 1984	Free
National Health and Nutrition Examination Survey (NHANES) *www.cdc.gov/nchs/nhanes.htm*	• First administered in 1971 • Health and nutritional status of adults and children in the U.S. • Contains interviews, physical examinations, and laboratory data • Complex multilevel statistical sampling of randomly selected households • Assess prevalence of health problems or examine factors associated with changes in prevalence • Data available from 1999	Free
National Immunization Survey (NIS) *www.cdc.gov/nis*	• Produce timely estimates of childhood immunization coverage rates as Advisory Committee on Immunization Practices (ACIP) recommended • Children 19 to 35 months • List-assisted random-digit-dialing telephone survey followed by mailed survey • Vaccinations: DTap, polio, MCV, Hib, Hep B, varicella zoster, PCV, Hep A, and FLU • Data available from 1995	Free
National Survey of Ambulatory Surgery (NSAS) *www.cdc.gov/nchs/nsas.htm*	• National data of ambulatory surgical care in hospital-based and freestanding ambulatory surgery centers • First conducted from 1994 to 1996, resumed again in 2006 • Patient demographics, sources of payment, information on anesthesia given, diagnoses, surgical and nonsurgical procedures	Free

TABLE 12-1 Examples of Publicly Available Data for Use in Health Services Research—cont'd

Data	Description	Fees
National Survey of Children with Special Health Care Needs (NS-CSHCN) *www.cdc.gov/nchs/slaits/cshcn.htm*	• To assess the prevalence and impact of special health care needs among children in the United States • To explore the extent to which children with special health care needs (CSHCN) have medical homes, adequate health insurance, access to needed services, and adequate care coordination • Other topics: functional difficulties, transition services, shared decision making, and satisfaction with care • Interviews conducted with parents or guardians • Data available in 2001, 2005-2006, and 2009-2010	Free
National Survey of Children's Health (NSCH) *www.cdc.gov/nchs/slaits/nsch.htm*	• Examines the physical and emotional health of children aged 0 to 17 years old. • Well-being of children including medical homes, family interactions, parental health, school and after-school experiences, and safe neighborhoods • To assess the awareness of, experience with, and interest in enrolling Medicaid and the State Children's Health Insurance Program (CHIP) for parents with uninsured children • Data available in 2003, 2007, and 2011-2012	Free

Agency for Healthcare Research and Quality (AHRQ)

Data	Description	Fees
Nationwide Inpatient Sample (NIS) *www.hcup-us.ahrq.gov/nisoverview.jsp*	• One of the Healthcare Cost and Utilization Project (HCUP) databases • Largest publicly available all-payer inpatient care database in the U.S. • Hospital inpatient stays database • Data available through HCUP central distributor from 1988	Fees vary
Kids' Inpatient Database (KID) *www.hcup-us.ahrq.gov/kidoverview.jsp*	• One of the HCUP databases • Only all-payer inpatient care database for children in the U.S. • Hospital inpatient stays for children • Conditions and procedures related to child health issues • Data available through HCUP central distributor in 1997, 2000, 2003, 2006, 2009	Fees vary
Nationwide Emergency Department Sample (NEDS) *www.hcup-us.ahrq.gov/nedsoverview.jsp*	• One of the HCUP databases • Largest all-payer emergency department database in the U.S. • Records from both the HCUP State Emergency Department Databases (SEDD) and the State Inpatient Databases (SID) • Data available through HCUP central distributor from 2006	Fees vary
State Inpatient Databases (SID) *www.hcup-us.ahrq.gov/sidoverview.jsp*	• One of the HCUP databases • Hospital databases from data organizations in participating states • Inpatient discharge abstract including clinical and nonclinical information • Data available through HCUP central distributor from 1990	Fees vary

Continued

TABLE 12-1 Examples of Publicly Available Data for Use in Health Services Research—cont'd

Data	Description	Fees
State Ambulatory Surgery Databases (SASD) www.hcup-us.ahrq.gov/ sasdoverview.jsp	• One of the HCUP databases • Ambulatory surgeries performed on the same day in which patients are admitted and released from data organizations in participating states • Data available through HCUP central distributor from 1997	Fees vary
State Emergency Department Databases (SEDD) www.hcup-us.ahrq.gov/ seddoverview.jsp	• One of the HCUP databases • Emergency department discharge information • Data available through HCUP central distributor from 1999	Fees vary
Medical Expenditure Panel Survey (MEPS) meps.ahrq.gov/mepsweb/	• First administered in 1996 • Large-scale surveys of families and individuals, their medical providers, and employers • Medical care use and expenditures • Major components: Household, insurance, medical provider, and nursing home (in 1996 only) components	Free
American Hospital Association (AHA)		
Annual Survey Database ams.aha.org/EWEB/ DynamicPage.aspx?WebCode =ProdDetailAdd&ivd_prc_ prd_key=95806632-0d48- 4819-bd7f-2b3c1343660b	• Comprehensive snapshot of U.S. hospitals based on primary survey data from the AHA Annual Survey of Hospitals, AHA membership data, and U.S. Census Bureau identifiers • Information on 6500 hospitals	Fees vary
American Nurses Association (ANA)		
National Database of Nursing Quality Indicators (NDNQI) www.nursingworld.org/Main MenuCategories/ThePractice ofProfessionalNursing/Patient SafetyQuality/Research -Measurement/Data-Access	• Managed by University of Kansas Medical Center School of Nursing • Collects unit-specific nurse-sensitive data from over 1500 hospitals across the nation • The NDNQI Research Council reviews proposals submitted to the ANA for access to NDNQI data	Fees vary
All-Payer Claims Database (APCD) Council		
All-Payer Claims Database (APCD) www.apcdcouncil.org/state/map (As of November 24, 2014 APCDs are currently available in 13 states: Colorado, Kansas, Maine, Maryland, Massachusetts, Minnesota, New Hampshire, Oregon, Rhode Island, Tennessee, Utah, Vermont, and Wisconsin)	• Large-scale databases that systematically collect health care claims from a variety of payer sources • Payers include private insurance carriers, pharmacy benefit managers, dental benefit administrators, Medicaid, Medicare, and Medicare Part D • APCD data can help to guide health reform policies such as payment reform and global payments • Emerging data source currently in development	Fees vary by state and years of data requested

plans and policymakers to advance nurse staffing legislation.

As a last example, using multiple national data sets including census and National Hospital Care Survey (NHCS) data, researchers found differences in life expectancy due to race and educational attainments (Olshansky et al., 2012). The researchers found that in 2008, adult men and women with less than a high school education had life expectancies not much better than those of all adults in the 1950s and 1960s. Furthermore, white men and women with 16 years or more of schooling had life expectancies far greater than black Americans with fewer than 12 years of education. The researchers concluded that educational enhancements for people of all ages and races were needed to reduce the large gap in health.

QUALITATIVE METHODS

Whereas quantitative research results have historically been used as evidence to support health care decision making by clinicians, hospital administrators, and policymakers, qualitative research methods can be used to address complex health care problems that require a collection of varied information. Qualitative HSR has not been used frequently in decision making to improve health services delivery (Rusinova et al., 2009). This may be in part caused by the long-held notion that the findings from qualitative research are anecdotal or subject to biases. However, the use of qualitative research methods (e.g., structured interview, focus groups, and participant observations) can produce contextual data on perceptions, beliefs, experiences, and behavior to create a rich understanding of a problem (Auerbach & Silverstein, 2003). These data can be used to create a more complete understanding of what interventions and/or strategies are necessary at the clinical, organizational, or policy level.

The use of rigorous qualitative research methods by HSR researchers has increased over the past decade. Qualitative methods may be used in mixed-methods research, in the development of survey questionnaires, and in research where the aim is to gain the perspective of stakeholders regarding a particular topic. For example, researchers (Elder et al.,

2007) conducted focus groups using a sample of African-American adults housed temporarily in South Carolina hotels following Hurricane Katrina to identify why New Orleans residents decided to either remain in their homes or heed local warnings to evacuate. The use of focus groups led to the discovery of a number of themes, including misperceptions about the severity of the hurricane because of miscommunication, and evacuation barriers related to poverty and concern about neighborhood crime. Future disaster preparedness plans targeted at underserved minority communities should consider the importance of culturally sensitive approaches.

PROFESSIONAL TRAINING IN HEALTH SERVICES RESEARCH

HSR has a tradition of training that emphasizes multidisciplinary education. Providing answers to complex health and health care problems requires a diverse research skill set. Traditional clinical research approaches (i.e., epidemiology, biology, chemistry) coupled with social and economic sciences use a combination of quantitative and qualitative methodologies to address health and health care problems. From randomized controlled trials to qualitative case studies, there is a strong emphasis on interdisciplinary research that addresses health service policy needs, is patient-centered, and addresses system-level problems.

COMPETENCIES

Fourteen core competencies for doctoral-prepared HSR researchers have been proposed (Forrest et al., 2009). Based on these, the authors of this chapter developed core curriculum and the associated competencies for nurse HSR scientists listed in Table 12-2. Nurse faculties may use this core curriculum to develop policy-related content in their doctoral programs. Aspiring nurse HSR scientists should review the competencies to self-assess their knowledge and expertise in these areas and strive to augment their education to gain competency in all areas.

A research doctorate (e.g., PhD) is the usual educational pathway to become a HSR researcher

TABLE 12-2 Nursing Health Services Research Doctoral-Level Core Competencies

Competency	CURRICULAR FOCUS	
	Analytic	Theory
1. Demonstrate breadth of comparative and cost-effectiveness research theoretical and conceptual knowledge by applying alternative models from a range of relevant disciplines including clinical epidemiology, biomedical informatics, health services research, biostatistics, and health economics.		C, I, H, B, E
2. Apply in-depth nursing disciplinary knowledge and skills relevant to comparative and cost-effectiveness research related to health promotion and/or disease prevention across the continuum of care in high-risk, underserved populations.	C, I, H, B, E, N	C, I, H, B, E, N
3. Apply knowledge of the structures, performance, quality, policy, and environmental context of health and health care to formulate value nursing solutions for health policy problems related to health promotion and/or disease prevention across the continuum of care in high-risk, underserved populations.	C, I, H, B, E	N
4. Pose innovative and important comparative and cost-effectiveness research questions informed by systematic reviews of the literature, stakeholder needs, and relevant theoretical and conceptual models to improve the care of high-risk, underserved populations.	C, I, H, B, E	C, I, H, B, E, N
5. Select appropriate interventional, observational, or qualitative study designs to address specific comparative and cost-effectiveness research questions to improve health promotion and/or disease prevention across the continuum of care in high-risk, underserved populations.	C, I, H, B, E	N
6. Know how to collect primary health outcome and health care utilization data obtained by survey, qualitative, or mixed methods.	C, I, H, B, E	
7. Know how to assemble and access secondary data from existing public and private sources.	C, I, H, B, E	
8. Use conceptual models and operational measures to specify study constructs for comparative and cost-effectiveness research questions and develop variables that reliably and validly measure these constructs.		C, I, H, B, E, N
9. Implement comparative and cost-effectiveness research protocols with standardized procedures that ensure reproducibility of the science.	C, I, H, B, E, N	
10. Ensure the ethical and responsible conduct of research in the design, implementation, and dissemination of comparative and cost-effectiveness research related to health promotion and/or disease prevention across the continuum of care in high-risk, underserved populations.	C, I, H, B, E	N, D
11. Work collaboratively in multidisciplinary teams.	C, I, H, B, E, N	
12. Use appropriate analytic methods in comparative and cost-effectiveness research to clarify associations between variables and to delineate causal inferences.	C, I, H, B, E	
13. Effectively communicate the findings and implications of comparative and cost-effectiveness research through multiple modalities to technical and lay audiences.	D	
14. Understand the importance of collaborating with stakeholders, such as policymakers, organizations, and communities to plan, conduct, and translate comparative and cost-effectiveness research into policy and practice.	D	

B, Biostatistics in comparative effectiveness research; *C*, clinical epidemiology; *D*, communication and dissemination; *E*, health economics; *H*, health services research; *I*, biomedical informatics; *N*, nursing.

The authors of this chapter (Stone, P. B., Smaldone, A. M., Lucero, R. J., and Choi, Y. J.) developed core curriculum and associated competencies for nurse HSR scientists by using competencies proposed by Forrest, C. B., Martin, D. P., Holve, E., & Millman, A. (2009, June 25). Health services research doctoral core competencies. *BMC Health Services Research, 9,* 107.

and develop knowledge that influences policymaking. Few schools of nursing have the capacity to train nurses to become HSR scientists; therefore, it is important to identify a university that has a HSR training program. HSR training takes place in a number of disciplines, including nursing, public health, business, and public policy. Schools of nursing that offer HSR training often provide interdisciplinary opportunities through partnerships with other disciplines. This is key to developing the competencies of the nurse HSR scientist.

FELLOWSHIPS AND TRAINING GRANTS

Funding for training in HSR comes from a variety of sources including government-funded institutional and individual training grants. In the past, the AHRQ was the primary funder of HSR. Nurses have successfully competed for individual HSR dissertation awards (R36) and postdoctoral research training awards.

Although not the primary mission of the National Institutes of Health (NIH), increasingly it is interested in funding HSR. The National Institute of Nursing Research (NINR) provides universities competitive funds for institutional training grants. These funds are given directly to schools of nursing to provide qualified students with stipends for living expenses, funds for tuition and fees, as well as limited travel to scientific meetings. Indeed, there are training grants that prepare predoctoral and postdoctoral students to conduct comparative effectiveness research. Additionally, doctoral students who have matriculated can apply for individual National Research Service Awards (NRSA), which provides similar funding for institutional training grants. The F31 funding mechanism is designed to support individual predoctoral students. Because the F31 is a training award, major considerations in the review are applicants' potential, their proposed research training plans, as well as institutional environment and commitment to training. The NIH RePORTER (*project reporter.nih.gov/reporter.cfm*) provides access to NIH-funded research projects. A list of NIH-funded F31 projects can be found on this website by

selecting the *F31 Predoctoral* activity code under the project details section.

LOAN REPAYMENT PROGRAMS

Along with concurrent funding for HSR training with predoctoral and postdoctoral fellowships, there are various mechanisms of federally qualified loan repayment programs. The NIH and Health Resources and Services Administration (HRSA) provide funding to encourage health professionals to pursue careers in health-related research at colleges and universities. The NIH Loan Repayment Programs (LRPs) (*www.lrp.nih.gov/index.aspx*) focuses on biomedical, behavioral, social, and clinical research. For at least a 1-year commitment of conducting qualified research, the NIH may repay up to $35,000 of student loan debt per year (National Institutes of Health Division of Loan Repayment, 2013). Unlike the HRSA Faculty Loan Repayment Program, the NIH LRP awards are based on a competitive peer-review process. There are two HRSA loan repayment programs (*www.hrsa.gov/loanscholarships/index.html*), the Faculty Loan Repayment Program (FLRP) and the NURSE Corps Loan Repayment Program (Health Resources and Services Administration, 2013). Individuals who participate in the FLRP can currently receive up to $40,000, plus a tax benefit, for 2 years of service at an accredited health professions college or university; or, if selected to participate in the NURSE Corps Loan Repayment Program, can receive up to 60% of their qualifying student loans repaid over 2 years plus the option for a third year to repay an additional 25%. More details about eligibility and service requirements can be found by visiting the websites listed above.

DISSEMINATION AND TRANSLATION OF RESEARCH INTO POLICY

There are a number of scientific journals that focus on HSR (e.g., *Health Affairs, Health Services Research, Medical Care,* and *Policy, Politics, & Nursing Practice*). As a source for scientific dissemination, AcademyHealth has become the primary interdisciplinary professional association for HSR researchers. As a component of AcademyHealth, the Interdisciplinary Research Group on Nursing Issues (IRGNI) provides a forum for researchers interested in promoting and supporting the development of HSR that focuses on nursing practice, workforce, and delivery of care. These venues have become important mechanisms to disseminate evidence for policy development and to guide the field of HSR.

DISCUSSION QUESTIONS

1. Based on Table 12-2, list any core competencies you have achieved. For those you have yet to achieve, develop a plan to achieve them.
2. Look up an existing data set listed in Table 12-1. Write a research question that could be answered using this data set and would be of interest to policymakers.
3. Review a current policy brief. What types of data were used in the evidence that informed the policy brief?

REFERENCES

AcademyHealth. (2008). What is HSR? Retrieved from *www.academy health.org/About/content.cfm?ItemNumber=831&navItemNumber=514*.

Aday, L. A., & Andersen, R. (1974). A framework for the study of access to medical care. *Health Services Research, 9*(3), 208–220.

Auerbach, C. F., & Silverstein, L. B. (2003). *Qualitative data: An introduction to coding and analysis*. New York: New York University Press.

Bleich, S. N., Wang, Y. C., Wang, Y., & Gortmaker, S. L. (2009). Increasing consumption of sugar-sweetened beverages among US adults: 1988-1994 to 1999-2004. *American Journal of Clinical Nutrition, 89*(1), 372–381.

Brownell, K. D., & Frieden, T. R. (2009). Ounces of prevention—The public policy case for taxes on sugared beverages. *New England Journal of Medicine, 360*(18), 1805–1808.

Committee on Comparative Effectiveness Research Prioritization, Institute of Medicine. (2009). Initial national priorities for comparative effectiveness research. Retrieved from *www.iom.edu/Object.File/Master/71/107/CER%20report%20brief%206%2030%2009.pdf*.

Conway, P. H., & Clancy, C. (2009). Comparative-effectiveness research—Implications of the Federal Coordinating Council's report. *New England Journal of Medicine, 361*(4), 328–330.

Donabedian, A. (1966). Evaluating the quality of medical care. *Milbank Memorial Fund Quarterly, 44*(Suppl. 3), 166–206.

Dougherty, D., & Conway, P. H. (2008). The "3T's" road map to transform US health care: The "how" of high-quality care. *Journal of the American Medical Association, 299*(19), 2319–2321.

Edwardson, S. R. (2007). Conceptual frameworks used in funded nursing health services research projects. *Nursing Economic$, 25*(4), 222–227.

Elder, K., Xirasagar, S., Miller, N., Bowen, S. A., Glover, S., & Piper, C. (2007). African Americans' decisions not to evacuate New Orleans before Hurricane Katrina: A qualitative study. *American Journal of Public Health, 97*(Suppl. 1), S124–S129.

Forrest, C. B., Martin, D. P., Holve, E., & Millman, A. (2009). Health services research doctoral core competencies. *BMC Health Services Research, 9*, 107.

Health Affairs. (2013). Health policy brief: Health gaps, health affairs. Retrieved from *www.healthaffairs.org/healthpolicybriefs/brief.php?brief_id=98*.

Health Resources and Services Administration. (2013). Loans & scholarships. Retrieved from *www.hrsa.gov/loanscholarships/index.html*.

Helping the Nation with Health Services Research. (2002). Retrieved from *www.ahrq.gov/news/focus/scenarios.pdf*.

Hospital Consumer Assessment of Healthcare Providers and Systems (HCAHPS). (2009). HCAHPS fact sheet. Retrieved from *www.hcahpsonline.org/files/HCAHPS%20Fact%20Sheet,%20revised1,%203-31-09.pdf*.

Iglehart, J. K. (2009). Prioritizing comparative-effectiveness research—IOM recommendations. *New England Journal of Medicine, 361*(4), 325–328.

Kutney-Lee, A., McHugh, M. D., Sloane, D. M., Cimiotti, J. P., Flynn, L., Neff, D. F., et al. (2009). Nursing: A key to patient satisfaction. *Health Affairs (Millwood), 28*(4), w669–w677.

Mark, B. A., Harless, D. W., McCue, M., & Xu, Y. (2004). A longitudinal examination of hospital registered nurse staffing and quality of care. *Health Services Research, 39*(2), 279–300.

The National Health and Nutrition Examination Survey. (n.d.) Retrieved from *www.cdc.gov/nchs/nhanes/about_nhanes.htm*.

National Institutes of Health Division of Loan Repayment. (2013). Retrieved from *www.lrp.nih.gov/index.aspx*.

Olshansky, S. J., Antonucci, T., Berkman, L., Binstock, R. H., Boersch-Supan, A., Cacioppo, J. T., et al. (2012). Differences in life expectancy due to race and educational differences are widening, and many may not catch up. *Health Affairs, 31*(8), 1803–1813.

Reason, J. (1990). *Human error*. Cambridge, UK: Cambridge University Press.

Rogers, E. (2003). *Diffusion of innovations* (5th ed.). New York: Free Press.

Rusinova, K., Frederic, P., Kentish-Barnes, N., Marine, C., & Azoulay, E. (2009). Qualitative research: Adding drive and dimension to clinical research. *Critical Care Medicine, 37*(1), S140–S146.

Volpp, K. G., & Das, A. (2009). Comparative effectiveness—Thinking beyond medication A versus medication B. *New England Journal of Medicine, 361*(4), 331–333.

ONLINE RESOURCES

Agency for Healthcare Research and Quality
www.campusrn.com/scholarships/768/a/ahrq_research_grants.html

CHAPTER 13

Using Research to Advance Health and Social Policies for Children

Louise Kahn   Freida Hopkins Outlaw   Sally S. Cohen

"There can be no keener revelation of a society's soul than the way in which it treats its children."

Nelson Mandela

Over the past decade, policymakers involved with children's issues have faced enormous challenges related to underperforming schools, overburdened health care systems, the increasing cost of public services, and fragmented approaches to the various problems. The importance of addressing these challenges has been recognized and they are now addressed using evidence-based research to inform both interventions and policy. New research findings have established the relationships among factors such as children's early brain development, poverty, other social determinants of health and well-being, and traumatic events. Researchers have also confirmed the influence of these factors on unrealized human potential and poor quality of life in the form of negative outcomes in later years (Felitti et al., 1998; Shonkoff & Phillips, 2000). Researchers and professionals who work with families with young children are noting the significance of conceptualizing child health policy more broadly, moving from individual approaches to a public health focus and encompassing the many aspects of social policy that affect children's well-being. The purposes of this chapter are to identify the major themes pertaining to social policies for children, explain how research has enhanced such policies, describe the remaining gaps in children's social policy and research, and explain how nurses can make meaningful contributions to the advancement of healthy social policies for children.

RESEARCH ON EARLY BRAIN DEVELOPMENT

Evidence regarding infant brain development in the 1990s propelled children's advocates and researchers to push for interventions with young children and families within the first few years of the life of the child. The groundbreaking report, *From Neurons to Neighborhoods: The Science of Early Childhood Development* (Shonkoff & Phillips, 2000), provided findings regarding the effects of genetics, environment, and early stress on brain architecture. In the 1990s collaborative research between the Centers for Disease Control and Prevention (CDC) and Kaiser Permanente demonstrated strong epidemiological evidence for the relationship between childhood trauma and long-term health and social outcomes (Felitti et al., 1998). This collaborative research on adverse childhood experiences (ACE), using data from 17,000 participants, is ongoing and continues to reveal the strong health, mental health, and social impacts of childhood adversity on their lives (Felitti & Anda, 2010).

In the 2000s, using neuroimaging technology and research, scientists demonstrated the impact of neurophysiologic and neurodevelopmental stress, trauma, and neglect on children. Their findings confirmed the need for safe, predictable, and enriched environments for young children (Perry, 2010).

In 2010 the Harvard Center for the Developing Child published *The Foundations of Lifelong Health are Built in Early Childhood*, a report that described how early life experiences manifest in the human body. The authors also described how significant adversity in childhood could undermine the body's stress response systems causing deleterious effects on the brain, immune system, cardiovascular system, and metabolism. They suggested that these effects on children could persist and lead to lifelong physical and mental health impairment (Center on the Developing Child, 2010).

RESEARCH ON SOCIAL DETERMINANTS OF HEALTH AND HEALTH DISPARITIES

Many national and international organizations have published reports with similar conclusions regarding the relationship between social determinants of health and health outcomes. Among them are the World Health Organization's (WHO, 2009) final report on health equity and social determinants of health, *Healthy People 2020* (U.S. Department of Health and Human Services [HHS], 2010), and a landmark Institute of Medicine study on health disparities entitled *Unequal Treatment: Confronting Ethnic and Racial Disparities in Health Care* (Smedley, Stith, & Nelson, 2003). All of these reports provide scientific evidence regarding how social determinants often play a larger role in determining health outcomes than clinical interventions.

Several themes emerge from recent reports in the area of children's health. Specifically, children of low socioeconomic status experience significant disparities in their health (Egerter et al., 2008). Economically disadvantaged and minority families in the United States have the highest rates of infant mortality. Children from poor racially segregated neighborhoods have more challenges than other children in accessing the services needed to maintain good health (Acevedo-Garcia et al., 2008).

ADVANCING CHILDREN'S MENTAL HEALTH USING RESEARCH TO INFORM POLICY

Approximately one in five children (13%-20%) in the United Sates has a serious mental illness that interferes with their functioning in the home, school, and community. Mental illness also harms children's relationships with their peers (CDC, 2013). Moreover, 21% of children between 9 and 17

years old have a diagnosable mental or addictive disorder that causes some level of impairment (National Alliance on Mental Illness [NAMI], 2013). Children's mental health needs accounted for $247 billion in health expenditures in the United States during 2007 (Miles et al., 2010).

Given the prevalence of mental health disorders in children, new approaches that integrate all child-focused systems are needed. Integrating systems in areas such as education, health, social welfare, juvenile justice, and mental health can provide a comprehensive framework for health promotion, disease prevention, and the use of evidence-based treatment when working with children, youths, and their families. These components are recognized as important aspects of a public health approach (Stiffman et al., 2010). Public health approaches to children's mental health services acknowledge that factors not traditionally associated with health can have major health implications. Public health models focus on community-wide variables rather than intervention with only the individual children and their families.

An initiative that focuses on children's mental health and is guided by a public health framework, supported by decades of research, is the System of Care Approach (SOC) to children's mental health (Miles et al., 2010). The SOC movement serves children and youths with serious mental health issues. It recognizes the importance of a community-based, nonfragmented, and coordinated network of child and youth services that is family-driven, youth-guided, and culturally and linguistically competent. It also recognizes the contribution of other supports for children and youths such as community recreation centers, church groups, coaches, and other community resources (Stroul, Blau, & Sondheimer, 2008). The American Academy of Pediatrics (2014) recently advocated care coordination as an essential element of health care for children and their families which includes a family-centered and collaborative approach with professionals.

Public health approaches impact children's mental health. At the turn of the 21st century, using a compilation of strong science-based research, the then Surgeon General urged all Americans to view mental health as an essential component of health, and advocated taking a public health approach to the identification, prevention, and treatment of mental illnesses. This approach also included removal of the stigma associated with mental health problems (HHS, 2001).

In 2013, the CDC released a report outlining a comprehensive approach to children's mental health. The report used research findings to inform health professionals of factors that increase children's risk of developing mental health problems such as poverty and trauma. It identified ways of promoting and tracking the effectiveness of children's mental health programs. The CDC (2013) advocated using systematic monitoring to increase the public's understanding of the mental health needs of children, the use of research findings to determine risk factors and prevention strategies, monitoring of children's early intervention and prevention programs, and the evaluation of the effectiveness of treatment programs.

RESEARCH ON CHILD WELL-BEING INDICATORS

A strategy that has been successful in forwarding policy that supports state-level progress in child health is the use of indicators of child well-being, called "childhood indicators," such as births to teen mothers, poverty rates, educational attainment, and immunization rates. The Annie E. Casey Foundation has been a leader in providing data in these areas for each state, and analyzing the extent to which these policies meet the needs of children and their families. The annual release of the *KIDS COUNT* data book which includes state data for 10 leading indicators receives extensive media attention and is often a catalyst for policy change (Annie E. Casey Foundation, 2013). Other foundations and organizations publish similar compilations of child and family indicators. An emerging technology that public health and other researchers are using to document population health disparities is Geographical Information Systems (GIS) mapping. GIS mapping can demonstrate disparities at census tract, zip code, neighborhood, and county levels, thereby identifying areas of need for community-level interventions.

RESEARCH ON "FRAMING THE PROBLEM"

Researchers and child advocates have become increasingly capable in communicating research findings and thereby advancing public policy, primarily by the use of framing theory. Framing theory suggests that people organize the world by using preexisting frames that guide their thoughts and feelings on an issue (FrameWorks Institute, 2001). Frames are strongly influenced by the media and can be very resistant to change. The FrameWorks Institute has been the leader in this area, conducting research to determine the current frames around child and family issues and designing strategic communications to change these frames to facilitate policy development. These efforts have advanced children's policy, particularly in the area of childcare, now reframed as "early care and education" (ECE).

One of the effective frames for policies relating to children is to evaluate the economic benefits current investments will yield in the future. A RAND study (Karoly et al., 1998) provided the impetus for other analyses of how funding ECE programs could be cost-effective. These studies led economists and researchers from the Minnesota Federal Reserve Bank to endorse such policies and to form partnerships with early childhood programs (Early Childhood Research Collaborative, 2010).

Nobel Prize winning economist James Heckman (2011) has undertaken groundbreaking work with economists, developmental psychologists, sociologists, statisticians, and neuroscientists to demonstrate that the quality of early childhood development heavily influences health, economic, and social outcomes for both individuals and society. Heckman (2011) wrote that the most efficient investment of limited economic resources is in the prevention of negative social and economic outcomes by promoting equity through the provision of high-quality early childhood parenting and education to disadvantaged families. He noted that every dollar invested in high-quality early childhood education produces a 7% to 10% return on investment per annum.

Heckman (2011) recommends investing in school readiness from birth through to the age of 5 by enriching home environments. He supports strong, high-quality, early childhood education programs and working with mothers by offering home visiting programs that seek to improve parenting skills.

One major success in linking research and policy is the Nurse Family Partnership (NFP) which partners low-income first-time mothers with nurses during pregnancy, continuing until the child's second birthday (Nurse Family Partnership, n.d.). Evaluations of the NFP and other home visitation models convinced President Obama to initiate a multibillion dollar federal program to expand early childhood home visitation. A home visitation provision was included in the Affordable Care Act (ACA). The national NFP office encourages nurses and others to advocate for increases in federal and state funding for home visitation.

GAPS IN LINKING RESEARCH AND SOCIAL POLICIES FOR CHILDREN

Although research findings have contributed to improvements in policies and programs for children and their families in areas such health care coverage and funding for early care and education, many children's outcomes remain unsatisfactory. For example, the reframing of childcare as early education and the expansion of prekindergarten services has not benefited infants and younger toddlers.

Large discrepancies exist between what research indicates is needed for healthy development, and what society delivers. We are unable to ensure that most children receive the quality of housing, food, and childcare that is commensurate with brain development, nor do all children have adequate health insurance coverage, even with the ACA and Medicaid expansions. Many children lack access to good, high-quality physical and mental health care.

Financial investments in programs for children are still relatively low. In 2008, only 10% of the U.S. federal budget was spent on children, compared to 38% on older adults and disabled persons (Isaacs et al., 2009). Moreover, the percentage of federal expenditures directed toward children has actually declined over time (from 20% in 1960, to 15% in 2008). During the first 2 years of the Obama presidency (2009-2010), laws were enacted that included substantial funding increases for the Child Care and Development Block Grant, home visiting programs, and the Child Health Insurance Program Reauthorization Act. This infusion of funding was an important start to the improvement of children's health and developmental outcomes, although current economic and political conditions put this progress at risk.

The backing of well-known economists has been tremendously valuable in garnering political support for many children's issues. Nonetheless, advocacy remains difficult because the constituents themselves—children and parents—are not easily mobilized because of the realities of daily life. Children from families with low socioeconomic resources and from racial and ethnic minority groups are particularly disadvantaged. Also, historically, issues associated with children and families have not had priority in the policy arena.

NURSING ADVOCACY

National and state nursing organizations have much untapped potential in terms of educating the public and policymakers by testifying on behalf of children and joining other coalitions working to influence child policy. It is important for nurses to be knowledgeable about findings from childhood research and subsequent policy implications and to keep abreast of the types of resources needed for improving the health of children. However, it is important to remember that evidence alone cannot change policies. In advancing children's policies other factors are important, such as careful framing, supporting interdisciplinary approaches, and working with community advocates toward common goals. Nurses and others who advocate for improved health and social policies for children must emphasize children's needs within their families and communities and the importance of coordinated care. It is important that they develop and implement strategies to widen the childhood policy community, and be persistent in advocating for policy change informed by high-quality research.

DISCUSSION QUESTIONS

1. Discuss the connections among child health, educational achievement, and social determinants of health.

2. Define a children's policy problem and describe how you might frame a social policy to ameliorate that problem.

3. How might nurses promote and implement public health approaches to children's mental health?

REFERENCES

Acevedo-Garcia, D., Osypuk, T. L., McArdle, N., & Williams, D. R. (2008). Toward a policy-relevant analysis of geographic and racial/ethnic disparities in child health. *Health Affairs (Millwood), 27*(2), 321–333.

American Academy of Pediatrics. (2014). Patient- and family-centered care coordination: A framework for integrating care for children and youth across multiple systems. *Pediatrics, 133*(5), e1451–e1460.

Annie E. Casey Foundation. (2013). The 2013 KIDS COUNT data book. Retrieved from *www.aecf.org/~/media/Pubs/Initiatives/KIDS%20COUNT/123/2013KIDSCOUNTDataBook/2013KIDSCOUNTDataBookr.pdf.*

Centers for Disease Control and Prevention. (2013). Mental health surveillance among children—United States, 2005-2011. Retrieved from *www.cdc.gov/mmwr/preview/mmwrhtml/su6202a1.htm?.*

Center on the Developing Child at Harvard University. (2010). The foundations of lifelong health are built in early childhood. Retrieved from *www.developingchild.harvard.edu.*

Early Childhood Research Collaborative. (2010). Retrieved from *www.earlychildhoodrc.org/partners.cfm.*

Egerter, S., Braverman, P., Pamuk, E., Cubbin, C., & Dekker, M. (2008). America's health starts with healthy children: How do states compare? Princeton, N.J.: Robert Wood Johnson Foundation Commission to Build a Healthier America. Retrieved from *www.commissiononhealth.org/Report.aspx?Publication=57823.*

Felitti, V. J., & Anda, R. F. (2010). The relationship of adverse childhood experiences to adult health, well-being, social function, and health care. In R. Lanius, E. Vermetten, & C. Pain (Eds.), *The effects of early life trauma on health and disease: the hidden epidemic.* London: Cambridge University Press.

Felitti, V. J., Anda, R. F., Nordenberg, D. F., Spitz, A. M., Edwards, V., Koss, M. P., et al. (1998). Relationship of childhood abuse and household dysfunction to many of the leading causes of death in adults. The Adverse Childhood Experiences (ACE) study. *American Journal of Preventive Medicine, 14*(4), 245–258.

FrameWorks Institute. (2001). A five minute refresher course in framing. Retrieved from *frameworksinstitute.org/assets/files/eZines/five_minute_refresher_ezine.pdf.*

Heckman, J. J. (2011). The economics of inequality: The value of early childhood education. *American Educator, Spring,* 31–47.

Isaacs, J. B., Vericker, T., Macomber, J., & Kent, A. (2009). Kids' share: An analysis of federal expenditures on children through 2008. Washington, DC: Urban Institute and Brookings. Retrieved from *www.brookings.edu/~/media/Files/rc/reports/2009/1209_kids_share_isaacs/1209_kids_share_isaacs.pdf.*

Karoly, L. A., Greenwood, P. W., Everingham, S. S., Hoube, J., Kilburn, R. M., Rydell, C. P., et al. (1998). Investing in our children: What we do and do not know about the cost and benefits of early childhood interventions. Washington, DC: RAND. Retrieved from *www.rand.org/pubs/monograph_reports/MR898.html.*

Miles, J., Espiritu, R. C., Horen, N. M., Sebian, J., & Waetzig, E. (2010). *A public health approach to children's mental health: A conceptual framework: Expanded executive summary.* Washington, DC: Georgetown University Center for Child and Human Development, National Technical Assistance Center for Children's Mental Health.

National Alliance on Mental Illness. (2013). Facts on children's mental health in America. Retrieved from *www.nami.org/Template.cfm?Section=Federal_and State_Policy_Lion&template=/Content Mangement/ContentDisplay.cfm&ContentID=43804.*

Nurse Family Partnership. (n.d.). Evidence-based public policy. Retrieved from *nursefamilypartnership.org.*

Perry, B. D. (2010). Effects of traumatic events on children. *The Guardian, 32,* 2–10.

Shonkoff, J. P., & Phillips, D. A. (Eds.), (2000). *From neurons to neighborhoods: The science of early childhood development.* Washington, DC: National Academies Press.

Smedley, B. D., Stith, A. Y., & Nelson, A. R. (Eds.), (2003). *Unequal treatment: Confronting racial and ethnic disparities in health care.* Washington, DC: National Academies Press. Retrieved from *www.nap.edu/openbook.php?isbn=030908265X.*

Stiffman, A. R., Stelk, W., Horwitz, S. M., Evans, M. E., Outlaw, F. H., & Atkins, M. (2010). A public health approach to children's mental health services: Possible solutions to current service inadequacies. *Administration Policy Mental Health, 37*(1–2), 120–124. doi:10.1007/s10488-009-0259-2.

Stroul, B. A., Blau, G. M., & Sondheimer, D. L. (2008). Systems of care: A strategy to transform children's mental health care. In B. A. Stroul & G. M. Blau (Eds.), *The system of care handbook transforming mental health services for children, youth, and families.* Baltimore, MD: Paul H. Brookes Publishing Co., Inc.

U.S. Department of Health and Human Services. (2010). *Healthy People 2020: The road ahead.* Retrieved from *www.healthypeople.gov/hp2020.*

U. S. Department of Health and Human Services. (2001). *Mental health: Culture, race and ethnicity—A supplement to mental health: A report of the Surgeon General.* Rockville: U. S. Department of Health and Human Services, Substance Abuse and Mental Health Services Administration, Center for Mental Health Services.

World Health Organization Commission on Social Determinants of Health. (2009). Final report: Closing the gap in a generation: Health equity through action on the social determinants of health. Retrieved from *www.who.int/social_determinants/thecommission/finalreport/en/index.html.*

ONLINE RESOURCES

Adverse Childhood Events on CDC
www.cdc.gov/ace
Nurse Family Partnership
nursefamilypartnership.org
Harvard Center for Developing Child
developingchild.harvard.edu/topics/science_of_early_childhood
Systems of Care
www.childwelfare.gov/pubs/soc

CHAPTER 14

Using the Power of Media to Influence Health Policy and Politics

Beth Gharrity Gardner · Barbara Glickstein · Diana J. Mason

"Power relations … as well as the processes challenging institutionalized power relations are increasingly shaped and decided in the communication field."

Manual Castells

In the 2008 Presidential campaign, social media did for the Obama campaign what the then new media of television did for John F. Kennedy in 1960. From the onset of his campaign, then U.S. Senator Barack Obama (D-IL) enlisted the support of Chris Hughes, a founder of Facebook, and David Axelrod, a former partner in the public relations firm ASK Public Strategies. Hughes and Axelrod built a team that marshaled every tool in the social media and marketing toolbox to create and sustain the Obama campaign. The campaign was ahead of competitors in using social media to connect with a growing audience of followers on Facebook, Twitter, and blogs. In the general election, then Senator Obama had 118,107 followers on Twitter, outpacing his opponent John McCain's 2865 followers by a factor of 40 to 1 (Lardinois, 2008). He used social media to build a grassroots movement that resulted in his historic victory (Talbot, 2008).

By the 2012 Presidential elections, the majority of social media users expected candidates to have a social media presence and stated that social media provided information that influenced their voting decisions (Steele, 2012). These trends among voters, and young voters in particular, were not lost on the Romney and Obama campaigns. By the eve of the 2012 conventions, both campaigns were regularly updating blogs on their websites and posting to Twitter, Facebook, and YouTube. As in 2008, Obama drastically outpaced all of his competitors in the

volume of messages sent, the number of followers or fans, and in social media response (e.g., shares, views, and comments) (Pew Research Center's Journalism Project Staff, 2012; Shaughnessy, 2012). Voters also played a larger role in communicating campaign messages. In 2012, the top five trending political topics on Facebook were "Barak Obama," "Mitt Romney," "voted," "four more years," and "Paul Ryan" (Groshek & Al-Rawi, 2013). Social media is now fully integrated into political campaigning and engagement (see Chapter 48).

The use of social media has not been limited to political campaigning. Launched immediately after Obama's 2008 win, Change.gov provided a website for people to share their ideas for improving legislation before it was signed into law. This sent the message that Obama had no intention of being limited by a traditional media operation as President. Rather, he was going to continue to engage people in supporting his agenda for the nation through multiple channels. When health care reform was teetering from a growing army of dissenters blocking its passage, he continued using social media to mobilize supporters to pressure Congress to act before the April 2010 recess. President Obama also took to the road and held town meetings in key communities because he knew that these meetings would garner reports on primetime television and radio and take a front-page position in newspapers. He could count on the primetime news including a sound bite and visual image of him speaking before a crowd of enthusiastic Ohioans. The personal appearances were a way to get his message to those who were not yet social media enthusiasts and to reinforce it with those who were already his followers on Twitter and

Facebook. In 2014, when the open enrollment window for signing up for health insurance drew to a close, Obama appeared on the show "Between Two Ferns," an online parody of celebrity interviews hosted by comedian Zach Galifianakis, to urge young adults to go to Healthcare.gov to sign up for health insurance. This unlikely appearance garnered coverage across traditional and social media platforms.

New digital information and communication technologies have dramatically changed how and what we think about communicating with others, whether connecting with family or building a grassroots political movement to push policymakers to pass new laws. Even traditional media outlets are now augmenting their work with all sorts of social media to extend their reach, impact, and, in some cases, survival. Legislators are routinely launching blogs, using Facebook, and tweeting to make their voices heard and to connect with their constituents. This chapter looks at the integration of traditional and social media as powerful tools for nurses to harness in shaping health policy and politics. Throughout, we draw insights from contemporary and past cases to highlight the role of media in influencing health policy and politics.

SEISMIC SHIFT IN MEDIA: ONE-TO-MANY AND MANY-TO-MANY

In the 21st century there has been a seismic shift in the way media is created and distributed. For many years, the dominant paradigm in media was a model in which one broadcaster sent a message out to a mass audience. This broadcast model is referred to as the one-to-many model. This model has been challenged by the Internet and user-generated content in which many people create media and distribute it to their individualized networks. This new model is sometimes referred to as the many-to-many model because it provides opportunities for feedback and interaction, features that have led to the ubiquitous use of the term "social media."

We now have convergence media, or the interweaving of traditional and social media. Rather than these platforms remaining separate, traditional and networked media are working side by side. For instance, even though the *New York Times* in print or even as an app is mostly a one-to-many broadcasting media model, the newspaper's blogs, videos, and comment sections reflect the digital side of the newspaper as a networked media platform. News organizations exclusive to the online environment have been created and some veteran print publications have moved entirely or mostly online, but the degree of convergence is unclear (Hindman, 2009).

MASS MEDIA: THE ONE-TO-MANY MODEL

Traditional media in radio, television, film, and newspapers was based on the idea that one broadcaster would try to reach as many audience members as possible. However, for those interested in influencing health policy and politics through the media there were many advantages and some significant disadvantages to the one-to-many model of broadcast media (Abramson, 2003).

Radio, film, and television have all been used to communicate messages about health to consumers and policymakers alike. What all these media share is the ability to broadcast a message to a mass audience, sometimes in the millions or tens of millions. When there were few media outlets it was possible to repeatedly broadcast a consistent message to a wide audience. The use of mass media has been a major tool in health promotion campaigns because it reaches a large audience and is capable of promoting healthy social change (Institute of Medicine, 2002; Wakefield, Loken & Hornik, 2010).

There are also disadvantages to mass media communications. Large corporations own media outlets and control what goes out through their channels and the expense of buying time or space in major media outlets can be prohibitive, especially for nonprofit organizations. Mass media campaigns, by definition, are intended to reach a wide audience but are not as effective at reaching target populations. For example, a mass media campaign about HIV prevention may reach a wide audience but fail to reach the specific population that is most vulnerable to infection. However, political operatives have developed increasingly sophisticated approaches to segmenting and targeting specific electoral districts with mass media when they want to pressure a policymaker who may hold a deciding vote on an important bill. Such organizations buy commercial time on the dominant television station in that policymaker's district. However, what no form of mass media does very well is allow users to create and distribute their own content with the messages they find most important.

MANY-TO-MANY: USER-GENERATED CONTENT AND THE "PROSUMER"

The rise of the Internet, and specifically websites that rely on users to generate content, are part of a new landscape of media creation and distribution. The early Internet featured websites that were one-way flows of information. The paradigm-shifting quality of the Internet began to emerge with the rise of Web 2.0, a term popularized by Tim O'Reilly (2005) at a conference in 2004. Web 2.0 refers to a range of Internet practices based on information-sharing, social networks, and collaborations, rather than the one-way communication style of the early era of the Internet. The key idea with the concept of Web 2.0 is that people are using the Internet to connect with other people, through their old face-to-face networks and through newly formed online social networks and communities of interest.

Prosumption is a term that some people use to describe this shift. Prosumption is the idea that producing and consuming are combined in this new many-to-many paradigm. Rather than an elite few who produce media for a mass audience to consume, now we are all both producers and consumers, or prosumers of media. The many-to-many paradigm refers not to a new form of technology but to a new way that people make use of that technology (Ritzer & Jurgenson, 2010). Social media tools may work best by enabling the development of communities of interest and social networks that successfully narrowcast, as opposed to broadcast, to like-minded individuals. Only time will tell how the many-to-many model will permeate the political communication landscape. Regardless, the collaborative, information-sharing Internet practices have broad implications for health media, policy, and politics, but they do not mean the end of mass media.

THE POWER OF MEDIA

A now classic example of the power of media in shaping health policy arose during the first months of William Jefferson Clinton's presidency when he tried but failed to enact health care reform legislation despite campaigning on a policy platform that sought to guarantee comprehensive health care coverage for every American. In 1993, he proposed the Health Security Act to Congress and the public with the hope that this would become a landmark legislation. Clinton's proposal initially had substantial public support, because many believed the country had a moral imperative to extend health care coverage to all who live in the United States. However, according to an analysis by the Annenberg Public Policy Center of the University of Pennsylvania (1995), one of the primary factors that unraveled the legislation's progress was the Harry and Louise campaign (a series of television advertisements about two fictional characters, Harry and Louise), which was sponsored by the Health Insurance Association of America (HIAA), an ardent opponent to the President's plan.

Actors portrayed a white, middle-class couple voicing grave concerns about the bill. They said, "Under the President's bill, we'll lose our right to choose our own physician," and "What happens if the plan runs out of money?" Although the ads were not the only reason for the demise of the Clinton plan, the Harry and Louise television spots encouraged fear and negativity within the span of 60 seconds. Suddenly, it seemed as though many of the Americans who had been concerned about the growing numbers of uninsured would become more concerned about how the bill would affect their own health care options and withdraw their support from the Act. What few people realize is that even though a large segment of the population remained convinced that the health care system needed major change, the commercials convinced decision makers that public sentiment was against the reforms. This is one of the things that make the media so powerful: media discourse impacts policymaking because policymakers "assume its pervasive influence" (Gamson, 2004, p. 243). The target audience for the Harry and Louise ads was not the public directly; rather, it was policymakers and those who could influence how the public perceived the issue, such as journalists. The ads originally aired in the country's major media centers: Washington, DC; Los Angeles; New York City; and Atlanta. They were seen and reported on by journalists. In fact, the ads and the issue under debate got more airtime by becoming part of the journalists' news stories (West, Heith, & Goodwin, 1996). Many people saw the ads or heard about them through viewing them on the evening news, not as a paid advertisement.

The Harry and Louise commercials are an example of the power of the media in policy and politics. It was a deliberate media strategy to reframe a public policy issue and mobilize a public constituency around it. The media saturate large numbers of people with images that directly or indirectly influence their opinions, shape their attitudes and beliefs, and transform their behavior (McLuhan, 1964). As such, understanding what is and is not shifting in the templates of message production, dissemination, and consumption is crucial for understanding media impacts.

Media campaigns such as these often rely on invoking viewer reactions through the use of misleading or extreme characterizations of legislation or opponents. Recent research suggests that such uncivil discourse is on the rise, especially in nontraditional media, such as talk radio and political blogs (Sobieraj & Berry, 2011; Jamieson, 2012). Given the traditional news values of controversy and conflict, such talk in new media channels may be especially likely to gain coverage from other media outlets. Another longstanding pathway to mass influence is through large media advertising expenditures. The amount of spending on political advertisements is often the largest segment of lobbying expenditure for sponsoring organizations. In 2014, an estimated $2.6 billion was spent on political advertising (Kantar U.S. Insights, 2014). Media advertising campaigns often conceal sponsorship with ambiguous or misleading names and may use cloaked websites to enhance the effectiveness of their deception. Cloaked websites are published by individuals or groups who conceal authorship to deliberately disguise a hidden political agenda

(Daniels, 2009). The lack of transparency of political advertising has a Machiavellian quality to it. Although advertisements for a political candidate are required to include a statement from the candidate that he or she authorized the ad, no such requirement exists for transparency of sponsorship of ads advocating policy positions.

WHO CONTROLS THE MEDIA?

The traditional media industry has been owned by six major corporations that, prior to the growth of social media, controlled 90% of the news Americans read, saw, or heard (Lutz, 2012). In 2003, the Federal Communications Commission voted to ease the restrictions on cross-ownership between different news entities, permitting one corporation to own the primary television, radio, and newspaper outlets in a community. This enabled a single corporation to control messages and put forth a particular perspective. CNN founder Ted Turner objected to this consolidation of corporate media power, arguing that allowing this cross-ownership "will extend the market dominance of the media corporations that control most of what Americans read, see, or hear" and "give them more power to cut important ideas out of the public debate" (Harris, 2005, p. 83).

The gap created by the declining revenue streams and reduced newsrooms for traditional or legacy media are starting to be filled by actors building new news operations and resuscitating longstanding ones. For instance, the Kaiser Family Foundation launched its own nonprofit news organization, Kaiser Health News, in 2009. Their content is now regularly carried in traditional news outlets. Newer digital news outlets are also gaining revenue and recruiting talent from traditional media news staffs. Revenue is recently coming from entrepreneurs who are investing in the media industry; for example, Amazon.com founder Jeff Bezos purchased the *Washington Post* in 2013. Although traditional news media continue to face revenue challenges, the largest numbers of journalists producing original reporting still come from the newspaper industry (Mitchell, 2013; 2014). In this more digital and diversified media field, the pathways to getting on the public's agenda may be more complex but many of the traditional media still adhere to familiar lines of influence.

Social media can actually drive traditional media to cover issues that major newsrooms may not deem worthy of their limited space and time, thus advancing political advocacy. One success story is that of the YouTube video campaign, *Kony 2012,* launched by Invisible Children, seeking to spur international awareness of the actions of Ugandan warlord Joseph Kony and his Lord's Resistance Army. Within a few days the video drew millions of viewers and spread to other social media such as Twitter, where it became the top story. Within weeks, the Senate introduced a bipartisan resolution condemning Kony. According to Senator Lindsey Graham (R-SC), "This is about someone who, without the Internet and YouTube, their dastardly deeds would not resonate with politicians. When you get 100 million Americans looking at something, you will get our attention" (Wong, 2012).

According to a survey conducted a week after the video's release, the way people learned about this story varied strikingly by age cohort. Around half of young adults (aged 18 to 29) who had heard about the video first did so through social media, compared with an even mix of social and traditional news sources for those aged 30 to 49. Traditional media, especially television, informed most adults aged 50 and over (Rainie et al., 2012b).

The ownership of the Internet (e.g., online infrastructures, operating systems, and search engines) is following consolidation patterns similar to traditional media, with a few large companies such as Apple, Google, Yahoo!, Facebook, and Microsoft dominating the field (Freepress.net, 2014). Nonetheless, the more decentralized structure of the Web may better enable citizens to not only break news, but shape it. This bodes well for nurses who have not always been able to garner media attention for their issues. A study commissioned by Sigma Theta Tau and published in 1998 documented nursing's invisibility in the media. The Woodhull Study on Nursing and the Media found that nurses were included in health stories in major print media (newspapers and news magazines published in September 1997) less than 4% of the time, even when they would have been germane to the story. And even more disturbing, nurses were represented in health care industry publications (such as *Modern Healthcare*) less than 1% of the time.

These findings may indicate a systematic journalistic bias against nursing. They also arise because nurses have not been proactive in accessing traditional media. Social media provides an opportunity for nurses to not wait for traditional media to value their perspectives. Nurses can use social media to create and distribute messages, to engage others to care about an issue, and to discuss issues from various vantage points. Given that the annual Gallup Poll continues to find that Americans rate the honesty and ethical standards of nurses higher than any other profession (e.g., in 2013, 82% for nurses, 69% for physicians, 21% for newspaper reporters, 8% for members of Congress), nurses have a unique opportunity to send persuasive messages (Gallup, 2014).

If nurses want visibility, they must become cyberactivists. Cyberactivists are people who want to create change in a variety of issues and have taken up the use of new media technologies and strategies that characterize Web 2.0 (McCaughey & Ayers, 2003), fusing the old and new media methods to allow for the widest range of engagement with the public. It has never been easier to become a cyberactivist because new digital technologies have lowered the motivational thresholds for activism, making it much easier to create, join, and coordinate groups (Shirky, 2008; Polletta et al., 2013). Nursing organizations are particularly well positioned to mount focused social media campaigns because they already have a list of people who can begin the spreading of messages. However, social networks are becoming crowded, so getting noticed requires a thoughtful strategy.

DISTRIBUTED CAMPAIGNS

Obama's social media campaign strategy was a distributed campaign, a bottom-up rather than a top-down approach to political campaigns that depends on a message spreading from the grassroots rather than broadcasting and control by the campaign staff (Ozimek, 2005). These campaigns are designed to involve more than core supporters. Distributed campaigns seek to engage swing voters and to provide opportunities for core supporters to craft messages that may appeal to these swing voters more effectively than messages created by campaign staff, thereby strengthening the commitment of core supporters to the campaign. E-mail, blogs, and other social media are used by campaign staff to initiate a dialogue that is subsequently developed by a broad community of supporters. Additionally, supporter-generated content such as more personalized Facebook groups and YouTube videos can be incorporated into the campaign.

Evidence supports the potential for distributed campaigns. In terms of shaping political communication, a 2012 Pew Internet and American Life Project survey found that 66% of social media users (estimated to be 39% of all American adults) are politically active on these sites, by posting links to political stories, encouraging others to vote, or encouraging others to take political action (Rainie et al., 2012a; Smith, 2013). In terms of consuming political information, a 2013 Pew survey indicates that approximately half of Facebook and Twitter users obtained news on those sites (Holcomb, Gottfried, & Mitchell, 2013).

Distributed campaigns provide people with tools for activism such as petitions to sign, e-mail scripts to send, or letters to sign and send to legislators. Organizations, such as Democracy in Action (*salsalabs.com/democracyinaction*), are available to help build the capacity of groups that want to develop action tools for reaching diverse audiences in distributive campaigns. Living in a media-saturated world can sometimes feel like being in a cacophony of conflicting voices. The challenge is how to use these powerful tools most effectively.

LINKING IN TO EXISTING COMMUNITIES

Most people regularly find information online from sources that are familiar or already aligned with their views (Hindman, 2009). Similarly, popular search engines such as Yahoo! and Google structure or filter links in a way that facilitates this return to the familiar and the mainstream. One way to work both with and around these patterns may be to link into existing communities of interest and social networks rooted in friends and family. In the Kony 2012 case discussed earlier, Senator Chris Coons (D-DE) told reporters that his 12-year-old twins and his 11-year-old daughter alerted him to the issue (Wong, 2012), which they and their peers most likely learned about through social media (Rainie et al., 2012b). Just as they have offline, the networked worlds of friendship, family, hobbies, and leisure groups may routinely overlap with political engagement and communication.

Such overlap is evident in data from the 2013 University of Southern California Annenberg School for Communication and Journalism's national digital future survey (Center for the Digital Future, 2013). In 2013, 16.7% of Internet users identified themselves as a member of an online community, defined as "a group that shares thoughts or ideas, or works on common projects, through electronic communication only." More than half of these groups were devoted to members' hobbies (62%). Other groups were social (39%) or professional (33%) with only 12% described as political. However, 85% of online community members said they used the Internet to participate in communities related to social causes (this was up 10% from 2007 and 40% from 2006); and nearly three quarters said they had participated in new social causes since they joined an online community.

Friends, family, and communities of interest may convince those who might not otherwise join a cause to join because they help to either create concern about the cause or motivate the individual to shift from concern to participation (Polletta et al., 2013). As these exchanges are increasingly enabled through social media networks, traditional media avenues for getting on the public's agenda are being restructured.

GETTING ON THE PUBLIC'S AGENDA

One of the most important roles that the media plays is getting issues on the agendas of the public and policymakers. What the mainstream media do or do not cover is equally powerful in determining which issues policymakers take into consideration. But the mainstream media's role in defining what is mainstream appears to be diminishing due to three interrelated factors: the abundance of new social media platforms, the lowered costs of producing media campaigns that can directly reach the public, and the downsizing among traditional news media outlets that may be undermining the quality of their reporting. The news-consuming public has responded to these interrelated trends. A survey conducted by the PEW Research Center early in 2013 found that nearly a third of people abandoned a particular news source because it was no longer providing the quality information they had come to expect (Enda & Mitchell, 2013). *The Digital Future Report* (Center for the Digital Future, 2013) also found that 30% of Internet users stopped a subscription to a newspaper or magazine because they could get the same information online. Additionally, more people are seeking out news stories they hear about via social media, even when they weren't looking (Mitchell, 2014). Most American adults (73%) get news from family and friends through word of mouth, but now around 15% are getting it from family and friends through social networking, and the percentage relying on social media is even higher for 18- to 29-year olds (nearly 25%) (Mitchell, 2013).

NEWS AS ENTERTAINMENT: INFOTAINMENT

The news media remain instrumental in getting issues onto the agenda of policymakers and generating the political campaign interest that encourages citizens to the voting booths (Groshek & Dimitrova, 2011), but non-news entertainment television programs can also mobilize public constituencies around an issue. Although the Internet has become a more important source for entertainment among Internet users, television remains the primary source for entertainment (Center for the Digital Future, 2013). This may be caused by the fact that television continues to be the dominant form of media in most people's lives, despite the rise of other forms of media online. In 2013, the television was on around 35 hours per week in the average American household (Nielsen Reports, 2013). Teenagers still spend more time watching TV than they do online (Rideout, Foehr, & Roberts,

2010). The Internet may be where people go to find out about a health issue, but they often first become aware of the issue through television and films.

Turow (1996) points out that non-news television entertainment that often stereotypes power relationships may be more successful than the news in shaping people's views of issues. Highly viewed TV presentations of health care hold political significance that should be assessed alongside news. Medical and nursing dramas on broadcast and cable television, such as *Grey's Anatomy*, *ER*, and *Nurse Jackie*, are often important sources of information about health and health policy for a wide audience. Researchers Turow and Gans (2002) systematically evaluated one television season of four hour-long medical dramas and found that health care policy issues appeared regularly in the programs. Evidence from a national telephone survey indicates that the percentage of regular viewers of the show *ER* who were aware that HPV is a sexually transmitted disease was higher (28%) one week after viewing an episode of the show about HPV than before seeing the show (9%). Even 6 weeks after viewing the episode, 16% had retained this knowledge. This capacity to quickly get a message out to millions of people through an hour-long drama is part of the reason that many health advocates work to get their particular issue included in a storyline of a major network drama.

DOCUMENTARY FILMS

Documentary films, in conjunction with online campaigns, are influencing health policy and politics while achieving mainstream commercial success. For example, two documentaries, *The Invisible War* (2012) and *Service: When Women Come Marching Home* (2011) were groundbreaking in creating public conversations about military sexual assault. Both were viewed by members of Congress and used as organizing tools nationally to get the public behind an agenda to change the military's practices. Kirsten Gillibrand (D-NY), Senator and Chairwoman of the Personnel Subcommittee on the Armed Services Committee, cited *The Invisible War* as shaping her decision to draft a bill to overhaul military sexual-assault policies by removing the chain of command from prosecuting sexual assaults. Although the bill was defeated in March of 2014, her yearlong campaign drew many supporters and put the issue firmly on the political agenda.

MEDIA AS A HEALTH PROMOTION TOOL

Media can promote health in three ways: public education, social marketing, and media advocacy. The first two are often used to help people change their health behaviors by acquiring important information they lacked (public education) or through visual or verbal messaging that can shift a person's attitudes and values (social marketing). Both can also be used in political campaigns and to shape public policy, but media advocacy specifically targets public policy.

MEDIA ADVOCACY

Media advocacy is the strategic use of media to apply pressure to advance a social or public policy initiative (Dorfman & Krasnow 2014; Wallack & Dorfman, 1996). It is a tool for policy change by mobilizing constituencies and stakeholders to support or oppose specific policy changes. It is a means of political action. It differs from social marketing and public education approaches to public health, as noted in Table 14-1. Media advocacy

TABLE 14-1 Media Advocacy Versus Social Marketing and Public Education Approaches to Public Health

Media Advocacy	Social Marketing and Public Education
Individual as advocate	Individual as audience
Advances healthy public policies	Develops health messages
Changes the environment	Changes the individual
Target is person with power to make change	Target is person with problem or is at risk
Addresses the power gap	Addresses the information gap

Adapted from Wallack, L., & Dorfman, L. (1996). Media advocacy: A strategy for advancing policy and promoting health. *Health Education Quarterly, 23*(3), 297. Copyright 1996 by Sage Publications. Reprinted by permission of Sage Publications.

defines the primary problem as a power gap, as opposed to an information gap, so mobilization of stakeholders is needed to influence the development of public policies.

The success of Mothers Against Drunk Driving (MADD) illustrates the power of media advocacy. MADD was formed in 1980 at a time when a drunk driver could kill a child and it would not be treated as a crime. MADD developed a policy agenda aimed at preventing drunk driving. It developed a Rating the States program to bring public attention to what state governments were and were not doing to fight alcohol-impaired driving. Then, just after Thanksgiving (the beginning of a period of high numbers of alcohol-related traffic accidents), MADD representatives held local press conferences with their state's officials and members of other advocacy groups to announce the state's rating. Local and national broadcast and print press brought the story to an estimated 62.5 million people. Subsequently, lawmakers in at least eight states took action to address drunken driving (Russell et al., 1995).

Today, MADD's website (*www.madd.org*) provides information in a number of areas: policies that people can endorse, a walk to raise funds to support the organization's work, a link to its Twitter page, and news about drunk driving initiatives. Getting on the news media's agenda is one of the functions of media advocacy (Dorfman & Krasnow, 2014). With numerous competing potential stories, media advocacy employs strategies to frame an issue in a way that will attract media coverage. For example, MADD often created media events by putting a wrecked car in front of a local high school a few days prior to a prom. Journalists flocked to these events and the visual impact of the wrecked car got people's attention. The news accounts and parental outrage that resulted from these media events eventually led to wide social support for the concept of the designated driver and harsher penalties for driving under the influence.

How a message is presented is as important as getting the attention of the news media. Debates surrounding the passage and implementation of the Affordable Care Act demonstrate this point. It certainly got on the media's agenda, but many important messages were lost in the news coverage that emphasized the controversies such as death panels and horror stories of individuals finding their insurance policies cancelled.

FRAMING

Getting an issue on the agenda of the public and policymakers and shaping the message requires framing. Framing "defines the boundaries of public discussion about an issue" (Wallack & Dorfman, 1996, p. 299). Even more simply put, a frame is a "thought organizer" (Gamson, 2004, p. 245). Reframing involves breaking out of the dominant perspective (or frame) on an issue to define a new way of thinking about it that can lead to very different ideas about potentially effective policy responses. Reframing requires working hard to understand the dominant frame, the values that underpin it as well as its limitations, and then exploring new frames.

Framing applies to all messaging and policy work, whether changing staffing policies in a hospital or promoting legislation that will remove soft drinks from schools. Framing for access to the media entails shaping the issue in a way that will attract media attention. It helps to attach the issue to a local concern, anniversaries, or celebrities or to make news by holding events that will attract the press, such as releasing new research at a press conference (Jernigan & Wright, 1996). Linking to issues already on the political agenda or the media's agenda (as newsworthy) can also be advantageous to gaining access. Most importantly, it requires some element of controversy (albeit not over the accuracy of an advocate's facts), conflict, injustice, or irony. The targeted medium or media will shape how the story is presented. For example, television requires compelling visual images. If a broad audience is to be reached, a powerful, brief message on television can provide a quick frame for an issue and influence how people will view it, but the interactive nature of social media provides the opportunity for others to continue to reframe a message, helping people to break out of a dominant frame.

Framing for content once you are in front of the media is more difficult than *framing for access.* A compelling individual story may gain visibility in some media, but there is no guarantee that the reporter or social media activists will focus on the public policy changes that are desired. Wallack and Dorfman (1996, p. 300) suggest that this reframing can be accomplished by the following:

- Emphasizing the social dimensions of the problem and translating an individual's personal story into a public issue
- Shifting the responsibility for the problem from the individual to the executive or public official whose decisions can address the problem
- Presenting solutions as policy alternatives
- Making a practical appeal to support the solution
- Using compelling images and symbols that resonate with the values of the audience
- Using the authentic voices of people who have experience with the problem
- Anticipating the opposition and knowing all sides of the issue

FOCUS ON REPORTING

Few journalists have the time and the editorial support or the breadth and depth of knowledge about science to provide thorough reporting on health issues that have policy implications. This often results in less-than-adequate reporting on important issues, such as how communities should respond to the West Nile virus. Roche (2002) examined print media coverage of the approaches to reducing the mosquito population to reduce the incidence of, and mortality from, West Nile encephalitis. None of the newspapers or magazines examined gave any information about risk of mortality from pesticide exposure or a cost analysis of this approach. Roche concluded that the public is "operating 'in the dark' in evaluating the question of whether pesticides should be deployed."

Nurses can assist journalists and cyberactivists by both reframing health policy issues and providing the depth of detail that others may lack. For example, a journalist covering a story on the nursing shortage has focused on the faculty shortage and the need to produce more nurses. You could help the journalist to see that framing the story as purely one of a supply issue, getting more people into the pipeline, misses the important issues of retention of existing nurses. While talking with this journalist does not ensure that your frame will be incorporated into the journalist's story, you can publicize the frame you believe is important through your blog, Facebook page, or Twitter account.

One strategy is to facilitate information exchange in the public arena by becoming news makers, aggregators, or curators of health news. Posting links to news articles and research on critical policy issues on social media sites, such as Facebook, makes the news easy to find. As searching for health information has become the third most popular online activity for all Internet users 18 and over (Zickuhr, 2010), nurses are positioned to explain complex health policy issues by breaking them down. This can be done not just for information sharing but also for civil engagement so that people will act, whether by having a conversation with a co-worker about the issue or contacting government representatives. Facebook friends, including other nurse colleagues, can share on Facebook, which reposts these articles to their personal networks to widen the community. Social networking can generate a buzz and create conversations about an issue or policy. It is digital activism and it has enormous potential to build networks, propagate power, and frame issues.

EFFECTIVE USE OF MEDIA

The following recommendations provide readers with a starting point for effectively using traditional and social media.

POSITIONING YOURSELF AS AN EXPERT

Health policy was once the domain of a limited field of experts setting the agenda for everyone else. The rise of user-generated content signals a radical departure from this approach. It signifies a profound transformation in what it means to be an expert and who is an expert. New media provides nurses with platforms to reach the public as media makers and aggregators of reliable health research information.

Gain Credentials. There are many types of credentials, although they are typically thought of as degrees from educational institutions, work titles, and affiliations. Some institutions require that their employees notify them of any interaction with the media, but this may be unnecessary if you don't name the institution in your interview or other communication. For example, you could be a nurse in women's health at a community hospital.

Become an Expert in Your Field. Becoming the go-to person who is the expert on a topic or particular field is another way to establish yourself as an expert. You can establish this by launching your own professional website, blog, and Twitter and Facebook pages, as well as by meeting with local journalists who cover health.

Use Personal and Clinical Experience. Part of why MADD's campaign has been compelling is their strategic use of stories from women whose children have been killed as a result of drunk driving. These bereaved mothers involved with MADD have transformed themselves into experts on the policy of driving while intoxicated and have used their experience to make this point with policymakers. Similarly, people who were infected with HIV/AIDS in the 1980s and believed that the federal government was acting too slowly to move treatment through clinical trials made themselves experts on the science of the disease and by using a variety of tactics including personal accounts of their illnesses, forced policymakers to speed up the time for drugs to reach the market. The Internet facilitates the rise of this kind of expertise.

GETTING YOUR MESSAGE ACROSS

Getting your message to the appropriate target audience requires careful analysis and planning. For example, you might want to target a message to local homeowners, many of whom watch a particular TV station's evening news. To get television coverage, you must have a visual story. California nurses staged a media event on a senior health issue by staging a "rock around the clock" marathon, with seniors in rocking chairs outside an insurance company. They received press coverage of the event, which elicited some supportive letters to the editor as well as some negative press from seniors who said that they were stereotyping older adults. See Box 14-1 for guidelines for getting your message across in traditional media, and Box 14-2 for ways to use social media tools to reach an audience.

BLOGGING AND MICROBLOGGING

Increasingly, blogs are used as ways to communicate personal experiences and opinions. Theresa Brown is an oncology nurse living and working in Pittsburgh. Her first career was as a doctorally prepared English professor before deciding that she wanted to work more closely with people. She wrote a narrative about a dying patient that was published on the first page of the *New York Times* Science section, which until then had been dominated by physicians' narratives. She was then invited to contribute to the *Times'* health blog, Well. As a result, issues of concern to practicing nurses received regular visibility through her posts. Her expertise as a nurse in cancer care is clearly valued by those who post responses to her blog entries.

Twitter, an example of microblogging, is a great way for nurses to listen as well as to talk to others on a very direct level. Twitter allows users to post short, 140-character messages (called tweets). For longer conversations, people use hashtags (# symbols) to track topics. People are very creative in the way they use Twitter and it holds a great deal of potential for nurses. For example, a Twitter Tweet-Chat is a prearranged chat that happens on Twitter through the use of Twitter posts (tweets) that include a predefined hashtag to link those tweets together in a virtual conversation. There is even a URL that provides a schedule of health-related TweetChats (*www.symplur.com/healthcare-hashtags/tweet-chats/*). When you can't attend a conference but know the hashtag that is being used by those in attendance, you can search for it on Twitter, read the live tweets, and join the discussion by tweeting from wherever you are. It represents both a media and a marketing tool. Each presenter's remarks and recommendations can reach a wider audience.

You can also use Twitter to convey a position on legislation that is up for a vote on the local, state,

or national level to inform public debate on how this policy will impact the health and well-being of individuals and communities. Also, you can use Twitter and other social media to link to relevant data supporting a particular position and to see what others are saying about this policy: Is it positive? Negative? Misinformed? Journalists frequently use Twitter to find sources of information on stories they are covering or to simply uncover new stories. Following key health journalists can provide opportunities for recommending yourself or other nurses as experts on specific topics or to help them to reframe their stories.

DIGITAL MEDIA AND SOCIAL NETWORKING SITES (SNS)

The development of Web 2.0 has meant increased participation and media attention on virtual communities, most frequently in social networking sites (SNS) such as Facebook, Twitter, LinkedIn, Pinterest, Google+, and MySpace. The impact that SNS will have on health policy is still emerging but there are some intriguing early examples of the advantage they may hold for advocacy. For instance, Facebook is emerging as an important venue for debate about health policy, and not just among people typically thought of as policymakers. The health care reform battle sparked a huge number of for- and against-themed pages, such as Ohio Against Health Care Reform (81 fans), Wyoming for Health Care Reform (247 fans), and the perennial Facebook meme, "I bet we can find 1,000,000 people who support/oppose" health care reform. Although measuring the effectiveness of such Facebook campaigns remains elusive, we will likely see more of this type of activity as health care reform is implemented.

Not everyone understands the potential of social media for shaping advocacy. Lovejoy and Saxon (2012) examined the content of tweets from the 100 largest nonprofit organizations in the United States, 24% of which were health-oriented. The authors identified three primary communication functions: information, community, and action. They found that the bulk of communications sent information (58%), 26% reinforced community via more interactive messages, and only 16% promoted some form of action such as donating, volunteering, or

BOX 14-1 Guidelines for Getting Your Message Across

The following guidelines will help you shape your message and get it delivered to the right media:

The Issue
- What is the nature of the issue?
- What is the context of the issue? (e.g., timing, history, and current political environment)
- Who is, or could be, interested in this issue?

The Message
- What's the angle or the "so what"? Why should anyone care? What is news?
- Is there a sound bite that represents the issue in a catchy, memorable way?
- Can you craft rhetoric that will represent core values of the target audience?
- How can you frame nursing's interests as the public's interests (e.g., as consumers, mothers, fathers, women, taxpayers, and health professionals)?

The Target Audience
- Who is the target audience? Is it the public, policymakers, or journalists?
- If the public is the target audience, which segments of the public?
- What medium is appropriate for the target audience? Does this audience watch television? If so, are the members of this audience likely to watch a talk show or a news magazine show? Or do they read newspapers, listen to radio, or surf the Internet? Or are they likely to do all of these?

Access to the Media
- What relationships do you have with reporters and producers? Have you called or written letters or thank-you notes to particular journalists? Have you requested a meeting with the editorial board of the local community newspaper to discuss your issue and what the members of the board might think about reporting on it?
- How can you get the media's attention? Is there a hot issue you can connect your issue to? Is there a compelling human interest story? Do you have a press release that describes your issue in a succinct, compelling way? Do you have other printed materials that will attract journalists' attention within the first 3 seconds of viewing it? Are there photographs you can take in advance and then send out with your press release? Can you digitalize the images and make them available on a website for downloading onto a newspaper?

- Whom should you contact in the medium or media of choice?
- Are you prepared? Are you news conscious? Do you watch, listen, clip, and track who covers what and how they cover it? What is the format of the program, and who is the journalist? What is the style of the program or journalist?
- Who are your spokespersons? Do they have the requisite expertise on the issue? Do they have a visual or voice presence appropriate for the medium? What is their personal connection to the issue, and do they have stories to tell? Have they been trained or rehearsed for the interview?

The Interviews
- Prepare for the interview. Obtain information on your interviewer and the program by reviewing the interviewer's work or talking with public relations experts in your area. Select the one, two, or three major points that you want to get across in the interview. Identify potential controversies and how you would respond to them, and rehearse the interview with a colleague.
- During the interview, listen attentively to the interviewer. Recognize opportunities to control the interview and get your primary point across more than once. What is your sound bite? Even if the interviewer asks a question that does not address your agenda, return the focus of the interview to your agenda and to your sound bite with finesse and persistence.
- Try to be an interesting guest. Come ready with rich, illustrative stories. Avoid yes or no answers to questions.
- Know that you do not have to answer all questions and should avoid providing comments that would embarrass you if they were headlines. If you don't know the answer to a question, say so and offer to get back to the interviewer with the information.
- Avoid being disrespectful or arguing with the interviewer.
- Remember that being interviewed can be an anxiety-producing experience for many people. This is a normal reaction. Do some slow deep-breathing or relaxation exercises before the interview, but know that some nervousness can be energizing.

Follow-up
- Write a letter of thanks to the producer or journalist afterward.
- Provide feedback to the producer or journalist on the response that you have received to the interview or the program or coverage.

BOX 14-2 Using Social Media

Mobile Text Messaging

Mobile and particularly text messaging is the ideal medium for communicating with everyone equally, regardless of their age, gender, or economic status. To get started, do the following:

- Create a subscriber base with zip codes so text alerts can be targeted to subscribers; you can then ask people in a specific Congressional district to contact their representative about an important issue.
- Send alerts about a news item, an action, or a "meet-up"—the calling of a gathering of people for a shared interest.
- Send a link to a website or local news item.
- Feature a text-alert campaign on your website homepage.

Blogging

Blogs are great ways for you to share your opinions and ideas on health and social topics and to bring attention to important issues. The following are some tips for blogging:

- Be creative.
- Engage your audience and invite readers to get involved.
- Tell important stories.
- Share your process (how your organization works).
- Share successes and challenges.
- Write short, action-oriented posts.
- Link to interesting local news.
- Find your niche.
- Be a subject matter expert.
- Be conversational.
- Write like you'd talk to your neighbor.
  One website that provides easy tools for starting a blog is *www.wordpress.com*.

Facebook *(www.facebook.com)*

Facebook provides a vehicle for building and growing a community. Lots of people are on Facebook to stay connected with friends and family. You can also create a Facebook page for your professional life, since mixing the two can be problematic if you're a clinician.

- Create a page for your organization or specific causes or issues; updates may include a new action item and a new goal.
- Upload relevant videos, photos, and articles.
- Turn your cause into a campaign.
- Set an achievable goal, and find a creative way to engage people to invite their friends.
- Host short-term causes.
- Use the announcements feature to keep followers informed.
- Always send new info.
- Keep it short.
- If one idea doesn't work too well, don't be afraid to shut it down and try a new idea!

Twitter *(www.twitter.com)*

Twitter asks one question, "What are you doing?" Answers must be under 140 characters in length and can be sent via mobile texting, instant message, or the Internet.

Photo and Video Sharing Sites: YouTube (*www.youtube.com*) and Flickr *(www.flickr.com)*

Photos and videos can provide important visual messages, enabling issues to get on the public's agenda by drawing attention to a cause. YouTube has created an online video community. Flickr is a way to manage and access photos.

---

engaging in advocacy. Guo and Saxton (2014) applied the same typology to investigate the tweets of 188 civil rights and advocacy organizations and had strikingly similar findings: 67% information, 20% community, and 12% action. Research on nonprofit organizations' use of social media has also shown that the interactive features of Facebook are often underused (Waters et al., 2009). These studies suggest that nonprofit organizations are not yet as successful at reinforcing and building an online community and then mobilizing it.

ANALYZING MEDIA

The first obligation that all nurses have is to be knowledgeable consumers of media. Nurses must seek out unbiased information before taking positions on policy issues and be able to critically evaluate media messages, assess who controls the media, and identify whose vested interests are being protected or promoted. Nurses should add *www.mediachannel.org* and *www.freepress.net* to their Internet favorites and evaluate their sources.

Getting to know the nature and quality of a particular journalist's or cyberactivist's work can help you to decide how much to trust it. Ask the following questions:

- Do they frequently misrepresent issues?
- Are their stories sensationalized or exaggerated?
- Do they present all sides of an issue with accuracy, fairness, and depth?
- Can you substantiate wild claims through sites such as *www.factcheck.org*, *www.snopes.com*, and *www.urbanlegends.about.com*?

WHAT IS THE MEDIUM?

The first step is to ask yourself from where you get your information and news.

- What is the reputation of the television or radio station, program, newspaper, or website? Is it known for balanced coverage of health-related issues? Is it partisan?
- Does it cover international and national, as well as state and local, issues?
- Is it a credible source of information about health issues and policies?

These questions provide a basis to judge whether or not the information and news you are getting is credible and representative of a broad sector of public opinion. You will need a sample of various media presentations of the issue to evaluate their messages and effectiveness.

WHO IS SENDING THE MESSAGE?

Part of understanding what the real message is about comes from knowing who is behind the message and why. You could interpret the real message behind the Harry and Louise commercials against President Clinton's health care reform legislation once you knew they were sponsored by the HIAA. If the legislation had passed, the majority of insurance companies would have been locked out of the health care market.

For news media, ask the following questions: Who owns this medium? Who sponsors the website? What are the owner's biases? In addition, more and more newspapers and online venues are using the Associated Press (AP), or other major national papers, as their source for stories. The AP does not investigate; they attend events, accept news releases, and file reports. If newspapers are using abridged stories from other papers, the news slant or bias of the other paper reflects the bias or slant of the paper you are analyzing. As newspaper and television newsroom budgets get slashed, few news outlets are able to afford investigative journalism. To preserve this important aspect of journalism, nonprofit investigative news organizations have arisen to fill the void, such as the online Kaiser Health News, founded and supported by the Kaiser Family Foundation, and ProPublica, supported by a major multiyear commitment of funding by the Sandler Foundation. While Kaiser Health News is specific to health, ProPublica is not but does cover health issues. For example, it published a series of reports on the excessive delays in the California State Board of Registered Nursing's actions on complaints against nurses who were found guilty of drug abuse, sexual assaults on patients, and homicides (*www.propublica.org/series/nurses*). The reporting by Pulitzer Prize-winning journalist Charles Ornstein and Tracy Weber resulted in the governor removing several board members who were up for reappointment and the executive secretary resigning.

WHAT IS THE MESSAGE, AND WHAT RHETORIC IS USED?

What is the ostensible message that is being delivered, and what is the real message? What rhetoric is used to get the real message across? In 2009, pollster Frank Luntz of the Luntz Research Companies leaked a 28-page memo of sound bites and rhetoric designed to stop the Washington takeover of health care to Politico. The memo, entitled "The Language of Health Care," is reminiscent of the analysis Luntz provided to Republicans for the 2004 presidential campaign and that was used by the Republicans to win legislative battles and political campaigns in 2006. His 2009 analysis provides insight into the language used to frame health care reform by federal policymakers. For example, he proposed that the phrase that "would 'scare people more' about the future of American healthcare" was: "That the government will decide what treatment I can or can't have" (Luntz, 2009, p. 24). *PolitiFact.com* chose "a government takeover of health care" as the 2010 Lie of the Year because it played a key role in public opinion about the ACA (Adair & Holan, 2010). Rhetoric relies on "words that work" and those that do not work based on polling results. One of the words not to say was: private health care/free market health care. Instead, the document advocated the phrase: patient-centered health care.

Every issue has spin doctors who develop believable messages based on focus groups and polling. As messages are repeated in the media, they become believable. It is essential to be attentive to the language used in media messages whether delivered directly by policymakers, pundits, or advocates, and to evaluate the credibility, bias, and intentions of these sources. What and whom should we believe?

Images also convey important messages. As Luntz's (2005) *New American Lexicon* notes, "Language is your base. Symbols knock it out of the park. The American people cannot always be expected to directly grasp the connection between your policies and your principles. Symbols bridge this gap, so use them" (Section 2, p. 2). The document promotes the obvious symbols of the American flag and Statue of Liberty. But consider the symbols used by health insurance companies to advertise to employed individuals and families. These ads use pictures of healthy active adults and bright-eyed children rather than images of obese individuals or people disabled by arthritis to attract new members to their insurance products. These are examples of targeted media messages in which images are symbols to augment carefully crafted rhetoric to sway a target audience to believe or act in a particular way.

IS THE MESSAGE EFFECTIVE?

Does the message attract your attention? Does it appeal to your logic and to your emotions? Does it undermine the opposition's position?

IS THE MESSAGE ACCURATE?

Who is the reporter or cyberactivist and what reputation do they have? Are they credible, with a reputation for accuracy and balanced coverage of an issue? What viewpoints are missing? Whose voice is represented in the message or article?

RESPONDING TO THE MEDIA

One of the most important ways to influence public opinion is to respond to what is read, seen, or heard in the media. Letters to the editor or call-ins to talk radio programs can be powerful ways to reframe an issue or put it on the public's agenda.

Op-eds (thought to be derived from opposite the editorial page or opinion editorial) allow a more in-depth response to current issues and provide a way to get an issue on the public's agenda. Although they may be solicited by a newspaper or magazine, local community papers often are eager to receive op-eds that describe an important issue, include a story that illustrates the local impact of the problem, and suggest possible solutions.

Tips for successful op-eds include:
- Keep it short and within the word limit specified by the publication.
- Hook it to a national event if the publication or website has a national focus, or to a local event for local publications.
- Have a timely topic, concisely and clearly written in a conversational style, and with an unexpected or provocative slant.
- Include details or clinical examples to bring the commentary alive.
- Use data to support your argument
- Define the problem, possible solutions and include a call to action.

Similarly, letters to the editor should be written immediately after the original story is published and follow the publication's guidelines for letters. They should be concise and make a specific point relevant to the article.

Calling in to talk radio provides another opportunity for sharing your perspectives. Identify yourself as a registered nurse and stay on the line while the host or program guest responds to your point or question. You may need to correct a misunderstanding or offer additional clarifying information.

Finally, it is always a good idea to contact a journalist to thank him or her for a good story. If you have a blog, be sure to link to the story in a post. If you see a tweet you like, you can retweet it to others who follow you. If you are on Facebook and like someone's posting, you can click on the *Like* icon and continue the spread of the posting.

CONCLUSION

Nurses have not always been taught how to use the media as a health promotion tool. Harnessing the traditional and new social media will provide opportunities to shape healthy public policies and engage in political activism.

DISCUSSION QUESTIONS

1. What are your major news sources? What are the potential biases of these sources?
2. How is framing and rhetoric shaping media discussions of a current health or social policy issue? What are the competing frames or rhetoric? How else might the issue be framed?
3. If you were to talk with a journalist about an issue of concern to you, how would you frame the issue? What language or images would you use for the frame?

REFERENCES

Abramson, A. (2003). *The history of television, 1942 to 2000.* New York: McFarland.

Adair, B., & Holan, D. B. (2010). PolitiFact's lie of the year: "A government takeover of healthcare." Retrieved from *www.politifact.com/truth-o-meter/article/2010/dec/16/lie-year-government-takeover-health-care/.*

Annenberg Public Policy Center of the University of Pennsylvania (1995). *Media in the middle: Fairness and accuracy in the 1994 health care reform debate.* Philadelphia: Annenberg Public Policy Center.

Barklow, T. K., Ziering, A. (producers), & Dick, K. (director). (2012). *The invisible war.* Sausalito, CA.: Distributed by Roco Films Educational.

Center for the Digital Future (2013). *The 2013 digital future report: Surveying the digital future, year eleven.* Los Angeles: USC Annenberg School. Retrieved from *www.digitalcenter.org/wp-content/uploads/2013/06/2013-Report.pdf.*

Daniels, J. (2009). Cloaked websites: Propaganda, cyber-racism, and epistemology in the digital era. *New Media & Society, 11*(5), 659–683.

Dorfman, L., & Krasnow, I. D. (2014). Public health and media advocacy. *Annual Review of Public Health, 35,* 293–306.

Enda, J., & Mitchell, A. (2013). Americans show signs of leaving a news outlet, citing less information. The Pew Research Center Project for Excellence in Journalism: The state of new media 2013. Retrieved from *stateofthemedia.org/2013/special-reports-landing-page/citing-reduced-quality-many-americans-abandon-news-outlets/.*

Freepress.net (2014). Who Owns the Media? Retrieved from *www.freepress.net/ownership/chart.*

Gallup, Inc (2014). Honesty/Ethics in Professions. *Gallup* [Survey conducted Dec. 5-8, 2013]. Retrieved from *www.gallup.com/poll/1654/honesty-ethics-professions.aspx.*

Gamson, W. A. (2004). Bystanders, public opinion, and the media. In D. A. Snow, S. A. Soule, & H. Kriesi (Eds.), *The Blackwell companion to social movements* (pp. 242–261). Malden, MA: Blackwell.

Groshek, J., & Al-Rawi, A. (2013). Public sentiment and critical framing in social media content during the 2012 U.S. Presidential campaign. *Social Science Computer Review, 31*(5), 563–576.

Groshek, J., & Dimitrova, D. (2011). A cross-section of voter learning, campaign interest and intention to vote in the 2008 presidential election: Did Web 2.0 matter? *Communication Studies, 9,* 355–375.

Guo, C., & Saxton, G. D. (2014). Tweeting social change: How social media are changing nonprofit advocacy. *Nonprofit and Voluntary Sector Quarterly, 43*(1), 57–79.

Harris, J. (2005). To be our own governors: The independent press and the battle for "popular information." In E. D. Cohen (Ed.), *News incorporated.* Amherst: Prometheus Books.

Hindman, M. (2009). *The myth of digital democracy.* Princeton, NJ: Princeton UP.

Holcomb, J., Gottfried, J., & Mitchell, A. (2013). News use across social media platforms. *Pew Research Journalism Project.* Retrieved from *www.journalism.org/2013/11/14/news-use-across-social-media-platforms/.*

Institute of Medicine (2002). *Speaking of health: Assessing health communication strategies for diverse populations.* Washington, DC: National Academies Press.

Jamieson, K. H. (2012). Cable news networks increase amount and public accessibility of incivility. *FlackCheck.org.* Retrieved from *www.flackcheck.org/press/press-release-incivility-in-public-discourse/.*

Jernigan, D. H., & Wright, P. A. (1996). Media advocacy: Lessons from community experiences. *Journal of Public Health Policy, 17*(3), 306–329.

Kantar, U. S. (2014). 2014 U.S. political ad spend & share. Retrieved from *us.kantar.com/public-affairs/politics/2014-political-media-projections/.*

Lardinois, R. (2008). Obama's social media advantage. ReadWriteWeb. Retrieved from *www.readwriteweb.com/archives/social_media_obama_mccain_comparison.php.*

Lovejoy, K., & Saxton, G. D. (2012). Information, community, and action: How nonprofit organizations use social media. *Journal of Computer-Mediated Communication, 17*(3), 337–353.

Luntz, F. (2005). *The new American lexicon.* Alexandria, VA: The Luntz Research Companies. Retrieved from *www.dailykos.com/story/2005/2/23/3244/72156.*

Luntz, F. (2009). The language of Healthcare in 2009. Retrieved from *content.time.com/time/nation/article/0,8599,1896597,00.html.*

Lutz, A. (2012, June 14). These 6 corporations control 90% of the media in America. *Business Insider.* Retrieved from *www.businessinsider.com/these-6-corporations-control-90-of-the-media-in-america-2012-6.*

McCaughey, M., & Ayers, M. (Eds.), (2003). *Cyberactivism: Online activism in theory and practice.* New York: Routledge.

McLuhan, M. (1964). *Understanding media: the extensions of man.* New York: McGraw Hill.

Mitchell, A. (2013). Overview. *Pew research center project for excellence in journalism: The state of new media 2013.* Retrieved from *stateofthemedia.org/2013/overview-5/.*

Mitchell, A. (2014). Overview. Pew Research Center Project for Excellence in Journalism: The state of new media 2014. Retrieved from *www.journalism.org/2014/03/26/state-of-the-news-media-2014-overview/.*

Nielsen Reports (2013, December 3). A look across media: The cross-platform report Q3 2013. Retrieved from *www.nielsen.com/us/en/reports/2013/a-look-across-media-the-cross-platform-report-q3-2013.html.*

O'Reilly, T. (2005, September 30). What is Web 2.0: Design patterns and business models for the next generation of software. *O'Reilly.*

Retrieved from *www.oreillynet.com/pub/a/oreilly/tim/news/2005/09/30/what-is-web-20.html?page=1*.

Ozimek, T. (2005). Distributed campaigns: Using the Internet to empower action. In D. Mason, J. Leavitt, & M. Chaffee (Eds.), *Policy & politics in nursing and health care* (5th ed.). St. Louis: Elsevier Saunders.

Pew Research Center's Journalism Project Staff. (2012, August 15). How the presidential candidates use the web and social media: Obama leads but neither candidate engages in much dialogue with voters. *Pew Research Center. Project for Excellence in Journalism.* Retrieved from *www.journalism.org/2012/08/15/how-presidential-candidates-use-web-and-social-media/*.

Polletta, F., Chen, P. C. B., Gardner, B. G., & Motes, A. (2013). Is the Internet creating new reasons to protest? In B. Klandermans, J. Steklenburg, & C. Roggeband (Eds.), *The future of social movement research: Dynamics, mechanisms, and processes.* Minneapolis: University of Minnesota Press.

Rainie, L., Hitlin, P., Jurkowitz, M., Dimock, M., & Neidorf, S. (2012b). The viral Kony 2012 video. Pew Research Internet Project. Retrieved from *www.pewInternet.org/2012/03/15/the-viral-kony-2012-video/*.

Rainie, L., Smith, A., Schlozman, K. L., Brady, H., & Verba, S. (2012a). Social media and political engagement. *Pew research Internet project.* Retrieved from *pewInternet.org/Reports/2012/Political-Engagement.aspx*.

Rideout, V. J., Foehr, U. G., & Roberts, D. F. (2010). *Generation M2: Media in the lives of 8- to 18-year-olds.* Menlo Park, CA: Kaiser Family Foundation.

Ritzer, G., & Jurgenson, N. (2010). Production, consumption, prosumption: The nature of capitalism in the age of the digital "prosumer." *Journal of Consumer Culture, 10*(1), 13–36.

Roche, J. P. (2002). Print media coverage of risk-risk tradeoffs associated with West Nile encephalitis and pesticide spraying. *Journal of Urban Health, 79*(4), 482–490.

Russell, A., Voas, R. B., DeJong, W., & Chaloupka, M. (1995). MADD rates the states: Advocacy event to advance the agenda against alcohol-impaired driving. *Public Health Reports, 110*(3), 240–245.

Shaughnessy, H. (2012). Will the US election be won on Facebook? *Forbes Online.* Retrieved from *www.forbes.com/sites/haydnshaughnessy/2012/02/02/will-the-us-election-be-won-on-facebook/*.

Shirky, C. (2008). *Here comes everybody: The power of organizing without organizations.* New York: The Penguin Press.

Smith, A. (2013). Digital politics: Pew research findings on technology and campaign 2012. *Pew research Internet project.* Retrieved from *www.pewInternet.org/2013/02/20/digital-politics-pew-research-findings-on-technology-and-campaign-2012/*.

Sobieraj, S., & Berry, J. M. (2011). From incivility to outrage: political discourse in blogs, talk radio, and cable news. *Political Communication, 28*(1), 19–41. doi:10.1080/10584609.2010.542360.

Steele, C. (2012). Election 2012: How social media will convert followers into voters. *PC News.* Retrieved from *www.pcmag.com/slideshow/story/293078/election-2012-how-social-media-will-convert-followers-into-v*.

Stotter, P. L. (producer), & Rock, M. (director). (2011). *Service: When women come marching home.* New York, NY: Distributed by Women Make Movies.

Talbot, D. (2008, September/October). How Obama really did it: The social-networking strategy that took an obscure senator to the doors of the White House. *Technology Review.* Retrieved from *www.technologyreview.com/web/21222*.

Turow, J. (1996). Television entertainment and the U.S. health-care debate. *Lancet, 347*(9010), 1240–1243.

Turow, J., & Gans, R. (2002). *As seen on TV: Health policy issues in TV's medical dramas.* Menlo Park, CA: The Henry J. Kaiser Family Foundation.

Wakefield, M. A., Loken, B., & Hornik, R. C. (2010). Use of mass media campaigns to change health behavior. *Lancet, 276*(9748), 1261–1271. doi:10.1016/S0140-6736(10)60809-4.

Wallack, L., & Dorfman, L. (1996). Media advocacy: A strategy for advancing policy and promoting health. *Health Education Quarterly, 23*(3), 293–317.

Waters, R. D., Burnett, E., Lamm, A., & Lucas, J. (2009). Engaging stakeholders through social networking: How nonprofit organizations are using Facebook. *Public Relations Review, 35*(2), 102–106.

West, D. M., Heith, D., & Goodwin, C. (1996). Harry and Louise go to Washington: Political advertising and health care reform. *Journal of Health Politics, Policy and Law, 21*(1), 35–68.

Wong, S. (2012). Joseph Kony captures Congress' attention. *Politico.* Retrieved from *www.politico.com/news/stories/0312/74355.html*.

The Woodhull Study on Nursing and the Media. (1998). *Healthcare's invisible partner: Final report.* Indianapolis, IN: Sigma Theta Tau.

Zickuhr, K. (2010). *Generations 2010.* Retrieved from *www.pewInternet.org/2010/12/16/generations-2010/*.

ONLINE RESOURCES

Center for Health Media and Policy
www.centerforhealthmediapolicy.com
Kaiser Health News
www.khn.org
Freepress
www.freepress.net
Media Channel
www.mediachannel.org
Pew Internet Research Project
www.pewInternet.org
Pew Research Center for People and the Press
www.people-press.org

CHAPTER 15

Health Policy, Politics, and Professional Ethics

Carol R. Taylor   Susan I. Belanger

"To see what is right and not do it is want of courage."
Confucius

Writing in the *Encyclopedia of Bioethics,* Dan Callahan, one of the founders of U.S. bioethics, states that three paramount human questions lie at the heart of bioethics:

- What kind of person ought I be to live a moral life and make good ethical decisions?
- What are my duties and obligations to other individuals whose life and well-being may be affected by my actions?
- What do I owe the common good or the public interest, in my life as a member of society?

The authors of this chapter believe that too few nurses take seriously their responsibilities as citizens, in spite of being frequently reminded that the sheer numbers as the largest group of health professionals (3.1 million) and as the most trusted professionals (Gallup's annual honesty and ethics survey), make us a formidable force (2013). Ethics may be defined as the formal study of who we ought to be, how we should make decisions and behave. This chapter centers around what is reasonable to expect of professional nurses as citizens in regard to designing and delivering a just health system that meets the needs of all, with special concern for the most vulnerable.

Designing a system for delivering health care that adequately meets the needs of a diverse public is a complex challenge. Health care planners have always worried about access, quality, and cost. Who should get what quality of care and at what cost? What you think about health care in the United States largely depends on your past experiences. If you are well insured or independently wealthy, you can access the best health care in the world. If you lack insurance and have limited financial resources, you may die of a disease that might have been prevented or treated at an early stage if you had had access to quality care. The U.S. system has been criticized for providing too little care to some and too much of the wrong type of care to others. Many now believe that a moral society owes health care to its citizens. Health care is like clean water, sanitation, and basic education. Others, however, believe that health care is a commodity, like automobiles, to be sold and purchased in the marketplace. If you lack the funds to buy a car, that may be sad, but society has no obligation to purchase a car for you. As you read this chapter, ask yourself what you believe about health care. Is it simply unfortunate if people cannot afford the health care they and their families need?

Daily nursing practice and people's health, well-being, and dying are directly affected by decisions made by governments, insurers, and health care institutions. Nursing needs a seat at these decision-making tables and nurses must be prepared and willing to take these seats. As the country's most trusted health care professionals, the nurses in these seats must be committed to ethical decision making. Drivers for much of human enterprise are power, position, prestige, profit, and politics (Barnet, n.d.). Strikingly absent from this list are people, patients, the public, and the poor! Nursing's challenge, as profits and politics increasingly dictate health priorities, is to keep health care strongly focused on the needs of patients, their families, and the public. Health care in the United States is a business, revenues need to be generated to make care possible, but health care can never be *only* a business. First and primarily, it is a service a moral society provides for its vulnerable members. Nurses play a critical role in keeping health care centered on the people it purports to serve.

This chapter opens with a description of the ethics of influencing policy and explores the professional ethics of nurses and their advocacy and health policy responsibilities. It offers a brief analyses of how nurses can use their voice to influence policy regarding scarce resource allocations and workplace issues. Throughout, short reflective practice vignettes invite readers to reflect on the adequacy of their moral agency in select advocacy challenges.

THE ETHICS OF INFLUENCING POLICY

An ethical critique of human behavior involves paying attention to the intention of the moral agent, the nature of the act performed, the consequences of the action, and the circumstances surrounding the act. Ethics has to do with right and wrong in this world, and policy and politics has everything to do with what happens to people in this world. Moreover, both ethics and politics have to do with making life better for oneself and others. Surely both deal with power and powerlessness, with human rights and balancing claims, with justice and fairness, and with good and evil. And good and evil are not the same as right and wrong. Right and wrong pertain to adherence to principles; good and evil pertain to the intent of the doer and the impact the deed has on other people. Surely policy and politics involves justice in the distribution of social goods; fairness and equity in relationships among and between people of different races, genders, and creeds; and access to education and assistance when one is in need. Although the goodness of an action lies in the intent and integrity of the human being who performs it, the rightness or wrongness of an action is judged by the difference it makes in the world. Therefore the principles applied in ethical analysis generally derive from a consideration of the duties one person owes another by virtue of commitments made and roles assumed,

and/or a consideration of the effects that a choice of action could have on one's own life and the lives of others.

In a perfect world, legislators would all intend the good of the public they serve and use ethical means to achieve good outcomes. In the real world, legislators and lobbyists intend many things other than the good of the public and some use unethical means to achieve dubious ends. A democracy with an increasingly heterogeneous public necessarily involves compromise. Which strategies to influence policy can nurses use without sacrificing personal and professional integrity? Each advocacy strategy involves a variation of the same question, that is, what means can be legitimately used to achieve an end that someone (or a political party or the electorate) believes to be good? The ends-and-means argument is often explained as follows. We can cut a man open (an evil means) to save his life (a good end). We can remove a perfectly healthy kidney from one person (an evil means) to transplant it to save the life and health of another (a good end). We admire the person who sacrifices his life (an evil means) to save the life of his friend (a good end). If our intention (to produce a good) can justify the means (doing an evil), then why can't we torture one man (an evil means) to gain information that might save another person's life or even the lives of many people (a good end)? Should we assure the passage of health care insurance reform (a good end) by strong-arm tactics (an evil means)?

It is important to note that cutting a person open, even to save his life, is not a good thing unless the person consents to it. Similarly one cannot steal one person's kidney even to save another; rather, the consent of both donor and recipient is required. The prisoner does not choose to be tortured; although it is very tempting to justify torture to protect innocent lives, if a man can be tortured on the suspicion that he may know something subversive, who is safe from governmental oppression? The price we pay for freedom and human rights is to grant them to all people, not just a favored few. And yes, it is risky, and yes, it may reduce our "efficiency" and in some cases it may even lead to loss of life. But the alternative is that no one has rights (i.e., just claims); rights become the privilege of a favored group, while all other individuals are utterly helpless before the power of the state.

Certainly the electorate does not consent to the corruption of the legislative process, and even if a majority did approve of bending the rules of fair engagement to ensure that a particular piece of legislation is passed, would that make it right? Would it not end up threatening the very foundations of a free society (because the foundation of a republic lies in the honesty of its processes)? What are the differences between normal legislative wrangling and abuse of power? What does it mean when political parties refuse to participate in the legislative process and/or use blatant scare tactics? What is legitimate dissent, and what is a refusal to accept democratic outcomes unless you happen to agree with them? Without civil disobedience, we would still have the Jim Crow laws. And without respect for the law, a society degenerates into either despotism or anarchy.

When people ask whether it is wrong to lie about something (e.g., the number of people affected by a particular disease) to get funding for research and/or treatment of patients with a particular disease, in a word the answer is yes. It is wrong. Why is lying wrong? It's wrong because it undermines the foundation of any relationship: trust. In like manner, lying to further a political agenda is wrong not only because it undermines trust, but also because it fosters further dishonesty. Judging by the amount of political dishonesty reported in the media, one is led to the conclusion that there is a lot of lying going on! Adding to it, telling more lies to further our own agenda, will only make matters worse.

REFLECTIVE PRACTICE: PANTS ON FIRE

Sarah Palin is famous for urging her supporters to oppose Democratic plans for health care using the scare tactic of death panels. She said the Democrats plan to reduce health care costs by simply refusing to pay for care:

And who will suffer the most when they ration care? The sick, the elderly, and the disabled, of course. The America I know and love is not one in which my parents or my baby with Down Syndrome will have to stand in front of Obama's death panel so his bureaucrats can decide, based on a subjective judgment of their level of productivity in society, whether they are worthy of health care. Such a system is downright evil.

In fact there was no panel in any version of the health care bills in Congress that judges a person's level of productivity in society to determine whether they are worthy of health care.

The truth is that the proposed health bill would have allowed Medicare, for the first time, to pay for optional doctors' appointments for patients to discuss living wills and other end-of-life issues with their physicians. PolitiFact awarded Palin with the 2009 Lie of the Year for the death panel claim, but the political impact of her statement is hard to overstate. In 2011, the Obama administration even deleted all references to end-of-life planning in a new Medicare regulation when opponents interpreted the move as a back-door effort to allow such planning. So even, in the regulations Palin achieved her goal (Holan, 2009).

DISCUSSION QUESTIONS

1. How do you judge Palin's quote? Effective strategy to oppose Democrats' plans for health care reform or unethical scaremongering?
2. Reflect on what informs your judgment: commitment to advance care planning, analysis of facts, political party loyalties?
3. Is it right for nurses to endorse health reform legislation even if the legislation is not perfect? (The answer is yes; it may indeed be the right thing to do.)

Remember, politics is about relationships, and relationships cannot prosper when one party insists that the other party must agree with them on every (or even any) issue. It is not wrong to compromise; compromise is part of the give and take of relationships, and it is part of the give and take of politics. What is critical is knowing when it is possible to compromise without sacrificing personal integrity. This prompts the question of whether it can be acceptable to distort an issue to manipulate public opinion or to win the support of a particular piece of legislation. It is usually, however, possible to frame a discussion in a manner that is more acceptable to a certain constituency without lying in this manner. For example, in the health care arena, one can use words that appeal to known values, words such as tradition and legitimate authority (words that tend to appeal to conservatives), and words such as autonomous and experimental (words that tend to appeal to liberals). Knowing the target audience and framing the issue in words that will help them listen (or at least not harden their opposition) is smart, not unethical. Now to return to the issue of nurses' (and others') lobbying activities: Here compromise is in order. Any professional group has a duty imposed on it by both its social role and its code of ethics, to push forward laws and policies that protect or advance the best interests of those whom they serve. And finally, any citizen, particularly a knowledgeable one, has a civic duty to speak out for the common good.

PROFESSIONAL ETHICS

A professional ethic is built around three essential components:

1. *Its purpose.* All professions develop in response to a social need, one that the members of the profession promise to meet. Put in legalistic terms, this need (along with the power and privileges society grants to the profession to help the professionals meet the need) and the profession's promised response to it constitute the profession's contract with society.

2. *The conduct expected of the professional.* The ethical code developed and promulgated by the profession, its code of ethics, describes the conduct society has a right to expect from professionals as they go about the business of the profession. However, it is not a list of prescribed do's and dont's but rather an articulation of those values that, in fact, outline the scope of the profession's practice and the relationships that ought to pertain between its members and the lay public, among the practitioners of this profession, between the practitioner and the profession itself, and between the professional

and the community within which he or she practices.

3. *The skills and outcomes expected in professional practice.* Nursing's standards of practice state with some precision the obligations of nurses in specific areas of practice. Clearly, each of these components is dynamic, that is, subject to change and reevaluation as the profession grows, as knowledge increases, and as social mores and expectations develop. This is not to claim that there are no constants (e.g., a general imperative to respect persons), but rather to say that the meaning and application of the imperatives change.

Professional ethics is the study of how personal moral norms apply or conflict with the promises and duties of one's profession. Society demands that professionals be held to a separate moral standard of conduct because the choices professionals make affect other people's lives more than their own. Nursing's foundational documents make each nurse's advocacy and health policy responsibilities clear. Although some may think that advocacy and health policy are an ethical ideal, they are rather a nonnegotiable moral obligation embedded in the nursing role. The ANA *Code of Ethics for Nurses* states: "The nurse promotes, advocates for, and strives to protect the health, safety, and rights of the patient" (2010). The 2015 revision of the *Code of Ethics* (soon to be published) places an even stronger emphasis on nursing's advocacy responsibilities. ANA's *Social Policy Statement: The Essence of the Profession* was published in 1980 and revised in 1995, 2003, and 2010. The introduction to the 2003 revision emphasizes nurses' central role in effecting health policy.

Nursing is the pivotal health care profession, highly valued for its specialized knowledge, skill, and caring in improving the health status of the public and ensuring safe, effective, quality care. The profession mirrors the diverse population it serves and provides leadership to create positive changes in health policy and delivery systems (p. 1).

The 2003 revision also included for the first time in its list of values and assumptions of nursing's social contract, "Public policy and the health care delivery system influence the health and well-being of society and professional nursing" (p. 4). This phrase appears again in the 2010 revision under the heading, "The elements of nursing's social contract" (p. 6). The 2010 revision also notes as a key social concern in health care and nursing "Expansion of health care resources and health policy" (p. 4).

REFLECTIVE PRACTICE: FOUNDATIONAL NURSING DOCUMENTS

The American Nursing Association publishes three documents packaged as the *Foundation of Nursing Package, 2010*. Included in the package are the *Code of Ethics for Nurses* and the revised *Nursing Social Policy Statement* and *Nursing Scope and Standards of Practice*. Together these documents describe what is reasonable for the U.S. public to expect of nurses. As this text goes to press, a newly revised *Code of Ethics* is being studied and may be available as early as 2015.

It is the responsibility of every professional nurse to be familiar with these foundational documents and to continually assess if her/his professional practice is congruent with what is expected.

PERSONAL QUESTIONS

1. When, if ever, did you read and reflect on these core documents?
2. In what ways do you expect your Code of Ethics to change? Do you support these changes?
3. Have you participated in discussions about how these documents pertain to your practice and what they suggest as growth opportunities for you or your colleagues?
4. What is reasonable to expect of every professional nurse in regard to advocacy and health policy?

MORAL AGENCY AND THE NURSE

Once professional nurses understand what is reasonable for the public to expect of them, the next step is to determine if one has the capacity to meet these expectations. In other words, one must ask, "Am I trustworthy?" Moral agency is quite simply the ability to be what is professed: a human, a parent, a professional nurse. Moral agency in any

specific situation requires more than knowing what is right to do; it also entails:

- *Moral character:* Cultivated dispositions that allow one to act as one believes one ought to act.
- *Moral valuing:* Valuing in a conscious and critical way which squares with good moral character and ethical integrity. For nurses this is a commitment to patient well-being and a degree of altruism.
- *Moral sensibility:* The ability to recognize the moral moment when an ethical challenge presents.
- *Moral responsiveness:* The ability and willingness to respond to the ethical challenge.
- *Ethical reasoning and discernment:* The knowledge of, and ability to use, sound theoretical and practical approaches to thinking through ethical challenges and to ultimately decide how best to respond to this particular challenge after identifying and weighing alternative courses of action; using these approaches to both inform and justify moral behavior. (See Box 15-1.)
- *Moral accountability:* The ability and willingness to accept responsibility for one's ethical behavior and to learn from the experiences of exercising moral agency.
- *Transformative moral leadership:* Commitment and proven ability to create a culture that facilitates the exercise of moral agency, a culture in which individuals are supported in doing the right thing simply because it is the right thing to do (Taylor, 2015).

Nurses who value their moral agency are familiar with the principles of bioethics which commit them, all things being equal, to: (1) respect the autonomy of individuals, (2) act so as to benefit (beneficence), (3) not harm (nonmaleficence), and (4) give individuals their due (justice). Other principles include keeping promises (fidelity) and responsiveness to vulnerability. A commitment to social justice and the common good has long characterized the profession of nursing. This commitment calls for the creation of a society in which all can flourish, not only the affluent, and the creation of a bottom floor beneath which no one can fall regarding access to basic nutrition, safe housing, education, health care, and employment.

BOX 15-1 Ethics Inventory

Think about a recent ethical challenge you encountered in practice.

- What signals you to an ethical challenge? Intellectual disconnect? Queasy feeling in the pit of your stomach? Discomfort or disappointment in the way you or your team are responding? Yuck factor?
- Pay attention to how you reason as you think about how you should and would respond.
  - What informs your judgment? Rephrased, how do you calibrate your moral compass?
  - Are there moral rules that apply?
  - Do you have a responsibility to respond? Are you personally able and willing to respond? Are there institutional or other external variables making it difficult or impossible to respond?
- What counts as a good response? What criteria/principles do you use to inform, justify, and evaluate your response?
  - Promotes human dignity and the common good
  - Maximizes good and minimizes harm
  - Justly distributes goods and harms
  - Respects rights
  - Responsive to vulnerabilities
  - Promotes virtue
  - Compatible with Code of Ethics for Nurses
  - Other

- What criteria/principles do you use to critique/evaluate your response?
  - We stayed out of trouble, not greatly inconvenienced.
  - We made money or at the very least didn't lose money!
  - Our patient satisfaction scores will be high, or at least not negative
  - Able to put my head on my pillow and fall asleep peacefully
  - My/our reputation is intact.
  - Transparency [Washington Post test; I could share how I/we responded with my children and feel proud.]
  - Consistency
  - Other
- Are there any universal (nonnegotiable) moral obligations that obligate all health care professionals?
- To whom would you turn if you were uncertain about how to proceed?
  - What agency resources exist to help you think through and secure a good response? How confident are you that these resources would facilitate a good resolution of your concern?
- Can you translate your moral judgments about how best to respond into action? If you believe that institutional or other variables are making it impossible to do what you believe is the ethically right thing to do, what are your options?

REFLECTIVE PRACTICE: NEGOTIATING CONFLICTS BETWEEN PERSONAL INTEGRITY AND PROFESSIONAL RESPONSIBILITIES

Shortly after the Department of Health and Human Services (HHS) announced the new federal rule that required all new private plans to cover prescribed FDA-approved contraceptive methods without cost-sharing, a number of corporations sued, claiming that this new requirement violates their religious rights. These lawsuits have worked their way through the federal courts and on November 26, 2013, the Supreme Court agreed to hear two cases that involved for-profit corporations. The Court agreed to hear a case from the Tenth Circuit Court of Appeals, which ruled in favor of Hobby Lobby, an Oklahoma-based chain of craft stores owned by a Christian family who claim that the contraceptive coverage requirement violates their company's religious freedom. The Court also agreed to hear a case from the Third Circuit Court of Appeals, which ruled against the corporation and its owners, finding that Conestoga Wood Specialties, a cabinet manufacturer, does not have religious rights. The Supreme Court decided to take these cases to resolve the conflict between the two decisions along with other U.S. Courts of Appeals' rulings (Sobel & Salganicoff, 2013).

PERSONAL QUESTION

1. You are a women's health nurse practitioner and are asked to collaborate on filing an amicus brief to the court supporting women's rights to free

approved contraceptive methods. From your practice you know how important women's accessibility to these methods are and have sat with many a tearful woman contemplating an unplanned pregnancy. You are Christian, however, and you support your church's stance on not using contraceptive methods. You feel torn between maintaining your personal integrity and fulfilling your nursing obligation to aid poor women without access to basic reproductive services. How will you reconcile your conflict?

It is important to note here that effecting the right courses of action is not merely within the scope of the moral agency of the nurse. Ethics happens in the realm of the individual, the institution, and society, and each can profoundly influence the others (Glaser, 1994). A nurse with strong moral agency who is committed to health policy reform can have a profound influence on the practice of nurses working in institutions and can also influence the public's health. Similarly, a nurse with strong moral agency who is practicing in an institution willing to sacrifice patient safety and well-being for financial profit in a society that has yet to guarantee basic health care for all may feel compromised at every turn. When a nurse knows the right course of action for a patient, family, or community and is prevented by internal or external variables from translating this knowledge into action, moral distress results, which, if unresolved over time, builds up moral residue (Epstein & Hamric, 2009; Rushton, 2006). Put yourself in the shoes of a nurse working in a busy inner city emergency room. Every day he discharges patients with instructions for follow-up treatment that he knows will never happen because of a lack of financial or personal resources. His choices seem to be to stop caring in order not to experience frustration or distress, to show up for work like a robot and do his job, or to find meaning and purpose in working collaboratively to change the system.

U.S. HEALTH CARE REFORM

A just and caring society provides for the health care needs of its people. The 2010 Commonwealth Fund International comparison of the U.S. health system concluded that despite having the most costly health system in the world, the United States consistently underperforms in most dimensions of performance relative to other countries. "Compared with six other nations—Australia, Canada, Germany, the Netherlands, New Zealand, and the United Kingdom—the U.S. health care system ranks last or next-to-last in five dimensions of a high-performance health system: quality, access, efficiency, equity, and healthy lives" (Davis, Schoen, & Stremkis, 2010). The report was hopeful that newly enacted health reform legislation in the United States would address these problems by extending coverage to those without and helping to close gaps in coverage, leading to improved disease management, care coordination, and better outcomes over time.

A discouraging 2013 Institute of Medicine report, *U.S. Health in International Perspective: Shorter Lives, Poorer Health,* concluded that although the United States is among the wealthiest nations in the world, it is far from the healthiest. Despite spending far more per person on health care than any other nation, the United States has more people dying at younger ages than people in almost all other high-income countries. Among 16 peer nations, all affluent democracies, the United States is at or near the bottom in nine key areas of health: infant mortality and low birth weight, injuries and homicides, teenage pregnancies and sexually transmitted infections, prevalence of HIV and AIDs, drug-related deaths, obesity and diabetes, heart disease, chronic lung disease, and disability. Included as factors linked to the U.S. disadvantage are inadequate health care, unhealthy behaviors, and adverse economic and social conditions. "The tragedy is not that the United States is losing a contest with other countries, but that Americans are dying and suffering from illness and injury at rates that are demonstrably unnecessary" (Woolf & Aron, 2013).

ACCESS TO HEALTH CARE

Any discussion of health care access must include a review of human rights and a discussion of whether or not there is such a thing as a human right to health care services, and whether or not a just society would provide a legal right to such services. A human right is a justice claim to an essential, universal human need. The justice of the claim is affected by (1) the universality of the need, (2) the extent to which a person can meet his or her own needs, and (3) the extent to which others can help meet these needs without compromising their own fundamental needs. Some argue that health care services, or at least illness care services, are not a human right; however, a far larger number think that such needs can easily meet each of these criteria, at least under a variety of circumstances. For almost a century, Presidents and members of Congress have tried and failed to provide universal health benefits to Americans. There are a few simple facts that are important: (1) the United States is the only industrialized country in the world that does not offer some type of universal health care; (2) each year tens of thousands of Americans lose their health care coverage caused by circumstances beyond their control; and (3) the main reason that Americans file bankruptcy is outstanding medical bills. The American Nurses Association website chronicles nurses' decades-long efforts to advocate for health care reforms that would guarantee access to high-quality health care for all.

REFLECTIVE PRACTICE: ACCEPTING THE CHALLENGE

The Affordable Care Act (ACA) has been challenged at every turn. In the 2014 State of the Union address, President Barack Obama reported:

One last point on financial security. For decades, few things exposed hard-working families to economic hardship more than a broken health care system. And in case you haven't heard, we're in the process of fixing that.

. . . Already, because of the Affordable Care Act, more than 3 million Americans under age 26 have gained coverage under their parents' plans.

More than 9 million Americans have signed up for private health insurance or Medicaid coverage— 9 million.

And here's another number: zero. Because of this law, no American, none, zero, can ever again be dropped or denied coverage for a preexisting condition like asthma or back pain or cancer. No woman can ever be charged more just because she's a woman. And we did all this while adding years to Medicare's finances, keeping Medicare premiums flat and lowering prescription costs for millions of seniors.

. . . That's why tonight I ask every American who knows someone without health insurance to help them get covered by March 31st. Help them get covered. . . . Citizenship demands a sense of common purpose; participation in the hard work of self-government; an obligation to serve to our communities (Obama, 2014).

PERSONAL QUESTION

1. You eagerly watched the State of the Union Address but you have mixed feelings about the ACA. You come from a family who greatly distrust big government and want the Act repealed. As a public health nurse you interact with families everyday who are complaining about difficulties enrolling in their state's online health insurance program. You've read about the successes some have had by contacting navigators in the governor's Office of Health Reform but you know that many don't know how to initiate this contact. Are you obligated to do all you can to get coverage for the public you serve even if this means setting aside your political commitments?

A 2013 U.S. Subcommittee on Primary Health and Aging reported that nearly 57 million people in the United States, one in five Americans, live in areas without adequate access to primary health care caused by a shortage of providers in their communities. The facts in this report are sobering:

- Fifty years ago, half of the physicians in the United States practiced primary care, but today fewer than one in three do.
- As many as 45,000 people die each year because they do not have health insurance and do not get to a physician on time.

- The average primary care physician in the United States is 47 years old, and one-quarter are nearing retirement.

In 2011, about 17,000 physicians graduated from American medical schools. Despite the fact that over half of patient visits are for primary care, only 7% of the nation's medical school graduates now choose a primary care career (Sanders, 2013).

REFLECTIVE PRACTICE: THE MEDICAID 5% COMMITMENT— AN APPEAL TO PROFESSIONALISM

More than one fifth of the U.S. population is ensured through Medicaid, a number that is growing rapidly as the ACA is implemented (The Kaiser Commission on Medicaid and the Uninsured, 2014). The Congressional Budget Office predicts that nine million additional people will gain coverage through Medicaid in 2014. One key concern is whether the increased demand will be adequately met, whether there will be a sufficient number of clinicians who accept new Medicaid patients. At the present about 30% of office-based physicians do not accept new Medicaid patients. In certain specialties, the percentage is considerably higher. The Medicaid reimbursement rates vary by state; in some cases they are so low that physicians regularly lose money on Medicaid patients.

In a recent article in the Perspective section of *The New England Journal of Medicine*, Lawrence Casalino proposed asking each physician to commit to providing care for enough Medicaid enrollees so that at least 5% of their practice consists of Medicaid patients (2013). Casalino concludes his short article with these words: "A 5%-commitment campaign would be a meaningful, highly visible demonstration of physician professionalism—of putting patients first."

DISCUSSION QUESTION

1. Nurses have always been at the forefront in ensuring that all have access to safe, effective, and appropriate care. How likely are today's advanced practice nurses to respond to Casalino's

challenge by ensuring that their practice commits to providing at a minimum care for enough Medicaid enrollees so that at least 5% of their practice consists of Medicaid patients? Will advanced practice nurses partnering with physicians be able to bring this issue to the practice and be skilled in effecting a positive response to Casalino's appeal to professionalism?

REFLECTIVE PRACTICE: YOUR STATE TURNED DOWN MEDICAID EXPANSION

As part of the ACA's broader effort to ensure health insurance coverage for all U.S. residents, the federal government from 2014 to 2017 has agreed to pay for 100% of the difference between a state's current Medicaid eligibility level and the ACA minimum. States that participate in the ACA expansion must provide Medicaid coverage to all state residents below a certain income level. As of January 2014, 26 states and the District of Columbia were expanding Medicaid (The Advisory Board Company, 2014). Every state that opted out has a Republican governor. Dickman and colleagues (2014) report that the Supreme Court's decision to allow states to opt out of Medicaid expansion will have adverse health and financial consequences. Based on recent data from the Oregon Health Insurance Experiment, they predict that many low-income women will forego recommended breast and cervical cancer screening; diabetics will forego medications; and all low-income adults will face a greater likelihood of depression, catastrophic medical expenses, and death. Disparities in access to care based on state of residence will increase. Because the federal government will pay 100% of increased costs associated with Medicaid expansion for the first three years (and 90% thereafter), opt-out states are also turning down billions of dollars of potential revenue, which might strengthen their local economy.

PERSONAL QUESTION

1. You practice in a mobile van that serves poor children and families in the inner city. You have

seen many media stories about families who are receiving badly needed health care for the first time in their lives because they now have coverage. You are exasperated with your state representatives who have repeatedly blocked efforts to expand Medicaid and worry about your state's ability to pay the costs of Medicaid in the future. You have personal knowledge of corruption within your state's current administration and are wondering if you should go public with your knowledge or feed it to the opposite party to ensure that current leaders will not be re-elected. What do you do?

ALLOCATING SCARCE RESOURCES

Health care resources are limited. No system has the financial resources to provide the best care, to everyone, in all situations (Hope, Reynolds, & Griffiths, 2002). Therefore, we look to the principles of distributive justice for answers.

Principles of Distributive Justice. Health care professionals, who are ideally situated to make microdistributive decisions and whose social role enables them to speak with authority to the general population about the impact of resource allocation decisions on the health and welfare of various segments of the population, must not allow social decisions to influence their clinical decisions. First, their ethical codes require, and for good reason, that health care professionals act in the best interests of the person on whom they are laying hands. Second, the will of the citizenry, as expressed through the votes of their elected representatives, should determine the distribution of the resources they have so diligently (if unwillingly) supplied to their governments. In general, the principles of distributive justice ought to be used to guide decision making at the sociopolitical levels. They are as follows:

1. *To each the same thing.* One of the simplest principles of distributive justice is that of strict or radical equality. The principle says that every person should have the same level of material goods and services. Even with this ostensibly simple principle, some of the difficult specification problems of distributive principles can be

seen, specifically construction of appropriate indexes for measurement and the specification of time frames. Because there are numerous proposed solutions to these problems, the principle of strict equality is not a single principle but a name for a group of closely related principles.

2. *To each according to his need.* The most widely discussed theory of distributive justice in the past three decades has been that proposed by John Rawls in *A Theory of Justice* (Rawls, 1971) and *Political Liberalism* (Rawls, 1993). Rawls proposes the following two principles of justice: (1) Each person has an equal claim to a fully adequate scheme of equal basic rights and liberties, and (2) social and economic inequalities are "to be to the greatest benefit of the least advantaged members of society" (Rawls, 1993, pp. 5-6). These principles give fairly clear guidance on what type of arguments will count as justifications for inequality. For example, the second principle would accept income disparities if these led to the greatest benefit to the least advantaged members of society (created job opportunities for the least well off) but would not support the rich getting richer at the expense of the poor.

3. *To each according to his ability to compete in the open marketplace.* Aristotle argued that virtue should be a basis for distributing rewards, but most contemporary principles owe a larger debt to John Locke. Locke argued that people deserve to have those items produced by their toil and industry, the products (or the value thereof) being a fitting reward for their effort. His underlying idea was to guarantee to individuals the fruits of their own labor and abstinence. According to some contemporary theorists (Feinberg, 1970), people freely apply their abilities and talents, in varying degrees, to socially productive work. People come to deserve varying levels of income by providing goods and services desired by others (Feinberg, 1970). Distributive systems are just insofar as they distribute incomes according to the different levels earned or deserved by the individuals in the society for their productive labors, efforts, or contributions.

4. *To each according to his merits (desserts).* Merit-based principles of distribution differ primarily according to what they identify as the basis for deserving. Most contemporary proposals regarding merit fit into one of three broad categories (Miller, 1976, 1989):

- *Contribution:* People should be rewarded for their work activity according to the value of their contribution to the social product.
- *Effort:* People should be rewarded according to the effort they expend in their work activity.
- *Compensation:* People should be rewarded according to the costs they incur in their work activity.

To illustrate some of the difficulties inherent in rationing decisions, we will discuss the case of Sarah Murnaghan. Sarah is an 11-year-old with cystic fibrosis. In June of 2013, Sarah received national media attention when her parents petitioned a federal judge to change the rules governing the allocation of organs to allow Sarah to be placed on the adult lung transplant list (Carroll, 2013). Sarah urgently needed a lung transplant. The family argued the severity of Sarah's illness, not her age, should be considered in deciding whether she receives an organ. Shortly thereafter, Sarah received two double lung transplants with adult lungs (Aleccia, 2013). Sarah's case raised questions about whether it was ethical to change the transplant allocation process based on one child's situation.

There were many concerns raised about Sarah's case, but the main one related to the judge's decision to allow Sarah to be listed on the adult transplant list. Many agree that politicians and judges should not intervene in this type of decision making, noting they rarely have all the information to make an informed judgment (Caplan, 2013; Tomlinson, 2013). Professional organizations and experts are better suited than government officials to decide such matters. In this situation, experts believed the decision should have been left to the United Network for Organ Sharing (UNOS), whose role is to oversee a fair and equitable process of organ allocation (UNOS, 2014). Clinicians with expertise in the area of transplantation for children agreed that if the usual process had been allowed,

Sarah would not have moved to the adult list (HRSA, 2013).

Another justice issue in Sarah's case concerned the displacement of adults from the transplant list. It is believed that children do better with child lungs than with adult lungs, so should Sarah have receive an adult lung? The transplant process is complex and the rules governing the process are meant to be fair and equitable for all. Placing Sarah on the adult list meant another recipient, with potentially a greater need, would not receive a lung.

Looking at Sarah's transplant from an ends and means argument, it can be said that receiving a transplant to allow Sarah to live is a good end. However, considering the means to that end, it could be said that Sarah's good end was obtained by an evil means. An ethical act is one that results in more benefits than harms to others. By displacing others from the transplant list, and by changing a previously established fair and equitable process, many would agree that Sarah's transplant was obtained by evil means, thereby making it an unethical act.

Nurses can often experience moral distress in situations such as Sarah's. Moral distress is experienced when nurses feel helpless to act in a way that benefits their patients. No one can fault Sarah's parents and medical team for wanting treatment to save her life. In the day-to-day care of patients, nurses can often cite a case when patients were not afforded the same level of material goods and services as others. Many would also say that benefits go to those who complain the loudest or pay the most. The least advantaged among us are the most often forgotten. Yet, in considering Sarah's case, nurses must be cognizant of the patients who were displaced by Sarah's movement to the top of the list. Should the way to procure a much-needed service be the result of a media frenzy, with the best politician winning? Of course not. However, gathering data, advocating for system changes when warranted, and raising awareness of the issues are all actions nurses can take to improve the situations of the patients they serve. Nurses can assist in promoting fair and compassionate treatment decisions by publishing their research, by raising awareness of allocation issues, and by remaining good stewards of available resources.

REFLECTIVE PRACTICE: BARRIERS TO THE TREATMENT OF MENTAL ILLNESS

Austin Deeds, the son of Virginia State Senator Creigh Deeds, was discharged home in November 2013 from a Virginia hospital emergency room because there were no open psychiatric beds. He then stabbed his father and killed himself. The tragedy focused national attention on the need for a major investment in the nation's mental health system. A 2008 report, Treatment Advocacy Center (TAC) found 17 public psychiatric beds per 100,000 U.S. citizens, down from 340 beds per 100,000 in 1955 (Torrey et al., n.d.). Although effective assisted outpatient treatment programs are available in 45 states, TAC reports that implementation of AOT is often incomplete or inconsistent because of legal, clinical, official, or personal barriers to treatment. The center lists the following clinical barriers to treatment: (1) hospitals, physicians, and mental health professionals who are unaware of the laws and/or don't know how to use them and (2) identification mechanisms that would enable hospital emergency rooms, law enforcement, and others to immediately recognize individuals under court-ordered outpatient treatment. Official barriers include perceived or projected fiscal impacts on local government, shortage of public personnel with knowledge or training in implementing the laws, opposition by the mental health officials charged with implementing the laws and standards, and opposition from tax-funded protection and advocacy groups (TAC, 2014).

PERSONAL QUESTION

1. You chair a local chapter of the Emergency Nurses Association and practice in an inner city hospital serving a large number of individuals with mental health impairments in a state without an outpatient treatment program. You would like your chapter to address everyday challenges procuring psychiatric care in your state. How can you leverage your health policy responsibilities for this population and bring about needed change?

ETHICS AND WORK ENVIRONMENT POLICIES

Politics, defined as "any activity concerned with the acquisition of power, gaining one's own ends," is not just for elected officials (Politics, n.d.). Politics are alive and well in every aspect of health care, from the operating room of a small community hospital to the board room of a multibillion-dollar pharmaceutical company. Every day, health care administrators make decisions that impact both nurses and the populations of patients they serve. Nurses are in key positions to influence hospital decision makers and to share the realities of the day-to-day care of patients. Nurses have the greatest influence when they are well-informed, open-minded, collaborative, and willing to do what is right even if there is a personal cost. Here we examine one workplace policy where nurses have the power to influence outcomes, the issue of mandatory flu vaccines.

MANDATORY FLU VACCINATION: THE GOOD OF THE PATIENT VERSUS PERSONAL CHOICE

In the opening paragraph, we asked, "What do I owe the common good or the public interest in my life as a member of society, or more specifically as a member of the nursing profession?" Discerning the right course of action is not always easy. For this discussion, we will consider the issue of mandatory flu vaccinations.

A Pennsylvania nurse was 3 months' pregnant when she was fired from a home infusion company for refusing a mandatory flu vaccine. She was fearful that receiving the vaccine might cause her to miscarry her baby (Lowes, 2014). She had previously experienced two miscarriages before becoming pregnant again. When she presented the required documentation from a physician recommending she not be vaccinated, the note was rejected. Her agency noted the physician failed to cite a medical reason for the exemption. Fear and anxiety were not considered valid reasons. The agency was unwilling to grant the nurse the option of wearing a mask because, as a home care nurse, it would have been difficult to enforce and doing so also placed her immunocompromised patients at risk (Lowes, 2014).

Although we as individuals might make the same decision as our colleague from Pennsylvania, as a profession we also have the responsibility to serve the good of our patients. How do we maintain that balance? When considering mandatory flu vaccination policies, nurses must consider the interests of the individual with those of the population, in this case, the population of patients served. Ethical arguments in this situation weigh personal choice (autonomy) against the best interests of patients. Many argue that a nurse's duty not to harm patients outweighs any restriction on personal choice (Antommaria, 2013; Tilburt et al., 2008). Likewise, fairness and promoting the good of patients compels nurses to consider ways to provide protection for their vulnerable patients and to keep them safe (Steckel, 2007).

Working though challenging issues is not easy. Using the Ethics Inventory to evaluate our personal approach to ethical issues is a good step toward improving our moral sensibility and moral valuing. Asking ourselves the question, "What counts as a good response?" can make us more aware of how we promote the common good and dignity of others. Do we maximize good and reduce harm for our patients? Do we act with virtue in difficult situations by speaking up when it may not be popular to do so? Do we act justly and/or advocate for justice in our work environments? Are we responsive to the vulnerabilities of others? Nurses are the most trusted of all professionals. Given our sheer numbers, think about the impact we could have if we shared one common voice to improve the care of the vulnerable.

CONCLUSION

Denise Thornby, former president of the American Association of Critical Care Nurses, always charged nurses to make waves. She exhorted nurses to

identify when health care was not working for people in need and to do whatever was necessary to address the need. She died in the summer of 2012. We cannot think of a better way to end this chapter than to repeat her charge to nurses everywhere.

Every day, every moment, you make choices on how to act or respond. Through these acts, you have the power to positively influence. As John Quincy Adams sagely said, 'The influence of each human being on others in this life is a kind of immortality.' So I ask you: What will be your act of courage? How will you influence your environment? What will be your legacy? (Thornby, 2001)

DISCUSSION QUESTIONS

1. Knowledge of ethical principles that support practice and policy can help nurses to recognize moral challenges and improve their ability to seek out the right thing to do when faced with a moral dilemma. Describe a recent clinical ethical dilemma and use the ethical terms discussed in the chapter to describe it.

2. In terms of ethnic and racial health disparities, what actions could nurses take to address these disturbing statistics from an ethical perspective?

3. Can you describe a situation in which you witnessed a health professional exhibit moral courage?

REFERENCES

The Advisory Board Company. (2014, September 4). Where states stand on Medicaid expansion. Retrieved from *www.advisory.com/daily-briefing/resources/primers/medicaidmap*.

Aleccia, J. (2013). After lung transplant that changed the rules, Sarah is doing fine. NBC News Health. Retrieved from *www.nbcnews.com/health/after-lung-transplant-changed-rules-sarah-doing-fine-2D11785542*.

American Nurses Association. (2010a). *Code of ethics for nurses with interpretive statements*. Silver Spring, MD: Author.

American Nurses Association. (2010b). *Nursing's social policy statement* (2010 ed.). Silver Spring, MD: Author.

American Nurses Association. (2010c). *Nursing: Scope and standards of practice* (2010 ed.). Silver Spring: Author.

Antommaria, A. H. (2013). An ethical analysis of mandatory influenza vaccination of health care personnel: Implementing fairly and balancing benefits and burdens. *American Journal of Bioethics, 13*(9), 30–37.

Barnet, R. (n.d). Dr. Bob Barnet's human drivers: 5 P's. From Taylor, C. R., Rethinking humane care for humans . . . trivial, superficial, unrealistic or essential? Presented at the American University of Beirut. Retrieved from *www.aub.edu.lb/fm/shbpp/ethics/public/Documents/Humane-care-presentation.pdf.*

Caplan, A. (2013). Who should decide if Sarah will get lungs? Not politicians or bureaucrats, bioethicist says. NBC News Health. Retrieved from *www.nbcnews.com/health/who-should-decide-if-sarah-will-get-lungs-not-politicians-6C10211522.*

Carroll, A. (2013, June 6). Why is everyone so sure they're right about transplant ethics? The Incidental Economist. Retrieved from *the incidentaleconomist.com/wordpress/why-is-everyone-so-sure-theyre-right-about-transplant-ethics/.*

Casalino, L. (2013). Professionalism and caring for Medicaid patients—The 5% commitment? *The New England Journal of Medicine, 369,* 1775–1777.

Davis, K., Schoen, C., & Stremkis, K. (2010). *Mirror, mirror on the wall: How the performance of the U.S. health care system compares internationally, 2010 update.* The Commonwealth Fund.

Dickman, S., Himmelstein, D., McCormick, D., & Woolhander, S. (2014). Opting out of Medicaid expansion: The health and financial impacts. Health Affairs Blog. Retrieved from *healthaffairs.org/blog/2014/01/30/opting-out-of-medicaid-expansion-the-health-and-financial-impacts/.*

Epstein, E. G., & Hamric, A. B. (2009). Moral distress, moral residue, and the crescendo effect. *The Journal of Clinical Ethics, 20*(4), 330–342.

Feinberg, J. (1970). *Justice and personal desert, doing and deserving.* Princeton, NJ: Princeton University Press.

Gallup. (2013, December). Honesty/ethics in professions. Retrieved from *www.gallup.com/poll/1654/honesty-ethics-professions.aspx.*

Glaser, J. W. (1994). *Three realms of ethics.* Kansas City, MO: Sheed & Ward.

Health Resources and Services Administration. (2013). Joint thoracic organ and pediatric transplantation committees: Meeting report. Retrieved from *optn.transplant.hrsa.gov/CommitteeReports/interim_main_Pediatric TransplantationCommittee_7_3_2013_13_58.pdf.*

Holan, A. D. (2009). Sarah Palin falsely claims Barack Obama runs a "death panel." Politifact.com. Retrieved from *www.politifact.com/truth-o-meter/statements/2009/aug/10/sarah-palin/sarah-palin-barack-obama-death-panel/.*

Hope, T., Reynolds, J., & Griffiths, S. (2002). Rationing decisions: Integrating cost-effectiveness with other values. In R. Rhodes, M. Battin, & A. Silvers (Eds.), *Medicine and social justice.* Oxford: University Press.

The Kaiser Commission on Medicaid and the Uninsured. (2014, June). *Medicaid moving forward.* Fact sheet. The Henry J. Kaiser Family Foundation.

Lowes, R. (2014). Pregnant RN fired for refusing flu vaccine: Not so simple? Medscape. Retrieved from *www.medscape.com/viewarticle/820234.*

Miller, D. (1976). *Social justice.* Oxford: Clarendon Press.

Miller, D. (1989). *Market, state, and community.* Oxford: Clarendon Press.

Obama, B. (2014). President Barack Obama's State of the Union address. Retrieved from *www.whitehouse.gov/the-press-office/2014/01/28/president-barack-obamas-state-union-address.*

Organ Procurement Organizations. (n.d.). 42 U.S. Code § 273. Findlaw. Retrieved from *codes.lp.findlaw.com/uscode/42/6A/II/H/273.*

Politics. (n.d.). Collins English dictionary—Complete & unabridged (10th ed.). Retrieved from *dictionary.reference.com/browse/politics.*

Rawls, J. (1971). *A theory of justice.* Harvard, MA: Harvard University Press.

Rawls, J. (1993). *Political liberalism.* New York: Columbia University Press.

Rushton, C. H. (2006). Defining and addressing moral distress: Tools for critical care nursing leaders. *AACN Advanced Critical Care, 17*(2), 161–168.

Sanders, B. (2013). Primary care access 30 million new patients and 11 months to go: Who will provide their primary care? A Report from Chairman Bernard Sanders Subcommittee on Primary Health and Aging U.S. Senate Committee on Health, Education, Labor & Pensions. Retrieved from *www.sanders.senate.gov/imo/media/doc/PrimaryCare AccessReport.pdf.*

Sobel, L., & Salganicoff, A. (2013). A guide to the Supreme Court's review of the contraceptive coverage requirement. Kaiser Family Foundation Women's Health Policy. Retrieved from *kff.org/womens-health-policy/issue-brief/a-guide-to-the-supreme-courts-review-of-the-contraceptive-coverage-requirement/.*

Steckel, C. M. (2007). Mandatory influenza immunizations for health care workers—An ethical discussion. *AAOHN Journal, 55*(1), 34–39.

Taylor, C. (2015). Values, ethics and advocacy. In C. Taylor, C. Lillis, & P. Lynn (Eds.), *Fundamentals of nursing: The art and science of nursing care* (8th ed.). Philadelphia: Wolters Kluwer.

Thornby, D. (2001). Make waves: The courage to influence practice. Speech given at American Association of Critical-Care Nurses, National Teaching Institute and Critical Care Exposition. Anaheim, CA. Retrieved from *www.aacn.org/wd/aacninfo/docs/board/presspeech2001.pdf.*

Tilburt, J. C., Mueller, P. S., Ottenberg, A. L., Poland, G. A., & Koenig, B. A. (2008). Facing the challenges of influenza in healthcare settings: The ethical rationale for mandatory seasonal influenza vaccination and its implications for future pandemics. *Vaccine, 26*(S4), D27–D30.

Tomlinson, T. (2013). Lungs for Sarah Murnaghan raise ethical questions. Bioethics in the News. Retrieved from *msubioethics.com/2013/06/27/lungs-for-sarah-murnaghan-raise-ethical-questions/.*

Torrey, E. F., Entsminger, K., Geller, J., Stanley, J., & Jaffe, D. J. (n.d.). The shortage of public hospital beds for mentally ill persons. A report of the Treatment Advocacy Center. Retrieved from *www.treatment advocacycenter.org/storage/documents/the_shortage_of_publichospital beds.pdf.*

Treatment Advocacy Center. (2014). Eliminating barriers to the treatment of mental illness. Retrieved from *www.treatmentadvocacycenter.org/problem/lack-of-implementation.*

United Network for Organ Sharing. (2014). Mission, vision & values. Retrieved from *www.unos.org/about/index.php?topic=vision_mission_values.*

Woolf, S. H., & Aron, L. (Eds.), (2013). U.S. Health in international perspective: Shorter lives, poorer health. National Research Council and Institute of Medicine. Washington, DC: The National Academies Press.

ONLINE RESOURCES

National Institutes of Health Bioethics Resources on the Web
bioethics.od.nih.gov
National Reference Center for Bioethics Literature
bioethics.georgetown.edu
Presidential Commission for the Study of Bioethical Issues
www.bioethics.gov/
The Markkula Center for Applied Ethics
www.scu.edu/ethics

CHAPTER 16

The Changing United States Health Care System

Barbara I.H. Damron   Demetrius Chapman   Freida Hopkins Outlaw

"America's health care system is neither healthy, caring, nor a system."

Walter Cronkite

The U.S. health care system is complex and pluralistic. It is a mix of private and public initiatives and institutions that employ millions of workers in a myriad of settings to provide a wide range of health-related services to the diverse U.S. population across geo-political environments that range from cities to rural areas. The purpose of this chapter is to provide an overview of the current major components of the American health care system, which is in the midst of dynamic change.

OVERVIEW OF THE U.S. HEALTH CARE SYSTEM

PUBLIC INSURANCE

The two principal health entitlement programs, Medicare and Medicaid, account for over one third of the nation's total health spending and $1 out of every $5 of federal spending goes to these programs (National Institute for Health Care Management Foundation [NIHCM], 2012).

Medicare. Medicare was created under Title XVIII of the 1965 Social Security Act as health insurance for the aged and disabled. The federal government funds it and in 2011 it cost $549 billion (23% of total health care expenditures for the United States) to provide care to the 49 million enrollees (Centers for Disease Control and Prevention [CDC], 2013). Medicare is divided into four parts: A, B, C, and D (Klees & Wolfe, 2013). The original two components were Part A, which pays for inpatient hospitalization, home health, hospice, and skilled nursing; Part B helps pay for physician appointments and outpatient hospital services; Part C is the Medicare Advantage Program, which expands beneficiaries' options for participation in private sector health care plans; and Part D helps pay for prescription drugs not otherwise covered by Parts A and B. Expenditures for the Medicare Drugs Program (Part D) was $67 billion in 2011 (CDC, 2013).

Medicare is reliant on financing from the nation's general revenue, which crowds out other uses of general revenue and substantially adds to annual deficits that accumulate debt and place upward pressure on taxes (NIHCM, 2012).

Medicaid. When Congress passed the 1965 legislation that established Medicaid, Title XIX of the Social Security Act, it was a response to the widely perceived inadequacy of welfare medical care (Klees & Wolfe, 2013).

151

In 2009, children aged under 21 years accounted for 48% of Medicaid recipients but only 20% of Medicaid expenditures; older adults, the blind, and people with disabilities made up 21% of Medicaid recipients and accounted for 63% of expenditures (CDC, 2013). Since its inception, the cost of Medicaid programs has increased at a faster pace than the U.S. economy. In 1970, Medicaid was 0.5% of the gross domestic product (GDP), by 2011 is was 2.8% of the GDP (Truffer et al., 2012). Medicaid is currently approximately 17% of the total health expenditure of the United States (CDC, 2013). The total Medicaid outlays in fiscal year 2011 were $432.4 billion, of which the federal government spent $275.1 billion (64%) and states spent $157.3 billion (36%) (Truffer et al., 2012).

Medicaid is financed by the combination of state general funds and federal matching funds and is now the largest single budget category for states (Trust for America's Health, 2011). All states except Vermont are required to have balanced budgets either through statutory law, constitutional requirement, or judicial decision (National Conference of State Legislatures [NCSL], 2010). Other authorities also exclude Wyoming and North Dakota as exceptions. When Medicaid spending increases, other state spending must be curtailed or taxes must be raised, creating a dilemma for states.

Originally, federal law mandated coverage for pregnant women, children under age 6 years from families at or below 133% of the federal poverty level (see Table 16-1 for federal poverty levels), children age 6 to 18 years at or below 100% of the federal poverty level, parents and relative caretakers of those who met the previous Aid to Families with Dependent Children cash assistance program, and older adults and the disabled who qualify for Supplemental Security Income (Kaiser Family Foundation [KFF], 2012). For states accepting the Medicaid expansion, people with household incomes at or below 133% of the federal poverty level will be eligible for coverage beginning in 2014. This expansion shifts the funding of all the participating states (100%) to the federal government for the first 3 years (2014 to 2017), and then incrementally the federal share will decrease to 90% by 2020 with each state paying the remaining 10%. With the

TABLE 16-1 Federal Poverty Guidelines*

Persons in Family/Household	Poverty Guideline	133% of Federal Poverty Level
1	$11,670	$15,521.10
2	$15,730	$20,920.90
3	$19,790	$26,320.70
4	$23,850	$31,720.50
5	$27,910	$37,120.30
6	$31,970	$42,520.10
7	$36,030	$47,919.90
8	$40,090	$53,319.70

*Federal Poverty Guidelines of the U.S. Department of Health and Human Services (January 22, 2014). Applicable to the 48 contiguous states and the District of Columbia.
From the Federal Register: *www.federalregister.gov/articles/2014/01/22/2014-01303/annual-update-of-the-hhs-poverty-guidelines.*

implementation of the Affordable Care Act (ACA), the eligibility for Medicaid beginning in 2014 became broader, increasing the expected overall enrollment to 77.9 million people by 2021 (Truffer et al., 2012); in 2011, Medicaid provided health care assistance to an estimated 55.7 million people.

When the ACA was signed into law, 26 states and another group of plaintiffs including the National Federation of Independent Businesses filed lawsuits that the Supreme Court agreed to consider (Liptak, 2012). The court ruled (7:2) that the requirement of broader Medicaid eligibility criteria required by the ACA was unconstitutionally coercive because states lacked adequate notice and because the Secretary of the U.S. Department of Health and Human Services (HHS) has the authority to withhold all Medicaid funds, a substantial part of the overall budgets of some states (Kaiser Family Foundation, 2012). As of 2014, when the federal funding of Medicaid expansion began, 25 states and the District of Columbia implemented the expansion, 6 states are debating expansion, and 19 states are not moving forward (KFF, 2014).

VETERANS ADMINISTRATION HEALTH SYSTEMS

Veterans benefits in the United States can be traced to the very first colonists. According to the U.S. Department of Veterans Affairs (n.d.), the Pilgrims of Plymouth Colony passed a law stating that disabled soldiers fighting the Pequot Indians would be supported by the colony. The first federal Veterans hospital was authorized in 1811. Since that time the U.S. Department of Veterans Affairs has expanded its health services to 820 clinics, 151 hospitals, and 300 Veterans Health Administration Veteran Centers (National Center for Veterans Analysis and Statistics, U.S. Department of Veterans Affairs, 2014), The Veterans Health Administration health care system currently provides care to 8.92 million people with the FY2015 Veterans Health Administration budget at $163.9 billion to care for the 21,973,000 U.S. veterans (National Center for Veterans Analysis and Statistics, U.S. Department of Veterans Affairs, 2014). Recently, the public admonished the Veterans Health Administration over its severe backlog of disability claims. Dao (2013) reported that in March 2013 there were more than 600,000 backlogged disability applications; backlogged by Veterans Health Administration standards means pending for 125 days or longer. Many people demanded the resignation of the Secretary of Veterans Affairs, Eric Shinseki, which took place on May 30, 2014. The organization Iraq and Afghanistan Veterans of America lobbies for reform and sent President Obama a letter signed by 67 senators. By March of 2014 the backlog of disability claims was reduced to 370,000. For a more detailed discussion of the U.S. Military and Veterans Health Administration System, see Chapter 39.

INDIAN HEALTH SERVICE

The Indian Health Service (IHS) (2014) is responsible for the provision of health services to members of federally recognized tribes. These obligations grew out of the special government-to-government relationships that the federal government has with Indian nations. In 1787, Article 1, Section 8 of the U.S. Constitution empowered the Congress "to regulate commerce with foreign Nations, and among the several States, and with the Indian Tribes" (National Archives, n.d.). Through numerous treaties, laws, executive orders, and Supreme Court decisions, the IHS came into existence to raise the health status of the 566 recognized tribes to parity with the general population (Shi & Singh, 2014).

The modern IHS was authorized and funded by the Indian Sanitation Facilities and Services Act of 1959 (Public Law [PL] 86-121), but not until the ACA (PL 111-148) was signed into law did the permanent reauthorization of the Indian Health Care Improvement Act (1976) (PL94-437) occur. It was the 1921 Snyder Act (PL 67-85) (Library of Congress, 2014) which made Indians citizens and created the basis of health care to American Indians and Alaska Native people (National Indian Health Board, 2009). American Indians have the worst health outcomes, with a life expectancy that is lower than all other Americans.

The IHS (2013) reports that American Indians and Alaska Natives born today have a life expectancy that is 4.1 years less than Americans of all races (73.6 years versus 77.7 years). When compared with Americans of all races, substantially higher death rates for American Indians and Alaska Natives exist for many diseases and preventable injuries. Infant, maternal, and pneumonia/influenza deaths are also higher in this population (Indian Health Service, 2013). It has been noted that many American Indians do not avail themselves of the health care services of the IHS for a number of reasons including a lack of American Indian health care providers (Shi & Singh, 2014). Since 1973, through funding from the National Institute of Mental Health and later transferred to the Substance Abuse and Mental Health Services Administration, the Minority Fellowship Program for Nursing was established to create a cadre of doctorally prepared minority nurses to provide leadership in research, practice, education, and policy in both private and public sectors. American Indian and Pacific Islander nurses are a part of this alumnae group who are focused on improving health care for this population.

INFRASTRUCTURE

Hospitals. The American Hospital Association (2014) reports that as of early 2014, there are 5723 hospitals that meet the agency's registered criteria for accreditation as a hospital by The Joint Commission or is a certified provider of acute services under Title 18 of the Social Security Act. Of these hospitals, 2894 (50%) are nonprofit community hospitals, 1068 (18%) are for-profit community hospitals, 1037 (18%) are state and local government community hospitals, 211 (3.6%) are federal government hospitals, 413 (7.2%) are psychiatric hospitals, 89 (1.5%) are long-term care hospitals, and 11 (<1%) are institutional hospitals (prison, college infirmaries). These hospitals have 920,829 beds with 36,156,245 admissions in 2012. As of 2010, North Dakota had the highest number of community hospital beds per capita (5.1 per 1000 people); Oregon and Washington had the lowest with 1.7 beds per 1000 people. The national average was 2.6 beds per 1000 people (CDC, 2013). Figure 16-1 summarizes the numbers and types of American hospitals.

According to Dafny (2014), hospitals are scrambling to shore up their positions in the health care market, consolidate resources, and improve operational efficiency and create health systems capable of managing the health of entire populations. Some of these consolidations, horizontal mergers of providers that supply similar services in the same geographic area, as well as vertical integration of services including urgent and long-term care, are beginning to get attention as potential violations of antitrust laws. In the fall of 2013, the Federal Trade Commission challenged the Idaho Medical Group's purchase of a rival medical group,

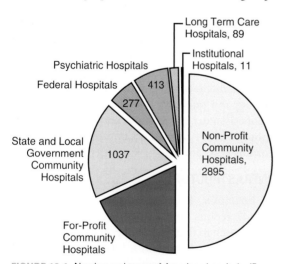

which would have created a combined 78% of the market in adult primary care (Dafny, 2014).

Academic hospitals, compared with community hospitals, are part of an academic health center and are referred to as teaching or university hospitals. An academic health center consists of one or more owned or affiliated teaching hospitals or health systems; an allopathic or osteopathic medical school; other health professional schools or programs, which may include nursing, dentistry, pharmacy, public health, veterinary medicine, allied health, and graduate studies; and a robust research program (Association of Academic Health Centers [AAHC], 2014). Academic health centers offer unique care that is not available elsewhere in the region. They also serve as a primary public safety net, providing almost $44 million in uncompensated patient care each year; one in seven provides more than $100 million per year (AAHC, 2014). The majority of the academic health centers belonging to the Association of Academic Health Centers (AAHC, 2014) have added clinical doctorates responding to changing educational and practice needs, with nursing being one of the common offerings (AAHC, 2009). Academic health centers lead in new interdisciplinary research models, nationally and globally, and in knowledge management and information technology. Nursing is in a prime position to lead in these academic health centers through education, administration, and building and sustaining programs of research.

Nursing Homes. As of 2011, America had 40.3 nursing home beds per 1000 people aged 65 years and older available to the 41.3 million Americans over age 64 years. According to the Centers for Medicare and Medicaid Services (CMS, 2012), the number of nursing homes participating in the Medicare and Medicaid programs has decreased steadily since 2002 with 15,671 remaining by the end of 2011. The trend has been a slight increase in larger nursing homes (100 to 199 beds) and a decrease in smaller nursing homes with fewer than 50 beds. The majority (69%) of nursing homes are for-profit. Another trend is an increase in dually participating nursing homes that are eligible for both Medicare and Medicaid funding. Only 4%

FIGURE 16-1 Number and types of American hospitals. (From AHA Hospital Statistics. [2014]. Retrieved from *www.aha.org/research/rc/stat-studies/fast-facts.shtml.*)

of nursing homes are Medicaid-only and they decreased by 6% to 785 in 2012.

The nursing home population at the end of 2011 was 2.9% of the over-65 and 10.7% of the over-85 population (CMS, 2012). Of those in nursing homes, 15% are under 65 years of age, whereas 7.6% are over 95 years of age. Women make up 67% of the residents, and nearly 4 out of 5 are non-Hispanic whites (78.9%).

PUBLIC HEALTH

The American Public Health Association defines public health as the practice of preventing disease and promoting good health within groups of people, from small communities to entire countries. Public health is provided by a variety of agencies, small and large, public and private. The CDC administers funding for many population-based prevention efforts (National Health Policy Forum [NHPF], 2010). State health departments are the agencies that most frequently get funding for programs associated with a specific disease or risk factor. Local health departments, such as city and county entities, can also be recipients of direct CDC funds. According to the NHPF (2010), most of the states (29; 58%) have established a decentralized public health organizational model, that is, local public health offices are independent of the state health department and are managed by local authorities. Six states have a centralized organization, in which all the local public health offices are managed from the state level, and 13 have a hybrid model. Two states, Hawaii and Rhode Island, do not have local public health agencies. The NHPF (2010) reports that there are 2794 local health departments in the United States, most of which serve counties (60%) and 9% serve multiple counties. Some health departments (18%) serve cities, towns, or townships. The American College of Physicians (2012) reports that in FY2010 to 2011, 40 states decreased their public health budgets. Of those, 29 had decreased their budgets for the second year in a row, and 15 had done it for a third year (2012). The HHS (2014) reported that the CDC will see a decrease of $432,461,000 in budget authority for FY2014 and operate with an overall budget of $6.665 billion.

Program investments that are scheduled to realize an increase in funding are infectious diseases; global disease protection; preventing the leading causes of disability, disease, and death; health monitoring; and environmental and work hazard prevention. Additional funds were allotted for Vaccines for Children and the World Trade Center Health Program.

Public health has finally become included in high-profile, tertiary care research centers. This includes the National Cancer Institute (NCI), the first and largest institute of the National Institutes of Health. The Cancer Control and Population Sciences division of the NCI is the bridge to public health research, practice, and policy. Through the NCI-designated cancer centers around the country, public health principles are the cornerstone of the departments within these centers that focus on community health, education, and the conducting of population-based research using community-based participatory approaches. An example is the NCI-designated University of New Mexico Cancer Center's Office of Community Partnerships and Cancer Health Disparities, which conducts community-based participatory research with Hispanic and Native American populations.

Building on the accelerating pace of discoveries in human genetic variation, epigenetic, molecular, biochemical, and cellular technologies for cancer care and prevention, public health genomics (PHG) has evolved as a "multidisciplinary field concerned with the effective and responsible translation of genome based knowledge and technologies to improve population health" (Burke et al., 2006). PHG at the NCI promotes the integration of genomics and personalized medicine into public health cancer research, policy, and control. The work of Anita Kinney, PhD, RN, exemplifies the contributions nurse scientists are making in this area through her work combining behavioral science, genomics, and cancer prevention strategies.

TRANSFORMING HEALTH CARE THROUGH TECHNOLOGY

Health care information technology (HIT) is the future, but the current systems have flaws that need major revisions. The advancement of HIT holds the promise of providing quality of care for patients and their families; increasing efficiency in the health care system; and reducing costs for payers, providers, and patients (Thune et al., 2013). The impact of technology on the transformation of health care is expanding rapidly, and billions of federal and private dollars are being spent. Health care providers and hospitals are benefitting from, and struggling with, software that can automate protocols, track medication, and transfer patients to different departments. The 2009 Congress passed legislation, through the Health Information Technology and Economic and Clinical Health Act (2009), allotting $35 billion to promote providers' adoption and use of federally certified HIT (Thune et al., 2013). Venture capital funding for HIT tripled from 2009 to 2012, skyrocketing to $955 million from $343 million (PricewaterhouseCoopers, 2013). Additionally, the federal government is spending up to $29 billion in incentives to motivate health care providers to digitize health care records (New-TechCity, 2012).

HEALTH INFORMATION TECHNOLOGY

Health information technology includes electronic health records (EHRs) and is aimed toward making it possible for health care providers to better manage patient care through the sharing of health information in a secure manner (Office of the National Coordinator for Health Information Technology [ONCHIT], n.d.). The main goal of HIT is to improve the quality and safety of patient care. Box 16-1 summarizes key terms used in health information technology. EHR adoption requires a significant investment of time and money. As of 2012, over 144,000 payments totaling $7.1 billion have already been issued to professionals and hospitals by the Centers for Medicare and Medicaid Services. Of concern is the lack of evidence of the effectiveness of the current health information technology system. During the 113th Congress, six senators summarized the deficiencies that exist with the current state of health information technology, including (1) lack of a clear path to interoperability, (2) increased costs associated with health information technology, (3) lack of

---

BOX 16-1 Health Information Technology Terms

Electronic Health Records (EHRs): A digital version of patients' paper charts. The EHR is a real-time, patient-centered record of patient information kept in a health care provider's office or in a hospital. Ideally, the EHR can link to hospital departments and to other health care providers.

Health Information Exchange (HIE): The movement of health information electronically across multiple organizations.

Interoperability: The ability of two or more electronic systems to communicate, or exchange, information and to use the information that has been exchanged. Interoperability is not the same thing as HIE. With interoperability, the information must be exchanged and usable.

Personal Health Record (PHR): Similar to the EHR, except the patient can set up and control the information. The PHR can be an electronic storage center for most of the patient's health information.

Source: *www.healthit.gov/policy-researchers-implementers/technologystandards-certification_glossary.*

---

oversight for the development of health information technology through the public sector, (4) the privacy of patients being put at risk, and (5) lack of clarity regarding costs of program sustainability (Thune et al., 2013).

Even in light of the challenges, the advantages of EHRs are evident in both the espousal of technology and the fact that 71% of users state they would purchase their EHR system again (Jamoom et al., 2012). Jamoom and colleagues also reported that nearly half of physicians without an EHR system are planning to purchase or use one already purchased within a year (Jamoom et al., 2012). Advantages of using EHRs for the provider include (1) accurate and complete information about a patient's health, (2) the ability to quickly provide care, (3) the ability to better coordinate the care that is given, and (4) an improved mechanism for sharing information with patients and their family caregivers (ONCHIT, n.d.).

In 1971, Lockheed engineers designed the first commercial electronic health record system for El

Camino Hospital (Thede, 2012). This system was very successful because it truly integrated physicians, nurses, and pharmacy processes and a respect for the nursing workforce was apparent in the system design (Thede, 2012). Nurses were freed from established tasks, such as multiple documentation, and thus had more time to spend with patients. This system that set a high standard was not replicated in informatics design in the U.S. health care system.

The changing U.S. health care system is dependent on the use of the EHR. Increasing numbers of providers who use this technology are reporting tangible improvements in their ability to make better decisions with more comprehensive information. Often when EHRs are discussed physicians are the focus; however, successful EHR systems have been found to be highly correlated with designs that respect nursing practice. A descriptive study of 100 nurses at a large Magnet hospital found that the majority of nurses studied (75%) thought that EHRs improved quality of documentation, whereas 76% believed patient safety and care improved (Moody et al., 2004). A number of years ago, the American Association of Colleges of Nursing and the National League of Nursing, the two nursing accrediting agencies, required that beginning informatics be added to the curriculum in all nursing schools (Thede, 2012). This requirement is in concert with the Institute of Medicine (IOM), which requires that informatics education be provided for all health care professionals (Thede, 2012). Nursing schools are now offering graduate degrees in informatics, which are largely focused on system design for hospitals, community health centers, and home care that are clinically directed (Moen & Knudsen, 2013). Intraprofessional and interprofessional collaboration is also a major component of the clinical system design by nurses. The practice, education, research, and policy implication for the purposeful use of nursing data will be fostered when the culture of health care delivery systems shifts from providing care in traditional ways to using tools such as the EHR to improve meaningful use of patient data. Thought leaders have published a new nursing informatics research agenda for 2008 to 2018. Specifically, Bakken,

Stone, and Larson (2008) noted that a nursing informatics research agenda for 2008 to 2018 must expand users of interest to include interdisciplinary researchers; build upon the knowledge gained in nursing concept representation to address genomic and environmental data; guide the reengineering of nursing practice; harness new technologies to empower patients and their caregivers for collaborative knowledge development; develop user-configurable software approaches that support complex data visualization, analysis, and predictive modeling; facilitate the development of middle-range nursing informatics theories; and encourage innovative evaluation methodologies that attend to human-computer interface factors and organizational context" (p. 206).

HEALTH STATUS AND TRENDS

It is common to evaluate the health care system on three dimensions: quality, access, and cost.

QUALITY

Quality of care is the degree to which health services for individuals and populations increase the likelihood of desired outcomes and are consistent with current knowledge. Some of the national health outcome measures most commonly cited are life expectancy, infant mortality, and vaccine preventable deaths. The IOM has identified members of the nursing profession as crucial for the changing health care system. In the seminal report of the IOM entitled *The Future of Nursing* (2011), four key messages were presented:

- Nurses should practice to the full extent of their education and training.
- Nurses should achieve higher levels of education and training through an improved education system that promotes seamless academic progression.
- Nurses should be full partners, with physicians and other health care professionals, in redesigning health care in the United States.
- Effective workforce planning and policymaking require better data collection and an improved information infrastructure.

Implementation of the four key messages of the IOM will enable nursing to take a leading role in the ever-challenging endeavor to improve quality while being cost-effective.

A few comparisons do help define the health systems of the United States. Squires (2011) reported on the findings of the Organization for Economic Cooperation and Development (OECD), which tracks and reports on more than 1200 health system measures across 34 industrialized countries. Some of the highlights of the U.S. system, when compared with 10 other industrialized nations that were reported by Squires (2011), include that the United States had the fewest practicing physicians per 1000 population (2.43); the OECD mean was 3 per 1000. U.S. hospital admission rates were lower, but the spending per discharge was the highest and more than double the median of the other countries being compared. Squires noted that Americans were the most likely to have a prescribed pharmaceutical and more likely to have four prescriptions per person and that the drugs in the United States were the most expensive of all the other nations being compared. The high rates of use and the high prices resulted in the highest drug spending per capita for the United States at $897 per person in 2008. The five most expensive health conditions are: heart disease, cancer, trauma, mental disorders, and pulmonary conditions (NIHCM, 2011).

Quality improvement in nursing was first introduced by Florence Nightingale during the Crimean War. Today, nursing quality is still involved with process, but has evolved to an emphasis on patient care outcomes. Every nurse plays a pivotal role in the measurement of quality.

ACCESS

Access is the ability to obtain needed, affordable, convenient, acceptable, and effective health care in a timely manner. Despite many initiatives, access to health care remains a serious problem. Although access has many dimensions in the current health care debate, it is a euphemism for adequate health insurance coverage, and there is a growing disparity between those who have insurance and those who are not covered. The number of people with health insurance increased to 260.2 million in 2011 from 256.6 million in 2010, as did the percentage of people with health insurance (84.3% in 2011, 83.7% in 2010) (U.S. Census Bureau, 2011).

COST

The cost of health care must be considered from several perspectives. For patients or consumers, cost is the price of purchasing needed health care goods and services and includes insurance premiums, co-pays, and deductibles; out-of-pocket health expenditures not covered by insurance; taxes (Social Security, federal, and state) that support health programs; in-kind services such as caring for aging parents or sick children; and voluntary contributions to health-related charities. For providers, the cost of health is producing health care products and services and delivering them to patients in a timely and convenient manner. The cost of health care is how much the state or nation spends on health care; the percentage of the total domestic production that health care consumes. Incentives and policy initiatives that address the cost of health may be beneficial to one, some, or none of these perspectives.

Most developed countries of the world have a health insurance system funded, subsidized, or managed by the national government, and with very few exceptions, the categorical delineation between countries with some type of national health system and those without is the country's economic development (Fisher, 2012). The great exception is the United States. According to the World Health Organization (2013), the United States spends 17.6% of its GDP on health care expenditures. It ranks second behind Sierra Leone in terms of percentage of GDP spent on health. Sierra Leone spends 20.8% of its GDP, but that amount per capita is $171 compared with the staggering amount of $8233 per person in the United States.

The United States is far from the healthiest society in the world despite having the most expensive care. The National Institute for Health Care Management Foundation (2011) reports some of the trends in American health care spending. The first trend is the disproportionate distribution of the costs, with just 5% of patients accounting for nearly 50% of health care spending; whereas nearly 50% of the U.S. population accounts for just 3% of spending on health care (NIHCM, 2011).

HEALTH STATUS OF THE UNITED STATES

For life expectancy (at birth and at age 65 years), *Healthy People 2020* reports that the United States is ranked 27th and 26th, respectively, out of the 33 peer countries determined by the OECD (Healthy People 2020, 2014). The other leading health indicators noted by Healthy People 2020 are: access to health services; clinical preventive services; environmental quality; injury and violence; maternal, infant, and child health; mental health; nutrition, physical activity, and obesity; oral health; reproductive and sexual health; social determinants; substance abuse; and tobacco. The CDC (2013) reports that the leading cause of death for men and women is heart disease, accounting for approximately 307,000 deaths for men and 290,000 deaths for women in 2010. The Institute of Medicine's Committee on the State of the USA Health Indicators identified a framework for health indicator development. Table 16-2 summarizes their findings.

CHALLENGES FOR THE U.S. HEALTH CARE SYSTEM

The challenges facing the U.S. health care system can be traced to the rise of professional sovereignty and the transformation of medicine into an

TABLE 16-2 Framework for Health and Health Indicator Development*

Social and Physical Environment		Health Outcomes
Socioeconomic status	→	Mortality
Race/ethnicity		Life expectancy at birth
Social support		Infant mortality
Health literacy		Life expectancy at age 65 years
Limited English proficiency		Injury-related mortality
Physical environments (where people live, learn, work, and play)		
Health-Related Behaviors		
Smoking	→	Health-related quality of life (morbidity)
Physical activity		Self-reported health status
Excessive drinking		Unhealthy days
Nutrition		
Obesity		
Condom use among youth		
Health Systems		
The health system is broadly defined as a set of institutions and players whose purpose is to maintain or improve people's health.	→	Condition specific outcomes
		Chronic disease prevalence
Cost		Serious psychological distress
Health care expenditures		
Access		
Insurance coverage		
Unmet medical, dental, and prescription drug needs		
Effectiveness of care		
Preventive services		
Childhood immunizations		
Preventable hospitalizations		

*No single measure can capture the health of the nation. Indicators are needed that reflect a broad range of factors such as health, risk for illness, and health system performance. The set of indicators presented here should not be viewed as perfect or permanent; rather, the committee identified potential indicators that met the data constraints and then applied the framework to determine the final selection of indicators.

From the Committee on the State of the USA Health Indicators; Institute of Medicine of the National Academies (2009). *State of the USA health indicators.* Washington, DC: The National Academies Press. Retrieved from*www.nap.edu/download.php?record_id=12534#.*

industry during the nineteenth and twentieth centuries, which Paul Starr so thoroughly described in his 1982 Pulitzer Prize–winning book, *The Social Transformation of American Medicine* (Starr, 1982). Although the advancements in biomedical science have been phenomenal, preventing the diseases that are the main reason for soaring costs in the health care system and increasing quality in health care delivery while lowering costs are still a struggle (American Association for Cancer Research, 2013).

CHRONIC DISEASES

One of the biggest and most costly aspects of health care is the treatment of chronic diseases. It is not possible to make insurance affordable without changing how chronic disease is treated. According to the Centers for Disease Control and Prevention (2009) chronic diseases are responsible for more than 75% of the $2.5 trillion spent annually on health care.

As a nation, 85% of health care dollars is spent on people with chronic conditions (Robert Wood Johnson Foundation [RWJF], 2010), many of which can be prevented. Yet, the majority of money, talent, and time continue to focus on tertiary care, with limited resources dedicated to prevention. The majority of costs in the U.S. health care system associated with preventable medical conditions and chronic diseases are associated with modifiable behaviors (CDC, 2009). Almost 50% of all Americans live with a chronic condition and the percentage of health care spending associated with people with chronic conditions has increased to 84% in 2009 from 78% in 2002 (RWJF, 2010). The number of Americans with chronic conditions will increase by 37% between 2000 and 2030, an increase of 46 million people (RWJF, 2010). Until, as a society, prevention is truly embraced as the most efficient approach to controlling the costs associated with chronic diseases, health care costs will continue to escalate. Nurses have a history of focusing on prevention even though it has not always been recognized in the health care environment. However, nurses are becoming much more visible in the health promotion and disease prevention field of research, as well as other areas associated with prevention, including chronic disease. For

example, Loretta Jemmott, PhD, FAAN, RN is nationally and internationally recognized for her research in the field of HIV/AIDS prevention among African-American adolescents. The Centers for Disease Control has designated several of her HIV prevention curriculums for national use in a variety of settings. Another example of an evidence-based nursing intervention that has had an impact on the management of chronic illness is the Transitional Care Model spearheaded by Mary Naylor, PhD, FAAN, RN. It is an interdisciplinary model that is providing high-quality cost-effective evidence-based care for vulnerable older adults living in the community. Her focus on prevention includes recognizing the unique needs of chronically ill older adults, improving the quality of their care, and thus preventing unnecessary hospitalizations while reducing cost. An important example of transformative work in an inpatient setting is Susan Hassmiller's and Patricia Rutherford's program, Transforming Care at the Bedside, which incorporates a number of nursing care factors including improving patient safety, improving the quality of patient care on medical surgical units, and retaining nurses. The program has improved safety by reducing patient falls, increased the time nurses can spend in direct care, and improved nurse retention, among other positive outcomes (Freda, 2008). Exemplars such as these inform nursing practice as well as providing models of care that can be used to educate students, influence health care policy, and improve practice while being cost-effective. (See the American Academy of Nursing website [*www.aannet.org*] to learn more about the Edge Runners, nurses whose work has changed health care systems.)

HEALTH CARE REFORM

Health care reform is a term used through the decades to discuss a variety of health policy changes. Health care reform has been riddled with debate and encompasses a vast array of legislation. Major milestones of health care policy include the Public Health Service Act of 1944, the Social Security Amendments of 1965, the Health Insurance Portability and Accountability Act of 1996, and the

Patient Protection and Affordable Care Act of 2010. Health care reform is driven by two major questions: (1) the cost of health care and (2) the right to health care.

Currently, health care reform is focused on the implementation of the ACA. This law addresses a vast array of health care delivery issues through 10 titles of the law. For more detail pertaining to the ACA, the reader is referred to Chapter 19.

Delivery system reforms are addressed in the ACA. An important aspect of delivery system reform in the law is the emphasis on comparative effectiveness research (CER). Evidence is provided on the effectiveness, benefits, and harms of different treatment options through CER; these studies compare ways to deliver health care, as well as comparing drugs, medical devices, tests, or surgeries (Agency for Healthcare Research and Quality, n.d.).

The Patient-Centered Outcomes Research Institute (PCORI) was established in the ACA and is a U.S.-based nongovernmental institute created to examine clinical effectiveness and the appropriateness of different medical treatments. It is based on the tenets of comparative clinical effectiveness research (CER) and ultimately aims to improve health care delivery and outcomes by helping people make informed health care decisions (PCORI, 2014). The overall goal of the PCORI is "to fund research that will assist patients, caregivers, clinicians, and others in making informed health decisions" (Barksdale, Newhouse, & Miller, 2014, p. 192). The engagement of people from within the community, including patients and their caregivers, is a major strength of the PCORI and aligns very much with those in the nursing profession, who have demonstrated expertise in the engagement process, both as generalists and specialists (Pearson et al., 2014). More than other agencies that fund research, PCORI has focused on meaningful involvement of patients, which means that patients and caregivers are included in all aspects of the research process (Barksdale, Newhouse, & Miller, 2014). No longer will they be excluded until the research process has been developed, but they will be part of the funding application helping to formulate the research questions and all other essential research processes, including dissemination of

findings as well as being a part of the research review panels (Barksdale, Newhouse, & Miller, 2014). PCORI is an agency where nursing leadership has the opportunity to flourish through active participation. Because nursing is culturally aligned with the principles of PCORI, it is positioned to provide thought leaders in all aspects of the institute.

The Patient-Centered Outcomes Research Trust Fund (PCORTF) was authorized by Congress as part of the ACA of 2010. It is through this trust fund that PCORI is funded. The PCORTF receives income from the general fund of the Treasury and from a fee assessed on Medicare, private health insurance, and self-insured plans. The PCORTF received $210 million in total in appropriations for FYs 2010 to 2012. For FYs 2013 to 2019, the PCORTF received $150 million from the general funding appropriation plus an annual $2 fee per individual assessed on Medicare, private health insurance, and self-insured plans, as well as an adjustment for increases in health care spending. The law mandates that each year, 20% of PCORTF funding is to be transferred to the HHS to support dissemination and research capacity-building efforts. Of that 20%, 80% is transferred to the Agency for Healthcare Research and Quality for these purposes (Patient-Centered Outcomes Research Institute, 2014).

OPPORTUNITIES AND CHALLENGES FOR NURSING

Many opportunities for nurses are unfolding, which are associated with the changing U.S. health care delivery system. Nurses are the providers with the greatest presence during health care delivery, and they provide the most holistic approach to patients. The evolving and collective nursing knowledge could solve a great many of the barriers and gaps in care for the American people if that knowledge was effectively channeled to health policies that address and solve these problems. Although nurses are very good at assessing the many systems impacting their patients' lives, they have been less visible in arenas where policy, politics, economic, social, and professional decisions regarding the U.S. health care system change are being made. The challenge is how to get the nursing profession's achievement recognized, not as separate accomplishments of individual nurses, selected nursing schools, or a particular hospital where nurses are making substantial contributions, but rather to create opportunities to let the public (with a focused emphasis on politicians and other decision makers and stakeholders) know that embedded in the fabric of nursing are the knowledge, skills, and desire to make significant contributions to the transformation of health care and that nursing is positioned to be part of meeting the challenges of the changing U.S. health care system.

DISCUSSION QUESTIONS

1. What change(s) in the changing U.S. health delivery system do you think will be an opportunity for nursing to improve health care? Please describe.
2. What challenges do you think the profession of nursing will face as the U.S. health delivery system changes? Do you think these changes are going to improve patient care? Do you think they will improve the visibility and status of nursing? Please support your answer with a rationale.
3. Do you think that the merger of some of the many delivery and payment sources of American health care would streamline care or increase its complexity?

REFERENCES

Agency for Healthcare Research and Quality. (n.d.). What is comparative effectiveness research. Retrieved from *effectivehealthcare.ahrq.gov/index.cfm/what-is-comparative-effectiveness-research1/*.

American Association for Cancer Research. (2013). AACR cancer progress report 2013. *Clinical Cancer Research, 19*(Suppl. 1), S1–S88.

American College of Physicians. (2012). Strengthening the public health infrastructure in a reformed health care system. Retrieved from *www.acponline.org/advocacy/current_policy_papers/assets/public_health.pdf*.

American Hospital Association. (2014). Fast facts on US hospitals. Retrieved from *www.aha.org/research/rc/stat-studies/fast-facts.shtml*.

Association of Academic Health Centers. (2009). Academic health centers: Providing health care services and expanding access. Retrieved from *http://www.aahcdc.org/Portals/0/pdf/FG_AHC_Providing_Health%20Care_Services_Expanding_Access.pdf*.

Association of Academic Health Centers. (2014). Mission of the AAHC. Retrieved from *www.aahcdc.org/About.aspx*.

Bakken, S., Stone, P., & Larsen, E. L. (2008). A nursing informatics research agenda for 2008–2018: Contextual influences and key components. *Nursing Outlook, 56*(5), 206–214.

Barksdale, D. J., Newhouse, R., & Miller, J. A. (2014). The Patient-Centered Outcomes Research Institute (PCORI). *Nursing Outlook, 62*(3), 192–200.

Burke, W., Khoury, M. J., Stewart, A., & Zimmern, R. L. Bellagio Group. (2006). The path from genome-based research to population health: Development of an international public health genomics network. *Genetics in Medicine, 8*(7), 451–458.

Centers for Disease Control and Prevention. (2009). Chronic diseases: The power to prevent, the call to control: At a glance 2009. Retrieved from *www.cdc.gov/chronicdisease/resources/publications/AAG/pdf/chronic.pdf*.

Centers for Disease Control and Prevention. (2013). Medicare, Medicaid, and CHIP: CMS National Training Program. Retrieved from *www.cdc.gov/stltpublichealth/Program/transformation/docs/chip-508.pdf*.

Centers for Medicare and Medicaid Services. (2012). Nursing home data compendium, 2012 ed. Retrieved from *www.cms.gov/Medicare/Provider-Enrollment-and-Certification/CertificationandCompliance/downloads/nursinghomedatacompendium_508.pdf*.

Dafny, L. (2014). Hospital industry consolidation—Still more to come? *The New England Journal of Medicine, 370,* 198–199.

Dao, J. (2013). Criticism of Veterans Affairs Secretary mounts over backlog of claims. *The New York Times.* Retrieved from *www.nytimes.com/2013/05/19/us/shinseki-faces-mounting-criticism-over-backlog-of-benefit-claims.html?_r=0*.

Fisher, M. (2012). Here's a map of the countries that provide universal health care (America is still not on it). *The Atlantic.* Retrieved from *www.theatlantic.com/international/print/2012/06/heres-a-map-of-the-countries-that-provide-universal-health-care-americas-still-not-on-it/259153/*.

Freda, M. C. (2008). Editorial: What are edge runners? *MCN. the American Journal of Maternal Child Nursing, 33*(3), 14.

Health Information Technology and Economic and Clinical Health Act. (2009). Congressional Research Service, Report No. R40101.

HealthIT. (n.d.). Glossary. Retrieved from *http://www.healthit.gov/policy-researchers-implementers/technology-standards-certification-glossary*.

Healthy People 2020. (2014). General health status. Retrieved from *www.healthypeople.gov/2020/about/genhealthabout.aspx#life*.

Indian Health Service. (2013). Indian health disparities. Retrieved from *www.ihs.gov/newsroom/includes/themes/newihstheme/display_objects/documents/factsheets/Disparities_2013.pdf*.

Indian Health Service. (2014). About IHS. Retrieved from *www.ihs.gov/aboutihs/*.

Institute of Medicine. (2011). *The future of nursing: Leading change, advancing health.* Washington, DC: National Academies Press.

Jamoom, E., Beatty, P., Bercovitz, A., Woodwell, D., Palso, K., & Rechtsteiner, E. (2012). *Physician adoption of electronic health record systems: United States, 2011.* NCHC data brief, no. 98. Hyattsville, MD: National Center for Health Statistics.

Kaiser Family Foundation. (2012). Medicaid eligibility, enrollment simplification, and coordination under the Affordable Care Act: A summary of CMS's March 23, 2012 final rule. Kaiser Commission on Medicaid and the Uninsured, Issue Paper. Retrieved from *kaiserfamilyfoundation.files.wordpress.com/2013/04/8391.pdf*.

Kaiser Family Foundation. (2014). How is the ACA impacting Medicaid enrollment? Retrieved from *kff.org/medicaid/issue-brief/how-is-the-aca-impacting-medicaid-enrollment/*.

Klees, B. S., & Wolfe, C. J. (2013). *Brief summaries of Medicare and Medicaid, Title XVIII and Title XIX of the Social Security Act as of November 1, 2013.* Office of the Actuary, Centers for Medicare and Medicaid Services, Department of Health and Human Services. Retrieved from *www.cms.gov/Research-Statistics-Data-and-Systems/Statistics*

-Trends-and-Reports/MedicareProgramRatesStats/Downloads/MedicareMedicaidSummaries2013.pdf.

Library of Congress. (2014). Voters. Retrieved from www.loc.gov/teachers/classroommaterials/presentationsandactivities/presentations/elections/voters9.html.

Liptak, A. (2012). Supreme Court uphold health care law, 5-4, in victory for Obama. *The New York Times.* Retrieved from www.nytimes.com/2012/06/29/us/supreme-court-lets-health-law-largely-stand.html?pagewanted=all&_r=0&pagewanted=print.

Moen, A., & Knudsen, L. (2013). Nursing informatics: Decades of contribution to health information. *Healthcare Informatics Research, 19*(2), 86–92.

Moody, L. E., Slocumb, E., Berg, B., & Jackson, D. (2004). Electronic health records documentation in nursing: Nurses' perceptions, attitudes, and preferences. *Computers, Informatics, Nursing, 22*(6), 337–344.

National Archives. (n.d.). The Constitution of the United States. Retrieved April 7, 2014, from www.archives.gov/exhibits/charters/constitution_transcript.html.

National Center for Veterans Analysis and Statistics, U.S. Department of Veterans Affairs. (2014). Department of Veterans Affairs statistics at a glance. Retrieved from www.va.gov/vetdata/docs/Quickfacts/Stats_at_a_glance_12_31_13.pdf.

National Conference of State Legislatures (NCSL). (2010). NCSL fiscal briefs: State balanced budget provisions, October 2010.Retrieved from www.ncsl.org/documents/fiscal/StateBalancedBudgetProvisions2010.pdf.

National Health Policy Forum (NHPF). (2010). Governmental public health: An overview of state and local public health agencies. Retrieved from www.nhpf.org/library/background-papers/BP77_GovPublicHealth_08-18-2010.pdf.

National Indian Health Board. (2009). Reauthorization of the Indian Health Care Improvement Act (IHCIA), Bringing Indian health services in to the 21st Century. Retrieved from www.nihb.org/docs/IHCIA/IHCIA%20Fact%20Sheet_March%2009.pdf.

National Institute for Health Care Management Foundation [NIHCM]. (2011). Understanding U.S. health care spending. Data brief, July 2011. Retrieved from www.nihcm.org/images/stories/NIHCM-CostBrief-Email.pdf.

National Institute for Health Care Management Foundation [NIHCM]. (2012). Government spending for health entitlement programs. Data brief, June 2012. Retrieved from www.nihcm.org/component/content/article/326-publications-health-care-spending/650-government-spending-for-health-entitlement-programs.

National Institute for Health Care Management Foundation [NIHCM]. (2013). Employer-sponsored health insurance: Recent trends and future directions. Data brief. Retrieved from www.nihcm.org/employer-sponsored-health-insurance-recent-trends-and-future-directions.

NewTechCity. (2012). Healthcare goes digital. Retrieved from www.wnyc.org/story/243822-healthcare-goes-digital.

Office of the National Coordinator for Health Information Technology (ONCHIT). (n.d.). Get the facts about electronic health records: advancing America's health care. Retrieved from www.healthit.gov/sites/default/files/pdf/fact-sheets/ehrs-advancing-americas-health-care.pdf.

Patient-Centered Outcomes Research Institute. (2014). What we do. Retrieved from www.pcori.org/content/what-we-do.

Pearson, G. S., Evans, L. K., Hines-Martin, V. P., Yearwood, E., York, J. A., & Kane, C. F. (2014). Promoting the mental health of families. *Nursing Outlook, 62*(3), 225–227.

PricewaterhouseCoopers. (2013). National Venture Capital Association. *MoneyTree™ Report.* Q4 2013/Full-year 2013. Data provided by Thomson Reuters. Retrieved from www.pwc.com/en_US/us/technology/assets/pwc-moneytree-q4-and-full-year-2013-summary-report.pdf.

Robert Wood Johnson Foundation. (2010). Chronic care: Making the case for ongoing care. Princeton, NJ: Robert Wood Johnson Foundation. Retrieved from www.rwjf.org/content/dam/farm/reports/reports/2010/rwjf54583.

Shi, L., & Singh, D. (2014). *Delivering health care in America: A systems approach* (6th ed.). Sudbury, MA: Jones & Bartlett Learning.

Squires, D. A. (2011, July). The U.S. Health System in perspective: A comparison of twelve industrialized nations. *Issues in International Health Policy.* The Commonwealth Fund. Retrieved from www.commonwealthfund.org/~/media/Files/Publications/Issue%20Brief/2011/Jul/1532_Squires_US_hlt_sys_comparison_12_nations_intl_brief_v2.pdf.

Starr, P. (1982). *The social transformation of American medicine.* New York: Basic Books, Inc.

Thede, L. (2012). Informatics: Where is it? *The Online Journal of Issues in Nursing, 17*(1), Retrieved from www.nursingworld.org/MainMenuCategories/ANAMarketplace/ANAPeriodicals/OJIN/TableofContents/Vol-17-2012/No1-Jan-2012/Informatics-Where-Is-It.html.

Thune, J., Alexander, L., Roberts, P., Burr, R., Coburn, T., & Enzi, M. (2013). Reboot: Re-examining the strategies needed to successfully adopt health IT. Washington, DC: United States Senate. Retrieved from www.amia.org/sites/amia.org/files/Reboot-Report-May-20-2013.pdf.

Truffer, C. J., Klemm, J. D., Wolfe, C. J., Rennie, K. E., & Shuff, J. F. (2012). 2012 Actuarial report on the financial outlook for Medicaid. Office of the Actuary, Centers for Medicare and Medicaid Services, U.S. Department of Health and Human Services. Retrieved from medicaid.gov/Medicaid-CHIP-Program-Information/By-Topics/Financing-and-Reimbursement/Downloads/medicaid-actuarial-report-2012.pdf.

Trust for America's Health. (2011). Investing in America's health: A state-by-state look at public health funding and key health facts. Retrieved from www.healthyamericans.org/assets/files/Investing%20in%20America%27s%20Health.pdf.

U.S. Census Bureau. (2011). Income, poverty, and health insurance coverage in the United States: 2011. Retrieved from www.census.gov/newsroom/releases/archives/income_wealth/cb12-172.html.

U.S. Department of Health and Human Services. (2014). Centers for Disease Control and Prevention. Justification of estimates for appropriation committees. Retrieved from www.cdc.gov/fmo/topic/Budget%20Information/appropriations_budget_form_pdf/FY2014_CJ_CDC_FINAL.pdf.

U.S. Department of Veterans Affairs. (n.d.). History—VA history. Retrieved from http://www.va.gov/about_va/vahistory.asp.

U.S. Department of Veterans Affairs. (2014). National Center for Veterans Analysis and Statistics. Retrieved from www.va.gov/vetdata/Veteran_Population.asp.

World Health Organization. (2013). World health statistics. Retrieved from www.who.int/gho/publications/world_health_statistics/2013/en/.

ONLINE RESOURCES

Trust for America's Health
www.healthyamericans.org
National Institute for Health Care Management
www.nihcm.org
The Office of the National Coordinator of Health Information Technology
www.healthit.gov
Patient-Centered Outcomes Research Institute (PCORI) Get Involved
www.pcori.org/get-involved

UNIT 2

CHAPTER 17

A Primer on Health Economics of Nursing and Health Policy

Len M. Nichols

"The price of light is less than the cost of darkness."
Arthur Nielsen

Economics is the study of how resources are allocated by people operating in the real world, that is, with constraints on their time, their money, and their knowledge. It can be summarized as the study of choices people make under constraints. Because some constraints are operable on everyone, economists say the real world is a world of scarcity, by which they mean no one, and certainly not everyone, can have everything they might want. Sometimes choices today can relax constraints in the future (e.g., studying for an advanced degree can enable someone to earn higher wages and have more income to spend on goods and services in the future). Sometimes choices today are extremely limited by effective constraints (e.g., when the only jobs available pay the minimum wage; no matter how hard one works or how much one makes, there are only 24 hours in a day and every human must sleep).

ECONOMICS AS A DISCIPLINE

Choices under constraints produce trade-offs, which usually boil down to the fact that you can have more of one desirable thing only if you give up another. Time for money is the classic trade-off and allocating a limited budget over competing priorities is something every manager (household or business) in the modern world is familiar with. This sets up the fundamental economic concept of opportunity cost, or what must be given up to get something else. This is a better definition of cost than price or out-of-pocket payment, both of which can be distorted by insurance, taxes, or subsidies from the true total cost of acquiring any good or service.

Economics is a social science, which means it uses logic and analytic tools to develop models which attempt to characterize and explain the essence of a human choice situation. Models must omit some details to be manageable, and the art of creating models is deciding which details are essential (and measurable) and which can be omitted. The results of the models are predictions or hypotheses about how the real world works, how choices will be made, or what the implications of choices already made will be. These predictions and hypotheses can then be tested against real world observations or data.

When the models are confirmed as correct, then the results are added to the body of economic knowledge and passed on to others. When the models and predictions are shown to be inaccurate then the models and thinking about the type of problem under study is revised. In that sense, economics is empirically driven or evidence based. Economics has evolved over time and continues to evolve, as new data emerge and new models, theories, and hypotheses are created; they compete with old models, theories, and hypotheses virtually all the time. This constant evolution is also partly why economists rarely reach unanimous consensus, but if a preponderance of evidence exists at a point in time then a majority of economists will lean in a certain direction, just like health or other professionals do as evidence evolves in their fields.

Why Health Care Is a Hard Economic Case.
Health care has some particular features that make

it different from most markets, even though economic analysis can still be applied with appropriate attention to these details. Number one is unavoidable information asymmetry. This means either buyers or sellers have knowledge the other does not about a good or service. This asymmetry violates one of the key tenets of competitive markets and creates the opportunity for some market participants to take advantage of others without safeguards and institutions to protect them. Health professionals know more than most patients will ever fully understand about the patient's condition and treatment options. This information gap is why the Hippocratic Oath and the Nursing Code of Ethics came into being and use long ago. In the extreme case, malpractice law and the procedures that health care organizations undertake to protect themselves from liability claims also protect patients. Plans and employers and consumer-oriented organizations try to act as agents on the patient's behalf, but they are almost always working from an informational disadvantage that affects market outcomes. The current movement toward transparent quality metrics is helping, but informational asymmetry is present in almost every health care transaction.

The second big difference in health care is the importance of third party payers compared with most markets. Public and private insurers (and sometimes employers, as self-insured organizations) pay the bulk of the cost of health care, but decisions about what services to deliver are made by clinicians and patients, sometimes far removed from knowledge of total cost. Therefore, direct market participants cannot weigh the true cost and benefit of choices, which again violates a key assumption of competitive markets.

Finally, the reality is that health care is sometimes a matter of life and death, and for humanitarian and professional ethics reasons, services are sometimes delivered regardless of a patient's ability to pay. This uncompensated care must be financed, and it is, by a combination of government subsidies, higher charges to private payers who can pay more, and some health care workers accepting little or no compensation for some of their efforts. Each of these three deviations from normal competitive

conditions means that market signals from health care transactions can be distorted, which can in turn distort investment and resource allocation decisions across the board. Distortions from competitive market norms require that economic analysis takes these features into account when analyzing health care markets.

A FUNDAMENTAL ECONOMIC TOOL

Supply and Demand. The first tool in the economists' tool kit is supply and demand analysis, which we apply to registered nurses (RNs) in a hospital setting to illustrate its use. This tool can explain wage and employment trends and help make predictions about the future.

Let's start with the demand curve for nurses. Centuries of evidence suggest that almost all demand curves are downward sloping, that is, as the price of whatever falls, consumers will want more of it, and vice versa. The price of a nurse to a consumer is the wage or salary, plus the costs of necessary benefits that an employer, the hospital, and consumer in this case must pay. Thus, economists postulate that the demand for nurses in the hospital setting looks something like what is shown in Figure 17-1.

U.S. Department of Health and Human Services (HHS), Health Resources and Services Administration (HRSA) (2010) provides the most recent

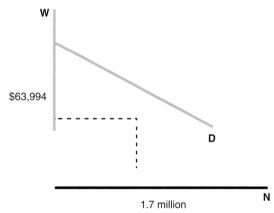

FIGURE 17-1 Demand for nurses in the hospital. The vertical axis is wage, **W**, which could be hourly, weekly, monthly, or annually, but must be specified to be precise. The horizontal axis is the number of nurses, **N**.

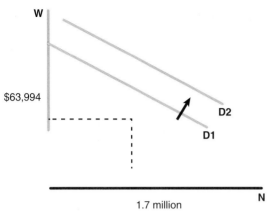

FIGURE 17-2 Demand for nurses in the hospital.

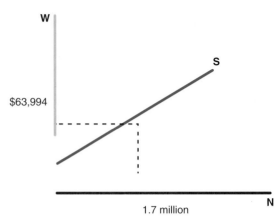

FIGURE 17-3 The supply of nurses in the hospital.

estimates at the annual level, so we will use annual figures for this illustration. The average wage was $63,994 and 1.7 million were employed in hospitals (2.8 million were working nurses in all fields).

As wages fall, more nurses would be demanded by hospitals, and conversely, as wages rise, fewer nurses will be sought after. We will discuss cycles of nursing wages and employment trends in a bit, but for now, we want to make clear what might shift the entire curve or demand schedule and thus change the number of nurses that would be demanded at each wage. Graphically, we are asking what might shift the curve from D1 to D2, as in Figure 17-2.

Factors that are assumed to be constant for each demand curve and, if they change, will shift the entire demand curve, include:

- The size and health of the population that might need hospital care, inpatient or outpatient
- The percentage of that population that is well managed and coordinated by an independent primary care group that minimizes the need for hospital care
- The number of hospitals, the number of beds in those hospitals
- The number of outpatient units
- The number of physicians and or advanced nursing practices, nursing homes, or home health agencies the hospitals own
- The production function of delivering care (substituting more or fewer other health professionals for RNs in the technology of care delivery)

- The prices/wages of potential substitutes or other complementary health professionals (e.g., licensed practical nurses, advanced practice nurses, or physicians)

Changes in any of these factors can shift the curve outward from D1 to D2, or inward (not shown). Changes in these factors help explain employment and wage trends for nurses over time.

The supply curve for hospital nurses is even more straightforward. The greater the wage, the more nurses are willing to work in the hospital setting or settings the hospital owns, as shown in Figure 17-3.

The factors that would shift the entire supply curve for nurses include:

- Net growth in qualified nursing personnel willing to work in hospitals, such as new entrants from nursing schools and programs minus retirements
- Working conditions in hospitals versus other employment alternatives (e.g., nursing homes, skilled nursing facilities, assisted living facilities, independent physician's offices, home health agencies, other ambulatory clinics, ambulatory surgery centers, diagnostic laboratories)
- Wages in alternative employment
- Other household income (either from a spouse or invested wealth)

Note the first supply-shifting factor, net growth in qualified nursing personnel, reflects the impact of nursing faculty, federal support for nursing education, and preceptor shortage realities. Combing the pieces of the tool, Figure 17-4 displays equilibrium in the market for hospital nurses. Figure 17-4 depicts an equilibrium in the economist's sense that the wage has no tendency to rise or fall, because the quantity demanded equals the quantity supplied. A change in the number of hospitals or the wages of nurses in nursing homes, for example, would shift demand or supply, respectively, and upset the equilibrium in this market over time.

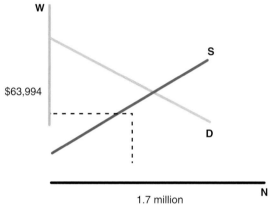

FIGURE 17-4 The demand and supply of nurses in the hospital.

Demand and supply curves, once stable, do engender forces that tend to push prices/wages to the market clearing levels, which is when the market reaches equilibrium and the demand equals supply and there is then no tendency to change.

One could construct supply and demand curves for each distinct market for nursing services, reflecting the employment levels in various RN workforce segments (Table 17-1) (HHS HRSA, 2013).

Pay attention to the fact that hospital employment is the largest single category, by far, and that it is growing fast enough to offset the considerable decline in employment in physician offices. This may be surprising to those who think hospital employment is shrinking along with admissions and readmissions. Nursing demand has increased because hospital outpatient growth plus hospital acquisition of physician practices has increased the ambulatory service mix of hospitals and the need for nurses that goes with that.

Vacancy Rates. The purpose of this primer is to use economics to explain key dimensions of the markets for nurses and their implications for health policy. All nurse managers know that hospitals usually face nursing vacancies, so they might be

TABLE 17-1 Estimated Number of Registered Nurses by Setting of Employment

	Census 2000 Estimate	ACS 2008-2010 Estimate	Estimated Growth/Decline	% Change in Growth
Hospitals	1,427,497	1,785,304	357,807	25.1%
Nursing care facilities	189,594	208,051	18,457	9.7%
Offices of physicians	156,559	134,231	−22,328	−143%
Home health care services	101,895	105,922	4027	40%
Outpatient care centers	70,224	131,022	60,798	866%
Other health care services	66,723	153,449	86,726	1300%
Elementary and secondary schools	51,495	61,323	9828	19.1%
Employment services	45,835	58,362	12,527	27.3%
Insurance carriers and related activities	22,919	25,155	2236	9.8%
Administration of human resource programs	20,509	38,136	17,627	85.9%
Justice, public order (and safety activities)	14,793	18,137	3344	22.6%
Offices of other health practitioners	13,346	7596	−5750	−43.1%
Colleges and universities, including junior colleges	12,637	16,320	3683	29.1%
Residential care facilities, without nursing	10,853	9928	−925	−8.5%
All other settings	70,397	71,706	1308	1.9%
Total	2,275,276	2,824,641	549,365	24.1%

wondering, how can there be a positive vacancy rate in hospitals and also strong tendencies to equilibrium wages? Doesn't the persistence of vacancy rates that never go away render the traditional tools of economics inaccurate for nursing markets? No, and here's why.

A vacancy rate, the percentage of nursing positions that are unfilled, is a reflection of a shortage, where demand exceeds supply. Shortages should not persist if wages adjust upward to market (equilibrium) clearing levels. The actual history of vacancy rates and nursing wage adjustments suggests that the standard economic model works reasonably well to explain movements in wages and employment, but with a lag for real world inertia. This inertia in raising wages is commonly caused by reluctance to raise nurses' pay until other options for recruitment are exhausted, as well as the time lag before information about higher wages and aggressive recruitment is well known enough to encourage more entry into nursing schools, reentry to work, or increasing hours of nursing work (Figure 17-5) (Feldstein, 2011).

One technical note about Figure 17-5; the blue line shows real wage growth, or wages adjusted for inflation. This is a relevant concept, because if wages do not rise as much as inflation, this amounts to a wage cut, because actual purchasing power of the wage level would have declined.

Two inferences should be drawn from Figure 17-5: (1) Real wage growth can be negative if vacancy rates are low enough or falling long enough and (2) vacancy rates have not ever fallen below 4% since 1979. This suggests there is a natural floor in vacancy rates below which hospital administrators are not comfortable hiring; that is, they do not really want the market for nurses to clear completely, possibly because they fear how high equilibrium wages might actually be at that moment, and those high wages would significantly increase hospital costs, very possibly forever. Thus, equilibrium in nursing markets is effectively reached when hospital vacancy rates are around 4%.

COST-EFFECTIVENESS OF NURSING SERVICES

In this era of hyper-cost consciousness, every part of the health care system is often required and wants to demonstrate its unique value. Cost-effectiveness is a technique that allows analysts to compare the costs and outcomes, in nonmonetary units such as body mass index reduction or quality adjusted life years (QALYs) saved, across two or more possible strategies. It differs from cost-benefit analysis in that the outcomes are not measured in monetary terms but in health-related terms. Thus, if intervention A is more cost-effective than

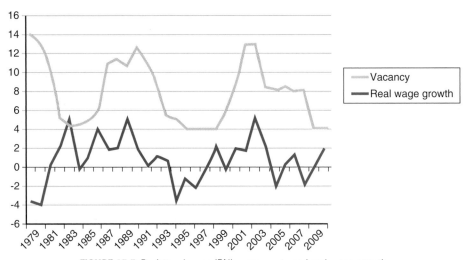

FIGURE 17-5 Registered nurse (RN) vacancy rate and real wage growth.

intervention B, either it yields the same health benefit for a lower cost or it delivers more health benefit per dollar cost. The relevant metric is usually cost per QALY saved.

Cost-effectiveness studies are surprisingly rarely done on alternative nursing staffing patterns and care delivery modalities. The literature is much more likely to report analyses of a small number of advanced practice nurses partially or wholly replacing physicians or being added to a physician-led team. It is far simpler, frankly, to investigate the impact on cost and outcomes from a specific *marginal* intervention, for example, adding a care-coordination nurse to a primary care practice, than to compare the cost-effectiveness of 7 : 1 versus 5 : 1 hospital patient to nurse staffing ratios across hospitals in the United States. The former requires only an accounting of changes in costs and outcomes, and marginal costs are typically just the nurses' salaries, whereas the marginal outcome effect might be reduced admissions, reduced emergency room visits, better hypertension control, and so on. The latter requires complete transparency of different hospital accounting systems, congruence on allocation of fixed costs and variable costs, and so on. This is why the few studies of the effect of nurse staffing patterns on cost that have been done have typically focused on the impact on quality or patient outcomes, not overall hospital costs. It is simply too difficult to compare costs across hospitals because of variable accounting practices.

A notable exception is the paper by Rothberg and colleagues (2005) that estimated the cost-effectiveness of moving the patient/nurse ratio from 8 : 1 to 4 : 1, using total hospital costs as the cost metric. Those costs depend on nursing wages, and how much they would have to rise to call forth the proposed increase in staffing ratios (acknowledging the supply curve for nursing labor is upward sloping, as we postulated and drew above); cost per hospital day; impact of more nursing hours on adverse events, mortality, and length of stay; and the risk of nurse dissatisfaction from high patient/nurse ratios and the cost of turnover. The most important feature of a good cost-effectiveness analysis is to do a complete inventory of existing and differential costs and impacts on outcomes.

Rothberg and colleagues (2005) used estimates of the range of these costs and impacts from the published literature and did sensitivity analyses of the values of the key variables along with a Monte Carlo technique, which essentially runs the experimental calculation (or gamble, hence the name) repeatedly to yield the range of possible outcomes and the best possible estimate of the most likely outcome from lower patient-to-nurse ratios.

Rothberg and colleagues (2005) found that reducing patient/nurse ratios from 8 : 1 to 4 : 1 reduced mortality and increased costs, but that the incremental mortality gain per dollar fell as the ratio got closer to 4 : 1. In other words, cost per life saved rose as the ratio fell toward 4 : 1. Moving from 8 : 1 to 7 : 1 cost $24,900 per life saved (in 2005 dollars), whereas moving from 5 : 1 to 4 : 1 cost $136,300 per life saved, more than 5 times as much. The former would clearly be within the $50,000 per life saved threshold typically used by U.S. insurers and government agencies around the developed world to decide if a treatment is worth covering (Grosse, 2008; Hirth et al., 2000; Neumann & Greenberg, 2009; Weinstein, 2008). The latter incremental gain in mortality would not pass this threshold test. Still, most states leave staffing decisions to hospitals, and they are, predictably, all over the map in the absence of a definitive empirical study and national regulation. Thus, the final decision is left to the market.

IMPACT OF HEALTH REFORM ON NURSING ECONOMICS

The Patient Protection and Affordable Care Act (ACA) has many features which impact nursing and the entire health care system, but the most far reaching for nursing are those which relate to payment and delivery reforms. The increasingly explicit aim of the ACA is to catalyze, through public programs and multipayer incentives, a transformation across the health care system from fee-for-service medicine (which is basically pay-for-volume) to more accountable health care that will be closer to pay-for-value. This approach is reflected in the ACA's shared savings programs, especially Pioneer Accountable Care Organizations, the ACA Patient-Centered Medical Home (PCMH) experiment, and the Comprehensive Primary Care Initiative, as well as with bundled payments. The underlying assumption, widely shared, is that enabling most health delivery organizations to provide high-value care is the only way the health system as a whole is going to be financially sustainable, while serving all of us, as the ACA also envisions, rather than some of us, as the U.S. health care system does now.

Although the new emerging models of care obviously differ in details, they share one common theme, which is to pay groups of providers for larger and larger units of service. For example, instead of paying physicians separately for each visit and associated tests with fee-for-service and then paying hospitals separately for each admission with a diagnosis-related group (DRG)–based payment, pay one lump sum to a team to take care of the patient for a given episode (bundled payment) or length of time (global capitation). The opportunity for nursing is that nurses' inherent skill set, patient-focused care, communication, and coordination across silos of care can help both physicians and hospitals deliver higher quality care more efficiently than today. The challenge for nursing is that the price is largely hidden, within the per visit charges of physicians and within the per diem charges of hospitals. This means that current data systems are unable to credibly estimate the value of nursing services and the optimal configuration of nurses within multidisciplinary clinical teams. Keeping a clear eye on nursing value to the team is essential for truly cost-effective and high-quality care to be priced and delivered, and not all managers are able to do this at the moment (Beurhaus, Welton, & Rosenthal, 2010).

These types of payment reforms are being adopted by private payers, in some cases faster than the government pilots can spread, such as with PCMHs. What they all have in common, for the first time in American health care (except for the closed staff model health maintenance organizations such as Kaiser Permanente and Group Health Cooperative), is that providers have powerful incentives to reorganize care delivery and coordination processes to seek the triple aim: cost-effective,

timely, and efficacious care. Although this transformation is likely to be good for nurses at the RN level and above in the medium and long term, the transformation is not without risks and probably bodes some pain for some nurses in the short term.

The first-order effect of these incentive changes will be to modernize the nation's nurse practice acts to reflect current standards. The intense battles in half of the state houses may become relatively moot, because now health delivery organizations will gain from using advanced practice nurses and others to the limit of their training, not the limit of their current scope of practice. Restrictive state nurse practice acts, even at this late date, too often are still intent on protecting physicians' short-run economic interests at the expense of higher-cost care and limited access to qualified providers for all concerned. The ACA and the incentives it unleashed will eventually lead physician groups to demand scope of practice liberalization or simply refuse to complain and prosecute its technical breach.

This general incentive realignment will then extend to reorganizing physician offices, starting with primary care because of the sheer number of PCMHs already in existence (attributable to public and private initiatives), but it will soon extend to specialists and hospitals also. Care-coordination nurses and nurses who can function well within and even lead team-based delivery of care will earn premium wages, because communication across former silos of care will be paramount to reduce the avoidable hospital admissions and readmissions that have been huge cost drivers for patients with multiple chronic conditions. Systems which learn how to lower the costs on high-cost patients who spend most of the 17% of gross domestic product without attaining satisfactory outcomes compared with other OECD (relatively rich) countries will be the systems that will flourish. It is very likely that effective nurses will be the backbone and sinew of care coordination and these new more efficient systems of care.

A short-run cost could materialize for those nurses who work for hospitals and physician groups who deny, delay, or resist this incentive realignment and do not clearly see the value of nursing services, long past the point of being behind their peers. Top-level managers of these organizations may not be doing appropriate cost-effectiveness analyses of how best to reorganize care to align with new incentive structures, but may rather be focused on preserving their top-level incomes even as overall revenue inevitably falls. The only solution they may see is to increase patient/nurse ratios by laying off relatively expensive RNs and either not replacing them or replacing them with lower trained and less expensive health professionals. And some small outlying hospitals will close owing to lack of demand for their services in a world focused on the ability of enhanced primary care to prevent hospitalizations and readmissions.

The marketplace will then have two strategies in competition: (1) a lower cost and more team-based approach and (2) a higher cost and more libertarian or traditional cowboy style go-it-alone health care. The lower cost and team-based approach will surely win, but it may take a while before the evidence is clear to the common public, and the traditional providers will, in the meantime, claim loudly that they are the only high-quality alternative left. Credible quality measurement infrastructures, price, and quality transparency for consumers to make comparison shopping possible will hasten the demise of the old school strategy, but even so it may take 10 years at least before it disappears altogether.

The ACA will then ultimately create a more welcoming environment for nurses and their many talents, but some might have a more painful transition to this better world than others.

DISCUSSION QUESTIONS

1. Describe at least three issues that make the health care market behave differently from other markets.
2. According to economic principles, what forces go into play as demand for nursing goes up?
3. What role could nurses play, enlarge, or expand in value-driven care delivery models such as Primary Care Medical Homes and Accountable Care Organizations?

REFERENCES

Beurhaus, P., Welton, J., & Rosenthal, M. (2010). Health care payment reform: Implications for nurses. *Nursing Economic$, 28*(1), 49.

Feldstein, P. J. (2011). *Health policy issues: An economic perspective.* Chicago, IL: Health Administration Press.

Grosse, S. (2008). Assessing cost-effectiveness in healthcare: history of the $50,000 per QALY threshold. *Expert Review of Pharmacoeconomics & Outcomes Research, 8*(2), 165–178.

Hirth, R., Chernew, M., Miller, E., Fendrick, A. M., & Weissert, W. G. (2000). Willingness to pay for a quality-adjusted life year: In search of a standard. *Medical Decision Making, 20*(3), 332–342.

Neumann, P., & Greenberg, M. (2009). Is the United States ready for QALYs? *Health Affairs, 28*(5), 1366–1371.

Rothberg, M., Abraham, I., Lindenauer, P., & Rose, D. (2005). Improving nurse to patient staffing ratios as a cost-effective safety intervention. *Medical Care, 43*(8), 785–791.

U.S. Department of Health and Human Services, Health Resources and Services Administration (HRSA), Bureau of Health Professions. (2010). The registered nurse population: Initial findings from the 2008 National Sample Survey of Registered Nurses. Retrieved from *bhpr.hrsa.gov/healthworkforce/rnsurveys/rnsurveyinitial2008.pdf.*

U.S. Department of Health and Human Services, Health Resources and Services Administration (HRSA), Bureau of Health Professions, National Center for Workforce Analysis. (2013). The U.S. nursing workforce: Trends in supply and education. Retrieved from *bhpr.hrsa.gov/healthworkforce/reports/nursingworkforce/nursingworkforcefullreport.pdf.*

Weinstein, M. (2008). How much are Americans willing to pay for a quality-adjusted life year? *Medical Care, 46*(4), 343–344.

CHAPTER 18

Financing Health Care in the United States

Joyce A. Pulcini   Mary Ann Hart

"There are more than 9000 billing codes for individual procedures and units of care. But there is not a single billing code for patient adherence or improvement, or for helping patients stay well."

Clayton M. Christensen

Health care financing in the United States is fragmented, complex, and the most costly in the world. The Affordable Care Act (ACA) of 2010 takes some steps to reshape how health care is paid for, but its primary purpose is to extend insurance coverage to approximately 30 million uninsured Americans through private insurance regulation, expansion of pubic insurance programs, and creation of health insurance marketplaces to foster competition in the private health insurance market. As the ACA is implemented, making health insurance more affordable and containing the rise in health care costs are significant ongoing policy challenges in system transformation. This chapter will provide an overview of the current system of health care financing in the United States, including the impact of the ACA.

HISTORICAL PERSPECTIVES ON HEALTH CARE FINANCING

Understanding today's complex and often confusing approaches to financing health care requires an examination of the nation's values and historical context. Some dominant values underpin the U.S. political and economic systems. The United States has a long history of individualism, an emphasis on freedom to choose alternatives and an aversion to large-scale government intervention into the private

realm. Compared with other developed nations with capitalist economies, social programs have been the exception rather than the rule and have been adopted primarily during times of great need or social and political upheaval. Examples of these exceptions include the passage of the Social Security Act of 1935 and the passage of Medicare and Medicaid in 1965.

Because health care in the United States had its origins in the private sector market, not government, and because of the growing political power of physicians, hospitals, and insurance companies, the degree to which government should be involved in health care remains controversial. Other developed capitalist countries, such as Canada, the United Kingdom, France, Germany, and Switzerland, view health care as a social good that should be available to all. In contrast, the United States has viewed health care as a market-based commodity, readily available to those who can pay for it but not available universally to all people. With its capitalist orientation and politically powerful financial stakeholders, the United States has been resistant to significant health care reform, especially as it relates to expanding access to affordable health insurance.

The debate over the role of government in social programs intensified in the decades after the Great Depression. Although the Social Security Act of 1935 brought sweeping social welfare legislation, providing for Social Security payments, workman's compensation, welfare assistance for the poor, and certain public health, maternal, and child health services, it did not provide for health care insurance coverage for all Americans. Also, during the decade following the Great Depression, nonprofit Blue Cross and Blue Shield (BC/BS) emerged as a private insurance plan to cover hospital and physician care. The idea that people should pay for their medical care before they actually got sick, through insurance, ensured some level of security for both providers and consumers of medical services. The creation of insurance plans effectively defused a strong political movement toward legislating a broader, compulsory government-run health insurance plan at the time (Starr, 1982). After a failed attempt by President Truman in the late 1940s to provide Americans with a national health plan, no progress occurred on this issue until the 1960s, when Medicare and Medicaid were enacted.

BC/BS dominated the health insurance industry until the 1950s, when for-profit commercial insurance companies entered the market and were able to compete with BC/BS by holding down costs through their practice of excluding sick (with pre-existing conditions) people from insurance coverage. Over time, the distinction between BC/BS and commercial insurance companies became increasingly blurred as BC/BS began to offer competitive for-profit plans (Kovner, Knickman, & Weisfeld, 2011. In the 1960s, the United States enjoyed relative prosperity, along with a burgeoning social conscience, and an appetite for change that led to a heightened concern for the poor and older adults and the impact of catastrophic illness. In response, Medicaid and Medicare, two separate but related programs, were created in 1965 by amendments to the Social Security Act. Medicare is a federal government-administered health insurance program for the disabled and those over 65 years (Kaiser Family Foundation [KFF], 2014c), and Medicaid, until recently, has been a state and federal government-administered health insurance program for low-income people, who are in certain categories, such as pregnant women with children.

GOVERNMENT PROGRAMS

CURRENT PUBLIC/FEDERAL FUNDING FOR HEALTH CARE IN THE UNITED STATES

In the United States, no single public entity oversees or controls the entire health care system, making the payment for and delivery of health care complex, inefficient, and expensive. Instead, the system is composed of many public and private programs that form interrelated parts at the federal, state, and local levels. The public funding systems, which include Medicare, Medicaid, the Children's Health Insurance Program (CHIP), the U.S. Department of Veterans Affairs (VA), and the Defense Health Program (TRICARE) for military personnel, their families, military retirees, and some others, continue to represent a larger and larger proportion of health care spending. Other examples of federal programs are the Indian Health Service, which covers American Indians and Alaskan Natives, and the Federal Employees Health Benefits (FEHB) Program, which covers all federal employees unless excluded by law or regulation.

Federal health expenditures for these programs totaled $731.6 billion or 26% of all health care expenditures in 2012 (Martin et al., 2014). Medicare outlays were $572.5 billion in 2012 and accounted for 20% of all national health care expenditures with Medicare Advantage (a Medicare-managed care program provided by insurance plans that can be chosen by beneficiaries instead of the traditional Medicare program) growing most rapidly (Martin et al., 2014). Medicaid outlays in 2012 were $412.2 billion and accounted for 15% of total national health care expenditures, and its spending growth also decelerated that year (Martin et al., 2014).

MEDICARE

Before the enactment of Medicare in 1965, older adults were more likely to be uninsured and more likely to be impoverished by excessive health care costs. Half of older Americans had no health insurance; but by 2000, 96% of seniors had health care coverage through Medicare (Federal Interagency Forum on Age-Related Statistics, 2000).

Medicare had a beneficial effect on the health of older adults by facilitating access to care and medical technology, and, in 2006, prescription drug coverage helped improve the economic status of older adults. The percentage of persons over age 65 years living below the poverty line decreased from 35% in 1959 (when older adults had the highest poverty rate of the population) to 9% in 2012 (U.S. Census Bureau, 2014).

Americans are eligible for Medicare Part A at age 65 years, the age for Social Security eligibility, or sooner, if they are determined to be disabled. Medicare Part A accounted for 31% of benefit spending in 2012 and covers 52 million Americans. Medicare Part A covers hospital and related costs and is financed through payroll deduction to the Hospital Insurance Trust Fund at the payroll tax rate of 2.9% of earnings paid by employers and employees (1.45% each) (KFF, 2014a). Medicare Part B, which accounted for approximately one third of benefit spending in 2012, covers 80% of the fees for physician services, outpatient medical services and supplies, home care, durable medical equipment, laboratory services, physical and occupational therapy, and outpatient mental health services. Part B is financed through subscriber premiums and general revenue funding as well as cost-sharing with beneficiaries.

Medicare Part C, or the Medicare Advantage Program, through which beneficiaries can enroll in a private health plan and also receive some extra services such as vision or hearing services, accounted for 23% of benefit spending in 2012 and had more than 14.1 million enrollees, or 28% of all Medicare beneficiaries in 2013 (Medpac, 2013). Medicare

Advantage enrollment has been increasing and is up 30% since 2010 (KFF, 2014a). Extra payments that the federal government has made to private Medicare Advantage Plans are due to be phased out by the ACA, raising concerns that insurers will drop their Medicare Advantage Plans as a result.

Medicare Part D is a voluntary, subsidized outpatient prescription drug plan with additional subsidies for low- and modest-income individuals. It accounted for 10% of benefit spending in 2012 and enrolled 39 million beneficiaries in 2013 (KFF, 2014a, 2014b). Figure 18-1 presents Medicare benefit payments by type of service in 2012 (KFF, 2014a). Medicare Part D is financed through general revenues and beneficiary premiums as well as state payments for recipients who get both Medicare and Medicaid, also known as "dual eligibles" (KFF, 2014b). The ACA phases out the Medicare Part D "donut hole," a period of noncoverage for prescription drugs that left many seniors unable to pay out-of-pocket for their medications.

The ACA authorized that certified nurse midwives (CNMs) be reimbursed at 100% of the physician payment rate. Other advanced practice registered nurses (APRNs), including nurse practitioners (NPs), are paid 85% of the physician rate

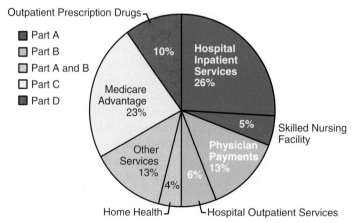

Total Benefit Payments = $536 billion

NOTE: Excludes administrative expenses and is net of recoveries. *Includes hospice, durable medical equipment, Part B drugs, outpatient dialysis, ambulance, lab services, and other services.
SOURCE: Congressional Budget Office (CBO) Medicare Baseline, February 2013.

FIGURE 18-1 Medicare benefit payments by type of service, 2012. (From Kaiser Family Foundation. [2014]. Retrieved from *kff.org/medicare/fact-sheet/medicare-spending-and-financing-fact-sheet/.*)

for the same services. In addition, Medicare will not pay for home care or hospice services unless they are ordered by a physician. And, unfortunately, the ACA required physician orders for durable medical equipment for Medicare beneficiaries.

MEDICAID

Medicaid is the public insurance program jointly funded by state and federal governments but administered by individual states under guidelines of the federal government. Medicaid is a means-tested program because eligibility is determined by financial status. Before changes by the ACA, only low-income people within certain categories, such as recipients of Supplemental Social Security Income (SSI), families receiving Temporary Assistance to Needy Families (TANF), and children and pregnant women whose family income is at or below 133% of the poverty level were eligible. To qualify for federal Medicaid matching grants, a state must provide a minimum set of benefits, including hospitalization, physician care, laboratory services, radiology studies, prenatal care, and preventive services; nursing home and home health care; and medically necessary transportation. Medicaid programs are also required to pay the Medicare premiums, deductibles, and copayments for certain low-income persons who are eligible for both programs. Medicaid is increasingly becoming a long-term care financing program of last resort for older adults in nursing homes. Many older adults have to spend down their life savings to become low income and be eligible for Medicaid. Family and pediatric NPs and CNMs are also required to be reimbursed under federal Medicaid rules if, in accordance with state regulations, they are legally authorized to provide Medicaid-covered services.

In keeping with its goal to expand health insurance coverage to more Americans, the ACA expands eligibility for the Medicaid program to any legal resident under the age of 65 years with an income up to 138% of the federal poverty level. The intent of the health reform law was to have one eligibility standard across all states and eliminate eligibility by specific categories (Commonwealth Fund, 2011; Rosenbaum, 2011). The federal government has agreed to pay for nearly all the expansion costs to insure more low-income people. The U.S. Supreme

Court, however, struck down the mandate to expand Medicaid and ruled that states could decide whether or not to expand the program. Figure 18-2 indicates that as of April 2014, 27 states had decided to expand Medicaid, 5 are still debating this, and 19 are not moving forward (KFF, 2014d). States that decide to opt out of the expansion can follow old federal guidelines for eligibility, leaving wide disparities in health insurance coverage between states and leaving uninsured large proportions of the population below 138% of the poverty level. Of the states that have opted out of expansion, all have Republican political leaders explicit in their opposition to the ACA, although Republican Governor Jan Brewer of Arizona pushed her state to expand Medicaid in 2013 so that 300,000 more poor and disabled residents of the state would have coverage (Schwartz, 2013). In many of the nonparticipating states, physicians, nurses, hospitals, and other health care organizations and stakeholders are pressuring their state governments to expand Medicaid as a way to improve access to health care for more low-income people.

CHIP was created in 1997 to help cover uninsured children whose families were not eligible for Medicaid. It has been funded through state and federal funds, but states set their own eligibility standards. The ACA commits the federal government to paying most of its costs, beginning in 2015, up to 100%. It also requires states to maintain their eligibility standards for CHIP (Emanuel, 2014). CHIP will be reauthorized in 2015, and, because it is expected that many more children will have gained coverage through family health insurance plans, debate is expected over the role of the program. CHIP is enrolling a record number of children now estimated to be one third of all children in the United States. Advocates want to maintain these high child health insurance rates until the ACA is fully implemented and full coverage for children under the provisions of the ACA is assured.

STATE HEALTH CARE FINANCING

State governments not only administer and partially fund some public insurance programs such as Medicaid and CHIP but they are also responsible for individual state public health programs.

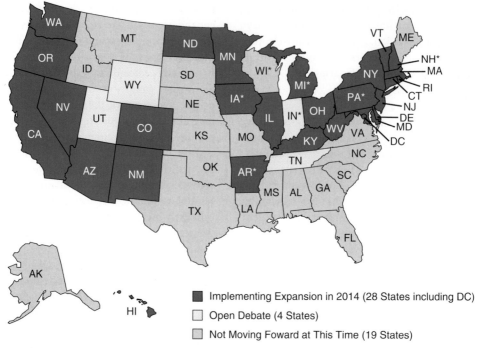

FIGURE 18-2 State Medicaid expansion, November 2014. (From FamiliesUSA. [2014]. Retrieved from *familiesusa.org/product/50-state -look-medicaid-expansion;* and Kaiser Family Foundation. [2014]. Retrieved from *kff.org/medicaid/fact-sheet/a-closer-look-at-the -impact-of-state-decisions-not-to-expand-medicaid-on-coverage-for-uninsured-adults/.*)

The definition of public health as compared with other types of health programs is not always well understood. The mission of public health as defined by the Institute of Medicine (IOM) is to ensure conditions in which people can be healthy (IOM, 1988). Whereas medicine focuses on the individual patient, public health focuses on whole populations. Medical care for the individual patient is associated with payment by health insurance, but population-based public health programs are funded by local, county, state revenues, often combined with grants from the federal government in areas such as maternal and child health, obesity prevention, HIV/AIDS, substance abuse, and environmental health. Even with a greater federal role in health care through the ACA, states will continue to have a major responsibility for the regulation of health insurance, health care providers and professionals, and public health activities.

Reduction of budgets for public health programs during times of fiscal constraint has resulted in the resurgence of infectious diseases such as tuberculosis and sexually transmitted diseases in some communities. A series of natural disasters such as tornados also brought to light gaps in the public health system, especially the ability to respond, for example, to mass casualty events. Although the ACA authorized $15 billion for the creation of a Prevention and Public Health Fund to invest in public health and disease prevention, Congress reduced by one third the amount of funding mandated by the law in 2012 and President Obama signed the legislation to pay for other initiatives (Health Policy Brief, 2012).

LOCAL/COUNTY LEVEL

Similar to state governments, local and county governments in many states also have the responsibility of protecting public health. Some provide indigent care by funding and running public hospitals and clinics, such as New York City's Health and Hospitals Corporation and Chicago's Cook County Hospital. Although receiving a subsidy from their local government, these hospitals, which have served primarily poor patients and those without health insurance, have gotten significant special payments, especially from Medicare to serve these populations. These disproportionate share hospital (DSH) payments are being gradually reduced under the ACA because it is presumed that eventually, under the ACA, many more people will gain health insurance coverage. Because public hospitals and clinics are so dependent on public funds, their budgets are historically squeezed during times of fiscal restraint by local, state, and federal governments, making them vulnerable to long-term sustainability. In fact, many public health hospitals have closed, and in many parts of the country, the populations they have served have been absorbed by other types of hospital providers (KFF, 2013).

THE PRIVATE HEALTH INSURANCE AND DELIVERY SYSTEMS

The U.S. health care system has been predominantly a private one that operates more like a business and, more or less, according to free market principles. Private health insurance has been the dominant payer and, for most Americans, it is obtained as a benefit of employment in the form of group health insurance. However, until the passage of the ACA employers have had no obligation to provide employee health insurance, leaving many Americans uninsured or underinsured, especially those working in lower-wage jobs. As private health insurance premiums have risen, employers asked employees to pay for a greater percentage of their insurance premium, and to enroll in plans that required more cost-sharing in the form of copayment, deductibles, and coinsurance. Approximately 15% of insured Americans have purchased their health insurance from the nongroup individual insurance market. Typically, these plans were more expensive and insurers in all but a few states had been able to deny insurance to applicants with pre-existing medical conditions, until the practice of discrimination based on medical history was outlawed by the ACA in 2010. Because private insurers are regulated by individual states, there are wide disparities in coverage from state to state, as private insurers are powerful political stakeholders who resist attempts at state or federal regulations to make insurance more accessible and affordable. Whereas private health insurance will continue to be a cornerstone of the U.S. health care financing system, public insurers such as Medicare and Medicaid are paying for an increasing percentage of health care costs.

It should be noted that health insurance is regulated by the states. Some states now mandate that NPs be considered primary care providers and eligible for credentialing and payment by private insurers. But there is wide variation in the extent to which APRNs are included in insurers' provider panels. This variation can be seen among states, among insurers within a given state, and among the plans offered by an insurer (Brassard, 2014).

Most care in the United States is provided by nonprofit or for-profit hospitals and health care systems and private insurance plans (Truffer et al., 2010). Pharmaceutical companies, suppliers of health care technology, and the various service industries that support the health care system in the United States are part of what has been called the medical industrial complex (Meyers, 1970), and there is little government regulation of these industries. Although the private delivery system is dependent on payment from private insurers as well as government insurers, it has usually been resistant to government-directed efforts to expand access to care or cost-containment measures. Well-financed special interest groups representing industry stakeholders have had a great deal of influence over the political process at both the state and federal levels. For example, the medical device industry is lobbying Congress hard to repeal or reduce the medical device tax that the ACA levied to help pay for the expansion of insurance coverage under the health care law and has gained significant support in Congress (Kramer & Kasselheim, 2013).

THE PROBLEM OF CONTINUALLY RISING HEALTH CARE COSTS

From the 1970s to the present, continually rising insurance premiums and health care delivery costs have strained government budgets, become a costly expense to businesses that offer health insurance to their employees, and put health care increasingly out of reach for individuals and families. Figure 18-3 depicts the annual percentage change in national health expenditures by selected sources of funds, 1960 to 2012 (KFF, 2014e).

Stakeholders in small and large businesses, government, organized labor, health care providers, and consumer groups have convened over the years to tackle the problem of rising health care costs, with little lasting success. Although a range of strategies was employed to curb rising health care costs over those 40 years, health care expenditures as a percentage of the gross domestic product (GDP) increased steadily over that time. Although multiple factors are responsible for rising health care costs as a percentage of GDP, the key one is that, unlike other capitalist democracies, the federal and state governments have little, if any, role in regulating what can be charged for health care services and supplies. Prices are largely negotiated between health insurances and providers, resulting in wide variances in prices for similar or exact services, largely based on the market clout of providers to negotiate higher prices. Other contributing factors to high health care costs include the complex administrative systems of insurers and providers, the use of expensive medical technology and medical specialists, and

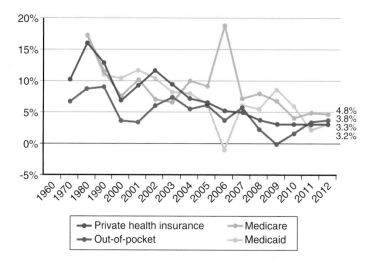

NOTE: This figure omits national health spending that belongs in the categories of Other Public Insurance Programs, Other Third Party Payers and Programs, Public Health Activity, and investment, which together represented about 20% of total national health spending in 2012. Medicare and Medicaid were enacted in 1965; by January 1970, all states but two were participating in Medicaid. Implementation of the Medicare Part D prescription drug benefit was the major cause of the 2006 increase in Medicare spending and decrease in Medicaid spending (Medicare replaced Medicaid drug coverage for dual eligibles).
SOURCE: Kaiser Family Foundation calculations using NHE data from Centers for Medicare and Medicaid Services, Office of the Actuary, National Health Statistics Group, at http://www.cms.hhs.gov/NationalHealthExpendData/ (see Historical; National Health Expenditures by type of service and source of funds, CY 1960-2012; file nhe2012.zip).

FIGURE 18-3 Annual percentage change in national health expenditures, by selected sources of funds, 1960 to 2012. (From Kaiser Family Foundation. [2014]. Retrieved from *kaiserfamilyfoundation.files.wordpress.com/2014/02/annual-percent-change-in-national -health-expenditures-by-selected-sources-of-funds-1960-2012-healthcosts.png*.)

the incentive in fee-for-service reimbursement for providers to increase their volume of services and provide unnecessary health care. Consumers have also lacked knowledge of the actual cost of their care, leading to an inability of the market to accurately respond to cost and differential health care prices by region, type of hospital, or health care facility.

Future costs will also be impacted by the aging of the population and increasing number of people with complex chronic illness who use a disproportionately high percentage of the health care dollars. For example, from 1977 to 2007, a very stable 5% of the population who had complex chronic illness accounted for nearly 50% of the health care expenditures (KFF, 2010; Stanton, 2006), despite efforts to control costs among this population. In 2009, the costliest 5% of beneficiaries accounted for 39% of all Medicare fee-for-service spending. The least costly 50% of beneficiaries accounted for 5% of all spending (Medpac, 2013). The majority of those in the high-expenditure group are not older adults but rather those with complex chronic illnesses (Stanton, 2006).

All other industrialized countries spend significantly less on health care but have better health outcomes and a longer life expectancy. For example, the United States ranks among the worst of industrialized nations on important health indicators such as infant mortality, maternal mortality, and life expectancy at birth (Squires, 2014). Yet, in 2012, it ranked first in health care costs per capita at approximately $8915 per person (Organization for Economic Co-operation and Development [OECD], 2013b). This amounted to close to 18% of its GDP, compared with The Netherlands, which ranked second at 12% of its GDP (OECD, 2013a).

COST-CONTAINMENT EFFORTS

Over time, several approaches have been used to contain costs, including the following.

Regulation Versus Competition. During the 1970s, modest government regulation attempted to contain health care costs through state rate-setting agencies and health planning mechanisms, such as Certificate of Need (CON) programs and regional Health Systems Agencies (HSAs), which evaluated and approved applications for the construction of new facilities, beds, and new technology. During the 1980s and early 1990s, when proponents of competition and free market health care became politically more influential, rate setting and CON programs were weakened and HSAs were eliminated. While free-market principles, as they apply to health care, have few similarities to a fully competitive market in economic terms, the rise of managed care programs and competition among health insurance plans in the 1980s may have temporarily slowed the growth of health costs before they began to rise again. As health insurers expanded the use of copayments, deductibles, and coinsurance as economic incentives to discourage care, the onus of cost-containment fell more heavily on the consumer/patient. However, ample research shows that low-income people may avoid necessary care because of copayments and deductibles. Chapter 17 more fully describes the mechanisms underlying the market system in health care.

Managed Care. The origins of today's managed care plans were in early prepaid health plans of the 1920s, which evolved into Health Maintenance Organizations (HMOs) in the 1970s, and into a variety of models in the subsequent 30 years, including Preferred Provider Organizations (PPOs). A managed care system shifts health care delivery and payment from open-ended access to providers, paid for through fee-for-service reimbursement, toward one in which the provider is a gatekeeper or manager of the patient's health care and assumes some degree of financial responsibility for the care that is given through a capitated budget in which to pay for the patient's care. Managed care implies not only that spending will be controlled but also that other aspects of care will be managed, such as quality and accessibility. In managed care, the primary care provider has traditionally been the gatekeeper, deciding what specialty services are appropriate and where these services can be obtained at the lowest cost. In the 1990s, negative media attention concerning the incentives to restrict care in the managed care model fueled a political backlash. Consumer and provider demands for greater choice for services and access to providers caused managed care plans to loosen gatekeeper requirements and provide more direct access to specialists. As a result, managed care became less effective in holding down expenditures and fueled a rise in health insurance premiums.

In addition, concerns of consumers and providers challenging the quality of care provided by some Managed Care Organizations (MCOs) resulted in state and federal laws to further regulate managed care plans (Kongstvedt, 2001). These laws included provisions related to grievance procedures, confidentiality of health information, requirements for informing patients of the benefits they will receive, antidiscrimination clauses, and assurances that various quality mechanisms were in place so that patient satisfaction was measured and efforts to control costs did not curtail needed care. In addition, most states adopted policies giving health plan enrollees a right to appeal plan determinations involving a denial of coverage to an independent medical review entity, which is often a private organization approved by the state (American Association of Health Plans, 2001). Efforts to pass into law the federal Patient's Bill of Rights, which contained many consumer protections related to managed care, were not successful.

Medicaid and Medicare also promoted managed care plans to control their expenditures for health care by using capitated payment and managing patient care. All 50 states offer some type of Medicaid-managed care plans, and states can decide if participation is voluntary or mandatory. Some states have created state-run Medicaid-only plans, but others enroll Medicaid recipients in private MCOs. By 2010, 70% of the Medicaid population received some or all of their services through Medicaid-managed plans (Kaiser Health News, 2010).

FINANCING MECHANISMS

Fee-for-Service Reimbursement. Until the 1980s, Medicare and private health insurers paid providers through fee-for-service (FFS) reimbursement. In FFS, providers charge a fee for each service, and then providers or patients submit claims to insurers for payment. There is a strong incentive under the FFS payment for providers to increase the volume of services and raise prices to increase their revenue. In addition, through the reimbursement mechanisms of their patients who are on Medicare, the federal government has paid hospitals according to the percentage of Medicare recipients, which has been inherently inflationary. Both health care organizations (such as hospitals) and individual providers (such as physicians) were historically paid through FFS reimbursement. By contrast, nursing services in hospitals continue to be grouped into an aggregate hospital fee or as part of the room fee, rendering nursing care to be in effect a cost center rather than a revenue generator. This mechanism makes it difficult to measure quality of nursing care in hospital situations.

Physician/Clinician Reimbursement Under Fee-for-Service. Payment for physician services is approximately 20% of total national health expenditures (Emanuel, 2014), a significant cost-driver in health care. FFS is still the predominant way of reimbursing for physician and clinician services. Public and private health insurers pay physicians through a complicated formula related to medical coding and medical billing to determine the final payment (Emanuel, 2014).

The American Medical Association (AMA) created Current Procedural Terminology (CPT), a coding system for visits to physicians and other providers. There are codes for evaluation and management, office visits, emergency room visits, prevention services, anesthesia, radiology, pathology, laboratory codes, and medicine codes, such as for dialysis (Emanuel, 2014). These codes are then linked to a specific diagnosis as outlined in the International Classification of Diseases IDC-9 (soon to be IDC-10) and then assigned payment levels.

Prospective Payment Systems. In the 1980s, the federal government replaced the old FFS system for Medicare Part A with a prospective payment system (PPS) for hospital care, establishing payment based on diagnosis-related groups (DRGs). DRGs set a payment level for each of the approximately 500 diagnostic groups typically used in inpatient care. The prospective payment approach helped to slow the rate of growth of payment for hospital care, shortening average length of stay, and increasing patient acuity in hospitals (Heffler et al., 2001).

In the past, insurers paid whatever physicians billed. But in 1992, under Medicare Part B physician payment reform, payment was linked to a Resource-Based Relative Value Scale (RBRVS). In this physician reimbursement system under Medicare, the relative value unit (RVU) for each service is based on the degree of physician work (time, skill, training, intensity), practice expertise (nonphysician labor and practice expenses), and the cost of malpractice for the specialty, as well as the geographic cost of living (Emmanuel, 2014). Its goal was not only cost savings but also to redistribute physician services to increase primary care services and decrease the use of highly specialized physicians. However, the RVU system has been criticized for still favoring specialist care and hospital-based care. The Centers for Medicare and Medicaid Services (CMS) adopts over 80% of the recommendations of the AMA's recommendations for RVUs for each service. This mechanism has been criticized as a conflict of interest, especially as specialists and surgeons comprise a significant proportion of the AMA committee making the recommendations (Emanuel, 2014). In addition, the same procedure done in a hospital is reimbursed at a higher rate than if done in a physician's office. Hence, the incentive is to do more procedures in hospital-owned facilities. The Medicare RVUs per service ratings have been adopted by private insurers, but they use different conversion factors, enabling them to pay more for each service.

Since 1997, the Medicare program has also attempted to contain costs by limiting how much physician payments can increase through the Sustainable Growth Rate (SGR), a target based on physician costs, Medicare enrollment, and the GDP (Emanuel, 2014). There is no incentive in the SGR for individual physicians to contain costs because the SGR is calculated for physician services for the entire country. The intent of the original law was to reduce Medicare payments to physicians if the SGR was exceeded. However, Congress regularly passes a so-called "doc-fix" bill to prevent SGR cuts from going into effect, enabling higher Medicare payment

rates for physicians, APRNs, and other providers (Lowrey, 2014). The SGR continues to be a controversial issue, and Congress has been unable to address the problem, except on an episodic basis.

Bundled Payments/Global Payments. An estimated 85% of payment to providers is still through an FFS payment system, creating an inherent incentive to increase volume and costs (Emanuel, 2014). More recently, policymakers are promoting bundled and global payments as a way to not only contain costs but to also provide an incentive for providers to better coordinate and manage patient care.

Under payment bundling, hospitals, doctors, and providers are paid a flat rate for an episode of care, rather than by individual service. Bundled payment is a form of prospective payment that is being tested by Medicare, private insurers, and provider systems, such as Accountable Care Organizations (ACOs). Global payment is a form of capitation in which the insurer is usually paid per member per month. Proponents of both argue that these payment models differ from traditional capitation in that payment is risk-adjusted and providers can share in savings if care is coordinated and managed and patients are kept healthy. Massachusetts is an example of a state that has provided incentives to insurers and providers to move to bundled and global payment reform.

THE ACA AND HEALTH CARE COSTS

Although improving access to care by enabling more Americans to gain health insurance coverage is the main objective of the ACA, the law is also expected to have a significant impact on containing health care costs. According to the Congressional Budget Office (2014), the ACA will reduce projected federal spending on health care by $109 billion between 2014 and 2024 (Jost, 2014). The ACA does this through reducing prices and controlling the use of services while maintaining quality (Emanuel, 2014). As of December 2014, there was evidence that spending was indeed decreasing. CMS reported that health care spending for 2013 increased by only 3.5%, the lowest rate of growth since 1960. This has been attributed at least in part to the ACA (Carey, 2014).

The ACA seeks to contain Medicare costs and pay for coverage expansion through:

- Medicare will phase out the extra payments it was making to insurers who offered Medicare Advantage Plans, the managed care private plans that older adults can choose instead of traditional FFS Medicare.
- Medicare will pay a lower annual increase in hospital, home, skilled nursing, and hospice care.
- Medicare will pay less for durable medical equipment such as wheelchairs, walkers, and oxygen equipment because of a mandated competitive bidding process for these supplies (Emanuel, 2014).

Additional provisions to control costs include:

- Reduction of special payments the federal government has historically made to hospitals serving disproportionate numbers of uninsured, with the expectation that more people will have health insurance under the ACA
- Taxing employers who offer high-cost private insurance plans to employees, encouraging them to redesign their health benefits and provide more affordable choices for their employees, scheduled to go into effect in 2018
- Encouraging the development of ACOs for Medicare recipients, integrated networks of providers responsible for managing and coordinating care of patients, especially those with costly chronic conditions
- Penalizing hospitals if they have excessive 30-day readmissions and hospital-acquired infections, by reducing their Medicare reimbursement and providing an incentive for them to improve the quality of care (Centers for Medicare and Medicaid Services, 2013)
- Implementing aggressive Medicare/Medicaid fraud and abuse prevention measures, which are projected to save the federal budget $7 billion over 10 years (McDonough, 2011)
- Establishing an Independent Payment Advisory Board (IPAB), which will recommend how to reduce the per capita growth of Medicare and reduce health care spending when health care inflation reaches a certain point

- Implementing administrative simplification measures that are aimed at the entire health sector and could save more than $11.6 billion in federal budget spending (McDonough, 2011)
- Conducting comparative effectiveness research, which will help physicians, other providers, and patients to determine which treatments work

Other provisions that have a major impact on nurses in primary care include some of the points that have been mentioned such as increases for reimbursement for primary care services, a strong focus on preventative health care (which is best delivered by nurses), and promotion of Patient-Centered Medical or Health Care Homes (PCMHs). As more and more Americans gain access to primary care services, nurses will be on the front lines of care. In addition, the Graduate Nursing Education (GNE) demonstration at five hospitals was part of the ACA. The demonstration is testing the use of Medicare funds to support clinical training of graduate nursing students, as is done with physicians (Graduate Medical Education, or GME). The outcomes of this demonstration may provide the evidence to move nursing's share of these funds from diploma nursing programs to graduate education. In another example, the Health Resources and Services Administration (HRSA) provided $250 million for nursing workforce demonstrations projects as well as ways to enlarge and refinance APRN workforce education.

DISCUSSION QUESTIONS

1. What forces have had an effect on increasing health care costs over the past 30 years?
2. What components of the ACA do you think will have a positive effect on improving health care outcomes and decreasing costs?
3. How has nursing fared in health care cost containment and what are the implications of the ACA on nursing?

REFERENCES

American Association of Health Plans. (2001). Independent medical review of health plan coverage decisions: Empowering consumers with solutions. Washington, DC: Author.

Brassard, A. (2014). Making the case for NPs as primary care providers. *The American Nurse*. Retrieved from *www.theamericannurse.org/index .php/2013/07/01/making-the-case-for-nps-as-primary-care-providers/*.

Carey, M. A. (2014, December 4). Growth in U.S. health spending is lowest since 1960. *Kaiser Health News*. Retrieved from *kaiserhealthnews .org/news/growth-in-u-s-health-spending-in-2013-is-lowest-since-1960/*.

Centers for Medicare and Medicaid Services. (2013). Fact sheets: CMS final rule to improve quality of care during hospital inpatient stays. Retrieved from *www.cms.gov/newsroom/mediareleasedatabase/fact -sheets/2013-fact-sheets-items/2013-08-02-3.html*.

Commonwealth Fund. (2011). Realizing health reform's potential. Retrieved from *www.commonwealthfund.org/~/media/Files/Publications/Issue %20Brief/2011/Jan/1466_Abrams_how_ACA_will_strengthen_primary _care_reform_brief_v3.pdf*.

Congressional Budget Office. (2014). Updated estimates of the effects of the insurance coverage provisions of the Affordable Care Act, April 2014. Retrieved from *www.cbo.gov/publication/45231*.

Emanuel, E. (2014). *Reinventing American health care*. New York: Public Affairs.

Federal Interagency Forum on Age-Related Statistics. (2000). *Older Americans 2000: Key indicators of well-being*. Federal Interagency Forum on Age-Related Statistics: Hyattsville, MD.

Health Policy Brief. (2012). Health policy brief: The prevention and public health fund. *Health Affairs*. Retrieved from *healthaffairs.org/health policybriefs/brief_pdfs/healthpolicybrief_63.pdf*.

Heffler, S., Levit, K., Smith, S., Smith, C., Cowan, C., Lazenby, H., et al. (2001). Health care spending growth up in 1999: Faster growth expected in the future. *Health Affairs*, *20*(2), 193–203.

Institute of Medicine. (1988). *The future of public health*. Washington, DC: National Academy Press.

Jost, T. (2014). Implementing health reform: CBO projects lower ACA costs, greater coverage. *Health Affairs Blog*. Retrieved from *healthaffairs.org/ blog/2014/04/15/implementing-health-reform-cbo-projects-lower-aca -costs-greater-coverage/*.

Kaiser Family Foundation. (2010). National health expenditures per capita and their share of gross domestic product, 1960–2008. Retrieved from *facts.kff.org/chart.aspx?ch=1344*.

Kaiser Family Foundation. (2013). Issue brief: How do disproportionate share hospital (DSH) payments change under the ACA? Retrieved from *kaiser familyfoundation.files.wordpress.com/2013/11/8513-how-do-medicaid -dsh-payments-change-under-the-aca.pdf*.

Kaiser Family Foundation. (2014a). Medicare spending and financing fact sheet. Retrieved from *kff.org/medicare/fact-sheet/medicare-spending -and-financing-fact-sheet/*.

Kaiser Family Foundation. (2014b). The Medicare prescription drug benefit fact sheet. Retrieved from *kff.org/medicare/fact-sheet/the-medicare -prescription-drug-benefit-fact-sheet/*.

Kaiser Family Foundation. (2014c). Medicare. Retrieved from *kff.org/ medicare/*.

Kaiser Family Foundation. (2014d). A closer look at the impact of state decisions not to expand Medicaid on coverage for uninsured adults. Retrieved from *kff.org/medicaid/fact-sheet/a-closer-look-at-the-impact -of-state-decisions-not-to-expand-medicaid-on-coverage-for-uninsured -adults/*.

Kaiser Family Foundation. (2014e). Annual percent change in National Health Expenditures, by selected sources of funds, 1960–2012. Retrieved from *kaiserfamilyfoundation.files.wordpress.com/2014/02/ annual-percent-change-in-national-health-expenditures-by-selected -sources-of-funds-1960-2012-healthcosts.png*.

Kaiser Health News. (2010). Research roundup: Medicare spending, community health centers, children's dental services. Retrieved from *www.kaiserhealthnews.org/Daily-Reports/2010/February/05/Research -Roundup.aspx*.

Kongstvedt, P. (2001). *The managed health care handbook* (4th ed.). Gaithersburg, MD: Aspen.

Kovner, A., Knickman, J., & Weisfeld, V. (2011). *Jonas and Kovner's health care delivery in the United States* (10th ed.). New York: Springer.

Kramer, D. B., & Kesselheim, A. S. (2013). The medical device excise tax– Over before it begins? *New England Journal of Medicine*, *368*, 1767– 1769. doi:10.1056/NEJMp1304175.

Lowrey, W. (2014). For 17th time in 11 years, Congress delays Medicare reimbursement cuts as Senate passes 'doc fix'. *Washington Post*. Retrieved from *www.washingtonpost.com/blogs/post-politics/ wp/2014/03/31/for-17th-time-in-11-years-congress-delays-medicare -reimbursement-cuts-as-senate-passes-doc-fix/*.

Martin, A. B., Hartman, M., Whittle, L., Catlin, A., & The National Health Expenditure Accounts Team. (2014). National health spending in 2012: Rate of health spending growth remained low for the fourth consecutive year. *Health Affairs*, *33*(1), 67–77. doi:10.1377/hlthaff.2013.1254.

McDonough, G. (2011). *Inside national health reform*. Berkley, CA: University of California Press.

MedPAC. (2013). A data book: Health care spending and the Medicare program. Retrieved from *www.medpac.gov/documents/Jun13DataBook EntireReport.pdf*.

Meyers, H. (1970). The medical-industrial complex. *Fortune*, *90-91*, 126.

Organization for Economic Co-operation and Development. (2013a). Health data, 2013. Retrieved from *www.oecd.org/health/health-systems/ oecdhealthdata.htm*.

Organization for Economic Co-operation and Development. (2013b). OECD factbook 2013: Economic and social statistics. Retrieved from *dx.doi .org/10.1787/factbook-2013-103-en*.

Rosenbaum, S. (2011). The basic health program: Health reform GPS. Retrieved from *healthreformgps.org/wp-content/uploads/basic-health -plan.pdf*.

Schwartz, D. (2013). Arizona governor Jan Brewer signs Medicaid expansion. Reuters. Retrieved from *www.reuters.com/article/2013/06/17/ us-usa-arizona-medicaid-idUSBRE95G12N20130617*.

Squires, D. (2014). Multinational comparisons of health systems data, 2013. Retrieved from *www.commonwealthfund.org/Publications/Chartbooks/ 2014/Multinational-Comparisons.aspx*.

Stanton, M. (2006). The high concentration of U.S. health care expenditures. In *Research in Action*, Issue 19. Washington, DC: Agency for Health Care Research and Quality.

Starr, P. (1982). *The social transformation of American medicine*. New York: Basic Books.

Truffer, C., Keehan, S., Smith, S., Cylus, J., Sisko, A., Poisal, J., et al. (2010). Health spending projections through 2019: The recession's impact continues. *Health Affairs*, *29*(3), 522–529.

U.S. Census Bureau. (2014). Income, poverty and health insurance in the United States: 2012—Highlights. Retrieved from *www.census.gov/ hhes/www/poverty/data/incpovhlth/2012/highlights.html*.

ONLINE RESOURCES

Kaiser Family Foundation
www.kff.org
Agency for Health Care Research and Quality
www.ahrq.gov
Commonwealth Fund
www.commonwealthfund.org

The Affordable Care Act: Historical Context and an Introduction to the State of Health Care in the United States

Andréa Sonenberg   Ellen S. Murray   Ellen-Marie Whelan

"So never lose an opportunity of urging a practical beginning, however small, for it is wonderful how often in such matters the mustard-seed germinates and roots itself."

Florence Nightingale

HISTORICAL, POLITICAL, AND LEGAL CONTEXT

Health care reform in the United States is an important issue, but since the 1930s, Presidents who have attempted to reform the system have faced significant political obstacles. The administrations of Presidents Franklin D. Roosevelt, Harry S. Truman, and John F. Kennedy all failed to garner enough political support to pass legislation for National Health Insurance programs through Congress. President Lyndon B. Johnson was able to gain enough congressional support to pass the 1965 Social Security Act, which established Medicaid and Medicare, two federal health care programs that were desperately needed at the time (Kaiser Family Foundation [KFF], 2009). Additional reforms, however, failed to pass during the administrations of Presidents Richard M. Nixon, Jimmy E. Carter, and William J. Clinton, and the need to address U.S. health care policy became increasingly imperative.

The lack of comprehensive health care reform in the United States has had harmful effects on the health of the U.S. population and has increased the cost of health care. Although the United States has the most expensive health care system in the world, far exceeding expenditures in other Organisation of Economic Co-operation and Development (OECD) countries, the United States ranks last among industrialized nations in preventable mortality (OECD, 2013) and ranks surprisingly low in other important health quality measures, such as maternal and child mortality. In 2010, there were 49.9 million uninsured people in the United States, and the U.S. Census Bureau reported a decline in employer-based health insurance coverage for the 11th year in a row (Physicians for a National Health Program [PHNP], 2011). Without action, these trends would have continued, and health care costs would have become prohibitively expensive for more and more of the population.

In an effort to address these issues, Congress passed the Patient Protection and Affordable Care Act (PPACA), and President Barack Obama signed it into law on March 23, 2010. A few days later, Congress negotiated and passed the Health Care and Education Reconciliation Act (HCERA). This legislation made significant amendments to the PPACA. The final, revised law, as amended by HCERA, is commonly referred to as the Affordable Care Act (ACA) (McDonough, 2011).

Some aspects of the law were put into effect immediately, whereas other portions will take effect in the years to come, with full implementation expected by 2023. One of the most significant pieces of the law, the creation of state health insurance exchanges and expansion of Medicaid, was implemented in January 2014 (U.S. Centers for Medicare and Medicaid Services [USCMS], 2014c).

The passage and implementation of the ACA, thus far, has been extremely controversial and politically divisive. In the days after President Obama signed the ACA law, lawsuits were filed by various groups challenging the constitutionality of the ACA, focusing specifically on the law's two major provisions: the minimum essential coverage provision, known as the individual mandate, and Medicaid expansion. The U.S. Supreme Court agreed to consider two of these cases: *Florida v. U.S. Dept. of Health and Human Svcs.* and *National Federation of Independent Business v. Sebelius.* In a 5 to 4 vote, the majority of the court ruled the individual mandate constitutional. However, the court ruled in a 7 to 2 vote that the mandated state Medicaid expansion under the ACA was unconstitutionally coercive to states, both because the law did not provide states with enough time for voluntary consent to the changes the law made to the structure of Medicaid, thus states were likely to be deemed noncompliant, and because the Secretary of the U.S. Department of Health and Human Services (HHS) held the power to withhold all existing Medicaid funds from noncompliant states. To remedy this, the court ruled in a 5 to 4 vote that the HHS Secretary would not be allowed to withhold existing Medicaid funds from noncompliant states, but all other Medicaid reforms under the ACA would remain intact and on schedule (KFF, 2012).

Although the Supreme Court voted largely in favor of the ACA, its decision to circumscribe the Secretary's power to withhold existing Medicaid funds renders the Medicaid expansion by states an optional element of the ACA. Analysts estimate that approximately 3 to 5 million fewer people will receive coverage owing to states that opt out of the Medicaid expansion funds (KFF, 2014b; Pear, 2012); as of February 2014, 26 states, including the District of Columbia, had decided to move forward with Medicaid expansion, 6 states were continuing to debate their decision, and 19 states had decided not to move forward with the expansion (KFF, 2014a). States that have decided against expansion may choose at any time to move forward with expansion and receive the full federal subsidies provided under

the law, which includes 100% of the cost of new Medicaid recipients for the first three years (through 2016) and no less than 90% coverage of costs through 2022 (Angeles, 2012). The ACA will transform the U.S. health care system by expanding health care access and coverage, reforming payment systems, and increasing the quality and coordination of care (McDonough, 2011).

CONTENT OF THE AFFORDABLE CARE ACT

EXPANSION OF ACCESS AND HEALTH INSURANCE COVERAGE

The provisions in the ACA related to insurance coverage are what most Americans think of as the Affordable Care Act, or Obamacare. Although providing health insurance to the previously uninsured does not guarantee improved access to care, it is a crucial first step. The insurance provisions in the ACA generally fall into three categories:

- Improves insurance coverage currently held by most Americans
- Expands insurance options for more Americans
- Increases the number of Americans with insurance

Improving Health Insurance Coverage. Much of what people know about the ACA are the changes to and expansion of health insurance coverage. Some improvements were made to the health insurance system immediately and others were phased in over time. Elimination of lifetime and unreasonable annual limits on benefits went into effect immediately and annual limits were prohibited in 2014. Other immediate provisions included the prohibition of cancellations of health insurance policies, prohibition of preexisting condition exclusions for children, and required coverage of preventive services. Prohibition of preexisting exclusion for adults went into effect in January 2014. Additional changes to public and private insurance coverage include:

- Insurers cannot discriminate when offering coverage based on an employee's wages, health status, medical condition or history, claims experience, genetic information, disability, or evidence of insurability, as well as other factors the HHS deems appropriate.

- Insurance rating variability (the variation in individual out-of-pocket premium rates) can be based only on age, family composition, geographic location, and tobacco use, with no rating based on health or gender.
- Full coverage without copayments is required for preventive services, including most screening tests and contraceptive methods, with a waiver of that last aspect for payers furnishing coverage to religiously observant organizations and employers.
- Quality reporting to the HHS is required in relation to coverage benefits and provider reimbursement structures that carry out patient safety initiatives through use of best clinical practices, evidence-based medicine, and health information technologies (ANA, 2010a, 2010b).

Minimum Essential Coverage. A minimum essential coverage provision (commonly referred to as the individual mandate) was established, requiring most individuals to obtain health care coverage for themselves and their dependents or face a shared responsibility payment (tax penalty) of either $95 or 1% of household income, starting in 2014 and increasing thereafter. Coverage can be obtained through employer-sponsored health insurance, new state health exchanges, government programs (Medicaid/Medicare), or grandfathered health plans, if the plan meets the ACA's minimum essential coverage insurance standards. The Minimal Essential Benefits coverage "must include items and services within at least the following 10 categories: ambulatory patient services; emergency services; hospitalization; maternity and newborn care; mental health and substance use disorder services, including behavioral health treatment; prescription drugs; rehabilitative and habilitative services and devices; laboratory services; preventive and wellness services and chronic disease management; and pediatric services, including oral and vision care" (USCMS, 2014b).

Insurance Amendments and the Indian Health Care Improvement Act. The ACA makes an additional series of amendments to the current health care system, which includes adjusting the implementation and structure of the ban on lifetime and annual insurance caps; continuation of federal exclusion of coverage for abortion services using federal funds; and permanently reauthorizing the Indian Health Care Improvement Act that provides legal authority for the provision of health care to Native Americans and Alaska Natives.

EXPANDING THE RECIPIENTS OF HEALTH INSURANCE

To cover more of uninsured people, the ACA includes the following three elements:

1. *Young adults:* The law requires third-party payers to cover dependents up until age 26 years.
2. *Individual mandate (everyone):* As of January 2014, individuals (and their dependents) were required to be protected by essential coverage (USCMS, 2014b). The only allowable exemptions are for hardship and religious reasons. The state exchanges are meant to provide competition among third-party plans to promote affordability (ANA, 2010a, 2010b).
3. *Making insurance more affordable (for low-income Americans):* To ease the burden of purchasing health insurance on consumers, premium tax credits will be made available to households and individuals with incomes between 100% and 400% of the federal poverty level (FPL) to offset the cost of purchasing insurance through state or federal health exchanges. Cost-sharing assistance will be made available for those at 250% FPL and under.

EXPANDING OPTIONS FOR HEALTH INSURANCE COVERAGE

Expanding Employer-Based Coverage. Employers with more than 50 employees are mandated to provide minimal essential benefits (USCMS, 2014d), and employers with more than 200 employees are mandated to automatically enroll new employees into third-party plans. There are penalties for noncompliance with these regulations ($750 per full-time employee, capped) for employers with more than 50 full-time employees that do not offer coverage or offer coverage deemed unaffordable or below the minimum essential coverage standard. The small business mandate to provide coverage has been delayed and is expected to be implemented between 2015 and 2016 (USCMS, 2014a). Employers are also permitted to reward participation in wellness programs (McDonough, 2011).

Medicaid and CHIP Expansion. Starting in January 2014, states were required to provide health coverage for all children, parents, and childless adults who are not entitled to Medicare and are at or below 133% FPL. The federal government is initially covering 100% of the cost of the expansion, with federal aid dropping to 90% starting in 2017. As per the Supreme Court's decision noted above, states may decide to opt out of the ACA's Medicaid expansion. States are required to maintain income eligibility levels for children covered by Medicaid and the Children's Health Insurance Program (CHIP) through September 30, 2019 to receive all federal matching funds.

The State and Federal Exchanges. State-based health insurance exchanges are a major component of the ACA, which will enable individuals, families, and small employers to shop for coverage in a competitive marketplace. States were required to begin enrollment through exchanges by October 1, 2013 and have fully operational exchanges by January 1, 2014. States had the options of partnering with the federal government to operate the exchange, defaulting to a federally facilitated exchange, or creating their own exchange, provided it meets or exceeds the federal government's minimum coverage standards. As of June 2014, 13 states had implemented their own exchange; 7 decided to partner with the federal government to implement and operated their exchange; and 19 decided to operate a federally facilitated exchange (The Commonwealth Fund, 2014).

Initially, enrollment through the federally facilitated exchange at Healthcare.gov and some state exchanges experienced a number of problems, largely dealing with technology and website issues. The state-run exchanges of Oregon, Minnesota, Massachusetts, and Maryland, in particular, had a number of technical difficulties (Ornstein, 2014).

This led to a smaller number of enrollees than expected, although the push for people to sign up by March 31, 2014 to avoid a tax penalty in 2015 resulted in more enrollments than the 6 million target. The KFF's website (*kff.org*) is a good source for up-to-date statistics and U.S. and state enrollment numbers and state exchange issues.

All exchanges must be accessible to potential enrollees via telephone, in person, and online. Nurses can play a key role in educating the public about the exchanges.

PAYMENT SYSTEMS REFORM

There are numerous payment reform provisions in the new law that will change how providers are reimbursed for the services they provide. These changes are often tied to increased provider accountability: moving from paying merely for quantity to paying more for quality of care and improved patient outcomes.

- *Enhanced payment for primary care providers:* There is a 10% increase in Medicare payments to primary care providers from 2011 through 2016. This provision includes nurse practitioners but not nurse midwives or other advanced practice registered nurses (ANA, 2014).
- *Value-based payments:* The law requires the Secretary to develop and implement a budget-neutral payment system that will use a value-based payment modifier to adjust Medicare physician payments based on the quality of care delivered. It will be phased in over time, starting with large practices (over 100 physicians) in 2015 and all eligible professionals by 2017. Payments will be based on quality measures in the Physician Quality Reporting System (PQRS) as a way to pay for value (value is quality relative to cost). Higher value gets higher reimbursement; lower value gets lower reimbursement.
- *Testing new payment models:* As a provision of the ACA, the Centers for Medicare and Medicaid (CMS) was also charged with starting a Center for Medicare and Medicaid Innovation (CMMI) to research, develop, and test effective payment and delivery models to improve the quality of care while lowering costs. Congress also granted

a new, unique authority to the Secretary of the HHS to expand the duration and scope of the testing for successful models (Shrank, 2013). Since its inception, the CMMI has initiated a wide variety of models that aim to realign incentives for providers to reward quality and the coordination of care instead of volume of services provided.

The following are examples of new payment initiatives.

Accountable Care Organizations. There are several regulations of the ACA that pertain to the eligibility, implementation, and quality monitoring of accountable care organizations (ACOs). ACO rules link the percentage of shared savings an entity is eligible to receive to its quality standards performance. Each new ACO model uses 32 quality measures to grade ACOs in five general areas that impact the beneficiary's care: patient/caregiver experience of care, care coordination, patient safety, preventive health, and at-risk population/frail older adult health (HHS, 2012). There is a defined set of performance standards and a scoring procedure in the regulation, including a methodology to account for more complex patients (HHS, 2012). Eligibility to be a member of an ACO that participates in the Shared Savings Program is dependent on the ACO's agreement to meet specific conditions including accountability to quality, cost, and comprehensive care of its assigned Medicare beneficiaries; a 3-year commitment to participate in the program; development of a legal structure to manage shared savings receipt and distribution; an adequate primary care workforce to care for the assigned number of beneficiaries; a management structure encompassing both clinical and administrative structures; and policies and procedures to implement evidence-based and coordinated care (Correia, 2011; HHS, 2012).

Advanced Primary Care Models. The CMMI created many different models of care to enhance and improve primary care. Medical homes (also known as patient-centered medical homes [PCMHs], primary care homes, or health homes) and nurse-managed health centers (NMHCs) are

well-known examples of models of delivery of comprehensive or advanced primary care. Given this diversity of developing advanced primary care models, the CMMI is testing a variety of approaches to enhanced primary care because there is no single, agreed-upon model (Baron, 2012).

Comprehensive Primary Care Initiative. This model of advanced primary care has both payment and system delivery reform components. Nearly 500 primary care practices were selected in seven markets where commercial and state health insurance plans agreed to join Medicare in providing increased access to data and bonus payments for increased care coordination.

Independence at Home. Home-based primary care allows clinicians to spend more time with their patients, perform assessments in a patient's home environment, and assume greater accountability for all aspects of the patient's care. In the Independence at Home program, practices led by physicians or nurse practitioners provide primary care home visits tailored to the needs of beneficiaries with chronic conditions and functional limitations.

Federally Qualified Health Center Advanced Primary Care. In this program, Federally Qualified Health Centers (FQHCs) that achieve a National Committee for Quality Assurance Level 3 PCMH Recognition receive additional funding to support care coordination for each of their Medicare patients. Nearly 500 FQHCs were accepted into this program to provide advanced primary care to approximately 195,000 patients with Medicare insurance (National Association of Community Health Centers, 2012).

Medicaid Health Home. The ACA created an option for states to permit Medicaid enrollees with at least two chronic conditions to designate a provider as a health home. States that implement this option will receive enhanced financial resources (90% federal matching payments for 2 years for health home related services) to support health homes in their Medicaid programs.

Transitional Models of Care. With the aim of decreasing readmission rates of the chronically ill discharged after hospitalization, the ACA has allocated $500 million to pilot transitional care projects for Medicare recipients. Transitional care has been described by many but the most well-known models are by Eric Coleman and Mary Naylor. Eric Colman's model pairs a transition coach with a patient with complex care needs. Patients learn self-management skills to ensure their needs are met during the transition from hospital to home (Coleman, 2003). Mary Naylor's model uses transitional care nurses to manage hospital discharge and follow-up in the home. Her research has documented its effectiveness in lengthening the time between Medicare recipient discharge and rehospitalization or death, as well as in reducing the overall number of readmissions and lowering health care costs (Brooten et al., 2002 and Naylor, 2000 as cited by Robert Wood Johnson Foundation [RWJF], 2014b). The CMMI's community-based care transitions program funds community-based organizations to use care transition services to effectively manage Medicare patients' transitions and improve their quality of care.

PAYMENT REFORM TO IMPROVE EQUITY FOR NURSING SERVICES

Nurse-Managed Health Center. Managed by an APRN, nurse-managed health centers (NMHCs) are another model of coordinated care and advanced primary care (Keeling & Lewenson, 2013). In addition to expanding primary care capacity, the ACA authorized, but did not mandate, funding for NMHCs to serve as training sites for students in primary care and enhance nursing practice.

Nurse Midwives. The ACA provides an enhanced Medicare reimbursement rate for certified nurse-midwives (CNMs) to 100% of the physician schedule; this had been 65% since CNMs were first designated primary care providers with the Omnibus Reconciliation Act of 1987 (U.S. Centers for Medicare and Medicaid, 2011). Since January 2011, the ACA has provided an enhanced Medicare reimbursement rate for certified nurse-midwives (CNMs) to 100% of the physician schedule (Title III, Section 3114) (Patient Protection and Affordable Care Act, 2010). This had been 65% since CNMs were first designated as primary care providers under the Omnibus Reconciliation Act of 1987 (U.S. Centers for Medicare and Medicaid, 2011).

Non-Discrimination in Health Care. Another payment issue, which directly improves access to nurse practitioner (NP) services, is that, effective in 2014, the ACA amended the Public Health Service Act entitled Non-Discrimination in Health Care. This Act mandates that neither group nor individual health plans shall discriminate against any health care provider's participation under the plan or coverage for their chosen provider, given that the health care provider is practicing within the scope of her or his applicable state license or certification (American Academy of Nursing, 2010). Once licensed, however, NP reimbursement under Medicaid continues to be determined by individual state regulations. Despite the disparity between the focus on expansion of an NP workforce and the regulatory barriers it faces in practice, both of these issues are significant concerns.

COORDINATION OF CARE AND PREVENTION

The ACA includes a variety of provisions to improve the performance of the health care system and the health status of the population through care coordination and prevention.

No Copays for Preventive Services. The ACA requires most health plans to cover recommended preventive services without copays or cost-sharing. This provision requires plans to cover the services listed in the HHS comprehensive list of preventive services. To assist in determining which preventive services should be covered for women, the HHS requested the Institute of Medicine (IOM) to examine the scientific evidence and identify critical gaps in preventive services for women as well as measures to further ensure women's health (IOM, 2011b). On August 1, 2011, the HHS adopted new guidelines for women's preventive services that are required to be covered without cost-sharing in most nongrandfathered health plans starting with the first plan or policy year beginning on or after August 1, 2012.

Federal Coordinated Health Care. The law establishes Federal Coordinated Health Care at the CMS to integrate care and improve coordination for "dual eligibles": those people who are covered by both Medicaid and Medicare.

Prevention and Public Health Investment Fund. The ACA creates a new Prevention and Public Health Investment Fund to support community and public health initiatives that aim to prevent injury and disease and eliminate access barriers to community health centers and clinical practices.

Home Visitation. The ACA expands and provides additional funding for evidence-based home visitation programs that foster health promotion and illness prevention. One of these programs is for at-risk pregnant women and children and is best represented by the Nurse-Family Partnership, a nationwide program with a substantial research base related to the short-term and long-term benefits for mothers and children. The evidence supports that home visits to low-income mothers, providing education and support during pregnancy and the early childhood years, result in a variety of social and health benefits to children and families (HHS, Administration for Children and Families, 2014; Mathematica, 2014). This program is run out of the Health Resources and Services Administration (HRSA), Bureau of Maternal and Child Health.

EXPANDING HEALTH CARE WORKFORCE CAPACITY

The ACA includes provisions to develop and expand a competent primary health care workforce. Approaches to expanding health care workforce capacity are: encourage models of care that promote use of all types of primary care providers and facilitate training and funding of services of all primary care providers, while expanding health care services access and improving quality of care.

The ACA enhances health care workforce education and training, particularly for primary care and mental/behavioral health education. It provides training grants to schools for the development, expansion, and enhancement of training programs in social work, primary care, graduate psychology, professional training in child and adolescent mental health, and preservice or inservice training to

paraprofessionals in child and adolescent mental health. Additionally, the ACA updates provisions in the Public Health Services Act and provides significant increases in discretionary funding for building the nurse workforce, including: funds for NMHCs; establishment of nurse education, training, and loan repayment grants; creation of a nurse faculty loan program; creation of a family NP training program; funds to support training in home visitation services for maternal and prenatal care; and funds for graduate nursing schools (Association of University Centers on Disabilities, 2010). Lastly, the ACA provides competitive grants for workforce planning and workforce development strategies at the state level, as well as competitive grants for coordinated and integrated care in mental and behavioral health.

Expanding the Nursing Workforce. Through a variety of funding and regulatory provisions, the ACA is indirectly focused on nursing by addressing: (1) the demand for a larger primary care workforce to improve access to care and (2) regulation of advanced nursing practice. Key elements of the ACA that address workforce shortages include funding for nursing education, reimbursement of nursing services, and reform of practice regulatory policy (e.g., Medicaid reimbursement, expanded CNM reimbursement under Medicare, allowance of NPs to own/manage NMHCs [and ultimately ACOs], and nondiscrimination in health care) (American Association of Nurse Practitioners, 2013b).

Expansion of funding for nursing education includes:

- Increased federal loan limits for nursing students, which increases the amounts nursing students can borrow from the federal government for their education. Narrowing the disparity between nursing students' educational costs and potential resources will facilitate increased enrollments and produce more nurses to address the health care demands of the nation (RWJF, 2014a).
- Expansion of the National Health Service Corps Loan Repayment Program will repay 60% of a student loan, including nursing, in exchange for

a commitment of 2 years of service in a critical health workforce shortage area.

- Establishing a Medicare Graduate Nurse Education (GNE) Demonstration, which is funded by the CMS and operated by the CMMI. The Demonstration Program, which will run for 4 years, will reimburse up to 5 hospitals (already in progress) the cost to clinically train APRN students. To be eligible, the hospitals had to partner with accredited schools of nursing and non-hospital community-based care settings (RWJF, 2014a).

- Expanding the Public Health Service Act to provide demonstration grants for family NP training programs, offering 1-year residencies for NPs in FQHCs and NMHCs (American Association of Colleges of Nursing [AACN], 2012; American Association of Nurse Practitioners, 2013a).

PUBLIC HEALTH PROVISIONS OF THE AFFORDABLE CARE ACT

According to Healthy People 2020 (HHS, 2014), a public health infrastructure "includes 3 key components that enable a public health organization at the Federal, Tribal, State, or local level to deliver public health services: (1) a capable and qualified workforce; (2) up-to-date data and information systems; and (3) public health agencies capable of assessing and responding to public health needs." These components enable the public health system to care for the nation's population health through a variety of services. A health care system reform that attempts to address improving access to care for a larger percentage of the population, cost (to the individual and system), and quality strives to improve the public's health. The provisions of the ACA aim to meet the health needs of the nation's population through such a framework.

IMPACT ON NURSING PROFESSION: DIRECT AND INDIRECT

The implications of the ACA for nursing fall into two categories: those that are related to the provisions directed specifically to nursing and those that

are related to the provisions that will either indirectly affect nursing or invite and demand nursing's involvement by affording new opportunities. It was the intention of the ACA to create a National Health Care Workforce Commission established under Title V (Health Care Workforce) of the ACA. The law aimed to monitor and influence national health workforce policy to further explore the health workforce needs of the nation (AACN, 2012; White House, n.d.). A nurse was appointed as Chair of this Commission, although, as of 2015, it remained unfunded by Congress, and thus has never met. Through a combination of training programs, loans, loan repayment programs, and scholarships (Commonwealth Fund, 2011), as previously summarized, the ACA will fulfill one of its other more direct roles, that of capacity building of the primary care workforce. It also eases criteria and expands the federal student loan program for schools and students focusing on primary care, increases funding of clinical education of APRNs through the GNE Demonstration, and increases funding to community health centers and the National Health Service Corps. In striving to expand workforce resources, the ACA addresses both the supply and regulation of practice of APRNs. Although the ACA does not directly address APRN practice regulation, it calls for modernization of scope of practice policies to facilitate the ability of APRNs to be a major source of primary care services.

INDIRECT IMPACT ON NURSING

An estimated 22 million of the 60 million uninsured people in America will be covered as a result of the ACA, with half of them covered through the private insurance markets and half covered through the expansion of Medicaid (Patel & Sanghavi, 2013). There is a growing concern regarding the existing capacity of primary care providers to meet the substantial and increasing demand for access to care that is emerging (Institute of Medicine, 2011a). One answer that has been put forth to assist in meeting this growing demand for primary care is to optimize use of APRNs, specifically NPs (Fairman et al., 2011; IOM, 2011a). Evidence supports that APRNs and NPs deliver high-quality health care and improved health outcomes at a lower cost than the traditional medical model (Newhouse et al., 2011). The expansion of the availability of primary care providers is an important rationale for continuing efforts to remove barriers to the scope of practice and payment of APRNs.

OVERALL COST OF THE ACA

COST TO THE NATION

At the time the ACA was signed into law, scorekeepers estimated the net cost of the ACA to equal $940 billion. In April 2014, the Congressional Budget Office (CBO) and the Joint Committee on Taxation (JCT) updated these numbers to reflect a number of implementation changes and to take into account the Supreme Court's decision on Medicaid expansion. In total, the ACA's coverage provisions will cost $1383 billion for the 2015 to 2024 period (CBO, 2014a, 2014b). The ultimate cost of the ACA will largely depend on the final implementation of the law and how closely it follows and resembles the original legislation. Owing to unforeseen challenges, the gross cost of the ACA could increase or decrease significantly, and it is best to keep apprised of accurate and up-to-date numbers by reviewing CBO updates and estimates at *www .cbo.gov/topics/health-care*.

COST FOR INDIVIDUALS AND HOUSEHOLDS

For individuals and families who do not fall under the Medicaid expansion (133% or less of the FPL), there are both premium tax credits and cost-sharing assistance available to lower the financial burden of purchasing health insurance. Subsidies for purchasing health insurance went into effect in January 2014 alongside the rollout of state health exchanges. Premium tax credits are available to all individuals and families with incomes between 100% and 400% of the FPL. In 2013, 100% FPL was $23,000 for a family of four, and 400% FPL was $94,000 for a family of four. Additionally, the ACA provides cost-sharing assistance for individuals and households with incomes under 250% FPL ($59,000 and under for a family of four in 2013).

Families and individuals have the option to purchase four types of plans, bronze, silver, gold, and platinum, on the state exchange market. Coverage and benefits in these plans vary, with bronze plans being the least comprehensive and platinum plans the most comprehensive. All premium credits are tax credits and will be delivered in advance directly to the insurers that a family or individual chooses in the health exchange. The remaining balance will be the responsibility of the family or individual. As an example, a family of four with an income of $47,000 who purchases a silver plan will end up paying approximately $247 a month to cover the entire family after factoring in premium credits and cost-sharing assistance (Angeles, 2013).

Owing to variability in state exchange models, the number of insurance options in state exchanges, and the implementation challenges several states faced in the fall and winter of 2014, individual and household insurance premiums and costs vary widely. The ACA aims to lower overall population health costs and ensure that individuals and households have insurance that adequately covers primary, preventative, and emergency health services. As of April 2014, over 8 million people had signed up for health insurance through the marketplace (state health exchanges), and the CBO estimated that an additional 5 million individuals have purchased ACA-compliant plans outside of the marketplace. Although comprehensive data on effectuated enrollments has not been obtained, initial public statements from issuers indicate that 80% to 90% of individuals who purchased a marketplace plan have made premium payments (Office of the Assistant Secretary for Planning and Evaluation, HHS, 2014).

POLITICAL AND IMPLEMENTATION CHALLENGES

The successful implementation and the realized benefits of the ACA will depend on a variety of factors, some of which are related to the political challenges the legislation has and will continue to face.

After the initial Supreme Court decision about the ACA, many states decided to forego Medicaid expansion. Public health officials fear that the very poorest populations living in noncompliant states will be left without support and without affordable health insurance options (Pear, 2012). As an example, Texas, a state that has refused to expand Medicaid, will leave 1.3 million uninsured people without viable health insurance options. In Florida, another nonparticipating state, 1 million people will be left without support (Kenney et al., 2012). Furthermore, the lack of Medicaid expansion in noncompliant states will have an even greater impact on rural communities where people are more likely to live in poverty and less likely to have employer-sponsored health coverage (Mueller et al., 2012). Many noncompliant states suggest that Medicaid expansion would overwhelm state budgets, but independent, nonpartisan analysis has shown that states would have an incremental cost of only 0.3% ($8 billion) more between 2013 and 2022 if they implement the Medicaid expansion than they would without it (Holahan et al., 2012).

In June 2014, the U.S. Supreme Court issued a ruling in *Burwell v. Hobby Lobby Inc. Stores* that further dismantled the law. Prior to the ruling, the ACA required health insurance plans to cover preventative reproductive health services for women, including all FDA-approved contraceptives, without cost-sharing (commonly referred to as the *contraception mandate*). Under the law, employers with 50 or more workers with insurance plans that did not meet this standard faced significant fines. In the Supreme Court case, Hobby Lobby Inc. argued that this mandate violated the Religious Freedom Restoration Act (RFRA), which states that the government must not "substantially burden a person's exercise of religion" unless there is a "compelling government interest" or if the law uses methods that are the "least restrictive way of furthering that interest." The Supreme Court, in a 5-4 decision, judged in favor of Hobby Lobby Inc., ruling that the government cannot force corporations to cover employees' birth control, effectively nullifying the contraception mandate. While this judgment directly impacts women's access to contraceptives, some analyst worry that employers will now use religious objections to opt out of other aspects of the ACA, which could have a significant impact on the future of the law (Carey, 2014).

Since the start of the implementation of the law, polling suggests that the overall public has both a lack of understanding of the ACA and mixed feelings on the law attributable to partisan politics and the ensuing misinformation. In 2013, a Kaiser Family Foundation poll found that 57% of individuals stated that they did not feel they had enough information about the ACA to understand how it will impact them personally. When filtered by income, this percentage increased to 68% for those with household incomes less than $40,000 (Kaiser Family Foundation, 2013). Furthermore, it is apparent that politics plays a significant role in the public's degree of approval of the law. In April of 2014, the CNN/ORC International Poll, which used the term the Affordable Care Act, released a poll that showed 61% of participants who were either in favor of the ACA or wished to see small changes in the law; 38% of participants wished to see it repealed. In comparison, a Washington Post/ABC Poll also released in April of 2014, and which used the term Barack Obama's health care plan, showed that only 36% of respondents felt the law was a good idea, and 49% felt that the law needed a major overhaul, or be repealed entirely (Fuller, 2014). Nonpartisan, clear messaging, and education campaigns are critical to the long-term success of the ACA.

CONCLUSION

Although there may be revisions throughout the period of implementation of this landmark legislation, as occurred with the Social Security Act, the ACA provisions aim to increase access to care; change the culture of health care from one of cure to one of health promotion and illness prevention; mitigate barriers to practice for primary care providers of all disciplines; capitalize on the skill and expertise of nursing in areas of leadership, practice, research, and innovation; and, through these mechanisms, improve population health outcomes. The challenge for nursing is to rise to the call and seize this moment of opportunity in becoming the leaders in health care that so many already recognize they should be. Understanding the reforms and realizing the potential implications to nursing are the first steps in achieving these roles.

DISCUSSION QUESTIONS

1. What are the key areas that the ACA provisions address and examples of each?
2. What are key opportunities for nursing leadership related to ACA implementation and monitoring?
3. What are specific provisions within the ACA that will directly impact the delivery and type or method of care you give to your patients?
4. Many of the payment reform changes in the ACA move away from physician fee-for-service payment to more value-based payment, taking into consideration improved quality measures and better patient outcomes. How will this change maximize the role of the entire health team, including nurses? How will this create new leadership opportunities for nurses?

REFERENCES

American Academy of Nursing. (2010). Implementing health care reform: Issues for nursing. Washington, DC: American Academy of Nursing. Retrieved from *www.aannet.org/assets/docs/implementinghealthcare reform.pdf*

American Association of Colleges of Nursing [AACN]. (2012). New AACN data show an enrollment surge in Baccalaureate and Graduate Programs amid calls for more highly educated nurses. Retrieved from *www.aacn.nche.edu/news/articles/2012/enrollment-data.*

American Association of Nurse Practitioners. (2013a). Provide sufficient funding for nurse practitioner education programs. Retrieved from *www.aanp.org/images/documents/federal-legislation/issuebriefs/ Issue%20Brief%20-%20Provide%20Sufficient%20Funding.pdf.*

American Association of Nurse Practitioners. (2013b). Recognize NP practices as Medicare shared savings accountable care organizations. Retrieved from *www.aanp.org/images/documents/federal-legislation/ issuebriefs/Issue%20Brief%20-%20Recognize%20NP%20Practices .pdf.*

American College of Nurse Midwives. (2013). Position statement: Midwives are primary care providers and leaders of maternity care homes. Retrieved from *www.midwife.org/ACNM/files/ACNMLibrary Data/UPLOADFILENAME/000000000273/Primary%20Care%20Position %20Statement%20June%202012.pdf.*

American Nurses Association. (2010a). ANA policy and provisions of health reform law April 27, 2010. Retrieved from *nursingworld.org/ MainMenuCategories/Policy-Advocacy/HealthSystemReform/Policy -and-Health-Reform-Law.pdf.*

American Nurses Association. (2010b). Health care transformation: The Affordable Care Act and more. Retrieved from *nursingworld.org/Main MenuCategories/Policy-Advocacy/HealthSystemReform/AffordableCare Act.pdf.*

American Nurses Association. (2014). Health care reform: Key provisions related to nursing. Retrieved from *www.rnaction.org/site/DocServer/ KeyProvisions_Nursing-PublicLaw.pdf?docID=1241&verID=1.*

Angeles, J. (2012). How health reform's Medicaid expansion will impact state budgets. Center on Budget and Policy Priorities. Retrieved from *www.cbpp.org/cms/?fa=view&id=3801.*

Angeles, J. (2013). Making health care more affordable: The new premium and cost-sharing assistance. Center on Budget and Policy Priorities. Retrieved from *www.cbpp.org/cms/?fa=view&id=3190.*

Association of University Centers on Disabilities. (2010). Title V of the Patient Protection and Affordable Care Act health care workforce provisions. Retrieved from *www.aucd.org/docs/policy/health_care/ Section%20by%20Section%20Summary%20of%20Health%20Care %20Workforce.pdf.*

Baron, R. (2012). New pathways for primary care: an update on primary care programs from the innovation center at CMS. *Annals of Family Medicine, 10*(2), 152–155. doi:10.1370/afm.1366.

Brooten, D., Naylor, M. D., York, R., Brown, L. P., Munro, B. H., Hollingsworth, A. O., et al. (2002). Lessons learned from testing the quality cost model of advanced practice nursing (APN) transitional care. *Journal of Nursing Scholarship, 34*(4), 369–375.

Carey, M. (2014). Hobby Lobby ruling cuts into contraceptive mandate. NPR. Retrieved from *www.npr.org/blogs/health/2014/06/30/327065968/ hobby-lobby-ruling-cuts-into-contraceptive-mandate.*

Coleman, E. (2003). Falling through the cracks: challenges and opportunities for improving transitional care for persons with continuous complex care needs. *Journal of the American Geriatrics Society, 51*(4), 549–555.

Commonwealth Fund. (2011). Realizing health reform's potential: How the affordable care act will strengthen primary care and benefit patients, providers, and payers. Retrieved from *www.commonwealthfund.org/ ~/media/Files/Publications/Issue%20Brief/2011/Jan/1466_Abrams _howACA_will_strengthen_primary_care_reform_brief_v3.pdf.*

The Commonwealth Fund. (2014). Health Insurance Marketplaces. Retrieved from *http://www.commonwealthfund.org/interactives-and-data/maps -and-data/state-exchange-map.*

Congress of the U.S. Congressional Budget Office. (2014a). Comparison of CBO's estimates of the net budgetary effects of the coverage provisions of the affordable care act. Retrieved from *www.cbo.gov/sites/default/ files/cbofiles/attachments/45231-ACA_Estimates.pdf.*

Congress of the U.S. Congressional Budget Office. (2014b). Updated estimates of the effects of the insurance coverage provisions of the affordable care act, April 2014. Retrieved from *www.cbo.gov/sites/ default/files/cbofiles/attachments/45231-ACA_Estimates.pdf.*

Correia, E. W. (2011). Accountable care organizations: The proposed regulations and the prospects for success. *American Journal of Managed Care, 17*(8), 560–568.

Fairman, J., Rowe, J. W., Hassmiller, S., & Shalala, D. E. (2011). Broadening the scope of nursing practice. *New England Journal of Medicine, 364,* 193–196.

Fuller, J. (2014). The most interesting number of the day is 61 percent. *The Washington Post.* Retrieved from *www.washingtonpost.com/blogs/ the-fix/wp/2014/05/12/the-most-interesting-number-of-the-day-is-61 -percent/.*

Holahan, J., Buettgens, M., Carroll, C., & Dorn, S. (2012). The cost and coverage implications of the ACA Medicaid expansion: National and state-by-state analysis. The Kaiser Commission on Medicaid and the Uninsured and The Urban Institute. Retrieved from *kaiserfamilyfoundation.files. wordpress.com/2013/01/8384.pdf.*

Institute of Medicine. (2011a). *Future of nursing: Leading change, advancing health.* Washington, DC: The National Academies Press.

Institute of Medicine. (2011b). *Clinical preventive services for women: Closing the gaps.* Washington, DC: The National Academies Press.

Kaiser Family Foundation. (2009). National health insurance—A brief history of reform efforts in the U.S. Retrieved from *kaiserfamily foundation.files.wordpress.com/2013/01/7871.pdf*.

Kaiser Family Foundation. (2012). A guide to the Supreme Court's Affordable Care Act decision. Retrieved from *kaiserfamilyfoundation.files .wordpress.com/2013/01/8332.pdf*.

Kaiser Family Foundation. (2013). Kaiser health tracking poll: March 2013. Retrieved from *kff.org/health-reform/poll-finding/march-2013-tracking -poll/*.

Kaiser Family Foundation. (2014a). Status of state action on the Medicaid expansion decision. Retrieved from *kff.org/health-reform/ state-indicator/state-activity-around-expanding-medicaid-under-the -affordable-care-act/*.

Kaiser Family Foundation. (2014b). The coverage gap: uninsured poor adults in states that do not expand Medicaid. Retrieved from *kff.org/health -reform/issue-brief/the-coverage-gap-uninsured-poor-adults-in-states -that-do-not-expand-medicaid/*.

Keeling, A., & Lewenson, S. (2013). A nursing historical perspective on the medical home: Impact on health care policy. *Nursing Outlook, 61*(5), 360–366.

Kenney, G., Zuckerman, S., Dubay, L., & Huntress, M. (2012). Opting in to the Medicaid expansion under the ACA: Who are the uninsured adults who could gain health insurance coverage? The Urban Institute. Retrieved from *www.urban.org/UploadedPDF/412630-opting-in-medicaid .pdf*.

Mathematica. (2014). Supporting evidence-based home visiting to prevent child maltreatment. Retrieved from *www.mathematica-pr.com/early childhood/evidencebasedhomevisiting.asp*.

McDonough, J. E. (2011). *Inside national health reform.* Los Angeles, CA: University of California Press.

Mueller, K., Coburn, A., Lundblad, J., MacKinney, A., McBride, T., & Watson, S. (2012). The current and future role and impact of Medicaid in rural health. Rural Policy Research Institute. Retrieved from *www .rupri.org/Forms/HealthPanel_Medicaid_Sept2012.pdf*.

National Association of Community Health Centers. (2012). Final Medicaid and exchange regulations: Implications for federally qualified health centers. Retrieved from *www.nachc.org/client/documents/4.12%20 IB%20-%20MCD%20and%20Exchange%20Final%20Rules%20-%20 FINAL.pdf*.

Naylor, M. D. (2000). A decade of transitional care research with vulnerable elders. *Journal of Cardiovascular Nursing, 14*(3), 1–14.

Newhouse, R. P., Stanik-Hutt, J., White, K. M., Johantgen, M., Bass, E. B., Zangaro G., et al. (2011). Advanced practice nurse outcomes 1990-2008: A systematic review. *Nursing Economics, 29*(5), 1–21.

Office of the Assistant Secretary for Planning and Evaluation, U.S. Department of Health and Human Services. (2014). Premium affordability, competition, and choice in the health insurance marketplace, 2014. Retrieved from *aspe.hhs.gov/health/reports/2014/Premiums/2014Mkt PlacePremBrf.pdf*.

Organization of Economic Co-operation and Development (OECD). (2013). *Health at a glance 2013: OECD indicators.* Paris: OECD Publishing. Retrieved from *dx.doi.org/10.1787/health_glance-2013-en*.

Ornstein, C. (2014). Epic fail: Where four state health exchanges went wrong. *ProPublica.* Retrieved from *www.propublica.org/article/epic -fail-where-four-state-health-exchanges-went-wrong*.

Patel, K., & Sanghavi, D. (2013). Ten questions about Obamacare you were too embarrassed to ask. *Brookings.* Retrieved from *www.brookings .edu/research/opinions/2013/09/30-ten-questions-about-obamacare -aca-patel-sanghavi*.

Patient Protection and Affordable Care Act, 42 U.S.C. § 18001. (2010).

Pear, R. (2012). Court's ruling may blunt reach of the health law. *New York Times.* Retrieved from *www.nytimes.com/2012/07/25/health/policy/ 3-million-more-may-lack-insurance-due-to-ruling-study-says.html*.

Physicians for a National Health Program. (2011). Number of uninsured climbs to highest figure since passage of Medicare, Medicaid. Retrieved from *www.pnhp.org/news/2011/september/number-of-uninsured -climbs-to-highest-figure-since-passage-of-medicare-medicaid*.

Robert Wood Johnson Foundation. (2014a). Health care reform law begins to have effect on nursing. Retrieved from *www.rwjf.org/en/about-rwjf/ newsroom/newsroom-content/2011/03/health-care-reform-law-begins -to-have-effect-on-nursing.html*.

Robert Wood Johnson Foundation. (2014b). The transitional care model. Retrieved from *thefutureofnursing.org/resource/detail/ transitional-care-model.*

Shrank, W. (2013). The Center for Medicare and Medicaid Innovation's blueprint for rapid-cycle evaluation of new care and payment models. *Health Affairs.* Retrieved from *content.healthaffairs.org/content/early/ 2013/03/21/hlthaff.2013.0216*.

U.S. Centers for Medicare and Medicaid. (2011). Payment for certified nurse-midwife services. *MLN Matters.* Retrieved from *www.cms. gov/Outreach-and-Education/Medicare-Learning-Network-MLN/MLN MattersArticles/downloads/mm7005.pdf*.

U.S. Centers for Medicare and Medicaid. (2014a). Do I have to offer health coverage to my employees? Retrieved from *www.healthcare.gov/do -i-have-to-offer-health-coverage-to-my-employees/*.

U.S. Centers for Medicare and Medicaid. (2014b). Essential health benefits. Retrieved from *www.healthcare.gov/glossary/essential-health-benefits/*.

U.S. Centers for Medicare and Medicaid. (2014c). Get covered: A one-page guide to the Health Insurance Marketplace. Retrieved from *www .healthcare.gov/get-covered-a-1-page-guide-to-the-health-insurance -marketplace/*.

U.S. Centers for Medicare and Medicaid. (2014d). What do small businesses need to know? Retrieved from *www.healthcare.gov/what-do-small -businesses-need-to-know/*.

U.S. Department of Health and Human Services. (2012). Accountable care organizations: Improving care coordination for people with Medicare. Retrieved from *www.healthcare.gov/news/factsheets/2011/03/ accountablecare03312011a.html*.

U.S. Department of Health and Human Services. (2014). Healthy people 2020: Public health infrastructure. Retrieved from *www.healthy people.gov/2020/topicsobjectives2020/overview.aspx?topicid=35*.

U.S. Department of Health and Human Services Administration for Children and Families. (2014). Home visiting evidence of effectiveness. Retrieved from *homvee.acf.hhs.gov/HomVEE_Executive_Summary _2013.pdf*.

White House. (n.d.). Affordable Care Act: The new health care law at two years. Retrieved from *www.whitehouse.gov/sites/default/files/ uploads/careact.pdf*.

ONLINE RESOURCES

Henry J. Kaiser Family Foundation
www.kff.org
U.S. Department of Health and Human Services, Information on Health Care
www.hhs.gov/healthcare
U.S. Department of Health and Human Services: About the ACA
www.hhs.gov/healthcare/rights
U.S. Health Insurance Marketplace
www.healthcare.gov/marketplace

UNIT 2

CHAPTER 20

Health Insurance Exchanges: Expanding Access to Health Care

Coral T. Andrews   Deborah B. Gardner

"Follow the path of the unsafe, independent thinker. Expose your ideas to the dangers of controversy. Speak your mind and fear less the label of 'crackpot' than the stigma of conformity. And on issues that seem important to you, stand up and be counted at any cost."

Thomas J. Watson

The health insurance exchange has been described "as arguably the single most important element of health care reform. It is the bridge between the current health care system we have and the system we want" (Klein, 2009, para. 3). Before the Affordable Care Act (ACA) went into effect, health insurance provided little security. Instead, it provoked apprehension and fear. As many as 129 million insured Americans, nearly one in two people, could be discriminated against because of preexisting conditions such as heart disease, diabetes, or cancer, or for that matter even pregnancy (Hilzenrath, 2009; U.S. Department of Health and Human Services [HHS], 2011). For other Americans, many knew that if they were diagnosed at some point with a serious illness it could leave them unable to access affordable coverage. This often resulted in people being trapped in ill-suited jobs or even dropped from their coverage. Vice President Biden stated in a recent speech about health care insurance before the ACA "... that every family was one job loss or one illness away from seeing the worst of the insurance system" (as cited in Simas, 2014). With the implementation of the ACA (Public Law [PL] 111-148, as amended) insurance access is changing. No longer are individuals with preexisting issues uninsurable. If you lose coverage or lose a job that had coverage, there will be a way to access

care. Now there is a new way for families to have access to affordable health insurance.

This chapter outlines the required functions of exchanges and differentiates exchange types, the coverage offered, and implementation challenges. The roles that nurses can play as the exchanges evolve are presented and an assessment of the impact of the health insurance exchanges after the first year is discussed.

WHAT IS A HEALTH INSURANCE EXCHANGE?

Section 1311 of the ACA requires each state to establish a health insurance exchange by January 1, 2014. The fundamental purpose of a health insurance exchange is to create an online marketplace for the sale and purchase of health insurance for customers (consumers). The exchange is required to serve two markets: the individual market and the small group market. The exchanges are structured to benefit customers by providing choice, transparency, and convenience, in which one chooses among competing health insurer providers (both public and private).

Marketplace competition is how everything is purchased, from books to shoes to food. Everything, that is, except health insurance. The health insurance exchanges were designed using this business model and current understanding of the economic drivers of health care. The benefits of using the marketplace model are obvious to anyone who has ever shopped at a Costco (Klein, 2009). The products are clearly priced, standardized for ease of comparison, and written in clear language to assess quality. Buying in bulk can lead to cost savings.

Health insurance exchanges are created to provide this same type of information and transactional opportunity. Essentially, the exchanges are designed to increase access for uninsured or underinsured Americans to quality and affordable health insurance by expanding the size of the insurance coverage pool. (The Henry J. Kaiser Foundation, 2013b)

Customers are also protected by ACA regulations that ensure insurance companies (issuers) that choose to sell their products (plans) through an exchange are not deceptive. Issuers are required to comply with other consumer protections, such as offering insurance to every qualified applicant and meeting the private market reform requirements in the ACA. However, exchanges are not issuers (insurance companies); rather, exchanges contract with the insurance companies who will provide insurance products available for purchase through exchanges (Fernandez & Mach, 2013).

EXCHANGE PURCHASERS

INDIVIDUAL PURCHASERS

The health insurance exchange is a marketplace that offers an individual the ability to compare health insurance plans. Each state was to create a market for the individual consumer to purchase health insurance, although states also had the options of partnering with the federal government to create an exchange or having the state's residents use a federal exchange. Individuals are required to have health insurance or face a fine (tax) imposed by the federal government. Dependent on an individual's income, he/she may qualify for a reduction in the overall cost of the health plan premium, known as federal subsidies. This is a way to reduce the overall out-of-pocket cost of the consumer and help to make insurance more affordable. Individuals may also qualify for Medicaid. Qualified health plans (QHPs) sold on the insurance exchanges cannot be priced differently outside of the insurance exchange (Peterson & Fernandez, 2010), but an insurance company can offer other plans off the exchange with different pricing.

Table 20-1 depicts scenarios of how individuals and those up to a family of six can potentially qualify for tax subsidies, Medicaid, and cost-sharing reductions (CSRs), which are additional out-of-pocket reductions.

Individuals and small businesses can also choose to continue any insurance coverage they already have. Plans that existed before the ACA are grandfathered and considered coverage that meets the terms of the law (Healthcare.gov, n.d.).

SMALL BUSINESS PURCHASERS

Currently, small businesses with 50 employees or less can shop for coverage for their employees in a different market. These exchanges are called small business health options programs (SHOPs). Starting in 2016, employers with up to 100 employees will be eligible to participate in the exchanges (Small Business Association, 2013). Moreover, all insurance companies participating in exchanges must offer plans that provide a core package of Essential Health Benefits. For some states, this may be equal to typical employer plans in the state.

Small businesses that purchase coverage through the insurance exchanges may also qualify for tax credits. The small business tax credit helps small businesses afford the cost of health care coverage for their employees and is specifically targeted for those businesses with low- and moderate-income workers. The credit is designed to encourage small employers to offer health insurance coverage for the first time or maintain coverage they already have. This makes health insurance more affordable for small employers who lack buying power in the market to negotiate price in the same way that a large employer can.

Before the ACA went into effect, small businesses paid on average 18% more than big businesses for health insurance. By pooling risks across small groups, larger pools can be created like large businesses to be cost-effective (Small Business Association, 2013).

OTHER HEALTH INSURANCE OPTIONS

Although the fundamental purpose of the exchanges is to facilitate the offer and purchase of health insurance, nothing in the law prohibits qualified

TABLE 20-1 Quick Check Chart: Do I qualify to save on health insurance coverage?

	NUMBER OF PEOPLE IN YOUR HOUSEHOLD					
	1	2	3	4	5	6
Private Marketplace Health Plans	You may qualify for lower premiums on a marketplace insurance plan if your yearly income is between ... *See next row if your income is at the lower end of this range.*					
	$11,490-$45,960	$15,510-$62,040	$19,530-$78,120	$23,550-$94,200	$27,570-$110,280	$31,590-$126,360
	You may qualify for lower premiums AND lower out-of-pocket costs for Marketplace insurance if your yearly income is between ...					
	$11,490-$28,725	$15,510-$38,775	$19,530-$48,825	$23,550-$58,875	$27,570-$68,925	$31,590-$78,975
Medicaid Coverage	If your state is expanding Medicaid in 2014: You may qualify for Medicaid coverage if your yearly income is below ...					
	$16,105	$21,707	$27,310	$32,913	$38,516	$44,119
	If your state isn't expanding Medicaid: You may not qualify for any Marketplace savings programs if your yearly income is below ...					
	$11,490	$15,510	$19,530	$23,550	$27,570	$31,590

From Healthcare.gov. (2014). Income levels that qualify for lower health coverage costs. Retrieved from www.healthcare.gov/how-can-i-save-money-on-marketplace-coverage/.

individuals, qualified employers, and insurance carriers from participating in the health insurance market outside of exchanges. Moreover, the ACA explicitly states that enrollment in exchanges is voluntary and no individual may be compelled to enroll in exchange coverage (Fernandez & Mach, 2013). Government plans, including federal, state, and local health insurance plans for employees, retirees, veterans, and other groups such as children (Children's Health Insurance Program [CHIP]), older adults (Medicare), and low-income households (Medicaid), continue to offer coverage to their participants (Healthcare.gov, n.d.).

FEDERAL OR STATE EXCHANGES

It is entirely up to each state to build their own exchange to meet the needs of its citizens or to have the federal government do it. Exchanges may be established either by the state itself as a state-based exchange (SBE) or by the Secretary of the U.S. Department of Health and Human Services (HHS) as a federally facilitated exchange (FFE). An FFE is operated solely by the federal government, or it may be operated by the federal government in conjunction with the state, as a partnership exchange. Fourteen states plus Washington, DC are running their own exchanges (both individual and small business [SHOP] markets). There are three states that only run SHOP markets and the marketplace for individuals is federally run. In 2014, 36 states had either state-federal partnerships or federally facilitated marketplaces. These decisions are highly politicized and will be changing and evolving in the years to come (National Conference of State Legislatures, 2014). No matter what type of exchange is established, all are subject to federal and state oversight. The ACA gives various federal agencies, primarily the HHS, responsibilities relating to the general operation of exchanges. Federal agencies are generally responsible for developing regulations, creating criteria and systems, and awarding grants to states to help them create and implement exchanges. All exchanges are required to carry out many of the same functions and adhere to many of the same standards (Fernandez & Mach, 2013). The primary functions relate to determining eligibility and enrolling individuals in appropriate plans, plan management, consumer assistance and accountability, and financial management.

STATE-BASED EXCHANGES

States had to declare their intentions to establish their own exchange no later than December 14, 2012 (Centers for Medicare and Medicaid Services [CMS], 2012). States intent on setting up their exchanges had to demonstrate their capabilities specific to basic functions set forth in the proposed rule released July 11, 2011 including enrollee support services, oversight of health plans offered through the exchange (QHPs), operation of websites, and risk management. However, there are other areas of program design in which a state has significant flexibility to customize its exchange to best meet the needs of its residents (Center for Budget and Policy Priorities, 2013).

DEVELOPMENT OF THE EXCHANGES

STATE OPTIONS

An SBE had the capacity to incorporate a brand design that uniquely fit its state's culture. Federal exchanges did not offer that same flexibility but did afford states an option to access an insurance marketplace without building it themselves. Some states had existing state laws that needed to be considered when making a choice about which model would be best for their population and their market. To pursue an SBE, a state was required to establish a statute (pass into law) and include in that law the accompanying governance structure that would oversee the marketplace (such as a board of directors). The state statute clarified the business structure, the governance structure, and the oversight. Exchanges, in their implementation, had to work with the federal government, state government, and legislatures. This required a high degree of collaboration.

The percentage of uninsured is variable from one state's market to the next. Because of this, an analysis of the benefits and risks of Medicaid expansion (as a policy decision and financial decision) had to be assessed. Strategic considerations contributed information to aid in making such policy decisions. For example: What change is the state seeking to effect by implementing the marketplace and expanding Medicaid? Will it increase access? Increase cost?

Understanding how the population is sorted into different groups by income was an important consideration in devising strategies to expand coverage. To address affordability, SBEs could implement a policy decision to actively purchase and negotiate with issuers or not negotiate directly but rather serve as a clearinghouse to display plans that met the qualifications established by the regulators. Each has merit. Medicaid expansion is just one of many variables taken into consideration as the insurance marketplace is conceptualized and sustained. Depending on the political climate at the state level and market dominance by issuers, the ability to advance any of the above policies could be enabled or disabled (The Henry J. Kaiser Family Foundation, 2013a).

ESTABLISHING STATE EXCHANGES

Once the key policy decisions were sorted out, funding was sought through the federal grant application process. The federal government made planning grants available to states that chose to convene and develop a plan to establish a health insurance exchange. SBEs had to complete and submit a blueprint application to the Secretary of the HHS. The blueprint served as a roadmap with timelines for building the exchange. Blueprints were due by November 2012. One notable ACA expectation was that SBEs would be self-sustaining by January 2015. There is flexibility in how states chose to generate revenue necessary to be self-sustaining, but many states did not want to take on this revenue challenge. The largest revenue source thus far, for federal and state exchanges, is being garnered from administrative fees on issuers who participate in the marketplace and leverage it in the sale of their products (Dash et al., 2013).

Once blueprints were completed, insurance exchanges received a certification by the federal government to start the build phase. The implementation phase began in October 2013. It is important to note that SBEs were phased in at different times. Early state innovators informed planning efforts. An initiative to identify and create early state innovators (incubators) was funded through federal grants to design and implement online health insurance exchanges. The participating states developed cutting edge and cost-effective technology components, intellectual property, and best practices for implementing insurance exchanges. These models served as a framework for adoption by other states. The knowledge gained from this initiative informed the statutory development (The Center for Consumer Information and Insurance Oversight, 2011).

THE FEDERAL EXCHANGE ROLLOUT: ACA SETBACK

At this time the federal health insurance exchange website has overcome its technical problems and is functioning well with enrollment numbers surpassing expectations. Unfortunately, when Healthcare.gov went live, there were so many problems plaguing the site that Congress held hearings demanding answers regarding its failure to launch (May 2013). A technical debacle, this event was a setback in the implementation of the ACA. The public became angry and fearful regarding personal health insurance access and government competence in leading health care reform. These fears were exacerbated as health policies for individual or small groups were being cancelled for millions of Americans around the same time.

Toward the end of 2013, as federal and state regulators were developing the marketplace to ensure ACA-compliant health coverage was available, the nation's health insurers focused on cancelling insurance policies that did not meet ACA standards. The cancellation notices came as a surprise to many Americans who relied on President Obama's repeated promise that "if you like your health plan, you can keep it." In retrospect, the Obama administration failed to explain the strict conditions required to keep your health plan. As this reality became apparent, a subsequent challenge arose when the federal marketplace failed to be accessible during its first 2 months of operation.

Because individuals would soon be required to have insurance, simultaneously their policies were being cancelled. Citizens in states without state-operated exchanges had no way to obtain insurance through the nonfunctioning marketplace website in time to avoid the 2014 penalties. Congressional leaders from both parties demanded resolution from regulators. This prompted President Obama to implement a "transitional policy" allowing insurers to renew previously cancelled policies through 2014 (McGarey, 2013).

NEW YORK'S SUCCESS STORY

The establishment and rollout of state health insurance exchanges have also been exceedingly complex and politically charged. There have been successes and failures as states that chose to develop their own exchanges met with many challenges. The state of New York is a success story. The state health care exchange surpassed its own expectations, with the state's enrollment efforts as one of the most effective in the nation. The New York health department reported that as of April 2014, 960,000 New Yorkers had signed up for health insurance through the state's exchange, and 70% had been uninsured the year before (Goldberg, 2014).

New York's success, in sharp contrast to the initial rollout of the national exchange, is attributed to the following factors: the state's exchange had few technical issues and ran smoothly after the first week; Governor Andrew Cuomo (Democratic governor) was a supporter of the law; an aggressive and highly visible advertising campaign was created that saturated the public airwaves and subways with enrollment reminders; and finally a majority of state residents supported the law in the first place (Goldberg, 2014). The New York Action Coalition that was formed in 2011 to implement in the state the recommendations of the Institute of Medicine's report on *The Future of Nursing* played a role in educating New Yorkers about the state exchanges, as did nurses in other parts of the country. Other state-run marketplaces have also prospered, including California's, Connecticut's, and Kentucky's (Goldstein, 2014).

THE OREGON STORY

The Cover Oregon exchange, once touted as a model for other states, is now described as "one of the worst in the country" (Viebeck, 2014a). The *Washington Post* reported that the website was so dysfunctional that "no resident has been able to sign up for coverage online since it opened early last fall" (Goldstein, 2014). How did this happen? The state received $304 million in federal grants, including $48 million for being one of the early innovator states. About $250 million was spent trying to get its website working but to no avail. Choosing between spending another $80 million in an effort to get the website functioning or about $5 million to have the federal government and Healthcare.gov take the lead, Cover Oregon's board made the decision to do the latter (Tennant, 2014).

An assessment of this failure was conducted (Cover Oregon Website Implementation Assessment, 2014). There were two themes identified as causes for the failed rollout: lack of communication and unrealistic optimism:

The lack of a single point of authority slowed the decision-making process and contributed to inconsistent communication, and collaboration across agencies was limited at best. In addition, communication with oversight authorities was inconsistent and at times confusing ... Although there are numerous sources of documented communication regarding project status, scope issues, and concerns about system readiness, there does not appear to be a formal acceptance by the Cover Oregon leadership of issues significant enough to affect the success of the October 1 launch until August 2013. (Cover Oregon Website Implementation Assessment, 2014, p. 2, p. 4)

Oregon is not the only state with technical troubles in the insurance marketplace, as Maryland and Massachusetts exchanges were faltering in 2014 and looking to partner with the federal government as well. Hawaii and Minnesota also experienced technical problems on the initial launch of their exchanges (Goldstein, 2014).

EXCHANGE FEATURES

PLANS/LEVELS

To achieve the overall ACA goals, there are several mechanisms included in the design of insurance exchanges that drive the intended outcomes of the law. The mechanisms include mandates, subsidies, guaranteed issue (requirement that insurance companies cover all applicants without discrimination for a preexisting condition), minimum benefits standards, and variable levels of cost-sharing.

The quality and affordability objective of the ACA is reflected in the marketplace design. The ACA ensures that health plans offer, in the individual and small group markets, the 10 identified minimum or essential health benefits (EHBs). The 10 categories are: ambulatory patient services; emergency services; hospitalization; maternity and newborn care; mental health and substance use disorder services, including behavioral health treatment; prescription drugs; rehabilitative and habilitative services and devices; laboratory services; preventive and wellness services and chronic disease management; and pediatric services, including pediatric oral and vision care. States did have some flexibility of adding to these benefits based on their population health priorities. Funding for additional benefits had to be reconciled at the state level. Consumers now have a standard benchmark by which plans are regulated (The Center for Consumer Information and Insurance Oversight, 2013).

MARKETPLACE INSURANCE CATEGORIES

There are five categories or metal level plans that must be offered through the health insurance marketplaces (Table 20-2). Each plan still includes the 10 essential health benefits but there is variable cost-share (the amount that the consumer pays vs. health plan) for each level. CSRs are also available for some consumers (based on their income).

TABLE 20-2 Marketplace Insurance Categories

Metal (Coverage) Levels	Consumer Payment Levels
Bronze Health Plan: pays 60% on average	You pay about 40%
Silver: health plan pays 70% on average	You pay about 30%
Gold: health plan pays 80% on average	You pay about 20%
Platinum: health plan pays 90% on average	You pay about 10%
Catastrophic: coverage plan pays less than 60% of the total average	Only available to people under 30 years old or have a hardship exemption

Source: *www.healthcare.gov.*

ROLE OF MEDICAID

Medicaid expansion was a key provision of the law. Along with the state health exchanges, another pathway for providing a continuum of affordable coverage to significantly reduce the number of uninsured is through Medicaid. In June 2012, the Supreme Court declared Medicaid expansion could not be mandated by the federal government; rather' it had to be offered as a choice for states. An analysis by the Urban Institute (Holahan et al., 2012) projected the impact of the ACA Medicaid expansion would vary across states depending on current coverage levels and number of uninsured. They anticipated that states implementing Medicaid expansion along with other provisions of the ACA could significantly reduce their number of uninsured. They also found that in looking at factors that reduce costs, states as a whole were likely to see net savings from the Medicaid expansion. However, this analysis provided little persuasion. As a result of each state's decision, a significant number of consumers who could qualify for Medicaid are not currently able to access this benefit (see Chapter 40).

NURSES' ROLES WITH EXCHANGES

Successful implementation of the state and federal insurance exchanges is dependent on accurate messaging by trusted professionals. Nursing remains the most trusted of the health professions. As such, this is an opportunity to help in educating the public on the purpose and function of the exchange being used by the state. Additionally, nurses need to look for opportunities to influence service coverage within the exchanges, including requirements for plans to cover critical nursing services. As health care exchanges are implemented and improved, nurses need to use their influence at the bedside and in the boardroom.

CONSUMER EDUCATION

Consumer outreach and education is a critical and challenging component of the health insurance exchange. Empowering consumers to make choices about their own health insurance coverage options is aided when they have access to information and resources that clearly explain their options. It is every nurse's responsibility to refer uninsured patients to the state or federal exchange for coverage, at the very least, and even better if nurses can articulate the basics, including that people may qualify for subsidies that can result in a very low per-month payment.

In addition to providing information and enrollment online, all exchanges are required to have a toll-free call center and in-person options that addresses the needs of consumers requiring assistance. Promoting health literacy is an area where nurses are particularly well positioned to contribute given they are educators, coordinators, and advocates. Nurses know that patient education needs to be adapted to different age, language (written and oral), and delivery preferences. The exchanges must provide the information to applicants and enrollees in plain language, written at a third grade level, and in an accessible and timely manner for individuals living with disabilities at no cost to the individual. Each exchange also provides navigators. These are usually community experts who can explain consumer eligibility, enrollment processes, and plan benefits (Brennaman, 2012).

The open enrollment periods of the health insurance marketplaces were focused on consumer education, in-person assistance, community

education, and outreach events into health care organizations. Social media has presented itself as a viable marketing channel for all ages but in particular those between the ages of 18 and 29 years who are less likely to perceive the need for health insurance. As noted earlier, the technology systems used for the health insurance exchanges is designed to create a user-friendly experience for the consumer.

The insurance exchange is an integrated system that leverages a "no wrong door" model to allow consumers and small businesses to shop and compare via one portal. Before health insurance exchanges, consumers would have to go to multiple places to search for information about health insurance options, prices, Medicaid entitlement, and so on. A streamlined marketplace supports a one-stop shopping experience for a small business or family. Families who have children, for example, who qualify for Medicaid or CHIP can be serviced through one portal (Medicaid.gov State Medicaid and CHIP Policies, 2014).

Likewise, small business employers can assess whether or not they qualify for tax credits, and the administrative burdens previously resulting in multiple invoices from different insurance subscribers are eased somewhat by aggregated billing through the insurance exchange. Employers receive one bill for their employees' coverage. Easing administrative costs supports small business viability.

While technology is critical, it is important to remember that business drives technology. The core business of the health insurance exchange is its ability to make the marketplace transparent for consumers through outreach and education efforts.

STATE REQUIREMENTS INCLUDE APRNS IN EXCHANGE PLANS

The ACA has provided an opportunity for advanced practice registered nurses (APRNs) to address long-standing barriers to practice, including reimbursement by third party payers. More states—in 2014, Minnesota, Connecticut, and Nevada—have passed legislation that supports full scope of practice for APRNs (American Association of Colleges of Nursing, 2014). In Oregon, insurers are now required to reimburse nurse practitioners in independent practices at the same rate as physicians, and Rhode Island was successful in removing their certified registered nurse anesthetist supervision requirement (Brassard, 2014). Much of this progress has come about in part by the success of the state and federal health insurance exchanges in extending coverage to millions of people who had been uninsured.

The high degree of autonomy provided to the states by the ACA in regulating their insurance markets creates many more governance tables for APRNs to be at. It is imperative that APRNs hold seats at these health exchange governance tables to bring nursing expertise to these decision-making bodies. This will require state and national nursing organizations to deploy their political capital to strategically place well-prepared APRN leaders to serve on these boards and commissions. This would ensure that the public has full access to a wide range of providers and promote interdisciplinary practices.

ASSESSING THE IMPACT OF THE EXCHANGES AND FUTURE PROJECTIONS

As the ACA's first individual market open enrollment period (OEP) has ended, the assessment of its impact is being closely watched. Enrollment numbers in the exchanges have been debated and there has been a lot of concern about whether those who signed up on the exchange would actually follow through in paying their premiums. A recent McKinsey survey report (Bhardwaj et al., 2014) shows that 83% of uninsured individuals have paid up. For previously insured individuals, the percentage of payers is 89%. Although this is progress for the health law, the survey also indicates that 74% of enrollees were previously insured.

Another closely watched aspect has been the ACA's impact on health care costs. Per capita health care costs have been rising at just under 3% a year since 2010, but that is less than half the average annual growth in the preceding 8 years. Some economists credit the ACA for a bit of the decline (Farley, 2014). A report by CMS (2014) estimated that

the premium rates for approximately 11 million people will increase and approximately 6 million people are expected to experience a premium rate reduction in 2015. This analysis included both individual and small employer groups. A primary cause of insurance premium rate hikes has been attributed to the requirement for insurers to cover high-risk consumers (Obamacarefacts.com, n.d.). The fact is that insurance companies can no longer deny coverage to Americans with preexisting conditions or charge higher rates based on health status or gender. Other analysts (Batley, 2014) attribute the rate increases to four factors: commercial underwriting restrictions, the age bands that do not allow insurers to vary premiums between young and old beneficiaries, the new excise taxes being levied on insurance plans, and new benefit designs. In 2015, health insurance premiums are expected to vary substantially by region, state, and carrier. Areas of the country with older, sicker, or smaller populations are likely to be hit hardest, whereas others may not see substantial increases at all (Viebeck, 2014b).

It will be several years before the success of the health insurance exchanges can be fully evaluated for their effectiveness in improving market competition (providing consumers with a diversity of choices and hopefully lower prices). However, a recent study by the Kaiser Family Foundation (Cox, et al., 2014) found that California and New York have significantly more competitive exchange markets compared with their individual markets in 2012. The study also found that Connecticut and Washington, DC states were very successful in enrolling more consumers and appear to have less competition than in their 2012 individual markets. Results from the remaining states show either similar levels of competition as pre-ACA markets or mixed signs. Another interesting trend noted was that although competition may not have increased in some states, enrollment across participating plans was significantly redistributed, suggesting a more dynamic market than indicated by statistics alone and the potential for greater price competition in the future (Cox et al., 2014).

If, over time, the exchanges prove to be effective and open to everyone, then workers and employers

UNIT 2

alike might well decide to use them. Recent projections from S&P Capital IQ, a financial research firm, are that 90% of American workers who now receive health insurance through their employers will be shifted to government exchanges by 2020 (as cited by Irwin, 2014). This reflects a very large and fast impact of the insurance exchanges on the current health care system. The S&P researchers estimate that big American companies could save approximately $700 billion between 2016 and 2025. It is envisioned that employers would provide their workers with a stipend to pay for health insurance on the exchanges rather than sponsor a plan themselves. The report concludes that the ACA will make a profound change in how employers offer health benefits and in how the average American employee purchases health insurance (Irwin, 2014).

CONCLUSION

In conclusion, the only way that health care reform will truly give a more efficient, more effective, more affordable health care system is if it begins to fundamentally change the inefficient, ineffective, unaffordable system currently in place. The strength of the health insurance exchanges is key to that transition. How the exchanges are governed will dictate how well the exchanges are patient-centered. Nurses must be involved in health exchange governance. It is also critical that nurses keep an eye on their respective state's insurance exchange progress. There are sources that can assist with this monitoring, including the consumer advocacy group, HealthInsurance.org, and the Kaiser Family Foundation.

DISCUSSION QUESTIONS

1. What barriers and opportunities do you believe impacted the implementation of the state health insurance exchanges?
2. What type of health insurance exchange does your state have? What were the factors that led to this choice?
3. How well is it meeting the needs of your state's citizens?

REFERENCES

American Association of Colleges of Nursing [AACN]. (2014). Connecticut and Minnesota pass legislation to recognize APRNs as full practice providers. AACN Policy Brief. Retrieved from *www.aacn.nche.edu/government-affairs/May-2014.pdf*.

Batley, M. (2014). Health premiums skyrocketing under Obamacare. Newsmax. Retrieved from *www.newsmax.com/Newsfront/obamacare-premiums-skyrocket/2014/04/08/id/564257/*.

Bhardwaj, A., Coe, E., Cordina, J., & Saha, R. (2014). Individual market: Insights into consumer behavior at the end of open enrollment. McKinsey Center for US Health System Reform. Retrieved from *http://healthcare.mckinsey.com/sites/default/files/McKinsey%20Reform%20Center_Individual%20Market%20Post%20OEP%20Trends.pdf*.

Brassard, A. (2014). Scope of practice wins in Iowa, Nevada, Oregon and Rhode Island. The American Nurse. Retrieved from *www.theamericannurse.org/index.php/2013/09/03/scope-of-practice-wins-in-iowa-nevada-oregon-and-rhode-island/*.

Brennaman, L. (2012). State health insurance exchanges: The critical role of nurses and nursing. American Nurses Association Issue Brief. Retrieved from *www.nursingworld.org/MainMenuCategories/Policy-Advocacy/Positions-and-Resolutions/Issue-Briefs/State-Health-Insurance-Exchanges.pdf*.

Center for Budget and Policy Priorities. (2013). State policy decisions in exchange implementation. Retrieved from *www.cbpp.org/files/state-policy-decisions-in-exchange-implementation-SBE.pdf*.

Center for Consumer Information and Insurance Oversight. (2011). States leading the way on implementation: HHS awards early innovator grants to seven states. Retrieved from *www.cms.gov/CCIIO/Resources/Grants/states-leading-the-way.html*.

Center for Consumer Information and Insurance Oversight. (2013). Essential health benefits standards: Ensuring quality, affordable coverage. Centers for Medicare and Medicaid Services. Retrieved from *www.cms.gov/CCIIO/Resources/Fact-Sheets-and-FAQ's/ehb-2-20-2013.html*.

Centers for Medicare and Medicaid Services [CMS]. (2012). Blueprint for approval of affordable state-based and state partnership insurance exchanges. Retrieved from *www.cms.gov/CCIIO/Resources/Files/Downloads/hie-blueprint-11162012.pdf*.

Centers for Medicare and Medicaid Services [CMS]. (2014). Report to Congress on the impact on premiums for individuals and families with employer-sponsored health insurance from the guaranteed issue, guaranteed renewal, and fair health insurance premiums provisions of the Affordable Care Act. Retrieved from *www.cms.gov/Research-Statistics-Data-and-Systems/Research/ActuarialStudies/Downloads/ACA-Employer-Premium-Impact.pdf*.

Cover Oregon Website Implementation Assessment. (2014). First data. Retrieved from *www.oregon.gov/DAS/docs/co_assessment.pdf*.

Cox, C., Ma, R., Claxton, G., & Levitt, L. (2014). Sizing up exchange market competition. Updated: May 1, 2014. The Henry J. Kaiser Family Foundation. Retrieved from *kff.org/health-reform/issue-brief/sizing-up-exchange-market-competition/*.

Dash, S., Lucia, K., Keith, K., & Monahan, C. (2013). Implementing the Affordable Care Act: Key decisions for state based exchanges. The Commonwealth Fund. Retrieved from *www.commonwealthfund.org/~/media/files/publications/Fund%20Report/*.

Farley, R. (2014). ACA impact on per capita cost of health care. FACTCHECK.ORG. Retrieved from *www.factcheck.org/2014/02/aca-impact-on-per-capita-cost-of-health-care/*.

Fernandez, B., & Mach, A. L. (2013). Health insurance exchanges under the Patient Protection and Affordable Care Act (ACA). Congressional Research Service 7-5700 R42663. Retrieved from *www.crs.gov*.

Goldberg, D. (2014). Why New York worked. Retrieved from *www.capitalnewyork.com/article/magazine/2014/04/8544390/why-new-york-worked*.

Goldstein, A. (2014). Obama administration prepares to take over Oregon's broken health insurance exchange. *Washington Post*. Retrieved from *www.washingtonpost.com/national/health-science/obama-administration-prepares-to-take-over-oregons-broken-health-insurance-exchange/2014/04/24/ff9aa220-cbc4-11e3-95f7-7ecdde72d2ea_story.html*.

Healthcare.gov. (n.d.). Health insurance marketplace. Retrieved from *www.healthcare.gov/*.

The Henry J. Kaiser Family Foundation. (2013a). State decisions for creating health insurance marketplaces. Retrieved from *kff.org/health-reform/state-indicator/health-insurance-exchanges/*.

The Henry J. Kaiser Family Foundation. (2013b). The youtoons get ready for Obamacare: Health insurance changes coming your way under the Affordable Care Act. Retrieved from *kff.org/health-reform/video/youtoons-obamacare-video/*.

Hilzenrath, D.S. (2009). Papers show insurers limited coverage for acne, pregnancy. *Washington Post*. Retrieved from *www.washingtonpost.com/wp-dyn/content/article/2009/09/18/AR2009091803501.html*.

Holahan, J., Buettgens, M., Carroll, C., & Dorn, S. (2012). The cost and coverage implications of the ACA Medicaid expansion: National and state-by-state analysis. The Urban Institute. Kaiser Commission on Medicaid and the Uninsured. Retrieved from *http://kaiserfamilyfoundation.files.wordpress.com/2013/01/8384.pdf*.

Irwin, N. (2014). Envisioning the end of employer-provided health plans. *The New York Times*. Retrieved from *www.nytimes.com/2014/05/01/upshot/employer-sponsored-health-insurance-may-be-on-the-way-out.html?_r=0*.

Klein, E. (2009). Health insurance exchanges: An overlooked key to reform's success. *Washington Post*. Retrieved from *www.washingtonpost.com/wpdyn/content/article/2009/07/28/AR2009072802114.html*.

May, A. (2013). What went wrong with HealthCare.gov—and what now. Retrieved from *www.benefitspro.com/2013/11/20/what-went-wrong-with-healthcaregov-and-what-now*.

McGarey, S. (2013). Market transitional policy—The latest setback in the implementation of ACA. Retrieved from *www.ascende.com/Insight-Knowledge/Advisories-Publications/Market-Transitional-Policy/*.

Medicaid.gov State Medicaid and CHIP Policies. (2014). State Medicaid and CHIP Policies for 2014. Retrieved from *www.medicaid.gov/Medicaid-CHIP-Program-Information/By-State/By-State.html*.

National Conference of State Legislatures. (2014). Healthcare reform—Affordable Care Act legislative database. Retrieved from *www.ncsl.org/research/health/new-health-reform-database.aspx*.

Obamacarefacts.com. (n.d.). Obamacare insurance premiums: How Obamacare impacts insurance premium rates. Retrieved from *http://obamacarefacts.com/obamacare-health-insurance-premiums.php*.

Peterson, C., & Fernandez, B. (2010). PPACA requirements for offering health insurance inside versus outside an exchange. Congressional Research Service. Retrieved from *www.ncsl.org/documents/health/inside-vs-outsideexchangepdf*.

Simas, D. (2014). Health coverage before the ACA, and why all Americans are better off now. *The White House Blog*. Retrieved from *www.whitehouse.gov/blog/2014/01/23/health-coverage-aca-and-why-all-americans-are-better-now*.

Small Business Association. (2013). Affordable Care Act 101: What the health care law means for small businesses. Retrieved from *www.sba.gov/sites/default/files/files/SBA%20ACA%20101%20Deck%20-%20Updated%20July%202013%20(Disclaimer).pdf*.

Tennant, M. (2014). After huge website crash, Oregon asks feds to run Obamacare exchange. New American. Retrieved from *www.thenewamerican.com/usnews/health-care/item/18157-after-huge-website-crash-oregon-asks-feds-to-run-obamacare-exchange*.

U.S. Department of Health and Human Services Report. (2011). At risk: Pre-existing conditions could affect 1 in 2 Americans. Retrieved from *aspe.hhs.gov/health/reports/2012/pre-existing/index.shtml*.

Viebeck, E. (2014a). Oregon to abandon O-Care exchange. *The Hill*. Retrieved from *thehill.com/policy/healthcare/204303-oregon-to-abandon-obamacare-exchange*.

Viebeck, E. (2014b). O-Care premiums to skyrocket. *The Hill*. Retrieved from *thehill.com/policy/healthcare/201136-obamacare-premiums-are-about-to-skyrocket*.

ONLINE RESOURCES

Federal Insurance Marketplace
www.healthcare.gov
National Academy for State Health Policy
www.nashp.org
The Commonwealth Fund
www.commonwealthfund.org

CHAPTER 21

Patient Engagement and Public Policy: Emerging New Paradigms and Roles

Mary Jo Kreitzer   Jane Clare Joyner[1]

"Even in an age of hype, calling something 'the block-buster drug of the century' grabs our attention. In this case, the 'drug' is actually a concept—patient activation and engagement—that should have formed the heart of health care all along."

Susan Dentzer

Over the past 5 years, there has been a significant shift in the role and expectations of people seeking health care. Historically, the role of the patient was to be passive and do what they were told to do. Patients who didn't follow orders were labeled as noncompliant. These roles were congruent with a hierarchical health care system where most often the physician was perceived to be in charge. According to the *Merriam-Webster Online Dictionary* (n.d.), the Latin word from which patient is derived literally means to suffer.

Although the language remains controversial, many people are more inclined to see themselves, along with their family members and caregivers, as consumers or clients of the health care system, and they seek relationships with health care providers that are on a par with other purchasing arrangements of goods and services in their lives. As purchasers of a service or product, they want choice, transparency of information, and data about quality and outcomes. They are also concerned about value.

The landmark Institute of Medicine report, *Crossing the Quality Chasm* (2001), was one of the first federal policy reports to describe the radical changes needed within the health care system to better meet the needs of patients. A set of new rules was identified that redefined the locus of control and relationships by emphasizing that care should be based on continuous healing relationships and be customized based on patient needs and values, that patients should be in control of health care decisions, that patients should have unfettered access to clinical knowledge and their own medical information, and that the health care system should anticipate needs rather than react to events.

Recognizing the critical role of the consumer in determining health outcomes, the Center for Advancing Health (2010) defines engagement as the actions we take to benefit from the health care available to us. Engagement behaviors range from finding good care to communicating with health professionals, organizing health care, paying for care, and making good treatment decisions.

There is evidence that patient engagement, also called patient activation, can be measured (Hibbard et al., 2004). Although much of the impetus for engagement comes from people's changing expectations, there is also growing evidence (Hibbard & Greene, 2013; Hibbard, Greene, & Overton, 2013; Katon et al., 1995; Robinson et al., 2008) that engagement is directly linked to health outcomes. It is estimated that 90% of people's health (Clymer et al., 2012) is unrelated to health care per se

---

[1]The opinions expressed are those of the authors and do not necessarily reflect the views of VA or the United States government.

(hospitals, health care providers, and drugs). Rather, an individual's health is more related to patterns of food consumption, exercise, sleep, and management of stress as well as social, environmental, and genetic influences. A framework developed by Carman and colleagues (2013) describes patient engagement as taking place at three levels: the direct care level, including engagement with clinicians as well as health-related groups and resources; the design and governance level, where the patient perspective is considered and integrated into the organization; and the policymaking level, including development of programs and policies at the local, state, and national level. Nielsen and colleagues (2012) also describe patient engagement as taking place in distinct spheres: at the clinical encounter level, the practice or organizational level, the community level, and the policy level.

Current efforts to redesign the health care system are focused on achieving what is called the triple aim. The Institute for Healthcare Improvement (n.d.) defines the triple aim as:

- Improving the patient experience of care (including quality and satisfaction)
- Improving the health of populations
- Reducing the per capita cost of health care

To achieve the triple aim, changes are needed within health care environments as well as in provider and consumer behavior. This chapter examines nursing and federal policy initiatives focused on patient engagement, highlights an exemplary model of patient engagement, and identifies critical strategies for hearing and embracing the patient's voice.

PATIENT ENGAGEMENT WITHIN NURSING

A core theme from the Institute of Medicine report entitled *The Future of Nursing: Leading Change, Advancing Health* (2011) is that nurses should be leaders in redesigning health care in the United States and be full partners in developing and shaping health policy and in implementing health care reform. Patient engagement initiatives, recently likened to a block-buster drug of the century (Dentzer, 2013), offer nurses the opportunity to

advance health policy and reform the health care system.

By definition, patient engagement involves individuals taking action to benefit from health care. Advancing patient engagement requires that nurses identify what will encourage patients (or others acting on the patient's behalf) to take action to benefit from available health care. Much of what is called patient engagement has been within the domain of nursing for decades. For example, in her *Notes on Nursing* published in 1860, Florence Nightingale advocated that the role of the nurse was to help the patient attain the best possible condition so that nature could act and self-healing could occur (Dossey, 2000). The American Nurses Association's *Code of Ethics for Nurses with Interpretive Statements* (2001) highlights nurses' commitment to the unique needs of the individual patient and the importance of engaging patients in planning their care.

Nurses are on the front line of delivering health care. They provide patient care across the health care spectrum and in more settings than any other health care profession. Also, for many patients, nurses hold a position of trust. Nurses have consistently been ranked as the most trusted profession (Gallup, 2013). As health reform advances, the health care environment is moving from a system in which the patient is passive to a system in which health care consumers are engaged and share accountability for health outcomes with health providers and the system as a whole. As the largest segment of the health care workforce, nursing is well positioned to promote this transition. Nursing competencies, such as fostering behavior changes through the use of patient education, case management, and aligning patient needs to the health care system, are assets to making this transition (O'Neil, 2009).

In 2013, the Nursing Alliance for Quality Care, a group composed of leading nursing organizations and consumer advocacy groups, published a paper addressing the role of the nurse in advancing patient and family engagement (Sofaer & Schumann, 2013). The paper identifies opportunities and strategies to further nursing's role in patient engagement. Several strategies, including aligning incentives to encourage patient engagement and enforcing regulatory expectations and standards that support patient engagement principles in practice, would require nurses to engage with other stakeholders to advance these public policy initiatives. As trusted providers of health care, nurses are in an optimal position to advance patient engagement through policy initiatives.

PATIENT ENGAGEMENT AND FEDERAL INITIATIVES

The federal government plays an important role in driving policy initiatives to foster patient engagement. Statutes passed by Congress become laws that are implemented and clarified by regulations issued by an executive branch agency. Federal advisory committees provide policy advice to agencies. The federal government can also affect patient engagement policy through awards of research grants. This section highlights examples of federal public policy initiatives.

THE AFFORDABLE CARE ACT

The Affordable Care Act (ACA) includes a number of elements that have the potential to impact and advance patient engagement initiatives.

Accountable Care Organizations. Section 3022 of the ACA created a new Medicare shared savings program: Medicare Accountable Care Organizations (ACO). A Medicare ACO consists of a group of providers (physicians, hospitals, and other health care providers) who are jointly responsible for the cost of care and the quality of care provided to their patient population. The law, which added a new section 1899 to the Social Security Act (42 U.S.C. 1395, et seq.), aims to incentivize providers to provide quality care at low cost, and penalize those who provide high cost or low quality care. The law requires groups of providers and suppliers to have a shared governance structure and stipulates a number of additional requirements to participate as a Medicare ACO. The statute requires ACOs to promote patient engagement and evidence-based medicine, to coordinate care, and to report cost and quality metrics.

Final regulations for the program were published in 2011 by the U.S. Department of Health and Human Services (HHS) (HHS Federal Register Notice, November 2, 2011). The Federal Register Notice emphasized that the new approach to delivering services to Medicare beneficiaries was designed to further a three-part aim to:

1. Provide better care for individuals
2. Promote better health for populations
3. Lower growth in expenditures for Medicare Parts A and B

The rule explained that the goal of the value-based purchasing is to reward better outcomes, innovations, and values. The notice further articulated the statutory requirement for ACOs to have a governing body with a mechanism for shared decision making and governance, including the authority to define processes that promote patient engagement. The rule explained that patient engagement, defined as "the active participation of patients and their families in the process of making medical decisions," is a necessary part of patient-centered care. The final rule describes four patient-centeredness requirements that overlap with patient engagement:

1. Evaluation of the health needs of the population assigned to the ACO
2. Effective communication of clinical knowledge to beneficiaries
3. Recognizing the patient's unique needs, preferences, values, and priorities, while engaging in shared decision making
4. Having written standards for communicating with patients and allowing patient access to their medical records

The final rule also describes ways to promote patient engagement, including shared decision-making methods and tools, methods to promote health literacy, use of a beneficiary experience-of-care survey, and the involvement of patients in the governing processes of the ACO.

Partnership for Patients. Another ACA innovation with a potential to impact patient engagement is the Center for Medicare and Medicaid Innovation (CMMI), which was established by section 3021 of the ACA. CMMI was created to test "innovative payment and service delivery models to reduce program expenditures…while preserving or enhancing the quality of care" for Children's Health Insurance Program, Medicare, or Medicaid beneficiaries. One initiative of CMMI is the Partnership for Patients, an organization consisting of more than 7500 partners, including organizations representing health care providers, consumers, and patients, as well as hospitals and health care systems and state and federal agencies (Center for Medicare and Medicaid Innovation: Report to Congress, 2012). Patient and family engagement is one focus of Partnership for Patients, which views the relationship between patients and families and health care providers as a key part of improving health care and reducing readmissions to hospitals (Partnership for Patients, 2013).

PCORI. The Patient Centered Outcomes Research Institute (PCORI), an independent, nonprofit health research organization, was created by section 6301 of the ACA. Washington and Lipstein (2011) explain that the organization, which focuses on patient-centered outcomes research, "will support many studies encompassing a broad range of study designs and outcomes that are relevant to patients, aiming to assist people in making choices that are consistent with their values, preferences, and goals." PCORI collaborates with federal agencies, such as the National Institutes of Health (NIH) and the Agency for Healthcare Research and Quality (AHRQ), to further patient-centered outcomes research, including patient engagement methods. PCORI's National Priorities for Research and Research Agenda (2012) states that its mission is "to fund research that offers patients and caregivers the information they need to make important health care decisions." Because it is a nongovernmental organization, opportunities to receive research funding (PCORI Funding Announcements) are posted on the organization's website rather than published in the Federal Register (PCORI Funding Opportunities, 2013). The organization established an Advisory Panel on Patient Engagement to provide scientific and technical expertise and prioritize research questions (PCORI Announcement of Advisory Panel, 2013).

HEALTH INFORMATION TECHNOLOGY

There is evidence that providing online access to electronic health records may empower patients to more fully contribute to their care (Woods et al., 2013) and that patients want to share access to their health information (Zulman et al., 2011). A section of the American Recovery and Reinvestment Act of 2009, the Health Information Technology for Economic and Clinical Health Act (HITECH Act) provisions, sought to stimulate the adoption of health information technology (HIT) by authorizing financial incentives for the adoption and meaningful use of electronic health records (EHR). The federal government's promotion of EHR technology and its use by providers to improve quality, safety, and efficiency are having an impact on patient engagement initiatives.

In explaining the EHR Incentive Program, also referred to as meaningful use, the Department of Health and Human Services, Health Resources and Services Administration (HRSA, 2013) identified the engagement of patients and families as a prominent goal of the program. The HRSA website explains that engaged patients communicate better, take a more active role in making health care decisions, are more compliant, and better manage their own care. HRSA also states that activated patients and families can lower health care costs by lowering both overuse and underuse of medical services, and that providers can benefit through reduced staff workloads and greater practice efficiency.

In testimony before the U.S. Senate Committee on Finance in July 2013, the Chief Medical Officer and Director of the Office of Clinical Standards and Quality, Centers for Medicare & Medicaid Services, explained that health information technology allows patients to participate in their health care and improve their overall health. The written testimony explained that stage 1 criteria of the EHR Incentive Program required "eligible professionals and hospitals to provide patients with an electronic copy of certain health information including diagnostic test results, problem lists, and medication lists upon request, and to provide patients with clinical summaries after each office visit." The criteria for stage 2 "require eligible professionals and hospitals to provide patients the ability to view online, download, and transmit certain health information." On November 12, 2012, the Health Information Technology Policy Committee, Office of the National Coordinator for Health Information Technology, announced the Committee's request for comments on its draft recommendations for stage 3 regulations (HHS Federal Register Notice, November 26, 2012). Comments collected through this process will be used to develop regulations to implement the next state of meaningful use regulations.

ADDITIONAL FEDERAL INITIATIVES

Federal advisory committees can inform public policy on health care initiatives like patient engagement. These entities, authorized by the Federal Advisory Committee Act of 1972 (Public Law 92-463), provide advice to the Executive Branch of the federal government (GSA, *FACA 101*). For example, the Health IT Policy Committee, the federal advisory committee that advises the HHS Office of the National Coordinator for Health IT, has established workgroups that discuss and evaluate topics and make recommendations to the full advisory committee (U.S. Department of Health and Human Services, Office of the National Coordinator for Health IT, 2014). One such workgroup, the Consumer Empowerment Workgroup, will "provide recommendations on policy issues and opportunities for strengthening the ability of consumers, patients, and lay caregivers to manage health and health care for themselves or others."

Other federal entities have also developed patient engagement policy initiatives. AHRQ developed an extensive policy document entitled Guide to Patient and Family Engagement in Hospital Quality and Safety (2013). The AHRQ publication is an evidence-based resource for hospitals that identifies strategies to promote patient and family engagement in the quality and safety of hospital care. AHRQ has also developed an online resource center on patient-centered medical homes, which includes resources to engage patients, families, and caregivers (www.pcmh.ahrq.gov/page/papers-briefs-and -resources). The federal government can also affect

patient engagement policy through awards of research grants focusing on patient engagement. For example, a number of funding opportunities offered by the National Institutes of Health have included references to patient engagement initiatives (HHS, NIH, 2012a, b).

THE VA SYSTEM: AN EXEMPLAR OF PATIENT-CENTERED CARE

The Veterans Health Administration, part of the United States Department of Veterans Affairs (VA), is the largest integrated health care system in the United States (Veterans Affairs, n.d.). A number of innovations at VA have the potential to significantly impact patient engagement.

VA is a leader in using electronic tools to engage patients by giving them access to their health information. One such tool is the Blue Button initiative. The appearance of the Blue Button icon signals that a patient is able to download his or her digital health record and share it with caregivers, family members, or other health care professionals. Such ready access to health information makes it easier for patients to monitor and engage in their health care. VA was the first organization to use Blue Button. Since its launch in VA in 2010, hundreds of organizations have joined the Blue Button Pledge Program, including Medicare and private health care insurers, as well as the Department of Defense (Ricciardi et al., 2013).

VA's implementation of patient-centered medical homes (PCMH) in primary care clinics across the nation also has the potential to improve patient engagement. The PCMH has been described by Nielsen and colleagues (2012) as "a model of primary care that is patient-centered, comprehensive, team-based, coordinated, accessible, and focused on quality and safety." They describe the empirical support for the PCMH model and identify data showing how PCMHs improve care and outcomes while lowering costs. Within VA, the aim of the PCMH initiative is to improve continuity of care and care management and coordination, improve patient access, and increase the use of preventative services (Kline, 2011; Rosland et al., 2013). The VA uses patient aligned care teams

(PACTs) to provide integrated health care. Implementation of the program is monitored through various metrics, including measures of patient engagement and satisfaction (Kline, 2011). Metrics used to measure patient engagement include patient compliance and satisfaction survey results; enrollment in VA's personal health record, My Healthe-Vet; and the number of patients who seek in-person authentication to use secure messaging (Kline, 2011).

VA, like many health care facilities in the private sector, has begun to offer complementary and alternative medicine (CAM), now often called integrative health or medicine. According to a 2011 survey (Ezeji-Okoye et al., 2013) by the VA's Health Care Analysis and Information Group, the use of CAM has grown significantly over the past decade. According to the survey, about 9 in 10 VA facilities directly provide CAM therapies or refer patients to outside licensed practitioners. CAM is used in the VA most commonly to help veterans manage stress, promote general wellness, and to treat problems including anxiety, posttraumatic stress disorder, depression, back pain, arthritis, fibromyalgia, and substance abuse. Offering integrative therapies is aligned with approaches in the VA to provide care that is personalized, proactive, and patient centered. This is consistent with broader trends in health care that reflect the incorporation of integrative therapies and healing practices into care models.

FROM PATIENT ENGAGEMENT TO CITIZEN HEALTH

Twenty years ago, in the book *Through the Patient's Eyes: Understanding and Promoting Patient-Centered Care*, Margaret Gerteis and her colleagues broke new ground in summarizing data obtained from thousands of patients through surveys and focus groups that advanced the perspective that "institutional" does not need to be synonymous with "impersonal." Seven areas were identified as important to improving the patient experience: respecting patients' values and preferences, coordinating care, providing information and education, attending to physical comfort, providing emotional support, involving family and friends in care, and ensuring

continuity among providers and treatment settings (Gerteis, 1993). As fundamental and basic as these core tenets of patient-centered care are, they have been largely ignored until recently with the reemergence of patient-centered care as an imperative, not an option.

Applying design thinking to the process of care redesign is a very helpful strategy to ensure that the consumer's voice is heard. As described by Tim Brown (2009) in *Change by Design*, design thinking is a human-centered planning process that includes three overlapping steps:
1. Inspiration (the search for solutions)
2. Ideation (the process of generating developing and testing ideas)
3. Implementation (the path leading from project room to market)

It is an iterative, nonlinear process that involves continuously testing and revisiting assumptions and adhering to a philosophy of fail earlier to succeed sooner. The foundation of design thinking is planning around three overlapping criteria:
1. *Desirability:* What makes sense to people, and what is needed or desired?
2. *Feasibility:* What is functionally possible?
3. *Viability:* What is likely to be sustainable?

Engaging people at the beginning of a planning process, whether the process focuses on care, education, or public policy, increases the likelihood that their voices and perspectives will be heard and the outcome will be desirable, or even optimal.

Citizen health care is a bold vision proposed by Doherty and Mendenhall (2006) that goes beyond the activated patient to the activated community. They argue that patients, families, and communities should be coproducers of health and health care with professionals acquiring community organizing skills to enable them to effectively work with people who see themselves as citizens of health care, builders of health in clinics and communities, rather than merely as consumers of medical services.

CONCLUSION

Although this chapter highlights governmental, professional (nursing), and organizational strategies aimed at shifting behavior to achieve patient engagement through policy initiatives, perhaps more thought and focus needs to be centered on what people can do for themselves and for each other to advance health and well-being. Determinants of well-being (Kreitzer, Delagran, & Uptmor, 2014) include health (physical, mental, emotional, and spiritual) as well as purpose, relationships, community, safety and security, and the environment.

In considering broader societal aspirations of human flourishing and economic sustainability, it is critical to consider ways to harness our cultural and democratic roots in service of advancing well-being and the common good. In *Healing the Heart of Democracy*, Parker Palmer notes that "when all of our talk about politics is either technical or strategic, to say nothing of partisan and polarizing, we loosen or sever the human connections on which empathy, accountability, and democracy itself reside" (2011). His central point is that we need to create a politics worthy of the human spirit, one that has a chance to serve the common good. This requires more than an engaged patient; it requires an engaged and informed citizenry.

DISCUSSION QUESTIONS

1. What is the role of the profession of nursing in creating an informed citizenry that is empowered to advance well-being within individuals, families, and communities?
2. What can you do in your practice to engage and empower patients and families?
3. What governmental, institutional, or private sector policies could enhance patient engagement and activation?

REFERENCES

Agency for Healthcare Research and Quality. (2013). Guide to patient and family engagement in hospital quality and safety. Retrieved from *www.ahrq.gov/professionals/systems/hospital/engagingfamilies/.*

American Nurses Association. (2001). *Code of ethics for nurses with interpretive statements.* Silver Springs, MD: Nursesbooks.org.

American Recovery and Reinvestment Act of 2009, Public Law 111–5. (2009). Retrieved from *www.gpo.gov/fdsys/pkg/PLAW-111publ5/content-detail.html.*

Brown, D. (2009). *Change by design: How design thinking transforms organizations and inspires innovation.* New York: Harper Business.

Carman, K., Dardess, P., Maurer, M., Sofaer, S., Adams, K., Bechtel, C., et al. (2013). Patient and family engagement: a framework for understanding the elements and developing interventions and policies. *Health Affairs, 32*(2), 223–231.

Center for Advancing Health. (2010). A new definition of patient engagement: What is engagement and why is it important. Retrieved from *www.cfah.org/file/CFAH_Engagement_Behavior_Framework_current.pdf.*

Clymer, J. M., Fielding, J. E., Rimer, B. K., & Pronk, N. P. (2012). The guidebook for healthy communities and healthy states. *America's health rankings: United Health Foundation,* Retrieved from *www.americashealthrankings.org/Reports.*

Dentzer, S. (2013). Rx for the "blockbuster drug" of patient engagement. *Health Affairs, 32*(2), 202.

Doherty, W. J., & Mendenhall, T. (2006). Citizen health care: a model for engaging patients, families and communities as coproducers of health. *Family, Systems and Health, 24,* 251–263.

Dossey, B. M. (2000). *Florence Nightingale: Mystic, visionary, healer.* Pennsylvania: Springhouse.

Ezeji-Okoye, S., Kotar, T., Smeeding, S., & Dufree, J. (2013). State of care: Complementary and alternative medicine in Veterans Health Administration—2011 survey results. *Federal Practitioner, 30*(11), 15–20.

Gallup. (2013). Honesty and ethics rating of clergy slides to new low. Retrieved from *www.gallup.com/poll/166298/honesty-ethics-rating-clergy-slides-new-low.aspx.*

Gerteis, M., Edgeman-Levitan, S., Daley, J., & Delbanco, T. L. (Eds.), (1993). *Through the patient's eyes: Understanding and promoting patient-centered care.* San Francisco, CA: John Wiley & Sons, Inc.

Hibbard, J., & Greene, J. (2013). What evidence shows about patient activation: better health outcomes and care experiences; fewer data on costs. *Health Affairs, 32*(2), 207–214.

Hibbard, J., Greene, J., & Overton, V. (2013). Patients with lower activation associated with higher costs; delivery systems should know their patients' scores. *Health Affairs, 32*(2), 216–222.

Hibbard, J., Stockard, J., Mahoney, E., & Tusler, M. (2004). Development of the patient activation measure (PAM): conceptualizing and measuring activation in patients and consumers. *Health Services Research, 39*(4/1), 1005–1026.

Institute for Healthcare Improvement. (n.d). The triple aim. Retrieved from *www.ihi.org/offerings/Initiatives/TripleAim/Pages/default.aspx.*

Institute of Medicine (U.S.). Committee on Quality of Health Care in America. (2001). *Crossing the quality chasm: A new health system for the 21st century.* Washington DC: National Academies Press.

Institute of Medicine. (2011). *The future of nursing: Leading change, advancing health.* Washington DC: National Academies Press.

Katon, W., Von Korff, M., Lin, E., Walker, E., Simon, G. E., et al. (1995). Collaborative management to achieve treatment guidelines: Impact on depression in primary care. *Journal of the American Medical Association, 273*(13), 1026–1031.

Kline, S. (2011). The Veterans Health Administration: Implementing patient-centered medical homes in the nation's largest integrated delivery system. Commonwealth Fund. Retrieved from *www.commonwealthfund.org/~/media/Files/Publications/Case%20Study/2011/Sep/1537_Klein_veterans_hlt_admin_case%20study.pdf.*

Kreitzer, M. J., Delagran, L., & Uptmor, A. (2014). Advancing wellbeing in people, organizations and communities. In M. J. Kreitzer & M. Koithan (Eds.), *Integrative nursing.* Chapter 10. New York: Oxford University Press.

Nielsen, M., Langner, B., Zema, C., Hacker, T., & Grundy, P. (2012). Benefits of implementing the primary care patient-centered medical home: A review of cost & quality results. *Washington: Patient-centered primary care collaborative*, Retrieved from *www.pcpcc.org/sites/default/files/media/benefits_of_implementing_the_primary_care_pcmh.pdf.*

O'Neil, E. (2009). Four factors that guarantee health care change. *Journal of Professional Nursing, 25*(6), 317–321.

Palmer, P. J. (2011). *Healing the heart of democracy.* New York: Jossey-Bass.

Partnership for Patients. (2013). Welcome to the Partnership for Patients. Retrieved from *partnershipforpatients.cms.gov/about-the-partnership/patient-and-family-engagement/the-patient-and-family-engagement.html.*

Patient. (n.d.). Merriam-Webster Online. Retrieved from *www.merriam-webster.com/dictionary/patient.*

Patient Centered Outcomes Research Institute. (2012). National priorities for research and research agenda. Retrieved from *www.pcori.org/assets/PCORI-National-Priorities-and-Research-Agenda-2012-05-21-FINAL1.pdf.*

Patient Centered Outcomes Research Institute. (2013). Announcement of an advisory panel on patient engagement. Retrieved from *www.pcori.org/get-involved/pcori-advisory-panels/advisory-panel-on-patient-engagement/.*

Patient Centered Outcomes Research Institute. (2013). Funding opportunities. Retrieved from *www.pcori.org/funding-opportunities/landing/.*

Ricciardi, L., Mostashari, F., Murphy, J., Daniel, J., & Siminerio, E. (2013). A national action plan to support consumer engagement via e-health. *Health Affairs, 32*(2), 376–384.

Robinson, J. H., Callister, L. C., Berry, J. A., & Dearing, K. A. (2008). Patient-centered care and adherence: Definitions and applications to improve outcomes. *Journal of the American Academy of Nurse Practitioners, 20*(12), 600–607.

Rosland, A., Nelson, K., Sun, H., Dolan, E., Maynard, C., et al. (2013). The patient-centered medical home in the Veterans Health Administration. *American Journal of Managed Care, 19*(7), e263–e272.

Sofaer, S., & Schumann, M. J. (2013). Fostering successful patient and family engagement: Nursing's critical role. Washington, DC: Nursing Alliance for Quality Care. Retrieved from *www.naqc.org/WhitePaper-PatientEngagement.*

U.S. Department of Health and Human Services, Center for Medicare and Medicaid Innovation. (2012). Report to Congress. Retrieved from *innovation.cms.gov/Files/reports/RTC-12-2012.pdf.*

U.S. Department of Health and Human Services, Centers for Medicare and Medicaid Services. Medicare Program; Medicare Shared Savings Program: Accountable Care Organizations. (2011). *Federal Register,* 76 Fed. Reg. 67802. Retrieved from *www.gpo.gov/fdsys/pkg/FR-2011-11-02/pdf/2011-27461.pdf.*

U.S. Department of Health and Human Services, Centers for Medicare & Medicaid Services. (2013, July 1). Health information technology: A building block to quality health care. Hearing before the U.S. Senate Finance Committee on Finance (testimony of Patrick Conway). Retrieved from *www.finance.senate.gov/imo/media/doc/HIT%20testimony%20%28P%20%20Conway%29%207%2017%2013.pdf.*

U.S. Department of Health and Human Services, Health Resources and Services Administration. (2013). Health IT Adoption Toolkit, meaningful use: Introduction. Retrieved from *www.hrsa.aquilentprojects.com/healthit/toolbox/HealthITAdoptiontoolbox/MeaningfulUse/intro2meaningfuluseandpatientandfamily.html.*

U.S. Department of Health and Human Services, National Institutes of Health. (2012a). Innovative health information technology for broad adoption by healthcare systems and consumers (R44). Retrieved from *grants.nih.gov/grants/guide/pa-files/PA-12-196.html.*

U.S. Department of Health and Human Services, National Institutes of Health. (2012b). Technology-based interventions to promote engagement in care and treatment adherence and for substance abusing populations with HIV (R34). Retrieved from *grants.nih.gov/grants/guide/pa-files/PA-12-118.html.*

U.S. Department of Health and Human Services, Office of the National Coordinator for Health IT. (2014). Consumer Empowerment Workgroup. Retrieved from *www.healthit.gov/policy-researchers-implementers/federal-advisory-committees-facas/consumer-empowerment-workgroup.*

U.S. Department of Health and Human Services, Office of the National Coordinator for Health Information Technology; Health Information Technology; HIT Policy Committee: Request for comment regarding the stage 3 definition of meaningful use of electronic records (EHRs) (2012). *Federal Register,* 77 Fed. Reg. 70444. Retrieved from *www.federalregister.gov/articles/2012/11/26/2012-28584/office-of-the-national-coordinator-for-health-information-technology-health-information-technology.*

U.S. Department of Veterans Affairs. (n.d.). Veterans Health Administration. Retrieved from *www.va.gov/health/.*

U.S. General Services Administration. FACA 101. Retrieved from *www.gsa.gov/portal/content/244333.*

Washington, A., & Lipstein, S. (2011). The Patient-Centered Outcomes Research Institute—Promoting better information, decisions, and health. *New England Journal of Medicine, 365,* e31.

Woods, W., Schwartz, E., Tuepker, A., Press, N., Nazi, K., et al. (2013). Patient experiences with full electronic access to health records and clinical notes through the My HealtheVet personal health record pilot: Qualitative study. *Journal of Medical Internet Research, 15*(3), e65.

Zulman, D., Nazi, K., Turvey, C., Wagner, T., Woods, S., & An, L. (2011). Patient interest in sharing personal health record information: A web-based survey. *Annals of Intern Medicine, 155*(12), 805–810.

ONLINE RESOURCES

Agency for Healthcare Research and Quality: Guide to Patient and Family Engagement in Hospital Quality and Safety
www.ahrq.gov/professionals/systems/hospital/engagingfamilies.
Center for Spirituality & Healing: Taking Charge of Your Health and Wellbeing
www.takingcharge.csh.umn.edu

CHAPTER 22

The Marinated Mind: Why Overuse Is an Epidemic and How to Reduce It

Rosemary Gibson

"Our minds have been marinated to believe more is better."

Rosemary Gibson

The Institute of Medicine has identified three health care quality challenges in the United States: underuse, misuse, and overuse. Overuse is when the potential for harm of a health care service exceeds the possible benefit. Dedicated clinicians, journalists, and public interest advocates are creating the urgency for policymakers to reduce it.

COMMONLY OVERUSED INTERVENTIONS

Commonly overused health care interventions in the United States were first identified in 2008 by the National Priorities Partnership, which was convened by the National Quality Forum. The interventions include: prescription drugs, laboratory tests, diagnostic imaging, procedures such as back surgery and prostatectomy, and treatments at the end of life. A frequent example of overuse is antibiotic treatment of a cold virus. It confers no benefit and reduces the effectiveness of antibiotics because bacteria mutate and develop resistance. The surge of antibiotic-resistant bacteria is a testament to the misuse of antibiotics, and the public health impact is rightly worrisome.

Other forms of overuse put patients at immediate risk of harm, disability, and death. Research on back surgery published in the Journal of the American Medical Association identified overuse of complex fusion procedures for spinal stenosis. Patients suffered more major complications and higher mortality compared with evidence-based, less-intensive surgical interventions (Deyo et al., 2010). A study of implanted cardiac defibrillators reported that 23% of patients who had surgery to implant the device did not meet evidence-based guidelines (Al-Khatib et al., 2011). The risk of in-hospital death was significantly higher in patients who received a nonevidence-based device than in patients who received an evidence-based device. Certain hospitals had especially high rates, 40% or more, of inappropriate use of defibrillators.

Studies such as these do not report the names of the hospitals performing unnecessary surgeries. The defibrillator study was funded by the National Institutes of Health and paid for by taxpayers. But the public is precluded from knowing the hospitals that are putting patients in harm's way. In addition to the human cost, overuse has a high financial cost. More than $210 billion is wasted every year on unnecessary treatments and tests (Institute of Medicine, 2014). The cost of overuse draws resources away from care that underserved populations desperately require. It contributes to the unsustainably high levels of health care spending that are a growing burden on families, employers, and federal and state governments.

REASONS FOR OVERUSE

Multiple reasons explain overuse. Uncertainty is a fundamental challenge in health care. In the face of uncertainty, a clinician may try to address a patient's concern. A provider's belief, rather than knowledge, may guide practice.

Physicians, nurses, and patients have different beliefs about the role of medical care. Some believe that medical interventions are risky and a "less is more" approach is desirable. Others believe in the possibilities of medicine and that they should be explored in a context of uncertainty. Beliefs may evolve and become dogma, which is authoritative and reinforced by habit rather than evidence. Clinicians and patients can become enthusiastic about a treatment even when evidence unequivocally points to its folly.

Fear of missing a diagnosis drives overuse. A physician or nurse practitioner does not want to miss a diagnosis of cancer or other serious disease. The risk of medical liability can propel overuse.

Providers' expectations of each other can prompt overuse. When a primary care physician refers a patient for a diagnostic imaging test, a radiologist may not believe the test is warranted, but performs it anyway because a colleague requested it. A specialist may not want to jeopardize future referrals. Also, it can be time consuming to contact the referring physician and explain why the test is not needed.

Patient expectations drive overuse. When a patient requests an inappropriate antibiotic or screening test, busy primary care providers may comply to save time or placate a patient, even though they know they should not.

A clinician's competence and diagnostic skills affect whether patients receive appropriate care. Young physicians in training, who have yet to hone their diagnostic skills, may order more tests than are necessary.

FINANCIAL INCENTIVES AS THE MAJOR CAUSE OF OVERUSE

Fee-for-service payment for health care services has been the main driver of overuse. With virtually no limit on the volume of services that providers can bill, the design of the payment system has propelled overuse to epidemic proportions and launched a highly lucrative business model.

When Medicare was established, no health care companies were on the Fortune 100 list. Today, there are fifteen. Publicly traded health care companies have a fiduciary duty to shareholders to increase revenue and profitability. Shareholder expectations can be met in a limited number of ways: raise prices, increase sales volume, and reduce expenses. Not-for-profit organizations are not immune from the incentive structure and are also at risk of overtreating patients.

Higher volume of prescription drugs, diagnostic imaging, hospital admissions, and surgery strengthens the financial bottom line. Manufacturers that sell products, equipment, and supplies to hospitals have the incentive to sell more, not to choose wisely. This is the reason why overuse remains the most neglected quality challenge in the United States. Fixing it will cause revenue reductions for providers and manufacturers. Not fixing it means that the health care enterprise is propped up by putting patients in harm's way.

Through this lens, overuse causes two additional harms. First, physicians, nurses, and pharmacists are required by their organizations to accommodate a faster workflow. They do more procedures, administer more medications, and fill more prescriptions in the same amount of time. Demands for higher productivity in a health care system that is yet to be free from faulty design and defects inevitably cause more patients to be harmed. When a clinician makes a mistake, his or her confidence can be shaken, creating a risk for more mistakes.

Even the most competent clinician is at risk of harming a patient when forced to work at a pace faster than human factors engineering suggests is feasible. Moral distress is heightened. Highly skilled clinicians desire to meet their professional duty to the patient while their employer's requirements preclude them from doing so. A clinician cannot serve two masters whose interests are diametrically opposed.

This profound and disturbing conflict can drive out highly skilled, caring professionals from patient care as they seek other ways to employ their skills.

Health care delivery systems are at risk of being caught in a downward spiral whose logical conclusion is not a safer system for patients and caregivers.

THE MARINATED MIND

The business model of health care requires consumers and patients to be high users of health care services. A steady stream of advertisements for drugs, medical devices, tests, and procedures creates public expectations for medical care that may be unrealistic, unnecessary, and harmful. Television medical dramas portray testing and surgery as the norm to an unsuspecting public whose mind has been marinated to believe that more treatment is better (Gibson & Singh, 2010). The benefits of treatment are extolled while risks are underplayed.

A subset of the public is becoming more aware of overuse. An analysis of cardiac bypass surgery trends in a California hospital conducted by Dartmouth Atlas researchers shone a light on communities where patients were at risk of overuse of unnecessary bypass surgery. The analysis identified a hospital in Redding, California as having the highest rate of cardiac bypass surgery in the country in 2001 and 2002 (Dartmouth Atlas of Health Care, 2005). The rate had nearly doubled during the preceding decade. A sudden outbreak of serious heart disease warranting the increase in surgery volume was unlikely to be the underlying cause of the upward trend. Although this information was publicly available, Medicare officials did not intervene.

The overuse trend was interrupted only when a patient who was diagnosed as having blockages that required bypass surgery obtained a second opinion elsewhere and was given a clean bill of health. After he contacted the Federal Bureau of Investigation, it was determined that more than seven hundred patients had had unnecessary heart procedures. The hospital and doctors paid nearly $500 million in fines and penalties.

More recently, large-scale overuse of cardiac procedures occurred at a Maryland hospital. A U.S. Senate investigation that was widely reported in the media found that about 600 patients had been given unnecessary cardiac stents (United States Senate Committee on Finance, 2010). A patient complaint launched the initial inquiry, which resulted in the doctor losing his medical license and the hospital paying fines.

Eliminating overuse can be one of the most effective ways to keep patients safe and to reduce costs. Relying on patients to pull the emergency brake when overuse is evident is not an effective strategy. Public policies that enable public reporting of providers who are performing unnecessary tests and procedures are needed.

PHYSICIAN AND NURSE ACKNOWLEDGMENT OF OVERUSE

A breakthrough in the recognition of overuse as a widespread patient safety concern occurred with the launching of the Choosing Wisely campaign by the American Board of Internal Medicine Foundation. The aim of the campaign is to encourage physicians, other health care providers, and patients to engage in conversations to reduce overuse of tests and procedures (American Board of Internal Medicine Foundation, 2014). Approximately fifty medical specialty societies and other organizations have identified top five lists of tests or procedures commonly used whose necessity should be questioned and discussed. The American Geriatrics Society, for example, recommends that antipsychotics should not be used as a first choice to treat behavioral and psychological symptoms of dementia (American Geriatrics Society, 2014). The American College of Radiology recommends that patients do not have imaging tests when they have a common headache without risk factors (American College of Radiology, 2014). Under the auspices of the American Academy of Nursing, nursing leaders are developing a list of nursing activities that should be questioned, as part of the Choosing Wisely initiative.

Consumer Reports joined the Choosing Wisely campaign to translate the information on overused tests and procedures for consumers to help them talk with their doctors so they can get the care they need, not the care they do not need (Consumer Reports Health, 2014). Consumer Reports is distributing information to the public through employer organizations, such as the National Business Coalition on Health and the Pacific Business Group on Health.

PUBLIC REPORTING TO REDUCE OVERUSE

Public reporting of hospital-specific information is a strategy to reduce overuse. As an example, the Leapfrog Group, an employer-driven hospital quality watchdog group, asked hospitals to voluntarily report their rate of elective deliveries before 39 completed weeks of pregnancy. Babies have a higher risk of morbidity and mortality, and mothers have a higher risk of postpartum complications, when delivery occurs before a full 39 weeks gestation.

The Leapfrog Group publicly reported these rates and they generated substantial media attention (Leapfrog Group, 2013). By highlighting hospitals' overuse of early elective deliveries, public awareness created urgency for reform and improvement. Since the first hospital rates were publicly reported, the rate of early deliveries without medical necessity has been declining significantly. Many organizations are working to reduce these high-risk births, including the American College of Obstetrics and Gynecology and the American College of Nurse-Midwives.

Public reporting of overuse of diagnostic imaging has also helped to reduce unnecessary testing. Medicare's Hospital Compare website reports the hospitals that perform double chest CT scans. These double scans occur when patients receive two imaging tests consecutively, one without contrast and a second with contrast. Experts say that patients should receive one or the other, not both, to avoid excess exposure to radiation.

Radiation exposure has risks. Researchers at the National Cancer Institute estimated that approximately 29,000 future cancers and 14,500 deaths could be related to CT scans performed in the United States in 2007. Chest CT scans are among the contributors to the increase risk (Berrington de González et al., 2009).

The New York Times and the Washington Post published the first round of data from Medicare's website using interactive maps that allowed readers to identify hospitals that performed high rates of double chest CT scans (Appleby & Rau, 2011; Bogdanich & McGinty, 2011). More than 75,000 Medicare patients had double scans. Because Medicare data excludes patients with private and other insurance, the number of people having unnecessary scans is likely to be higher.

Members of the public are consumers of this data, as are hospital leaders and board members whose hospitals are overusing these scans. A hospital's visibility in the mainstream media can be a powerful stimulus for improvement. The reporting of overuse has encouraged some hospitals to reduce double chest CT scans (Chedekel, 2013).

JOURNALISTS ADVOCATE FOR MORE TRANSPARENCY ABOUT OVERUSE

Enterprising journalists have provided the public with valuable information about overtreatment. In addition, they have helped to change public policy to enable more data transparency on overuse.

The Wall Street Journal published a series of articles in 2010 that used Medicare claims data to identify billing patterns of individual doctors who participate in the program. The claims data is a computerized record of the bills Medicare pays. The journalists' analysis revealed clear cases of overtreatment. However, the journalists could not use the Medicare data to publish details of individual doctors' billings because of a 1979 court order barring disclosure of that information. Using additional sources, journalists pieced together profiles of physicians who were putting their patients at risk. For example, they identified a neurosurgeon who had the highest rate of multiple spinal-fusion surgeries among his peers and operated on some of his patients' spines as many as seven times (Carreyrou & McGinty, 2011).

The newspaper's parent company, Dow Jones, filed a lawsuit in 2011 to overturn a long-standing prohibition against the release of information on individual doctors' Medicare billing practices. In a major step toward transparency, a Florida judge ruled in May 2013 that the federal government should make the information available. In 2014, the Centers for Medicare and Medicaid Services (CMS) made Medicare data on physician payment information more transparent and accessible, while maintaining the privacy of beneficiaries (Blum, 2014). Journalists and researchers, along with the public, now have greater access to data to shine a light on overuse.

The wise use of health care resources is an imperative. The amount of money available for health care services is not unlimited. With proper stewardship, the nation can ensure that all Americans will receive the care they need, not the care they do not.

DISCUSSION QUESTIONS

1. Have you had medical care that you thought was unnecessary?
2. What is your top five list of most overused interventions in medicine and nursing?
3. What public policies can reduce overuse?

REFERENCES

Al-Khatib, S. M., Hellkamp, A., Curtis, J., Mark, D., Peterson, E., Sanders, G. D., et al. (2011). Non-evidence-based ICD implantations in the United States. *Journal of the American Medical Association, 305*(1), 43–49.

American Board of Internal Medicine Foundation. (2014). Choosing Wisely. Retrieved from *www.choosingwisely.org/about-us/*.

American College of Radiology. (2014). Choosing Wisely. Retrieved from *www.choosingwisely.org/doctor-patient-lists/american-college-of-radiology/*.

American Geriatrics Society. (2014). Choosing Wisely. Retrieved from *www.choosingwisely.org/doctor-patient-lists/american-geriatrics-society/*.

Appleby, J., & Rau, J. (2011). Many hospitals overuse double CT scans, data show. *Washington Post*. Retrieved from *www.washingtonpost.com/national/health-science/many-hospitals-overuse-double-ct-scans-data-shows/2011/06/16/AGvpTAaH_story.html*.

Berrington de González, A., Mahesh, M., Kim, K., Bhargavan, M., Lewis, R., Mettler, H. F., et al. (2009). Projected cancer risks from computed tomographic scans performed in the United States in 2007. *JAMA Internal Medicine, 169*(22), 2071–2077.

Blum, J. (2014). CMS modifies policy on disclosure of physician payment information. CMS Blog. Retrieved from *blog.cms.gov/2014/01/14/cms-modifies-policy-on-disclosure-of-physician-reimbursement-information/*.

Bogdanich, W., & McGinty, J. C. (2011). Medicare claims show overuse for CT scanning. *New York Times*. Retrieved from *www.nytimes.com/2011/06/18/health/18radiation.html?pagewanted=all&_r=0*.

Carreyrou, J., & McGinty, T. (2011). Hospital bars surgeon from operating room. *Wall Street Journal*. Retrieved from *online.wsj.com/news/articles/SB10001424052748704336504576259142044058726*.

Chedekel, L. (2013). Dempsey Hospital makes progress reducing double CT scans, *Connecticut Health I-Team*. Retrieved from *c-hit.org/2013/04/04/dempsey-hospital-makes-progress-reducing-double-ct-scans-2/*.

Consumer Reports Health. (2014). About the Choosing Wisely campaign. Retrieved from *consumerhealthchoices.org/campaigns/choosing-wisely/*.

Dartmouth Atlas of Health Care: Studies of Surgical Variation. (2005). Cardiac surgery report. Retrieved from *www.dartmouthatlas.org/downloads/reports/Cardiac_report_2005.pdf*.

Deyo, R. A., Mirza, S. K., Martin, B. I., Kreuter, W., Goodman, D. C., & Jarvik, J. G. (2010). Trends, major medical complications and charges associated with surgery for lumbar spinal stenosis in older adults. *Journal of the American Medical Association, 303*(13), 1259–1265.

Gibson, R., & Singh, J. P. (2010). *The treatment trap*. Chicago, Illinois: Ivan R. Dee.

Institute of Medicine. (2014). U.S. health care costs: Where is the money going? Retrieved from *resources.iom.edu/widgets/vsrt/healthcare-waste.html*.

Leapfrog Group. (2013). New data: Early elective deliveries decline at hospitals as health leaders caution against unnecessary deliveries. Retrieved from *www.leapfroggroup.org/policy_leadership/leapfrog_news/4976192*.

United States Senate Committee on Finance. (2010). *Staff report on cardiac stent usage at St. Joseph Medical Center*. S. PRT. 111–157.

ONLINE RESOURCES

Leapfrog Group
www.leapfroggroup.org
Medicare Hospital Compare
www.medicare.gov/hospitalcompare/search.html
ProPublica (a public interest investigative journalism group)
www.propublica.org

CHAPTER 23

Policy Approaches to Address Health Disparities

Carmen Alvarez   Antonia M. Villarruel

"Inequality is as dear to the American heart as liberty itself."

William Dean Howells

Health disparities refer to differences in the incidence, prevalence, mortality, and burden of diseases and other adverse health conditions that may exist among specific population groups (U.S. Department of Health and Human Services [HHS], 2000). Health disparities continue to persist by race and gender and social determinants of health (SDH) such as socioeconomic status (Braveman et al., 2010), English language proficiency (Lim, 2010), and insurance status (Chou et al., 2013). Collectively, these factors impact on a person's predisposition to illness, quality of life, and longevity. There have been many policy initiatives to address health disparities in general as well as specific priority areas, such as infant mortality (Underwood & Villarrueal, 2007). In the context of the rapid changes occurring in health care, we discuss policy opportunities, such as the Affordable Care Act (ACA), to reduce health care disparities.

HEALTH EQUITY AND ACCESS

Health equity can be defined as the "attainment of the highest level of health for all people" (HHS, 2010). If equity is described as fairness and opportunity, health equity refers to a person's opportunity to obtain optimal health and not be denied this opportunity based on social status or other such factors (Braveman, 2011). Health inequities in the United States remain a problem for, among others, racial and ethnic minorities, as well as low-income populations. An established contributor to poor health outcomes is a lack of access to health care. An increase in access to health care services is anticipated as a result of the implementation of the ACA.

POLICY APPROACHES TO ADDRESS HEALTH DISPARITIES

The provisions in the ACA hold great promise for reducing health disparities. African American women, for example, are more likely to be diagnosed with advanced-stage tumors and die from breast cancer more frequently compared with white women (Centers for Disease Control and Prevention [CDC], 2011). African Americans are more likely to be uninsured and underinsured (Duckett & Artiga, 2013). Upon implementation of the ACA, researchers estimate a 60% decrease in the number of uninsured women aged 18 to 64 in 2014 (Levy, Bruen, & Ku, 2012). This increase in insured women suggests that more women will be able to obtain timely screenings and have access to early treatment.

Another health disparity is infant mortality, with African American infants more likely to be born preterm and have almost three times the mortality rate as white babies (Hauck, Tanabe, & Moon, 2011). At greatest risk for these outcomes are low-income and uninsured women. Access to health insurance may support women obtaining health care before and between pregnancies (Markus et al., 2013).

In support of greater access to care is Medicaid expansion to include not only greater population coverage, but also greater preventative health coverage without cost-sharing, and more funding to state

Medicaid programs that choose to cover preventative services for patients (Mitchell & Baumracker, 2013). The expanded preventative services now covered by Medicaid include the successful Nurse Family Partnership (NFP) program, an evidence-based program designed to improve pregnancy outcomes, improve child health and development, and improve parental life course (Olds, 2006).

Not all states will participate in expanding Medicaid programs, particularly the Deep South states (Kaiser Family Foundation, 2013). This is an opportune time for nursing innovation to reach populations that will continue to have limited access to care. Nurses have exemplified innovation through education programs, such as the Family Farm Worker Health Program (Nichols, Stein, & Wold, 2014). It is an established 2-week service-learning opportunity where nurse practitioner students provide primary care services for migrant workers. Nurse practitioners hone their primary care skills, but more importantly a marginalized population obtains access to health care. Jill Rollet (2008) provided another example of a nurse leader and innovator. The author tells the story of how a nurse practitioner, who saw the need for home health care services for the elderly in her community, rose to the challenge to meet the demand.

The ACA has focused on policies that improve quality and increase access. Quality health care is as critical as access to health care. Research has established that low-income and minority groups often receive lower quality care than their wealthier white counterparts (Agency for Healthcare Research and Quality, 2013). The ACA calls for elevating quality of primary care for patients and funding the testing of models of care, such as the patient-centered medical home (PCMH).

The PCMH has been the model of care with the most promise to improve receipt of quality care and health outcomes. Using data from the National Survey of Children's Health, researchers demonstrated that children with access to medical homes were more likely to receive timely preventative services and less likely to have unmet medical needs (Strickland et al., 2011). Among a Latino population, those who had a PCMH were more likely to receive preventative services (Beal, Hernandez, &

Doty, 2009). Within the PCMH model, coordination between primary care, specialized providers, ancillary staff, and other health care establishments is improved and patients are thought to receive more patient-centered care (Bitton, Martin, & Landon, 2010). Although PCMH holds promise in reducing health disparities, findings from studies suggest that low-income and minority groups are less likely to have access to a PCMH (Strickland et al., 2011).

Already aligned with the PCMH model are community health centers (CHCs), such as federally qualified health centers and nurse-managed health centers. These types of health centers are part of the health care safety net that provides comprehensive, patient-centered, quality care to low-income, uninsured, and underserved populations (Esperat et al., 2012). Recognizing the unique contributions of CHCs to community health, the ACA has allocated $11 billion over 5 years for the expansion, operation, and development of CHCs (Shin et al., 2013). The Health Resources and Services Administration (HRSA) allocated another $150 million in grants to support CHC outreach and enrollment activities (Shin et al., 2014). With the implementation of health reform and Medicaid expansion in select states, CHCs will be providing more primary care to low-income populations. Payment strategies that adequately compensate CHC for providing patient-centered primary care to a high burdened clientele is needed. Given that CHCs often provide non-medical services (i.e., nutrition, dental services) for a community and not individuals, criteria that account for community-centered care need to be developed to guide payment for the comprehensive care provided (Ku et al., 2011).

Under the PCMH model, data on the health status and needs of a community would be more readily available. Based on the National Committee for Quality Assurance, PCMHs are required to have the capacity to collect and use data for their population management. They should be incentivized to explore how their patients' outcomes may be associated with social determinants of health, and supported to collaborate with local entities to address these challenges. For example, obesity remains a leading cause of morbidity, especially among

Blacks and Mexican-Americans. Contributing to the problem of obesity, particularly in low-income communities, are limited options for walking and purchasing fresh fruits and vegetables (CDC, 2010). PCMHs that recognize obesity as a major problem among their clientele could collaborate with local farmers and farmers' markets to provide fresh produce for the clientele and address food desserts in impoverished areas.

Although standards exist for classifying PCMHs, there remains a lack of clarity on standards of patient-centered care. Quality measures have largely focused on receipt of services, as indicated by standards of care and patient satisfaction (Bitton, Martin, & Landon, 2010). However, in striving to emphasize health promotion and preventative care there is a need to expand on these quality measures. Preventable diseases related to health behavior are significant contributors to the high cost of health care (Dower, 2013). Therefore, as PCMH strives to improve primary care and support health promotion, evaluation of patient-centered care, care in which providers work with patients to encourage healthy lifestyles, is warranted.

EVALUATING PATIENT-CENTERED CARE

Nurse-managed health centers have demonstrated expertise in providing quality care (Barkauskas et al., 2011) where patients report receiving continuity of care, being listened to, and feeling as though their needs are being met (Pohl et al., 2007). Potential indicators of patient-centered care are patient engagement and patient activation. Patient engagement is not solely about how one uses health care, but more about how providers work to include and empower individuals to be involved in, and aware of, health promotion and risk reduction. Patient activation refers to a person's "knowledge, skill, and confidence" in managing their health and health care (Hibbard, 2009). Level of patient activation has demonstrated a positive association with the management of chronic disease. Low levels of patient activation are associated with higher health care costs (Hibbard, 2009, 2013). Evaluation and reporting of engagement strategies, patient

activation, and health outcomes may better inform solutions for addressing social determinants of health and health disparities.

SUMMARY

This is an opportune time for nurse practitioners and nurse researchers to highlight the unique contributions of nursing to health promotion, particularly for low-income populations. Nursing expertise will be critical to implement the needed health system reforms, and our continued professional involvement with research, advocacy, community outreach, and policy will help ensure that underserved populations' health challenges are addressed. However, to successfully eliminate health disparities, a broad range of policy solutions must be developed. Nurses should continue their advocacy for eliminating scope-of-practice restrictions that prohibit nurses from practicing to the extent of their education and consequently decreasing access to care.

DISCUSSION QUESTIONS

1. One could argue that it is possible to provide patient-centered quality care outside of a PCMH designated clinic. What can nurses and nurse practitioners do to ensure such quality care regardless of the environment in which they practice?
2. What can nurses do to support looking beyond health care to address social determinants of health?

REFERENCES

Agency for Healthcare Research and Quality. (2013). 2012 National healthcare disparities report. Retrieved from *www.ahrq.gov/research/findings/nhqrdr/nhdr12/2012nhdr.pdf*

Barkauskas, V. H., Pohl, J. M., Tanner, C., Onifade, T. J. M., & Pilon, B. (2011). Quality of care in nurse-managed health centers. *Nursing Administration Quarterly, 35*(1), 34–43.

Beal, A., Hernandez, S., & Doty, M. (2009). Latino access to the patient-centered medical home. *Journal of General Internal Medicine, 24*(3 Suppl.), S514–S520.

Bitton, A., Martin, C., & Landon, B. E. (2010). A nationwide survey of patient centered medical home demonstration projects. *Journal of General Internal Medicine, 25*(6), 584–592.

Braveman, P. A. (2011). Monitoring equity in health and healthcare: A conceptual framework. *Journal of Health, Population, and Nutrition, 21*(3), 181–192.

Braveman, P. A., Cubbin, C., Egerter, S., Williams, D. R., & Pamuk, E. (2010). Socioeconomic disparities in health in the United States: What the patterns tell us. *American Journal of Public Health, 100*, S186–S196.

Centers for Disease Control and Prevention (2010). *DNPAO state program highlights. Improving retail access for fruits and vegetables.* Unpublished manuscript.

Centers for Disease Control and Prevention. (2011). CDC health disparities and inequalities report, United States, 2011. *Morbidity and Mortality Weekly Report, 60*(14), 11–37.

Chou, C., Tulolo, A., Raver, E., Hsa, C., & Young, G. (2013). Effect of race and health insurance on health disparities: Results from the national health interview survey 2010. *Journal of Health Care for the Poor & Underserved, 24*(3), 1353–1363.

Dower, C. (2013). Health policy brief: Health gaps. *Health Affairs.* Retrieved from *healthaffairs.org/healthpolicybriefs/brief_pdfs/healthpolicybrief_98.pdf.*

Duckett, P., & Artiga, S. (2013). Health coverage for the Black population today and under the Affordable Care Act. The Kaiser Family Foundation. Retrieved from *kff.org/disparities-policy/fact-sheet/health-coverage-for-the-black-population-today-and-under-the-affordable-care-act/.*

Esperat, M. C. R., Hanson-Turton, T., Richardson, M., Tyree Debisette, A., & Rupinta, C. (2012). Nurse-managed health centers: Safety-net care through advanced nursing practice. *Journal of the American Academy of Nurse Practitioners, 24*(1), 24–31.

Hauck, F. R., Tanabe, K. O., & Moon, R. Y. (2011). Racial and ethnic disparities in infant mortality. *Seminars in Perinatology, 35*(4), 209–220.

Hibbard, J. (2009). Improving the outcomes of disease management by tailoring care to the patient's level of activation. *The American Journal of Managed Care, 15*(6), 353.

Hibbard, J. H. (2013). Patients with lower activation associated with higher costs; delivery systems should know their patients' "scores". *Health Affairs (Millwood, Va.), 32*(2), 216–222.

Kaiser Family Foundation (2013). Characteristics of poor uninsured adults who fall into the coverage gap. Retrieved from *kff.org/health-reform/issue-brief/characteristics-of-poor-uninsured-adults-who-fall-into-the-coverage-gap/.*

Ku, L., Shin, P., Jones, E., & Bruen, B. (2011). Transforming community health centers into patient-centered medical homes: The role of payment reform. The Commonwealth Fund, Retrieved from *www.commonwealthfund.org/publications/fund-reports/2011/sep/transforming-community-health-centers.*

Levy, A. R., Bruen, B. K., & Ku, L. (2012). Health care reform and women's insurance coverage for breast and cervical cancer screening. *Preventing Chronic Disease, 9*(10).

Lim, J. (2010). Linguistic and ethnic disparities in breast and cervical cancer screening and health risk behaviors among Latina and Asian American women. *Journal of Women's Health, 19*(6), 1097–1107.

Markus, A. R., Andres, E., West, K. D., Garro, N., & Pellegrini, C. (2013). Medicaid covered birth, 2008 through 2010, in the context of the implementation of health reform. *Women's Health Issues, 23*(5), e273–e280.

Mitchell, A., & Baumracker, E. (2013). Medicaid's federal medical assistance percentage (FMAP), FY2014. *Congressional Research Service, Report for Congress.* Retrieved from *fas.org/sgp/crs/misc/R42941.pdf.*

Nichols, M., Stein, A. D., & Wold, J. L. (2014). Health status of children of migrant farm workers: Farm worker family health program, Moultrie, Georgia. *American Journal of Public Health, 104*(2), 365–370.

Olds, D. L. (2006). The nurse–family partnership: An evidence-based preventive intervention. *Infant Mental Health Journal, 27*(1), 5–25.

Pohl, J. M., Barkauskas, V. H., Benkert, R., Breer, L., & Bostrom, A. (2007). Impact of academic nurse-managed centers on communities served. *Journal of the American Academy of Nurse Practitioners, 19*(5), 268–275.

Rollet, J. (2008). 2008 NP entrepreneur of the year. Advance Health Care Network for NPs and PAs. Retrieved from *nurse-practitioners-and-physician-assistants.advanceweb.com/Article/2008-Nurse-Practitioner-Entrepreneur-of-the-Year.aspx.*

Shin, P., Sharac, J., Alvarez, C., & Rosenbaum, S. (2013). Community health centers in an era of health reform: An overview and key challenges to health center growth. Kaiser Commission on Medicaid and the Uninsured, Kaiser Family Foundation. Retrieved from *kff.org/health-reform/issue-brief/community-health-centers-in-an-era-of-health-reform-overview/.*

Shin, P., Sharac, J., Zur, J., Alvarez, C., & Rosenbaum, S. (2014). Assessing the potential impact of state policies on community health centers' outreach and enrollment activities. RCHN Community Health Foundation. Retrieved from *www.rchnfoundation.org/wp-content/uploads/2014/01/GG-policy-brief-CHC-OE-FINAL-unembargoed.pdf.*

Strickland, B. B., Jones, J. R., Ghandour, R. M., Kogan, M. D., & Newacheck, P. W. (2011). The medical home: Health care access and impact for children and youth in the United States. *Pediatrics, 127*(4), 604–611.

U.S. Department of Health and Human Services (2000). *Healthy people 2010: Understanding and improving health* (2nd ed.). Washington, DC: U.S. Government Printing Office.

U.S. Department of Health and Human Services (2010). National partnership for action to end health disparities. Retrieved from *www.minorityhealth.hhs.gov/npa/files/Plans/NSS/NSS_05_Section1.pdf.*

Underwood, L., & Villarrueal, A. (2007). Policy approaches to address health disparities. In D. Mason, J. Leavitt, & M. Chaffee (Eds.), *Policy & politics in nursing and health care* (6th ed.). St. Louis, MO: Elsevier.

ONLINE RESOURCES

The Kaiser Family Foundation Disparities Policy
kff.org/disparities-policy
The National Association for Community Health Centers
www.nachc.com
Agency for Healthcare Research and Quality Patient-Centered Medical Homes
www.pcmh.ahrq.gov/portal/server.pt/community/pcmh__home/1483

CHAPTER 24

Achieving Mental Health Parity

Freida Hopkins Outlaw   Patricia K. Bradley   Marie Davis Williams

"Of all the forms of inequality, injustice in health [mental health] is the most shocking and the most inhuman."

Martin Luther King, Jr., at the Second National Convention of the Medical Community for Human Rights, Chicago, March 25, 1966

The fight for mental health parity has been protracted and marked by many challenges, disappointments, and victories. Mental health parity refers to the equivalence of coverage for mental health treatment and clinical visits within insurance plans (Peters, 2006). Historically, many insurance plans have placed limits on services for patients with mental health and/or substance abuse diagnoses, while requiring the patients to pay more out-of-pocket costs for selected services than are required to be paid by patients who have medical conditions such as diabetes, asthma, or heart disease (Harvard Mental Health Letter [HMHL], 2009). Insurers and employers have been guarded about offering mental health and substance abuse coverage because of many factors; these include the stigma associated with mental illnesses and substance abuse and that many believe these disorders are untreatable or are otherwise too expensive to treat (Barry, 2006; Smaldone & Cullen-Drill, 2010). This disparity has had grave implications for those with mental health and substance abuse health care needs such as late or missed diagnosis, inadequate care, or individuals not seeking treatment for financial or social stigma reasons. Individuals, families, and society as a whole are impacted by this substantial disparity. It has been estimated that annually 26.2% of Americans aged 18 and over (1 in 4) experience a mental health disorder (National Institute of Mental Health [NIMH], 2014). Further, about 6% of this population (1 in 17) suffers from a serious mental illness (SMI). It has also been estimated that 45% of individuals with a mental disorder meet criteria for having two or more diagnosable mental illnesses. The cost of these mental disorders is estimated at $100 billion annually and is calculated by factoring in the cost of care as well as the lost productivity by those affected including absenteeism, short-term disability absences, and on-the-job productivity (Burton et al., 2008; Marth, 2009).

This chapter describes the historical struggle to achieve mental health and substance abuse parity, passage of the Mental Health Parity Act (MHPA), the Mental Health Parity Addiction Equity Act (MHPAEA), and the influence of the Affordable Care Act (ACA) on expanding parity requirements. It also describes gaps in the parity laws and challenges of implementing the law at both state and national levels. Recommendations for all psychiatric nurses with specific attention to Advanced Practice Psychiatric Nurses are offered.

HISTORICAL STRUGGLE TO ACHIEVE MENTAL HEALTH PARITY

Since the early 1970s, mental health advocates have been working in conjunction with federal legislators to secure the passage of mental health parity legislation (United States Department of Health and Human Services [HHS], 1999). Senators Paul Wellstone (D-WI) and Pete Domenici (R-NM) led the effort to achieve mental health parity. They spearheaded legislation in the U.S. Senate and were able to insert partial parity language into a bill, preventing insurance plans from being able to pay less to treat mental health disorders compared with what they paid to treat physical health conditions

(Levinson & Druss, 2000). This first incremental step toward mental health parity was enabled by the passage of the Mental Health Parity Act (MHPA) of 1996, which went into effect on January 1, 1998. The MHPA applied to two types of coverage: large group self-funded health plans and large group fully insured group health plans.

One of the flaws of the 1996 Mental Health Parity Act was that it did not contain a substance abuse benefit, in spite of the fact that substance abuse and mental health conditions often occur together (Kuehn, 2010). In 2002, the National Survey on Drug Use and Health estimated 17.5 million adults from a representative survey of 68,000 individuals in the United States had a serious mental illness, with about 23% of them either abusing or dependent on alcohol or illicit drugs (Kuehn, 2010). Researchers have determined that when only one of the cooccurring disorders (mental illness or substance abuse disorder) is treated, both disorders usually get worse. In addition to the tremendous suffering that the individual with an untreated or poorly treated cooccurring disorder and their family experience, these individuals also use the most costly services, such as emergency rooms and inpatient facilities, and have the worse clinical outcomes (New Freedom Commission on Mental Health [NFCMH], 2003).

In 2008 a more expansive parity bill, the Wellstone and Domenici Mental Health Parity and Addiction Equity Act of 2008 (MHPAEA) was passed. This bill included a substance abuse benefit. Also, in 2008, Congress passed the Medicare Improvements for Patients Act (MIPA), which supplemented the mental health parity laws for Medicare recipients in every state except Idaho and Wyoming (HMHL, 2009). Currently, 49 states and the District of Columbia have some form of legislated mental health parity law, although they vary significantly (see National Conference of State Legislatures [NCSL], 2014 for a list of Fully Parity, Minimum Mandated Benefit, and Mandated Offering State Laws).

MEANING OF PARITY FOR MENTAL HEALTH AND ADDICTION TREATMENT

The MHPAEA, signed into law by President George W. Bush in October 2008, affects large employers, Medicaid managed care plans, and some State Children's Health Insurance Program (SCHIP) plans (HMHL, 2009; Smaldone & Cullen-Drill, 2010). Specifically, it amended the Mental Health Parity Act (MHPA) of 1996 by stipulating businesses with 51 or more employees, who offer a health insurance plan with mental health and substance abuse coverage, offer these benefits at the same level as their medical and surgical coverage. It means that deductibles, copayments, out-of-pocket expenses, outpatient visits, inpatient stays, and treatment limits must be the same for mental health and substance abuse treatment as they are for medical and surgical services (Melek, 2009; United States Department of Labor, 2010).

In the 2008 MHPAEA, there were no requirements as to which mental health or substance abuse conditions must be covered, but whatever was covered had to be at parity with medical coverage. This was a huge improvement for mental health and substance abuse treatment because historically there has been strict limitations placed on patient visits. Additionally, flexibility in the scope and duration of treatment has been associated with positive treatment outcomes in substance abuse as well as mental health conditions (Swanke & Zeman, 2011). Benefits offered to out-of-network coverage were extended so that insurance plans had to offer out-of-network coverage for mental health and substances abuse services if it did so for medical or surgical services. This legislation also put into place an oversight mechanism to determine if insurers were discriminating against certain conditions. It allowed a cost-based exemption if the insurer could prove that parity raised their total plan costs by greater than 2% or more in the first year after enactment (Melek, 2009; U.S. Department of Labor, 2012).

The Wellstone-Domenici Act of 2008 became law on January 1, 2010 and the interim final rules became effective on April 5, 2010. The new federal rules providing mental health parity were effective for insurance plans whose renewal date began on or after July 1, 2010 and covered 82 million individuals in self-insured employer health plans that were not governed by state parity laws, and an additional 31 million employees in plans that were subject to state regulations (HMHL, 2009). On November 8, 2013 the Departments of Treasury, Labor, and Health and Human Services issued a final rule specifying how to apply the Paul Wellstone and Pete Domenici MHPAEA to insurance plans. The Wellstone-Domenici Parity Act still does not require that insurance plans provide mental health or substance use benefits if they are not already offered in their insurance plan, but it does require that plans which do offer mental health and substance abuse coverage to their participants provide parity in their medical, mental health, and substance abuse coverage and care management.

GAPS IN THE MENTAL HEALTH PARITY LAWS

Clearly the MHPA of 1996 and the MHPAEA of 2008 represent steps forward. There are, however, gaps in the laws that need to be addressed. For example, the bills do not mandate mental health and substance abuse coverage, and services provided through most commercial plans do not include evidence supported recovery services for persons with severe and persistent mental illness. recovery-based services for persons with severe and persistent mental illness. Presently recovery services are not mandated in the parity laws but states can include them as a covered service if they choose to do so.

Recovery is defined by the New Freedom Commission on Mental Health (NFCMH, 2003) as the "process in which people [with serious mental illnesses] are able to live, work, learn, and participate fully in their communities" (p. 5). Recovery-based services in mental health treatment include those that encompass self-direction and empowerment, are holistic and strength-based, provide peer support, and develop responsibility and hope. For example, researchers have noted that individuals with serious emotional illnesses who have hope, usually linked with peer and family support, have higher rates of recovery from their symptoms (Substance Abuse and Mental Health Services Administration [SAMHSA], 2006).

Recovery-based services such as supportive housing and supported employment are not usually covered by the Medicaid program or commercial insurances as many of these services do not meet medical necessity criteria. As a result, there is limited payment for services identified as essential for the treatment of the person's illness, injury, or condition. Medical necessity criteria often exclude anything deemed experimental or not yet proven.

MENTAL HEALTH PARITY AND ADDICTION EQUITY ACT AND THE ACA

Many mental health and addiction experts have recognized the passing of the parity laws as a critical step toward moving the treatment of mental health and addiction disorders into the mainstream of medical care in the United States (Barry and Huskamp, 2011). Most also agree that although the fight is not over, the passage of the Affordable Care Act (ACA) has been an important vehicle for improving the access and fragmentation issues that impact the delivery of effective mental health and addiction services. The ACA ensures that people will be provided health care including equitable mental health treatment as well as evidence-based mental health and addiction services (Lieberman, 2013). It specifically improves access for many people who would otherwise not have coverage as it requires most insurance plans to cover both mental health and addiction services at parity with medical and surgical services (Barry and Huskamp, 2011). The ACA also addresses long-standing delivery system issues such as fragmentation of services, including the lack of integration of primary care and mental health and addiction services, lack of coordination of services, and the very limited use of evidence-based practices to treat cooccurring mental health and substance use disorders (Barry and Huskamp, 2011). Coordinated services are important as it has been established that people with serious mental illnesses die from mostly modifiable risk factors such as smoking, obesity, substance use including alcohol abuse, and poor medical care (Barry and Huskamp, 2011) at least 25 years earlier than the general population (National Association of State Mental Health Program Directors [NASMHPD], 2006)

STATE-LEVEL IMPLEMENTATION

Wide variances exist at the state level with some states limiting the benefit expansion to specific mental illnesses; however, the new federal law replaces less comprehensive state laws while the more comprehensive state laws remain intact (HMHL, 2009). Garfield (2009) found in her research that states are primarily influenced by their own problems and the resources available to them, and are only guided by national efforts if they are congruent with their particular state's idiosyncrasies. Most insurers were concerned with the passage of parity legislation as they feared that health care costs would rise at an unsustainable rate. In fact, this has not been the case; health care costs have not increased significantly.

Mental health parity legislation is a critical step toward ameliorating many of the negative economic conditions for the states by increasing the work productivity of employees who need, but have not been able to receive, mental health and substance abuse services because of discrimination in benefit design and plan administration associated with mental health and addiction treatment compared with other health conditions (NASMHPD, 2012). As a result of the passage of the MHPAEA, effective and adequate treatment can be accessed enabling employees to remain in the workforce, thus eliminating lost time at work and other negative aspects associated with untreated mental health and addiction disorders.

CHALLENGES IN IMPLEMENTING THE LAW

As insurers begin to provide mental health and addiction services they will be wise to implement those services that have been found to be evidence based. The Institute of Medicine (IOM, 2001) defines evidence-based medicine as the integration of best researched evidence and clinical expertise with patient values. States can advance evidence-based practices by using dissemination and demonstration projects and creating public-private partnerships to guide this implementation (NFCMH, 2003).

The Bringing Science to Service initiative is intended to make approaches that are supported by research widely available to patients and families (Isett et al., 2007). The first group of disseminated evidenced-based practices that support and enhance recovery-based psychiatric rehabilitation included assertive community treatment, supported employment, illness management and recovery, integrated treatment for cooccurring mental illness and substance abuse, family education, and medication management. Although by no means an exhaustive list of evidence-based practices, these represent those practices that the Center for Medicare and Medicaid Services (CMS) believes have undergone rigorous research and study and have proven outcomes. Yet to date, the implementation of these initiatives has been inconsistent in mental health and substance abuse treatment.

A major challenge to implementation is the lack of public awareness of the Mental Health and Substance Use Health Coverage Law. A recent survey conducted by the American Psychological Association (2014) found that only 4% of adults were aware of the Mental Health Parity and Addiction Equality Act of 2008 and the benefits it provides. Lack of knowledge of the benefits these laws provide is a major barrier to people with mental health and addiction disorders getting the care that they need.

IMPLICATIONS FOR NURSING: MENTAL HEALTH RELATED ISSUES AND STRATEGIES

Nurses can influence the knowledge, beliefs, and attitudes toward mental health and substance use illnesses, as well as the creation and implementation of evidence-based culturally competent interventions for people with mental health, substance use, and cooccurring disorders, through their involvement with politics and policy at the community (local), state, and national levels. One example of this is the formation of collaborative coalitions among leading psychiatric nursing entities such as the psychiatric nursing and substance use disorders expert panel of the American Academy of Nursing, American Nurses Association, American Psychiatric Nurses Association, International Society of Psychiatric Mental-Health Nurses, and The International Nurses Society on Addictions. Furthermore, advanced practice psychiatric nurses (APPNs) are educated as psychiatric mental health-clinical nurse specialists

(PMH-CNS) or psychiatric mental health-nurse practitioners (PMH-NP). Unlike other specialty groups in nursing where the CNS role was more system oriented, the PMH-CNS role developed as direct providers (Hanrahan, Delaney, & Merwin, 2010), with established roles as nurse psychotherapists in health care agencies and independent practice.

Issue: The Mental Health Parity and Addictions Equity Act of 2008 provides new mental health and substance abuse benefits. Consumers of mental health and substance abuse services and their families may not know or understand the extent of what mental health parity and addiction equity means for their health care.

Strategy: Psychiatric nurses at all levels of preparation and experience are in a strong position to provide leadership in achieving mental health and addiction equity for those individuals who need these services as they are excellent in engaging patients to become and stay involved in their treatment (Pearson et al., 2014). Psychiatric nurses are also trusted consumer advocates and educators. Becoming knowledgeable about the law and regulations and developing proficiency in disseminating this information to ensure that consumers are receiving the full benefits to promote recovery is an imperative for nurses.

Issue: Gaps in the law remain relative to the vital services that are needed to support people with severe and persistent mental illness and substance abuse disorders.

Strategy: Psychiatric nurses need to be involved in policy development at the local, state, and national levels mandating a array of services that are not covered by the parity law or the ACA but that are effective for individuals with severe mental illness and substance abuse disorders.

Issue: As result of the new Mental Health Parity and Addictions Equity Act of 2008 and the Affordable Care Act of 2010 an increased number of diverse individuals will have access to services which will put a strain on the existing inadequate network of providers.

Strategy 1: APPNs as proven expert frontline mental health providers skillful in engaging diverse populations can take the lead in providing evidence-based and culturally competent mental health and substance abuse services to a diverse population of patients, thus expanding the provider network.

Strategy 2: Psychiatric nurse educators must include emerging evidence-based practices and health policies in curriculums that support and enhance recovery-based psychiatric rehabilitation services.

Strategy 3: Doctorally prepared psychiatric nurse researchers must be in the forefront of generating science that informs both the treatment and policy initiatives associated with mental health, substance abuse, and cooccurring disorders.

DISCUSSION QUESTIONS

1. Are your state's mental health parity laws more comprehensive or less comprehensive than the federal laws and in what ways?
2. How are consumers in your workplace (hospital, community mental health center, etc.) educated about the benefits that they are entitled to as a result of the 2008 MHPAEA?
3. What components would you include in an educational program for consumers about the benefits of the 2008 MHPAEA?
4. How important is it for psychiatric nurses at all levels to be involved in mental health policy such as the MHPAEA of 2008? Please describe.

REFERENCES

American Psychological Association. (2014). 2014 Mental health parity survey. Retrieved from *www.apa.org/helpcenter/parity-survey-2014.pdf.*

Barry, C. L. (2006). The political evolution of mental health parity. *Harvard Review of Psychiatry, 14*(4), 185–194.

Barry, C. L., & Huskamp, H. A. (2011). Moving beyond parity—Mental health and addiction care under the ACA. *New England Journal of Medicine, 365*(11), 973–975.

Burton, W. N., Schultz, A. B., Chen, C.-Y., & Edington, D. W. (2008). The association of worker productivity and mental health: A review of the literature. *International Journal of Workplace Health Management, 1*(2), 78–94.

Garfield, R. L. (2009). Mental health policy development in the states: The piecemeal nature of transformational change. *Psychiatric Services, 60*(10), 1329–1335.

Hanrahan, N. P., Delaney, K., & Merwin, E. (2010). Health care reform and the federal transformation initiatives: Capitalizing on the potential of advanced practice psychiatric nurses. *Policy Politics & Nursing Practice,* *11*(3), 235–244.

Harvard Mental Health Letter [HMHL]. (2009). Benefiting from mental health parity: Determining coverage, understanding the limits, and appealing decisions. *Harvard Mental Health Letter, 25*(7), 4–5.

Institute of Medicine [IOM]. (2001). *Crossing the quality chasm: A new health system.* Washington, D.C.: National Academies Press.

Isett, K. R., Burnam, M. A., Coleman-Beattie, B., Hyde, P. S., Morrissey, J. P., Magnabosco, J., et al. (2007). The state policy context of implementation issues for evidence-based practices in mental health. *Psychiatric Services, 58*(7), 914–921.

Kuehn, B. M. (2010). Integrated care key for patients with both addiction and mental illness. *JAMA: The Journal of the American Medical Association, 303*(19), 1905–1907.

Levinson, C. M., & Druss, B. G. (2000). The evolution of mental health parity in American politics. *Administration and Policy in Mental Health, 29*(2), 139–145.

Lieberman, J. A. (2013). How will healthcare reform affect psychiatry coverage? *Medscape Psychiatry,* WebMD, LLC. Retrieved from *www.medscape.com/viewarticle/810906.*

Marth, D. (2009). Mental Health Parity Act of 2007: An analysis of the proposed changes. *Social Work in Mental Health, 7*(6), 556–571.

Melek, S. (2009). Preparing for parity: Investing in mental health. Retrieved from *www.milliman.com/expertise/healthcare/publications/rr/pdfs/preparing-parity-investing-mental-WP05-01-09.pdf.*

National Association of State Mental Health Program Directors (NASMHPD). (2006). NASMHPD Medical Directors Council technical report: Morbidity and mortality in people with serious mental illness. Alexandria, VA. Retrieved from *www.nasmhpd.org/docs/publications/MDC docs/Mortality%20and%20Morbidity%20Final%20Report%208.18.08.pdf.*

National Association of State Mental Health Program Directors. (2012). Fact sheet on implementing mental health parity: The SBHA role. Retrieved from *www.nasmhpd.org/docs/Policy/Parity_Fact%20Sheet%20on%20Implementing%20MH%20Parity.pdf.*

National Conference of State Legislatures [NCSL]. (2014). State laws mandating or regulating mental health benefits. Retrieved from *www.ncsl.org/IssuesResearch/Health/StateLawsMandatingorRegulatingMenatlHealthB/tabid/14352/Default.aspx.*

National Institute of Mental Health [NIMH]. (2014). The numbers count: Mental disorders in America. Retrieved from *www.nimh.nih.gov/health/publications/the-numbers-count-mental-disorders-in-america/index.shtml.*

New Freedom Commission on Mental Health [NFCMH]. (2003). Achieving the promise: Transforming mental health care in America. Final report. DHHS Pub. No. SMA-03-3832. Rockville, MD: United States Department of Health and Human Services. Retrieved from *www.michigan.gov/documents/NewFreedomMHReportExSum_83175_7.pdf.*

Pearson, G. S., Evans, L. K., Hines-Martin, V. P., Yearwood, E., York, J. A., & Kane, C. F. (2014). Promoting the mental health of families. *Nursing Outlook, 62*(3), 225–227.

Peters, J. (2006). Mental health parity: Legislation and implications for insurers and providers. *The Heinz Journal, 3*(2), 1–9.

Smaldone, A., & Cullen-Drill, M. (2010). Mental health parity legislation: Understanding the pros and cons. *Journal of Psychosocial Nursing & Mental Health Services, 48*(9), 26–34.

Substance Abuse and Mental Health Services Administration (SAMHSA). (2006). National consensus statement on mental health recovery. Rockville, MD: USDHHS, CMHS. Retrieved from *www.power2u.org/downloads/SAMHSA%20Recovery%20Statement.pdf.*

Swanke, J. R., & Zeman, L. D. (2011). Parity not perfect: Making sense of substance addiction equity for case managers. *Case Management Journals, 12*(3), 101–107.

United States Department of Health and Human Services. [HHS]. (1999). *Mental health: A report of the Surgeon General.* Rockville, MD: National Institute of Mental Health. Retrieved from *profiles.nlm.nih.gov/ps/access/NNBBHS.pdf.*

United States Department of Labor. (2010). Mental health parity. Retrieved from *www.dol.gov/ebsa/mentalhealthparity/.*

United States Department of Labor. (2012). Report to Congress: Compliance with requirements of the Mental Health Parity and Addiction Equality Act of 2008. Retrieved from *www.dol.gov/ebsa/publications/mhpaeareporttocongress2012.html.*

ONLINE RESOURCES

Department of Treasury, Labor and Health and Human Services final rule governing the implementation of the Paul Wellstone and Pete Domenici MHPAEA

www.dol.gov/ebsa/pdf/mhpaeafinalrule.pdf

State Laws Mandating or Regulating Mental Health Benefits

www.ncsl.org/IssuesResearch/Health/StateLawsMandatingorRegulatingMenatlHealthB/tabid/14352/Default.aspx

Fact Sheet: The Mental Health Parity and Addiction Equity Act of 2008 (MHPAEA)

www.cms.gov/CCIIO/Programs-and-Initiatives/Other-Insurance-Protections/mhpaea_factsheet.html

FAQs about ACA Implementation Part XVII and Mental Health Parity Implementation

www.dol.gov/ebsa/faqs/faq-aca17.html

Breaking the Social Security Glass Ceiling: A Proposal to Modernize Women's Benefits[1]

Carroll L. Estes   Terry O'Neill   Heidi Hartmann

"We must begin by insuring that the Social Security system is beyond challenge. [It is] a vital obligation each generation has to those who have worked hard and contributed to it all their lives."

Gerald R. Ford

Although Social Security is a program that is vitally important to all Americans, it is especially critical to the financial security of women. Women live longer than men and on average women today who reach the age of 65 outlive men by 2.3 years (Social Security Administration, 2014). These additional years of longevity increase the risk that women may outlive their savings or that their pensions may lose their purchasing power. For women of color, greater longevity is particularly challenging.

Women, and especially women of color, are less likely than men to have employer pensions. On average, only 28% of women age 65 to 74 receive a pension income compared with 42% of men age 65 to 74 (Institute for Women's Policy Research, 2011). Where women do have pensions, they tend to be smaller on average than those earned by men. The picture is even more dismal for individuals from communities of color, where less than half of employed African Americans and less than

one-third of employed Latinos are covered by employer-sponsored retirement plans (Rhee, 2012).

Women depend substantially in retirement on the benefits they receive from Social Security. These benefits last a lifetime and unlike many private pensions, Social Security benefits are adjusted for increases in inflation. In 2010, 46% of elderly unmarried men and 58% of elderly unmarried women of color relied on Social Security for 90% or more of their total income (United States Census Bureau, 2012).

As women have increased their participation in the workforce, the number of women insured to receive Social Security benefits has grown. Although men are still more likely than women to be insured for Social Security retirement and disability benefits, the gender gap is shrinking. Both Social Security retirement and disability benefits require older adult workers to have 40 quarters of coverage (work credits) to be fully insured for benefits. These can be earned at any time during a worker's life. To be fully insured for disability benefits, a worker must have what is called a current connection with the workforce which means that in addition to having a total of 40 quarters, an individual must also have worked for 5 of the 10 years preceding the start of the disability to qualify for disability benefits.

Constituting a majority of all Social Security beneficiaries, women depend more than men on the program for their support in retirement and old age. Women live longer than men, have a history of lower earnings during their working years, take more time out of the work force to care for family

---

[1]This chapter is adapted from the report *Breaking the Social Security Glass Ceiling: A Proposal to Modernize Women's Benefits,* with permission from the National Committee to Preserve Social Security and Medicare Foundation.

members, and live in more difficult economic circumstances (Rockeymoore & Meizhu, 2011). As a result, they enter retirement with little or no protection from private pensions, inadequate retirement savings, and smaller Social Security benefits than those received by men.

The effects of these disparities are magnified for women of color. They are disproportionally lower earners and are more likely to have worked in part-time positions (Rockeymoore & Meizhu, 2011). A substantial segment of women of color, especially if single, approach retirement with little or no retirement savings and little access to private pensions (Insight Center for Community and Economic Development, 2010). The absence of alternative financial support has the effect of leaving women of color primarily dependent on what is usually a very modest Social Security retirement income. Further, families of color are more dependent than other families on survivor and disability benefits under Social Security (Rockeymoore & Meizhu, 2011).

BENEFITS FOR WOMEN

Since Social Security began paying monthly benefits in 1939, the program has offered a broad array of benefits for women. Women who are insured on their own earnings records can qualify for either retirement or disability benefits based on those earnings. If married, a woman may also be eligible for a spouse's or widow's benefit based on a husband's earnings record. A married woman who is eligible both for her own Social Security benefit and a spousal benefit can receive more from Social Security if the amount payable as a spouse is higher than her benefit. In other words, she can receive her benefit plus the difference between her benefit and the spouse's or widow's benefit.

Women who have been married more than once might be eligible on one or more spouses' records in addition to their own. To qualify for divorced wife's or divorced widow's benefits, the marriage must meet the duration of marriage test. Under the current test, a marriage must have lasted for a minimum of 10 years. If divorce occurs before 10 years of marriage, a woman is not eligible for

benefits on that husband's work record. If divorce occurs after 10 or more years of marriage, a woman can qualify for the same spousal benefit she would have received had there been no divorce.

Early retirement also reduces benefits. A disabled or older widow with no work experience may have no choice but to apply for a reduced benefit at the earliest age of eligibility. For those who are not disabled, the earliest age of eligibility for a widow's benefit is 60. Social Security offers little incentive for widows to defer filing for benefits because, if the deceased spouse retired early as is often the case, her benefits will be reduced based on the husband's decision to claim early retirement.

The average woman generally receives a substantially smaller Social Security check than a male worker. In 2009, the average annual Social Security income of a retired man was $15,620, while the average yearly income of a retired woman was $12,155. This disparity is explained in part because women generally have lower earnings than men. For example, in 2009, the median earnings of full-time working age women was $35,000 annually, compared with $46,800 for men (Institute for Women's Policy Research, 2011). Additionally, women are more likely to spend years outside the workforce providing uncompensated care to children and other family members.

In 2009, more than 20 million women over the age of 65 received Social Security benefits (Joint Economic Committee, 2010). A woman who reaches age 65 today can expect to live an additional 20.7 years (The Board of Trustees, Federal Old-Age and Survivors Insurance and Federal Disability Insurance Trust Funds, 2012). For these women, Social Security represents a critical source of income and is often their only available hedge against inflation. Without it, over half of these women would be living in poverty. Even with Social Security, 12% of older women and 15% of widows still live in poverty. This is 50% higher than the poverty rate for all people aged 65 and older.

The problem is even greater for women of color. In 2009, 26.1% of African American women who were 75 or older and who were receiving Social Security were living in poverty. For Hispanic women of the same age, 21.4% were living in poverty, despite the fact that they were receiving Social Security (Hartman, Hayes, & Drago, 2011).

A husband's death can lead to enormous financial hardship. Currently when a woman's husband dies, the total amount of Social Security benefits paid to the household is reduced by as much as 33% to 50%. The reduction is larger for households in which both spouses have had nearly equal earnings. As more women entered the workforce in the second half of the twentieth century, their contribution to total household income increased; however, Social Security rules have not been updated to reflect this change. Consequently this increased contribution to household income by wives may not result in higher Social Security benefits.

As increasing numbers of women earn wages that equal or exceed those of their husbands, more of them will experience a benefit reduction approaching 50% of household Social Security benefits when the husband dies. To illustrate this point consider the case of a couple where both husband and wife worked. Each receives $1500 per month for a combined family benefit of $3000. When the husband dies, the woman's monthly Social Security benefit remains $1,500, while the husband's benefit ends. She receives no widow's benefit because her own Social Security benefit is equal to her husband's benefit. Thus, the effect of the husband's death is to reduce the total family benefit by 50%. By contrast, if this same woman had no Social Security on her own record and instead received a wife's benefit of $750, the total family benefit would be $2,250. Upon the husband's death, the widow would receive a benefit of $1,500, the same amount that was being paid to her late husband. In this case, the reduction in the total family benefit would be 33%. The effect of this reduction can be devastating, especially for women living alone after age 65, for women of color who are more likely to be poor, and for women from low-earning or wealth-depleted households.

STRENGTHENING THE PROGRAM

The following proposals would improve benefit equity and safeguard benefits for women.

IMPROVING SURVIVOR BENEFITS

Women living alone often are forced into poverty because of benefit reductions stemming from the death of a spouse. Widows from low-earning or wealth-depleted households are particularly at risk of poverty. Providing a widow or widower with 75% of the couple's combined benefit treats one-earner and two-earner couples more fairly and reduces the likelihood of leaving the survivor in poverty. The new benefit would be capped at the benefit level of a lifelong average earner (about $1584 for an individual retiring at age 66 in 2012).

Proposal: Increase the benefit paid to a surviving spouse to an amount that is equal to 75% of the total combined benefits that were paid to the couple prior to the spouse's death, capped at the benefit level of a lifelong average earner.

PROVIDING CREDITS FOR CAREGIVERS

One of the principal reasons women have fewer assets and less income in retirement than men is that they often interrupt their participation in the labor force to care for children and, increasingly, elderly parents, parents-in-law, and other family members. Because of the nature of the formula used in its calculation, these temporary interruptions can lead to a significant reduction in the amount of Social Security benefit payable. These interruptions occur for unmarried women as well as married women since women increasingly have children outside marriage and many adults, whether married or not, care for other family members. Until now, spousal benefits have been the only way women were partially compensated for caregiving.

Accordingly, we recommend a revision in the computation of the Average Indexed Monthly Earnings (AIME) primary insurance amount (PIA). The AIME PIA is the amount that a worker can receive if application for benefits is deferred until reaching the normal retirement age (NRA). Imputed earnings for up to 5 family service years would be granted to a worker who leaves or reduces his/her participation in the work force to provide care to children under the age of 6 or to elderly or disabled family members. This proposal would also help women who are not eligible for spousal benefits because they never married or else had marriages that lasted for fewer than 10 years.

Proposal: Compute the AIME PIA by imputing an annual wage for each family service year so that total earnings for the year would equal 50% of that year's average annual wage index. Family service years would be those in which an individual provides care to children under the age of 6 or to elderly or disabled family members. Up to 5 family service years could be granted to any worker.

ENHANCING THE SPECIAL MINIMUM PIA

In addition to computing the AIME PIA, Social Security also calculates a worker's monthly benefit based on an alternative computational method known as the Special Minimum PIA. If this method results in a higher benefit then the worker's payment is based on this computation. The intent is to provide a more adequate benefit to those who have spent the preponderance of their working lives in low-wage employment. However, because the Special Minimum Benefit has been indexed for many years to inflation rather than to growth in wages it now requires updating. The computation should also incorporate the concept of providing years of coverage to those who must leave the workforce to provide care to family members.

Proposal: Improve the Special Minimum Benefit, by increasing the benefit to equal 150% of the aged poverty level for workers with 30 years of credit, indexing future increases in the minimum benefit to growth in wages rather than the CPI, and providing up to 10 family service years of credit toward the computation of the benefit.

EQUALIZING RULES FOR DISABLED WIDOWS AND WIDOWERS

Widows and surviving divorced spouses can qualify for disabled widow's benefits beginning at age 50. They are the only disabled persons whose benefits are subject to an actuarial reduction (most individuals who apply for Social Security benefits prior to attaining their full retirement age have their benefits reduced to make sure that, on average, there is no increase in the total lifetime benefits paid as a result of the early claiming of benefits. The

resulting adjustment is called an actuarial reduction.) The amount of this reduction is 28.5% of the deceased spouse's full retirement age (FRA) benefit. In contrast, the benefits paid to disabled workers are not actuarially reduced. Instead, they receive 100% of the full retirement age benefit.

Proposal: Treat disabled widows and surviving divorced spouses in the same manner as other disabled individuals in determining their eligibility for benefits by eliminating: (1) the provision that restricts eligibility to widows who are age 50 or older, (2) the actuarial reduction that currently accompanies eligibility for disabled widow's benefits, and (3) the 7-year time limit for when widows must become disabled to qualify for benefits.

BENEFIT EQUALITY FOR WORKING WIDOWS AND SURVIVING DIVORCED HUSBANDS

Under current law, the benefit for widows and surviving divorced spouses is capped at the amount the deceased husband would have received if he were still alive. If a husband retires before normal retirement age his widow inherits his early retirement reduction; however, the amount of the reduction is limited to no more than 82.5% of the wage earner's full benefit. Apart from that limited protection, a widow can neither cancel her husband's early retirement reduction nor enhance her widow's benefit by delaying her own retirement. We believe that the widow's benefit, including benefits for surviving divorced spouses, should no longer be tethered to the reduction her deceased spouse elected to receive when he applied for retirement benefits.

Proposal: Eliminate the pass-through to widows and surviving divorced spouses of the actuarial reduction that stems from their husbands' decisions about when to apply for retirement benefits. The only factor that should be relevant in determining a widow's benefit should be the actuarial reduction that results from the surviving spouse's own decisions about when to retire.

STRENGTHENING THE COLA

When automatic cost of living adjustments (COLAs) for Social Security benefits were enacted in the 1970s there was only one Consumer Price

Index (CPI), the CPI-W, which reflects price increases based on the purchasing patterns of urban wage earners and clerical workers. The purpose of the COLA is to adjust the Social Security benefit so that inflation does not erode its purchasing power. In 1987, the Bureau of Labor Statistics developed, and has since maintained, an experimental CPI known as the CPI-E, that is specifically based on the purchasing patterns of America's seniors.

Historically, the CPI-E has reflected a rate of inflation that has been between 0.2 and 0.3 percentage points higher than inflation as measured under the CPI-W. This is primarily attributable to the greater weight placed on health expenditures in this index, which reflects the fact that seniors devote a higher percentage of their monthly spending to health care costs than do younger consumers. The current CPI-W formula does not keep pace with the increasing cost of health care.

Although it is still an experimental index and has not yet been fully developed, we believe the CPI-E is a more accurate measure of inflation than the CPI-W. This is because it is based on a market basket of goods and services that better reflects the purchasing patterns of seniors, especially their greater consumption of health care services.

Proposal: Adopt the CPI-E for the purpose of determining the amount of the COLA adjustment for Social Security benefits.

RESTORING STUDENT BENEFITS

Social Security pays benefits to children until the age of 18, or 19 if they are still attending high school, if a working parent has died, has become disabled, or has retired. In the past, those benefits continued until the age of 22 if the child was a full-time student in college or a vocational school. Congress ended post-secondary students' benefits in 1981. Research has shown that recipients of this benefit were disproportionately children of parents in blue-collar jobs, African Americans, and with lower incomes than other college students (Hertel-Fernandez, 2010). This benefit would help women who must defer saving for their retirement because they are assisting their children with college.

Proposal: Reinstate benefits for children of disabled or deceased workers until the age of 22 while the child is attending a college or vocational school on a full-time basis.

IMPROVING THE BASIC BENEFIT

After years of operating under a COLA which does not reflect the higher inflation attributable to health expenditures and the fact that seniors devote a higher percentage of their monthly expenditure to health care costs, seniors need to have their increased costs offset by an across-the-board benefit increase. Women, especially those who have worked a lifetime on low pay (often the result of sex-based wage discrimination), are financially vulnerable in retirement because they are less likely to have private pensions or discretionary income that would allow for saving.

Proposal: Increase the basic benefit of all current and future beneficiaries by 5% of the average benefit (approximately $55 per month).

EQUAL BENEFITS FOR SAME-SEX MARRIED COUPLES AND PARTNERS

Gay and lesbian same-sex couples, whether married or not, are denied a host of benefits under state and federal law that are routinely provided to heterosexual married couples (The Sage Foundation, 2010). These laws confer rights, protections, and benefits to married couples. However, partners in same-sex relationships cannot receive these benefits, usually because federal laws do not recognize any form of same-sex relationship in determining eligibility for family benefits.

The Social Security Act should be revised to provide benefits to domestic partners and the members of same-sex marriages. Further, the children of these relationships should receive Social Security benefits under the same terms and conditions as the children of heterosexual couples.

Proposal: Amend the Social Security Act to define wife and husband so that they no longer rely on gender-specific pronouns; provide eligibility to spousal benefits to individuals who are members of same-sex marriages, domestic partnerships, civil unions, or any other such relationship according to the states by law; and extend to the children of these relationships benefits under the same terms as children of heterosexual couples.

TABLE 25-1 Proposals to Improve Social Security Benefits for Women

Proposal	Cost as a Percent of Taxable Payroll	Cost as a Percent of Increase in Shortfall
1. Improving Survivor Benefits	0.06%	2.3%
2. Providing Social Security Credits for Caregivers	0.24%	9%
3. Enhancing the Special Minimum Benefit	*	*
4. Equalizing Rules for Disabled Widows	0.02%	1%
5. Benefit Equality for Working Widows	No estimate available	No estimate available
6. Strengthening the COLA	0.34%	13
7. Restoring Student Benefits for Children of Disabled or Deceased Workers up to Age 22	0.07%	3%
8. Improving the Basic Benefit of all Current and Future Beneficiaries	0.75%	28%
9. Equal Benefits for Same-Sex Married Couples and Partners	0%	Negligible
10. Improving Benefits for Disabled Adult Children	No estimate available	No estimate available

Estimates for proposals 1, 2, 4, 6, 7, and 8 are from the National Academy of Social Insurance, *Fixing Social Security: Adequate benefits, adequate financing,* published in October 2009.

Estimate for proposal 9 is from the *Adequacy Committee recommendations to the Save Social Security Coalition for a Plan to Strengthen and Improve Social Security and SSI (c.a. 2011).*

*An estimate for this proposal is not available. However, a similar proposal by NASI, increasing the benefit to 125% of poverty and including 8 years of coverage based on credit for a child under age 5, costs 0.26% of taxable payroll and increases the actuarial shortfall by 13% (2009).

IMPROVING BENEFITS FOR DISABLED ADULT CHILDREN

One of the categories of childhood benefits that is payable on a worker's record are benefits to an adult child who became disabled before reaching the age of 22. In addition to being disabled the child must be unmarried at the time the application for benefits is filed. Eligibility continues as long as the child remains disabled and unmarried. Benefits may be affected if the child becomes employed. Marriage at any time ends entitlement to this benefit, unless the child's husband or wife is receiving benefits either as a disabled adult child or as a disabled widow or widower. Marriage to anyone else permanently ends a disabled adult child's eligibility unless the marriage is annulled. Marriages ending in divorce preclude reentitlement. These rules are not well understood and result in great hardship to the affected individuals.

When a disabled adult child qualifies on a parent's record, benefits for the child and for other family members may be adjusted subject to the family maximum. If all eligible family members live in the same household, expenses and income are usually shared; however, people with disabilities are increasingly living independently. A consequence of doing so is a substantial reduction in total family income from Social Security. A remedy is to compute the benefit for a disabled adult child without regard to the family maximum as is already the case when calculating the benefit for a divorced spouse.

Proposal: Improve benefits for disabled adult children by (1) allowing beneficiaries to reestablish entitlement to benefits after divorce and (2) by computing the benefit for these individuals without regard to the provisions of the family maximum.

See Table 25-1 for the cost impact of these various proposals.

CHANGES WE OPPOSE

We believe the following proposals would weaken the protections offered by Social Security for all Americans, male as well as female, and should not be incorporated into the Social Security program.

PRIVATIZING SOCIAL SECURITY

Over the years, some policymakers and politicians have proposed plans that would offer a privatized Social Security option for workers under age 55. Plans of this nature usually call for diversion of payroll taxes out of Social Security into private accounts. These diversions put additional strains on the system and would result in benefit reductions. Women and minorities, who are frequently on the lower end of the wage scale and rely more heavily on Social Security, would be particularly vulnerable to privatization schemes. Today's Social Security system replaces a higher percentage of salary for low-income wage earners and thus is of particular benefit to women and minorities (Estes, 2004).

INCREASING THE RETIREMENT AGE

The 2010 National Commission on Fiscal Responsibility and Reform has proposed increasing the retirement age. This and other commissions argue that people are living longer and can therefore work longer. Although on average people are living longer, these longer life expectancies are by no means across the board. Over the last quarter-century, the life expectancy of lower-income men increased by 1 year compared with 5 years for upper-income men. Lower-income women have actually experienced a decline in longevity over the same period. Moreover, lower-income workers are far more likely than higher earners to be employed in occupations that require hard manual labor and the performance of duties that compromise their health and their ability to work.

MEANS TESTING THE BENEFIT FORMULA

Several proposals have been offered to change the benefit computation formula in an effort to make it less generous for moderate to high-wage earners; however, these proposals have been drafted so that they reduce benefits for virtually all workers, even those earning as little as $11,000 per year. With women and minorities disproportionately represented in occupations that pay lower wages, introducing means testing into the current benefit formula should be avoided because of the adverse impact it would have on their lives.

STRENGTHENING FINANCING

Social Security is not bankrupt or in crisis and it can pay all promised benefits in full for the next 20 years, through to 2033. After that, the program will still be able to pay 75% of all benefits that are owed to Social Security beneficiaries in subsequent years (The Board of Trustees of the Federal Old-Age and Survivors Insurance and Federal Disability Trust Funds, 2012). According to the Social Security Trustees, the program's funding shortfall, known as an actuarial deficit, is 2.67% of taxable payroll (The Board of Trustees of the Federal Old-Age and Survivors Insurance and Federal Disability Trust Funds, 2012). In our view, this shortfall is manageable and resolvable. There are a number of straightforward reforms that, if adopted, would increase Social Security's funding by more than enough both to close the actuarial deficit and pay for most of the costs associated with the program improvements called for by this chapter. We have compiled a list of options which fall within the traditional actions that Congress has adopted in the past when strengthening the financial condition of the Social Security program.

ELIMINATE CAP ON PAYROLL CONTRIBUTIONS

Currently, there is a cap of $110,100 on the amount of a worker's wages that are subject to Social Security contributions. One option is to eliminate this cap and modestly adjust the benefit formula when determining benefits for high-wage earners. Under current law, the benefit formula is based on the average indexed monthly earnings (AIME). Eliminating the cap and adjusting the AIME would eliminate most of Social Security's current actuarial deficit by producing revenue equal to about 2.17% of taxable payroll (Reno & Lavery, 2009).

SLOWLY INCREASE THE CONTRIBUTION RATE BY 0.05% OVER 20 YEARS

Scheduling a gradual increase in the Social Security payroll tax rate by a very small percentage and phasing it in over a long period of time would significantly strengthen Social Security's financial position now and into the future, providing revenue equal to 1.34% of taxable payroll.

TREAT ALL SALARY REDUCTION PLANS IN THE MANNER OF 401(k)s

Currently, workers pay Social Security and Medicare taxes on their contributions to retirement accounts, such as 401(k), 403(b), and 527 plans, but do not pay these taxes on their contributions to flexible spending accounts such as health care, transit, and dependent care plans. Adopting this change provides revenue equal to about 0.48% of taxable payroll.

In total, the above set of proposals provides a combined saving of 3.99% of taxable payroll. This would close the current actuarial deficit (2.67% of payroll) and at the same time fund the modest set of program improvements recommended in this chapter. They are modest in their effect on individual workers, consistent with the approaches that have been employed by Congress in the past, and illustrate what can be achieved when Social Security is reformed.

DISCUSSION QUESTIONS

1. To what extent are women in your family affected by inequities in the rules related to Social Security benefits? What impact do these have on their health, quality of life, and well-being?

2. If you were a member of Congress, what policy options would you support to ensure that women have Social Security benefits equal to those of men and which take account of the work performed by stay-at-home moms?

3. Which of the options for ensuring the financial health of Social Security would you support?

REFERENCES

Board of Trustees, Federal Old-Age and Survivors Insurance and Federal Disability Insurance Trust Funds. (2012). The 2011 annual report of the board of trustees of the old age and survivors insurance and disability insurance trust funds. Retrieved from *www.ssa.gov/oact/tr/2011/tr2011.pdf*.

Estes, C. L. (2004). Social Security privatization and older women. *Journal of Aging Studies*, *18*(1), 9–26. Retrieved from *urpe.org/ec/SS/SSOlderWomenEstes.pdf*.

Hartman, H., Hayes, J., & Drago, R. (2011). Social Security: Especially vital to women and people of color, men increasingly reliant. Washington DC: Institute for Women's Policy Research. Retrieved from *policylinkcontent.s3.amazonaws.com/SocialSecurityVitalToWomenPeopleOfColor_IWPR_2.pdf*.

Hertel-Fernandez, A. (2010). A new deal for young adults: Social Security benefits for post-secondary school students. Washington, DC: National Academy of Social Insurance. Retrieved from *www.nasi.org/research/2010/new-deal-young-adults-social-security-benefits-post*.

Insight Center for Community and Economic Development. (2010). Lifting as we climb: Women of color, wealth, and America's future. Retrieved from *www.cunapfi.org/download/198_Women_of_Color_Wealth_Future_Spring_2010.pdf*.

Institute for Women's Policy Research. (2011). Six key facts on women and Social Security. Retrieved from *www.iwpr.org/publications/pubs/six-key-facts-on-women-and-social-security*.

Joint Economic Committee, United States Congress. (2010). Social Security provides economic security to women. Retrieved from *www.jec.senate.gov/public/?a=Files.Serve&File_id=d0036901-2da3-4387-b77f-d33afffe6f7f*.

Reno, V., & Lavery, J. (2009). Fixing Social Security: Adequate benefits, adequate financing. Washington, DC: National Academy of Social Insurance. Retrieved from *www.nasi.org/research/2009/fixing-social-security*.

Rhee, N. (2012). Black and Latino retirement (in)security. University of California Berkeley Center for Labor Research and Education. Retrieved from *laborcenter.berkeley.edu/pdf/2012/retirement_in_security2012.pdf*.

Rockeymoore, M. M., & Meizhu, L. (2011). Plan for a new future: The impact of Social Security reform on people of color. Washington, DC: Commission to Modernize Social Security. Retrieved from *www.insightcced.org/uploads/CRWG/New_Future_Social_Security_Commission_Report_Final.pdf*.

Social Security Administration. (2014). Social Security is important to women. Retrieved from *www.ssa.gov/women*.

The Sage Foundation. (2010). Improving the lives of LGBT older elders. Washington, DC. Retrieved from *www.lgbtmap.org/file/improving-the-lives-of-lgbt-older-adults.pdf*.

United States Census Bureau. (2012). Current population survey annual social and economic supplement. Retrieved from *www.census.gov/hhes/www/poverty/publications/pubs-cps.html*.

ONLINE RESOURCES

Social Security Administration
www.ssa.gov
National Committee to Preserve Social Security & Medicare Foundation
www.ncpssm.org
Institute for Women's Policy Research
www.iwpr.org
NOW Foundation
www.now.org

CHAPTER 26

The Politics of the Pharmaceutical Industry

Douglas P. Olsen

"There's a better way to do it…find it."

Thomas Edison

Prescription medications have been a mainstay of modern medical therapy since the 1920s, starting with insulin for diabetes and followed by the development of vaccinations and antibiotics. This trend accelerated in the 1950s with the development of drugs to treat chronic and incipient conditions such as hypertension, heart disease, type II diabetes, psychiatric disorders, and cancer. When physicians were surveyed in 2001 about the most important innovations in medical treatment since 1976, 11 of the top 20 were medications (Fuchs & Sox, 2001). However, the pace of this innovation may be slowing. Olfson and Marcus (2013) found that the effect size (i.e., degree of benefit) demonstrated in clinical trials of medications has been in decline since 1966, and in a summation of annual ranking of new drugs for 2001 to 2010, the journal *Prescrire International* (2012) found 7.5% (69 out of 918 drugs) offered an advantage and only 1.7% were a real advance (17 out of 918 drugs).

Today, 47.5% of Americans take at least one prescription drug (National Center for Health Statistics [NCHS], 2012), and 71% of all outpatient visits result in a prescription (Cherry et al., 2008). Despite slowed innovation, the prominence of medications in treatment is increasing with an overall 235% increase in the prescribing rate for the most widely used drugs from 1988 to 1994, 1999 to 2002, and 2007 to 2010 (Center for Disease Control [CDC], 2012) (Figure 26-1).

This demand fuels a large, profitable industry where the top 12 companies had $311 billion in

revenues and $49 billion in profits in 2012 (CNNMoney, 2012). Health care is expected to be 20% of the U.S. GDP by 2021. In 2011, $263 billion, approximately $830 per person, was spent on retail prescription drugs (Centers for Medicare and Medicaid Services [CMS], 2012). Although overall spending on drugs was down slightly from 2011 to 2012, it is expected to rise by more than 5% by 2014 in part because of increased health care coverage with the implementation of the Affordable Care Act (CMS, 2012). Market demand combined with large sums of money in the pharmaceutical industry translates into political clout. The Center for Responsive Politics reports that the pharmaceutical industry spent $117 million in 2013 in lobbying which was chiefly focused on patent reform, research funding, and Medicare. An additional $46.5 million was spent in 2013 on political contributions, including to individual candidates and through Political Action Committees, with 42% going to Democrats and 58% going to Republicans (Center for Responsive Politics, 2013).

As part of a public relations campaign, the U.S. pharmaceutical industry emphasizes the money it generates is for research and development which was estimated at $67.4 billion in 2010 by the Pharmaceutical Research and Manufacturers of America (PhRMA) 2012 Annual Report. However, critics claim that research funded by the National Institutes of Health (NIH) and buyouts of drugs-testing from small enterprises make up an increasing proportion of development spending and that the amount of basic research by the large pharmaceuticals is shrinking (Angell, 2004). Others claim that drug companies are shifting away from research and development toward patent and market

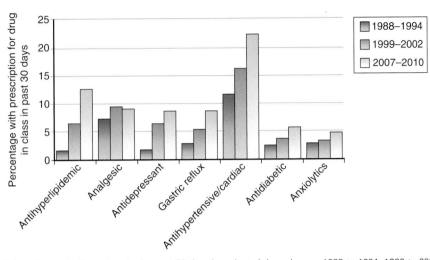

FIGURE 26-1 Selected prescriptions given in the past 30 days by selected drug classes, 1988 to 1994, 1999 to 2002, and 2007 to 2010 (Data from the CDC. Retrieved from *www.cdc.gov/nchs/hus/contents2012.htm#092.*)

manipulation (Kotze, 2012). One common such practice in which drug companies paid generic manufacturers to delay production was recently banned by the Supreme Court (Wyatt, 2013).

These numbers reveal an industry driven by market forces to maximize return on investment. Some industry analysts express concern that over-emphasis on low-hanging fruit in the form of me-too drugs, drugs with effects similar to available medications, and increasing market share by advertising and legal maneuvering have deemphasized basic research, resulting in less innovation (Public Citizen's Congress Watch, 2002).

GLOBALIZATION CONCERNS

Increasing globalization of the pharmaceutical industry adds pressure to remain competitive and also adds complexity to regulatory efforts. The U.S. health care system has developed a deep dependence on foreign manufacturers to provide generic drugs, over-the-counter drugs, and the ingredients used in U.S. drug production. Concerns have been raised about the quality of overseas manufacturing and ingredients as well as the Food and Drug Administration's (FDA's) ability to ensure quality and safety. These concerns arise at a time when generic drugs are being increasingly seen as one way

to control health care costs. The generic drug industry claims that use of generic drugs saved over $1 trillion dollars from 1999 to 2012 (Generic Pharmaceutical Association, 2011).

The FDA estimates that foreign manufacture of drugs and drug-related ingredients has doubled since 2002, with China and India accounting for the majority of the increase (U.S. Government Accountability Office [GAO], 2011). Currently, the Indian pharmaceutical industry produces 40% of generic and over-the-counter medication sold in the United States (Harris, 2014). FDA Commissioner Margaret Hamburg has said that 80% of ingredients used in the United States are imported from India and China (The Times of India, 2014). The *New York Times* (Harris, 2014) reports that, "The crucial ingredients for nearly all antibiotics, steroids and many other lifesaving drugs are now made exclusively in China." (Drug companies consider the source of their ingredients proprietary, so publically available figures are estimates.)

Quality problems have been reported in India and China. Half of the 21 warning letters sent to manufacturers by the FDA last year went to India (Harris, 2014; The Times of India, 2014). The World Health Organization (2014) estimates that 20% of medications sold in India are counterfeit. In 2008, the deaths of 81 Americans were linked to contaminated heparin whose main ingredient was made in China. The form of the contamination suggested cost reduction motivation rather than accidental happenstance (Mundy, 2011; GAO, 2011).

In 2012, a law was passed allowing the FDA to collect user fees from foreign manufacturers of foreign drugs to fund increased levels of inspection. Inspections are supposed to occur every 2 years, but the FDA lacks the staff to maintain this pace (GAO, 2011). Also, increased inspections could reduce supplies. While the FDA insists that foreign manufacturers meet U.S. standards, the Indian government's top regulator of the pharmaceutical industry, G.N. Singh, says, "If I follow U.S. standards, I will have to shut almost all drug facilities." (Dey, 2014).

The United States is highly dependent on foreign drug manufacturers, and the FDA struggles to monitor production. Until a stronger regulatory framework is in place globally, nurses prescribing and dispensing drugs, as well as nurses counseling patients on the use of generics, must be prepared to answer patient questions and remain alert for unusual reports of adverse effects.

VALUES CONFLICT

The industry is designed to produce profits, and like the manufacture of most other products in the United States, market forces shape the manufacture of medications. However, medications, essential to health care, are also held to be a public good. The dual private-enterprise/public-good nature of drug manufacturing helps explain some of the industry's more controversial aspects including industry-funded education and advertising campaigns aimed at both clinicians and patients. Reinhardt (2001) states, "On some occasions, lawmakers and the general public seem to expect pharmaceutical firms to behave as if they were community owned, non-profit entities. At the same time, the firms' owners... always expect the firms to use their market power and political muscle to maximize the owners' wealth" (p. 137).

A free enterprise system that lacks the ability to patent new items discourages innovation because inventions that can be freely copied confer little

economic incentive for developing novel products (Taylor, 2007). The industry puts the expense of bringing a new drug to market at $1.2 billion (PhRMA, 2012), so, to offset development expenses and encourage innovation, new medications are patented with exclusive marketing rights for 7 years. This creates an incentive to deliver new drugs to market, while striving for rapid clinical acceptance. Financial assessments of a pharmaceutical company typically include the pipeline or the drugs in development. Companies are often on a boom-bust cycle with profits soaring when a new drug emerges and falling when the pipeline dries up (Ekelund & Persson, 2003).

Drug companies increase profits in two ways: (1) bringing new medications to market, especially for conditions where there are no equivalent generic drugs available, and (2) increasing the market for existing medications. Firms increase market share by advertising to prescribers and the public, as well as through promotion activities that include sponsorship of clinical education and assistance to patient advocacy groups. However, precise and reliable marketing figures are difficult to identify because industry reporting combines marketing and administration costs. The total marketing budget for the industry was estimated at $29.9 billion in 2005, up from $11.4 billion in 1997 (Donohue, Cevasco, & Rosenthal, 2007).

One of the chief promotion methods to clinicians, called detailing, combines education-like activity with traditional advertising. In detailing, a company representative provides clinicians with educational materials, free samples, meals, and reminder items, including mugs, pens, or toys. In 2005, an estimated $6.8 billion dollars (22% of promotion spending) went to detailing. In addition, $18.4 billion (58% of promotion spending) went to free drug samples (Donohue, Cevasco, & Rosenthal, 2007).

The search for blockbuster drugs results in drug development focused on those classes of medication producing large profits. The profitability of a drug is a combination of perceived patient need together with patent exclusivity. Therefore, drug development based on potential profit will differ from development based on dispassionate assessment of public need. Classes of drugs with the highest sales include psychotropics, drugs for acid reflux, statins for cholesterol reduction, and most recently drugs for autoimmune disorders (IMS Institute for Healthcare Informatics, 2012). The Orphan Drug Act of 1983 provides financial incentives to develop treatments for rare diseases, and represents an attempt to mitigate the effects of the industry's dual nature on development of new drugs. In FY 2011 the FDA approved 10 medications for orphan conditions (FDA, 2011).

DIRECT TO CONSUMER MARKETING

Direct to consumer (DTC) advertising began in earnest in 1997, 6 months after David Kessler, who opposed easing regulations to allow more DTC, left his post as commissioner of the U.S. FDA. At that time, it was made easier to comply with the regulatory requirement that DTC broadcast advertising contain a major statement of the drug's risks and adequate provision for consumers to obtain full information about the drug. These conditions are now satisfied with a risk statement and referral to concurrent print advertisements, websites, or toll-free telephone numbers (Bradford et al., 2010). Industry spending on DTC advertising is estimated to have increased from $579 million in 1996 to a high of $5.5 billion during 2006 before falling to 4.2 billion in 2010 (Bradford et al., 2010; Mintzes, 2012). Profit spurred the growth of DTC marketing, and it is estimated that money spent on DTC advertising produces a fourfold return in sales (Rosenthal et al., 2003).

The heated debate about DTC advertising highlights the ambivalence over medications as both a public good and a lucrative product. Both sides in the debate frame arguments in terms of DTC's effect on public health, passing over profitability as a rationale for favoring DTC advertising. Ethical and policy reasons favoring DTC advertising include increased public awareness of treatment options and enhanced ability for informed choices by consumers. One argument against DTC advertising is that the information disseminated by the advertisements is biased and designed to build profit rather than being a dispassionate account of the risks, benefits, and alternatives which are essential to informed choice.

Research shows that, although awareness has increased, information received by the public through advertising is problematic. A series of FDA surveys (Aikin, Swasy & Braman, 2004) indicates that the public and physicians view DTC advertising as raising awareness of treatment options and stimulating clinical discussion but also note that the advertisements tend to overemphasize the benefits of a particular drug. Consistent with the FDA's findings regarding awareness, Bradford and colleagues (2010) found that among osteoarthritis patients "advertising tends to encourage more rapid adoption among patients who are good clinical candidates for the therapy and leads to less rapid adoption among some patients who are poor clinical candidates." However, consistent with the potential for bias, Woloshin, Schwartz, and Welch (2004) found that consumers, when given data concerning the effectiveness of a drug, perceived drugs as less beneficial than when given the qualitative data typical of most drug advertising. Wilkes, Bell, and Kravitz (2000) reported that 43% of consumers believed that only completely safe drugs could be advertised, and 21% believed that advertising was restricted to extremely effective drugs. In adolescents, Leader and colleagues (2011) found that although teenage girls remembered the tag line of HPV vaccine advertising, they did not understand the medical information. In a review of research on the clinical effect of DTC marketing Mintzes (2012) concluded that there was no positive effect on adherence, treatment quality, or earlier provision of care. In addition, Mintzes (2012) found no shifting to less appropriate, more costly forms of treatment related to DTC.

The industry largely confines advertising to a few classes of drugs that generate the greatest profit rather than focus on distributing information on the basis of public need (Donohue, Cevasco, & Rosenthal, 2007) (Figure 26-2). Currently the prescription drug classes with the most DTC spending treat hyperlipidemia, asthma, depression, and erectile dysfunction (Mintzes, 2012). Past leaders included heartburn and sleep disturbance (Donohue, Cevasco, & Rosenthal, 2007). There are also indications that prescribing patterns are influenced in ways inconsistent with health priorities. Weissman and colleagues (2003) found that 25% of patients who asked clinicians about an advertised drug received a new diagnosis, erectile dysfunction being the most common.

Another concern about DTC marketing is disease mongering, that is, promoting exaggerated perceptions of the seriousness of known disorders or even inventing new diseases to open new markets and improve sales. Examples include female sexual dysfunction, erectile dysfunction, acid reflux, insomnia, and allergies (Appelbaum, 2006).

CONFLICT OF INTEREST

The large quantity of money spent promoting drugs to clinicians raises conflict-of-interest concerns that arise from the industry's dual nature. Public interest is served when treatment is based solely on a clinical assessment of the patient's best interests, not on personal or monetary considerations tied to specific medications. However, industry's primary interest in profitability is served by promoting particular drugs. There is evidence

indicating that this may occur specifically among nurse prescribers. In a survey of more than 500 nurse practitioners, Blunt (2005) reported that 80% altered their prescribing practice after interaction with a drug company, and Ladd, Mahoney, and Emani (2010) found that 48% of nurse practitioners were more likely to prescribe the highlighted drug following an industry-sponsored educational event coupled with lunch or dinner. The trend to target nurses may increase due to the omission of nurse prescribers in the new sunshine laws requiring physicians to report gifts and payments from industry (Gorlach & Pham-Kanter, 2013).

EDUCATION

Drug companies are a major sponsor of medical continuing education. Between 1998 and 2003, commercial sponsorship of continuing medical education went from $302 million to $971 million, reached a high of $1.25 billion in 2007, and fell to $846 million in 2010, possibly caused by reform measures (Accreditation Council for Continuing Medical Education [ACCME], 2011; Steinbrook, 2005). Industry marketing has become so integral to clinical education that PhRMA (2008b) claims, "Restricting pharmaceutical marketing would

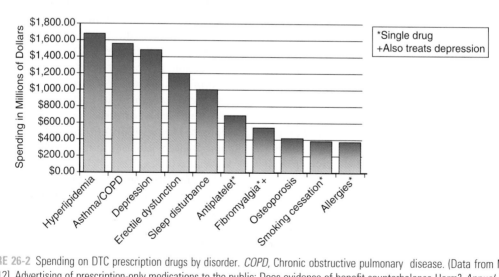

FIGURE 26-2 Spending on DTC prescription drugs by disorder. *COPD,* Chronic obstructive pulmonary disease. (Data from Mintez, B. [2012]. Advertising of prescription-only medications to the public: Does evidence of benefit counterbalance Harm? *Annual Review of Public Health, 33,* 259-277.)

likely significantly reduce the dissemination of information about new treatments…." In a report in the *New England Journal of Medicine*, Steinbrook (2008) concluded, "Continuing medical education has become so heavily dependent on support from pharmaceutical and medical device companies that the medical profession may have lost control over its own continuing education." In 2008, the Association of American Medical Colleges (AAMC) identified the conflict between medical treatment as a social good and medical treatment as a commodity. In their report, Industry Funding of Medical Education, the AAMC states "these conflicts can have a corrosive effect on three core principles of medical professionalism: autonomy, objectivity, and altruism" (AAMC, 2008). The pervasive potential for conflict of interest in continuing medical education prompted the Institute of Medicine (IOM, 2009) to recommend developing "a new system of funding accredited continuing medical education that is free of industry influence…."

Both the American Nurses Association, through the American Nurses Credentialing Center (ANCC), and the American Medical Association (AMA), through the Accreditation Council for Continuing Medical Education (ACCME), have attempted to eliminate conflicts of interest via strict guidelines for commercial sponsorship of accredited continuing education. The guidelines emphasize independence of content, transparency through conflict of interest disclosures by content developers, separation of promotion from educational activity, and appropriate use of funds (ACCME, 2007; ANCC, n.d.). The AMA Council on Ethical and Judicial Affairs recommends that physicians, medical schools, and professional associations stop accepting industry funding for education, and the American Psychiatric Association announced its intention to phase out industry-funded education (Kuehn, 2009).

The amount of commercial money directed at nursing education is not known, but it appears to be increasing as more nurses earn prescriptive authority. Advanced practice nurses represent a relatively untapped resource for pharmaceutical marketing/education (Jutel & Menkes, 2008).

Although not all nurses prescribe, nurses influence the use and purchase of drugs in other ways, including suggesting the use of particular medications to physicians and patients, distributing medications, reporting adverse effects, conducting research, as well as managing clinical trials.

Whatever value industry-sponsored education has in the overall education of clinicians, for the industry itself it is primarily a form of marketing. Drugs are so integral to modern health care that comprehensive education in almost all areas involves extensive discussion of medications, and even unbiased appraisals may favor one drug over another. However, when commercial interests sponsor education, it cannot be discerned where unbiased evaluation ends and promotion begins. For example, if two experts have an honest disagreement about treatments and the company sponsors the one that holds their drug superior to the lifestyle change favored by the other expert, then the discourse is biased by giving one side resources to magnify their opinion. Social justice is better served through fair and equal access to all forms of discourse (Horster, 1992). Distortion of the discourse on health care in the public and professional community occurs through marketing techniques applied to products with the potential to generate revenue. And so, in market-driven public discourse, health practices with modest or little profit potential such as exercise and moderate eating are unlikely to receive the attention accorded to highly profitable pharmaceuticals.

GIFTS

The giving of explicit or disguised gifts also creates potential conflicts of interest for clinicians. After years of anecdotal denial by clinicians that gifts carry influence there is now evidence to the contrary. After reviewing research on the effect of drug company representatives on physician practice, the IOM (2009) concluded that the evidence indicated an influence on both "prescribing patterns and requests for additions to hospital formularies." And so, voluntary guidance from the industry (PhRMA, 2008a), the government (Office of

Inspector General, U.S. Department of Health and Human Services [HHS]., 2003), and the AMA (2005) limits the practice of giving gifts. PhRMA guidelines prohibit both the most egregious types of gifts given in the past by drug companies (including cash kickbacks, event tickets, and fees for bogus consultations) as well as those once considered benign, including mugs or pens. Voluntary PhRMA guidelines suggest gifts be limited to educational or clinically useful items of less than $100. Provision of meals is still allowed at clinical sites when in conjunction with educational presentations.

In addition to voluntary guidance, the federal Physician Payment Sunshine Act (PPSA) was enacted in 2010 and took effect August 2013. The act improves transparency by requiring manufacturers to track and report to Centers for Medicare & Medicaid Services (CMS) payments and items of value given to physicians and hospitals but with some notable exceptions including money for CMEs and drug samples. Nurse prescribers are not included in the law although some states have similar laws which do include nurses including Massachusetts, Vermont, and Minnesota (AMA, n.d.; AMA, 2013; Gorlach, & Pham-Kanter, 2013).

Although the AMA has issued ethical guidance for physicians, guidance for nurses is notably absent. Most major U.S. nursing organizations say little about relations with the pharmaceutical industry. The American Association of Nurse Anesthetists (ANA) provides criteria for the ethical endorsement of products and services in its code of ethics (American Association of Nurse Anesthetists, 2005). However, the ANA has issued no guidance specific to relations with industry, and neither has any other major specialty association, despite calls for ethical guidance on this topic (Crigger, 2005; Gleason & Schaffer, 2013; Olsen, 2009).The need for ethical guidance for nurse practitioners was shown by Ladd, Mahoney, and Emani (2010), who found that a majority of nurses consider industry-sponsored meals, speakers, and gifts ethically acceptable while acknowledging the influence of such on education. In addition, 93% stated that gifts had no influence despite evidence to contrary among physicians (Ladd, Mahoney, & Emani, 2010; IOM, 2009).

SAMPLES

Providing free samples of drugs is another controversial form of gifts given to clinicians. The claim is often made that prescribers use these to benefit the economically disadvantaged. The free samples are usually of new, expensive drugs that the patient may not be able to afford once the samples have run out. However, research shows that recipients of sample medications are more likely the wealthy rather than the poor or uninsured (Cutrona et al., 2008) and that any economic advantage associated to receiving the free sample is short-lived (Alexander, Zhang, & Basu, 2008). Ladd, Mahoney, and Emani (2010) found that 62% of nurse practitioners dispensed samples and that of these practitioners, 62% acknowledged that the samples encouraged their prescribing of the "new highly marketed medications." In addition, 81% of nurse practitioners stated that it is ethical to give samples to *anyone* (emphasis added) (Ladd, Mahoney, & Emani, 2010). Despite their widespread use, samples are excluded from reporting requirements in the federal sunshine laws.

CONCLUSION

In addition to tangible safety concerns emerging with increasingly globalized pharmaceutical production, a more subtle yet pervasive effect of having a market-driven industry expected to deliver a public good may be a subtle shift in the nature of the public benefit expected. The sum effect of the vast amount of money spent to promote drug sales through education and advertising to clinicians and advertising directly to the public may be to alter the public's concept of life and health to conform to the interests of the pharmaceutical industry. This means a worldview where life's problems are medical conditions visited on us through no fault of our own and whose solutions require external interventions, most often a pill. In this view, personal responsibility means recognizing and admitting to having a disorder and then being compliant with treatment.

Medications are a miracle of modern health care but the tradition will continue only if unbiased information regarding their benefits and uses is distributed in accordance with rational decisions about the public's health, rather than the effect on industry profits.

DISCUSSION QUESTIONS

1. Many of the controversial aspects of the pharmaceutical industry arise because society expects the industry to compete as a profit-motivated industry as well as to provide an essential public good. Can these two missions be accomplished without conflict?

2. The industry spends a great deal of money to influence the prescribing practices of providers, and available data show that clinicians, including nurses, are influenced. What are the ethical issues that emerge from this finding?

3. Professional continuing education is heavily dependent on funding from the pharmaceutical industry. Medicine may be attempting to extricate itself, but nursing shows no signs of this. What are the pros and cons of this?

REFERENCES

Accreditation Council for Continuing Medical Education. (2007). ACCME standards for commercial support: Standards to ensure the independence of CME activities. Retrieved from *www.accme.org/dir_docs/doc_upload/68b2902a-fb73-44d1-8725-80a1504e520c_uploaddocument.pdf*.

Accreditation Council for Continuing Medical Education. (2011). Annual report. Retrieved from *www.accme.org/sites/default/files/630_2011_Annual_Report_20130807.pdf*.

Aikin, K., Swasy, J., & Braman, A. (2004). Patient and physician attitudes and behaviors associated with DTC promotion of prescription drugs—Summary of FDA survey research results. U.S. Department of Health and Human Services, Food and Drug Administration, Center for Drug Evaluation and Research. Retrieved from *www.fda.gov/downloads/Drugs/ScienceResearch/ResearchAreas/DrugMarketingAdvertisingandCommunicationsResearch/UCM152860.pdf*.

Alexander, G., Zhang, J., & Basu, A. (2008). Characteristics of patients receiving pharmaceutical samples and association between sample receipt and out-of-pocket prescription costs. *Medical Care, 46*(4), 394–402.

American Association of Nurse Anesthetists. (2005). Code of ethics for the certified registered nurse anesthetist. Retrieved from *www.aana.com/resources2/professionalpractice/Pages/Code-of-Ethics.aspx*.

American Medical Association (AMA). (2005). Ethical guidelines for gifts to physicians from industry. Retrieved from *www.ama-assn.org/ama/pub/category/5689.html*.

American Medical Association. (n.d.). Physician Payments Sunshine Act—Overview and key provisions. Retrieved from *www.ama-assn.org/*

resources/doc/washington/physician-payments-sunshine-act-overview-key-provisions.pdf*.

American Medical Association. (2013). State "sunshine" laws. Retrieved from *www.ama-assn.org/resources/doc/washington/state-sunshine-laws-chart.pdf*.

American Nurses Credentialing Center. (n.d.). Standards for disclosure and commercial support. Retrieved from *www.nursecredentialing.org/ContinuingEducation/Accreditation/How-to-Apply/CommercialSupport/CommercialSupportStandards.aspx*.

Angell, M. (2004). *The truth about the drug companies: How they deceive us and what to do about it.* New York: Random House.

Association of American Medical Colleges. (2008). Industry funding of medical education: Report of an AAMC task force. Retrieved from *www.aamc.org/publications*.

Appelbaum, K. (2006). Pharmaceutical marketing and the invention of the medical consumer. *PLoS Medicine, 3*(4), e189.

Blunt, E. (2005). The influence of pharmaceutical-company-sponsored educational programs, promotions, and gifts on the self-reported prescribing beliefs and practices of certified nurse practitioners in three states. 16th International Nursing Research Congress, Sigma Theta Tau, Hawaii. Retrieved from *stti.confex.com/stti/inrc16/techprogram/paper_23835.htm*.

Bradford, W., Kleit, A., Nietert, P., & Ornstein, S. (2010). The effect of direct to consumer television advertising on the timing of treatment. *Economic Inquiry, 48*, 306–322. doi:10.1111/j.1465-7295.2009.00215.x.

Center for Disease Control. (2012). Health. United States: U.S. Department of Health and Human Services. Retrieved from *www.cdc.gov/nchs/hus.htm*.

Centers for Medicare and Medicaid Services. (2012). National health expenditure projections 2012-2022. Retrieved from *www.cms.gov/Research-Statistics-Data-and-Systems/Statistics-Trends-and-Reports/NationalHealthExpendData/Downloads/Proj2012.pdf*.

Center for Responsive Politics. (2013). Retrieved from *www.opensecrets.org/lobby/indusclient.php?id=H04&year=2013*.

CNNMoney. (2012). Fortune 500 industries 2012: Pharmaceuticals. Retrieved from *money.cnn.com/magazines/fortune/fortune500/2012/industries/21/*.

Cherry, D., Hing, E., Woodwell, D., & Rechtsteiner, E. (2008). *National ambulatory medical care survey: 2006 summary national health statistics reports. Number 3.* Hyattsville, MD: National Center for Health Statistics.

Crigger, B. (2005). Pharmaceutical promotions and conflict of interest in nurse practitioner's decision making: The undiscovered country. *Journal of the American Academy of Nurse Practitioners, 17*(6), 207–212.

Cutrona, S. L., Woolhandler, S., Lasser, K. E., Bor, D. H., McCormick, D., & Himmelstein, D. U. (2008). Characteristics of recipients of free prescription drug samples: A nationally representative analysis. *American Journal of Public Health, 98*(2), 284–289.

Dey, S. (2014). If I follow U.S. standards, I will have to shut almost all drug facilities: G N Singh. *Business Standard*, Retrieved from *www.business-standard.com/article/economy-policy/if-i-follow-us-standards-i-will-have-to-shut-almost-all-drug-facilities-g-n-singh-114013000034_1.html*.

Donohue, J. M., Cevasco, M., & Rosenthal, M. B. (2007). A decade of direct-to-consumer advertising of prescription drugs. *New England Journal of Medicine, 357*(7), 673–681.

Ekelund, M., & Persson, B. (2003). Pharmaceutical pricing in a regulated market. *The Review of Economics and Statistics, 85*(2), 298–306.

Food and Drug Administration [FDA]. (2011). FY 2011 Innovative drug approvals. Retrieved from *www.fda.gov/downloads/aboutfda/reportsmanualsforms/reports/ucm278358.pdf*.

Fuchs, V. R., & Sox, H. C. (2001). Physicians' views of the relative importance of thirty medical innovations. *Health Affairs, 20*(5), 30–42.

Generic Pharmaceutical Association. (2011). SAVINGS: An economic analysis of generic drug usage in the U.S. Retrieved from *www.tevagenerics.com/assets/base/pdf/Savings,AnEconomicAnalysis.pdf*.

Gleason, R., & Schaffer, S. (2013). There is no free lunch: Strategies to prevent industry influence. *Journal for Nurse Practitioners, 9*(2), 71–76. Retrieved from *dx.doi.org/10.1016/j.nurpra.2012.12.009*.

Gorlach, I., & Pham-Kanter, G. (2013). Brightening up: The effect of the physician payment sunshine act on existing regulation of pharmaceutical marketing. *The Journal of Law, Medicine and Ethics, 41*(1), 315–322.

Harris, G. (2014). Medicines made in India set off safety worries. *New York Times*, Retrieved from *www.nytimes.com/2014/02/15/world/asia/medicines-made-in-india-set-off-safety-worries.html*.

Horster, D. (H. Thompson, trans). (1992). *Habermas: An introduction*. Philadelphia: Pennbridge.

IMS Institute for Healthcare Informatics. (2012). The use of medicines in the United States: Review of 2011. Retrieved from *www.imshealth.com/ims/Global/Content/Insights/IMS%20Institute%20for%20Healthcare%20Informatics/IHII_Medicines_in_U.S_Report_2011.pdf*.

Institute of Medicine. (2009). Conflict of interest in medical research, education, and practice. Retrieved from *www.iom.edu/Reports/2009/Conflict-of-Interest-in-Medical-Research-Education-and-Practice.aspx*.

Jutel, A., & Menkes, D. (2008). Soft targets: Nurses and the pharmaceutical industry. *PLoS Medicine, 5*(2), e5.

Kuehn, B. (2009). Associations say no to industry funding. *Journal of the American Medical Association, 301*(18), 1865–1866.

Kotze, A. (2012). Reining in patent term extensions for related pharmaceutical products post-photocure and Ortho–McNeil. *Northwestern University Law Review, 106*(3), 1419–1450.

Ladd, E., Mahoney, D., & Emani, S. (2010). "Under the Radar": Nurse practitioner prescribers and pharmaceutical industry promotions. *The American Journal of Managed Care, 16*(12), e358–e362.

Leader, A. E., Cashman, R., Voytek, C. D., Baker, J. L., Brawner, B. M., & Frank, I. (2011). An exploratory study of adolescent female reactions to direct-to-consumer advertising: The case of the human papillomavirus (HPV) vaccine. *Health Marketing Quarterly, 28*(4), 372–385. doi:10.1080/07359683.2011.630289.

Mintzes, B. (2012). Advertising of prescription-only medicines to the public: Does evidence of benefit counterbalance harm? *Annual Review of Public Health, 33*, 259–277.

Mundy, A. (2011). House investigates heparin crisis. *The Wall Street Journal*, Retrieved from *online.wsj.com/news/articles/SB10001424052748703775704576162450111643240*.

National Center for Health Statistics. (2012). Health, United States, 2012. Hyattsville, MD. Retrieved from *www.cdc.gov/nchs/data/hus/hus12.pdf*.

Office of Inspector General, U.S. Department of Health and Human Services [HHS]. (2003). *OIG compliance program guidance for pharmaceutical manufacturers*. Washington, D.C. Federal Register 68, No. 86.

Olfson, M., & Marcus, S. (2013). Decline in placebo-controlled trial results suggests new directions for comparative effectiveness research. *Health Affairs, 32*(6), 1116–1125.

Olsen, D. (2009). Nurses and the pharmaceutical industry: Part 1. *American Journal of Nursing, 109*(1), 36–39.

PhRMA. (2008a). Code on interactions with healthcare professionals. Washington, D.C. Retrieved from *www.phrma.org/files/PhRMA%20Marketing%20Code%202008.pdf*.

PhRMA. (2008b). Pharmaceutical marketing in perspective: Its value and role as one of many factors informing prescribing. Retrieved from *www.phrma.org/files/attachments/PhRMA%20Marketing%20Brochure%20Influences%20on%20Prescribing%20FINAL.pdf*.

PhRMA. (2012). 2012 Annual report. Retrieved from *www.phrma.org/sites/default/files/pdf/phrma_2011_annual_report.pdf*.

Public Citizen's Congress Watch. (2002). United Seniors Association: Hired guns for PhRMA and other corporate interests. Retrieved from *www.citizen.org/documents/UnitedSeniorsAssociationreport.pdf*.

Reinhardt, U. (2001). Perspectives on the pharmaceutical industry. *Health Affairs, 20*(5), 136–149.

Rosenthal, M. B., Berndt, E. R., Donohue, J. M., Epstein, A. M., & Frank, R. G. (2003). *Demand effects of recent changes in prescription drug promotion*. Menlo Park, CA: Kaiser Family Foundation.

Prescrire International (Staff). (2011). New drugs and indications in 2010: inadequate assessment; patients at risk. *Prescrire International, 20*(115), 105–110.

The Times of India (Staff). (2014). If you want our market, meet our standards, US FDA chief says. *The Times of India*, Retrieved from *timesofindia.indiatimes.com/business/india-business/If-you-want-our-market-meet-our-standards-US-FDA-chief-says/articleshow/30639993.cms*.

Steinbrook, R. (2005). Commercial support and continuing medical education. *New England Journal of Medicine, 352*(6), 534–535.

Steinbrook, R. (2008). Financial support of continuing medical education. *Journal of the American Medical Association, 299*(9), 1060–1062.

Taylor, T. (2007). *Principles of economics: Economics and the economy*. St. Paul, MN: Freeload Press.

U.S. Government Accountability Office. (2011). FDA faces challenges overseeing the foreign drug manufacturing supply chain. Retrieved from *www.gao.gov/assets/130/126943.pdf*.

Wilkes, M. S., Bell, R. A., & Kravitz, R. L. (2000). Direct-to-consumer prescription drug advertising: Trends, impact, and implications. *Health Affairs, 19*(2), 110–128.

Weissman, J. S., Blumenthal, D., Silk, A. J., Zapert, K., Newman, M., & Leitman, R. (2003). Consumers' reports on the health effects of direct-to-consumer drug advertising. *Health Affairs Web Exclusive*. Retrieved from *content.healthaffairs.org/cgi/reprint/hlthaff.w3.82v1.pdf*.

Woloshin, S., Schwartz, L., & Welch, H. (2004). The value of benefit data in direct-to-consumer drug ads. *Health Affairs Web Exclusive*. Retrieved from *content.healthaffairs.org/cgi/content/abstract/hlthaff.w4.234*.

World Health Organization. (2014). Counterfeit medicines. Retrieved from *www.who.int/medicines/services/counterfeit/impact/ImpactF_S/en/index1.html*.

Wyatt, E. (2013). Supreme Court lets regulators sue over generic drug deals. *New York Times*, Retrieved from *www.nytimes.com/2013/06/18/business/supreme-court-says-drug-makers-can-be-sued-over-pay-for-delay-deals.html*.

ONLINE RESOURCES

Pharmaceutical Research and Manufacturers of America (PhRMA)
www.phrma.org
Food and Drug Administration (FDA)
www.fda.gov/default.htm
The Pew Charitable Trusts website on pharmaceutical policy
www.prescriptionproject.org

CHAPTER 27

Women's Reproductive Health Policy

Carol F. Roye

"You cannot have maternal health without reproductive health."

Hillary Clinton

Reproductive health is a foundation of public health. In 2002, the countries of the United Nations sought to determine the highest priorities for promoting health and reducing poverty globally. As a result, they agreed to a broad set of targets: the Millennium Development Goals. Of the eight goals, one addresses reducing child and infant mortality and a second addresses reducing maternal mortality (United Nations, 2008). Fertility control, or a woman's ability to time her pregnancies, is widely considered to be a vital element in reducing both infant and maternal mortality (Donovan & Wulf, 2002; National Research Council, 1995.)

WHEN WOMEN'S REPRODUCTIVE HEALTH NEEDS ARE NOT MET

INFANT MORTALITY

Three critical factors influencing pregnancy outcomes are:

1. *Age at which women conceive.* For biological reasons, teenage mothers and mothers in their forties are more likely than women in their twenties and thirties to have infants who do not survive.
2. *Spacing of pregnancies.* The chance of dying in infancy increases by 60% to 70% for a child born less than 2 years after an older sibling.
3. *Having too many children.* Children born fourth or higher in birth order have a threefold greater risk of dying than those lower in birth order.

Clearly, one easily implemented solution to these problems is to provide women with contraception and access to safe abortions. It is important to note that infant mortality rates among black infants have typically been twice as high as those for white infants, though the gap is narrowing slightly (Goodnough, 2013). Even when you consider socioeconomic status (SES), black women are more likely to have low birth-weight babies, a factor which can lead to infant mortality.

The infant mortality rate (IMR) in the United States is much lower than it is in the world's poorest countries; however, in 2010 the United States ranked 32nd among the 34 Organization for Economic Cooperation and Development (OECD) nations for infant mortality (CDC, 2013). Furthermore, although much more attention has been paid to infant and maternal mortality in resource-poor countries, in the United States access to birth control (defined as whether or not a state pays for comprehensive contraceptive services for poor women through Medicaid) influences the IMR. A state's failure to allow Medicaid to pay for comprehensive contraceptive services is a statistically significant predictor of a higher infant mortality rate (Roye, 2014). In addition, large family size and unplanned pregnancies and births place children at risk for physical abuse and neglect (Zuravin, 1991).

Access to safe, legal abortions also improves public health. Infant mortality rates declined when abortion was legalized by a Supreme Court decision in January 1973 with the case of Roe v Wade. In the early 1980s, researchers recognized there had been a striking decrease in the infant mortality rate in the decade since the Roe v Wade decision. One study sought to understand this precipitous decline by analyzing the role of four public policies: Medicaid, subsidized family planning services for poor women, maternal and infant care projects, and the legalization of abortion. The researchers found that the increase in legal abortions was the single most important factor in reducing infant mortality rates (Grossman & Jacobowitz, 1981).

MATERNAL MORTALITY

Although the United States saw a sevenfold reduction in maternal mortality in the 20th century, deaths related to pregnancy and childbirth persist even though many are preventable. There has been a recent upturn in maternal deaths in the United States, some of which are related to preexisting maternal chronic conditions, such as diabetes and obesity (Edwards & Hanke, 2013). And recent evidence shows that maternal mortality is greatly underestimated. As with infant mortality, the global ranking of the United States on maternal mortality is dismal, worse than a number of lower-resource Eastern European nations (WHO, 2010).

Predictors of maternal mortality are similar to those for infant mortality. For example, one predictor is a higher number of previous live births. Despite racial disparities in infant and maternal mortality (black women and infants suffer greater mortality), for both white and black women, pregnancy-related mortality was approximately twice as high for women after delivering a fifth or higher order live birth than for women after a first live birth. Furthermore, a little more than half of pregnancies in the United States are unintended (Alan Guttmacher Institute, 2013). Clearly, access to reproductive health care for all women would have a significant effect on public health by improving health outcomes for mothers and children.

ABORTION POLICY

There are thoughtful people on both sides of the abortion debate today. Many of those who oppose legal abortion earnestly believe that abortions are tantamount to infanticide, and therefore abortions should be outlawed. Among those who hold this view, however, there remains debate about whether abortion should be allowed in cases of incest, rape, or threat to the life of the mother. This is a key point because if women in need of an abortion were not able to get that care and were thus fated to die as a result of a severe complication of pregnancy (such as preeclampsia) or because of the mother's preexisting condition (such as heart disease), then there

is room for legitimate discussion among them about whether policy banning or allowing abortion is also tantamount to killing. Indeed, as noted above, access to safe abortions reduces maternal and infant mortality significantly.

WHY DO WE NEED POLICY SPECIFICALLY DIRECTED AT WOMEN?

One might wonder why women's reproductive health deserves special attention from policy experts; after all, women make up one-half the population. Firstly, women's unique reproductive health needs have been targeted by politicians because of the potential for pregnancy. Over the years, as reproductive medicine has advanced (including contraception and abortion techniques), it has become a focus of political rhetoric and a hot button issue. This has extended to political battles over who has control over a pregnant woman's body, the woman or legislators. Secondly, women's reproductive health needs are a nexus where health and sex (thus sexual taboos) meet. With our history of Puritanism, sex has always been a particularly sensitive topic in the United States. Moreover, there is a misguided concern that any discussion of sex will lead to promiscuity.

The context of the issue of women's health is the resurgence of orthodox religion, particularly the Religious Right, in the 1970s. Indeed, Randall Balmer, an evangelical Christian and religious historian, said that after holding a 2-year seminar on fundamentalist religions, an Ivy League university determined that: "the defining feature of fundamentalism, across religions, is an attempt to control women and their sexual behavior" (Roye, 2014). This religious influence has increased over the years, making it more difficult for women to access needed health care. It has, in many ways, overtaken the discussion of women's health and affected policymakers who now may feel that by preventing access to reproductive health care, they are taking a moral stand. However, as we have seen, there are serious public health consequences for everyone when women are not able to access reproductive health care. As a result of this religious influence over legislators in some states, there were more abortion-restrictions enacted by states between 2011 and 2013 than in the previous decade: 205 restrictions from 2011 to 2013, compared with 189 from 2001 to 2010 (Alan Guttmacher Institute, 2014).

WOMEN'S HEALTH AND U.S. POLICY

In the second half of the 20th century, women's health (defined here as access to the full range of reproductive health services, including contraception and abortion care) became a controversial topic that was viewed through a religious lens. However, this had not been the case earlier in American history. Until the middle of the nineteenth century, legal abortion, like so much else in this country, was governed by British common law. This held that abortion was criminal only if performed without due cause, after the woman felt fetal movement, which usually occurs at about the 16th week of pregnancy. This was known as the quickening doctrine after the medical term for the mother's perception of fetal movement. It is not even clear that late abortions were prosecuted. In fact, in 1800 there was no American legislation at all on the subject of abortion. Of course, there was similarly no legislation on contraception as there were no medically recognized means of preventing conception (Mohr, 1979).

In the early 19th century, there were no laboratory tests to reliably diagnose pregnancy. Common signs and symptoms of early pregnancy, such as absence of menstruation and nausea, can be caused by other factors. Thus a physician, or a woman herself, could take steps to correct her blocked menstrual flow. There were widely advertised products and medicines to help women restore menstruation or cure blocked or delayed menstruation. The fine print stated that the products should not be used by married women because they could cause miscarriages; this served as a signpost to women who wanted to end a pregnancy. Such was the nonchalant view of abortion that these ads could be found not only in newspapers, but also in the religious press (Brodie, 1994).

Many of those drugs and practices were unscientific and ineffective. Some, such as douching with carbolic acid, were downright dangerous. It was actually the concern about the danger of these methods that led to the first antiabortion laws in some states in the 1820s.

Other objections came from physicians who wanted to ban abortion unless a physician said it was needed. This was a move to improve their income because at the time anybody could advertise themselves as abortion providers. Abortion was a lucrative business that physicians wanted for themselves (Mohr, 1979).

It should also be noted that abortion is safer than carrying a pregnancy to term (Raymond & Grimes, 2012). Furthermore, women have always been so distressed by an unwanted pregnancy, and often so desperate to terminate it, that they have knowingly risked their lives to end the pregnancy. Not surprisingly, then, women were accessing illegal abortions before it was legal in the United States and were dying from conditions, such as gas gangrene, which can result from an unhygienic abortion. Survivors of these procedures often became so scarred that they lost their fertility.

The story of abortion policy in the United States. is long and tangled (Roye, 2014). By 1880 most states had antiabortion laws and by 1910 every state had them except Kentucky, where the courts had outlawed the practice. Some of the laws enacted in the late 1800s remained on the books until the 1973 Roe v Wade decision.

In the mid-20th century, physicians began to agitate to legalize abortion, this time out of concern for their patients' health. Religious bodies, such as the Southern Baptist Convention, advocated for the legalization of abortion to help women who were at risk of being maimed and killed by illegal, unsafe procedures. Indeed, members of the clergy banded together and formed networks to help women access safe abortions. The best known of these, the Clergy Consultation Service on Abortion, was formed by Reverend Howard Moody, a Texas-born Baptist minister (Moody, 1971).

For complex reasons, having primarily to do with politics, power, and money rather than women's health or public health, abortion became a hot button political issue after Roe v Wade. Today the introduction of laws limiting women's access to reproductive health care, and the fate of those laws, depends on who is in power in a given state and in the federal government.

Roe v Wade has been attacked by state and federal legislators who want to overturn the law. For example, in 2000, in the case of Stenberg v Carhart, a sharply divided Supreme Court struck down a Nebraska statute banning so-called partial birth abortion because the law placed an undue burden on a woman's right to have an abortion since it did not allow for an exception when the mother's health is threatened by continuing the pregnancy. Yet an almost identical federal law, the Partial-Birth Abortion Ban Act of 2003, was upheld by the Supreme Court in 2007 (Mears, 2007). A partial-birth abortion, which is a late term abortion, is properly called intact dilation and evacuation. It is very rare procedure typically performed to protect the mother's health or when a fetus is found to have a severe, often life-limiting congenital defect.

Despite this legal success, abortion opponents realized that it would be very difficult to have Roe v Wade struck down, so they turned their efforts to the states. In 2011, 162 state bills were signed into law restricting abortion rights, and similar legislation continues to be introduced. In some states abortion is very difficult to access, especially for poor women, because of a mandated waiting period between a required visit to the abortion facility and the procedure. This entails 2 days off from work, and finding transportation and childcare twice. Other states are likely to have no abortion providers in the near future because of onerous and medically unnecessary requirements being placed on these facilities, such as a requirement that the physical building where abortions are performed meet the same standards as an ambulatory surgery center, and a requirement that the abortion doctor have admitting privileges at a local hospital. Today, women's access to abortion varies widely by the state in which they reside and remains contentious. For example, in 2012, Virginia introduced a bill mandating a vaginal ultrasound for women prior to a first trimester abortion (involving inserting a probe in the vagina). However, there was such an outcry that they made the vaginal penetration optional, allowing an abdominal ultrasound (with the wand over the abdomen). The bill passed.

ACCESS TO CONTRACEPTION

Until the full implementation of the Affordable Care Act (ACA), which mandates comprehensive preventive health care for women, including contraceptive services without copays, access to contraception, particularly for poor women, will also continue to vary by state. Women who can afford to get health care and pay for contraception have always been able to purchase it. However, for poor women who rely on Medicaid access may again depend on the state in which they reside. Some states allow full access to contraception (and abortion) for poor women, although other states do not. Although laws are always in flux, as of 2015, only 21 states mandated comprehensive insurance coverage for contraception. Poor women in states that do not require payers (including Medicaid) to cover contraceptives often cannot access the means to prevent pregnancy, resulting in the unfortunate consequences discussed above.

Another public health issue related to contraception that became a political football is approval of over the counter (OTC) access to emergency contraception (EC): the morning-after pill. EC had been used successfully for years overseas before it became available in the United States. It is a very safe medication (usually 1 or 2 doses of a common birth control pill formulation), which may prevent pregnancy if taken within 3 to 5 days of unprotected intercourse. Despite the FDA's scientific panel overwhelmingly agreeing that EC should be available to women over the counter, it took years to receive approval because of political opposition. The objection stemmed, in part, from the erroneous belief by some that EC causes an abortion by preventing implantation of a fertilized ovum. Although it is not clear exactly how EC works, the evidence suggests that it does not prevent implantation but may work by suppressing ovulation, particularly if taken during the first half of the menstrual cycle, or by other mechanisms that have not as yet been well studied, such as the thickening of cervical mucus (Trussell, Raymond, & Cleland, 2014). EC first became available OTC for women aged 18 and older, despite the evidence demonstrating that it is a safe medication for all women. In

2013 a judge's ruling finally made it legally available for adolescent and adult women of all ages.

THE AFFORDABLE CARE ACT

The ACA stands to dramatically improve the reproductive health landscape for women who have insurance. As noted, it mandates comprehensive preventive health care for women, including contraceptive services, without copays (White House Blog, 2013). This care was included in the ACA because of a recommendation in the Institute of Medicine's (IOM's) 2011 report *Clinical Preventative Services for Women: Closing the Gaps* that women's health services be covered without copays when a network provider delivers them. It should be noted that religious organizations, with a specific religious mission, are exempt from this regulation (Liptak, 2013). However, other employers, who have for-profit, non-religious businesses, such as Hobby Lobby, a chain of craft shops with stores across the country, sued to exempt themselves from this regulation because the employers have personal objections to contraception. In 2014, the Supreme Court ruled that the owners of "closely-held" profit-making corporations (with company shares held by one person or a small group of people) cannot be forced by the ACA to provide their employees with contraceptives that offend their religious beliefs.

DISCUSSION QUESTIONS

1. Thinking about the national conversation about women's reproductive health policies today, how would you respond to those who wish to limit women's access to contraception or abortion?

2. Investigate your state's policies on access to contraception and abortion for women with insurance and those without. What are your state's infant and maternal mortality rates? Discuss the possible relationship between these factors.

REFERENCES

Alan Guttmacher Institute. (2013). Fact Sheet: Unintended pregnancy in the United States. Retrieved from *www.guttmacher.org/pubs/FB -Unintended-Pregnancy-US.html.*

Alan Guttmacher Institute. (2014). More state abortion restrictions were enacted in 2011–2013 than in the entire previous decade. Retrieved from *www.guttmacher.org/media/inthenews/2014/01/02/ index.html.*

Brodie, J. F. (1994). *Contraception and abortion in nineteenth-century America.* Ithaca, NY: Cornell University Press.

Center for Disease Control [CDC]. (2013). CDC grand rounds: Public health approaches to reducing U.S. infant mortality. *Morbidity and Mortality Weekly Report, 62*(31), 625–628.

Donovan, P., & Wulf, D. (2002). Family planning can reduce high infant mortality levels. *Issues in Brief, Apr*(2), 1–4. Series 2.

Edwards, J. E., & Hanke, J. C. (2013). An update on maternal mortality and morbidity in the United States. *Nursing For Women's Health, 17*(5), 376–388.

Goodnough, A. (2013). U.S. Infant mortality rate fell steadily from '05 to '11. *The New York Times,* A21. Retrieved from *www.nytimes.com/2013/04/ 18/health/infant-mortality-rate-in-us-declines.html?_r=0.*

Grossman, M., & Jacobowitz, S. (1981). Variations in infant mortality rates among counties of the United States: the roles of public policies and programs. *Demography, 18*(4), 695–713.

Institute of Medicine. (2011). *Clinical preventive services for women: Closing the gaps.* Washington, DC: National Academy of Sciences.

Liptak, A. (2013). Court confronts religious rights of corporations. *New York Times,* Retrieved from *www.nytimes.com/2013/11/25/us/court-confronts -religious-rights-of-corporations.html.*

Mears, B. (2007). Justices uphold ban on abortion procedure. *CNN.com,* Retrieved from *www.cnn.com/2007/LAW/04/18/scotus.abortion/.*

Mohr, J. (1979). *Abortion in America: The origins and evolution of national policy.* New York: Oxford University Press.

Moody, H. (1971). Abortion: Woman's right and legal problem. *Theology Today, 28*(3), 337–346.

National Research Council. (1995). *The best intentions: Unintended pregnancy and the well-being of children and families.* Washington, DC: The National Academies Press.

Raymond, E. G., & Grimes, D. A. (2012). The comparative safety of legal induced abortion and childbirth in the United States. *Obstetrics and Gynecology, 119*(2/1), 215–219.

Roye, C. (2014). *A woman's right to know.* Pleasantville, NY: Frances Price Enterprises.

Trussell, J., Raymond, E. G., & Cleland, K. (2014). Emergency contraception: a last chance to prevent unintended pregnancy. Retrieved from *ec .princeton.edu/questions/ec-review.pdf.*

United Nations. (2008). Delivering on the Global Partnership for Achieving the Millenium Development Goals. *MDG Gap Task Force Report,* Retrieved from *www.un.org/millenniumgoals/pdf/MDG%20Gap%20 Task%20Force%20Report%202008.pdf.*

White House Blog. (2013). How the Affordable Care Act improves the lives of American women. Retrieved from *www.whitehouse.gov/blog/ 2013/10/24/how-affordable-care-act-improves-lives-american-women.*

World Health Organization. (2010). Maternal mortality: Maternal mortality ratio. Retrieved from *apps.who.int/gho/data/node.wrapper.MATERNAL MORT1?lang=en.*

Zuravin, S. J. (1991). Unplanned childbearing and family size: Their relationship to child neglect and abuse. *Family Planning Perspectives, 23*(4), 155–161.

ONLINE RESOURCES

United States Health Resources and Services Administration
www.hrsa.gov/womensguidelines
Alan Guttmacher Institute
www.guttmacher.org
The Henry J. Kaiser Family Foundation
www.kff.org

CHAPTER 28

Public Health: Promoting the Health of Populations and Communities

Mary Mincer Hansen

"Health care is a right for everyone, in every country, rich or poor. Not providing health, education, and social protection is fundamentally unjust—in addition to being a bad economic and political strategy."

World Bank President Jim Yong Kim

THE STATE OF PUBLIC HEALTH AND THE PUBLIC'S HEALTH

Public health's mission is to protect and promote the health of populations and the communities in which these populations live, learn, and labor. One of the major raisons d'etre of public health is to influence and implement policy (Figure 28-1).

To understand the complexity of the public health system that works to fulfill this mission and influence policy, one must first understand that public health is performed by a tapestry of organizations with a workforce that is comprised of numerous professions (Figure 28-2). Nurses are major players in the public health workforce. The history of nursing is grounded in prevention. As Wright (2010) points out, Florence Nightingale viewed the role of nursing not only as care of the sick, but also as helping individuals to keep their constitutions and environments healthy. Therefore, it is imperative that nurses, regardless of their practice arena, be aware of and advocate for evidence based public health policy.

Public health has a distinguished history that includes major achievements in improving longevity and the quality of life. "During the twentieth century, life expectancy at birth among U.S. residents increased by 62%, from 47.3 years in 1900 to 76.8 in 2000, and unprecedented improvements in population health status were observed at every stage of life" (Centers for Disease Control and Prevention [CDC], 2011). In the first 10 years of this century, the U.S. annual death rate plummeted from 881.9 deaths per 100,000 population to 741. These impressive outcomes can be directly linked to public health interventions (CDC, 2011).

Unfortunately, during its recent history, the United States has focused primarily on treatment of illness rather than prevention, which has led to underfunding of the public health system and the specter of a reversal of these positive health achievements. A recent Institute of Medicine (IOM) report highlighted the abysmal health statistics for Americans compared with their counterparts in other high-income countries and warns that this has significant implications for our country (National Research Council and Institute of Medicine, 2013). The case for ecological, population-based, and community-focused interventions to address the socioeconomic drivers of poor health outcomes is beginning to be recognized as essential to reversing this downward spiral (IOM, 2012).

Two consequences of this downward spiral that are gaining attention are in the areas of defense and the economy. In 2011, the aggregate effects of obesity on members of the military were identified as decreased ability to perform physical activities, increased cost of health care for this population, and potential increased risk of psychological problems as found in the civilian population (Sanderson, Clemes, & Biddle, 2011). In fact, a publication by an association of retired generals and admirals

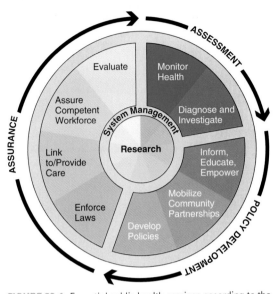

FIGURE 28-1 Essential public health services according to the Centers for Disease Control and Prevention (CDC). (From *www.cdc.gov/nphpsp/essentialservices.html.*)

went so far as to assert that obesity is a threat to national security and advocate for public health policy to address obesity in American youth (Mission Readiness, 2010).

The second consequence is the effect of poor population health on the economy. "The failure ... to develop and deliver effective preventive strategies is taking a large and growing toll on the nation's economy" (IOM, 2012). The incongruency of the United States spending less than 5% of all health care expenditures on public health and prevention activities is mind boggling (Mays & Smith, 2011). It is not as if investing in prevention has not been shown to be cost effective. It has been postulated that a modest investment in public health that led to a 1% reduction in chronic disease health care spending could potentially realize an $11 return for each $1 invested (IOM, 2012).

This lack of investment in public health has limited its ability to implement and advocate for evidence-based prevention strategies. One tactic that governmental public health is initiating to increase its effectiveness and credibility in the eyes of the public and policymakers is accreditation. Accreditation is viewed as a driver of quality

improvement and a tangible demonstration that certain standards have been met. Meeting these standards is viewed as a major step in assuring that a basic package of quality services will be provided to populations and that this will be accomplished through healthy community transformation (Riley, Bender, & Lownik, 2012).

IMPACT OF SOCIAL DETERMINANTS AND DISPARITIES ON HEALTH

A growing body of research has found that your zip code can be a greater contributor to your health status than your genetic code. "People who are poor and powerless have worse health and longevity than those with money, power, and prestige" (Flaskerud & DeLilly, 2012, p. 494). According to the CDC (2013a, p. 184), "[there are] persistent disparities between some population groups in health outcomes, access to health care, adoption of health promoting behaviors, and exposure to health-promoting environments." There is a link between these disparities and social determinants of health. These determinants can be categorized as socioeconomic (e.g., education and income), social structure (e.g., gender and ethnic discrimination), and environmental (social, built, and natural) (IOM, 2011).

The health disparities are stark. Black adults are at a 50% greater risk of dying prematurely from cardiovascular disease when compared with their white counterparts. Adult diabetes prevalence is higher among individuals without a college degree and with lower incomes. An estimated 40% of households do not have access to stores where they can easily purchase fresh fruit and vegetables (CDC, 2013a).

The public health approach to successfully moderate the social determinants leading to health disparities is grounded in policy. Reutter and Kushner (2010) make the case that nurses are perfectly positioned to act to influence policy and indeed have this as a professional mandate. Nurses have the experiences with clients to be able to use powerful stories, based on true-life situations, and to raise the

UNIT 2

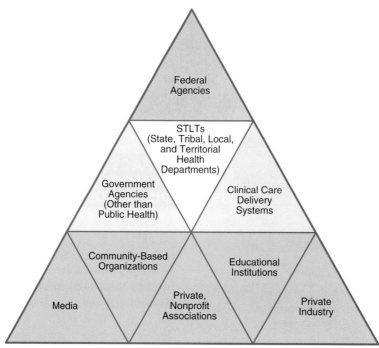

FIGURE 28-2 Components of the public health system. (From Chapman, K. Weaver, G. & Taveras, S. [2013]. Building capacity of the public health system to improve population health through national, nonprofit organizations. Centers for Disease Control and Prevention. Retrieved from *www.cdc.gov/stltpublichealth/funding/rfaot13.html*.)

awareness of the public, policymakers, and health care providers regarding the role of social determinants in health disparities. Individually, and through engagement with their professional organizations, nurses have the responsibility to advocate for policies such as fair wages and early childhood education for the disadvantaged to have the opportunity to improve their chances for a healthy life.

MAJOR THREATS TO PUBLIC HEALTH

OVERWEIGHT AND OBESITY

The incidence, causes, and effects of overweight and obesity are well documented. The most recent CDC data indicates that more than one-third of adults and almost 17% of youth are obese with the highest incidence being in the over-60 population (Ogden et al., 2012). Equally concerning is the fact that another 30% of adults are overweight (Fryar,

Carroll, & Ogden, 2012). Current research has linked obesity to major causes of death, such as cardiovascular disease and cancer, as well as psychosocial effects, such as depression. An emerging issue is the stigmatization of the obese individual that may approximate the prevalence rate of racial discrimination in the United States (Puhl & Heuer, 2010). Another extremely troubling by-product for overweight children is that they feel stigmatized and may experience decreased academic and social success (Karnik & Kanekar, 2012).

Public health policy interventions to address obesity are increasingly being viewed as the most effective way to have a positive impact on its causes (Dodson et al., 2012). Policy interventions for obesity target social, environmental, and economic aspects of the lived experience of populations. An example of current public health policy efforts to address obesity is legislation related to types of healthy and so-called competitive foods, those consumables that are not provided as part of the school feeding programs, available in the school setting. A recent analysis of legislation introduced to promote healthy eating in schools highlighted the example where parents and community members review food contracts for nutritional value of foods that will help students learn and lead a more healthy life (Shroff et al., 2012).

MENTAL HEALTH

Similar to its broad definition of physical health, the World Health Organization has defined mental health as "a state of wellbeing in which every individual realizes his or her own potential, can cope with the normal stresses of life, can work productively and fruitfully, and is able to make a contribution to her or his community" (Herrman, Saxena, & Moodie, 2005, p. 2). Research has found a connection between mental health and lifestyle behaviors that either promote or detract from physical health and longevity (Perry, Presley-Cantrell, & Dhingra, 2010). In addition, mental illness and cardiovascular disease account for 70% of the global reduction in economic output from noncommunicable diseases (Bloom et al., 2012).

As with other chronic diseases, public health interventions to promote mental health and prevent and treat mental illness require a multifaceted approach. This approach includes policy interventions to provide the opportunity for income equity, safe housing and neighborhoods, and sanctions against discrimination rooted in the social stigma inherent in mental illness (Perry, Presley-Cantrell, & Dhingra, 2010). In addition, parity and access to coverage of behavioral health services similar to the coverage of medical conditions is critical. Historically, behavioral health services have been either excluded from insurance or drastically limited in coverage. The Affordable Care Act demonstrates the use of policy to improve mental health services by mandating behavioral health coverage as one of the essential health services (Aggarwal & Rowe, 2013).

CLIMATE CHANGE

According to the CDC, environmental changes due to climate change, such as rising sea levels, extreme temperatures and storms, and poor air quality are impacting human health (CDC, 2013b). These impacts include food insecurity and threats to food safety (Lake et al., 2012); increases in infectious diseases, injury and violence, heat-related and respiratory illnesses; and mental health disorders (Ebi, 2011).

Public health and health care professionals must take an active role in addressing this potentially catastrophic public health threat. Actions that should be undertaken include research, education, and mitigation. Research is needed to provide the data to educate health professionals, policymakers, and populations about the causes and approaches to prepare for and mitigate the consequences (McMichael & Lindgren, 2011). Advocating for practices and policies to reduce the human contribution to climate change and to have in place plans to respond to it are essential public health responsibilities.

CHALLENGES FACED BY GOVERNMENTAL PUBLIC HEALTH

Governmental public health is composed of the CDC, a state Public Health Department in each state and territory, and local health departments within the states. Even though the roles and services outlined at the beginning of this chapter have been agreed upon as essential, there is no uniformity in structure of, or services offered by, state and local health departments. In fact there is a saying among public health professionals that "once you have seen one health department you have seen one health department." This has hindered efforts to obtain adequate funding, collect data and measure health outcomes, and to fully use the promise of technology to improve communication, efficiency, and effectiveness.

As previously discussed, funding prevention yields a good return on investment. Since public health is devoted to prevention, it makes sense to invest in it to realize this return. However, "the public health infrastructure is not funded adequately to carry out its mission" (IOM, 2012). A major drawback of this underfunding of infrastructure and capacity to fulfill its mission is an inadequate workforce, of which nursing makes up the largest percentage of professionals (Swearingen, 2009). Compounding this issue is the recent finding that a significant percentage of state and local health departments report difficulty in recruiting registered nurses to fill position vacancies (University of Michigan Center of Excellence in Public Health Workforce Studies, 2013). This lack of adequate funding is even more perplexing based on the findings of Mays and Smith (2011) that death rates for selected causes of mortality were reduced by 3% to 6.9% with each 10% incremental increase in local public health spending.

Another challenge to public health is that policy development should be based on scientific evidence, yet public health research has not been funded to the degree that medical care research has been. In addition, conducting this research is more complex and must be interpreted in the context of multiple population variables as well as concerns of inequality in implementation. From a practical sense there are barriers to evidence-based policy decision making. These barriers include: not translating research into a format that is easily understood by policymakers and the media, competing political pressures by special interest groups, and mistrust of research findings that can be spun (Orton et al., 2011). One compelling way to present research to politicians that has proven effective is to embed it in the context of a powerful personal story told in person by a constituent. An example of this could be having a son whose father died of lung cancer related to smoking come and talk to his state representative prior to a vote on banning smoking from all public places.

Underlying all major challenges to public health is the fact that our system "lacks a coherent template for population health information that could be used to understand the health status of Americans and to assess how well the nation's efforts and investments result in improved population health" (IOM, 2011, p. 2). Without data to guide the three public health mandates of assessment, assurance, and policy development, the public's health in the United States will continue to fall behind its peer countries in health outcomes. Confounding this challenge is the Health Information Technology

for Economic and Clinical Health Act (HITECH), which mandates that care providers and public health have the interconnectivity to be able to transmit and receive data. Public health departments must build an integrated information technology (IT) system that connects a variety of provider types, communicates with multiple IT platforms, and is updated continuously to meet the changing information landscape (Lenert & Sundwall, 2012).

CHARTING A BRIGHT FUTURE FOR PUBLIC HEALTH

There are many innovative public health strategies to promote population health and reduce disparities. Three areas that will be discussed are technology, partnerships, and a health in all policies approach to policymaking.

Technology has spawned a plethora of social media communication venues. Use of these innovative communication tools for health purposes has inherent benefits and risks. Moorhead et al. (2013) identified the benefits as increased health information access, social support, opportunity for public health surveillance, and an additional tool to advocate for health policy. Limitations included threats to confidentiality and privacy, as well as concerns regarding the accuracy and appropriateness of information for the consumer.

An example of the application of social media in public health is the use of a Facebook site developed by community health nurses to educate teens and young adults about the causes, treatment, and prevention of chlamydia. The page also has links to providers and other educational resources (see Caryn Forya at https://www.facebook.com/CarynForya). The nurses studied the outcomes of use of this social media tool and found a "23% self-reported increase in condom use, and 54% reduction in positive Chlamydia cases among 15- to 17-year-olds" (Jones, Baldwin, & Lewis, 2012, p. 106).

Public health has long realized that partnering is critical to success in a resource-constrained and multifarious milieu. A sustained transformation of communities and the health environment requires a network of committed entities. An exemplar of the power of public health partnerships is the Alameda County Place Matters Policy Initiative (http://www.acphd.org/social-and-health-equity/policy-change/place-matters.aspx). Led by the local public health department and a champion county supervisor, a multisector partnership was formed to influence health polices related to social determinants of health and equity. One example of success was that their testimony highlighting the link between health and housing, requested by a local environmental and economic justice organization, brought together policymakers with diverse political ideologies to support affordable housing (Schaff et al., 2013).

Another example of a potential partnership that holds great promise for improving health outcomes is the Accountable Care Organization (ACO) aspect of the Affordable Care Act. As part of this health reform law, ACOs are incentivized to manage a patient population and nonprofit hospitals are required to conduct community health-needs assessments. Given that public health already has the expertise in these areas, it behooves ACOs and public health to forge a partnership.

A broader initiative to improve the health status of all Americans is a health in all policy (HiAP) approach to policy formulation. This approach is grounded in the assumptions that the policies controlling the social determinants of health and health equity are under the purview of nonhealth care professionals and that the health outcomes influenced by these policies are critical to a "strong economy and vibrant society" (Rudolph et al., 2013, p. 1). Mandating that the health implications, both positive and harmful, be considered when formulating all policies promotes intersectoral collaboration and can reduce unintended consequences and improve their efficiency and effectiveness.

Even though public health in the United States faces daunting issues and challenges, it is still a beacon of hope if we as a country nurture its potential. This can be done through partnerships, policies, and political will. It is up to all health professionals to be aware of major issues facing their clients, whether they be physical, mental, or social, and advocate for a society that provides the resources for individuals and populations to practice healthy behaviors, and communities to build an infrastructure that promotes health.

DISCUSSION QUESTIONS

1. What are specific actions that health professionals can take regardless of their practice area and site to promote population and community health?
2. How should health professionals proactively plan to update their knowledge and skills to respond to the major public health issues and challenges facing them and their clients?
3. How will the rapid advances in technology and health-system reform affect the public's health?

REFERENCES

Aggarwal, N. K., & Rowe, M. (2013). The individual mandate, mental health parity, and the Obama Health Plan. *Administration and Policy in Mental Health*, *40*(4), 255–257. doi:10.1007/s10488-011-0395-3.

Bloom, D. E., Cafiero, E., Jané-Llopis, E., Abrahams-Gessel, S., Bloom, L. R., et al. (2012). *The global economic burden of noncommunicable diseases*. Geneva: World Economic Forum.

Centers for Disease Control and Prevention [CDC]. (2011). Ten great public health achievements, United States, 2001-2010. Retrieved from *www.cdc.gov/mmwr/preview/mmwrhtml/mm6019a5.htm*.

Centers for Disease Control and Prevention [CDC]. (2013a). Introduction: CDC Health disparities and inequalities report. United States, 2013. *MMWR*, *62*(Suppl 3), 1–187.

Centers for Disease Control and Prevention [CDC]. (2013b). CDC Features: Public health response to a changing climate. Retrieved from *www.cdc.gov/Features/ChangingClimate/*.

Chapman, K., Weaver, G., Taveras, S., & [CDC]. (2013). Building capacity of the public health system to improve population health through national, nonprofit organizations. Centers for Disease Control and Prevention., Retrieved from *www.cdc.gov/stltpublichealth/funding/rfaot13.html*.

Dodson, E. A., Eyler, A. A., Chalifour, S., & Wintrode, C. G. (2012). A review of obesity-themed policy briefs. *American Journal of Preventive Medicine*, *43*(3 Suppl 2), S143–S148. doi:10.1016/j.amepre.2012.05.021.

Ebi, K. (2011). Climate change and health risks: Assessing and responding to them through "adaptive management." *Health Affairs (Project Hope)*, *30*(5), 924–930. doi:10.1377/hlthaff.2011.0071.

Flaskerud, J. H., & DeLilly, C. R. (2012). Social determinants of health status. *Issues in Mental Health Nursing*, *33*(7), 494–497. doi:10.3109/01612840.2012.662581.

Fryar, C. D., Carroll, M. D., & Ogden, C. L. (2012). Prevalence of overweight, obesity, and extreme obesity among adults: United States, trends 1960–1962 through 2009–2010. Hyattsville, MD: National Center for Health Statistics. Retrieved from *www.stevesaenz.com/uploads/1/0/6/4/1064 2571/prevalence_of_overweight_obesity_and_extreme_obesity_among _adults.pdf*.

Herrman, H., Saxena, S., & Moodie, R. (2005). *Promoting mental health: Concepts, emerging evidence, practice: A report of the World Health Organization, Department of Mental Health and Substance Abuse in collaboration with the Victorian Health Promotion Foundation and the University of Melbourne.* Geneva: World Health Organization.

Institute of Medicine [IOM]. (2011). For the public's health: The role of measurement in action and accountability. Washington, DC: National Academies Press. Retrieved from *site.ebrary.com/id/10466003*.

Institute of Medicine [IOM]. (2012). For the public's health: Investing in a healthier future. Washington, DC: National Academies Press. Retrieved from *www.iom.edu/Reports/2012/For-the-Publics-Health -Investing-in-a-Healthier-Future.aspx*.

Jones, K., Baldwin, K. A., & Lewis, P. R. (2012). The potential influence of a social media intervention on risky sexual behavior and Chlamydia incidence. *Journal of Community Health Nursing, 29*(2), 106–120. doi :10.1080/07370016.2012.670579.

Karnik, S., & Kanekar, A. (2012). Childhood obesity: A global public health crisis. *International Journal of Preventive Medicine, 3*(1), 1–7.

Lake, I. R., Hooper, L., Abdelhamid, A., Bentham, G., Boxall, A. B. A., et al. (2012). Climate change and food security: Health impacts in developed countries. *Environmental Health Perspectives, 120*(11), 1520–1526. doi:10.1289/ehp.1104424.

Lenert, L., & Sundwall, D. N. (2012). Public health surveillance and meaningful use regulations: A crisis of opportunity. *American Journal of Public Health, 102*(3), e1–e7. doi:10.2105/AJPH.2011.300542; Retrieved from *ajph.aphapublications.org/doi/pdf/10.2105/AJPH.2011.300542*.

Mays, G. P., & Smith, S. A. (2011). Evidence links increases in public health spending to declines in preventable deaths. *Health Affairs, 30*(8), 1585–1593.

McMichael, A. J., & Lindgren, E. (2011). Climate change: Present and future risks to health, and necessary responses. *Journal of Internal Medicine, 270*(5), 401–413. doi:10.1111/j.1365-2796.2011.02415.x.

Mission Readiness. (2010). *Too fat to fight.* Washington, DC: Mission Readiness.

Moorhead, S. A., Hazlett, D. E., Harrison, L., Carroll, J. K., Irwin, A., & Hoving, C. (2013). A new dimension of health care: Systematic review of the uses, benefits, and limitations of social media for health communication. *Journal of Medical Internet Research, 15*(4), e85.

National Research Council and Institute of Medicine. (2013). US health in international perspective: Shorter lives, poorer health. National Academies Press. Retrieved from *www.ncbi.nlm.nih.gov/pubmed/24006554*.

Ogden, C. L., Carroll, M. D., Kit, B. K., & Flegal, K. M. (2012). Prevalence of obesity in the United States, 2009-2010. U.S. Department of Health and Human Services, Centers for Disease Control and Prevention, National Center for Health Statistics. Retrieved from *wood-ridge.schoolwires .net/cms/lib6/NJ01001835/Centricity/Domain/175/Obesity%20Article .pdf*.

Orton, L., Lloyd-Williams, F., Taylor-Robinson, D., O'Flaherty, M., & Capewell, S. (2011). The use of research evidence in public health decision making processes: Systematic review. *PLoS ONE, 6*(7), e21704.

Retrieved from *ajph.aphapublications.org/doi/pdf/10.2105/AJPH.2011 .300542*.

Perry, G. S., Presley-Cantrell, L. R., & Dhingra, S. (2010). Addressing mental health promotion in chronic disease prevention and health promotion. *American Journal of Public Health, 100*(12), 2337.

Puhl, R. M., & Heuer, C. A. (2010). Obesity stigma: Important considerations for public health. *American Journal of Public Health, 100*(6), 1019–1028. doi:10.2105/AJPH.2009.159491.

Reutter, L., & Kushner, K. E. (2010). "Health equity through action on the social determinants of health": Taking up the challenge in nursing. *Nursing Inquiry, 17*(3), 269–280.

Riley, W. J., Bender, K., & Lownik, E. (2012). Public health department accreditation implementation: Transforming public health department performance. *American Journal of Public Health, 102*(2), 237–242.

Rudolph, L., Caplan, J., Mitchell, C., Ben-Moshe, K., & Dillon, L. (2013). Health in all policies: Improving health through intersectoral collaboration. Institute of Medicine, Retrieved from *www.iom.edu/Global/ Perspectives/2013/HealthInAllPolicies.aspx*.

Sanderson, P. W., Clemes, S. A., & Biddle, S. J. H. (2011). The correlates and treatment of obesity in military populations: A systematic review. *Obesity Facts, 4*(3), 229–237. doi:10.1159/000329450.

Schaff, K., Desautels, A., Flournoy, R., Carson, K., Drenick, T., et al. (2013). Addressing the social determinants of health through the Alameda County, California, Place Matters policy initiative. *Public Health Reports (Washington, DC: 1974), 128*(Suppl. 3), 48–53.

Shroff, M. R., Jones, S. J., Frongillo, E. A., & Howlett, M. (2012). Policy instruments used by states seeking to improve school food environments. *American Journal of Public Health, 102*(2), 222–229.

Swearingen, C. D. (2009). Using nursing perspectives to inform public health nursing workforce development. *Public Health Nursing, 26*(1), 79–87. doi:10.1111/j.1525-1446.2008.00756.x.

University of Michigan Center of Excellence in Public Health Workforce Studies. (2013). Enumeration and characterization of the public health nurse workforce. Retrieved from *www.rwjf.org/en/about-rwjf/ newsroom/features-and-articles/public-health-nursing.html*.

Wright, J. (2010). The concept of public health. *British Journal of School Nursing, 5*(4), 206.

ONLINE RESOURCES

Centers for Disease Control and Prevention
www.cdc.gov
World Health Organization
www.who.int/en
Institute of Medicine
www.iom.edu
American Public Health Association
apha.org

CHAPTER 29

TAKING ACTION:

Blazing a Trail...and the Bumps Along the Way—A Public Health Nurse as a Health Officer

Gina Miranda-Diaz

"Do not go where the path may lead, go instead where there is no path and leave a trail."

Ralph Waldo Emerson

After accumulating 225 credits, spanning more than 3 decades from Bachelor of Science in Nursing to Doctor of Nursing Practice, I was unemployed. Armed with credentials and a passion for public health I went to the local town hall to speak to Brian P. Stack, the Mayor of Union City and a New Jersey State Senator, who had often called upon me to volunteer at health fairs. During our conversation, the Mayor offered me a position as Health Officer, which required state licensure. I wondered exactly what the role and functions of a Health Officer were. According to the New Jersey State Department of Health (NJSDOH), a Health Officer is defined as:

… the public health chief executive officer of a municipal, regional, county, or contractual health agency. This individual is responsible for evaluating health problems, planning appropriate activities to address these health problems, developing necessary budget procedures to finance these activities, and directing staff to carry out these activities efficiently and economically. (NJSDOH, n.d., a.)

This is a position that has not traditionally been held by nurses. When I became a Health Officer, I was only the second nurse in the history of the state to hold this title, and the first Latina.

GETTING THE JOB: MORE DIFFICULT THAN YOU MIGHT THINK

But before I could do the job, I had to get licensed. My next of many challenges was to answer a very important question: How do I prepare for the licensing examination? After logging onto the NJSDOH website, I read the details of the two-part exam, the first of which consists of 100 true/false questions across the topic areas of management and administration, environmental and occupational health, chronic diseases, and communicable disease (NJDOH, n.d., a.). You had to pass this before you could go on to take the second part of the exam. I began preparing for the exam long before receiving my eligibility notice. Over a 60-day period, I reviewed more than 500 pages of study materials from various sources. I also sought additional advice from individuals who had taken the exam in previous years; however, their advice was quite unexpected. Many told me to keep my expectations low for passing the exam and to expect to need multiple attempts. With this in mind, I was more determined than ever to succeed, and channeled all my energy and efforts into passing.

Two months later, on a warm, sunny day in May, I entered the lobby at the New Jersey Fire Academy in Sayreville and discovered that was I the only nurse there, and the oldest individual taking the exam. Feeling slightly terrified, I picked up my pencil and proceeded to answer the 100 true/false questions within the allotted 90 minutes. After waiting an agonizing hour for the results, I was notified that I was eligible to advance to the second half of the examination. Thirty days afterward, on June 9, 2012, I received my Health Officer license. I was exhilarated by the promise of beginning a new chapter of my life and treading a new career path.

With license in hand, I was now qualified to accept the offer of employment extended to me. "This should be a cakewalk," I thought. Upon meeting with Mayor/Senator Stack to discuss the employment offer, I realized that the exam was not the only hurdle I had to clear. Unfortunately, Union City was designated a fiscally stressed municipality and the salary offer was equivalent to that of a part-time Health Officer. There was no possibility of earning a living wage in that city, and, sadly, I had to turn down the offer.

After exhaustive searches on the Internet, I met with Mayor Felix E. Roque, MD, of West New York, New Jersey. Once he learned of my desire to become a Health Officer, Mayor Roque told me about his many health goals for the community. He believed in the importance of having an advanced practice nurse experienced in public health to lead the local Department of Health. After consideration of the current workload of the veteran Health Officer (seven towns), the Mayor offered me a part-time position as Health Officer in his town. I eagerly accepted for three reasons: My pay for this part-time position would be nearly as much as I would have made in the full-time position in Union City; I would have the title of Director; and Mayor Roque was a physician who embraces health promotion and disease prevention.

Finally, despite all the difficulties, I was thrilled to begin my new role as a leader in public health and make my mark in my newly adopted community. I believed that this would be the height of my career as the first Latina nurse to be appointed as a Health Officer in New Jersey. I believed the path ahead was clear for me to take up the reins and move this Department of Health in the right direction. But soon that belief would be tested.

CREATING ACCESS TO PUBLIC HEALTH CARE IN WEST NEW YORK

For the first time, the town of West New York had a bilingual Registered Nurse as its Health Officer, who was able to provide access to public and

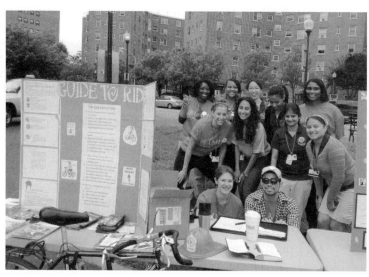

FIGURE 29-1 Nursing students from the University of Medicine and Dentistry of New Jersey College of Nursing brought their poster on bike safety to the fair.

community health services to its residents. Nearly 80% of the population speaks Spanish (U.S. Census Bureau, 2012). My bilingual skills are a huge asset for helping inhabitants who speak only Spanish. They now have access to a public health official who is both linguistically and culturally competent.

I started by establishing goals for the community of West New York that were consistent with Healthy New Jersey 2020 (NJSDOH, n.d., b.). This plan outlines health goals for New Jersey residents and is modeled on the federal government's *Healthy People 2020*. Community strategies include efforts to improve access to public health providers and create organizational partnerships for improving health for all residents of West New York.

ON-THE-JOB TRAINING

No one in the Health Department was even remotely interested or willing to provide any on-the-job training for me. Baptism by fire would be a more appropriate description of my orientation. On the first day on the job, April 1, 2013, I was filled with excitement as well as anxiety about the unknown. Following an introduction to the staff, I was escorted to a nondescript desk in the corner of the room and eagerly awaited an orientation. I waited … and waited … but no orientation would ever materialize. There was absolutely no desire to assist me in any way in my new role. In danger of feeling defeated on my first day, I realized I had to find my own way forward. Clearly, there was very little comprehension about the role of a public health nurse, much less a public health nurse in the role of Health Officer. Gaining any understanding would necessitate a paradigm shift for everyone in the Health Department and town hall.

What I lacked in confidence in my role as a Health Officer, I had in abundance as a public health nurse. On the second day at work, I put on my public health nurse hat and conducted an assessment of the community. West New York is truly a tale of two cities: waterfront properties, high-end restaurants, and supermarkets are juxtaposed with a blue-collar community filled with tenements and bodegas, with food vendors lining the streets.

Several health concerns had been plaguing many of the less affluent residents of West New York, such as lead poisoning, mold, and safety. According to a recent report authored by the Division of Highway and Traffic Safety (DHTS) (n.d., a.), there was also an increase in pedestrian and cycling accidents, despite a revision of the traffic laws in New Jersey. To that end, the DHTS (n.d., b.) launched a campaign, *Safe Passage: Moving Towards Zero Fatalities*. Revisions in the law mandate that cars stop, instead of yield, to pedestrians crossing a state marked crosswalk. Despite the new laws, however, pedestrian accidents and fatalities continue to rise as pedestrians are distracted (for instance, by texting), dart out into traffic, or ignore traffic signals.

Head trauma for children under 18 years of age not wearing a protective helmet when cycling is another issue. Of the 500,000 plus individuals who suffered bicycle-related injuries in the United States in 2010, 26,000 were children under the age of 17 (Centers for Disease Control and Prevention [CDC], 2013). The CDC reported that bicycle safety laws are often ignored by more than 50% of cyclists. New Jersey had established its own bicycle and pedestrian safety law in 2005 mandating that "all children under the age of 17 must wear a helmet while riding a bicycle, skateboarding, roller skating, and inline skating" (New Jersey Department of Transportation, 2005).

After reviewing this data, it suddenly beame crystal clear to me that my first goal at the West New York Department of Health should be to organize a safety fair. I had a conversation with the Mayor who offered his support and agreed to mobilize resources for me.

POLITICAL CHALLENGES

It soon became apparent that everyone, from the town administrator to the director of public affairs, wanted to place their imprimatur on the project. I just wanted to move forward with my project without any limitations, but working in municipal government does not allow for purely independent anything. There are multiple layers and players and each one has an idea about how things should be done. I provided every department head in the town hall with a copy of the evidence on bicycle safety and the law, optimistic that the evidence would garner support from the powers that be. However, no one seemed very eager to collaborate with me and I realized I was on my own.

According to the Mayor, I was authorized to direct members of my department, a fact that was not documented in writing, which contributed to a culture of resistance among staff. Since the Mayor worked in the town hall a mere 8 to 10 hours a week, I was at the mercy of the town administrators and other individuals indifferent to my purpose. Following weeks of preparation, I was ready to create and distribute flyers and began visiting every public and parochial school in town. When it was time to advertise the fair, I had to summon assistance from the Department of Public Affairs, but that was met with yet more indifference and bureaucratic red tape. Finally at the end of my rope, I contacted the Mayor, and he instructed the staff from public affairs to advertise the safety fair in the local newspaper and on cable television. Even though there were individuals who did not value the merits of the safety fair, they agreed, albeit reluctantly, to support the fair.

With only 20 working days to prepare, I had to work quickly. I immediately rolled up my sleeves to begin preparations. First, I had to contact the New Jersey Division of Highway Traffic Safety in the state capitol of Trenton and inquire about resources. On the following day, I was provided with two resources: a local trauma medical center and the Automobile Association of America (AAA). I spoke to a veteran Health Officer about seeking donations from different sources for the purchase of bicycle helmets. My excitement waned with the mocking tone of his voice and that of another staff member who insisted, "No one gives anything away for free, any more." Later, I would gladly prove them wrong. Between the medical center and the AAA, 125 bicycle helmets were donated. In fact, they also gave me coloring books and pamphlets on bicycle safety and pedestrian safety. I was so happy for the children and could not believe my good fortune. Seeing the wide-eyed stares on the faces of the staff as I carted in all of the free helmets was priceless.

SAFE KID DAY ARRIVES

My defining moment as a Health Officer has to be the holding of the inaugural Safe Kids Day (SKD) in West New York. Every year, on May 18, SKD is celebrated around the globe, but it had never been celebrated in West New York, until now. Safe Kids Day seemed the perfect opportunity to put on a safety fair for the community that is evidence based. Hosting the SKD fair meant that I would be able to highlight a number of safety issues: wearing of bicycle helmets, pedestrian issues, fire, medication, and driving safety.

Despite the clouds that dominated the sky and the threat of rain on the morning of the fair, more than 200 children and parents attended. There were nursing students presenting posters on correctly fitting a bicycle helmet, use of hand signals, and pedestrian safety. The American Red Cross provided emergency and disaster information for all those who participated. Community leaders focused on traffic safety. The Rebeka Verea Foundation arrived with backpacks and information on the perils of texting, distracted driving, and speeding. Local firefighters brought their shiny fire engine, plastic helmets for the children, fire-safety coloring books, and fire detectors for everyone. The first West New York SKD fair was a resounding success.

NURSES SHAPING POLICY IN LOCAL GOVERNMENT

My initial months in the role of Health Officer were very busy. I was able to influence policy on the municipal level. For example, I extended the office's hours of operation by 30 minutes to afford residents and business owners more access. I also discovered that my department was deviating from the state regulations on obtaining a marriage license. Upon careful review of the regulations, I noted many inconsistencies in the documentation that was being requested by the vital statistics registrar on my staff. Hispanic immigrants and individuals from outside the country were being asked for additional documents, such as passports, birth certificates, and licenses. Requesting documentation beyond the required license was arbitrary and not based on the state's regulations. Often individuals had to return with the additional documents and lose another morning or afternoon from work. Our procedures are now in compliance with the state's regulations.

Another health issue I have dealt with is lead poisoning in children residing in Hudson County (including West New York). Lead poisoning has been documented as the leading environmental health problem in children under the age of 6 (CDC, 2013). Elevated lead levels are related to the age of the dwellings in West New York. Half of the 240,000 tenement apartments were built before 1950 (NJSDOH, 2010) and 70% of the paint used during that era contained lead. Lead paint can be also found on cracked windowsills and in playgrounds. Other sources of lead are chili powder, candy, and improperly glazed pottery often sold in the local bodegas from various Latin American countries (Medlin, 2004). Part of my role at the Health Department is to assign health and sanitation inspectors to randomly scrutinize supermarkets, groceries, and 99-cent stores to make sure lead-based products are not on the shelves. In 2013, I became actively involved with the Partnership for Maternal Child Health in Northern New Jersey to become part of the solution in the battle for Healthy Homes, an initiative to reduce lead poisoning.

Collaborating with a large organization, such as this one, is often helpful for introducing legislation, in this case to ensure that every child has the opportunity to live in a healthy home. Membership in professional organizations, such as the New Jersey State Nurses Association and the New Jersey Chapter of the National Association of Hispanic Nurses (where I served as vice president), is also important. Professional organizations unite nurses pursuing a common goal and use their political know-how and strength in numbers to influence policy. Do not leave advocacy for someone else to do. Be the individual who is part of a collective voice.

SUCCESSES AND CHALLENGES

I never dreamed that I would be faced with so many hurdles during my first year as a Health Officer, but each day I feel more confident and secure in my abilities. Success is sweeter when I am able to plow ahead toward goals for the community despite the bureaucracy of local government. I can overcome challenges if I remain open to inclusiveness and flexibility in my new role and adapt to the workings of local government. Each obstacle becomes a teachable moment, and that affords me the opportunity to grow into my role. I have forged alliances with local organizations, public health nurses, and municipal town hall employees. And I have advocated for the health of the residents of West New York. Each success strengthens my credibility and each failure helps me prepare better for the next experience. I plan to be an integral part of the health department by engaging in advocacy and influencing policy while continuing to define the Advanced Public Health Nurse as a Health Officer.

REFERENCES

Centers for Disease Control and Prevention. (2013). Head injuries and bicycle safety. Retrieved from *www.cdc.gov/healthcommunication/toolstemplates/entertainmened/tips/headinjuries.html.*

Division of Highway and Traffic Safety, New Jersey Office of the Attorney General. (n.d., a.). Safe bicycle riding. Retrieved from *www.nj.gov/oag/hts/downloads/Safe_Bicycle_Riding_in_NJ.pdf.*

Division of Highway and Traffic Safety. (n.d., b.). Safe Passage: Moving to zero fatalities. Retrieved from *www.nj.gov/oag/hts/index.html.*

Medlin, J. (2004). Lead: Sweet candy, bitter poison. *Environmental Health Perspectives, 112*(14), A803.

New Jersey State Department of Health. (n.d., a.). Licensure for health officers. Retrieved from *www.state.nj.us/health/lh/hofficer.shtml.*

New Jersey State Department of Health. (n.d., b.). Healthy New Jersey. Retrieved from *www.state.nj.us/health/chs/hnj2020/.*

New Jersey State Department of Health. (2010). Lead poisoning control-family health services. Retrieved from *www.nj.gov/health/fhs/documents/childhoodlead2010.pdf.*

New Jersey State Department of Transportation. (2005). Biking in New Jersey: Regulations. Retrieved from *www.state.nj.us/transportation/commuter/bike/regulations.shtm.*

U. S. Census Bureau. (2012). State and county quickfacts. Retrieved from United States Department of Commerce. *quickfacts.census.gov/qfd/states/34000.html.*

CHAPTER 30

The Politics and Policy of Disaster Response and Public Health Emergency Preparedness

Tener Goodwin Veenema   Clifton P. Thornton   Roberta P. Lavin

"By failing to prepare, you are preparing to fail."
Benjamin Franklin

PURPOSE STATEMENT

The United States has experienced a dramatic increase in the frequency and intensity of natural and man-made disasters. Disasters and major public health emergencies (PHEs) garner aggressive and sustained media coverage regardless of their scope and impact. The coverage often results in a mandate for a political response, which may drive the creation of disaster health policies by Congress. These policies, while addressing the public outcry from the most recent disaster, may have unexpected consequences, both positive and negative. This chapter will focus on the challenges the United States and communities face in disaster and emergency preparedness and the policy responses to these challenges.

BACKGROUND AND SIGNIFICANCE

Disaster health policies affect all of those impacted by a disaster, including health and human service responders, hospital-based receivers, suppliers, and community members. The passage of policies that alter scope of practice and standards of care can ensure greater access to care or be a barrier to care. Disasters and PHEs provide a unique environment that allows nurses and physicians to care for people and save lives, tasks for which they have been trained. Because of their intimate involvement in responding to all levels of disasters, they must be involved in the planning and policymaking phase of disasters to avoid unintended consequences and ensure effective policy and planning that maintains human dignity and is guided by social justice (American Medical Association [AMA], 2004; American Nurses Association [ANA], 2010).

PRESIDENTIAL DECLARATIONS OF DISASTER AND THE STAFFORD ACT

Recognizing that disasters have the potential to cause loss of life, property damage, human suffering, income loss, and great financial burdens to all levels of government, the United States enacted the Robert T. Stafford Disaster Relief and Emergency Assistance Act in 1988. This act amends the Disaster Relief Act of 1974 and describes how the federal government will assist local and state organizations in preparing for, responding to, and recovering from disasters (Robert T. Stafford Disaster Relief and Emergency Assistance Act [Stafford Act], 2013). Under the Stafford Act, the President of the United States has the authority to issue major declarations regarding disaster, emergency, and fire management services to be allocated to the state and local government when the need arises (Bea, 2010). Figures 30-1 and 30-2 show how these provisions of the act are carried out.

The Stafford Act is composed of several titles that outline the responsibilities of the federal government in preparation for disasters, mitigation efforts, administrative provisions, major disaster assistance, emergency assistance, and emergency preparedness (Stafford Act, 2013). The cornerstone of disaster preparedness is to ensure that local and state organizations are prepared for the event. These local groups are responsible for dealing with the immediate consequences of the disaster. The Stafford Act outlines how the federal government will assist local, state, and tribal organizations in disaster response by coordinating with them and facilitating a unified command (Stafford Act, 2013). By working through shared personnel, infrastructure, and resources, the federal and local governments divide the burden of the disaster and support each other through the response and recovery process.

POLICY CHANGE AFTER SEPTEMBER 11

The extended media coverage of the terrorist attacks of September 11 contributed to policy changes that

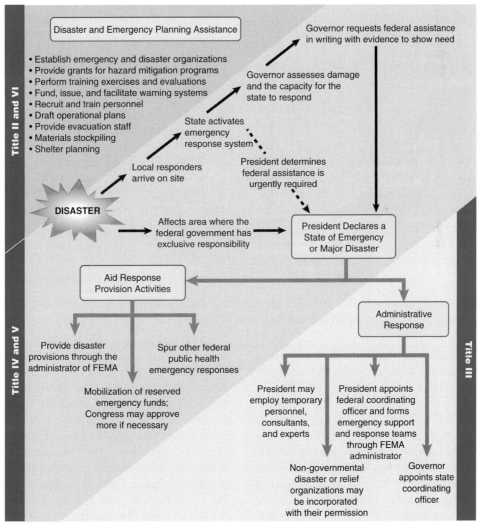

FIGURE 30-1 Flowchart of the provisions of the Stafford Act. *FEMA,* Federal Emergency Management Agency.

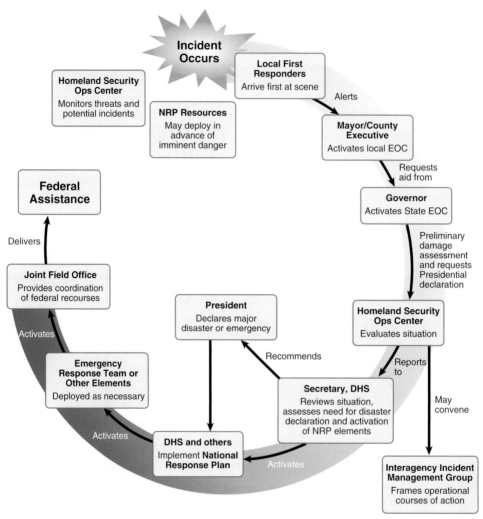

FIGURE 30-2 Overview of federal involvement through the Stafford Act. *DHS*, Department of Homeland Security; *NRP*, National Response Plan. (U.S. Army Combined Arms Center, 2012).

significantly increased the individual authoritative power that the President holds (Sylves, 2008). Congress expanded the ability of the President to declare a state of emergency within the previously existing Stafford Act and to use this as a security measure for the United States. One of the first new policies drafted after 9/11 was the Homeland Security Act that was signed into law on November 25, 2002. It created the U.S. Department of Homeland Security (DHS) headed by the Secretary of Homeland Security, established a directorate for Information Analysis and Infrastructure Protection, created

the Critical Infrastructure Information Act of 2002, established the Cyber Security Enhancement Act, and moved many programs involved in disaster response to new leadership under DHS (Homeland Security Act, 2002, Section 102).

Two days after the Homeland Security Act was signed, Congress and the President finalized the National Commission on Terrorist Attacks Upon the United States. This was enacted through Public Law (PL) 107-306 and is more commonly known as the *9/11 Commission Report*. It contains a chilling recount of the events surrounding the hijacking of the commercial aircrafts along with the data concerning the preparedness, management, and response to the terrorist attacks, which was published in 2004. The report determined that the perpetrators were vastly underestimated and that the institutions involved in border protection, civilian aviation, and national security were not aware of the threat or did not understand the power that they had amassed (Kean & Hamilton, 2004). The purpose of the report, however, was not to place blame on organizations, but rather to make observations about the actions that were taken to prepare for these events and use them to guide future endeavors. The implementation of the recommendations of the report is detailed in *Implementing 9/11 Commission Recommendations* (DHS, 2011a) and in various testimonies since 2011.

THE POLITICS UNDERLYING DISASTER AND PUBLIC HEALTH EMERGENCY POLICY

Disaster policy in the United States has been performed in a predominately retrospective manner. The government develops policy and procedures for handling disasters after one has occurred. For instance, the formation of the DHS followed the 9/11 terrorist attacks, Project BioShield was introduced after the anthrax attacks, and the Post-Katrina Emergency Management and Response Act (PKEMRA) resulted from Hurricane Katrina. Disaster plans were created in response to those policies and/or disasters. For a more comprehensive list of disaster policies that followed national disasters and large-scale public health emergencies, see Figure 30-3 and Table 30-1. The implementation of disaster health policies created in direct response to a previous disaster often results in a knee-jerk response characterized by shining a laser focused upon correcting one glaring deficit while frequently overlooking another.

THE HOMELAND SECURITY ACT

The Homeland Security Act was designed to address potential shortcomings in the preparation and

protection of the United States to future attacks. It was believed that the Homeland Security Act, which restructured current federal government resources and bodies to enable a more centralized and cohesive organization, would improve not only the communication of potential threats but also the response to disasters. It was quickly realized that one of the unintended consequences of this Act included the move of the Strategic National Stockpile (SNS) to the DHS. In doing so, the SNS lost the advantage of the medical and scientific expertise at the Centers for Disease Control and Prevention (CDC) and the relationship that existed between state and local public health authorities that was built on a relationship of trust. It took a legislative fix to eventually move the SNS back to the U.S. Department of Health and Human Services (HHS) in the Project BioShield Act.

An additional unintended consequence of the policy was the move of the National Disaster Medical System (NDMS) to the DHS. The NDMS was created in 1984 and had been managed by the U.S. Public Health Service with the HHS to provide medical services in a disaster when the state and local capabilities became overwhelmed. It comprised highly trained and exercised medical personnel and others needed for the response, mortuary service, and patient transport. Despite the expressed concerns of many individuals within the NDMS and personnel within the Government Accountability Office the move was made. The result was that access to the DHS Secretary was limited, and while the NDMS budget remained unchanged, almost two thirds of it was used for other purposes. By 2005, the NDMS had lost a large proportion of their staff, furniture, and supplies. Action reports following the Gulf Hurricanes of 2005 revealed a story of serious and systemic problems. The NDMS had gone from being a national asset to national tragedy that ranged from no medical supplies for the teams to the inability to transport equipment or rent vehicles (Leonard, 2009). Ultimately, the NDMS was transferred back to the HHS on January 1, 2007 as part of the Pandemic All-Hazards Preparedness Act (PL 109-417, 2006). The original policy had been driven by an act of terrorism. The revisions to correct the unintended consequences

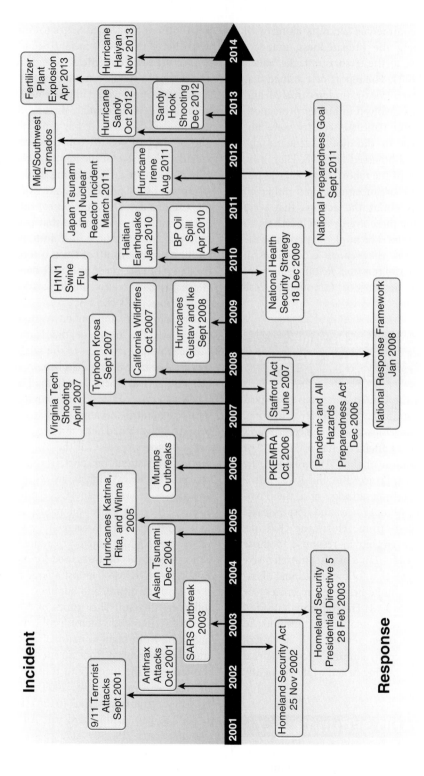

FIGURE 30-3 Recent major national and international disasters.

TABLE 30-1 U.S. Disaster Policies Enacted Since 9/11

Policy	Date Enacted	Description
Homeland Security Act (HSA)	November 2002	Created the U.S. Department of Homeland Security (DHS), this is the first new federal executive department since 1989 in response to the terrorist attacks of September 11, 2011. The act aims to restructure the departments responsible for protecting the United States from terrorist attacks into a single department. It functions to prevent terrorist attacks within the United States, decrease the susceptibility to attacks, and to respond to attacks if they occur. The department combines the U.S. Citizenship and Immigration Services, U.S. Coast Guard, U.S. Customs and Border Protection, Federal Emergency Management Agency, U.S. Immigration and Customs Enforcement, and the Transportation Security Administration together to integrate their individual regulatory responsibilities into carrying out the provisions outlined by the DHS. (Homeland Security Act, 2002, Section 102)
Homeland Security Presidential Directive-5 (HSPD5)	February 2003	Established the National Incident Management System (NIMS) to fill the need for a comprehensive approach to managing crises and their consequences as a single entity through all levels of government across the nation. Under this act, the Secretary of Homeland Security is responsible for preventing, preparing for, response to, and recovering from terrorist attacks, major disasters, and other emergencies that occur in the United States. The secretary will initiate coordination of the government's resources if a federal department or agency requests the assistance of the secretary; federal assistance has been requested by state and local authorities whose resources have been depleted; more than one federal department or agency has become involved in response to an event; or the President has directed the secretary to begin management. The directive is not designed to shift the responsibility of planning for and responding to disasters away from the local and state organizations to the federal government, but rather provide the secretary as a tool for local and state organizations to use if they become overwhelmed by an event (U.S. Department of Homeland Security, 2003).
Post-Katrina Emergency Management Reform Act (PKEMRA)	July 2006	This act began as a bill proposed to the 109th Congress to amend the Homeland Security Act and aimed to keep the Federal Emergency Management Agency (FEMA) within the DHS while establishing new provisions to plan, respond, and recover from disasters. It also implemented an all-hazards strategy for preparedness and promoted planning for the protection and postdisaster restoration of necessary infrastructures and resources. Most notably, the act redefined the role of the administrator of FEMA and added provisions ranging from outlining the Presidential roles and responsibilities in disasters to providing counseling for victims. The Post-Katrina Emergency Management and Reform Act (PKEMRA) also addressed staffing issues; education regarding planning, preparedness, and training; and addressed fraud, waste, and abuse within the system. (S.3721, 2006).
Pandemic and All-Hazards Preparedness Act (PAHPA)	December 2006	Amended the Public Health Service Act within the U.S. Department of Health and Human Services (HHS) with the goal to improve upon the public health and medical preparedness and response capabilities of the United States for all disasters and emergencies. The act also established a new Assistant Secretary for Preparedness and Response (ASPR) as well as new authorities for other programs. The act established new construction and acquisition of medical countermeasures and strives to develop a quadrennial National Health Security Act. The secretary is responsible for organizing a nationwide public health situational awareness communication network that will allow the rapid detection and response to public health issues. The legislation also required the HHS and ASPR to disseminate novel and best practices of outreach to and care of at-risk individuals before, during, and following public health emergencies (Public Law 109-417).

Continued

TABLE 30-1 U.S. Disaster Policies Enacted Since 9/11—cont'd

Policy	Date Enacted	Description
National Response Framework (NRF)	January 2008 May 2013	Replacing the older National Response Plan, the National Response Framework (NRF) serves as the nation's all-hazards response guide to handling natural and man-made disasters. Its guidelines detail how leaders at all levels of government along with private sector partners and health care providers must prepare for and provide a unified domestic response through enhanced coordination and integration. The Framework is scalable and adaptable to a variety of different events and works to align key roles and responsibilities across the United States. The priorities of response are to save lives, protect property and the environment, stabilize the incident, and provide for basic human needs. The Framework is always in effect, and elements of the plan can be implemented at any time as they are needed. Besides the main body of the document, the NRF also comprises Emergency Support Function (ESF) Annexes, Support Annexes, and Incident Annexes. ESF Annexes assign resources and capabilities that are most frequently needed in a national response into functional areas. Support Annexes detail the essential supporting processes and considerations that are most common to the majority of incidents. Last, Incident Annexes describe the unique response aspects of incident categories. The second edition of the framework was released in May 2013 (DHS, 2008; DHS, 2013b).
National Health Security Strategy (NHSS)	December 2009	A society that is able to manage and function well during large-scale incidents that affect the health of workers who are responsible to provide food, water, and health care to the greater population helps strengthen security and stability for the United States. The National Health Security Strategy (NHSS) was designed to minimize the consequences from these incidents by coordinating the stakeholders responsible for providing these important resources. The strategy offers a framework in which to improve relevant portions of the Pandemic and All-Hazards Preparedness Act, legislation meant to improve the preparedness and response of the country to emergencies. Developed by the HHS, the two stated goals of the NHSS are to build community resilience and to strengthen and maintain health and emergency response systems (HHS, 2009).
Homeland Security Presidential Directive-8 (HSPD8)	March 2011	In recognition that emergency preparedness is an effort that requires input from multiple sectors of government as well as input from civilians, President Barack Obama drafted PPD-8 in 2011. This directive aims to strengthen the security and resilience of the United States through preparation for acts of terrorism, cyber attacks, pandemics, and natural disasters. It views preparation for these events as a shared responsibility among the private and nonprofit sector, government, and individuals. The directive itself is aimed at the responsibilities of the government in establishing safeguards against the aforementioned threats, but it also addresses the fact that complete preparedness is an all-of-nation effort. This directive serves as a call to action to prepare the nation to establish an effective national preparedness system. Once this system is established, it will allow evaluation and tracking of the efforts made to prevent, protect against, dampen the effects of, or respond to and recover from threats to the nation's security. Coordinating this preparedness system is the responsibility of the Assistant to the President for Homeland Security and Counterterrorism, while the Secretary of Homeland Security is responsible for developing the preparedness goal (Presidential Policy Directive/PPD-8, 2011c)

TABLE 30-1 U.S. Disaster Policies Enacted Since 9/11—cont'd

Policy	Date Enacted	Description
National Preparedness Goal	September 2011	Outlines the approach of the United States to preparation for all types of disasters through a shared-responsibility model. The directive describes the responsibilities of the population and emphasizes that the individual, community, private and nonprofit sectors, faith-based organizations, and federal, state, and local governments should be involved in national security. The focus of the directive is to use individual and community preparedness to contribute to national security to provide benefit to all. The National Preparedness Goal aspires to involve all of these individuals and groups in the five mission areas of prevention, protection, mitigation, response, and recovery with regard to disasters. The directive outlines specific core capabilities for each of these mission areas that must be achieved to meet the goal (DHS, 2011d).
National Preparedness System	November 2011	The National Preparedness System holds the same view of an all-of-nation approach to preparing for and managing disasters. The system outlines an organizational process for all community members to use while moving forward in preparing to achieve the National Preparedness Goal. The National Preparedness System is composed of six parts. These include identifying and assessing risk, estimating capability requirements, building and sustaining capabilities, planning to deliver capabilities, validating capabilities, and reviewing and updating the plans developed through these processes (Federal Emergency Management Agency, 2014).
Homeland Security Presidential Directive-21 (HSPD21)	February 2013	This directive addresses the need for a critical infrastructure of security and resilience which aims to advance a national unity of effort in strengthening and maintaining a secure, functioning, and resilient critical infrastructure. The directive recognizes the importance of infrastructure that is essential to the nation's safety, prosperity, and well-being. The directive also recognizes the vast complexity of this infrastructure, noting that it includes both physical and cyber space that is controlled by government, business, private, and individual owners. All components of this infrastructure must be secure and be able to withstand or recover from threats to safety. Because these components of the infrastructure share ownership among federal, state, local, tribal, territorial, public, and private owners, a team effort must be used to establish security. An all-hazards approach to identifying possible threats and planning for these events is taken to begin preparation for security. The federal government functions to help direct and guide planning for the remaining sectors and owners, with a particularly large role to be performed by the Secretary of Homeland Security (Office of the Press Secretary, 2013).

were driven by evidence-based decisions and pressure from professional organizations.

PROJECT BIOSHIELD 2004

In reaction to the 2001 anthrax attacks, President George W. Bush introduced Project BioShield to prepare for future bioterrorism attacks, signing it into law on July 21, 2004 (Cohen, 2011; Gottron & Shea, 2011). Protection of the general population was thought to be best achieved by obtaining medical countermeasures (MCMs) against chemical, biologic, radiologic, and nuclear (CRBN) threats (Gottron & Shea, 2011). A sum of $5.6 billion was approved for 10 years to be used for the development and purchase of MCMs (DHS, 2013a). Evaluation of the progress of BioShield, however, reveals excessive spending for a vaccine that has limited commercial value and unintended consequences (Sell & Watson, 2013).

Through BioShield, the federal government had the authority to create a market and enter into contracts with companies promising the purchase of certain products if developed (Gottron & Shea, 2011; Kadlec, 2013). The first BioShield contract was with VaxGen, paying $877.5 million for the acquisition of 75 million doses of a new anthrax vaccine (Kadlec, 2013). VaxGen had never produced a vaccine licensed with the U.S. Food and Drug Administration (FDA) and 2 years later, VaxGen still had no vaccine. The government had to terminate the contract despite already paying $1.5 million to the company (Cohen, 2011; Kadlec, 2013). Later, $2.696 billion dollars were awarded to seven pharmaceutical companies, yet only eight MCMs were produced and only five have been licensed (Kadlec, 2013).

In 2014, the HHS biodefense budget has been proposed to be increased to $4.1 billion, and Project BioShield has been reapproved with a suggested budget of $2.8 billion to use until 2018 (Sell & Watson, 2013). BioShield has yet to produce any vaccine to the threats President Bush discussed as most ominous when he introduced the program (Cohen, 2011) and in 2010 the Commission on the Prevention of Weapons of Mass Destruction Proliferation and Terrorism graded the federal government an F in their abilities to readily respond and prevent biologic attacks (Cohen, 2011).

PKEMRA 2006 AND DISASTER CASE MANAGEMENT

Before PKEMRA there was no federal authority to fund disaster case management (DCM) through the federal government. All previous DCM had been provided through Volunteer Organizations Active in Disaster (VOADs) and essentially addressed social services related issues and unmet needs. After Hurricanes Katrina and Rita it became apparent that individuals and families impacted by disaster needed case management to help them return to a state of self-sufficiency and it needed to address the human services needs of the most vulnerable.

Passing the PKEMRA legislation did not result in the immediate creation of a program, and a year after passage no efforts had been made to create a deployable case management program within the

Federal Emergency Management Agency (FEMA). The Administration of Children and Families (ACF) had proposed providing DCM in the immediate aftermath of Hurricane Katrina and was rejected. In 2007, they again proposed DCM be run by the ACF and implemented in the field through a partnership with faith-based organizations. The ACF pilot was successful and led to the publication of the first *Disaster Case Management Implementation Guide* in 2009 (Lavin & Menifee, 2009).

Simultaneously, FEMA undertook another pilot in Texas to provide support for the same hurricane victims ACF was addressing in Louisiana including the people still lingering in FEMA temporary housing. It was implemented in the fall of 2009 with the Louisiana Recovery Authority. RAND analyzed the program in 2010 and found that there were significant problems with the implementation (Acosta, Chandra, & Feeney, 2010). Because of the vagueness of the original legislation it was not clear where the program was to be located within the government or what it was to include.

NATIONAL COMMISSION ON CHILDREN AND DISASTERS 2009

Each major disaster event has had a significant impact on our nation's children and yet little attention was given to them in the legislation until the National Commission on Children and Disasters (the Commission) was established pursuant to the Kids in Disasters Well-being, Safety, and Health Act of 2007 as provided in Division G, Title VI of the Consolidated Appropriations Act of 2008. One of the major objectives of the Commission was to examine and assess the needs of children in all phases of a disaster and to make policy recommendations at the local, state, and federal levels. The intended consequence was to be the most comprehensive review of the impact of disaster on children that had been undertaken to date and the recommendation of policies to address the gaps. It was hoped that the public attention would drive significant changes. An unintended consequence of a Commission made up predominately of academics and social activists is that there is sometimes inadequate understanding of the realities in the field during a disaster and the issues faced by all socioeconomic groups. A discussion surrounding the need for baby bathtubs in shelters went on for months, yet many of the Commissioners lacked an appreciation for the logistic challenge to maintain such a supply and the ability to transport it during a disaster. The repulsion by some at the thought of washing a baby in a sink demonstrated a lack of cultural understanding and the realities of living in a disaster shelter. Many questioned if this debate was the best use of resources and the political clout of the Commission. The compromise was that basins would be provided as soon as possible after a need was identified rather than keeping a stockpile for delivery within 3 hours.

THREAT LEVEL SYSTEM OF THE U.S. DEPARTMENT OF HOMELAND SECURITY

The signing of Homeland Security Presidential Directive-3 in 2002 established the Homeland Security Advisory System (HSAS) to communicate information concerning the threat of terrorist attacks to the federal, state, and local organizers (Homeland Security Presidential Directive-3, 2002; Sharp, 2013). The system was composed of five levels of perceived threat and a color to accompany each: green (low), blue (guarded), yellow (elevated), orange (high), and red (severe) (Homeland Security Presidential Directive-3, 2002). By assigning a color to each level, the federal government was aiming to quickly and clearly communicate the threat level to the general population and key organizations involved in protecting the United States from terrorist attacks (DHS, 2011b). An important part of preparing for disasters involves communicating information to the state and local organizations about the threats of attack so they are motivated to respond accordingly. This was the purpose of establishing HSAS, but the information communicated was greatly misunderstood. It contained little record as to what caused the change in threat level and what people should do in response (Sharp, 2013). Very few states incorporated HSAS threat level information into their disaster plans or

even addressed the topic (Sharp, 2013). There was no documented protocol to follow for providing threat information to federal or state organizations (Sharp, 2013). A 2004 study revealed that 38% of people surveyed thought the system had evolved into a tool that conveyed political ideas, only 2 years after it started (Shapiro & Cohen, 2007).

The program became the subject of comedians, the Internet became riddled with mockery of the program, and many Americans became desensitized to the threat level. Throughout the 10 years that the HSAS was used, the threat level changed only 16 times but remained almost constantly yellow and never reduced to the low or guarded level (U.S. Department of Homeland Security, 2013). It has been thought that politicians were afraid to reduce the terror threat below yellow and advertise to the world that the United States was not paying attention. A consistent state of threat level yellow desensitized the American people, and news corporations stopped running updates.

CONCLUSION

Disaster health policies should be thoughtfully designed and drafted in anticipation of the next event. Policies and the resultant plans they inspire should be constructed through collaboration and in coordination with the planned stakeholders of the policy, community, and organizational members and the health care personnel responding to the event. Nurses and physicians are in a unique position to contribute to these policy discussions. To fulfill this role, nurses and physicians must be aware of challenges faced in disaster planning and to previous policy successes and failures.

DISCUSSION QUESTIONS

1. How can the evaluation of policies be better incorporated into the planning phase of policy? Consider which aspect of policymaking would be involved, funding requirements, personnel needs, and timing for evaluation of programs.
2. What can be done to direct the planning of disaster policy to be more proactive instead of retroactive?

3. How can the involvement of a community of interest be used to avoid the unintended consequences?

REFERENCES

Acosta, J., Chandra, A., & Feeney, K. C. (2010). *Navigating the road to recovery: Assessment of the coordination, communication, and financing of the disaster case management pilot in Louisiana*. Santa Monica, CA: Rand Corporation.

American Medical Association. (2004). AMA code of medical ethics. Retrieved from *www.ama-assn.org/ama/pub/physician-resources/medical-ethics/code-medical-ethics.page*.

American Nurses Association. (2010). Code of ethics for nurses with interpretive statements. Retrieved from *www.nursingworld.org/MainMenuCategories/EthicsStandards/CodeofEthicsforNurses/Code-of-Ethics.pdf*.

Bea, K. (2010). *Federal Stafford Act disaster assistance: Presidential declarations, eligible activities, and funding*. Congressional Research Service. Retrieved from *www.hsdl.org/?view&did=27383*.

Cohen, J. (2011). Biodefense: 10 years after: Reinventing project BioShield. *Science, 333*(6047), 1216–1218. doi:10.1126/science.333.6047.1216.

Gottron, F., & Shea, D. A. (2011). Federal efforts to address the threat of bioterrorism: Selected issues and options for congress. Congressional Research Service. Retrieved from *digital.library.unt.edu/ark:/67531/metadc103084/m1/1/high_res_d/R41123_2011Feb08.pdf*.

Homeland Security Act. (2002). Public Law No. 107-296, S. 102, 107th Congress, 2002.

Homeland Security Presidential Directive-3. (2002). Retrieved from *georgewbush-whitehouse.archives.gov/news/releases/2002/03/20020312-5.html*.

Kadlec, R. (2013). Renewing the project BioShield Act: What has it brought and wrought? Center for a New American Security. Retrieved from *www.cnas.org/files/documents/publications/CNAS_RenewingTheProjectBioShieldAct_Kadlec.pdf*.

Kean, T. H., & Hamilton, L. H. (2004). The 9/11 Commission report. Retrieved from *www.9-11commission.gov/report/911Report.pdf*.

Lavin, R., & Menifee, S. (Eds.), (2009). *Disaster case management implementation guide*. Washington, DC: Administration for Children and Families.

Leonard, B. (Ed.), (2009). *Decline of the National Disaster Medical System: Report by the Committee on Government Reform, Minority Staff, US House of Representatives*. Darby, PA: Diane Publishing.

Pandemic All-Hazards Preparedness Act. (2006). Public Law 109-417. 109th Congress, 2006.

Robert, T., & Stafford Disaster Relief and Emergency Assistance Act. (2013). Public Law 93-288 as amended, U.S.C. 5121 et seq.

S.3721, 109th Congress. (2006). Post-Katrina Emergency Management Reform Act of 2006. (enacted).

Sell, T. K., & Watson, M. (2013). Federal agency biodefense funding, FY2013-FY2014. *Biosecurity and Bioterrorism: Biodefense Strategy, Practice, and Science, 1*(3), 196–216.

Shapiro, J. N., & Cohen, D. K. (2007). Color bind: Lessons from the failed Homeland Security Advisory System. *International Security, 32*(2), 121–154.

Sharp, V. H. (2013). *Faded colors: From the homeland security advisory system (HSAS) to the national terrorism advisory system (NTAS)*. Master's thesis. Monterey, CA: Naval Postgraduate School.

Sylves, R. (2008). *Disaster policy and politics: Emergency management and homeland security*. Washington, DC: CQ Press.

U.S. Army Combined Arms Center. (2012). National Incident Management System (NIMS). Retrieved from *usacac.army.mil/cac2/call/docs/06-08/ch-2.asp*.

U.S. Department of Health and Human Services. (2009). National Health Security Strategy of the United States of America. Retrieved from *www.phe.gov/preparedness/planning/authority/nhss/strategy/documents/nhss-final.pdf*.

U.S. Department of Health and Human Services. (2013). Project BioShield acquisitions. Public health emergency: Public health and medical emergency support for a nation prepared. Retrieved from *www.phe.gov/about/amcg/Pages/projectBioShield.aspx*.

U.S. Department of Homeland Security. (2003). Homeland Security Presidentail Directive 5. Retrieved from *http://www.dhs.gov/publication/homeland-security-presidential-directive-5*.

U.S. Department of Homeland Security. (2008). National Response Framework. Retrieved from *www.fema.gov/pdf/emergency/nrf/nrf-core.pdf*.

U.S. Department of Homeland Security. (2011a). Implementing 9/11 Commission recommendations: Progress report 2011. Retrieved from *www.dhs.gov/xlibrary/assets/implementing-9-11-commission-report-progress-2011.pdf*.

U.S. Department of Homeland Security. (2011b). National terrorism advisory system public guide. Retrieved from *www.dhs.gov/xlibrary/assets/ntas/ntas-public-guide.pdf*.

U.S. Department of Homeland Security. (2011c). Presidential Policy Directive/PPD 8: National Preparedness. Retrieved from *www.dhs.gov/presidential-policy-directive-8-national-preparedness*.

U.S. Department of Homeland Security. (2011d). National Preparedness Goal (1st ed.). Retrieved from *www.fema.gov/media-library-data/20130726-1828-25045-9470/national_preparedness_goal_2011.pdf*.

U.S. Department of Homeland Security. (2013a). Chronology of changes to the homeland security advisory system. Retrieved from *www.dhs.gov/homeland-security-advisory-system*.

U.S. Department of Homeland Security. (2013b). National Response Framework, 2nd edition. Retrieved from *www.fema.gov/media-library-data/20130726-1914-25045-1246/final_national_response_framework_20130501.pdf*.

U.S. Federal Emergency Management Agency. (2014). National Preparedness System. Retrieved from *www.fema.gov/national-preparedness-system*.

U.S. Office of the Press Secretary. (2013). Presidential Policy Directive-Critical Infrastructure Security and Resilience. Retrieved from *www.whitehouse.gov/the-press-office/2013/02/12/presidential-policy-directive-critical-infrastructure-security-and-resil*.

ONLINE RESOURCES

Center for Disease Control and Prevention: Emergency Preparedness and Response
emergency.cdc.gov

Federal Emergency Management Agency
www.fema.gov

Overview of the National Response Framework through the Federal Emergency Management Agency
www.fema.gov/national-response-framework

The Robert T. Stafford Disaster Relief and Emergency Assistance Act
www.fema.gov/pdf/about/stafford_act.pdf

U.S. Department of Labor—Office of the Assistant Secretary for Policy
www.dol.gov/dol/aboutdol/history/carter-asper.htm

CHAPTER 31

Chronic Care Policy: Medical Homes and Primary Care

Susan Apold

"Change will not come if we wait for some other person or some other time. We are the ones we've been waiting for. We are the change that we seek."

President Barack Obama

Chronic conditions are the leading cause of death in the world and have replaced specific acute episodic disease as the number one cause of mortality and morbidity in the United States (Centers for Disease Control and Prevention [CDC], 2014). Almost half of all adults in the United States are living with at least one chronic condition (Robert Wood Johnson Foundation, 1996) and one in four Americans is living with multiple chronic disease (Ralph et al., 2013). This tectonic shift has evolved over the past century as a result of an aging population; advances in public health; increasing knowledge of genetics; and improvements in pharmacology, research, and technology.

This changing epidemiology of the nation and its impact on the cost of health care became one of the major drivers of health care reform in the United States and resulted in the passage of the Affordable Care Act (ACA) on March 23, 2010. This historic legislation brought the most sweeping changes to the U.S. health care system since the passage of amendments to the Social Security Act in 1965 (which created Medicare and Medicaid). The ACA supports initiatives from the public and private sectors that seek to improve quality of care and support a reimbursement model that compensates for quality, not quantity, of care. It is widely believed that a shift in focus from a fee-for-service model of care, where revenue is generated on the number of patients seen and the number of

procedures and diagnostic tests ordered, to payment for comprehensive patient-centered care evaluated by outcomes will result in lower cost and higher quality. Comprehensive patient-centered care is the focus of the profession of nursing.

THE EXPERIENCE OF CHRONIC CARE IN THE UNITED STATES

Chronic illness is a condition that continues indefinitely, limits activity, and requires ongoing actions and responses from patients and caregivers (Larsen, 2009; Robert Wood Johnson Foundation, Partnership for Solutions, 2002). It is a relatively new phenomenon. In the early 1900s, the leading causes of mortality in the United States were tuberculosis, pneumonia, and gastritis/enteritis. The average life expectancy then was 47 years (National Center for Health Statistics, 1909). Health care was an oxymoron as diagnosis and treatment of disease were the only tools in the health care armamentarium. With only a rudimentary comprehension of the major causes of mortality and without antibiotics, insulin, and imaging ability, the sick were identified late in their illness (or not at all) and either got better or died. The system developed to handle disease was based on face-to-face encounters with physicians who provided a service in exchange for a fee. That fee-for-service system with an emphasis on illness management remains central to health care policy today.

A century later, life expectancy is 78.9 years (Social Security Online Actuarial Tables, 2010); the first baby boomers are Medicare-eligible; and in 2014 the youngest baby boomers turned 50, a continuing challenge to the nation's ability to effectively and efficiently manage the growing prevalence of chronic illness (Anderson, 2005). Treatment of chronic disease accounts for more than 75% of the nation's health care budget. The financial impact on the U.S. economy of treatment and lost productivity caused by chronic illness is more than $1.3 trillion per year, with projections of an increase to $5.7 trillion by 2050 (Bloom et al., 2011). Increases in health care spending have not translated into improvements in health care quality. In a fee-for-service episodic care model, research shows that care is fragmented and illness-based; patients frequently do not get the care that they want or need (Coleman et al., 2009; Mattke, Seid, & Ma, 2007). Fee-for-service models of care do not provide for the management of chronic illness. Payment for services is based upon face-to-face encounters with health care providers for acute and episodic illness, and much needed aspects of care management, such as coordinating services between and among providers, managing multiple providers across chronic illness problems, or transitioning from one type of care and care provider to another, are not reimbursed and therefore not done. Neither federal entitlement programs nor private insurances have traditionally provided coverage for prevention or care management.

MEDICAL HOMES

One initiative which blends comprehensive care with quality and reimbursement is the Patient-Centered Medical Home (PCMH). The concept of a medical home was first advanced by the American Academy of Pediatrics (AAP) in 1967 as a place where all medical information about a patient would be located (Sia et al., 2004). The National Committee for Quality Assurance (NCQA), which has the largest PCMH program, defines a medical home as "…a model or philosophy of primary care that is patient-centered, comprehensive, team-based, coordinated, accessible, and focused on quality and safety" (NCQA, 2014). The PCMH is built on the Chronic Care Model (CCM) proposed by Gerteis and colleagues (2003), which requires a whole-person orientation and a relationship between patient and provider which is regular,

accessible, and mutual. The eight dimensions of patient-centered care can be found in Table 31-1. The American College of Physicians (ACP) expanded the PCMH model to include reimbursement incentives for the management and coordination of care (Barr & Ginsburg, 2006). Reimbursement in this model would support system-based versus volume-based care, that is, payment based on a process of care delivery that assures positive outcomes rather than the volume of patients seen by a given provider. Furthermore, reimbursement would acknowledge the value of providing coordinated care in a system that incorporates the elements of the CCM. In addition, the ACP model requires that a medical home must be team-based and led by a physician.

In 2006, led by IBM and major national medical associations (American College of Physicians, American Academy of Family Physicians, American Osteopathic Association, AAP), the Patient-Centered Primary Care Collaborative (PCPCC) was established to promote the widespread implementation of the medical home concept as a major force in the provision of health care. In 2007, the aforementioned medical societies developed the Joint Principles of the Patient-Centered Medical Home. These principles included such concepts as whole-person orientation to care, care coordination, voluntary focus on quality and safety, enhanced access to care, and payment which recognizes the value added to care. In addition, the principles included

---

TABLE 31-1 Dimensions of Patient-Centered Care

1. Respect for patients' values, preferences, and expressed needs
2. Information and education
3. Access to care
4. Emotional support to relieve fear and anxiety
5. Involvement of family and friends
6. Continuity and secure transition between health care settings
7. Physical comfort
8. Coordination of care

From Gerteis, M., Edgman-Levitan, S., Daley, J., & Delbanco, T.L. (2003). *Through the patient's eyes: Understanding and promoting patient-centered care.* San Francisco, CA: Jossey-Bass.

the necessity that a PCMH has, at its core, a physician-patient relationship and that the PCMH occurs within a physician-led practice setting. The PCPCC has evolved in their definition of a PCMH and has adapted their definition from the Agency for Healthcare Research and Quality (AHRQ). The current position of the PCPCC is that a PCMH is an approach to care that is "patient-centered, comprehensive, coordinated, accessible, and committed to quality and safety" (PCPCC, 2013). The requirement of the PCPCC that the model be implemented in a physician-led team remains a principle in this group's definition.

In 2008, the NCQA, the Utilization Review Accreditation Commission (URAC), The Joint Commission, and the Accreditation Association for Ambulatory Health Care implemented medical home accreditation programs.

Since its introduction the PCMH concept has proliferated and studies are under way to evaluate the effect this model has on the Institute for Healthcare Improvement's (IHI) Triple Aim: improving the patient care experience, improving the health of populations, and reducing the per capita cost of health care. The National Academy for State Health Policy reports that more than 47 states have adopted policies to advance the PCMH initiative. The NCQA reports that 10% (approximately 7000) of primary care practices are credentialed as PCMHs (NCQA, 2014). Quality data, reported annually by the Milbank Memorial Fund, indicate that PCMHs "demonstrate improvements in the areas of cost, utilization, population health, prevention, access to care, and patient satisfaction" (Nielsen et al., 2014). This report highlights 20 studies of PCMHs in 2012 to 2013. Although the data represent early results and have not been subjected to a peer-review model, they do indicate that primary care practices engaged in this model demonstrate consistent positive outcomes on a variety of measures, specifically:

- Decreases in cost of care
- Reductions in the use of unnecessary or avoidable services
- Improvements in population health and access to care
- Increases in patient satisfaction
- Decreases in income-based disparities

THE ROLE OF NURSING IN MEDICAL HOMES

The concept of a medical home is a natural fit with nursing. Nursing has always held the core values inherent in patient-centered care: an orientation to the whole person; consideration of the patient's emotional, social, and educational needs; and coordination of care across multiple community and health care agencies are fundamental nursing skills. The American Nurses Association's definition of nursing provides the best evidence that the profession of nursing has both opportunities and responsibilities as a driving force in health care reform, chronic care policy, and implementation of new models of care delivery:

"Nursing is the protection, promotion, and optimization of health and abilities, prevention of illness and injury, alleviation of suffering through the diagnosis and treatment of human response, and advocacy in the care of individuals, families, communities, and populations." (American Nurses Association, 2003, p. 3)

The natural fit between the nursing profession and the concepts underpinning the chronic care model led the advanced practice nursing community to lobby for a name change from *medical home* to *health home*. A health home reframes the context of care from pathology (medicine) to health and supports the Institute of Medicine (1996) focus on the process of care and not on any one type of provider. However, legislation requiring the implementation of demonstration projects designed to test this method of health care delivery (Tax Relief and Health Care Act [S.1796], 2006) codified the term *medical home* in federal statute. Curiously, the ACA refers to medical homes in relation to Medicare and health homes in relation to Medicaid.

An additional point of controversy for the nursing community was the PCPCC premise that a PCMH be led by a physician and exist only within physician-led practices. Because of that principle, PCMH credentialing organizations were unable to certify practices led by nurses whose practices otherwise met the criteria for a medical home. Leaders within nurse practitioner (NP) associations and nurse-managed health centers engaged in a variety of strategies to influence policy on the implementation of the medical home model and the appropriate health care provider leadership of medical homes. The message to patients and other stakeholders was clear: Nurses and NPs have the capacity to serve as both leaders and participants in PCMH models of care delivery.

Organizational and grassroots strategies to influence policy on NPs and PCMHs were somewhat successful. NPs influenced members of the Senate Finance Committee to recognize NPs as leaders of medical home demonstration projects. Support for a technical amendment to the S.1796 emerged from Senators Bingaman (D-NM), Harkin (D-IA), Murkowski (R-AK), and Collins (R-ME), who read a colloquy on the Senate floor that spoke of the inclusion of NPs as leaders of medical homes (Congressional Record, 2008).

In July 2008, the ACP worked with NP representatives to discuss the ACP's policy on NPs. As a result of this meeting, the ACP published a policy monograph that recognizes the role of NPs in primary care and advocates for testing NP-led medical homes (ACP, 2009). After subsequent conversations, the PCPCC adopted the AHRQ's definition of a PCMH, which uses provider-neutral language. Because of PCPCC's adoption of this language, the NCQA updated the criteria for consideration for practices to be certified as PCMHs to include NPs, physician's assistants, and a variety of providers who practice primary care. A number of NP practices and nurse-managed health centers have met the criteria put forth by the NCQA and have been certified as medical homes, making them eligible for reimbursement subsidies for care management and coordination.

Nonetheless, organized medicine remains dedicated to a definition of a medical home that includes physicians as the leaders, and major physician organizations hold fast to the original Joint Principles adopted by the PCPCC in 2007, specifically requiring that a medical home must include a "personal physician in a physician-directed team-based medical practice" (American Academy of Family Physicians, AAP, ACP, and American Osteopathic Association, 2011).

PATIENT-CENTERED MEDICAL HOMES: THE FUTURE

Preliminary data speak to the emerging success of this model of care. Any care model which seeks to understand patients and their health as a whole within the context of their lives places the patient at the center of care, precisely where they should be. Patient-centered versus illness-centered approaches to health make intuitive sense and are central to the science of nursing. The future of PCMHs depends on a variety of factors. Practices must have economic support for the transformation from traditional fee-for-service models to true outcome-based patient-centered units. In addition to economic support for all health care providers, those who provide both direct and indirect care must undergo training in true nonhierarchical interprofessional teamwork. With the patient at the center of this system, all members of the health care team must be available and able to take leadership roles that best meet patient needs. This will require education, training, and patience for the change process.

The nursing profession continues to play a pivotal role in the development of successful PCMHs. Nursing education focuses on patient centeredness, team building, team membership, and managing change and conflict. These are principles found in nursing curricula from baccalaureate through doctoral education. Nurses need to encourage providers to adopt the principles of PCMHs and develop their own practices within that model. Finally, professional nurses have an obligation to be informed about best practice models, funding sources, and legislation and policy around new models of health care delivery.

The ACA identifies NPs as lead providers in medical home demonstration projects and allows for provider-neutral language in the definition of health homes. The PCPCC has revised its definition of a medical home to include patient-centered, comprehensive, and coordinated care that is accessible and committed to quality and safety.

The NCQA provides for recognition of medical homes led by NPs. Additional work is necessary to eliminate barriers to NP practice to maximize the NP workforce in the pursuit of access to safe, affordable care within the health home model.

DISCUSSION QUESTIONS

1. In 2006, organized medicine developed Joint Principles for a Patient-Centered Medical Home. The first two principles mandated physician practices and physician-led teams as a condition of PCMHs. Do these principles hinder the advancement of PCMHs? How should organized nursing respond, if at all, to these principles?

2. Select a PCMH accrediting body (NCQA, URAC, The Joint Commission, and the Accreditation Association for Ambulatory Health Care). Review the criteria for certification of PCMHs. Identify the strategies that medical practices would implement to transform from a traditional fee-for-service model to a PCMH model. What role can nursing play in this transformation?

3. Critique nursing's strategy on influencing PCMH policy. What lessons can be learned from the strategies that were implemented? What additional strategies might have been employed?

REFERENCES

American Academy of Family Physicians, American Academy of Pediatrics, American College of Physicians, and American Osteopathic Association. (2011). Guidelines for patient-centered medical home recognition and accreditation programs. Retrieved from *www.acponline.org/running _practice/delivery_and_payment_models/pcmh/understanding/ guidelines_pcmh.pdf*.

American College of Physicians. (2009). Nurse practitioners in primary care. Policy monograph. Washington, DC: American College of Physicians. Retrieved from *www.acponline.org/advocacy/current_policy _papers/assets/np_pc.pdf*.

American Nurses Association. (2003). *Nursing's social policy statement* (2nd ed.). Silver Springs, MD: American Nurses Association.

Anderson, G. F. (2005). Medicare and chronic conditions. *New England Journal of Medicine, 353*(3), 305–309.

Barr, M., & Ginsburg, J. (2006). The advanced medical home: A patient-centered, physician-guided model of health care. Washington, DC: Policy Monograph of the American College of Physicians. Retrieved from *www .acponline.org/advocacy/current_policy_papers/assets/adv_med.pdf*.

Bloom, D. E., Cafiero, E. T., Jané-Llopis, E., Abrahams-Gessel, S., Bloom, L. R., Fathima, S., et al. (2011). The global economic burden of noncommunicable diseases. Geneva: World Economic Forum. Retrieved from *www3.weforum.org/docs/WEF_Harvard_HE_GlobalEconomic BurdenNonCommunicableDiseases_2011.pdf*.

Centers for Disease Control and Prevention. (2014). Chronic diseases and health promotion. Retrieved from *www.cdc.gov/chronicdisease/ overview/index.htm?s_cid=ostltsdyk_govd_203*.

Coleman, K., Austin, B., Brach, C., & Wagner, E. (2009). Evidence on the chronic care model in the new millennium. *Health Affairs, 28*(1), 75–85.

Congressional Record. (2008). S6485-S6486.

Gerteis, M., Edgman-Levitan, S., Daley, J., & Delbanco, T. L. (2003). *Through the patient's eyes: Understanding and promoting patient-centered care.* San Francisco, CA: Jossey-Bass.

Institute of Medicine. (1996). *Primary care: America's health in a new era.* Washington, DC: National Academy Press.

Larsen, P. D. (2009). Chronicity. In P. D. Larsen & I. M. Lubkin (Eds.), *Chronic illness: Impact and intervention* (7th ed.). Sudbury, MA: Jones & Bartlett.

Mattke, S., Seid, M., & Ma, S. (2007). Evidence for the effect of disease management: Is $1 billion a year a good investment? *Am J Manag Care, 13*(12), 670–676.

National Center for Health Statistics. (1909). Mortality statistics 1909, tenth annual report. Retrieved from *www.cdc.gov/nchs/products/vsus.htm*.

National Committee for Quality Assurance. (2014). The future of patient centered medical homes: Foundation for a better health care system. Retrieved from *www.ncqa.org/Portals/0/Public%20Policy/2014%20 Comment%20Letters/The_Future_of_PCMH.pdf*.

Nielsen, M., Olayiwola, J. N., Grundy, P., & Grumbach, K. (2014). The patient-centered medical home's impact on cost & quality: An annual update of the evidence 2012-2013. Washington, DC: Patient-Centered Primary Care Collaborative. Retrieved from *www.pcpcc.org/resource/ medical-homes-impact-cost-quality*.

Patient-Centered Primary Care Collaborative. (2013). Defining the medical home. Retrieved from *www.pcpcc.org/about/medical-home*.

Ralph, N., Mielenz, T., Parton, H., Flately, A. M., & Thorpe, L. (2013). Multiple chronic conditions and limitations in activities of daily living in community-based sample of older adults living in New York City. *Preventing Chronic Disease, 10*, 130–159.

Robert Wood Johnson Foundation. (1996). *Chronic care in America: A 21st century challenge.* San Francisco, CA: The Institute for Health & Aging, University of California. Retrieved from *www.rwjf.org/files/ publications/other/ChronicCareinAmerica.pdf*.

Robert Wood Johnson Foundation, Partnership for Solutions. (2002). Chronic conditions: Making the case for ongoing care. Retrieved from *www .rwjf.org/reports/npreports/betterlives.htm*.

Sia, C., Tonniges, T. F., Osterhus, E., & Taba, S. (2004). History of the medical home concept. *Pediatrics, 113*(Suppl. 5), 1473–1478.

Social Security Online Actuarial Tables. (2010). Retrieved from *www .ssa.gov/OACT/STATS/table4c6.html*.

Tax Relief and Health Care Act. (2006). Section 204 of HR 6111, Baucus, M. (D-MT), Retrieved from *www.thomas.gov*.

ONLINE RESOURCES

National Committee on Quality Assurance: Patient-Centered Medical Home Recognition
www.ncqa.org/Programs/Recognition/PatientCenteredMedicalHomePCMH .aspx
The Institute for Healthcare Improvement
www.ihi.org/Engage/Initiatives/TripleAim/Pages/default.aspx
The Patient-Centered Primary Care Collaborative
www.pcpcc.org

UNIT 2

CHAPTER 32

Family Caregiving and Social Policy

Karen M. Robinson   Susan C. Reinhard

"There are four kinds of caregivers in this world: Those who have been caregivers, those who currently are caregivers, those who will be caregivers, and those who will need caregivers."

Rosalynn Carter

It is well established that the American population is aging. With the graying of the population, family caregivers will be needed more than ever to provide services to persons with chronic illness for increasingly long periods of time (Stevenson, 2008).

Persons most likely to need long-term services and support (LTSS) are in their 80s and older. Understanding the effects of the size of the baby boom generation compared with preceding and succeeding age cohorts is important to predict the demand for LTSS. When the oldest of 79 million baby boomers reach their 80s, the supply of available caregivers will experience a drastic shift in ratio as the demand for caregivers outpaces the supply. The projected ratio of potential caregivers to persons aged 80 years and over will decline between 2010 and 2030 in all states; the current ratio of more than seven potential caregivers for every person age 80 and over will fall 4 to 1 by 2030 and less than 3 to 1 by 2050 (Redfoot, Feinberg, & Houser, 2013). This declining ratio stems from changes in family size and composition, notably in fertility rates of successive cohorts of baby boomers. Only 11.6% of women in their 80s in 2010 were childless compared with a projected 16.0% of women in their 80s in 2030 (Kirmeyer & Hamilton, 2011).

Rising demand for caregivers with projected shrinking supply suggests improved social policy is needed to better serve the needs of older persons with disabilities. Family caregivers play this valuable, irreplaceable role in our society by supporting people who have LTSS needs.

WHO ARE THE FAMILY CAREGIVERS?

National estimates indicate that 52 million Americans over the age of 18 years provide support to older adults with chronic illnesses who live in the community (Coughlin, 2010; Family Caregiver Alliance [FCA], 2012). The average caregiver is a 49-year-old woman who works outside the home but also provides care for her mother, spending nearly 20 hours per week in unpaid care. This time spent in unpaid caregiving is almost equivalent to another part-time job. Caregivers are themselves aging; one third of caregivers who care for a person 65 years or over are 63 years of age themselves. Most recipients live in their own home (58%) with another 20% living in the home of their caregiver (FCA, 2012; National Alliance for Caregiving [NAC] and American Association of Retired Persons [AARP], 2009). More than one in six American employees who work full or part time reported caring for a family member (Cynkar & Mendes, 2011; FCA, 2012). Employees who worked at least 15 hours per week reported that caregiving significantly interfered in their work life. A total estimate of $3 trillion in lost wages, pensions, retirement funds, and benefits was calculated for the ten million caregivers over age 50 years caring for their parents (MetLife Mature Market Institute, NAC, & Center for Long Term Care Research and Policy at New York Medical College, 2011).

UNPAID VALUE OF FAMILY CAREGIVING

Family caregivers' contributions have enormous value to their loved ones and also to the nation. Caregivers provide high-quality care at low cost that is consistent with consumer preferences. In 2009, the economic value of family caregiving reached $450 billion; more than the total national spending for Medicaid, including federal and state contributions and medical and long-term care, which totaled $361 billion in 2009 (Feinberg et al., 2011).

Among noninstitutionalized persons needing assistance with activities of daily living such as bathing, dressing, and eating, families remain the most important source of help. Yet many do not identify themselves as caregivers but describe their support in terms of the relationship with the other person, such as spouse, daughter, son, partner, or friend. An estimated 83% of Americans identify a feeling of obligation to provide assistance to their parent(s) in times of need (Pew Research Center, 2010). The work of family caregivers is essentially irreplaceable, mainly because providing an alternate source of care is difficult and costly. The value of this unpaid care is stunning, but it exacts a high, often hidden cost on the quality of life for family caregivers. The health risk related to caregiving is enormous, even to caregivers who are initially in good health.

CAREGIVING AS A STRESSFUL BUSINESS

Caregivers make great sacrifices to provide this care, enduring negative effects on their physical and mental health, as well as burnout and depletion of financial resources. More than half of caregivers caring for someone 50 years of age and older spend more than 10% of their income on expenses. One in three family caregivers are forced to use some of their savings to cover caregiving expenses (NAC, 2009).

The association between physical and mental health and being a family caregiver is well established (Pinquart & Sorensen, 2007). Caregiving has all the features of a chronic stress experience as it creates physical and psychological strain over an extended period of time. Among family caregivers of persons with dementia, more than four out of five of them reported at least one chronic illness, and nearly two out of three reported multiple chronic illnesses. The proportion of chronic illnesses was especially high for caregivers aged 65 years and older as well as for spouse caregivers. This important research finding identified an increased

health risk for older female spouse caregivers compared with older male spouse caregivers (Wang et al., 2013).

High levels of unpredictability and uncontrollability accompany family caregiving situations. Thus, caregiving can create secondary stress in multiple domains of life, such as work and family relationships. Caregiving fits the definition for chronic stress so well that it is used as a model for studying its health effects (Schulz & Sherwood, 2008).

Evidence indicates that most family caregivers are not prepared for caregiving and often provide care with little or no support (NAC & AARP, 2009). Family caregivers are now performing tasks at home that previously were provided only in hospitals by nurses and other health care professionals. Findings from the first national survey that focuses on the medical/nursing tasks that family caregivers are expected to perform found that almost half (46%) of them are performing a wide range of tasks with little to no training or support from health care professionals (Reinhard, Levine, & Samis, 2012). Of these caregivers, most (78%) manage medications, including complex medication schedules, injections, and intravenous therapy. Unpaid family caregivers are performing wound care, including colostomy care and postsurgical site care, preparing food for special diets, helping with assistive devices, and managing ventilator care. More than half of family caregivers providing this care reported they had no other choice because there was no one else to do it or insurance would not cover professional help.

Despite their critical role in providing care coordination and complex care, and the new Affordable Care Act (ACA) health reform priority of preventing unnecessary rehospitalizations, these family caregivers get very little training or support. For example, nearly half (47%) of family caregivers who administered medications said they never received training from any source. Even many of those expected to provide wound care did not get the type of instruction they needed to provide this specialized care.

This is the new normal for family caregivers, with both positive and negative consequences. On the positive side, family caregivers who performed five or more medical/nursing tasks reported they were an important factor in preventing nursing home admission that neither they nor their family members desired. On the negative side, they were also more likely to report feeling stressed and worried about making a mistake. More than half reported feeling depressed and more than one third reported fair or poor health (Reinhard, Levine, & Samis, 2012). Caregivers consistently report higher levels of depressive symptoms and mental health problems when compared with their non-caregiving peers. Estimates identify that between 40% and 70% of family caregivers have clinically significant symptoms of depression, with approximately a quarter to a half of them meeting the diagnostic criteria for major depression (FCA, 2009).

Savundranayagam and Brintnall-Peterson (2010) found that family caregivers often become secondary patients because they do not adhere to their own medication schedules or keep track of their own health appointments. Lack of time given to meet self-care needs had detrimental effects on the caregivers' health (Nikzad-Terhune et al., 2010). The strain of caring for family members with dementia results in their family caregivers using 25% more health care services compared with non-caregivers of the same age (NAC, 2011).

SUPPORTING FAMILY CAREGIVERS

Demographic projections inform us that for the foreseeable future, we will never have as many caregivers per person for those who need care at 80 years and older than we have today. We are sliding down the caregiver ratio curve, and families are already beyond their capacity to serve. Caregivers are expected to prevent hospitalizations and nursing home admissions. They are expected to juggle their jobs and their complex caregiving responsibilities. To accomplish these expectations, unpaid caregivers need support from health care professionals, social networks, employers, and public policymakers.

Public policy initiatives have been slow to be developed and implemented but there are opportunities to speed progress. Table 32-1 summarizes several high-priority recommendations that can be taken at the federal and state levels to support

the work of family caregivers. Of six national policies and programs (tax credits, vouchers to pay minimum wage for some caregiving hours, respite services, transportation, family caregiver assessment, and paid leave of absence from work) presented to caregivers as potential help, the most popular was a tax credit of $3000. The majority of caregivers (56%) rated the tax credit as their preferred policy strategy (NAC & AARP, 2009). There are, however, many other options to support family caregivers, some of which can be embedded in larger changes in health care delivery.

HEALTH CARE DELIVERY REFORMS THAT HOLD PROMISE

The ACA explicitly uses the term "caregiver" 46 times and contains a number of new models of care that hold promise for better support for family caregivers (Feinberg & Reamy, 2011). A few are offered here for illustration, but funding through the Center for Medicare and Medicaid Innovation can fuel other models.

Patient-Centered Medical Homes and Health Homes. Patient-Centered Medical Homes (PCMHs), a term that is captured in the ACA, continues to promote new state options to provide Health Homes for people with chronic conditions. The core feature of PCMHs and Health Homes is that each patient has a health care professional (who could be a nurse) who leads a coordinated and integrated team, where the patient and family caregiver are viewed holistically with complete inclusion in the care system instead of as individual parts (FCA, 2009). Care coordination is receiving priority to make this Health Home model work and nurses have always taken on this central role (Robinson, 2010). A team of health and social service professionals is organized to address the specific needs of the individual and family caregiver. All health professionals involved talk to one another (and with the individual and caregiver) about existing care needs, preferences, and potential solutions. The online medical and social history of the individual and the caregiver is available at any time of the day or night to all involved, permitting them to keep in touch about ongoing needs.

TABLE 32-1 High-Priority Policy Recommendations to Support Family Caregivers

Categories of Support	Federal	State
Direct Services, such as Respite, Information, and Referral		
Ensure that all publicly funded long-term care programs cover services, such as respite care and adult day services, that supplement caregiving by family, friends, and others	X	X
Provide adequate funding for the Lifespan Respite Care Program	X	
Expand funding for the National Family Caregiver Support Program	X	
Increase state and federal funding for respite care	X	X
Offer additional services geared to special needs of caregivers, such as support groups and mental health counseling	X	X
Ensure that services and supports reflect needs of diverse caregiver populations	X	X
Assessment of Caregivers' Needs		
Stimulate development and delivery of family caregiver assessment protocols across all care settings to develop effective support plans for both the care recipient and the family caregiver	X	X
Require assessment of family caregiver's willingness and ability to provide care prior to hospital discharge; provide training, especially for medical/nursing tasks the family caregiver is expected to perform	X	X
Reimburse health care professionals for family caregiver assessment, care management, and training	X	X
Education and Training		
Create appropriate training opportunities and direct family caregivers to these training resources, particularly to ensure a safe transition from hospital to home or nursing home to home; fund training for family caregivers	X	X
Financial Relief		
Establish and coordinate policies to pay relatives and friends who care for people with disabilities as part of a plan of services and supports	X	X
Permit payment of family caregivers through consumer-directed models in publicly funded programs	X	X
Expand programs that permit family caregivers to direct the services that are offered to them (consumer direction for caregivers' services)	X	X
Amend Supplemental Security Income rules so they do not reduce benefits for caregivers living with family members	X	
Assure continued health insurance benefits for family caregivers forced to leave employment or during leaves of absence attributable to caregiving duties	X	X
Create incentives for increased public awareness about existing programs and policies		X
Tax Implications		
Provide a refundable Long-Term Services and Supports tax credit for caregivers to give some relief from the high costs of caregiving	X	X
Encourage employers to take advantage of existing tax incentives, such as flexible spending accounts for dependent care, to provide dependent- or family-care benefits	X	X
Workplace Flexibility, Including Family and Medical Leave Act		
Extend the Family and Medical Leave Act to provide paid leave and cover more workers for longer periods	X	
Provide paid family leave for caregiving	X	X
Provide paid sick leave for family caregiving		X
Caregiver Rights; Legal Protection		
Ensure that caregivers as well as patients are aware of the patient's right to appeal hospital discharge, skilled nursing facility, and Medicare home health care decisions	X	X

Independence at Home Demonstration. This program makes the person's home the Health Home. Costly, high-need Medicare beneficiaries and their family caregivers have primary care delivered in their homes, and the evaluation will test whether this new model achieves patient and family caregiver satisfaction. Expectations include lower health care costs as institutionalization is avoided (Feinberg & Reamy, 2011).

Community-Based Care Transition Program. The Centers for Medicare and Medicaid Services (CMS) is testing models to improve the transition from hospital to home for high-risk Medicare beneficiaries and their family caregivers. Patient and family activation measures are in development to help evaluate this program, although most transitional care models do not yet explicitly include a focus on family caregivers (Gibson, Kelly, & Kaplan, 2012). The research and advocacy communities in this field are urging a more systematic inclusion of family caregivers in the design, implementation, and evaluation of transitional programs.

HOME AND COMMUNITY-BASED SERVICES

Caregivers need education and support services to sustain their critical role as providers. Frequently, caregivers do not know where to turn for help. When assistance is sought, many community agencies cannot provide assistance because of budget constraints and outdated policies. The federal government can ensure that all family caregivers have access to caregiver assistance and to practical, high-quality, and affordable home and community-based services. The Medicare and Medicaid programs must be updated to support family caregivers through home and community-based services. Supporting family caregivers is one of the most cost-effective long-term care investments. When caregivers can continue as providers, they are often able to delay costly nursing home admission and reduce reliance on programs such as Medicaid (Reinhard, Montgomery, & Gibson, 2008).

FAMILY CAREGIVER ASSESSMENT

To support more people with chronic illnesses in the community, the needs of the individual and the family caregiver must be assessed and must be made part of a "safe and adequate discharge" (FCA, 2009, p. 1). Assessment of the family caregiver's health, willingness to provide care, and training and support needs will promote person- and family-centered care and ensure the health and safety of Medicaid beneficiaries served in the community rather than in nursing homes.

In 2005, nationally recognized health and LTSS experts achieved consensus on the principles and guidelines for effective family caregiver assessment in practice. A second panel of national and state experts recognized support for family caregivers, including assessing their needs, as one of five key dimensions in a high-performing state LTSS system (Reinhard et al., 2011). The 2013 federal Commission on Long-Term Care called for CMS to require assessment of family caregivers' needs and to include those needs in care plans (or hospital discharge plans) that depend on the participation of that family caregiver (Commission on Long-Term Care, 2013).

Some states are already including family caregiver assessment in their home and community-based services and other federal or state-funded family caregiver support programs. Rhode Island enacted the Family Caregivers Support Act of 2013 as part of the state's Medicaid LTSS reform efforts (Family Caregivers Support Act, 2013). The new state policy requires a family caregiver assessment if the plan of care for the Medicaid beneficiary involves a family caregiver.

Requiring a family caregiver assessment is one part of the support plan. Paying for it is another. No federal or state funding streams exist to pay for assessment of caregivers. Programs such as Medicare and Medicaid should pay providers to conduct family caregiver assessments if family caregivers are expected to provide substantial care, particularly during hospital discharge and transitional and postacute care (FCA, 2009).

Unpaid family caregivers most likely will continue to be the largest provider of LTSS in the United States. ACA legislation includes several provisions to improve quality of life for caregivers and individuals with chronic illnesses for whom they provide care. The ACA does not provide as much support for caregivers as was expected or is needed; however, the plans summarized here provide a platform on which to launch additional policy initiatives to aid caregivers.

DISCUSSION QUESTIONS

1. What are the most severe physical and emotional risks experienced by caregivers?
2. What health care delivery reforms hold the most promise to help caregivers?

REFERENCES

Commission on Long-Term Care (2013). Report to the Congress. (GPO No. 052-071-01565-5). Washington, DC: Commission on Long-Term Care. Retrieved from *bookstore.gpo.gov/products/sku/052-071-01565-5.*

Coughlin, J. (2010). Estimating the impact of caregiving and employment on well-being. *Outcomes Insight Health Manag, 2*(1), 1–7.

Cynkar, P., & Mendes, E. (2011). More than one in six American workers also act as caregivers. Gallup Wellbeing. Washington, DC: Gallup World Headquarters. Retrieved from *www.gallup.com/poll/148640/one-six-american-workers-act-caregivers.aspx.*

Family Caregiver Alliance (2009). 2009 National policy statement. San Francisco, CA: Family Caregiver Alliance. Retrieved from *www.caregiver.org/caregiver/jsp/content_node.jsp?nodeid=2279.*

Family Caregiver Alliance. (2012). Fact sheet: Selected caregiver statistics. Retrieved from *www.caregiver.org/caregiver/jsp/publications.jsp?nodeid=345.*

Family Caregivers Support Act. (2013). Rhode Island Public Law No. 2013-469.

Feinberg, L., & Reamy, A. M. (2011). Health reform law creates new opportunities to better recognize and support family caregivers. Washington, DC: American Association of Retired Persons Public Policy Institute. Retrieved from *www.aarp.org/relationships/caregiving/info-10-2011/Health-Reform-Law-Creates-New-Opportunities-to-Better-Recognize-and-Support-Family-Caregivers.html.*

Feinberg, L., Reinhard, S. C., Houser, A., & Choula, R. (2011). Valuing the invaluable: 2011 update—The growing contributions and costs of family caregiving. Washington, DC: American Association of Retired Persons Public Policy Institute. Retrieved from *www.aarp.org/relationships/caregiving/info-07-2011/valuing-the-invaluable.html.*

Gibson, M. J., Kelly, K., & Kaplan, A. K. (2012). Family caregiving and transitional care: A critical review. San Francisco, CA: Family Caregiver Alliance. Retrieved from *www.caregiver.org/jsp/content_node.jsp?nodeid=2603.*

Kirmeyer, S. E., & Hamilton, B. E. (2011). *Childbearing differences between three generations of U.S. women (NHCS Brief No. 68).* Washington, DC: National Center for Health Statistics.

MetLife Mature Market Institute, National Alliance for Caregiving, and Center for Long-Term Care Research and Policy at New York Medical College (2011). The MetLife study of caregiving costs to working caregivers: Double jeopardy for baby boomers caring for their parents. Westport, CT: MetLife. Retrieved from *www.caregiving.org/archives/1773.*

National Alliance for Caregiving (2009). The Evercare Survey of the economic downturn and its impact on family caregiving. Bethesda, MD: National Alliance for Caregiving. Retrieved from *www.caregiving.org/data/EVC_Caregivers_Economy_Report%20FINAL_4-28-09.pdf.*

National Alliance for Caregiving (2011). Caregiving costs: Declining health in the Alzheimer's caregiver as dementia increases in the care recipient. Bethesda, MD: National Alliance for Caregiving. Retrieved from *www.caregiving.org/pdf/research/Alzheimers_Caregiving_Costs_Study_FINAL.pdf.*

National Alliance for Caregiving and American Association of Retired Persons (2009). Caregiving in the US: A focused look at those caring for someone age 50 or older. Bethesda, MD: National Alliance for Caregiving. Retrieved from *assets.aarp.org/rgcenter/il/caregiving_09.pdf.*

Nikzad-Terhune, K. A., Anderson, K. A., Newcomer, R., & Gaugler, J. E. (2010). Do trajectories of at-home dementia caregiving account for burden after nursing home placement? A growth curve analysis. *Social Work in Health Care, 49,* 734–752. doi:10.1080/00981381003635296.

Pew Research Center (2010). Social and demographic trends: The decline of marriage and rise of new families. Washington, DC: Pew Research Center. Retrieved from *www.pewsocialtrends.org/files/2010/11/pew-social-trends-2010-families.pdf.*

Pinquart, M., & Sorensen, S. (2007). Correlates of physical health of informal caregivers: A meta-analysis. *J Gerontol B Psychol Sci Soc Sci, 62*(2), 126–137.

Redfoot, D., Feinberg, L., & Houser, A. (2013). The aging of the baby boom and the growing care gap: A look at future declines in the availability of family caregivers. Washington, DC: American Association of Retired Persons Public Policy Institute. Retrieved from *www.aarp.org/home-family/caregiving/info-08-2013/the-aging-of-the-baby-boom-and-the-growing-care-gap-AARP-ppi-ltc.html.*

Reinhard, S., Kassner, E., Houser, A., & Mollica, R. (2011). Raising expectations: State scorecard on long-term services and supports for older adults, people with physical disabilities, and caregivers. Washington, DC: American Association of Retired Persons Public Policy Institute. Retrieved from *www.aarp.org/home-family/caregiving/info-09-2011/ltss-scorecard.html.*

Reinhard, S., Levine, C., & Samis, S. (2012). Home alone: Family caregivers providing complex chronic care. Washington, DC: American Association of Retired Persons. Retrieved from *www.aarp.org/home-family/caregiving/info-10-2012/home-alone-family-caregivers-providing-complex-chronic-care.html.*

Reinhard, S. C., Montgomery, R., & Gibson, M. J. (2008). Informal caregivers: Sustaining the core of long-term services and supports. Washington, DC: Academy Health. Retrieved from *www.academyhealth.org/files/ltc/2008/colloquium/materials/Reinhard.pdf.*

Robinson, K. M. (2010). Care coordination: A priority for health reform. *Policy Polit Nurs Pract, 11*(4), 266–274. doi:10.1177/1527154410396572.

Savundranayagam, M. Y., & Brintnall-Peterson, M. (2010). Testing self-efficacy as a pathway that supports self-care among family caregivers in a psychoeducational intervention. *J Fam Soc Work, 13,* 149–162. doi:10.1080/10522150903487107.

Schulz, R., & Sherwood, P. C. (2008). Physical and mental health effects of family caregiving. *The American Journal of Nursing, 108*(9), 23–27.

Stevenson, D. G. (2008). Planning for the future-long term care and the 2008 election. *New England Journal of Medicine, 358*(19), 1985–1987.

Wang, X. R., Robinson, K. M., & Carter-Harris, L. (2013). Prevalence of chronic illnesses and characteristics of chronically ill informal caregivers of persons with dementia. *Age and Ageing, 43*(1), 137–141. doi:10.1093/ageing/aft142.

ONLINE RESOURCES

Caregiving Resource Center at American Association of Retired Persons (AARP)
www.aarp.org/home-family/caregiving
Family Caregiving Alliance
www.caregiver.org
National Alliance for Caregiving
www.caregiving.org
Top 20+ Websites for Caregivers-Caregiving Café
www.caregivingcafe.com

CHAPTER 33

Community Health Centers: Successful Advocacy for Expanding Health Care Access

Alice Sardell   Carmina Bernardo

"I mean, everybody should have access to medical care, and, you know, it shouldn't be such a big deal."

Paul Farmer

COMMUNITY HEALTH CENTERS DEMONSTRATE THE ADVOCACY PROCESS FOR INNOVATION

In 2013, 1200 community health centers (CHCs) served more than 22 million people at 9000 clinical sites all over the United States (National Association of Community Health Centers [NACHC], 2013). These programs provide medical, dental, mental health and substance abuse services, nutrition counseling, outreach, transportation, and other social services to uninsured patients as well as those with Medicaid, Medicare, Children's Health Insurance Program (CHIP), and even private health insurance. CHCs also include programs serving migrant workers and the homeless.

CHCs are located in areas designated by the federal government as medically underserved and provide care without regard to insurance status or ability to pay. They are primarily funded by a mix of public insurance and federal grants. About half of the patients receiving primary health care at CHCs live in rural areas, 72% have incomes at or below the federal poverty level, three quarters are either uninsured or covered by Medicaid, and most are members of racial and ethnic minorities (NACHC, 2013). Patients served by CHCs are sicker than patients seen by other providers and tend to have higher levels of chronic illness, yet independent federal government evaluations find that these patients receive high-quality care (NACHC, 2011).

CHCs are unique health service institutions in several important ways. First, they are a community-oriented, culturally sensitive model of health care services integrated with social and educational services. Second, they are governed by consumer boards that, by federal law, must have a majority of members who are patients at the health center. Third, they are safety net providers, caring for people who do not have health insurance. Fourth, the 2010 enactment of the Patient Protection and the Affordable Care Act and its accompanying legislation, the Health Care and Education Affordability Reconciliation Act (referred to as the ACA or health reform in this chapter), gave CHCs the opportunity to play a critical role on the front lines of health reform: helping uninsured individuals enroll in new health coverage options, while meeting the health service needs of the newly insured.

These health care institutions were first funded as neighborhood health centers as part of the War on Poverty in 1965, one aspect of President Lyndon B. Johnson's Great Society Program. They were created by activist physicians and federal government officials, "policy entrepreneurs" who believed that disparities in health status were intimately linked to social, economic, and political inequalities. Health centers were to treat whole communities, not just individuals, and to provide jobs as well as health services. Although these programs were products of the policy environment of the 1960s, they survived the end of the War on Poverty and subsequent political challenges during the more conservative Nixon and Reagan administrations. Not only did they overcome these challenges but they also became institutionalized as part of the federally funded health care system. In fact, health centers were the only domestic social program (other than abstinence-only health education) that was expanded during President George W. Bush's tenure in office.

The policy history of the CHC program explains how a program providing care to communities with very few political resources, and therefore little political influence, was able to survive and grow in an era in which less and less attention was paid to problems such as poverty and inequality. This occurred because supporters within federal executive agencies and Congress nurtured the program during its first decade until an effective national advocacy organization was built. This national organization, its state partners, and local health centers then successfully created broad support for health centers that is bipartisan and exists across ideological boundaries. The story of the survival of the CHC program is a story about the creation of a policy network supportive of CHCs. The story of its expansion is a tale of skilled policy advocates who have been able to frame the argument for health center funding in a way that fits within a political environment vastly different from the one in which it was born.

THE CREATION OF THE NEIGHBORHOOD HEALTH CENTER PROGRAM

The first neighborhood health centers were funded in 1965 as demonstration programs by the Community Action Program established by the Economic Opportunity Act (EOA) of 1964. The goal of this legislation was to eliminate the causes of poverty in the United States. Health was not initially one of the areas in which programs were to be established, but early on it became clear that participants in the educational and training programs that were established, such as Head Start and the Jobs Corps, suffered from lack of access to health care. The very first health programs were created by two medical educators, Dr. H. Jack Geiger and Dr. Count Gibson, of Tufts University Medical School (Sardell, 1988).

The model of the two centers that they established, one in a Boston housing project and one in a poor rural area of Mississippi, was based on a public health/social medicine approach. It combined comprehensive health services, community development, and the training and employment of community residents. Health center staff in Mississippi found that children in the community had recurring episodes of malnutrition and dysentery. In response they organized residents who decided to construct wells and establish a farm cooperative to feed themselves and their children. Other health centers funded under this program, which was authorized by an amendment to the EOA by Senator Edward Kennedy (D-MA), also provided community development and employment opportunities as well as health care services. For example, a neighborhood health center in Brooklyn, NY gave preference in hiring to local residents, and health center staff facilitated the creation of a community organization to rehabilitate housing in the area.

By the end of 1971, 100 neighborhood health centers had been funded under Kennedy's 1966 amendment. The original neighborhood health center model contained four elements: social medicine, community-based care, community economic development, and community participation. From a social medicine perspective, health status is shaped by the physical and social environment, and treatment includes intervention in that environment. Health care was to be community based by offering services to all of the residents of a specific geographic catchment area (rather than to those who fit within certain disease or health insurance categories) and by employing community residents to serve as a bridge between patients and professional staff. These workers, often called family health workers, made home visits and provided health education and advocacy services along with health care. The recruitment, training, and employment of these workers was also an example of the way in which neighborhood health centers were venues for community economic development. Finally, maximum feasible participation of the poor was required of all programs funded under the EOA. As we discuss later, when health centers received a separate federal program authorization in 1975 community governance became a central component that defined the program (Sardell, 1988).

Policy innovation in the United States most often requires that one or more individuals "invest their resources—time, energy, reputation, and sometimes money" in advocating for a new policy idea. John Kingdon calls these advocates "policy entrepreneurs" (Kingdon, 1995). Policy advocacy is most successful when entrepreneurs in and outside of government work together to support a new policy or program. This is what happened in the case of the creation of the neighborhood health center program. Activist physicians and federal Office of Economic Opportunity (OEO) officials worked together to create a policy that would increase health care access to low-income populations and to provide services that were different from those offered by mainstream medical institutions. In addition, Senator Edward M. Kennedy (D-MA) acted as an advocate for the program within Congress, deflecting opposition to both antipoverty programs and to socialized medicine.

When President Nixon took office the political environment changed; Nixon was not supportive of the social programs initiated by the Johnson administration. Yet during the Nixon administration, sympathetic federal agency officials protected the program until its advocates outside of government grew stronger (Sardell, 1988).

PROGRAM SURVIVAL AND INSTITUTIONALIZATION

Beginning in 1968 the public health service (PHS) within the U.S. Department of Health, Education, and Welfare (DHEW) also provided funding for the establishment of about 50 comprehensive health centers in low-income areas. The involvement of the PHS in primary health services had been historically limited to the funding of categorical disease programs. However, the 1960s was a period in which socially concerned health professionals, administrators, and social scientists joined the agency as an alternative to serving in the military

during the Vietnam War. Some of these individuals became policy entrepreneurs within the PHS for comprehensive health service programs for underserved populations. They were supported in their efforts by top DHEW officials appointed by President Johnson.

Although the Nixon administration did not support the neighborhood health center program, there were civil servants in the PHS, as well as the OEO, who acted to protect it. As the OEO was phased out, decisions as to the timing of the transfers of individual programs to the PHS were made in ways that would protect more politically vulnerable programs, such as those in the South. In addition, agency officials awarded technical assistance grants to newly formed state health center associations and (in 1973) to the National Association of Neighborhood Health Centers, an organization created in 1970. Key congressional leaders such as Senator Kennedy and Congressman Paul Rogers (D-FL) also supported the health center program during the presidencies of Richard Nixon and Gerald Ford.

In 1972, the DHEW announced that it planned to phase out federal grants to health centers on the assumption that they would be funded through Medicaid. However in 1974 and 1975 Congress, in opposition to the Nixon and Ford administrations, enacted legislation that specifically described community health centers and authorized grant funding for them. The legislation was vetoed by both presidents, but in 1975 Congress overrode President Ford's veto. The creation of the program took place within the wider context of intense conflict between presidents who aimed to reduce the role of the federal government in social policy and a liberal democratic Congress that wanted to preserve the social programs of the Great Society. This congressional action was a critical point in the history of the program because it now had its own legislative authority that defined its characteristics.

A CHC has to have a governing board with a consumer majority. This board establishes general policies for the center, has fiduciary responsibility, and appoints its executive director. A majority of board members have to be consumers who use its services. When enacted, this was the most rigorous community participation provision in any health service program up to that time. This legislative provision, reaffirmed many times, has meant that community-based primary care programs that do not have this governing board structure, such as those run by hospitals, cannot receive federal grants as CHCs. This provision has also enabled advocates to frame CHCs as embodying local control, an aspect of the program that has appealed to Republicans as well as Democrats.

The Ford administration (1974 to 1977) attempted to reduce CHC program funding and to end categorical grant programs in health. Within that political environment, federal program officials initiated changes that helped to expand congressional support. New program monitoring systems were established that provided measurable performance criteria for the health centers so that congressional concern with efficiency was addressed. In addition, rural health initiatives and smaller-scale, basic medical programs were funded. More centers could be funded because they required fewer resources than the large urban centers. And rural, white congressional districts could potentially become a part of the health center constituency. These changes were part of the institutionalization of the health center program (Sardell, 1988). Over time, the cost-effectiveness of CHCs has been one of the major arguments made for increasing support for this model of care. Further, since the 1980s, members of Congress from rural districts and states have been important health center champions.

At the same time federal agency officials were making programmatic decisions that would ultimately strengthen congressional support for CHCs, the National Association of Community Health Centers began to educate members of Congress about the value of CHCs. A policy analyst was hired, a weekly newsletter on policy events was published, and the association initiated an annual policy and issues forum in Washington, DC, which brought together health center consumers and staff to learn about policy issues and the policy process. In 1976, a Department of Policy Analysis was created. During the following decades, membership in the NACHC grew, as did the organizational infrastructure. Today, this organization is one of the most effective advocacy organizations in Washington, DC.

CONTINUING POLICY ADVOCACY

During the next 2 decades, under both Republican and Democratic presidents, the health center community strengthened its advocacy efforts and Congress continued to increase funding for the program. While Jimmy Carter was President (1977 to 1981), the rural health initiative concept of smaller centers was extended to urban areas and the focus on management efficiency continued. President Ronald Reagan's attempt to end the CHC program as a separate federal grant program was rejected by Congress in 1981. An important shift in the source of health center funding occurred during the 1990s as a result of legislation initiated by the staff of Senator John Chafee (R-RI) and the NACHC to deal with the problem of low Medicaid and Medicare reimbursement rates for services delivered at CHCs. Under the Federally Qualified Health Center (FQHC) Program, which became part of Medicaid in 1989 and Medicare in 1990, CHCs and look-alikes (clinics that did not get federal grant monies under the CHC program but had the characteristics of CHCs) would have special Medicaid and Medicare reimbursement rates that were closer to actual costs than regular per-visit rates paid by Medicaid in many states. As a result, health centers were able to collect higher reimbursements for Medicaid and Medicare patients and Medicaid replaced federal grants as the major source of revenue for health centers. From 1990 to 1998, the proportion of health center revenues from federal grants substantially decreased from 41% to 26%.

THE EXPANSION OF COMMUNITY HEALTH CENTERS UNDER A CONSERVATIVE PRESIDENT

Republican George W. Bush was elected president in 2000 as a conservative, yet he embraced CHCs, a program created by a liberal Democratic president in the 1960s. In 2001, in his first year in office, Bush proposed a 5-year initiative to expand health center sites to serve 6.1 million new patients. Congress supported funding for this initiative and throughout his two terms in office President Bush acted to fulfill his promise to expand the CHC program. Each time that Congress did not approve his full request for health center funding, the President would add the missing funds to his request for the following year (Hawkins, 2009). While the Bush administration was promoting the expansion of health centers, it was slashing spending for a wide variety of domestic programs including food stamps, home energy assistance, training grants for health professions, veterans' benefits, and Medicaid (Pear, 2005). In addition, during the effort to reauthorize the CHC program during 2007 and 2008, the Bush administration quietly helped to gain support from Republican members of Congress in spite of conservative opposition to the expansion of social programs at the federal level (Hawkins, 2009). What explains the support that CHCs, programs serving ethnic minorities and the poor, had from President Bush?

First are the data-based policy arguments that show that health centers provide access to high-quality health care for underserved populations in a cost-effective way and are central in efforts to reduce ethnic and racial disparities in health status (NACHC, 2011). Second is the expansion of the policy network to include conservative members of Congress, so that now that network includes an ideologically diverse set of policymakers. In addition to the liberal Democrats and moderate Republicans who were program supporters in its formative years, health center champions in Congress during Bush's first term in office included powerful Republican conservatives such as Senators Orrin Hatch of Utah (R), Christopher "Kit" Bond of Missouri (R), and Representative Henry Bonilla (R) of Texas. In fact, Senator Bond and Congressman Bonilla educated George W. Bush on the value of the health center model during his first campaign for the presidency (Hawkins, 2005). Third, it is the long experience and high levels of skill of the officials and staff of the CHC advocacy community that has successfully wedded policy arguments with

grassroots political activity. Primary care associations at the state and regional levels, together with the NACHC, have successfully met a series of policy challenges to the program's continued existence and growth and have helped to create the very broad support enjoyed by the CHC program almost 50 years after its creation.

COMMUNITY HEALTH CENTERS IN THE ERA OF OBAMACARE

The 2008 election of a Democratic President who began his professional life as a community organizer (and was endorsed during the Democratic Presidential primary by Senator Edward M. Kennedy, the long-time champion of CHCs) suggested that the CHC program would continue to enjoy Presidential support.

The American Recovery and Reinvestment Act (ARRA) of 2009, federal legislation designed to respond to the steep recession in the American economy, included an almost $2 billion investment in CHCs for both new sites and the expansion of existing sites (Bureau of Primary Health Care, 2010). The CHC program was the only direct health services program to receive money under the ARRA.

When Congress was beginning to consider this legislation, two CHC champions, Congressman David Obey (D-WI), Chair of the House Appropriations Committee, and Senator Tom Harkin (D-IA), Chair of the Senate Appropriations Subcommittee for Labor-Health and Human Services, Education, and Related Agencies programs, included funding for CHCs in the House and Senate bills. Health centers presented data to members of Congress about the many newly unemployed workers seeking care at CHCs, the cost savings achieved when disparities in access to care were reduced and chronic disease was effectively managed, and the fact that health centers were themselves engines of job creation and community economic development.

The $2 billion authorized for CHCs in the ARRA was more than that recommended by either the House ($1.5 billion) or the Senate ($1.87 billion.) Usually, when the Senate and House negotiate on final legislation, the amount of funding for a program is a compromise. But in the case of funding for CHC expansion in the Recovery Act, those negotiating the final bill, Democratic party leaders from both Houses, Representatives from the Obama administration, and a small group of Republicans supporting the stimulus package, agreed to actually raise the amount (Hawkins, 2009). Clearly, support for CHCs came from both parties and from members of Congress across the liberal/conservative ideological spectrum, from Socialist Bernie Sanders to Conservative Orrin Hatch.

CHC advocates were very active in the process of formulating health care reform legislation during 2009, arguing that expanding health insurance alone is not sufficient to create access to high-quality preventive and primary health care. Senator Bernard Sanders (I-VT) and the House Majority Whip James Clyburn (D-SC) were key congressional champions for including funding for health centers in the health reform bills (Hawkins, 2009; McDonough, 2011, pp. 204-205). The health reform legislation enacted in March 2010 emphasizes public health initiatives and preventive and primary health services as means to improve health outcomes, reduce health care disparities, and save money. The legislation continues federal support for expansion of the numbers of CHCs and the services that they provide. Eleven billion dollars in new funding is authorized for the CHC program over a period of 5 years, beginning in fiscal year 2011, both to serve an additional 20 million patients and to increase medical, dental, and mental health services. While most of the funds will be spent on providing services, $1.5 billion of the authorization is for new construction and renovation of existing facilities.

Other provisions of the new health reform legislation also affect the operations of health centers. Federal eligibility for Medicaid is expanded (to all those with an annual income less than 133% of the federal poverty level) and that will provide health insurance coverage to 16 million more people, some of whom were previously treated as self-pay patients at CHCs, and some of whom probably did not seek primary care. However, the national impact of expanding Medicaid is now uncertain.

The 2012 U.S. Supreme Court decision in National Federation of Independent Business v Sebelius meant that the Medicaid expansion is essentially optional for states (Kaiser Family Foundation, 2012). By the end of 2013, only 25 states and the District of Columbia moved ahead with implementing the expansion (Ku et al., 2013). More states may decide to opt in at a later date.

The legislation also seeks to protect the financial viability of health centers within the new health insurance system. In addition to the $11 billion to establish the Health Center Trust Fund mentioned previously, $1.5 billion in new funding from 2011 to 2015 is authorized for the National Health Service Corps (NHSC), which provides educational scholarships and loans to primary care providers who agree to serve in provider shortage areas. Funding expansions for the NHSC is expected to improve CHC recruitment efforts (Kaiser Family Foundation, 2013). In addition, new grant programs are established for the development of teaching and residency programs at CHC sites (NACHC, 2010).

Another ACA provision that benefits CHCs is the increased reimbursement rates for Medicaid primary care services to the same levels as Medicare payments in 2013 and 2014 (Health Care Education and Reconciliation Act, 2010). Combined with the Medicaid eligibility expansion, the enhanced Medicaid rate should potentially increase Medicaid revenue at CHCs (Ku et al., 2013). The ACA has also given CHCs the opportunity to broaden their safety net role through new federal funding for outreach and enrollment assistance for CHC patients who are newly eligible for Medicaid or subsidized private health insurance. In May of 2013, the Health Resources and Services Administration announced that over 1000 CHCs across the United States were granted $150 million to educate their patients about the new health insurance options available under health reform and to assist any eligible patient with enrolling in these programs (U.S. Department of Health and Human Services, Human Resources and Services Administration, 2013).

In spite of new federal funding and the Medicaid expansion, challenges to the sustainability of CHCs remain. Funding for CHCs remains as critical as ever, because millions of people are expected to remain uninsured after the ACA is implemented, particularly in states that ultimately decide not to expand Medicaid. A recent analysis projects that if only half the United States ultimately takes up the Medicaid expansion, more than 30 million people will remain uninsured (Nardin et al., 2013). In addition, through the newly created insurance marketplaces under the ACA, many CHC patients will be newly enrolled in private health insurance, known as qualified health plans (QHPs). CHCs must have the capacity, knowledge, and experience to successfully navigate the complexities of private health insurance, such as ensuring they are included in provider networks, negotiating reasonable reimbursement rates, and understanding the out-of-pocket cost-sharing rules among the different levels of QHP coverage.

The result of 5 decades of advocacy by health care activists, federal officials, members of Congress, and organized health center patients and staff has been the recognition and support of CHCs as critically important parts of the U.S. health care delivery infrastructure. A social medicine model originally funded as a poverty program is now viewed as a cost-effective way to focus on the social, economic, and environmental variables that influence the health status of all Americans.

DISCUSSION QUESTIONS

1. What does the creation of the CHC program tell us about the conditions necessary for policy innovation?
2. Who were the policy entrepreneurs supportive of the institutionalization and continuation of the federal CHC program at key junctures in its history?
3. Research the policy history of a CHC or FQHC program in your local community or region. Who were/are the individuals/institutions acting as policy entrepreneurs supportive of this program?

REFERENCES

Bureau of Primary Health Care. (2010). The Health Center Program: Recovery Act Grants. Retrieved from *www. bphc.hrsa.gov/recovery.*

Hawkins, D. R., Jr. (2005). Phone interview with Daniel R. Hawkins, Jr., Senior Vice President, Public Policy and Research, National Association of Community Health Centers.

Hawkins, D. R., Jr. (2009). Phone interview with Daniel R. Hawkins, Jr., Vice President for Federal, State, and Public Affairs, National Association of Community Health Centers.

Health Care Education and Reconciliation Act. (2010). Pubic Law No. 111-152, 124 Stat. 1052. Sec. 1202. Retrieved from *www.gpo.gov/fdsys/pkg/PLAW-111publ152/pdf/PLAW-111publ152.pdf.*

Kaiser Family Foundation. (2012). *A guide to the Supreme Court's Affordable Care Act decision.* Washington, DC: Kaiser Family Foundation. Retrieved from *kaiserfamilyfoundation.files.wordpress.com/2013/01/8332.pdf.*

Kaiser Family Foundation. (2013). *Community health centers in an era of health reform: An overview and key challenges to health center growth.* Washington, DC: Kaiser Family Foundation. Retrieved from *kaiser familyfoundation.files.wordpress.com/2013/03/8098-03.pdf.*

Kingdon, J. (1995). *Agendas, alternatives, and public policies* (2nd ed.). New York: HarperCollins.

Ku, L., Zur, J., Jones, E., Shin, P., & Rosenbaum, S. (2013). *How Medicaid expansions and future community health center funding will shape capacity to meet the nation's primary care needs.* Washington, DC: The George Washington University School of Public Health and Health Services. Retrieved from *sphhs.gwu.edu/pdf/elR/GGRCHN_PolicyResearch Brief_34.pdf.*

McDonough, J. E. (2011). *Inside national health reform.* Berkeley, CA: University of California Press and Milbank Memorial Fund.

Nardin, R., Zallman, L., McCormick, D., Woolhandler, S., & Himmelstein, D. (2013). The uninsured after implementation of the Affordable Care Act: A demographic and geographic analysis. Health Affairs Blog. Retrieved from *healthaffairs.org/blog/2013/06/06/the-uninsured-after-implementation-of-the-affordable-care-act-a-demographic-and-geographic-analysis/.*

National Association of Community Health Centers. (2010). Community health centers and health reform. Retrieved from *www.nachc.com/client/Summary%20of%20Final%20Health%20Reform%20Package.pdf.*

National Association of Community Health Centers. (2011). Community health centers: The local prescription for better quality and lower costs. Retrieved from *www.nachc.com/client/A%20Local%20Prescription%20Final%20brief%203%2022%2011.pdf.*

National Association of Community Health Centers. (2013). America's health centers fact sheet. Retrieved from *www.nachc.com/client//America's_Health_Centers2013.pdf.*

Pear, R. (2005). Domestic programs subject to Bush's knife: Aid for food and heating. *New York Times*, A22.

Sardell, A. (1988). *The U.S. experiment in social medicine: The community health center program, 1965–1986.* Pittsburgh, PA: The University of Pittsburgh Press.

U.S. Department of Health and Human Services, Health Resources and Services Administration. (2013). Health center outreach and enrollment assistance fiscal year 2013; HRSA-13-279, CFDA# 93.527. Retrieved from *bphc.hrsa.gov/outreachandenrollment/hrsa-13-279.pdf.*

ONLINE RESOURCES

Bureau of Primary Health Care
www.bphc.hrsa.gov
National Association of Community Health Centers
www.nachc.com
National Rural Health Association
www.ruralhealthweb.org

CHAPTER 34

Filling the Gaps: Retail Health Care Clinics and Nurse-Managed Health Centers

Tine Hansen-Turton   Jamie M. Ware   Brian Valdez   Sarah Hexem

"The innovation point is the pivotal moment when talented and motivated people seek the opportunity to act on their ideas and dreams."

W. Arthur Porter

According to the Congressional Budget Office (CBO), the Affordable Care Act (ACA) will increase the number of insured Americans by more than 30 million through 2016 (CBO, 2012). In fact, with 7 million people expected to sign up for insurance through the exchanges, and another 13.1 million accessing coverage through state Medicaid expansion, 2014 will bring the biggest surge in health coverage the United States has seen in decades (Cowley, 2013). But does expanded coverage equal improved care? The experience in Massachusetts suggested not. Shortly after Massachusetts enacted legislation guaranteeing near universal health coverage, the state's primary care physicians were overwhelmed by an influx of newly insured patients. As a result, in 2008 the average wait time to see a primary care physician in Boston was 49.6 days, the longest in the United States (Thompson, 2009).

There is already a shortage among U.S. primary care physicians. Recent research suggests it would take 15,000 primary care physicians just to fill the current gap, and 45,000 to care for the people who will gain health coverage by 2025 (Cowley, 2013). To avoid a repeat of what happened in Massachusetts, the Institute of Medicine (IOM) has stated, "Advanced practice registered nurses (APRNs) should be called upon to fulfill and expand their potential as primary care providers" (IOM, 2011, pp. 1-2). Across the United States, nurses in retail

clinics and nurse-managed health clinics (NMHCs) are already stepping in to fill gaps in care. This chapter discusses how these two innovative models of care can expand access for newly insured individuals, the challenges they face, and the policy implications for nursing and health care.

RETAIL HEALTH CLINICS

Retail-based convenient care clinics are small health care facilities located in high-traffic retail outlets with pharmacies that provide affordable and accessible nonemergency care to individuals who otherwise would have to wait for appointments with a traditional primary care provider. The majority of these clinics are staffed by APRNs, although some clinics also use physician assistants. The first retail clinics appeared in the mid-2000s. Since then, the industry has expanded across the United States, growing from 150 clinics in 2006 to approximately 1500 in 2013. By 2016, the number of clinics is expected to double to nearly 3000 (Accenture, 2013). Popularity of the model has grown so rapidly that 30% of all Americans now live within a 10-minute drive of a clinic (Rudavsky, Pollock, & Mehrotra, 2009). Clinic operators include hospitals, health systems, and for-profit corporations.

The retail clinic model is designed to make care convenient and affordable for all patients. Therefore, the patient population represents a cross-section of income brackets, age groups, and payer mixes including insured, uninsured, and self-pay patients. Unlike traditional primary care providers, most retail clinics are open 7 days a week, with extended weekday hours; no appointments are

293

necessary; and visits generally take 15 to 20 minutes. Retail clinics also practice transparent pricing. Patients without insurance typically pay $40 to $75 for a clinic visit (Convenient Care Association [CCA], n.d.b).

The services offered at retail clinics include acute and chronic disease care, immunization, physical examinations, health screenings and health education such as EpiPen instruction and prescription, and preventative care. Some of the most common treatments are sore throat, common cold, flu, allergy, sinus infection, immunization, and blood pressure testing. The clinics distribute thousands of flu shots annually. Many retail clinics have expanded their services to also include chronic disease care.

ACCESS AND QUALITY IN RETAIL CLINICS

Along with providing care at more convenient times and locations, retail clinics expand access by reaching a high percentage of people without a regular source of care. Recent research suggests as many as 60% of all retail clinic patients do not have a regular primary care provider (Mehrotra & Lave, 2012). Visits to retail clinics grew fourfold from 2007 to 2009, and according to a study in Health Affairs, some of the retail clinics operated by hospitals have become the largest entry point for patients entering the hospital health care system (Mehrotra & Lave, 2012).

In terms of quality, 93% of patients report being highly satisfied with the convenience of retail clinics (CCA, n.d.a). A 2011 study also found that the clinics had a 92.7% compliance with quality measure for appropriate testing of children with pharyngitis, which was well above the Healthcare Effectiveness Data and Information Set (HEDIS) average of 74.7%. The compliance score for appropriate testing of children with upper respiratory infection was 88.3%, again well above the HEDIS average of 83.5% (Jacoby et al., 2011). Quality scores and rates of preventive care offered at retail clinics are similar to the care delivered at other settings, as is the return visit rate. This suggests that the quality of the care in retail clinics is high and

does not generate additional follow-up use (Rohner, Angstman & Garrison, 2012).

RETAIL CLINICS AND COST

The potential cost savings associated with retail clinics is substantial. A study conducted by the Rand Corporation found that the cost of care at retail clinics is significantly lower than the average cost at urgent care centers, primary care offices, and emergency rooms (ERs) (Mehrotra et al., 2009). In another study, retail clinics were able to lower costs by reducing ER use for pediatric patients and hospital admissions for patients with chronic illnesses (Parente, n.d.). Finally, Blue Cross and Blue Shield of Minnesota recently eliminated copays for enrollees who used a retail clinic, stating that the clinics have produced a $1.2 million cost savings (Blue Cross and Blue Shield of Minnesota, 2008).

CHALLENGES AND REACTIONS TO THE MODEL

The reaction of consumers and APRNs to retail clinics has been largely positive. As stated earlier, consumers have been overwhelmingly satisfied with the convenience of retail clinics, and nurse practitioner associations are pleased with the way retail clinics are expanding career opportunities for APRNs. However, the reaction has not all been positive. Physicians worry that the quality of care in retail clinics is not adequate and that retail clinics might interfere with the continuity of care. Neither of these objections holds much weight in light of the research. Studies such as the ones cited earlier show that the quality of care in retail clinics is high. In terms of care continuity, retail clinics routinely forward primary care providers electronic records of the care they provide to their patients.

Despite the actions taken to address physicians' concerns, retail clinic advocates still spend much of their time responding to legislation sponsored by organized medicine, which seeks to place overly burdensome regulations on retail clinics. The same is true of nurse-managed health clinics (NMHCs).

NURSE-MANAGED HEALTH CLINICS

The ACA defines an NMHC as "a nurse practice arrangement, managed by advanced practice nurses, that provides primary care or wellness services to underserved or vulnerable populations and that is associated with a school, college, university or department of nursing, federally qualified health center, or independent nonprofit health or social services agency" (Hansen-Turton, 2013, p. 1). Unlike retail clinics, all of the care in NMHCs is directed by nurse practitioners or other APRNs. There are approximately 250 NMHCs operating in rural, urban, and suburban communities across the United States (Hansen-Turton, 2013). NMHCs are not confined to retail settings. They can be found in schools, senior centers, housing developments, and other easily accessible locations. Approximately 60% are affiliated with a school of nursing; the rest operate as independent nonprofit organizations.

Another difference is that NMHCs are safety-net providers catering almost exclusively to low-income, uninsured individuals and those on Medicaid. Therefore, NMHC patients tend to be sicker and disproportionately experiencing health disparities. The most common diagnoses at NMHCs include chronic diseases such as hypertension, diabetes, hypercholesterolemia, obesity, depression, upper respiratory infection, and asthma.

Because they are safety-net providers, NMHCs offer care regardless of the patient's ability to pay. Services typically include basic primary care, diagnostic testing, and wellness care designed to promote chronic disease management and prevention through patient education, lifestyle change, and counseling. Depending on the model, some clinic directors choose to focus exclusively on either primary or wellness care; others offer a combination of the two. A small number of NMHCs also provide behavioral health and dental services onsite. Finally, although the care is APRN-directed, it is also team-based and fully integrated. This means the nurses work with other providers such as social workers, behavioral health specialists, and physicians to ensure care is well coordinated and patient-centered. To facilitate this process, NMHCs use established referral networks.

QUALITY AND COST IN NMHCs

APRNs and NMHCs have a 30-year track record of delivering high-quality care. In 2012, the National Governors Association conducted a review of the literature around APRN care quality and cost. The study concluded that APRNs can perform many primary care services as well as physicians can, with equal or higher patient satisfaction rates (Schiff, 2012). Another literature review looking specifically at NMHC quality of care stated that breast cancer screenings, immunizations, and smoking cessation advising in NMHCs exceeded the HEDIS 75th percentile (Barkauskas et al., 2011). A third study examining outcomes for 500 children treated for viral infections at an NMHC concluded that the quality and efficiency of care provided by the NMHC exceeded expectations and surpassed national benchmarks (Coddington et al., 2011).

Similar results were found when evaluating cost. Within 6 months of establishing an NMHC, one city experienced a cost savings of $26,000 as a result of decreased use of emergency services (Coddington & Sands, 2008). Another NMHC providing care to patients who were HIV positive was able to reduce hospital charges by $785,744 over 1 year (Coddington & Sands, 2008).

NMHCs AND WORKFORCE DEVELOPMENT

Because so many NMHCs are affiliated with schools of nursing, they play a key role in clinical education and workforce development. In 2012, the National Nursing Centers Consortium (NNCC) conducted a survey of 28 NMHCs and found that 99% of the clinics served as clinical education sites for health professions students. All together, the clinics educated a total of 1500 students with a mean of 55 at each site. The largest percentage of students trained were bachelor-level nurses (61%), followed by advanced practice nurses (29%); other students included medical residents and social work, physician assistant, and pharmacy students.

CHALLENGES TO THE MODEL

Despite their well-documented benefits in terms of expanding access and strengthening workforce development, NMHCs face a number of challenges that threaten the sustainability of the model. First, unlike other safety-net providers such as federally qualified health centers (FQHCs), NMHCs do not have access to a stable source of federal funding. Because FQHCs, rural health clinics, and other safety-net providers see a high percentage of uninsured patients, the federal government provides these clinics with grant funding intended to cover the cost of caring for the uninsured. Even through NMHCs also see a high percentage of uninsured (35% to 40%), many nurse-led clinics are prohibited from obtaining federal funding attributable to: (1) the inability of academically affiliated NMHCs to meet the FQHC program's community governance requirements and (2) lack of support from existing FQHCs.

To address this problem, the ACA officially recognized NMHCs as safety-net providers and created a $50 million federal grant program to specifically fund these clinics. Although inclusion in the ACA represented a major victory for NMHCs, Congress has never appropriated funding to the grant program. In 2010, the administration distributed $15 million in grant funding to 10 NMHCs in the United States, but these grants have since expired, and the funding has not been renewed. The lack of a stable source of federal funding has and will continue to cause NMHCs to close. Each time a clinic closes, thousands of underserved patients lose access to a critical point of care. If policymakers value the contribution NMHCs are making to expanding primary care capacity and workforce development, it is vital that Congress move to place NMHCs on the same footing as other safety-net providers, by supporting the reauthorization of the NMHC grant program with renewed funding.

Second, even though APRNs are qualified to act as primary care providers in all 50 states, many of the U.S. Managed Care Organizations (MCOs) still refuse to contract with APRN primary care providers. According to a 2011 study involving 258 of the U.S. Health Maintenance Organizations (HMOs), 25% of the HMOs surveyed did not permit APRNs to serve as primary care providers. Of the plans responding, Medicare plans were the most likely to permit APRNs to serve as primary care providers at 83%, followed by Medicaid plans at 75%, and commercial plans at 67% (Hansen-Turton et al., 2013).

The fact that a significant number of MCOs continue to prohibit APRNs to serve as primary care providers is especially disturbing considering millions of Americans are poised to receive health coverage through state Medicaid expansion. As discussed earlier, the research demonstrates that the care offered by APRNs is as good as or better than that of other primary care providers. Therefore, the restriction on managed care participation unnecessarily limits the potential of APRNs to fill gaps in care. Additionally, some of the MCOs that do allow APRNs to serve as primary care providers reimburse them at a rate that is less than physician primary care providers.

The ACA includes anti-discrimination language that could be used to prohibit these practices and encourage MCOs to contract with APRN primary care providers. However, in early 2014 the U.S. Department of Health and Human Services declined to publish regulations enforcing the provision. To avoid a repeat of what happened in Massachusetts, policymakers must reverse this trend and move to ensure the full and fair participation/reimbursement of APRNs in managed care.

Third, there are a variety of state laws and policies that can impact NMHCs and their ability to serve patients. Because they are managed and staffed by APRNs, state-level scope of practice, licensing, and physician collaboration laws can either promote or hinder the expansion of the NMHC model. On the positive side, 18 states and the District of Columbia now permit APRNs to practice without any physician supervision. In 2013 alone, Nevada and Rhode Island both passed legislation allowing APRNs to practice independent of physician supervision. The fact that more states are granting APRNs greater independence is an indication that policymakers are coming to the realization that using APRNs is the best way to deliver high-quality care to those covered under the ACA.

However, there continues to be pushback from organized medicine. In recent years, the NNCC, which represents the NMHCs, has seen a new trend emerging in the United States. Doctors are pushing for laws that force APRNs to practice as part of a physician-directed health care team. Although the NMHC model recognizes the benefits of team-based care and its ability to improve patient outcomes, there is no reason the health care team has to be physician-led. APRNs are capable of managing 80% to 90% of the care provided by primary care physicians without referral or consultation (Mundinger, 1994). Additionally, a seminal study in the *Journal of the American Medical Association* concluded that patients of primary care APRNs have outcomes comparable to those of primary care physicians (Mundinger et al., 2000).

Rather than improving health care access, forcing APRNs to practice as part of physician-directed teams could potentially limit the health care options open to vulnerable patients. For example, APRNs serving rural areas of Virginia are concerned that the state's new team-based care law, which requires APRNs to consult with a physician on all complex cases, is overly restrictive. The low-income, vulnerable patients using NMHCs suffer from multiple chronic and complex conditions. Requiring an APRN to consult with a physician on every patient presenting complex symptoms could lead to hundreds of additional hours of consultation and reduce the time APRNs actually spend seeing patients. In light of the fact that there is no difference in the quality of care delivered by APRNs and primary care physicians, excess consultation seems like an unnecessary burden on the time available to APRNs and physicians alike.

Another area where the team-based care concept is presenting problems is in patient-centered medical home (PCMH) programs. Some states have published regulations requiring PCMHs to be led by a physician. NMHCs around the United States are already acting as PCMHs. In fact, in 2010 eight NMHCs became the first nurse-led practices in the United States to be officially recognized as PCMHs by the National Committee on Quality Assurance (NCQA). The requirement that PCMHs be physician-led effectively bars the participation of NMHCs in medical home programs. If NMHCs cannot participate in these programs, they will not be eligible for reimbursement incentives available to other providers, and clinics recognized by the NCQA could lose their certification.

To ensure that all patients can enjoy the benefits of team-based and patient-centered care, states need to support the inclusion of APRNs. APRNs in NMHCs have the ability to bring the advantages of team-based, patient-centered care to low-income, medically underserved patients other providers may not be able to reach. But if they are tied to physicians, or unable to participate in PCMH programs, the capacity of APRNs to provide care is limited.

FUTURE DIRECTIONS FOR RETAIL CLINICS AND NMHCs

The future for retail clinics is largely bright. All indications are that the industry will continue to expand rapidly. A recent study predicts that the number of clinics will grow to nearly 3000 by 2016 (Accenture, 2013). More hospital systems are opening retail clinics that should serve as a catalyst for growth. Also, more clinic operators are expanding the services they provide to include chronic disease care, which will drive up patient volumes. All and all, the relatively young retail clinic industry is a success story that has used APRNs and public-private partnerships to expand and transform access to care.

The biggest ongoing policy issue for retail clinics is the push to get the services of the clinics reimbursed through managed care. Even though retail clinics have been shown to lower managed care costs (discussed earlier), many MCOs have not established a method of reimbursement for the clinics. The Convenient Care Association, which represents retail clinics around the United States, is working with retail clinic operators and managed care companies to overcome this barrier.

By contrast, NMHCs will most likely continue to face challenges. One positive trend is that in recent years more NMHCs have been able to access federal funding by obtaining FQHC recognition. However, only about 10% of the U.S. NMHCs are FQHCs. The fact that more states are passing legislation to grant APRNs greater independence of practice should also encourage NMHC growth. But unless state and national policymakers move to address the challenges listed earlier, this opportunity will be missed. Considering the primary care shortage, and the passage of the ACA, it is imperative that the United States take full advantage of this important health care resource. Failure to do so will limit access to care, especially for the underserved.

Groups such as the NNCC and other nursing organizations are working with national and state policymakers to offer potential solutions to the issues NMHCs face. But for progress to be made, nurses need to remain engaged in the political process so they can influence the creation of an environment that supports NMHC growth.

DISCUSSION QUESTIONS

1. Why are retail and nurse-managed clinics important in light of the ACA, and what opportunities do they offer to expand the role of nurses?
2. How are retail and nurse-managed clinics different from traditional primary care providers and are they in competition with traditional primary care providers?
3. What are the challenges facing retail and nurse-managed clinics and how can they be overcome?

REFERENCES

Accenture. (2013). Retail medical clinics: From foe to friend? Retrieved from *www.accenture.com/SiteCollectionDocuments/PDF/Accenture-Retail-Medical-Clinics-From-Foe-to-Friend.pdf?vm=r*.

Barkauskas, V., Pohl, J., Tanner, C., Onifade, J., & Pilon, B. (2011). Quality of care in nurse-managed health centers. *Nursing Administration Quarterly, 35*(1), 34–43.

Blue Cross and Blue Shield of Minnesota. (2008). Blue Cross offers no copay for use of retail clinics. Retrieved from *www.bluecrossmn.com/bc/wcs/.idcplg?IdcService=GET_DYNAMIC_CONVERSION&Revision SelectionMethod=Latest&dDocName=POST71A_12162*.

Coddington, J., & Sands, L. (2008). Cost of health care and quality outcomes of patients at nurse-managed clinics. *Nursing Economics, 26*(2), 75–83.

Coddington, J., Sands, L., Edwards, N., Kirkpatrick, J., & Chen, S. (2011). Quality of health care provided at a pediatric nurse-managed clinics. *Journal of the American Academy of Nurse Practitioners, 23*(12), 674–680.

Congressional Budget Office. (2012). Updated estimates for the insurance coverage provisions of the Affordable Care Act. Washington, DC: U.S. Government Printing Office. Retrieved from *www.cbo.gov/sites/default/files/cbofiles/attachments/03-13-Coverage%20Estimates.pdf*.

Convenient Care Association. (n.d.a). Convenient care clinics: Increasing access [fact sheet]. Retrieved from *www.ccaclinics.org/images/stories/downloads/factsheets/ccafactsheet_increasing_access.pdf*.

Convenient Care Association. (n.d.b). Convenient care clinics: Reducing costs for consumers and third-party payers [fact sheet]. Retrieved from *www.ccaclinics.org/images/stories/downloads/factsheets/ccafactsheet_affordable_care.pdf*.

Cowley, G. (2013). Millions are about to get health insurance. Will they get care? Retrieved from *www.msnbc.com/msnbc/doctor-gap-next-hurdle-health-care*.

Hansen-Turton, T. (2013). Testimony of the National Nursing Centers Consortium regarding fiscal year 2014 appropriations for the nurse-managed health clinic grant program. Retrieved from *www.nncc.us/site/images/pdf/testimonyhouselhhs_2013.pdf*.

Hansen-Turton, T., Ware, J., Bond, L., Doria, N., & Cunningham, P. (2013). Are managed care organizations in the United States impeding the delivery of primary care by nurse practitioners? A 2012 update on managed care organization credentialing and reimbursement practices. *Population Health Management, 16*(5), 306–309.

Institute of Medicine. (2011). The future of nursing: Leading change, advancing health. Retrieved from *thefutureofnursing.org/sites/default/files/1%20Key%20Messages%20of%20the%20Report%20(19-42).pdf*.

Jacoby, R., Crawford, A., Chauhari, P., & Goldfarb, N. (2011). Quality of care for 2 common pediatric conditions treated by convenient care providers. *American Journal of Medical Quality*, January-February, 53–58.

Mehrotra, A., & Lave, J. (2012). Visits to retail clinics grew fourfold from 2007 to 2009, although their share of overall outpatient visits remain low. *Health Affairs, 31*(9), 2123–2129.

Mehrotra, A., Hangsheng, L., Adams, J., Wang, M., Lave, J., Thygeson, N.M., et al. (2009). Comparing costs and quality of care at retail clinics with that of other medical settings for 3 common illnesses. *Annals of Internal Medicine, 151*(5), 321–328.

Mundinger, M. (1994). Advanced practice nursing—Good medicine for physicians. *New England Journal of Medicine, 330*(3), 211–214.

Mundinger, M., Kane, L., Lenz, R., Totten, M., Tsai, Y., Cleary, P.D., et al. (2000). Primary care outcomes in patients treated by nurse practitioners or physicians: A randomized trial. *Journal of the American Medical Association, 283*(1), 59–68.

Parente, S. (n.d.). The impact of retail clinics on cost and utilization [PowerPoint slides]. Retrieved from *www.slideserve.com/niveditha/the-impact-of-retail-clinics-on-cost-utilization-are-they-1217413*.

Rohner, J., Angstman, K., & Garrison, G. (2012). Early return visits by primary care patients: A retail nurse practitioner visit versus standard medical office care. *Population Health Management, 15*(4), 216–219.

Rudavsky, R., Pollock, E., & Mehrotra, A. (2009). The geographic distribution, ownership, prices, and scope of practice at retail clinics. *Annals of Internal Medicine, 151*(5), 321–328.

Schiff, M. (2012). *The role of nurse practitioners in meeting increasing demand for primary care*. Washington, DC: National Governors Association.

Thompson, E. (2009). Wait times to see doctors are getting longer. USA Today. Retrieved from *usatoday30.usatoday.com/news/health/2009-06-03-waittimes_N.htm*.

ONLINE RESOURCES

Convenient Care Association
www.ccaclinics.org/?vm=r
MSNBC
www.msnbc.com/msnbc/doctor-gap-next-hurdle-health-care
National Nursing Centers Consortium
www.nncc.us/site/?vm=r

CHAPTER 35

Developing Families

Lisa Summers

"The happiness of any society begins with the well-being of the families that live in it."

Kofi Annan

If one simply looks at the numbers, there is no doubt that maternal-child health (MCH) care deserves attention from health care policymakers. There were almost 4 million babies born in the United States in 2012 (Martin et al., 2013). Childbirth is a high-volume, high-cost health care event in the United States. Childbirth-related hospitalizations totaled $16.1 billion in 2008. Maternity care is a particularly important topic for federal and state government policymakers, because the Medicaid program pays for about half of all births nationwide.

The perinatal period presents an important opportunity to impact lifelong health. There is a growing body of knowledge suggesting that the care provided to expectant mothers and new families can help limit the burden of chronic disease decades later. The opportunities for building strong families from the outset may be even greater than the potential to impact physical health.

Indeed, policymakers are beginning to take note of the importance of providing access to quality care for developing families. For example, in 2011, the President of the Association of State and Territorial Health Officials (ASTHO) issued a challenge in the form of a healthy babies initiative, with a specific goal to decrease prematurity in the United States by 8% by 2014 (ASTHO, 2014). In 2012, the National Governors Association announced a learning network on improving birth outcomes that eventually included 13 states that focused on demonstrated best practices (National Governors Association, 2014). And the W. K. Kellogg Foundation launched the Best Babies Zone (*www*

.bestbabieszone.org) initiative in four pilot cities. This unprecedented attention to MCH prompted the Association of Maternal Child Health Programs (AMCHP) to provide a summary table of national and state initiatives and call 2012: The Year of National Initiatives to Improve Birth Outcomes (Calahan, 2013). This chapter focuses on some of the innovative models that nurses and others have demonstrated to be effective in supporting developing families. It addresses some of the policy barriers to spread and scale up these innovative models and underscores the need for an approach to health care that looks far beyond clinical care.

THE NEED FOR IMPROVEMENT

Much of the increased interest in maternity care is driven by a growing realization that, as a country, we perform poorly on many health indicators, particularly when it comes to infant mortality. According to rankings by the World Health Organization and other organizations (Organization for Economic Co-operation and Development, 2013), the United States has a rate of infant mortality much higher than that of European nations, largely because of a high percentage of preterm births (Barfield et al., 2013). Each year, in honor of Mother's Day, Save the Children presents a State of the World's Mothers report that shines a spotlight on the fact that more than half of all first-day deaths in the industrialized world are in the United States, attributable in large part to preterm birth (Save the Children, 2013). Although the emotional and psychosocial cost of giving birth preterm is immeasurable, the financial cost of prematurity has been estimated at $26 billion (Institute of Medicine [IOM], 2007). On the heels of that report came the health care reform debate, and although the need to bend the cost curve had long been an important driver of reform efforts, the recession served to underscore what an impact health care spending was having on America's economy and ability to be competitive in a global marketplace. There is a growing realization that the American way of birth is the costliest in the world (Rosenthal, 2013).

These data are concerning, but when we look at racial and ethnic health disparities, the picture becomes even more disturbing (Centers for Disease Control and Prevention, 2013; Halfon, 2009). The most recent statistics show that although the infant mortality rate has declined slightly, the non-Hispanic black rate is 2.2 times the non-Hispanic white rate (MacDorman & Mathews, 2014). Fortunately, the national conversation about racial equity is increasingly looking beyond housing, education, and employment and focusing on inequities in access to health care, the quality of care, and outcomes such as infant mortality (Turner, 2013).

SOCIAL DETERMINANTS AND LIFE COURSE MODEL

Why does the United States, a country that claims some of the best health centers, cutting-edge research, and most highly developed health care technology in the world, spend so much yet fare so poorly? Many would suggest the cause lies in challenges addressing the social determinants of health. In MCH, the Life Course Theory (LCT) or Life Course Health Development (LCHD), models for better understanding the development of disease and the promotion of health across populations and over time, speak to the importance of addressing these social determinants.

LCHD has been called "a revolution in our understanding of health development" (Halfon, 2009). LCHD models have been supported through hundreds of population-level studies that demonstrate the link between early life events and chronic diseases that develop later in life (Kuh & Shlomo, 2004). Although understanding of the mechanisms by which early events affect neurologic, endocrine, or other systems is far from complete, studies are beginning to explain how factors that impact fetal development can lead to increased risk of conditions such as diabetes or obesity in adulthood. This

provides advocates for population health a compelling argument for preventing disease by addressing upstream issues. Obviously, MCH offers the ultimate opportunity for upstream interventions, and key MCH policymakers have embraced this conceptual framework. In an effort to bridge theory, research, and practice, the Health Resources and Services Administration's (HRSA) Maternal and Child Health Bureau (MCHB) has integrated the LCT Model into its strategic planning. A concept paper summarizes the key concepts of LCT and proposes how the agency can redirect current programs for greater impact (Fine & Kotelchuck, 2010).

LCT is a framework for learning why health disparities persist, even when there have been significant improvements across all groups (as is the case with infant mortality). LCT offers several key concepts, such as early programming (how early experiences program an individual's future development), critical or sensitive periods (when the impact is greatest, e.g., during fetal development), and cumulative impact (although individual episodes of stress may have minimal impact, the cumulative impact over time may have a profound impact). These key concepts are summarized in Box 35-1. An approach that incorporates these concepts is increasingly reflected in policies and programs.

INNOVATIVE MODELS OF CARE

Long before the development of LCT, nurses have been attuned to the social determinants of health and have taken a holistic approach to care. The profession of nursing includes many practical innovators who have developed care models that integrate a life course perspective. The national dialogue about health care reform has focused attention on such innovation and provided a platform for scale-up of local and small-scale innovations. The American Academy of Nursing created the Raise the Voice campaign as a platform to showcase nurse innovators (called Edge Runners) who have developed innovative, evidence-based care models. Among the Edge Runners that have taken a holistic approach to care for developing families are the Nurse-Family Partnership (*www.nursefamily partnership.org*) and three others highlighted in this chapter: birth centers, Centering Health Care, and the Chicago Parent Program.

BIRTH CENTERS

A birth center is a homelike facility that provides family-centered care for healthy women before, during, and after pregnancy, labor, and birth. The Patient Protection and Accountability Act (2010, p. 454) defines a freestanding birth center as a health facility:
- that is not a hospital;
- where childbirth is planned to occur away from the pregnant woman's residence; and
- that is licensed or otherwise approved by the state to provide prenatal labor and delivery or postpartum care and other ambulatory services that are included in the plan.

The American Association of Birth Centers has established national standards and an accreditation program through the Commission for the Accreditation of Birth Centers.

A compelling body of evidence to support the safety of birth center care began with the publication of the first National Birth Center Study in 1989 (Rooks et al., 1989), a prospective study of 11,814 women admitted for labor and delivery to 84 freestanding birth centers in the United States. The most recent study, a prospective cohort study of 15,574 women, confirmed previous studies of birth center care (Stapleton, Osborne, & Illuzzi, 2013). In addition to good outcomes, the lower rates of intervention and fewer cesarean births associated with birth center care lead to a significant cost savings (Truven Healthcare Analytics, 2013).

The birth center movement began in the 1970s with a demonstration project by the Maternity Center in New York City, and initially served primarily well-educated women seeking an alternative to hospital care. Edge Runner Ruth Watson Lubic, a founder of that movement, wanted to make birth center care available to all women, including low-income mothers who are more likely to experience poor birth outcomes, so the next step in innovation was replication of the model in the southwest Bronx. The Childbearing Center of Morris Heights demonstrated not only improved outcomes but also, to a greater extent than anticipated, the expressed empowerment of the African-American and Hispanic families using the center. With the help of a MacArthur genius award, she went on to establish the Family Health and Birth Center in a low-income community in Washington, DC in 1994. Being in the shadow of the capitol, where African-American women experience some of the worst birth outcomes in the nation, has allowed the facility to showcase this model of care (and the potential to address the worst of the worst health disparities) for a host of government officials.

Lubic's work has evolved beyond the concept of the birth center to reenvision and redefine perinatal care. The Developing Families Center was born in an attempt to place health care in its social context through integrating case management, social supports, and infant and toddler education. As a result of this experience, Lubic suggests the perinatal period begins before intended conception, encompasses the childbearing and early child-rearing experiences, and concludes at the third birthday of the child.

CENTERING HEALTH CARE

Just as birth centers have been a disruptive innovation in birth care, Centering Pregnancy has been a dramatically disruptive innovation in prenatal care. Centering Pregnancy replaces the traditional model of one-on-one prenatal care, bringing women out of the exam room into a group of 8 to 12 women with similar due dates. In addition to routine health assessment, women experience interactive learning (as opposed to typical health education) and community building in a group setting.

Centering was first described in the literature in 1998 as an "interdisciplinary model of empowerment." Edge Runner Sharon Schindler Rising built on her experience of group care to develop a model that involves women in self-care, encourages socializing and building of community, and, by its very design, addresses social determinants of health. This initial pilot program emphasized the evaluation of outcomes. In part because of initial positive outcomes, Centering had already achieved significant uptake when a randomized controlled trial was published in 2007 (Ickovics et al., 2007). This study, which found women assigned to group care were significantly less likely to deliver preterm, prompted increased interest in the model. Similar results have been found in subsequent studies.

The model is defined by 13 essential elements, listed in Box 35-2. Only a couple of these elements, the involvement of family support and ongoing evaluation, are common components of traditional perinatal care, although involvement in self-care activities is becoming the norm in health care. Most of the essential elements that form the foundation of group care require a significant departure from the current delivery model. The elements (e.g., adequate space for health assessment to occur and for everyone in the group to sit in a circle) often require redesign of physical space. Yet, each of these elements corresponds with the 10 rules of system redesign suggested by the IOM in *Crossing the Quality Chasm* (IOM, 2001). They also demonstrate how relatively abstract rules (e.g., care is customized according to patients' needs and values, or knowledge is shared and information flows freely) can be applied in the provision of everyday care.

Perhaps most crucial to the success of the model is the facilitative leadership style (Novick et al., 2013). For many health care providers, the nonhi-

---

BOX 35-2 Essential Elements of Centering Care

There are 13 elements which define the Centering model of care:
1. Health assessment occurs within the group space.
2. Participants are involved in self-care activities.
3. A facilitative leadership style is used.
4. The group is conducted in a circle.
5. Each session has an overall plan.
6. Attention is given to the core content, although emphasis may vary.
7. There is stability of group leadership.
8. Group conduct honors the contribution of each member.
9. The composition of the group is stable, not rigid.
10. Group size is optimal to promote the process.
11. Involvement of support people is optional.
12. Opportunity for socializing with the group is provided.
13. There is ongoing evaluation of outcomes.

From Centering Healthcare Institute. Retrieved from *centeringhealthcare.org/pages/centering-model/elements.php.*

---

erarchical nature of group interaction and time spent listening, providing education and guidance only when appropriate, requires a significant shift from their usual practice. Basic and advanced training for providers to facilitate or co-facilitate Centering groups is an important component of successful implementation of Centering.

Women who receive prenatal care in groups are highly satisfied, socialized to receiving care in a group, and want to continue that model of care with their babies. Centering Parenting is a continuity model that combines well-woman care and well-baby care during the first year of life (Bloomfield & Rising, 2013).

CHICAGO PARENT PROGRAM

Although not a redesigned model of health care delivery, the Chicago Parenting Program provides another example of an innovative approach to integrating the LCT and addressing social determinants of health. Working in collaboration with parents and acting on the growing understanding that preventive interventions in the first 5 years are the most cost-effective strategy to promote children's mental health, the Chicago Parent Program was specifically designed for ethnic minority parents from low-income neighborhoods. The Chicago Parent Program uses videotaped scenes in 11 weekly group sessions, led by trained group leaders, to help parents understand a variety of topics such as child-centered time, praise and encouragement, and using time-outs. Parents also learn how to manage stress and have weekly practice assignments to use what they are learning at home. It is now spreading to other cities in the United States.

HEALTH CARE REFORM

The ACA has had a significant impact on care to developing families, in general, and the ability of these innovators to bring these models to scale.

PRIMARY CARE AND PREVENTION

The ACA contains many provisions that directly target primary care, including increasing reimbursement rates, investing in the primary care workforce, and expanding the reach of Federally Qualified Health Centers (Abrams et al., 2011). Maternity and newborn care is listed as 1 of 10 essential health benefits (Association of Maternal and Child Health Programs, 2013). There are specific provisions addressing prevention in pregnancy, such as the mandated coverage of tobacco cessation services for pregnant women. Some provisions, such as requiring that women receive insurance coverage for all U.S. Food and Drug Administration-approved methods of birth control without cost-sharing, have been challenged in the courts (see Chapter 53 for a discussion of some of these legal challenges).

FOSTERING INNOVATION

The Center for Medicare and Medicaid Innovation (CMMI), or The Innovation Center, was established by the ACA for the purpose of testing "innovative payment and service delivery models." The goal is to advance best practices that will preserve or improve the quality of care, while reducing costs.

In 2012, the U.S. Department of Health and Human Services (HHS) Secretary Sebelius announced (in an event at the Developing Families Center) the Strong Start Initiative, a public campaign to reduce early elective deliveries and a grant program that would test the effectiveness of "enhanced prenatal care approaches" to reduce preterm births among Medicaid beneficiaries. The CMMI chose three evidence-based approaches: Centering/group visits, birth centers, and Maternity Care Homes (these are sites that assume responsibility for coordinating quality, evidence-based, woman-centered perinatal care and social services). The Strong Start Initiative has highlighted prenatal care as a significant issue with the HHS and brought increased recognition of problems facing MCH. Across the United States, key MCH advocates (some of whom had never sat at the table together) came together to submit proposals. In some states where those proposals were not chosen for funding, advocates have continued to work together with birth centers and Centering is on the radar as never before. For those sites that were funded, data collection is under way, including an evaluation that includes both outcomes and evaluation.

PAYMENT REFORM

The ACA contains many provisions that are an attempt to change the existing perverse payment incentives that drive the provision of more intervention. For example, despite the cost savings, the scale-up of birth centers has been hampered by lack of payment for the facility services. The ACA included a provision that would mandate Medicaid payment for facility services. Unfortunately, many states have not yet implemented that provision (Stapleton, Osborne, & Illuzzi, 2013). And yet it is estimated that if 10% of U.S. births occurred in birth centers, the potential savings in facility service payments alone compared with hospital facility service payments could reach $800 million per year.

BARRIERS TO SUSTAINING, SPREADING, AND SCALING-UP MODELS

There are many forces that can drive innovation or stifle it. There is a growing emphasis on the need to provide innovators with the tools and support to scale up proven innovation (Agency for Healthcare Research and Quality, n.d.).

PLAYERS

The health care industry is made up of many stakeholders, with competing (and sometimes unclear) interests. Although the landscape is changing, nurses have not always been strong players. In particular, nurse midwives, who have been the innovators behind both Centering and the birth center movement, have not always been in a powerful position to effect change. One clear advantage for Centering has been that it is an interdisciplinary model that has enjoyed uptake from physicians (both obstetricians and family physicians) as evidenced by an editorial in an obstetric journal where two physicians conclude, "We believe it is time to start thinking of group prenatal care as the default model for prenatal care" (Garreto & Bernstein, 2014). But the women and families served by these models can be strong advocates and persuade policymakers to support policies that remove the barriers to sustaining these MCH services.

SCOPE OF PRACTICE

Lifting barriers to practice is a necessary step for scaling up nurse-led innovations that use certified nurse midwives, clinical nurse specialists, and nurse practitioners. See Chapters 54 and 66 for more on scope of practice.

FUNDING

Any innovative model that relies on a new and/or separate funding stream is at risk. Birth centers and Centering are innovations that have been able to grow in part because they are within the existing payment system. Because a midwife, physician, or nurse practitioner credentialed to provide prenatal care is performing the routine prenatal assessment in the group space, it is billed as any other prenatal visit. Likewise, credentialed providers can bill for services provided in a birth center, although they have faced a greater challenge contracting with payers. In addition, a birth center requires a significant capital investment. Centering also requires an initial investment in system redesign, training, and, often, redesign of space.

PAYMENT

The fact that the ACA provision mandating adequate payment to birth centers has not yet been fully implemented is evidence of how difficult it is to effect change. There are other barriers to birth center facility services payment by both commercial and Medicaid payers, including lack of recognition of and contracting with nurse midwives by Medicaid and commercial managed care organizations, and inadequate reimbursement by many state Medicaid agencies.

REGULATION

The regulatory process can aid or hinder innovation. For example, in the case of payment for birth centers, many states have not yet completed the regulatory process that implements the new payment mandate.

CONCLUSION

Not since the creation of the Children's Bureau in 1912 has there been such attention to MCH care and openness to reform. Although significant barriers exist, nurses are becoming increasingly effective advocates for change by building collaborative relationships with key allies and stakeholders, applying new science, engaging families, and having a clear message for the media, all key components of effective advocacy for developing families.

DISCUSSION QUESTIONS

1. Why has the U.S. health care system paid so little attention to social determinants of health, and what evidence do you see of this changing?
2. How have you seen "perverse payment incentives" impact health care delivery, and do you see that changing?
3. How has the group care model been applied to health care outside maternal and child health, for example, diabetes or other chronic diseases?

REFERENCES

Abrams, M., Nuzum, R., Mika, S., & Lawlor, G. (2011). Realizing health reform's potential: How the ACA will strengthen primary care and benefit patients, providers and payers. New York: The Commonwealth Fund. Retrieved from *www.commonwealthfund.org/publications/issue-briefs/ 2011/jan/strengthen-primary-care.*

Agency for Healthcare Research and Quality. (n.d.). Taking innovations to scale. Retrieved from *www.innovations.ahrq.gov/takingInnovations ToScale.aspx.*

Association of Maternal and Child Health Programs. (2013). The Patient Protection & Affordable Care Act: Summary of key maternal and child health related highlights with updates on status of implementation. Retrieved from *www.amchp.org/Policy-Advocacy/health-reform/ resources/Documents/The%20Patient%20Protection%20and%20 Affordable%20Care%201-20-12.pdf.*

Association for State and Territorial Health Officials [ASTHO]. (2014). ASTHO healthy babies initiative. Retrieved from *www.astho.org/ healthybabies.*

Barfield, W., D'Angelo, D., Moon, R., Lu, M., Wong, B., & Iskander, J. (2013). CDC grand rounds: Public health approaches to reducing U.S. infant mortality. *MMWR. Morbidity and Mortality Weekly Report, 62*(31), 625–628.

Bloomfield, J., & Rising, S. S. (2013). Centering parenting: An innovative dyad model for group mother-infant care. *Journal of Midwifery and Women's Health, 58*(6), 683–689.

Callahan, T. (2013, January/February). 2012: The year of national initiatives to improve birth outcomes. *Pulse.* Retrieved from *www.amchp.org/ AboutAMCHP/Newsletters/Pulse/Archive/2013/JanFeb2013/Pages/ Feature4.aspx.*

Centers for Disease Control and Prevention. (2013). CDC health disparities and inequality report—United States, 2013. *MMWR. Morbidity and Mortality Weekly Report, 62*(3), 1–189.

Fine, A., & Kotelchuck, M. (2010). Rethinking MCH: The Life Course Model as an organizing framework. Washington, DC: U.S. Department of Health and Human Services, Maternal Child Health Bureau. Retrieved from *mchb.hrsa.gov/lifecourse/rethinkingmchlifecourse.pdf.*

Garreto, D., & Bernstein, P. S. (2014). Centering pregnancy: An innovative approach to prenatal care delivery. *American Journal of Obstetrics and Gynecology, 210*(1), 14–15.

Halfon, N. (2009). Life course health development. Expert voices. Retrieved from *www.nihcm.org/pdf/ExpertVoices_Halfon_FINAL.pdf.*

Ickovics, J. R., Kershaw, T. S., Westdahl, C., Magriples, U., Massey, Z., Reynolds, H., et al. (2007). Group prenatal care and perinatal outcomes: A randomized controlled trial. *Obstetrics & Gynecology, 110*(2 Pt. 1), 330–339.

Institute of Medicine. (2001). Crossing the quality chasm: A new health care system for the 21st century. Washington, DC: National Academies Press. Retrieved from *www.iom.edu/Reports/2001/Crossing-the-Quality -Chasm-A-New-Health-System-for-the-21st-Century.aspx.*

Institute of Medicine. (2007). Preterm births: Causes, consequences and prevention. Washington, DC: National Academies Press. Retrieved from *www.iom.edu/Reports/2006/Preterm-Birth-Causes-Consequences-and -Prevention.aspx.*

Kuh, D., & Shlomo, Y. B. (2004). *Life course approach to chronic disease epidemiology.* New York: Oxford University Press.

MacDorman, M., & Mathews, T. J. (2014). QuickStats: Infant mortality rates, by race and Hispanic ethnicity of mother—United States, 2000, 2005 and 2010. *MMWR. Morbidity and Mortality Weekly Report, 63*(1), 25.

Martin, J. A., Hamilton, B. H., Osterman, M., Curtin, S., & Matthews, T. (2013). Births: Final data for 2012. *National Vital Statistics Report, 62*(9).

National Governors Association. (2014). Maternal and child health 2013 learning network: Improving birth outcomes. Retrieved from *www .nga.org/cms/home/nga-center-for-best-practices/meeting–webcast -materials/page-health-meetings-webcasts/col2-content/main-content -list/maternal-and-child-health-2013-l.html.*

Novick, G., Reid, A. E., Lewis, J., Kershaw, T. S., Ickovics, J. R., & Rising, S. S. (2013). Group prenatal care: Model fidelity and outcomes. *American Journal of Obstetrics and Gynecology, 209*(2), 112.e1–112.e6.

Organization for Economic Co-operation and Development. (2013). Infant mortality. Retrieved from *www.oecd-ilibrary.org/social-issues -migration-health/infant-mortality_20758480-table9.*

Patient Protection and Accountability Act. (2010). Retrieved from *demo.tizra.com/phj6t/454.*

Rooks, J. P., Weatherby, N. L., Ernst, E. K., Stapleton, S., Rosen, D., & Rosenfield, A. (1989). Outcomes of care in birth centers. The National Birth Center Study. *New England Journal of Medicine, 321*(26), 1804–1811.

Rosenthal, E. (2013, June 30). American way of birth: Costliest in the world. *New York Times,* Retrieved from *www.nytimes.com/2013/07/01/health/ american-way-of-birth-costliest-in-the-world.html?pagewanted=all.*

Save the Children. (2013). Surviving the first day: State of the world's mothers, 2013. Retrieved from *www.savethechildrenweb.org/SOWM -2013/?_ga=1.17470137.1499728326.1393445991.*

Stapleton, S. R., Osborne, C., & Illuzzi, J. (2013). Outcomes of care in birth centers: Demonstration of a durable model. *Journal of Midwifery & Women's Health, 58*(1), 3–14.

Truven Healthcare Analytics. (2013). The cost of having a baby in the United States. Retrieved from *transform.childbirthconnection.org/ reports/cost/.*

Turner, A. (2013). The business case for racial equity. Ann Arbor, MI: Altarum Institute. Retrieved from *altarum.org/publications/the-business -case-for-racial-equity.*

ONLINE RESOURCES

Agency for Healthcare Research and Quality
www.innovations.ahrq.gov/takingInnovationsToScale.aspx
American Academy of Nursing's Raise the Voice and Edge Runners
www.aannet.org/raisethevoice
American Association of Birth Centers
www.birthcenters.org
Centering Healthcare Institute
www.centeringhealthcare.org
Maternal and Child Health Bureau
mchb.hrsa.gov

CHAPTER 36

Dual Eligibles: Issues and Innovations

Susan C. Reinhard

"These programs were never designed with the idea of people getting both (Medicare and Medicaid). They were not designed to work together, and we are seeing that. There are different systems for enrollment, grievances, financing, misaligned incentives, cost shifting. … All these things can result in poor care, poor outcomes."

Melanie Bella

National and state policymakers are focusing serious attention on a small but significant category of people who have both Medicare and Medicaid coverage and are known as "dual eligible," a term that does little to capture their historically high-cost, poor-care experiences. Reducing costs is a major driver of this attention. But so too is the growing recognition that the duals need better care. Nurses are in a position to shape new initiatives. We know these people. They are our patients. They are our families. One was my father.

WHO ARE THE DUALS?

There are 9.6 million people who are eligible for both Medicare and Medicaid (Young et al., 2013). These duals are the poorest and sickest of all Medicare beneficiaries, but they are not a homogeneous group and there are large state variations.

Six out of ten duals fall into the frail older adult subgroup. My father fell into this group 2 months after he entered a nursing home after suffering a stroke at 80 years of age. A retired dentist with six children whom he and my mother sent through college, he entered the world of the duals because the high cost of a nursing home depleted all his economic resources. He spent down to Medicaid.

This is a very common route to becoming a dual. Almost three quarters (73%) of all Medicare beneficiaries living in long-term care facilities are duals (Jacobson, Neuman, & Damico, 2012). Fortunately, because nurses helped to create New Jersey policy to permit people like my father to get care outside of a nursing home, he was able to move to a wonderful assisted living community that supported a private studio apartment and daily choices on what to eat, wear, and do. Policy makes a difference. At that time, had he lived in my sister's state of Pennsylvania, as a dual he would have only had a nursing home choice, with a stranger for a roommate.

While older frail adults comprise 60% of the duals population, people with a disability under the age of 65 years comprise the other 40% (Jacobson, Neuman, & Damico, 2012). These individuals may have a physical disability, a behavioral or substance abuse condition, or some combination of all of three. Almost half (49%) have mental or cognitive conditions (Kasper, Watts, & Lyons, 2010).

But age differences are not the only reason this is a heterogeneous group (Coughlin, Waidman, & Phadera, 2012). About 17% live in a nursing home, another one out of five uses community-based long-term services and supports (LTSS), and one out of four has multiple chronic conditions, but no need for LTSS. Surprisingly, two out of five have one or no chronic conditions or LTSS, but as extremely low-income people, they face a host of social and environmental challenges. Clearly, their health and social needs vary substantially.

Despite their heterogeneity, compared with people who are not on both Medicare and Medicaid (the nonduals), the duals are more vulnerable. Figure 36-1 provides important comparisons. It shows that more than half of duals have a cognitive

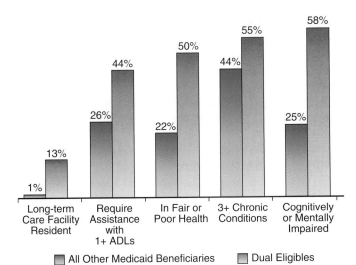

FIGURE 36-1 Dual eligible beneficiaries account for a disproportionate share of Medicare and Medicaid spending. (Source: Jacobson, G., Neuman, T. & Damico, A. [2012]. Medicare's role for dual eligible beneficiaries. *Medicare Policy Issue Brief.* Kaiser Family Foundation. Retrieved from *kaiserfamilyfoundation.files.wordpress.com/2013/01/8138-02.pdf.*)

or mental impairment, compared with 25% of non-duals. They are more than twice as likely to be in fair or poor health, and more likely to require help with activities of daily living (ADL), such as bathing, dressing, and eating.

The number of duals varies by state, not just because of state demographics but also because of their Medicaid policy. In part because states vary in their Medicaid eligibility rules, the share of total Medicaid enrollees ranges from 9% in Utah to 26% in Maine; spending on duals as a percentage of total Medicaid spending varies from 20% in Arizona to 55% in North Dakota (Young et al., 2013).

WHAT ARE THE CHALLENGES?

From a care perspective, the greatest challenge is delivering services and supports to these vulnerable groups within the duals population. Many need complex health care. But many also need long-term supportive services, such as housing and transportation. And most desperately need help coordinating all of these services, some of which are covered by Medicare, some covered by Medicaid, and some offered through other public and private sources. Most existing delivery models for Medicare and Medicaid do not coordinate services. These individuals live in an unmanaged care world:

- If they are getting LTSS, their LTSS provider (paid by Medicaid) gets little information about

the inpatient, clinician, and prescription services paid by Medicare.
- Data linking Medicare and Medicaid service use and expenditures at the individual level are lacking.
- Services that both Medicare and Medicaid cover, such as home health, hospice, and durable medical equipment, intersect in complex ways that few understand.
- If a person wants to appeal a denial for services, there are two different appeal processes.

These are just a few examples of the silos that are created by separate administration of two complex programs at the state and individual levels. The disconnects can range from annoying and costly to lethal. For example, inadequate information about medications prescribed in the hospital under Medicare, and medications prescribed in the nursing home under Medicaid, can lead to complications from polypharmacology (Walsh et al., 2010).

What do the duals experience? In a series of focus groups with older adults who are duals, most expressed interest in having care coordination (Reinhard, 2013). They felt supported when a case manager or others called to see how they were doing and if they got what they needed to take care of their condition, for example, checking their blood sugar. Family caregivers, the primary coordinators of care, want to be included in care planning and execution, especially when they have a regular role in that execution. Also, consumers really want their clinicians and providers to communicate with one another so everyone is on the same page.

From a cost perspective, the current uncoordinated care situation is untenable. The dual eligible population represents a relatively small proportion of the total population, while accounting for a higher part of total system costs. For Medicaid, the duals account for 15% of enrollment but 39% of the expenditures. For Medicare, duals account for 20% of the enrollment but 31% of the expenditures (The Henry J. Kaiser Family Foundation, 2013) (Figure 36-2).

Even within the duals population, two cost facts stand out. First, some duals have lower than average care costs, while fewer than 20% account for almost 60% of all expenditures (Coughlin, Waidman & Phadera, 2012). High-cost duals tend to live in institutions, have three or more ADL limitations, and are substantially more likely to have diabetes or Alzheimer's disease. And second, 69% of Medicaid spending on duals goes to long-term care (Young et al., 2013).

Given the heterogeneity of this relatively small group of people spread across the United States it is very important to develop financing and care models that target expert care and coordination for people and their families who may be dealing with multiple physical conditions, serious behavioral health conditions, and LTSS needs that include crucial social aspects of care, particularly housing. People cannot choose home and community care options for LTSS unless they have a place to live.

The separation between health care and housing support is a chasm. Some states have recognized this dilemma and have tried (unsuccessfully) to use Medicaid funds for supportive housing.

HEALTH CARE DELIVERY REFORMS THAT HOLD PROMISE

After decades of trying to get federal and state policymakers to pay attention to this high-cost, vulnerable population, advocates are hopeful that change is possible. There is growing consensus that providing quality care for duals needs to be more efficient in terms of both the cost and delivery of care. Duals need better care coordination, with a particular focus on high-cost individuals who receive many services without sufficient attention to the quality of those services. We need to measure quality of life as well as quality of care. Many duals need access to more integrated primary, acute, behavioral health, and LTSS, with a particular focus on blending health and social services. Families should be engaged and supported whenever possible. And people who are on both Medicare and Medicaid need harmony between the two sets of programs in terms of rules and procedures.

The Affordable Care Act (ACA) is creating a path for these goals. The ACA created the Medicare-Medicaid Coordination Office in the Centers for Medicare and Medicaid Services (CMS). The goal of this new office is to improve the integration of Medicare and Medicaid benefits for duals. In addition, the Center for Medicare and Medicaid

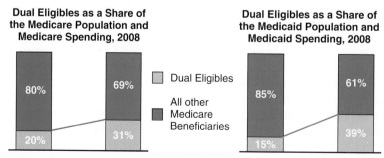

FIGURE 36-2 A larger share of dual eligibles than other Medicare beneficiaries has multiple chronic conditions and functional or cognitive impairments. (Source: Jacobson, G., Neuman, T. & Damico, A. [2012]. Medicare's role for dual eligible beneficiaries. *Medicare Policy Issue Brief.* Kaiser Family Foundation. Retrieved from *kaiserfamilyfoundation.files.wordpress.com/2013/01/8138-02.pdf.*)

Innovation has a new demonstration authority to test innovative payment and service delivery models.

One of the most significant demonstration projects emerging from the new center is known as the Financial Alignment Demonstration (Musumeci, 2012, 2013). This is a federal-state partnership to develop service and payment models that will better integrate care and align financial incentives across the Medicare and Medicare programs. Currently, if a state invests resources to improve care of people who are on Medicaid but also on Medicare, the state may incur Medicaid costs while the federal government saves money. These new models offer a pathway to focus resources across the two programs in a way that may improve the quality and coordination of care, while reducing costs for both.

In most cases, demonstration states are experimenting with managed care plans to accomplish these goals. The plans receive a prospective blended rate for all primary, acute, behavioral health, and LTSS. Under this capitated approach, states and the CMS can share savings. A few states are exploring a managed fee-for-service financial alignment model that does not involve capitation. The state is responsible for care coordination and the delivery of fully integrated Medicare and Medicaid benefits. They will receive a retrospective performance payment if a target level of Medicare savings is achieved.

It is too soon to say how these new models are working. Two out of three states are trying to do something about integrating Medicare and Medicaid services for the duals (Walls et al., 2013), but only eight have applied to the CMS and have been approved to be demonstrations that started in 2013. More are on the way. It takes time to build capacity in the states to serve these populations and an infrastructure to integrate both Medicare and Medicaid services and financing (Neuman et al., 2012). Yet some states are pursuing new models even without applying for this financial alignment demonstration or waiting for results. And many are focusing on LTSS, a major cost-driver for state Medicaid programs (Burwell & Saucier, 2013).

State movement toward managed LTSS is accelerating. Managed LTSS is not integrated care in that it does not integrate primary, acute, and LTSS services, and it does not integrate Medicaid and

Medicare. It is worth including here because many LTSS users are duals, and managed LTSS can be a step toward more fully integrated care models. Sixteen states had a managed LTSS program in 2013, serving a total of 389,000 people (Saucier, Burwell, & Halperin, 2013). Preliminary research suggests they are effective at protecting consumer choices and continuity of care (Saucier, Burwell, & Halperin, 2013).

IMPLICATION FOR NURSES

Nurses and other advocates need to monitor the state and federal shift from fee-for-service models to managed care for duals. One should not be deluded into thinking that the fee-for-service world was wonderful and the managed care world will be dreadful. In fact, there are some success stories.

The Program for All-Inclusive Care of the Elderly (PACE), a capitated managed care program, started in the early 1970s when the Chinatown-North Beach community of San Francisco responded to the pressing LTSS needs of their community. They created On Lok Senior Health Services to create a community-based system of LTSS. On Lok is Cantonese and means peaceful, happy abode (National PACE Association, 2014). PACE has integrated health and social services for frail, older adults in the community for as long as desirable and feasible.

Nurses have been an integral part of this model. In fact, American Academy of Nursing Edge Runner Jennie Chinn Hansen founded On Lok and the University of Pennsylvania's School of Nursing has a nurse-run PACE program for duals known as the Living Independently for Elders (LIFE) program. There are now 82 PACE sites in 29 states, usually with fewer than 500 duals in each capitated program. As of 2011, PACE had enrolled fewer than 22,000 duals (Neuman et al., 2012). Evaluations have shown that PACE successfully integrates acute and long-term care and reduces hospitalizations, although evaluators debate the extent to which savings can be accrued (Brown & Mann, 2012).

The Evercare model was founded in 1987 by two geriatric advanced practice nurses who had a vision for how better care might be delivered to frail older adults in nursing homes. The target population was Medicare beneficiaries in nursing homes, who, as noted earlier, quickly spend down their resources paying for their nursing home stay and become dually eligible for Medicaid. Nurse practitioners were placed in the nursing homes to monitor changes in health, make early diagnoses and interventions, and coordinate better communication and appropriate services. Eight years later, Evercare became a federal demonstration project that was evaluated by the University of Minnesota with excellent results, including a 50% reduction in emergency room visits and a 40% reduction in hospitalizations without changes in mortality (Kane et al., 2003). With these findings, federal policy moved this program into permanent status, converting them to Special Needs Plans offered throughout the United States.

While the nursing literature is not robust in this area, there is evidence that nurses can make a significant contribution to the quality of care provided to older adults in plans targeted to duals. For example, using a nurse care manager model in a community-based dual-eligible Special Needs Plan can improve patient outcomes (Roth et al., 2012). These nurse care managers are skilled at complex psychosocial assessments and behavior interventions that can address the social determinants so often neglected in traditional medical practices.

Evidence suggests some common features of successful care coordination programs (Brown & Mann, 2012): regular (monthly) face-to-face contact between the care coordinator and the consumer; strong rapport with the patient's primary clinician; an effective communication hub for providers and patients with the ability to know when patients are hospitalized so transition support can be provided; access to reliable information about prescriptions, with access to prescribers and pharmacists; and use of behavior change techniques to help people create and adhere to self-care plans, including medication adherence.

POLICY IMPLICATIONS

Care coordination is in the limelight, and nurses are in a position to make a critical contribution. We need to be careful how we are defining and executing care coordination because the evidence is not strong that it will save money, at least for Medicare (Brown & Mann, 2012). Much has to do with how capitation rates are set and where the savings go.

State experimentation is proceeding, and more evidence will emerge from the demonstrations years from now. In the meantime, states are advancing certain elements of care coordination: use of care assessments, person-centered focus, comprehensive care plans, inclusion of the patient and family in care decisions, and the use of multidisciplinary teams. Some states are more prescriptive than others in how care coordination is to be defined and delivered and what entity should be designated the primary care coordinator, whereas others give much flexibility to managed care plans. Thus, there is a great deal of flux at this time. But the best advice for policymakers at this time, as it has been in the past, is to target high-risk cases and pay attention to subgroup differences. Everyone does not need, nor can we afford, one-to-one close care coordination. And one size will not fit all.

As we design new systems of care, and people move from one program to another, we need to provide sufficient transition periods to avoid abrupt changes to the consumer's provider network, care manager, and other key aspects of care (Saucier, Burwell, & Halperin, 2013). Advocates also need to keep the attention on the adoption of clear, transparent public goals for what the new programs are designed to do, particularly in relation to the consumer's experience, population health, and cost-reduction expectations (Burwell & Saucier, 2013). We need to build sufficient state and federal capacity to oversee the programs being created, especially to monitor quality and areas that might need improvement.

This is a period of substantial change that brings opportunities for improved care, better use of resources, and important roles for nurses and other members of the team. But it also brings a clarion call for research and advocacy. We need more evidence to help us move in the right direction, and we need advocacy to keep a watchful eye on what is happening to those who most need the right changes: the people called duals, the people we know, the people we care for.

DISCUSSION QUESTIONS

1. How are patient and family care affected by having two different payment sources (Medicare and Medicaid)?
2. What are some current efforts to develop more coherent policies and programs to support people who have both Medicare and Medicaid coverage?
3. What are some key areas to monitor as new policies and programs are developed for the duals?

REFERENCES

Brown, R., & Mann, D. (2012). Best bets for reducing Medicare costs for dual eligible beneficiaries: Assessing the evidence. Menlo Park, CA: The Henry J. Kaiser Family Foundation. Retrieved from *kaiserfamilyfoundation.files.wordpress.com/2013/01/8353.pdf*.

Burwell, B., & Saucier, P. (2013). Managed long-term services and supports programs are a cornerstone for fully integrated care. *Generations: Journal of the American Society on Aging, 37*(2), 33–38.

Coughlin, T. A., Waidman, T., & Phadera, L. (2012). The diversity of duals eligible beneficiaries: An examination of services and spending for people eligible for both Medicare and Medicaid. Menlo Park, CA: The Henry J. Kaiser Family Foundation. Retrieved from *kff.org/medicaid/issue-brief/the-diversity-of-dual-eligible-beneficiaries-an/*.

Henry J. Kaiser Family Foundation. (2013). Faces of dually eligible beneficiaries: Profiles of people with Medicare and Medicaid coverage. Menlo Park, CA: The Henry J. Kaiser Family Foundation. Retrieved from *kaiserfamilyfoundation.files.wordpress.com/2013/07/8446-faces-of-dually-eligible-beneficiaries1.pdf*.

Jacobson, G., Neuman, T., & Damico, A. (2012). Medicare's role for dual eligible beneficiaries. Menlo Park, CA: The Henry J. Kaiser Family Foundation. Retrieved from *kaiserfamilyfoundation.files.wordpress.com/2013/01/8138-02.pdf*.

Kane, R. L., Keckhafer, G., Flood, S., Bershadsky, B., & Saidaty, M. S. (2003). The effect of Evercare on hospital use. *Journal of the American Geriatric Society, 51*, 1427–1434.

Kasper, J., Watts, M., & Lyons, B. (2010). Chronic disease and co-morbidity among dual eligible: Implications for patterns of Medicaid and Medicare service use and spending. Menlo Park, CA: The Henry J. Kaiser Family Foundation. Retrieved from *kff.org/health-reform/report/chronic-disease-and-co-morbidity-among-dual/*.

Musumeci, M. (2012). Explaining the state integrated care and financial alignment demonstrations for dual eligible beneficiaries. Washington, DC: The Henry J. Kaiser Family Foundation. Retrieved from *kaiserfamilyfoundation.files.wordpress.com/2013/01/8368.pdf*.

Musumeci, M. (2013). Long-term services and supports in the financial alignment demonstrations for dual eligible beneficiaries. Washington, DC: The Henry J. Kaiser Family Foundation. Retrieved from *kaiserfamilyfoundation.files.wordpress.com/2013/11/8519-long-term-services-and-supports-in-the-financial-alignment-demonstrations.pdf*.

National PACE Association. (2014). What is PACE? Retrieved from *www.npaonline.org/website/article.asp?id=12&title=Who,_What_and_Where_is_PACE*.

Neuman, P., Lyons, B., Rentas, J., & Rowland, D. (2012). Dx for a careful approach to moving dual-eligible beneficiaries into managed care plans. *Health Affairs, 37*(6), 1186–1194.

Reinhard, S. C. (2013). What do older adults want from integrated care? Generations. *Journal of the American Society on Aging, 37*(2), 68–71.

Roth, C. P., Ganz, D. A., Nickels, L., Martin, D., Beckman, R., & Wenger, N. S. (2012). Nurse care manager contribution to quality of care in dual-eligible Special Needs Plan. *Journal of Gerontological Nursing, 38*(7), 44–54.

Saucier, P., Burwell, B., & Halperin, A. (2013). Consumer choices and continuity of care in managed long-term services and support: Emerging practices and lessons. Washington, DC: AARP Public Policy Institute. Retrieved from *www.aarp.org/content/dam/aarp/research/public_policy_institute/ltc/2013/consumer-choices-report-full-AARP-ppi-ltc.pdf*.

Walls, J., Scully, D., Fox-Grage, W., Ujvari, K., Cho, E., & Hall, J. (2013). Two-thirds of states integrating Medicare and Medicaid services for dual eligibles. Washington, DC: AARP Public Policy Institute. Retrieved from *www.aarp.org/content/dam/aarp/research/public_policy_institute/health/2013/states-integrating-medicare-and-medicaid-AARP-ppi-health.pdf*.

Walsh, E., Freiman, M., Haber, S., Bragg, A., Ouslander, J., & Wiener, J. (2010). Cost drivers for dually eligible beneficiaries: Potentially avoidable hospitalizations from nursing facility, skilled nursing facility, and home and community based services waiver programs. Washington, DC: Centers for Medicare and Medicaid Services. Retrieved from *www.cms.gov/Research-Statistics-Data-and-Systems/Statistics-Trends-and-Reports/Reports/downloads/costdriverstask2.pdf*.

Young, K., Garfield, R., Musumeci, M., Clemons-Cope, L., & Lawton, E. (2013). Medicaid's role for dual eligible beneficiaries. Menlo Park, CA: The Henry J. Kaiser Family Foundation. Retrieved from *kaiserfamilyfoundation.files.wordpress.com/2013/08/7846-04-medicaids-role-for-dual-eligible-beneficiaries.pdf*.

ONLINE RESOURCES

AARP.
www.aarp.org/research/ppi
Center for Health Care Strategies: Integrating Care for Dual Eligibles: An Online Toolkit
www.chcs.org/publications3960/publications_show.htm?doc_id=606732
The Henry J. Kaiser Family Foundation
kff.org/tag/dual-eligible
The Scan Foundation
www.thescanfoundation.org/categories/dual-eligibles-1

CHAPTER 37

Home Care and Hospice: Evolving Policy

Elaine D. Stephens

"There are no limits to what you can do when you know how to be a leader."

Val Halamandaris

Home care and hospice in the United States has both a long history and a dynamic evolving future. The origins of home care go back to the 1880s although political and public policy interest in home care significantly increased when Medicare was passed in 1965 and included a home care benefit for enrollees. The number of Medicare certified home health agencies in 1967 was 1753, and by 2009, that number had grown to 10,581 (Centers for Medicare and Medicaid Services [CMS], 2009a).

Hospice care has experienced similar growth. In 1967, a nurse in London, Dame Cicely Saunders, founded St. Christopher's Hospice, the first institution of its kind. The first hospice in the United States, The Connecticut Hospice, opened in 1974 in Branford Connecticut. Congress created the hospice benefit in 1982, and from 1984 to 2010 the number of hospices participating in Medicare rose from 31 to 3407. In addition, it is estimated there are 200 additional volunteer agencies that are not Medicare-certified (National Association for Home Care & Hospice [NAHC], 2010).

Policymakers have continued their interest in home care and hospices as health care delivery mechanisms, and reimbursement continues to shift toward population management and risk-based capitated payment models. These models appear to be inevitable given the current trends within health care spending. Health care spending consumed 17.6% of GDP in the United States during 2010 and is predicted to consume 34% of GDP by 2040

(CMS, 2009b). The number of Accountable Care Organizations (ACOs), collaborative efforts among groups of health care organizations from different parts of the sector who work together to ensure every patient is getting coordinated care (Brashears, 2013), has been growing, and the success of such new health care delivery systems will depend heavily on the availability of home and community based service systems. These services are key to preventing unnecessary and expensive institutionalization. Home care and hospices and all of their component programs are the bridge between the various health care sectors: hospitals, physicians, advanced practice nurses (APNs), and nursing homes.

The need for quality home-based care will continue to grow because of a growing and aging population. Dr. Ken Dychtwald, gerontologist and founder and CEO of Age Wave, a benchmark research company that advises major corporations in the United States on product development and branding for our growing aging demographic, states, "Our health care challenge is, without a doubt, a demographically-driven phenomenon. And this challenge will steadily spiral upward with the aging boomer generation" (Dychtwald, 2011). More than 45% of Americans have at least one chronic disease, and many home care patients have five to six chronic conditions. To meet the changing health care needs of this burgeoning aging and chronically ill population, we will need to embrace new models of service delivery, with home care and hospices playing a significant role. The challenge for home care will be to design programs and service delivery mechanisms as part of new models of care, and to promote its value to policymakers.

DEFINING THE HOME CARE INDUSTRY

The home care industry is composed of five segments: home health, hospices, home medical equipment (HME), home infusion pharmacy (HIP), and private duty. These home-based services make up the care delivery system that other health care segments such as hospitals, long-term care providers, APNs, and physicians use to bring health care delivery into the community.

Home care is governed by a highly complex patchwork of state and federal mandates as well as private sector practices. Certain states require that all home care segments be licensed and others have licensure for some but not all segments. Payment is generally dictated by Medicare, Medicaid, commercial insurance companies (HMOs, PPOs, and indemnity programs), long term care insurance, and private pay. Accrediting organizations such as the Joint Commission and the Community Health Accreditation Program provide enhanced standards that complement state licensure and federal payment regulations.

HOME HEALTH

Perhaps the most commonly known and most widely used segment, home health services, are provided to individuals of all ages although most clients are either older adults or children with chronic and debilitating diseases.

Policymakers have not focused on approaches to care at home until relatively recently. Steven H. Landers, MD, MPH, and President and CEO of the Visiting Nurse Association and Health Group in Red Bank, New Jersey notes, "Maybe this is because academic centers and American medicine became so focused on acute institutional care in the past half century that home care has been overlooked" (Landers, 2013). Until recently, home care services have been organized with a focus on postacute rehabilitation with Medicare and commercial insurance companies focused on limiting home care coverage to individuals who are defined as homebound and require the skilled services of a nurse or physical, occupational, or speech therapist.

The cost advantages of the use of home care when compared with other institutional settings has fueled interest, however, and government and insurance companies are increasingly interested in using home care services with fewer restrictions.

HOSPICE

Hospice and palliative care programs continue to grow for adults and children with advanced life-limiting illnesses, and hospices are currently the fastest growing segment of the Medicare program (Forster & Simione, 2011). In 1979 the Health Care Financing Administration (now CMS) initiated demonstration programs at 26 hospices across the country to assess the cost-effectiveness of hospice care and to determine what services hospices should provide. In 1982, Congress included a provision to create a Medicare hospice benefit which was made permanent in 1986. By 2011, an estimated 1.65 million patients received services from hospices annually (National Hospice and Palliative Care Organization [NHPCO], 2011).

Hospice care is provided in settings that are considered equivalent to a patient's home. This can include skilled nursing facilities and assisted living facilities. Where the patient meets certain qualifying criteria, hospice care can also be delivered in inpatient settings including hospitals where the hospital and hospice contract with each other. The hallmark of a hospice is an interdisciplinary approach to care delivery for the myriad of issues patients and caregivers are confronted with. Physicians, nurses, social workers, spiritual care workers, bereavement experts, therapists, home care aides, and volunteers work together to coordinate a plan of care for the patient and family. Medicare, Medicaid, and private insurers pay for hospice care and generally follow the framework outlined in the Medicare conditions for coverage which include the physician attesting that the patient has a life-limiting illness, and, if the illness follows its normal course, will result in death within 6 months or less (CMS, 2008a). Patients must agree to being in the hospice care program, which does not support curative methods (CMS, 2008b).

Although the growth of hospice care is desirable, it has fueled increased scrutiny and interest by government policymakers. The Medicare Payment Advisory Commission (MEDPAC) is expected to include the following recommendations in its upcoming report: accelerating the implementation of new payment models, reducing reimbursement for patients in nursing facilities, and including hospice care as part of the benefits included in Medicare Advantage plans.

HOME MEDICAL EQUIPMENT

Home medical equipment (HME, also known as durable medical equipment, or DME) includes mobility devices, oxygen equipment, and incontinence, orthotic, and nutrition products. HME providers deliver equipment to the home or institutional residence, which is paid for out of pocket by the patient, Medicare, or private insurer. A controversial competitive bidding process was implemented in 2009 for DME, prosthetic, orthotic, and other supplies and now covers 99 areas of the country (DMEPOS). The goal of competitive bidding for DME is to save money, ensure access, and limit fraud (CMS, 2014). Medical equipment including such items as home blood glucose monitors require an order from a physician with their signature following a face-to-face visit. This represents a major challenge to the scope of current practice of APRNs who have been able to do this for patients in the past and creates an unnecessary barrier for patients (American Nurses Association [ANA], 2014).

HOME INFUSION PHARMACY

Home infusion pharmacy involves the administration of medications using intravenous, subcutaneous, and other relevant interventions in the home. Therapies now commonly administered in the home include antibiotics, chemotherapy, pain management, and parenteral nutrition. An increasing range of these services are covered by commercial insurers for individuals of all ages, enabling patients to leave hospital settings or avoid them altogether. Services are also sometimes covered under Medicare Part D, while products, supplies, and nursing services are paid for under Medicare Part A. Home care providers have expanded clinician education, expertise, and availability to provide an increasing range of services in the home. Managed care companies have been a key influence in promoting the delivery of these services in the home as a cost-effective option for care provision. As technology improves the equipment that delivers these medications and treatments, patients and families are less intimidated by the concept of receiving these treatments in the home. These technologies are enabling more patients to remain independent and in the comfort of their own surroundings during treatment.

PRIVATE DUTY

Private Duty companies provide a broad range of services from medical and nursing care, personal care, to bill paying and transportation. Their goal is to provide whatever is needed to keep an aged, ill, or disabled individual independent and at home (Private Duty Home Care Association [PDHCA], 2007). Some states require licensure if nursing or therapy services are provided. Services are most frequently paid out of pocket or through long-term care policies. Often family members pool their resources, sharing the cost of services for their parents. The National Family Caregivers Association estimates that 65 million people (29% of the U.S. population) provide care for a chronically ill, disabled, or aged family member or friend at some point during any given year and caregivers spend an average of 20 hours a week providing care for a loved one (Marsh & Brown, 2011). Although caring for a loved one can be rewarding, it also brings many challenges. Caregivers can experience depression, anger, and exhaustion as they attempt to juggle their care delivery, jobs, and the care of their own children or spouses.

REIMBURSEMENT AND REIMBURSEMENT REFORM

Historically, private insurers and Medicaid have generally followed Medicare's lead in terms of qualifications for home care reimbursement. Reimbursement for services in the home focused only on home care until 1982 when the Medicare hospice benefit became available. In 1986, states were given the option to include hospice care under Medicaid. In a response to rapidly rising home health costs, the Balanced Budget Act of 1997 had a very negative impact on home health providers as a result of the authorization of the temporary Interim Payment System. This was followed by the Home Health Prospective Payment System (PPS) launched in 2000 and which had a positive impact on providers until 2008. The Medicare home health benefit has been cut through legislative and regulatory action by $110 billion for the period 2009-2019 according to the Congressional Budget Office (NAHC, 2013). Competitive bidding was implemented in 2009 for HME, decreasing the number of vendors who could provide equipment and increasing the regulatory requirements. Hospice providers underwent smaller incremental changes between 1984 and 2009 but are now poised for major reimbursement changes in 2014 which will decrease reimbursement for hospice care. Under the provisions of health reform, all segments will be impacted by the Medicare savings strategies and new models of care delivery which will require providers to modify their programs and services.

The focus on home care in the ACA was driven largely by overall growth in: (1) the numbers of Medicare providers, (2) related net income margins or profitability, (3) use, and (4) concerns about fraud and abuse. The need for new delivery models such as chronic care management, ACOs, patient-centered medical homes, and postacute bundling initiatives will all drive reimbursement reforms for home health. Other reimbursement reforms will include expansion of telehealth pilot programs and decreasing the base rates currently existing under the Medicare home care prospective payment system that pays for home care services. ACA provides the Secretary of Health and Human Services (HHS) significant discretionary authority in implementing its provisions and does not require reductions in home health payments. However, a pattern of continued downward provision of Medicare home care payments has occurred. Perhaps the biggest burden for home health and hospice providers today is increasing regulatory changes requiring more transparency, reporting, and documentation. These new requirements have become

the focus of intense audits and are resulting in extensive denials of claims. Government contracted auditing focused on documentation of physician face-to-face appointments, homebound status, medical necessity, and therapy assessments has resulted in the industry needing to invest significant additional administrative resources. This in turn impacts their ability to be as efficient as possible during a period of declining reimbursement.

HOSPITAL USE AND READMISSIONS AND THE FOCUS ON CARE TRANSITIONS

Since the announcement of readmission penalties on hospitals' Medicare reimbursement, home care providers have implemented aggressive measures, in collaboration with hospitals, to move patients from the acute to the home setting more quickly, and to implement care planning and delivery that is designed to prevent readmission. The dysfunction of our health care system and the resultant unmet need is most apparent at the point of discharge from hospital (Andrews, 2014). MedPAC has stated that the burden of unmet needs at hospital discharge is primarily driven by hospital admissions and readmissions (MedPAC, 2008). Although there is disagreement on what percentage of readmissions are preventable, there is broad agreement that more effective models of care transition are needed. Robert Wood Johnson Foundation researchers indicate that inadequate care coordination, including inadequate management of care transitions, can be responsible for $25 to $45 billion of expenditure per year (Burton, 2012). The pioneering work of Mary D. Naylor, PhD, RN, and Eric A. Coleman, MD, MPH, have identified care transition models that are leading to improved transition planning and changes in practice (Naylor, 2009).

QUALITY AND OUTCOME MANAGEMENT

Home care and hospice care are also engaged in CMS's triple aim to improve patients' care and care quality, as well as lower costs. Up until 2000, home care was paid for on a fee-for-service basis under Medicare. In 2000, when CMS changed the payment system to a prospective payment system, they also implemented a data collection tool called the Outcome and Assessment Information Set (OASIS). This tool enables standardized data to be collected through assessment of home care patients by nurses and therapists at defined periods of time, namely admission, transfer, and discharge. These data are then transmitted to CMS and are used to establish the basis for reimbursement and monitoring of patient outcomes. There were improvements to the system in 2010 (OASIS-C) and there are proposed improvements for 2014 (OASIS C-1) and for the first time, home care outcome results were made available for consumers on the CMS website. Patient satisfaction scores have also been added (U.S. Department of Health and Human Services [HHS], 2009). These data have improved the capacity to understand and make transparent the impact of home health on certain disease conditions, and enable consumers and purchasers to compare home care providers based on outcomes and patient satisfaction. From 2008, providers who did not participate in this system were subject to a 2% penalty.

THE IMPACT OF TECHNOLOGY ON HOME CARE

Changes in the types and availability of technology have impacted every aspect of home care delivery. Electronic health records (EHRs) are widely used in home care, enhancing documentation of the care provided. EHR facilitates communication with members of the home care team and with APNs and physicians overseeing the care provided. The availability of evidence-based clinical pathways has helped assure the standardization of care and the quality of information available to the clinicians delivering the care. By March of 2014, 78% of home health agencies were using electronic medical record systems (Brennan, 2014).

Telehealth has also become a standard mode of care enabling the patient to better understand the connection between their health choices and behaviors and the impact on health outcomes. Telehealth is expanding to enable both clinicians and patients easier access to experts in chronic disease management and nutrition and to clinical specialists. Uti-

lization patterns are enhanced by replacing in-person visits with electronic interventions. Continuing development and availability of technology is key to home care's future in helping to control use, promote quality, control cost, and manage labor expense (Suter & Hennessey, 2011).

CHAMPIONING HOME CARE AND HOSPICE AND THE ROLE OF NURSES

Early champions of home care were Senator Claude Pepper (D-FL), Senator Ted Moss (D-UT), Senator Robert Dole (R-KS), and John Heinz (R-PA), who pushed for the Medicare hospice benefit. While policymakers focused primarily on acute care delivery, the pendulum began to shift, especially in the early 2000s. Institutions dedicated to research began to release studies underscoring the economic and quality benefits of home care (Sutherland, Fisher, & Skinner, 2009; Gozalo, Miller, & Mor, 2002; Martin et al., 2008; Cole, 2006). These studies documented the increasing need and desire by Americans for home care, the cost savings of home care, and the minimization of rehospitalization that can be prevented with earlier home care interventions. On March 10, 1982, the National Association of Home Health Agencies and the Council of Home Health Agencies, an affiliate of the National League of Nursing, agreed to come together and formed what is now the largest home care and hospice association, the National Association for Home Care & Hospice (NAHC). They hired Val Halamandaris, a health policy expert who worked for Senator Claude Pepper to lead them. Today, with more than 6000 members, they advocate for the patients, families, providers, nurses, therapists, and home care aides who all serve a growing home care and hospice population. Other trade associations followed, including the Visiting Nurse Association of America and National Hospice and Palliative Care Organization. There are many examples of these associations coming together to advocate for change and for the mission and vision of home and hospice care.

In May 2011, the NAHC launched the Home Health Care Nurses Association in an effort to unify the voices of nurses working in home and hospice care. Each year they publish stories of home care and hospice nurses in all 50 states. Nurses, as chief executives of many home care organizations, continue to lobby members of Congress, take congressional representatives on home visits, and spearhead campaigns to influence decision-makers. The predominance of nurses as trustees of national trade associations enables nurses to have an enormous influence on decision making and to champion change, a power underused in the past.

Home care is the hospital without walls, the extension of the clinical office visit, and brings health care to millions of homes each day. The desire of this and the coming generations will be to remain in their homes, although the challenges in achieving this will be multiple, including: reimbursement reform, the fight for talent, chronic and transitional care management, the need for technology, and better end-of-life care. Home care and hospice care are the solution for U.S. health care policy in controlling costs, quality, and access, and this undertaking must largely be carried by nurses.

DISCUSSION QUESTIONS

1. How can nursing education prepare nurses for both the clinical roles in care delivery and leadership roles in delivery and policy formulation?
2. What are effective ways nurses can engage policymakers to sustain a focus on home care and hospice care?
3. What technology innovation do you see as a disruptive innovation in home and hospice care that nurses could take the lead on?

REFERENCES

American Nurses Association (ANA). (2014). Letter to Marilyn Tavenner, RE: DME Face-to-Face Encounter Rule. Retrieved from *www.nursing world.org/DocumentVault/ANA-Comments/DME-2013Letter.pdf*.

Andrews, J. (2014). Patients key to reducing readmissions. *Healthcare Finance News*. Retrieved from *www.healthcarefinancenews.com/news/ patients-key-reducing-readmissions*.

Brashears, S. (2013). Examining the future of the home care industry in ACOs. *Caring Magazine, May*, 43. Retrieved from *digitalcaringmagazine .nahc.org/Vizion5/viewer.aspx?issueID=49&pageID=44*.

Brennan, R. (2014). Health information exchange through health IT: What's working. Presentation to the ONC Health IT Summit for Nurses. *Informat-ics Enabling Patient-Centered Care Across the Continuum*. University of Maryland-Baltimore, July 16–18, 2014.

Burton, R. (2012). Improving care transitions. Health Affairs/Robert Wood Johnson Foundation. *Health Policy Brief Series*. Retrieved from *www.healthaffairs.org/healthpolicybriefs/brief.php?brief_id=76*.

Centers for Medicare & Medicaid Services [CMS]. (2008a). 42 CFR Part 418, Medicare and Medicaid Programs hospice conditions of participations; final rule. Retrieved from *www.cms.hhs.gov/center/hospice .asp*.

Centers for Medicare & Medicaid Services [CMS]. (2008b). 42 CFR Part 418.58, Hospice conditions of participation: Quality assessment and performance improvement.

Centers for Medicare & Medicaid Services [CMS]. (2009a). Center for Information Systems, Health Standards and Quality Bureau.

Centers for Medicare & Medicaid Services [CMS]. (2009b). National Health Expenditure Data; Executive Office of the President, Council of Economic Advisors: The Case for Health Care Reform.

Centers for Medicare & Medicaid Services [CMS]. (2014). Home health quality initiative. Retrieved from *www.cms.gov/Medicare/Quality-Initiatives-Patient-Assessment-Instruments/HomeHealthQualityInits/ index.html?redirect=/HomeHealthQualityInits*.

Cole, C. S. (2006). Improving the quality of long-term care. The Robert Wood Johnson Foundation. Retrieved from *www.rwjf.org/en/research-publications/find-rwjf-research/2006/12/improving-the-quality-of-long-term-care.html*.

Dychtwald, K. (2011). Riding the age wave: How America can stay afloat and enjoy the ride. *Caring Magazine*, 27. Retrieved from *digital caringmagazine.nahc.org/Vizion5/viewer.aspx?issueID=30&pageID=29*.

Forster, T. M., & Simione, R. J. (2011). Hospice payment reform: A look into the future. *Caring Magazine*. Retrieved from *digitalcaringmagazine .nahc.org/Vizion5/viewer.aspx?issueID=29&pageID=10*.

Gozalo, P., Miller, S., & Mor, V. (2002). Hospice in nursing homes: Factors influencing hospitalization and choice of hospice. *Academy for Health Services Research and Health Policy, 19*, 5.

Landers, S. (2013). Medicine's future: Helping patients stay healthy at home. *Cleveland Clinic Journal of Medicine*. Retrieved from *www.ccjm .org/content/80/e-Suppl_1/e-S1.full*.

Marsh, A. G., & Brown, S. (2011). Family care giving: The issue of our time. *Caring Magazine*, 28. Retrieved from *digitalcaringmagazine.nahc.org/ Vizion5/viewer.aspx?issueID=25&pageID=24*.

Martin, J. P., English, D., Musial, C., & Corridor Group. (2008). Collaborative care: Improving the hospice-nursing home relationship. *California HealthCare Foundation Issues Brief*. Retrieved from *www.chcf.org/ publications/2008/09/collaborative-care-improving-the-hospicenursing -home-relationship*.

Medicare Payment Advisory Commission [MedPAC]. (2008). Report to the Congress: Medicare payment policy. Retrieved from *medpac.gov/ documents*.

National Association for Home Care & Hospice [NAHC]. (2010). *Basic statistics about home care*. Retrieved from *www.nahc.org*.

National Association for Home Care & Hospice [NAHC]. (2013). Medicare home health patients suffer from $110 billion in cuts. *NAHC Legislative Blueprint for Action*. Retrieved from *www.congressweb.com/ nahc/2014MarchResources.htm*.

National Hospice and Palliative Care Organization [NHPCO]. (2011). Hospice: A historical perspective. NHPCO National Data Set, Retrieved from *www.nhpco.org*.

Naylor, M. D. (2009). United States Senate Committee on Finance, April 21, 2009. Washington DC, 2, Retrieved from *www.nursing.upeen.edu/news/ Documents/Mary_Naylor_statement_4-17-09f.pdf*.

Private Duty Home Care Association (PDHCA). (2007). Home page. Retrieved from *www.pdhca.org*.

Remington, L. (2014a). Healthcare technology trends 2014. *The Remington Report, 22*(1), 9–12.

Remington, L. (2014b). Is the growth of ACOs slowing down? *The Remington Report, 22*(1), 4–8.

Remington, L. (2013). MedPAC Report: Home health and hospice. *The Remington Report, 21*(3), 14–18.

Suter, P., & Hennessey, B. (2011). Effective use of technology to engage both patients and provider partners. *Caring Magazine*, 20–25.

Sutherland, J. M., Fisher, E. S., & Skinner, J. S. (2009). Getting past denial: The high cost of health care in the United States. *New England Journal of Medicine, 361*(13), 1227–1230.

U.S. Department of Health and Human Services [HHS]. (2009). Home health compare. Retrieved from *www.medicare.gov/HHCompare*.

ONLINE RESOURCES

National Home Infusion Association (NHIA)
www.nhia.org/resource/medicare_ptd
National Association for Home Care and Hospice
www.nahc.org

CHAPTER 38

Long-Term Services and Supports Policy Issues

Charlene Harrington   Caroline Stephens   Laura M. Wagner

"A policy is a temporary creed liable to be changed, but while it holds good it has got to be pursued with apostolic zeal."

Mahatma Gandhi

The U.S. population is aging, with the number of adults aged 65 and over projected to almost double between 2012 and 2060, from 43.1 million to 92 million (one in seven people). Moreover, the number of the oldest old (aged 85 years and over) is projected to triple from 5.9 million to 18.2 million, reaching 4.3% of the total population (US Census Bureau, 2012). The demand for long-term services and supports (LTSS) and the need for nurses and other personnel to provide those services is growing rapidly. The Institute of Medicine (IOM, 2008) predicts a major shortage of health workers with geriatric training to address the growing needs of the aging population. With total expenditures of $233 billion in 2012, projected to increase to $403 billion in 2012 (Keehan et al., 2012), LTSS is a critical sector (representing 9% of total health spending), but one that receives little attention from the nursing profession.

This policy chapter focuses on some of the policy and political issues facing nursing in long-term care. First, it reviews the problems of poor quality of nursing home care, weak enforcement of federal quality regulations, and profit-making nursing homes. Second, it examines nursing home staffing and reimbursement policies. Third, it discusses the need for expanding home and community-based service (HCBS) programs. Finally, nurses are urged to become advocates for older and disabled people who need long-term care services.

POOR QUALITY OF CARE

Poor nursing home quality has been documented since the early 1970s and culminated in the passage of the Omnibus Budget Reconciliation Act (OBRA) of 1987 to reform nursing home regulation. The federal law requires comprehensive assessments of all nursing home residents and assurance that residents maintain the highest possible mental and physical health. Although the federal government sets the standards, state survey and certification agencies conduct annual surveys and complaint investigations to verify compliance for a nursing home to be certified to receive federal funds.

Although the federal regulations are clear, many nursing homes provide poor quality of care. In 2010, over 94% of nursing homes received a total of about 150,000 deficiencies for failure to meet federal regulations (Harrington et al, 2011a). Many formal complaints were made to state regulatory agencies about poor nursing home quality, and 23% of nursing homes were cited for causing actual harm or immediate jeopardy to nursing home residents in 2010. Many nursing homes failed to provide adequate infection control (43%), a safe environment (43%), adequate food sanitation (39%), and quality standards (34%). Others received deficiencies for failure to meet professional standards (30%), failure to provide comprehensive care plans (28%), and giving unnecessary drugs (23%) (Harrington et al., 2011a).

WEAK ENFORCEMENT

Many studies have documented that the federal and state survey and enforcement system as well as the complaint investigation processes are weak (U.S. Government Accounting Office [GAO], 1999, 2011). State surveyors are often unable to detect serious problems with the quality of care. Some state survey agencies improperly downgrade the scope and severity of the deficiencies observed and do not refer nursing homes for intermediate sanctions. The timing of state surveys continues to be predictable and consumer complaint investigations are not timely (U.S. GAO, 2011). Poor state investigations and documentation of deficiencies, large numbers of inexperienced state surveyors, and weak federal oversight of state activities continue.

When violations are detected, few facilities have follow-up enforcement actions or sanctions taken against them (Harrington et al., 2008). The continued widespread variation in the number and type of deficiencies issued by states shows that states are not using the regulatory process consistently and are not following federal guidelines (U.S. GAO, 2011). More importantly, state enforcement problems are related to inadequate federal and state resources for regulatory activities, which have not kept pace with inflation.

One study documented the benefits of strong regulation in those states that more rigorously implemented federal regulations. Regulatory stringency was significantly associated with better quality for four of the seven measures studied and the regulations were found to be cost effective (Mukamel et al., 2012). To ensure the safety of residents, strong enforcement and increased funding for the survey and certification program are needed and poorly performing facilities need to be cut from the Medicare and Medicaid programs.

INADEQUATE STAFFING LEVELS

Low nurse staffing levels are the single most important contributing factor to poor quality of nursing home care in the United States. Over the past 25 years, numerous research studies have documented the important relationship between nurse staffing levels, in particular registered nurse (RN) staffing, and the outcomes of care (Bostick et al., 2006; Castle, 2008; Spilsbury et al., 2011; Schnelle et al., 2004; CMS, 2001). The benefits of higher staffing

levels, especially RN staffing, can include lower mortality rates; improved physical functioning; and reduced antibiotic use, pressure ulcers, catheterized residents, urinary tract infections, hospitalization rates, physical restraint and side-rail use, weight loss, and dehydration. States that have introduced higher minimum staffing standards for nursing homes have higher nurse staffing levels, lower deficiency citations, and improved quality of outcomes (Harrington, Swan, & Carrillo, 2007; Mukamel et al., 2012; Wagner, McDonald, & Castle, 2013a; Wagner, McDonald, & Castle, 2013b).

The average U.S. nursing home provided a total of 3.9 hours per resident day (HPRD) of total RN and Director of Nursing, licensed vocational or practical nurse (LVN/LPN), and nursing assistant (NA) time in 2010 (Harrington et al., 2011a). Of the total time, most (62% or 2.4 HPRD) is provided by NAs, who care for an average of 11 residents and are only required to have 2 weeks of training. RNs provide only 42 minutes (0.7 hour) of time per patient day. Although the average staffing hours have increased over time, there are wide variations, and some facilities have dangerously low staffing.

A Centers for Medicare and Medicaid Services (CMS) (2001) report found that staffing levels for long-stay residents that are below 4.1 HPRD result in harm or jeopardy for residents. (The total should consist of at least 1.3 HPRD for licensed nurses and 2.8 HPRD of NA time.) NA time should range from 2.8 to 3.2 HPRD depending on the care residents need, and this is just to carry out basic care activities (CMS, 2001). This amounts to 1 NA per 7 residents on both the day and evening shifts and 1 NA per 12 residents at night. On average, nonprofit and government nursing homes are more likely to meet the recommended standards than for-profit homes (Harrington et al., 2012). Establishing higher staffing levels should have the highest policy priority at both the state and federal levels.

CORPORATE OWNERSHIP

Many studies have shown that for-profit nursing homes operate with lower costs and staffing compared with nonprofit facilities which provide higher staffing, higher quality of care, and have more trustworthy governance (Comondore et al., 2009). Nevertheless, for-profit companies owned 69% of the nation's nursing homes, compared with non-profit (26%) and government-owned facilities (6%) in 2010 (Harrington et al., 2011a). For-profit corporate chains emerged as a dominant organizational form in the nursing home field during the 1990s and they increased from 39% in the 1990s to 55% of all nursing homes in 2010 (Harrington et al., 2011a). The largest nursing home chains are publicly traded companies with billions of dollars in revenues. Many large nursing home chains own a number of related companies including residential care/assisted living facilities, home health agencies, hospices, pharmacies, therapy organizations, and staffing organizations. These related companies refer patients to each other and use their corporate interrelationships to maximize revenues.

Private equity companies have purchased many of the largest nursing home chains and these companies have few reporting requirements. Many large chains have multiple investors, holding companies, and multiple levels of companies involved such that property companies are separated from the management of facilities largely to avoid litigation (Wells & Harrington, 2013). The lack of transparency in the ownership responsibilities has made regulation and oversight by state survey and certification agencies problematic. To address these issues, the Affordable Care Act included provisions for reporting corporate ownership information on the Medicare Nursing Home Compare website along with information regarding expenditures on staffing and direct care (Wells & Harrington, 2013). These changes arose from advocacy by consumer organizations and unions.

The 10 largest for-profit chains had residents with the highest acuity and the lowest nurse staffing hours compared with nonprofit and government nursing homes between 2003 and 2008 (Harrington et al., 2012). The study also showed that the 10 largest for-profit chains had the highest numbers of violations of federal quality regulations and the most serious deficiencies that caused harm or jeopardy compared with nonprofit and government nursing homes (Harrington et al., 2012). In addition, the four largest for-profit nursing home chains

purchased by private equity companies between 2003 and 2008 had more deficiencies after being acquired.

Regulators need to undertake stronger enforcement actions when chains fail to meet the nursing home staffing requirements and quality regulations. Chains should be targeted for regulatory oversight by state survey agencies rather than the current procedure of focusing on individual facilities. Greater financial accountability for chains and private equity companies would address the quality problems.

FINANCIAL ACCOUNTABILITY

U.S. nursing home expenditures increased from $85 billion in 2000 to $143 billion in 2010 (CMS, 2012). Medicare covers up to 100 days of nursing home care after a medically necessary hospital stay of at least three days and Medicaid generally pays for those with low incomes who need long-term nursing home care. Medicare, Medicaid, and other government sources paid for 63% of total nursing home expenditures in 2010, and the remainder was paid by individuals out-of-pocket (28%) or private insurance (9%).

Nursing home reimbursement methods and per diem reimbursement rates are of great importance because they influence the costs and quality of care. State Medicaid reimbursement policies have primarily focused on cost containment at the expense of quality and have established very low payment rates. Facilities tend to respond by cutting nurse staffing levels and quality of care (Grabowski, Angelelli, & Mor, 2004). Nursing homes also keep wages and benefits low, which results in high employee turnover rates (Castle, Engberg, & Men, 2007; CMS 2001). Nursing home wages and benefits are substantially lower than those of comparable hospital workers and lower than many of those with jobs in the fast food industry and other unskilled jobs, and are generally well below the level of a living wage (CMS, 2001).

Congress passed Medicare, the prospective payment system (PPS) for reimbursement that was implemented in 1998 to control overall payment rates to skilled nursing homes (Medicare Payment

Advisory Commission [MedPac], 2012). Under the PPS, Medicare rates are based in part on the resident case mix (acuity) in each facility to take into account the amount of staffing and therapy services that residents require. Skilled nursing homes however do not need to demonstrate that the actual amount of staff and therapy time provided is related to the payments allocated under the PPS rates. Funds can be shifted from staffing into profits.

Excess profits have grown dramatically over time because Medicare does not limit the profit margins of nursing homes. In 2010, the profit margins on Medicare payments in for-profit nursing homes were 21% while profit margins in nonprofit nursing homes were 9.5% (MedPac, 2012). A recent study of total revenues and expenditures for all payers in California nursing homes found that administrative expenses grew only slightly, although profits grew by 80% of total revenues from 2007 to 2010. It also found that direct care expenditures have been steadily declining, and for-profit nursing homes had substantially higher administrative costs and profit levels three times greater than nonprofit facilities (Harrington et al., 2013).

One policy option is to revise the Medicaid and Medicare payment systems to specify the minimum proportion of the payments that must be used for nurse staffing and therapy services and the maximum payments for profits and administration costs. If the minimum amount of payments were regulated, nursing homes would be prevented from cutting nurse staffing and using the funds for profit making. If profits and administrative costs were capped at 20% for all payers (Medicare, Medicaid, private insurance, and self-pay), there could be a large savings in the United States (Harrington et al., 2013). Thus quality could be improved and costs reduced by increasing nursing home financial accountability.

OTHER ISSUES

A large and growing percentage of older people are admitted and often readmitted to hospitals and emergency departments (EDs). Estimates suggest nursing home residents have more than 2.2 million ED visits annually, half of which result in a hospital admission (Wang et al., 2011). In addition, studies indicate that 24% to 67% of nursing home resident ED visits and 47% of hospitalizations are potentially preventable or could be managed in an ambulatory care setting, resulting in more than $1.9 billion in unnecessary health care spending (Grabowski, O'Malley, & Barhydt, 2007; Stephens et al., 2012). Unfortunately, these potentially preventable ED visits and hospitalizations unnecessarily expose individuals to the risks associated with care transitions, such as higher morbidity and mortality, delirium, and functional decline, among others (Creditor, 1993; Ouslander et al., 2010).

Many of these unnecessary visits are caused by inadequate assistance with activities of daily living and instrumental activities of daily living, deficient monitoring and treatment of chronic conditions, and inadequate responses to acute conditions that could, at least under optimal conditions, be addressed within the facility (Ouslander et al., 2010). Lack of access to timely and appropriate primary care, appropriate RN care, and adequately trained staff and clinical resources appear to significantly contribute to inappropriate use. The structure of Medicare and Medicaid's coverage of acute and long-term care creates conflicting incentives regarding dually eligible beneficiaries, leading to increased rates of hospitalizations without accountability for care coordination (Grabowski, 2007). New financial penalties given to hospitals for 30-day readmissions and new CMS demonstration projects to integrate payments for acute and long-term care have been designed to give incentives to improve the quality of care.

HOME AND COMMUNITY-BASED SERVICES

LTSS services that are needed for more than 90 days are focused on providing assistance with limitations in activities of daily living and supporting those with cognitive limitations and mental illness. About 11 million people living in the community receive assistance with activities of daily living; 92% of those individuals received informal help from family and friends, and only 13% received paid help (Kaye, Harrington, & LaPlante, 2010).

There are increased pressures to expand HCBS, especially in the Medicaid program which pays for most LTSS. The public increasingly reports a preference for LTSS provided at home over services in institutions. The 1990 Americans with Disability Act (ADA) and the subsequent legal judgment in the 1999 Olmstead Supreme Court decision require that states must not discriminate against persons with disabilities by refusing to provide community services when these are available and appropriate (Kaye, Harrington, & LaPlante, 2010).

In response to the increased demand, Medicaid HCBS programs grew by 52% (from 2.1 million to 3.2 million) and expenditures increased by 170% (from $19.5 to $52.7 billion) between 2000 and 2010 (Ng, Harrington, & Musumeci, 2013). In spite of the growth in HCBS, there are wide variations in access to services and expenditures across states. Moreover, states do not provide equitable access to groups such as those with developmental disabilities, the aged and disabled, individuals with mental health problems, children, and other groups (Ng, Harrington, & Musumeci, 2013). In 2012, only 32 states had Medicaid personal care attendant programs, and many states have limited services under their HCBS waiver programs. States have begun to shift individuals in HCBS programs to Medicaid managed care programs, even though most managed care programs have little or no experience providing LTSS.

Some states have rapidly expanded their HCBS programs, whereas others still lag behind, relying heavily on institutional services. The percentage of LTSS participants receiving HCBS increased from 56% in 2005 to 65% in 2010, and the percentage of LTSS expenditures for HCBS increased from 30% to 45% in the same period. Although progress has been made, the increased adoption of state cost control policies has led to large increases in persons on waiver wait lists. The waiting lists for Medicaid HCBS have increased from 192,000 reported in 2002 to more than 524,000 in 39 states in 2012, with waiting periods averaging 27 months for services across the country (Ng, Harrington, & Musumeci, 2013). Access could be improved by standardizing and liberalizing state HCBS policies, but state fiscal concerns are barriers to rebalancing between HCBS and institutional services.

The Affordable Care Act included important new provisions to expand HCBS through a Medicaid state plan rather than a waiver. It also established the Community First Choice Option in Medicaid to provide personal care services to individuals, created the State Balancing Incentive Program to provide enhanced federal matching payments to eligible states, and extended the Medicaid Money Follows the Person Rebalancing Demonstration program. It also continued the Aging and Disability Resource Center initiatives. All these provisions to expand HCBS under Medicaid were advocated by ADAPT (*www.adapt.org*), an advocacy organization for individuals with disabilities, along with a coalition of consumer advocacy groups. It will be important to determine whether states take advantage of the new options to expand HCBS.

Although the cost of nursing home care is almost six times as much as HCBS (Harrington, Ng, & Kitchener, 2011b), the main opposition to expanding Medicaid HCBS has been the potential for increased costs to states if additional Medicaid participants request new LTSS services. However, studies show that states offering extensive HCBS had spending growth comparable to those states with low HCBS spending (Kaye, 2012). States that had well-established HCBS programs had much less overall LTSS spending growth compared with those with low HCBS spending because these states were able to reduce institutional spending.

PUBLIC FINANCING

In the long run, the United States needs a comprehensive mandatory public long-term care insurance system for everyone. Currently, the only segment of the U.S. population whose cost of LTSS is covered is individuals who live below the poverty-threshold enrolled in Medicaid. Except for short-term postacute care, the rest of the U.S. population must either pay for care out-of-pocket or resort to privately purchased long-term care insurance. The financially crippling cost of nursing home care (as much as $90,000 per year) is one of the great fears confronting persons who are otherwise self-supporting. Yet relatively few individuals have either the means or motivation to insure themselves privately. Only about 7 million private long-term care policies were in force covering 3% of the population aged 20 and over in 2005 (Feder, Komisar, & Friedland, 2007). Few older adults can afford to purchase private long-term care insurance, so this does not appear to be a viable financing mechanism for the future (Wiener, 2009).

A mandatory social insurance program for LTSS offers distinct advantages over the current means-tested system. If everyone paid into the system, individuals would have access to coverage when they are chronically ill or disabled without the humiliation of having to become poor to receive services. By expanding the Medicare program to include LTSS, the payment of LTSS contributions early in a worker's life could prefund LTSS services that generally are required late in life, spreading the risk across the entire population. Countries in Scandinavia, Germany, and Japan have adopted mandatory public long-term insurance systems that can serve as models for the United States. These countries generally provide protection and coverage for persons who need LTSS (Wiener, 2009). The nation should focus on public financing of LTSS insurance that would ensure that all citizens have access to high-quality LTSS.

CONCLUSION

We need a vision for advocacy in LTSS that is multidimensional and long range. Political efforts are needed at the local, state, and national levels. Community mobilization, public education, legislative reform, and legal actions are all needed to bring about policy changes to ensure access to high quality LTSS services. Consumer advocates and organizations such as The Consumer Voice, ADAPT, and the AARP have taken a lead in reform efforts, but they need help to make progress. Nurses and nursing organizations should form joint alliances with consumer organizations to advocate for needed changes in the long-term care system.

Organized nursing needs to place its considerable political influence into LTSS reform, including improving the quality of nursing home care and expanding HCBS. These efforts could improve the lives of residents in nursing homes as well as those who need HCBS. Nurses should act not only because of a concern for all those individuals who need LTSS but also to ensure that they, their families, and friends will have access to high-quality, appropriate LTSS in the future.

DISCUSSION QUESTIONS

1. What are the most important steps needed to improve the poor quality of nursing home care in the United States and the inadequate nurse staffing levels (RNs, LVNs, and NAs)?
2. Because consumers prefer HCBS, what policy changes are needed to ensure an adequate supply of services and a high quality labor force?
3. What strategies can nurses use to effectively advocate for a higher quality of care, greater access to LTSS services, and adequate public funds to pay for LTSS?

REFERENCES

Bostick, J. E., Rantz, M. J., Flesner, M. K., & Riggs, C. J. (2006). Systematic review of studies of staffing and quality in nursing homes. *Journal of the American Medical Directors Association, 7*(6), 366–376.

Castle, N. (2008). Nursing home care giver staffing levels and quality of care: A literature review. *Journal of Applied Gerontology, 27*(4), 375–405.

Castle, N. G., Engberg, J., & Men, A. (2007). Nursing home staff turnover: Impact on nursing home Compare quality measures. *The Gerontologist, 47*(5), 650–661.

Centers for Medicare & Medicaid Services [CMS]. (2001). Appropriateness of minimum nurse staffing ratios in nursing homes. In *Report to Congress: Phase II Final* (vol. I to III). Baltimore: CMS.

Centers for Medicare and Medicaid Services [CMS]. (2012). National health expenditures historical data for 2010. Baltimore, MD: CMS. Retrieved from *www.cms.gov/Research-Statistics-Data-and-Systems/Statistics -Trends-and-Reports/NationalHealthExpendData/NationalHealth AccountsHistorical.html*.

Comondore, V. R., Devereaux, P. J., Zhou, Q., Stone, S. B., Bussey, J. W., Ravindran, N. C., et al. (2009). Quality of care in for-profit and not-for-profit nursing homes: Systematic review and meta-analysis. *British Medical Journal, 339*, b2732.

Creditor, M. C. (1993). Hazards of hospitalization of the elderly. *Annals of Internal Medicine, 118*(3), 219–223.

Feder, J., Komisar, H. L., & Friedland, R. B. (2007). Long-term care financing: Policy options for the future. Washington, DC: Georgetown University. Retrieved from *ltcfinalpaper061107.pdf*.

Grabowski, D. C. (2007). Medicare and Medicaid: Conflicting incentives for long term care. *Millbank Quarterly, 85*(4), 579–610.

Grabowski, D. C., Angelelli, J. J., & Mor, V. (2004). Medicaid payment and risk-adjusted nursing home quality measures. *Health Affairs, 23*(5), 243–252.

Grabowski, D. C., O'Malley, A. J., & Barhydt, N. R. (2007). The costs and potential savings associated with nursing home hospitalizations. *Health Affairs, 26*(6), 1753–1761.

Harrington, C., Carrillo, H., Dowdell, M., Tang, P. P., & Blank, B. W. (2011a). Nursing facilities, staffing, residents and facility deficiencies, 2005 through 2010. San Francisco, CA: University of California, Department of Social and Behavioral Sciences. Retrieved from *ualr.edu/seniorjustice/uploads/2011/11/FACILITY%20DEFICIENCIES.pdf.*

Harrington, C., Ng, T., & Kitchener, M. (2011b). Do Medicaid home and community based services save money? *Home Health Care Services Quarterly, 30*(4), 198–213.

Harrington, C., Olney, B., Carrillo, H., & Kang, T. (2012). Nurse staffing and deficiencies in the largest for-profit chains and chains owned by private equity companies. *Health Services Research, 47*(1), Part I, 106–128.

Harrington, C., Ross, L., Mukamel, D., & Rosenau, P. (2013). Improving the financial accountability of nursing facilities. Washington, DC: Kaiser Commission on Medicaid and the Uninsured, June. Retrieved from *kaiserfamilyfoundation.files.wordpress.com/2013/06/8455-improving-the-financial-accountability-of-nursing-facilities.pdf.*

Harrington, C., Swan, J. H., & Carrillo, H. (2007). Nurse staffing levels and Medicaid reimbursement rates in nursing facilities. *Health Services Research, 42*(3 Pt. I), 1105–1129.

Harrington, C., Tsoukalas, T., Rudder, C., Mollot, R. J., & Carrillo, H. (2008). Study of federal and state civil money penalties and fines. *The Gerontologist, 48*(5), 679–691.

Institute of Medicine [IOM], Committee on the Future Health Care Workforce for Older Americans. (2008). *Retooling for an aging America: building the health care workforce.* Washington, DC: National Academy of Science Press.

Kaye, H. S. (2012). Gradual rebalancing of Medicaid long-term services and supports saves money and serves more people, statistical model shows. *Health Affairs, 31*(6), 1195–1203.

Kaye, H. S., Harrington, C., & LaPlante, M. P. (2010). Long-term care in the United States: Who gets it, who provides it, who pays, and how much does it cost? *Health Affairs, Special issue, 29*(1), 11–21.

Keehan, S. P., Cuckler, G. A., Sisko, A. M., Madison, A. J., Smith, S. D., Lizonitz, J. M., et al. (2012). National health projections: Modest annual growth until coverage expands and economic growth accelerates. *Health Affairs, 31*(7), 1600–1612.

Medicare Payment Advisory Commission [MedPAC]. (2012). Report to Congress: Medicare payment policy. In Skilled nursing facility services, chapter 7 (pp. 171–208). Washington, DC: MedPac, March 2012. Retrieved from *www.medpac.gov/documents/Mar12_EntireReport.pdf.*

Mukamel, D. B., Weimer, D. L., Harrington, C., Spector, W. D., Ladd, H., & Li, Y. (2012). The effect of state regulatory stringency on nursing home quality. *Health Services Research, 47*(5), 1791–1813.

Ng, T., Harrington, C., & Musumeci, M. (2013). *Medicaid home and community based service programs: 2010 data update.* Washington, DC: Kaiser Commission on Medicaid and the Uninsured.

Ouslander, J. G., Lamb, G., Perloe, M., Givens, J. H., Kluge, L., Rutland, T., et al. (2010). Potentially avoidable hospitalizations of nursing home residents: Frequency, causes, and costs. *Journal of the American Geriatrics Society, 58*(4), 627–635.

Schnelle, J. F., Simmons, S. F., Harrington, C., Cadogan, M., Garcia, E., & Bates-Jensen, B. (2004). Relationship of nursing home staffing to quality of care. *Health Services Research, 39*(2), 225–250.

Spilsbury, K., Hewitt, C., Stirk, L., & Bowman, C. (2011). The relationship between nurse staffing and quality of care in nursing homes: A systematic review. *International Journal Nursing Studies, 48*(6), 732–750.

Stephens, C., Blegen, M., Newcomer, R., Miller, B., & Harrington, C. (2012). Emergency department use by nursing home residents: Effect of severity of cognitive impairment. *The Gerontologist, 52*(3), 383–393.

U.S. Census Bureau. (2012, December 12). U.S. Census Bureau projections show a slower growing, older, more diverse nation a half century from now. *News Room.* Washington, DC. Retrieved from *www.census.gov/newsroom/releases/archives/population/cb12-243.html.*

U.S. General Accounting Office [GAO]. (1999). *Nursing homes: Additional steps needed to strengthen enforcement of federal quality standards.* Report to the Special Committee on Aging, U.S. Senate. GAO/HEHS-99-46. Washington, DC: GAO.

U.S. Government Accountability Office [GAO]. (2011). *More reliable data and consistent guidance would improve CMS oversight of state complaint investigations.* GAO-11-280. Washington, DC: GAO. Apr 7, 2011.

Wagner, L. M., McDonald, S. M., & Castle, N. G. (2013a). Staffing-related deficiency citations in nursing homes. *Journal of Aging and Social Policy, 25*(1), 83–97.

Wagner, L. M., McDonald, S. M., & Castle, N. G. (2013b). Nursing home deficiency citations for physical restraints and side rails. *Western Journal of Nursing Research, 35*(5), 546–565.

Wang, H. E., Shah, M. N., Allman, R. M., & Kilgore, M. (2011). Emergency department visits by nursing home residents in the United States. *Journal of the American Geriatrics Society, 59*(10), 1864–1872.

Wells, J., & Harrington, C. (2013). Implementation of Affordable Care Act provisions to improve nursing home transparency, care quality, and abuse prevention. Washington, DC: Kaiser Commission on Medicaid and the Uninsured. Retrieved from *www.kff.org/medicare/upload/8406.pdf.*

Wiener, J. M. (2009). *Long-term care: Options in an era of health reform.* Washington, DC: RTI International.

ONLINE RESOURCES

Medicare Nursing Home Compare
www.medicare.gov/nursinghomecompare/search.html
Medicare Home Health Compare
www.medicare.gov/homehealthcompare/search.html
The Henry J. Kaiser Family Foundation
kff.org

CHAPTER 39

The United States Military and Veterans Administration Health Systems: Contemporary Overview and Policy Challenges

John S. Murray

"No one who fights for this country should ever have to fight for a job, or a roof over their head, or the care that they have earned."

President Barack Obama

The U.S. Military Health System (MHS) provides a number of important health care services to as many as 8.3 million service members, military retirees, and their families (Murray & Chaffee, 2011; The Kaiser Foundation, 2012). Military health care is provided by approximately 140,000 military, civilian, and contract personnel working around the globe at 59 military treatment facilities (MTFs) capable of providing diagnostic, therapeutic, and inpatient care. Additionally, care is delivered at hundreds of military outpatient clinics and by private sector civilian providers (Government Accountability Office [GAO], 2012; Murray & Chaffee, 2011).

Military nursing consists of several components: active duty, reserve, National Guard, enlisted medical technicians, and federal civilian registered nurses. The Army Nurse Corps is comprised of 40,000 nursing team members, whereas the Air Force has 18,000 and the Navy approximately 5,800 (U.S. Senate Committee on Appropriations, 2012). Active duty military nurses in all armed forces must have a bachelor's degree in nursing (BSN) from an accredited school to serve in the military.

The MHS has two missions (Figure 39-1):

- A military readiness mission: supporting wartime and other deployments (GAO, 2012; Murray & Chaffee, 2011).
- A health care benefits mission: providing medical services and support to members of the armed forces, retirees, and their dependents (GAO, 2012; Murray & Chaffee, 2011).

The Veterans Health Administration (VHA) is home to the United States' largest integrated health care system consisting of 152 medical centers, nearly 1,400 community-based outpatient clinics, community living centers, Vet Centers, and residential homes for disabled veterans. More than 239,000 staff, including 53,000 licensed health care clinicians, work to provide comprehensive care to more than 8.3 million veterans each year at these facilities. The VHA nursing team consists of 77,000 personnel nationwide composed of registered nurses, licensed practical/vocational nurses, and nursing assistants. Of these, approximately 5440 are advanced practice nurses (Certified Registered Nurse Anesthetists, Nurse Practitioners, and Clinical Nurse Specialists). A BSN degree is not a requirement to work for the VHA (U.S. Department of Veterans Affairs Office of Nursing Services, 2010). The VHA's primary mission is to honor America's veterans by providing exceptional comprehensive care that improves their health and well-being. It accomplishes this benchmark of excellence by

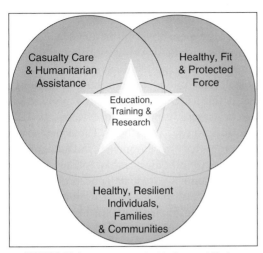

FIGURE 39-1 The Military Health System Mission.

providing exemplary services that are both patient centered and evidence based (U.S. Department of Veterans Affairs, 2013a).

THE MHS AND VHA BUDGETS

The National Defense Authorization Act (NDAA) is passed by Congress annually and specifies the overall budget for the Department of Defense (DoD), which includes funding for the MHS. Funding supports the delivery of health care to service members and their families as well as supporting education and training of military medical personnel, research, and purchasing medical equipment and supplies for MTFs and clinics (Murray & Chaffee, 2011). Each year, senior military nursing leaders speak before Congress regarding accomplishments and challenges over the previous year as well as identifying what new programs and policies are needed. In 2012 the Chief of the Army Nurse Corps presented information to support the need for a new trauma-training program for nurses. This program would allow the nurses to continue to develop their full capability to manage critical trauma patients across the battlefield. In response, Congress provided funding to support the development of the Army's first Trauma Nurse Course that prepares nurses for the ever-changing traumatic

injuries treated on the battlefield (U.S. Senate Committee on Appropriations, 2012). Patient outcomes from advanced treatment of traumatic injuries on the battlefield that have resulted from this training will inform policy regarding what nurses need to know to provide this specialty care.

As with U.S. health care costs over the past decade, expenses for the MHS have also significantly increased, more than doubling from $19 billion dollars in 2001 to a projected budget of $49.4 billion in 2014, equivalent to approximately 9.5% of the entire DoD budget. Although reasons for this large increase are many, two in particular receive great attention from Congress. There currently exists a vast amount of duplication and redundancy within the current three service medical departments (Air Force, Army, and Navy). This includes personnel, processes, and equipment, which add to growing defense health care costs. Additionally, wartime requirements have led to increased expenditures. When military health care personnel are deployed, patient care is often shifted to civilian care, which is more expensive (Beasley, 2012). To be fiscally responsible, the DoD has completed a comprehensive analysis of military health care spending. Strategic planning is aimed at eliminating duplication and redundancy as well as controlling costs, while continuing to provide optimal care (Office of the Under Secretary of Defense, 2013). Since 2007, military nurses have taken the lead role in standardizing health care policies and procedures related to education, training, and research for the DoD (Murray, 2009; Murray & Chaffee, 2011). For example, instead of creating new simulation programs to meet training needs in the National Capital Region, nurses brought together the three military services and civilian academic and health care institutions to create a robust platform reducing duplication of services. This initiative met the directive set forward by the Deputy Secretary of Defense for the three branches of the military to partner on education and training initiatives to reduce defense health care costs (Murray, 2010).

Historically, the VHA has been underfunded. However, for 2014, the VHA requested and received $64 billion dollars to provide reliable and timely resources to support the delivery of accessible and high-quality medical services to veterans. This is a 4.5% increase over the 2012 budget and approximately 40% of the total Department of Veterans Affairs budget (Merlis, 2012). One reason for escalating costs is the financial outlay required to cover the increased number of veterans seeking care from the VHA as a result of physical and mental injuries to personnel who have been deployed multiple times in Iraq and Afghanistan. Funding will support acute hospital, rehabilitative, psychiatric, nursing home, noninstitutional extended state home domiciliary, and outpatient care. The budget also supports upgrading of treatment facilities as well as the purchase of equipment and supplies. In addition, the VHA is the United States' largest provider of graduate medical and nursing education as well as a major contributor to medical research which is supported by the annual budget (U.S. Department of Veterans Affairs, 2013b; 2013c).

Like the MHS, the VHA is expected to provide exceptional care while controlling costs, and has implemented a number of performance measures aimed at continually monitoring the provision of high-quality care, access to care, revenue cycle improvement to improve efficiency and accuracy, as well as partnering with the MHS to improve collaboration and sharing of resources. In fact, for many years the VHA was considered an industry leader because of its safety and quality measures (U.S. Department of Veterans Affairs, 2013c).

ADVANCED NURSING EDUCATION AND CAREER PROGRESSION

The MHS places great importance on advanced nursing education. During war, health care continues to evolve based on the nature of combat as well as the challenges posed by working in the austere environments characteristic of the battlefield (Spencer & Favand, 2006). Military nurses must possess the advanced practice specialty skills needed during conflict. Additionally, master's degrees are required to be obtained before being promoted to more senior military ranks. Professional growth and development is continuously provided throughout a nurse's career in the MHS by way of leadership experiences, on-the-job training, and continuing education. A variety of educational programs, including postgraduate opportunities, are available. Full funding, in addition to continuing to receive full salary and benefits, is provided for nurses earning advanced practice degrees as well as those pursuing doctoral studies. The armed services are committed to advancing military nursing science to optimize the health of military members and their families. Graduate education in civilian programs is available for selected promising nurse researchers. Additionally, to further advance the nursing research needs of the MHS, in 1992 Congress established the TriService Nursing Research Program (TSNRP), which is the only program funding and supporting rigorous scientific research in the field of military nursing (Duong et al., 2005).

TSNRP funds a wide range of studies to advance military nursing science. For example, in 2011 a pilot study was conducted to determine the sensitivity and specificity of small animal positron emission tomography-computed tomography (PET-CT) in identifying metabolic changes in muscle tissue surrounding simulated shrapnel injuries, and comparing this imaging with traditional x-ray images. Results showed the PET-CT to be more sensitive in identifying tissue changes. Military nurses now have a unique opportunity to educate patients and military health care providers, as well as to inform policy changes, about the possibility of early tissue changes around embedded shrapnel fragments and the use of PET-CT imaging as a possible surveillance tool. Another study supported by TSNRP in 2010 sought to understand how posttraumatic stress symptoms (PTSS) affect couple functioning in Army soldiers returning from combat. Findings included that almost 50% of couples had at least one person in the relationship with a high level of PTSS. Based on these results, development of interventions and policies designed to mitigate, or even prevent, negative outcomes such as divorce, violence, and suicide for military couples facing combat deployment are under way (TSNRP, 2013).

The VHA, like the MHS, also places great emphasis on the role of advanced practice nurses and currently employs approximately 5300 (4267 NPs, 533

CNSs, and 500 CRNAs) (U.S. Department of Veterans Affairs Office of Nursing Services, 2010; United States Government Accountability Office, 2008) to deliver care. The VHA also recognizes the importance of providing educational benefits for nurses, thus permitting them to participate in graduate education. Additionally, VHA facilities provide some of the best platforms for clinical education and experience which many nurses use in their advanced studies (Caroselli, 2011). For example, VHA health care facilities provide a broad spectrum of primary, medical, surgical, behavioral health and rehabilitative care, and diagnostic services that serve as excellent clinical training sites. The VHA has also established the VHA Nursing Academy to address the growing national shortage of nurses. Although not a nursing school, the Academy establishes partnerships with academic institutions to expand the number of nursing faculty, enhance the professional and scholarly development of nurses, and increase student enrollment in nursing programs. For instance, advanced practice nurses and nurse researchers from the VHA serve as clinical instructors and faculty. The Academy provides excellent experiences for nurses and thus serves as a recruitment source. Following graduation, many nurses seek employment at VHA hospitals to focus on the health care needs of veterans (Caroselli, 2011; U.S. Department of Veterans Affairs, 2012).

CONTEMPORARY POLICY ISSUES INVOLVING MHS AND VHA NURSES

POSTTRAUMATIC STRESS DISORDER

The problem of posttraumatic stress disorders in veterans has existed for centuries; however, the condition is attracting high levels of current attention caused by the conflicts in Iraq and Afghanistan and the disorder now impacts up to 22% of veterans (Johnson et al., 2013; Murray & Garbutt, 2012; Sabella, 2012). VHA and MHS nurses, along with their behavioral health counterparts, have collaboratively developed evidence-based guidelines on assessment and effective treatments which include

multiple treatment modalities such as trauma-focused psychotherapies (e.g., exposure therapy), anxiety management, stress reduction, guided imagery, relaxation techniques, cognitive processing and behavioral therapy, and social support (Johnson et al., 2013; Murray & Garbutt, 2012; Murray & Smith, 2013; Sabella, 2012).

Current policies highlight requirements related to the timely assessment, treatment, and follow-up care of PTSD in both DoD and VHA clinical settings (U.S. Department of Veterans Affairs & Department of Defense, 2010). However, most military service members and veterans do not seek treatment for PTSD because of stigma, barriers to care, and negative perceptions associated with receiving mental health care (Hoge, 2011; Murray & Garbutt, 2012; U.S. Department of Veterans Affairs & Department of Defense, 2010). Policy issues requiring high priority include better understanding of the barriers to low mental health service use in the MHS and VHA (Hoge, 2011). Nurses are highly instrumental in understanding obstacles to care as well as working to develop and implement collaborative care models to increase outreach to veterans in need of mental health services.

SEXUAL ASSAULT

Although the DoD and VHA continue to address military sexual trauma (MST; sexual assault or repeated, threatening sexual harassment that occurs during military service) and to describe what is being done to tackle this issue, many members of Congress believe there is an epidemic in the armed forces. It is estimated that 6.1% of women and 1.2% of men serving in the armed forces experienced and reported unwanted sexual contact in 2012. These numbers are believed to be much higher given that incidents go unreported as a result of fear of retaliation which could impact careers and the lack of trust that appropriate action will be taken against the offender (Johnson et al., 2013). Most experiences (67%) happened at work on military installations (Department of Defense, 2012). This is not a new issue for the military. For over two decades senior military officials and members of Congress have proposed recommendations to address sexual assault and harassment. Despite these efforts, the incidence of such events continues to increase annually. This creates substantial financial and emotional cost that affects several generations of veterans and lasts long after a victim leaves the military. At this point, the VHA picks up the costs associated with a variety of physical and mental health problems (primarily posttraumatic stress disorder and depression), which sexual assault and harassment can trigger.

In 2013, Congress required a response to this ongoing problem. NDAA 2013 mandated immediate policy changes to include investigation of all occurrences of sexual misconduct, requiring an independent review of all legal proceedings and investigations surrounding MST, and improving victim protections and reporting policies (U.S. Department of Defense, 2013). VHA mental health providers, including nurses, are developing and evaluating therapies specific to MST. Furthermore, nurses are using telehealth technology to reach out to veterans in remote areas of the country.

SUICIDE

Veteran suicide in the United States continues to remain an underreported epidemic and the most critical health issue facing the MHS and VHA. It is estimated that approximately one service veteran dies by suicide every hour (Murray & Smith, 2013). Veteran suicide rates have been reported to be as high as 20 per 100,000 people, or almost twice that of the United States in general (Murray & Smith, 2013; U.S. Department of Veterans Affairs, 2012). Several factors are associated with these alarming numbers. For example, many veterans suffer from comorbid mental health disorders such as PTSD, depression, impulsive behaviors, and substance abuse (Sher, Braquehais, & Casas, 2012). Suicide risk is also greater in veterans experiencing relationship problems, social isolation, difficulty reintegrating into the civilian community, and financial difficulties related to unemployment (Murray & Smith, 2013).

Efforts must be expanded to connect more veterans to the mental health resources needed to combat any suicidal tendencies. Concerns about confidentiality, stigma associated with mental illness, and limited availability of mental health services in some locations continue to be the major barriers to veterans seeking appropriate mental health care (Merlis, 2012). Another problem is delayed access to care. It is VHA policy that veterans seeking mental health care are seen within 14 days. The reality is that the wait for many is closer to 50 days on average before treatment is received. Although backlog has been identified as an issue, a greater problem is scheduling procedures not being followed. Instead of veterans receiving an appointment within 14 days, they are oftentimes given the next available appointment, which could be months away, placing a veteran's well-being at risk (Office of the Inspector General, 2012).

The MHS and VHA continually strive to improve upon suicide prevention programs. Current priorities include a national suicide prevention hotline with free access to trained counselors 24 hours a day, 7 days a week, 365 days a year (Figure 39-2). Since 2007, response has been provided to more than 825,000 callers with more than 28,000 lifesaving rescues. In 2009, the VHA initiated an anonymous on-line chat service. To date, this service has provided help to more than 94,000 individuals (U.S. Department of Veterans Affairs, 2013d). The hotline and online chat system are just two approaches within a more comprehensive plan developed by the VHA to prevent suicide but are not enough to tackle the problem since not all veterans are aware of the hotline, on-line chat, and other available mental health services (U.S. Department of Veterans Affairs, 2013d). VHA nurses are working to provide outreach programs to educate

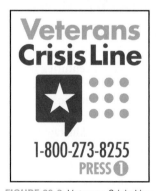

FIGURE 39-2 Veterans Crisis Line.

veterans and their families about the Veterans Crisis Line and online chat as well as collaborating with communities and partner groups nationwide (e.g., community-based organizations, Veteran Service Organizations, and local health care providers) to spread the word about the mental health services available through the VHA (Johnson et al., 2013; Mason & Schwartz, 2014).

Treatment plans for veterans who have suicidal thoughts and behaviors include somatic therapies (e.g., medications) as well as psychosocial and psychotherapies (e.g., cognitive behavioral processing). Equally important is addressing the spectrum of challenges confronting veterans. Although many are related to mental health, others include difficulties with reintegrating into family and community life as well as finding employment (Murray & Smith, 2013).

ACCESS TO CARE

More recently, it has come to light that access to care for veterans is worse than previously thought. In May 2014, the Veterans Affairs (VA) Inspector General began to investigate patient wait times and scheduling practices on the basis of concerns that veterans were not receiving timely care. Preliminary findings showed that systemic patient safety issues and possible wrongful deaths occurred as a result of gross mismanagement of resources, unethical behavior, and possible criminal misconduct by VHA senior hospital leadership. Before the 2014 investigation, a 2013 U.S. Government Accountability Office (GAO) report determined that at least 50 veterans experienced delayed gastroenterology consultations for colon cancer, some of whom later died of the disease. Findings such as this provided evidence that delayed access to health care is associated with negative health outcomes (Chokshi, 2014), and these scheduling practices are not in compliance with VHA policy (U.S Department of Veteran Affairs Office of the Inspector General, 2014). Kizer and Jha (2014) noted that almost 20 years ago the VHA had to implement sweeping reforms to increase both quality and accountability. The reforms of the 1990s improved quality and increased access and efficiency (Kizer & Jha, 2014). The successes of the past reforms in the VHA

provide clear evidence that the problems are fixable (Kizer & Jha, 2014) and new reforms are again needed to fix current challenges. One such attempt at reform is the VA Management Accountability Act of 2014, which has passed the U.S. House of Representatives and gives the Secretary of the VA greater authority to fire senior administrators. In addition, Senator Bernie Sanders (I-VT) along with John McCain (R-AZ) introduced a bipartisan comprehensive bill that supports veterans having access to community as well a federal health care providers. The bill also provides emergency funding for the VHA to hire more physicians, nurses, and other health care workers.

POST-DEPLOYMENT HEALTH-RELATED NEEDS

During World War II, the likelihood of surviving battlefield injuries was approximately 70%; during the Vietnam War survivability improved to 76%; and survival of service members wounded in the wars in Iraq and Afghanistan has increased to over 90%. Greater survivability is related in part to advances in medical care, improved protective gear (e.g., Kevlar vests), new medications (e.g., clotting agents), and significantly improved medical evacuation transport systems so that the wounded receive emergency surgeries within 30 to 90 minutes of injury. Despite these good survivability statistics, injured service members have significant physical, emotional, and cognitive injuries requiring attention for decades afterward (Manring et al., 2009; Tanielian & Jaycox, 2008).

Posttraumatic stress disorder, depression, and traumatic brain injury continue to be high-level policy interests for the MHS and VHA because these health-related issues often go unrecognized (Merlis, 2012). Additionally, a gap remains in the state of the science related to traumatic brain injury and the most effective way to address this problem (Murray & Chaffee, 2011; Tanielian & Jaycox, 2008). Each of these conditions has wide-ranging and harmful consequences if untreated. Employment, family relationships, social functioning, and parenting are severely impacted. Additionally, recurring problems such as substance abuse, homelessness, and suicide can occur. These invisible wounds of war will continue to require high priority to ensure they are appropriately recognized. Effort is needed to ensure policies and programs are consistent across the military services, within the VHA, and in collaboration with the civilian sector if they are to realize care-seeking behaviors and result in improvements in the delivery of high quality care for veterans (Tanielian & Jaycox, 2008). Policy discussions at the national congressional level are essential to determine if the MHS and VHA have the capacity to address the needs of the veteran population and how non-VHA health care settings can help address the rapidly growing needs of America's veterans (Johnson et al., 2013).

Additionally, the American Academy of Nursing has created an awareness campaign as another avenue to improve health care for veterans. Have You Ever Served? encourages all health care providers to identify veterans in their patient population to ensure they receive the appropriate type and level of care for military-related conditions (Collins, Wilmoth, & Schwartz, 2013). See Box 39-1 for more information on Have Your Ever Served?.

SEAMLESS TRANSITION

Although major strides have been made in tertiary care, little progress has been made with reentry of veterans into the civilian world. The lack of seamless transition and continuity of care from MHS to VHA care continues to be an ongoing challenge faced by veterans and has received considerable

---

BOX 39-1 Have You Ever Served?

by Diana J. Mason

Despite the crisis that occurred in the spring of 2014 over excessive wait times for veterans seeking care in the VHA system, and cover-ups by administrators at some VHA health care facilities (Veterans Health Administration, 2014), VHA clinicians are nonetheless experts in assessing and managing health conditions that arise from service-related exposures and injuries. These exposures vary by service period, location, and role the veteran played.

The 2014 crisis resulted in calls for increasing veterans' access to care in the private sector. Only about one fourth of veterans receive their care in the VHA health system with the remainder either not accessing any care or getting it from the private sector. A 2011 survey of community mental health and primary care providers revealed that only about 44% ask their patients whether they are veterans (Kilpatrick et al., 2011). Linda Schwartz, PhD, RN, FAAN, U.S. Assistant Secretary of Veteran Affairs for Policy and Planning, has noted that veterans may present to clinicians in the private sector with symptoms that clinicians may not recognize as service-related. As a result, veterans can live in chronic pain or be misdiagnosed for years.

As part of First Lady Michelle Obama's Joining Forces initiative *(www.whitehouse.gov/joiningforces)*, the American Academy of Nursing developed an initiative to increase clinicians' awareness of the importance of assessing every patient's veteran status, including whether the patient is a child of a veteran, since some exposures during war can cause genetic changes for offspring and some families have been exposed to toxins on military bases. The initiative is called "Have You Ever Served in the Military?" and aims to have all clinicians ask patients, "Have you ever served? If so, when and where did you serve and what did you do?" In addition, the initiative aims to embed in the electronic health record an algorithm that begins with this question and then links the responses to potential exposures, symptoms, and health problems.

The initiative was endorsed by the National Association of State Directors for Veteran Affairs. More information about the initiative can be found at *www.haveyoueverserved.com*.

References

Kilpatrick, D. G., Best, C. L., Smith, D. W., Kudler, H., & Cornelison-Grant, V. (2011). *Educational needs of health care providers working with military members, veterans and their families*. Charleston, SC: Medical University of South Carolina Department of Psychiatry.

Veterans Health Administration. (2014). Interim report: review of patient wait times, scheduling practices, and alleged patient deaths at the *Phoenix Health Care System*. Retrieved from <www.va.gov/oig/pubs/VAOIG -14-02603-178.pdf>.

congressional attention. In fact, it is estimated that only 52% of service members transitioning their care successfully make their way into the VHA system (Merlis, 2012). Many of these veterans wait for almost 1 year to gain access to the VHA because of backlog related to the vast number of claims for care, changing policies to cover a broader type of claims, and the continuing need to digitize paper health records (Bresnick, 2013). Even more troublesome, many veterans are not even being placed on wait lists. Compliance with VHA policy is needed to mitigate further access delays to health care services, which veterans have earned and deserve (U.S Department of Veteran Affairs Office of the Inspector General, 2014).

In 2008, Congress mandated that the DoD and VHA jointly develop a comprehensive management and transition policy to ensure service members received seamless behavioral health care. In response DoD and the VHA collaboratively developed an inTransition program. In this program service members are assigned a support coach, an experienced, licensed behavioral health provider, who is responsible for providing individual assistance with mental health support during the transition process. The support coach serves as a bridge to provide help between behavioral health care systems and providers. InTransition is not case management. The program is designed to assist the service member during the transition period only by encouraging the individual to continue their behavioral health care. The VHA provides a case manager who monitors the veteran over time. The program serves as an added resource to care delivered by health care providers and case managers (Office of the Assistant Secretary of Defense, 2010).

Finally, DoD and the VHA were charged with developing an integrated, interoperable electronic health record (EHR) which could be used by both agencies (Merlis, 2012). The VHA and MHS currently keep entirely different records, making it difficult for health care information to be shared and transferred when a service member transitions to the VHA. However, efforts to develop a mutually agreed upon interoperable, integrated EHR have come to a standstill because of disagreements regarding how to merge systems (Bresnick, 2013).

CONCLUSION

As our nation faces an increasing need to provide health care to military service members, policymakers will need to provide continuous support to strengthen the MHS and VHA. Although both health care systems function in parallel and in conjunction with each other, greater attention needs to focus on ensuring that service members transitioning from the MHS to the VHA do so in a seamless manner.

DISCUSSION QUESTIONS

1. Are current MHS and VHA policies effective in addressing the needs of military service members and veterans?
2. What major policy issues do the MHS and VHA most need to address to improve health care services for veterans?
3. What major reforms are needed within the VHA to improve health care for veterans?

REFERENCES

Beasley, K. (2012). Innovative solutions will reduce DOD health care costs. Retrieved from *www.moaa.org/uploadedFiles/MOAA_Main/Main_Menu/Take_Action/Top_Issues/Innovative%20Solutions.pdf.*

Bresnick, J. (2013). VA contractor digitizes benefits backlog, talks joint HER. Retrieved from *ehrintelligence.com/2013/07/10/va-contractor-digitizes-benefits-backlog-talks-joint-ehr/.*

Caroselli, C. (2011). The Veterans Administration Health System: An overview of major policy issues. In D. J. Mason, J. K. Leavitt, & M. W. Chaffee (Eds.), *Policy & politics in nursing and health care.* St. Louis, MO: Elsevier.

Chokshi, D. A. (2014). Improving health care for veterans—A watershed moment for the VHA. Retrieved from *www.nejm.org/doi/full/10.1056/NEJMp1406868.*

Collins, E., Wilmoth, M., & Schwartz, W. (2013). "Have You Ever Served in the Military?" Campaign in partnership with the Joining Forces Initiative. *Nursing Outlook, 61*(5), 375–376. doi:10.1016/j.outlook.2013.07.004.

Department of Defense. (2012). Department of Defense annual report on sexual assault in the military. Retrieved from *www.ncdsv.org/images/DOD_Annual-report-on-sexual-assault-in-the-military-FY2012_Exec Summ_5-7-2013.pdf.*

Duong, D. N., Schempp, C., Barker, E., Cupples, S., Pierce, P., Ryan-Wenger, N., et al. (2005). Developing military nursing research priorities. *Military Medicine, 170*(5), 362–365.

Government Accountability Office [GAO]. (2012). Defense health care: Applying key management practices should help achieve efficiencies within the military health system. Retrieved from *www.gao.gov/assets/600/590090.pdf.*

Hoge, C. W. (2011). Interventions for war-related post-traumatic stress disorder: Meeting veterans where they are. *Journal of the American Medical Association, 306*(5), 549–551. doi:10.1001/jama.2011.1096.

Johnson, B. S., Boudiab, L. D., Freundl, M., Anthony, M., Gmerek, G. B., & Carter, J. (2013). Enhancing veteran-centered care: A guide for nurses in non-VHA settings. *American Journal of Nursing, 113*(7), 24–39.

The Kaiser Foundation. (2012). Military and veterans' health care. Retrieved from www.kaiseredu.org/Issue-Modules/Military-and-Veterans-Health-Care/Background-Brief.aspx. doi:10.1097/01.NAJ.0000431913.50226.83.

Kizer, K. W., & Jha, A. K. (2014). Restoring trust in VHA health care. Retrieved from www.nejm.org/doi/full/10.1056/NEJMp1406852.

Manring, M. M., Hawk, A., Calhoun, J. H., & Andersen, R. C. (2009). Treatment of war wounds: A historical review. *Clinical Orthopaedics and Related Research, 467*(8), 2168–2191. doi:10.1007/s11999-009-0738-5.

Mason, D. J., & Schwartz, L. (2014). To the Editor New York Times: Veterans' health care, under scrutiny. Retrieved from www.nytimes.com/2014/05/23/opinion/veterans-health-care-under-scrutiny.html?ref=todayspaper&_r=1.

Merlis, M. (2012). The future of health care for military personnel and veterans. Retrieved from www.academyhealth.org/files/publications/AHMilitaryVetBrief2012.pdf.

Murray, J. S. (2009). Joint task force national capital region medical: Integration of education, training & research. *Military Medicine, 174*(5), 448–454.

Murray, J. S. (2010). Walter Reed National Military Medical Center: Simulation on the cutting edge. *Military Medicine, 175*(9), 659–663.

Murray, J. S., & Chaffee, M. W. (2011). The U.S. Military Health System: Policy challenges in wartime and peacetime. In D. J. Mason, J. K. Leavitt, & M. W. Chaffee (Eds.), *Policy & politics in nursing and health care.* St. Louis, MO: Elsevier.

Murray, J. S., & Garbutt, S. (2012). Meeting the health care needs of America's military veterans. Retrieved from ce.nurse.com/.

Murray, J. S., & Smith, D. (2013). Veteran suicide: Addressing the intensifying battle. Retrieved from ce.nurse.com/content/ce695/veteran-suicide/.

Office of the Assistant Secretary of Defense. (2010). HA Policy: 10-001: Department of Defense *inTransition* Program. Retrieved from www.health.mil/libraries/HA_Policies_and_Guidelines/10-001.pdf.

Office of the Inspector General. (2012). Veterans Health Administration: Review of veterans' access to mental health care. Retrieved from www.va.gov/oig/pubs/VAOIG-12-00900-168.pdf.

Office of the Under Secretary of Defense. (2013). Overview: United States Department of Defense fiscal year 2014 budget request. Retrieved from comptroller.defense.gov/budget.html.

Sabella, D. (2012). PTSD among our returning veterans: How to recognize and assist veterans with this increasingly common mental health disorder. *American Journal of Nursing, 112*(11), 48–52. doi:10.1097/01.NAJ.0000422255.95706.40.

Sher, L., Braquehais, M. D., & Casas, M. (2012). Post-traumatic stress disorder, depression, and suicide in veterans. *Cleveland Clinic Journal of Medicine, 79*(2), 92–97.

Spencer, B., & Favand, L. (2006). Nursing care on the battlefield. Retrieved from www.americannursetoday.com/article.aspx?id=5138.

Tanielian, T., & Jaycox, L. H. (2008). Invisible wounds of war: Psychological and cognitive injuries, their consequences, and services to assist recovery. Retrieved from www.rand.org/content/dam/rand/pubs/monographs/2008/RAND_MG720.pdf.

TriService Nursing Research Program [TSNRP]. (2013). Funded studies. Retrieved from www.usuhs.mil/tsnrp/FundedStudies/funded.php.

U.S. Department of Defense. (2013a). Department of Defense annual report on sexual assault in the military. Retrieved from www.sapr.mil/media/pdf/reports/FY12_DoD_SAPRO_Annual_Report_on_Sexual_Assault-volume_two.pdf.

U.S. Department of Defense. (2013b). Sexual Assault Prevention and Response (SAPR) Program. Retrieved from www.sapr.mil/public/docs/directives/649501p.pdf.

U.S. Department of Veterans Affairs & Department of Defense. (2010). VHA/DoD clinical practice guideline for the management of post-traumatic stress. Retrieved from www.healthquality.va.gov/ptsd/CPGSummaryFINALMgmtofPTSDfinal021413.pdf.

U.S. Department of Veterans Affairs Office of Nursing Services. (2010). About the office of nursing services. Retrieved from www.va.gov/NURSING/About_ONS.asp.

U.S. Department of Veterans Affairs. (2012). VA Nursing Academy. Retrieved from www.va.gov/oaa/vana/.

U.S. Department of Veterans Affairs. (2013a). About the VHA. Retrieved from www.va.gov/health/aboutVHA.asp.

U.S. Department of Veterans Affairs. (2013b). Funding highlights: The budget for fiscal year 2013. Retrieved from www.whitehouse.gov/sites/default/files/omb/budget/fy2013/assets/veterans.pdf.

U.S. Department of Veterans Affairs. (2013c). Veterans Health Administration: Federal funds for medical services. Retrieved from www.whitehouse.gov/sites/default/files/omb/budget/fy2013/assets/vet.pdf.

U.S. Department of Veterans Affairs. (2013d). Veterans crisis line. Retrieved from www.mentalhealth.va.gov/suicide_prevention/.

U.S. Department of Veterans Affairs Office of the Inspector General. (2014). Review of patient wait times, scheduling practices, and alleged patient deaths at the Phoenix health care system. Retrieved from www.va.gov/oig/pubs/VAOIG-14-02603-178.pdf.

United States Government Accountability Office. (2008). Recruitment and retention challenges and efforts to make salaries competitive for nurse anesthetists. Retrieved from www.gao.gov/assets/120/119575.pdf.

U.S. Senate Committee on Appropriations. (2012). Hearing on Defense Department Health Programs. Retrieved from www.appropriations.senate.gov/ht-defense.cfm?method=hearings.view&id=de73767a-6390-484e-9281-ef68d4fd1343.

ONLINE RESOURCES

American Academy of Nursing "Have You Ever Served in the Military?" campaign
www.haveyoueverserved.com
Defense Centers of Excellence for Psychological Health and Traumatic Brain Injury
www.dcoe.health.mil
Military Health System
www.health.mil
National Center for PTSD
www.ptsd.va.gov/about
Veterans Health Administration
www.va.gov/health
inTransitions Program
www.health.mil/inTransition

CHAPTER 40

Contemporary Issues in Government

Deborah B. Gardner

"At every stage, and under all circumstances, the essence of the struggle is to equalize opportunity, destroy privilege, and give to the life and citizenship of every individual the highest possible value both to himself and to the commonwealth. That is nothing new."

Teddy Roosevelt

CONTEMPORARY ISSUES IN GOVERNMENT

Tremendous pressures face our government at national, state, and local levels. We have entered an age where the gap between rich and poor is rapidly widening. Prospects for federal legislative remedies to most political issues appear slim. Political dysfunction in Washington, DC has pushed responsibility for hard choices down to the states, both red and blue, exacerbating the differences between them (Holland, 2014). The public has taken notice of these trends and their opinion of Washington leadership is at an all-time low (Gallup, 2014). Almost two thirds of the public believe their government is controlled by a handful of powerful interests. Confidence in the Courts as a check on abuses of power and defender of the public interest is divided (Pew Research Center, 2013).

Against this backdrop, the story of the United States' historic health care reform is still unfolding.

Predictably, implementation of the Affordable Care Act (ACA) has sparked numerous controversies. This chapter highlights how the economics of health care legislation are interrelated with many federal and state issues. The interconnected policy issues presented include fiscal policy or budgetary spending and debt management, demographic shifts, immigration reform, economic inequality, and climate change. The simple nature of media sound bites and Twitter feeds fails to adequately capture or educate the public regarding the complexity of the issues facing U.S. policymakers and citizens. To help close this knowledge gap for nurses and other health care providers, it is critical to examine how the current political climate impacts decision making on these complex national policy issues and undermines public trust in the democratic process.

THE CENTRAL BUDGET STORY

Politicians and the media often focus on the U.S. annual budget as *the* key issue regarding the fiscal health of our country. This focus obscures many of the underlying issues and masks the fact that politicians are avoiding hard choices about what programs to cut or taxes to levy. At present, while government spending increases, many programs are experiencing deep funding cuts. Why? The basic reason is that costs for entitlement programs are

335

increasing leaving less money for discretionary spending. Projections suggest that over the next decade growth in government spending will be directed at caring for an increasingly large and politically powerful older adult population (Figure 40-1). As baby boomers age, retire, and live longer, the number of Social Security, Medicare, and Medicaid beneficiaries continue to grow. This growth will place increasing pressure on the federal budget. In conjunction with these factors, the ratio of U.S. workers supporting every Social Security recipient diminished from the 1940s ratio of 159 workers for every recipient to fewer than three workers in 2014 (Social Security Online, 2014). Between 2014 and 2024, the number of Social Security beneficiaries is projected to increase three times as fast as the number of workers paying taxes to support the program (Congressional Budget Office [CBO], 2014b).

Despite the ACA showing initial cost savings, Medicare, Medicaid, and Children's Health Insurance Program (CHIP) costs are expected to rise (CBO, 2014b). By 2024, spending on Social Security, health care, and interest payments on the national debt will leave less than 8% of the national income available to pay for all other discretionary needs: defense, education, medical research, and transportation (CBO, 2014a) (Figure 40-2). As a result, the government's ability to respond to other national problems and priorities is increasingly being compromised. This reality has been called the central budget story (Samuelson, 2014).

The impact of such cost-cutting decisions is felt strongly at both state and local levels. This will be a hard trend to reverse as the constituencies for mandatory benefits, led by Social Security's 57 million, are more numerous and powerful than other interest groups needing federal support. Politicians from both parties are loath to take on reforming Social Security and Medicare, in particular, because of their stakeholders. In his testimony before Congress in 2014, Douglas Elmendorf, the director of the nonpartisan CBO, noted there are various ways to proceed (Elmendorf, 2014):

So we have a choice as a society to either scale back those programs relative to what is promised under current law; or to raise tax revenue above its historical average to pay for the expansion of those programs; or to cut back on all other spending even more sharply than we already are. ... They tend to be unpleasant in one way or another, and we have not, as a society, decided how much of that sort of unpleasantness to inflict on whom. But some combination of those three choices will be needed. (Jones, 2014)

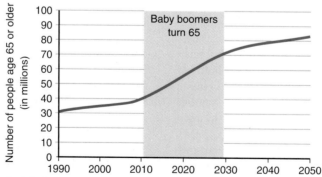

FIGURE 40-1 The aging of the baby boom generation will boost the number of Americans age 65 or older. The highlighted period represents the timespan between the oldest and the youngest of the baby boom generation reaching 65. (From U.S. Census Bureau. *Historical national intercensal estimates and 2012 national population projections.* Compiled as part of the Peter G. Peterson Foundation analysis, "CBO's New Budget Projection Shows More Action Needed to Tame Debt and Deficits," released February 2014. Retrieved from *pgpf.org/Chart-Archive/0181_aging_baby_boom.*)

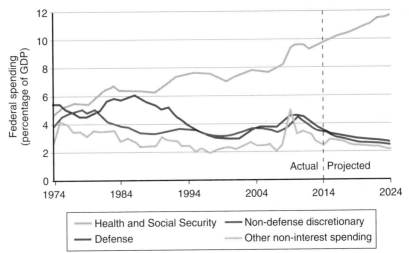

FIGURE 40-2 Health and Social Security are the major drivers of non-interest spending. Health programs include Medicare (net of offsetting receipts), Medicaid, Children's Health Insurance Program, and health insurance subsidies for the exchanges. (From Congressional Budget Office. [2014, February]. The budget and economic outlook: Fiscal years 2014 to 2024; Office of Management and Budget. [2013, April]. *Budget of the United States government, fiscal year 2014*; and Bureau of Economic Analysis. [2014, January]. *National income and product accounts tables*. Compiled by PGPF.)

FISCAL POLICY AND POLITICAL EXTREMISM

One of the key responsibilities of Congress is to pass an annual budget that funds the government. Budgets are the linchpin of economic policy because decisions on how revenues are spent to meet the country's competing needs, such as providing a strong defense, funding education, and improving the health care system, validate political commitments (International Budget Partnership, 2014). As with all budgets, deficits and debt are of key importance to this decision making (Box 40-1).

Since the Great Recession of 2008, budget debates have dominated congressional activity. Conflicts over the powers to tax, spend, and borrow have always been at the heart of American politics. However, since 2009, rigid posturing, caustic rhetoric, and costly political actions taken regarding the federal deficit and national debt have made a compromise over the annual budget unachievable. This has resulted in Continuing Resolutions (CRs), bills that simply continue preexisting appropriations, becoming the norm.

Political tensions over the budget rose to a new level in 2011. The Republican-led House (with strong Tea Party influence) threatened to vote against raising the debt ceiling and to shut down the government if a long-term plan was not developed to further reduce the budget deficit. Legislative agreement was reached in a last-minute deal, but the delay in voting to raise the debt ceiling led to a downgrade in the credit rating of the United States for the first time in history (Kogan, 2012).

It is important to note some facts regarding this fiscal battle. There is a significant difference between a government shutdown and not increasing the debt ceiling. In a government shutdown, day-to-day operations are frozen. Government agencies are forced to stop or reduce functioning; for example, federal workers are furloughed, losing productivity and tax dollars (Klein, 2013a). However, failing to raise the debt ceiling is even more devastating. In this situation, the federal government can no longer pay any of its employees' salaries or benefits. Those receiving Social Security, Medicare, and Medicaid payments would go without. Federal services would grind to a halt. Failing to increase the debt ceiling could result in the Treasury either defaulting on

---

BOX 40-1 Budget Basics

- **Mandatory Spending** is federal spending based on existing laws rather than the budgeting process. For instance, spending for Social Security and Medicare is based on the eligibility rules for that program. Mandatory spending or entitlement programs are not part of the annual appropriations process.
- **Discretionary Spending** is the portion of the budget that the President requests and Congress appropriates every year. Examples include education, defense, and the Environmental Protection Agency.
- The **fiscal year** is the accounting period of the federal government. It begins on October 1 and ends on September 30 of the next calendar year. For example, FY 2014 began October 1, 2013 and ends September 30, 2014.
- **Revenues**, also known as receipts, are the funds collected from the public. Most of the federal government's revenues consists of receipts from individual income taxes, social insurance (payroll) taxes, and corporate income taxes.
- The **Federal or Budget Deficit** is the amount of spending (outlays) that exceeds total revenues (income) in *1* fiscal year. (From Congressional Research Service 7-5700 [*www.crs.gov 98-410*].)
- The **National Debt** is the total amount of money the federal government owes and the result of *accumulated budget deficits* over the years. The link between the budget deficit and national debt is that a large part of deficit bills is incurred through previous tax and spending policies that created deficits and long-term debts in the first place.
- The **Debt Limit**, also known as the debt ceiling, is how much total debt the government can accumulate or owe. Raising the debt limit enables the government to pay for things it has legally committed to funding in the past. Raising the debt limit does not authorize new spending commitments.

Sources: Amadeo, K. (n.d.). *Discretionary fiscal policy: Budget, taxation and how it differs from monetary policy. Retrieved from usecomony.about.com/od/glossary/g/discretionary.htm;* Amadeo, K. (n.d.). U.S. debt ceiling. What it is, and what happens if it's not raised? Retrieved from *usecomony.about.com/od/glossary/g/discretionary.htm*

U.S. debt or paying it late. The dollar value would plummet and a destabilization of financial markets felt across the world. Either scenario undermines the trust that the American people, other nations, banks, and businesses place in the U.S. government honoring its financial obligations (U.S. Department of the Treasury, 2013). This may be at least one reason why no other major industrialized nation sets a total debt limit on its central government (Ruffing & Stone, 2013).

2013 DEBT CEILING CRISIS: CONTINUED POLITICAL DYSFUNCTION

Although a legislative agreement was reached to avert the 2011 debt ceiling crisis (The Budget Control Act of 2011, Public Law 112-25, S.365, 125 Stat. 240), it was far from congenial. The legislation included a package of automatic spending cuts (known as sequestration) that would begin in 2013 if an annual budget compromise could not be reached. While the intent of the Act was to force Congress to compromise on budget funding choices, this was not the outcome. In 2013, both a debt ceiling crisis and a shutdown were on the table once again (Khimm, 2012).

Known as the United States Fiscal Cliff, the controversy over defunding the ACA resulted in a 16-day federal shutdown. Standard & Poor's, a national financial rating agency, estimated the cost of this shutdown at $24 billion (Johnson, 2013). A CR for fiscal year (FY) 2014 was passed in December of 2013. Then, in January, after a bipartisan compromise was reached, a budget was finally approved. This agreement ended the last-minute, crisis-driven budget battles that had consumed Congress for much of the previous 3 years (Krasney, 2013). Historically, the debt ceiling has been raised with little controversy between Congress and the President (Amadeo, n.d.a). Thus, what may sound like politics as usual to those who do not closely follow national policy actually represents a new type of challenge for policy agreement and implementation.

THE CURRENT BUDGET DEFICIT

The year 2014 was the fifth consecutive year in which the deficit has declined as a share of gross domestic product (GDP) since peaking at 9.8% in 2009; it is projected to decline further in 2015. The Congressional Budget Office (CBO) estimates that the 2014 deficit will equal 3% of the nation's economic output, or GDP—close to the average seen during the past 40 years (CBO, 2014a).

Although the budget deficit is decreasing, there is concern that deficits will start to rise again after 2015. Should deficits grow, either additional debt or hotly disputed spending cuts and tax hikes will be required. Timely action will need to be taken. Thus work must be done to put fiscal policy on a sustainable course. According to former Senator Alan Simpson (R-WY), co-chair of the presidential debt commission created in 2010, "The tragic part of it is, all the anguish we're going through isn't dealing with two-thirds of the American budget" (Kuhnhenn, 2014). Barring reform, these programs will be forced to reduce benefits.

Health professionals need to understand that in such an adversarial political climate important issues including health care reform are being marginalized rather than debated for success. In the past, the government has successfully controlled growing deficits with collaboratively developed strategies. Legislation was developed through both debate *and* compromise. Unfortunately, compromise has become a negative term. According to Mann and Ornstein (2012), authors of *It's Even Worse Than It Looks,* the budget battles are a symptom of the United States' larger problem, that of a dysfunctional political climate. Is it any surprise that the public is apathetic and discouraged?

HOW WILL THE NATION'S ECONOMIC HEALTH BE ADDRESSED?

While Republicans voice alarm over large deficits and the national debt, partisan opinions remain strongly divided regarding the most effective approach to balancing the federal budget to reduce budget deficits and debt. Democrats take a traditionalist approach, which proposes a mix of spending cuts as well as increasing revenue by raising taxes and reducing tax loopholes. However, the majority of congressional Republicans have strongly

rejected the idea of raising taxes and have focused on discretionary spending cuts and reforming the large entitlement programs, such as Social Security and Medicare (Amadeo, n.d.b).

Unfortunately, both sides are guilty of having talked about these issues for more than 20 years without significantly addressing them in terms of policy change. Historically, our country has frequently operated with heavy deficits. Deficits often occur during times of war or economic downturns and, in the past, decreased military spending and stimulus packages have spurred economic recovery. But the current situation is different. The government is no longer spending to grow the economy. Instead, increased spending will be the result of rising mandatory expenses or entitlements, such as Medicare and Social Security. This spending, when combined with tax cuts and the impact of the Great Recession, makes the situation unsustainable. Can congressional leaders strike a smart compromise? As partisan posturing is being placed ahead of cooperative problem solving, the majority of U.S. citizens are not holding their breath (McCarthy, 2014).

THE IMPACT OF POLITICAL DYSFUNCTION

Unprecedented gridlock in Congress is preventing the government from getting business done, having a destructive effect on domestic and foreign policy (Hass, 2013). The Pew Research Center reported the passage of only 55 substantive bills by the 113th (2013 to 2014) Congress. That is fewer than any Congress in the 20 years since the institution began keeping such records. Substantive legislation excludes bills that are purely ceremonial legislation (e.g., post-office renamings). There is speculation that the 114th Congress could be even less productive (DeSilver, 2013). Given the negative impact on legislation, it is important to review the forces creating this power struggle.

POLARIZATION

The gridlock in Congress is often attributed to political polarization. Polarization is the idea that

Republicans and Democrats represent such disparate worldviews that the gaps between them rule out the possibility of finding a common ground. Much of the tension may lie in answering the proverbial question: What is the role of government in protecting the rights of all of its citizens? This is a question both political parties take seriously and view differently. It can certainly be found at the heart of the health care reform battle. However, political scientist Gregory Koger (2012) argues that partisanship, not polarization, is the primary cause of gridlock. He asserts that while the Republican and Democratic parties tend to nominate candidates with different views on major issues, partisan conflict in Congress is largely a strategic choice. He reframes polarization as teamwork within parties. Legislators work to restrain their internal party differences to compete with the opposing party. According to Koger (2012), rather than actually striving to make the United States a stronger nation, posturing in Congress (seeking to improve the reputation of one party at the expense of the other party) reigns supreme. This congressional partisanship has negative consequences for public policy efforts.

LOSS OF CONGRESSIONAL MODERATES

Building on Koger's argument that partisanship has become stronger, there are data that reflect a large decrease in congressional moderates. Sometimes referred to as bridge builders, moderates tend to transcend partisan politics, voting on an issue regardless of affiliation. The National Journal's 2013 vote ratings report reflects a Congress more partisan in voting than ever before (Kraushaar, 2014):

For the fourth straight year, no Senate Democrat was more conservative than a Senate Republican—and no Senate Republican was more liberal than a Senate Democrat. In the House, only two Democrats were more conservative than a Republican—and only two Republicans were more liberal than a Democrat. Contrast this lack of ideological overlap with 1994, when 34 senators and 252 House members voting

records put them between the most liberal Republican and the most conservative Democrat. (Kraushaar, 2014)

Outside conservative groups, such as the Club for Growth and the Senate Conservatives Fund, are enforcing ideologic purity among members as well as primary candidates. The move to the extreme right is clearly seen as House Speaker John Boehner faces constant revolt from a growing number of Tea Party–affiliated members. In the 2014 elections some of the most conservative senators had primary challengers from the right (Kraushaar, 2014).

GERRYMANDERING

The U.S. Constitution specifies that seats in Congress be apportioned according to the U.S. Census. Individual states create congressional districts, which then elect members of the U.S. House of Representatives. Each decade, as new census numbers are presented, redistricting occurs at the federal, state, and local levels. Gerrymandering is a negative label for redistricting. It is a process historically riddled with political finagling as politicians redraw the boundaries of electoral districts so as to create an unfair advantage for a particular political party or faction (McNamara, 2014). Both parties have participated in this practice since the process began, but the influence of gerrymandering on election outcomes over the past decade has renewed concern. For instance, despite the Democratic support that brought President Barack Obama to a second term in 2012, Republicans achieved a 33-seat majority in the House. This was a significant achievement given that Republican candidates, as a group, received 1.4 million *fewer* votes than their Democratic opponents. It is only the second time since World War II that the party receiving the most votes failed to win a majority of House seats (Ohlemacher, 2014).

It is also argued that representatives from sharply gerrymandered districts feel less compelled to pay attention to broad-based public opinion, because what they are really concerned about is the opinions of their specific constituencies. While some assert that gerrymandering is a red herring (Cohn,

2013), the current focus and money spent by both parties to dominate in the redistricting progress suggest otherwise.

CONGRESSIONAL GRIDLOCK: WHERE IS THE PRESIDENT'S POWER?

So wherever and whenever I can take steps without legislation to expand opportunity for more American families, that's what I'm going to do. (Excerpt from 2014 State of the Union Address)

Throughout history, Presidents have exercised their authority by using executive orders, proclamations, and memorandums. Reasons for Presidential executive orders are: to direct government officials and agencies to take a specified action; to clarify or further existing law; to respond to an emergency, such as a natural disaster; or to bypass congressional gridlock.

In his 2014 State of the Union Address, President Obama unveiled his plan to sign an executive order raising the minimum wage of federal contractors to $10.10 per hour. He also pledged to move forward on implementing his Climate Action Plan via executive order. Republican members of Congress responded by announcing plans to challenge the legality of these executive orders (Weatherford, 2014).

The President's recess appointments have also come under fire. The Supreme Court is expected to rule on the constitutional provision that allows the President to make recess appointments of high-level government officials when the Senate is not in session (Barnes, 2014). Representative Tom Rice (R-SC) has also proposed a resolution, entitled Stop This Overreaching Presidency (STOP), directing the House of Representatives to file a civil suit to challenging the President's directive to the U.S. Department of Health and Human Services to extend health coverage that would have been terminated or cancelled as a result of provisions in the ACA (Weatherford, 2014).

The outrage voiced by conservative members of Congress at President Obama about his misuse of the executive power may be more strategic than substantive. President Obama, to date, has issued 170 executive orders since taking office in January 2009. This is fewer than most Presidents holding office in the past 100 years (Weatherford, 2014). Since the Courts have rarely invalidated an executive order, Congress is unlikely to win a legal challenge (Barnes, 2014). While the President has been targeted for his use of executive powers, nothing he has undertaken has met with more opposition that his health reform efforts.

BELEAGUERED HEALTH CARE REFORM

The Affordable Care Act (ACA) was signed into law in 2010. Yet this contentious and long-awaited legislation continues to be the focus of endless news stories. By 2014, the Republican-majority House had voted more than 54 times without success to have the ACA repealed (O'Keefe, 2014). Supreme Court challenges continue. The health reform debate has large overtones symbolic of what some have called a culture war between proponents of different visions for America's future. Leflar (2013, p. 1) aptly describes it as a "saga of polarized ideology, vicious politics, perverse economics, and a high-level legal battle against the background of a health care system in disarray." As the complex and poorly understood ACA initiatives are implemented, the ongoing criticism of the legislation has affected public perceptions. A 2014 Kaiser Family Foundation poll found that 46% of the public still holds a negative view of the law and only 38% view it favorably. However, when asked about repealing the ACA, 59% of Americans wanted to see the program improved, not repealed (Hamel, Firth, & Brodie, 2014).

Although the full impact of this legislation on the U.S. health care system is not known, the conversation regarding health care has fundamentally changed since its passage. As a highly visible national and local conversation, new expectations are being placed on a deeply entrenched health care system. Stakeholders, from patients to providers to politicians, are seeing access to care in new ways, clarifying true costs and identifying incentives to sustain successful systemic changes. The role of the federal and state governments in partnering with private partners to implement health care reform is likely to be an ongoing discussion as health care will be in a constant state of reform and modification for years to come.

IMPLEMENTATION CHALLENGES

Policy implementation involves complex regulations issued by federal agencies, such as the U.S. Departments of Health and Human Services, Labor, and the Treasury. Implementation also involves policy choices by the 50 states, with a majority of Republican governors (30) and Republican-controlled legislatures (27) (Sullivan, 2013). Among the major implementation issues are: the expansion of the Medicaid program to cover more low-income people, the formation of state exchanges (health insurance marketplaces), the establishment of an Independent Payment Advisory Board for Medicare tasked with reducing Medicare costs while retaining quality of care, the adoption of new payment models, the coverage of contraceptives as part of the essential benefits package, and the founding of the Patient-Centered Outcomes Research Institute (Leflar, 2013). These new programs at the federal and state levels are designed to improve research dissemination to enhance patient outcomes and control costs through the development of new payment models that incentivize better care coordination. They are also broadly designed to enhance access to health care and improve population health. (See Chapter 19.)

INCREASING ACCESS

The ACA, despite a rocky rollout and determined opposition from critics, has spurred the largest expansion in health coverage in America in half a century (Levey, 2014). Exclusion of patients with preexisting conditions is now a thing of the past. Curbs have been placed on insurance industry profit levels and, for the first time, millions of low-income Americans can afford to seek treatment for chronic illnesses such as cancer and diabetes. As the first deadline for coverage in 2014 passed, it was estimated that 8 million people signed up for private insurance nationally (Morgan, 2014). Three million

young people remain on their parent's health care plans (U.S. Department of Health and Human Services, 2012). More than 8 million uninsured people are eligible for Medicaid and more than 71 million additional Americans are receiving preventive services coverage (e.g., colonoscopy, flu shots) without cost sharing (Skopec & Sommers, 2013).

These gains have been achieved amid intense political resistance. Although the opposition seems unprecedented, when Medicare and Medicaid became law in 1965, President Lyndon Johnson faced the hostility of the insurance industry and the American Medical Association. Both groups declared the programs to be the start of socialized medicine. The media argued that hospitals faced unbearable burdens and predicted that older adults would flood the facilities in great numbers. Such predictions did not come to pass. Medicare, providing health insurance for all Americans over 65 years, proved popular almost immediately. After the rollout, about 19 million people signed up (Kliff, 2013b). Medicaid was harder to implement. Financed jointly by the federal government and the states, Medicaid provides medical assistance for certain individuals and families with low incomes and resources. In its first year, only 26 states agreed to participate in Medicaid. The program did not include all 50 states until 1982 (Kaiser Family Foundation, 2009).

MEDICAID EXPANSION: STATE-DRIVEN ADOPTION

Aimed at creating greater health care equity, the expansion of the Medicaid program to cover more low-income adults is one of the ACA's most notable measures. However, the number of Americans who will gain this health insurance depends on the number of states that agree to expand Medicaid coverage. Twenty-five states, the same number that originally resisted Medicaid in 1965, have chosen to opt out and refused their share of the funds (Kaiser Family Foundation, 2014). As the ACA begins to take effect, the ramifications of the Supreme Court's Medicaid ruling are becoming clearer. In states that chose to opt out of the Medicaid expansion, a coverage gap is developing. It is estimated that 5.8 million American adults living in opt-out states will not be able to obtain health insurance because they earn too little to qualify for federal exchange subsidies but too much to qualify for Medicaid (Urban Institute, 2014). The Urban Institute also found that the rate of uninsured is almost 50% higher in states that refused the expansion than in those that embraced the policy (Holland, 2014).

As reasons for opting out, states cite ideological opposition or concern that paying for even part of the expanded program will burden future state finances. "Ironically, taxpayers in states refusing to implement the Medicaid expansion (such as Texas) will be subsidizing the expansions in other states (such as Arkansas), through a portion of their federal income taxes" (Leflar, 2013, p. 8.) In fact, the state of Arkansas took a unique approach that other states may model (e.g., Iowa). Led by a Democratic governor and a Republican legislature, they expanded coverage by gaining an exemption to use federal funding to purchase insurance for new recipients from private insurance firms, rather than through a publicly run program. This hybrid Medicaid approach is appealing to many states facing similar ideologic conflicts (Kliff, 2013a). Unfortunately, this is only a partial Medicaid expansion program and federal funding will decline each year for Arkansas and likely to generate further budget battles. (See Chapter 19.)

FEDERAL INSURANCE EXCHANGE: CRASHING DEBUT

The debut of the federal exchange website, a centerpiece of the law, was riddled with problems. Labeled a debacle in the headlines, millions of Americans were left frustrated and justifiably suspicious when they tried to sign up for coverage online. The Healthcare.gov rollout was a political disaster for the President. Dr. Ezekiel Emanuel, former advisor to the White House on health care reform, diagnosed three mistakes that led to this implementation fiasco. First, that the Obama administration waited too long to release specific regulations and guidance on how the exchange would work and got a late start in building the physical website. Second, the Centers for Medicare and Medicaid Services (CMS), responsible for coordinating the project, had little expertise in creating a complex e-commerce

website. No one senior person in the agency was tasked with running the exchange rollout. Finally, CMS did not review best practice models. Massachusetts had years of experience with its exchange. States such as California, Connecticut, and Kentucky spent several years building their exchanges, gaining experience, and providing a good consumer experience (Emanuel, 2013).

Former U.S. Health and Human Services Secretary Kathleen Sebelius took responsibility for the initial failure of the Healthcare.gov website. She became the administration's point person for taking questions from Congress during October 2013 hearings. The White House called in a team of management and technology experts to fix the site. By December 2013, they had it working more or less smoothly. Secretary Sebelius officially resigned in April of 2014 and was replaced by President Obama's former budget director, Sylvia Mathews Burwell, who was confirmed without controversy (Rampton, 2014). (See Chapter 20.)

AFFORDABLE CARE ACT COSTS AND SAVINGS

While the ACA continues to spark diverse views regarding its effectiveness, everyone agrees that we have to find ways to get more health care for our health care dollars. There is reason for optimism. Recent studies suggest that Medicaid expansions are resulting in health and financial gains (Baicker et al., 2013; Sommers, Baicker, & Epstein, 2012). These studies also document an increase in the use of most health care services. The industry appears to be moving, albeit slowly, toward a system that rewards outcomes and quality, not just volume.

New estimates show that the ACA's coverage provisions will result in lower net costs to the federal government. The Congressional Budget Office and the staff of the Joint Committee on Taxation released estimates in April of 2014 on the budgetary effects of the provisions of the ACA that relate to health insurance coverage. The agencies currently project a net cost of $36 billion for 2014, $5 billion less than the previous projection for the year. They also project a cost reduction of $104 billion for the 2015 to 2024 period. Considering all of the provisions, including coverage, the most recent comprehensive estimates by the Congressional Budget Office and the Joint Committee on Taxation indicate that the ACA will reduce federal deficits (Congressional Budget Office, 2014b).

LEGAL CHALLENGES TO THE ACA

The Supreme Court's decisions are impacting health care reform and the tenor of debate that surrounds it. The first challenge came in 2012 when the Supreme Court ruled that states could opt out of the Medicaid expansion. A second major challenge focused on the ACA contraception mandate. Two cases, Sebelius v Hobby Lobby Stores, Inc. and Conestoga Wood Specialties Corp. v Sebelius, dealt with the ACA, religious freedom, and women's access to contraception by for-profit business owners (The Economist, 2014). A closely divided Supreme Court ruled in favor of family-owned for-profit businesses being treated as individuals and therefore could not be required to pay for insurance coverage of contraception (Richy, 2014). (See Chapters 19 and 53.)

Finally, the newest challenge under review by the Supreme Court is the case of King v Burwell. The plaintiffs point to a passage in the ACA that suggests the federal government can only offer premium subsidies to the state exchanges. Only 16 states and the District of Columbia have state-based exchanges; the other states have an exchange run by the federal government. If the Court rules in favor of the plaintiff, it would mean about 8 million people could no longer afford health insurance, and as the number of people enrolled drops, insurance premiums would go up for all. The Court is expected to rule in the summer of 2015 (Ydstie, 2015).

IMMIGRATION REFORM: WILL HEALTH CARE BE INCLUDED?

Generations of immigrants have been and continue to be essential to the U.S. economy and cultural diversity. In 2011, the Hispanic Pew Center estimated that over 11 million undocumented immigrants were living in the United States including 1

million children (Passel and Cohn, 2012). Conservative estimates identify at least 5100 children in U.S. foster care, their parents having been detained or deported (Wessler, 2011). We are at a point in time when the need for immigration reform has never been more pressing and our country more ready. Amid growing bipartisan and public support for comprehensive immigration reform, how immigration reform will connect to health care reform has been a very divisive issue.

A confluence of factors, from the role of the Latino vote in the 2012 Presidential election to a broad coalition of immigrant rights activists, galvanized debate in Congress and culminated in the Senate's passage of large-scale comprehensive bipartisan immigration reform legislation: The Border Security, Economic Opportunity and Immigration Modernization Act of 2013 S.744 (National Immigration Law Center, 2013). The proposal falls short, denying immigrants access to affordable health care for up to 15 years. With a polarized Congress current immigration reform legislation remains in limbo.

CURRENT HEALTH CARE ACCESS

Living as an undocumented immigrant in the United States provides limited options for health care. If injured, sick, or chronically ill an undocumented immigrant can experience days, weeks, or even months of pain, with the emergency room usually the only available remedy. Lack of progress on immigration reform over the past two decades has placed financial pressures on safety-net health care organizations and created ethical challenges for health care professionals seeking to provide quality care to all patients. Undocumented immigrants are currently ineligible for the major federally funded public insurance programs: Medicaid, Medicare, and CHIP. The publicly funded health care safety net provides some access for undocumented immigrants. State-level Emergency Medicaid covers hospitalization for emergency medical treatment and Federally Qualified Health Centers provide some primary care. Health care professionals must often resort to using emergency treatment provisions to help undocumented patients manage health problems. This is recognized as the most expensive and medically problematic way to treat chronic disease (Fitz, Wolgin, & Oakford, 2013).

THE ETHICS AND ECONOMICS OF ACCESS

The Hastings Center (Berlinger & Gussmano, 2013) provides an indepth overview of the ethical issues that are key to guiding legislative development. Their report notes that excluding the undocumented while health care reform is being implemented undermines the health-related rights of citizen children whose access to health care depends on their parents, and it works against the goals of reducing health disparities affecting vulnerable populations (Berlinger & Gussmano, 2013). How to integrate undocumented immigrants and other new immigrants into the country's comprehensive efforts to improve the health care system is a challenging problem.

Immigrant advocacy groups strongly support allowing undocumented immigrants access to basic affordable health care. The purpose of the ACA is to eliminate the need for the poor and uninsured to seek uncompensated health care from emergency rooms. Advocacy groups argue that the health of future citizens or the ability to control health care costs should not be compromised. "Ensuring that every person in this country has access to high-quality preventive care enhances public health, improves individuals' lives, curbs health costs and reduces uncompensated care for doctors and hospitals" (Rome, 2013).

More conservative advocacy groups argue they are not being anti-immigrant. Instead, they claim that it is about following the rules and not rewarding those who break them. They argue that we cannot afford to include this population in the ACA plan and that taxpayers should not have to foot the bill for health care to anyone who manages to establish illegal residence (Camarota, 2011; Longmire, 2013; Rector, 2007). With sequestration cuts, shrinking budgets, and smaller incomes this has been an effective message.

However, the Center for American Progress (Fitz Wolgin, & Oakford, 2013) challenges the stereotype of immigrants as takers and presents an array of strong research findings that demonstrate immigrants are a net positive for the economy and pay more into the system than they take out. The Social Security Administration released projections regarding the impact of unauthorized immigrants' contributions and also found they have played a key role in prolonging the solvency of the Social Security Trust Fund (Goss et al., 2013). Other findings emphasize that the gains to legalizing the nation's undocumented immigrant population and reforming our legal immigration system would add a cumulative $1.5 trillion to U.S. GDP over a decade (Hinojosa-Ojeda, 2010). A study by the Institute on Taxation and Economic Policy (2013) found that undocumented immigrants pay a significant amount of money in taxes each year. This data challenges the perception that immigrants are a drain on the U.S. economy.

IMMIGRATION HEALTH CARE REFORM OPTIONS

The main sources of health coverage for illegal or non-qualified immigrants are through an employer or the private, individual coverage market. However, immigrants often work in jobs that do not offer coverage or are unable to afford coverage on the individual market without access to tax credits. Currently, eight states (CA, FL, IL, MA, NJ, NY, WA, WI) and the District of Columbia have fully funded programs that provide coverage to immigrants regardless of their citizenship status. However, programs for illegal immigrants are limited to specific groups (such as children or pregnant women) or provide limited services (The Kaiser Family Foundation, 2013a). The Kaiser Family Foundation (2013b) suggests several policy options for increasing access to affordable coverage for immigrants. The options include expanding access to Medicaid by either eliminating or reducing the five-year waiting period for adults who are in a lawful status. The other option is to consider granting all immigrants on the pathway to citizenship, including those in provisional status, the same access as

UNIT 3

citizens to affordable health coverage options (e.g., Medicaid, CHIP, and exchanges).

Although there are increased costs associated with expanding coverage to individuals with provisional status, there are also offsetting savings. For one, reductions in the number of uninsured contribute to savings in programs and services for this population. As with other populations, access to affordable health coverage enables individuals to obtain medical care when needed. Waiting for care can both exacerbate the problem(s) and raise costs through greater emergency room use. Access to health care, including prevention, can facilitate earlier diagnosis and treatment of conditions as well as improve care management. Additionally, because immigrants tend to be younger and healthier, they help spread the risk in an insurance pool, which lowers overall premium costs. Lastly, by supporting an individual's ability to focus on employment and providing for their family, health coverage also contributes to long-term economic benefits (Kaiser Family Foundation, 2013b).

As immigration reform awaits legislative action, it will be important for nurses and other health professionals to communicate the importance of including access to health care in immigration reform. An immigration bill that makes people wait so many years for guaranteed affordable insurance and care just makes no sense.

RISING ECONOMIC INEQUALITY

Extreme economic inequality not only limits economic growth in the communities and in the nation as a whole, it impairs family well-being (Shapiro, Meschede, & Osoro, 2013). Economic inequality is the financial disparity between entities (e.g., individuals, groups, countries). Two primary measures are used to evaluate economic inequality. One is wealth, a measure of the money and material possessions or assets people own, and the other is income (Bernstein, 2013). Wealth and income disparities affect peoples' access to basic items and services that should be available to everyone, such as food, housing, and health care. Individual and population health disparities are highly associated with economic inequality in this country.

TABLE 40-1 Economic Inequality Facts

Fact #1	U.S. income inequality is the highest it has been since 1928.
Fact #2	The collective earnings of the top 1% increased from 10% of total earnings in 1980 to 20% today. In contrast, the bottom 90% received 65% of the earnings in 1980. Today the share is less than 50%.
Fact #3	The black/white income gap in the U.S. has persisted. In 2011, median black household income was 59% of median white household income.
Fact #4	Wealth inequality is even greater than income inequality. The highest-earning fifth of U.S. families earned 59.1% of all income; the richest fifth held 88.9% of all wealth.

Source: DeSilver, D. (2014). 5 facts about income inequality. Pew Research Center. Retrieved from *www.pewresearch.org/fact-tank/2014/01/07/5-facts-about-economic-inequality/*.

Recent research from Thomas Piketty (2014) and Emmanuel Saez (2013), two highly regarded economists, provides strong evidence of growing inequality in the United States from 2009 to 2012. While income for the top 1% rose by 31.4%, the bottom 99% saw income growth of just 0.4% (Saez, 2013). The gap between rich and poor also rose in emerging economies, for example, India and China (The Economist, 2011). President Obama as well as other world leaders cite rising economic inequality as a threat to social mobility and economic stability. In his 2013 State of the Union Address, President Obama called "economic inequality the defining challenge of our time" (The White House, 2013). The Pew Research Center summarizes current facts regarding economic inequality in the United States (Table 40-1).

MEASURING WEALTH

Economic inequality has been rising in similar ways around the world since 1980 (Galbraith, 2012). This trend appears to be strongly driven by the financial markets of a global economy. As stated earlier, as a standard measure of economic inequality, income provides an easy gauge for comparing the gains of the very wealthy with those of the middle class and the poor (Bernstein, 2013). However, wealth is more encompassing than income because assets and debts can modify the impact of income on economic outcomes. Wealth allows families to be more upwardly mobile by supporting them to move into better and safer neighborhoods, investing in businesses, saving for retirement, and supporting their children's college aspirations. Having a financial cushion also provides a measure of security when a job loss or other crisis strikes. Some people have little or no accumulated wealth (what one owns minus what one owes) because they have little or no income. Some people may have a substantial income, but be in debt because of student loans or health care expenses and therefore have little wealth.

Sadly, another factor impacting contemporary wealth outcomes is historical wealth accumulation. Policies and taxation preferences from previous eras in our country's history continue to unfairly impact wealth along lines of race and favor the already affluent. Notably, there is an enormous and long-standing wealth gap between white households and households of color. The Institute on Assets and Public Policy reports the number of years families owned their homes was the largest predictor of the gap in wealth growth by race (Shapiro Meschede, & Osoro, 2013). Including wealth-assets and debt is key because even small amounts of wealth can ensure some economic security and opportunity. The unprecedented wealth destruction during the 2008 financial crises and recession that followed, accompanied by long-term high unemployment, underscores the critical importance wealth plays in weathering emergencies and helping families achieve long-term financial security.

THE GREAT RECESSION RESHAPED THE ECONOMY

Inequality highlights distribution patterns and reveals who actually benefits from economic growth (Reich, 2014). Recent events have borne this out and made growing economic inequality part of the debate over whether our nation is on a sustainable economic path. Just before the 2008 financial crisis,

Congress was cutting taxes for the highest earners in an effort to stave off a depression. In the wake of the financial crisis that created the Great Recession of 2008, the credibility of such free market and trickle-down economic ideologies is increasingly being challenged (Piketty, 2014; Stiglitz, 2012). Leading economists guided fiscal policy responses to the crises, including the highly controversial bank bailouts and economic stimulus package.

However, since the recovery began, the richest have rebounded the fastest and median incomes have dropped (Fox, 2014). Beginning with the 2011 Occupy Wall Street protests that voiced the plight of the bottom 99% of income and wealth holders, inequality has quickly moved to the top of the political agenda. One of the richest businessmen in America, Warren Buffet, is even crusading for a higher inheritance tax. He argues that the United States risks becoming a plutocracy as inherited wealth is making heredity, rather than merit, determine one's ability to command resources (Roche, 2011). Many perceive the impact of recent economic shifts in wealth disparities as having an unprecedented impact on both economic security and political equality.

COSTS OF ECONOMIC INEQUALITY

New research is challenging the traditional economic view that inequality is a necessary evil for an efficient capitalist society (Galbraith, 2012; Piketty, 2014). Nobel Prize winner Joseph E. Stiglitz (2012) argues that unequal societies are not only inefficient but also tend to have unstable and unsustainable economies. Technological change and globalized markets are identified as key reasons for the problem of growing global and U.S. economic inequity. Google Chairman Eric Schmidt notes that companies, in their drive to compete with one another on a global level, are focused on cutting wages and replacing workers with technology. As a result, wages as a percentage of the economy are near an all-time low. In his perspective, this has led to the stagnation in middle-class wages and slow global economic growth (Blodget, 2014).

Economic inequality is not only bad for the economy and the pocket book but also negatively influences economic mobility and opportunities to improve one's life (Schmitt, 2014). The American Dream of being able to succeed regardless of the economic circumstances in which one was born is increasingly untenable. The United States is not as socially mobile as was once thought. A study of 22 countries found that the United States ranked 15th in social mobility. In countries such as the United States, where income inequality is high, it was also found that intergenerational income gains are very low (Corak, 2013). Other studies support these findings. For instance, a report from the Center for American Progress found that income inequality diminishes economic mobility between generations (Bernstein, 2013).

Finally, research suggests that as the rich accumulate more of the country's total income and wealth, they also gain political power (Reich, 2014; The Economist, 2012). This results in a cycle of greater political influence and increased inequality. The cycle can be described as: (1) increased inequality yields greater resources for the rich that (2) the rich can then apply resources to political contributions, which (3) leads parties to move their platforms to favor the positions of wealthier individuals, and (4) increases the wealth divide; then back to (1) (O'Neil, 2012; Schmitt, 2014). However, many conservatives argue there are little data to support these concerns (Nichols & McChesney, 2013). They assert that candidates cannot buy campaigns, no matter how much money they garner (e.g., Ross Perot, Steve Forbes, and Mitt Romney). Angus Deaton, a Princeton economist, does not agree: "The political equality that is required of a democracy is always under the threat from economic inequality, and the more extreme the inequality, the greater the threat to democracy" (Reich, 2014).

IMPACT OF ECONOMIC INEQUALITY ON HEALTH EQUITY

In considering the social determinants of health, nurses know that employment and working conditions, which provide income, have powerful effects on health and health equity. We also know that quality of life is determined by more than income,

such as health, housing, the environment, financial security, and social connectedness. Highly unequal societies do worse overall on such quality of life indicators. High levels of inequality are strongly associated with poor social and human development outcomes (Edsall, 2012; Wilkinson & Pickett, 2009).

Recent studies are deepening our understanding of what drives economic and health inequality (Chettyet et al., 2014; Piketty, 2014). Chetty and colleagues (2014) found that geography is a significant factor in upward mobility in the United States. For example, the odds of increasing income (upward mobility) were considerably lower in Atlanta and Memphis and higher in northeastern cities such as New York and Boston. The study also found that fairly poor children in Seattle (bottom 25th percentile of income) do as well financially as middle-class children (50th percentile of income) who grew up in Atlanta. However, the influence of geography on mobility varies by where one starts on the social class ladder. Geography was less of a significant influence on children born to high-income families than for middle-class and poor children.

EFFECTIVELY ADDRESSING ECONOMIC INEQUALITY

A recent Pew Research Center survey found that the majority of Democrats (68%) and Republicans (61%) believe economic inequality in the United States has grown, but they disagree about its causes and solutions (Pew Research Center, 2014). Only 45% of Republicans say that the government should do something about it, compared with 90% of Democrats (Wade, 2014). Republicans tend to endorse an individualist explanation for poverty (e.g., people are poor because they do not work hard), whereas Democrats tend to support a more structural explanation (e.g., where you start on the social class ladder). Many Republicans strongly believe that government aid to the poor does more harm than good. Notably, the answers to these questions on the Pew survey diverged much more by political affiliation than social class (Wade, 2014). For example, responders who identified as having low incomes and Republican affiliation did not support government intervention on the issue. Such is the power of ideology inherent in political affiliation.

Economists are also divided about what to do about economic inequality. Two ideological frames seem to underlie the policy approaches recommended by economists. Those with a more conservative view argue that the policy response needs to focus on removing government regulation to enable a more free market. Lawson Bader, president of the Competitive Enterprise Institute, a nonprofit libertarian think tank, agrees that the U.S. economy is performing at a subpar level. However, he argues that government attempts to fix the problems in some mechanistic way are not the answer (Reich, 2014).

The second frame is more Keynesian, or regulatory, in its approach. Joseph Stiglitz and New York University Professor of Economics Nouriel Roubini, among others, argue that legislative action is needed. They suggest that higher taxes, particularly for the upper-middle class and top 1%, would help with the redistribution issue and release the U.S. economy's growth potential in a sustainable way. Stiglitz and Roubini also agree that the government should limit the tax breaks, subsidies, and loopholes allowed to the major energy, agribusiness, pharmaceutical, and financial companies (Fischl, 2013). Some argue that we should focus on the poor and poverty (Schmitt, 2014), while others point to joblessness (Klein, 2013b).

PROPOSED POLICY STRATEGIES

In his 2013 State of the Union Address, President Obama proposed increasing the minimum wage as a way to decrease income inequality (White House, 2013). The majority of Americans agree with this strategy (Drake, 2014). He also stressed the need to create economic mobility opportunities through funding better education, job opportunities, and new retirement plans (White House, 2013). The Republican response to his message was twofold: the real problem is the inequality of opportunity caused by President Obama's administrative policies, yet they do not want to be seen as undermining the American working population (Vanic, 2014).

Republicans have introduced bills in the House and the Senate proposing the formation of a Monetary Commission to evaluate the core issues of income inequality and to make policy recommendations (Benko, 2014). These policy actions align with the Republican belief that regulation and redistribution work against America's economic system of free market capitalism. More specifically, they argue that redistribution undermines economic growth opportunities as the rich have fewer incentives to start new businesses or hire new employees (Debate.org, 2014).

There does appear to be one consensus strategy seen as viable to reducing economic inequality: investing in education reform. Both conservatives and liberals agree that to make the United States more competitive in the future, education reform is needed. It is also well understood that allocating more resources does not automatically lead to better results (Fischl, 2013).

To date, the congressional response to the current economic disparities and the budget situation has been to implement austerity measures, such as decreasing spending in the budget for social programs. Many other countries have followed a similar path of austerity with few positive results. While there is overwhelming evidence that severe inequality makes our country more vulnerable to economic stagnation and volatility, there is no agreement on the causes or the solutions. Like all complex problems, real solutions will be multifaceted and require bipartisan effort. Inequality is shaped by the rules of the current system and those rules can be remade.

CLIMATE CHANGE: IMPACTING GLOBAL HEALTH

Another contemporary issue that is impacting the health and economy of our nation is climate change. Although climate change is one of the most serious public health threats, few people are aware of how it can directly affect them. This may be the reason why few Americans are concerned about environmental issues. A 2014 Gallup poll indicates that only 24% of Americans worry a great deal about this issue (Riffkin, 2014). This puts climate change, along with the quality of the environment, near the bottom of a list of 15 top issues. Not surprisingly, Americans from the two major political parties express different levels of worry about climate change and the environment. Many more Democrats (45%) said they worry a great deal about the quality of the environment compared with Republicans (16%).

The factors of climate and local environment intersect with health status. This makes improving the health of populations a thorny problem because of the interacting influence of social, environmental, and economic systems. Research indicates that social and economic conditions are stronger determinates of health and sickness than access to medical care or genetic endowment (Galea et al., 2011). Additional evidence suggests that the greatest public health challenges of today include air quality; climate change; the safe management of chemicals; and adequate, safe sources of water, food, and energy. These are the multifaceted conditions that create the "social determinants of health" (Koh et al., 2010). As public health is a core component of the nurse's role, it is morally imperative that nurses cultivate a professional understanding of climate change as well as a personal commitment to acting on environmental issues.

CLIMATE CHANGE: IT'S HAPPENING

Many scientists argue that current human activity, specifically the production of greenhouse gases, is a key factor in global warming and, thus, climate change (Hansen, Sato, & Ruedy, 2014). This human-induced warming and the overuse of fossil fuels are closely linked to climate change (National Oceanic and Atmosphere Association, 2014). Two reports on climate change have received a great deal of public notice. The 2014 United Nations report completed by the Intergovernmental Panel on Climate Change (IPCC WGII AR5; Intergovernmental Panel on Climate Change, 2014) and The National Climate Assessment report (Melillo, Richmond, & Yohe, 2014) offer strong evidence that climate change is here and now. The United Nations report warns that the impacts of global warming are likely to be "severe, pervasive and irreversible." The controver-

sial report states that natural systems are currently bearing the bulk of the burden of climatic changes (Watts, 2014). As changes continue, there will be a stronger negative impact on humans.

The negative impacts of climate change are especially visible in relation to the water supply. On one hand, there is a higher risk of flooding in lowland areas. On the other hand, as drought expands in other areas, water availability is compromised and crop yields decrease. The report emphasizes that no one on the planet will be untouched by the impacts of climate change. It further cautions that humans may be able to adapt to some but not all of these changes and only within limits (Intergovernmental Panel on Climate Change, 2014).

Although climate change has the potential to harm everyone, children, older adults, and communities living in poverty are among the most vulnerable. The poor will likely be hit the hardest. Food shortages, flooding, the destruction of property, and malnutrition are some of the many ways climate change can mean disaster for the poor. As temperatures rise, so will health risks. As access to food and water become inconsistent, a host of chronic health issues will be exacerbated. Climate change-related injury and illness will increase the demand for and cost of health care, meaning even less access for many impoverished people (Goldenburg, 2014).

The poor in less developed countries are not the only populations threatened by rising sea levels. While sea levels worldwide are expected to rise an average of two to three feet by 2100, they could surge more than six feet along the Atlantic seaboard. A recent study named Boston, New York, and Norfolk, VA the three most vulnerable metropolitan areas (Davenport, 2014). "Another study found that just a one point five-foot rise in sea level would expose about six trillion dollars worth of property to coastal flooding in the Baltimore, Boston, New York, Philadelphia, and Providence, RI areas" (Gillis, 2014).

MITIGATION VERSUS ADAPTATION

While the predictions for climate change are dire, the United Nations 2014 report offers a great deal of information on managing climate change. Historically, the climate-policy community has debated about whether to focus on reducing emissions (mitigation) or managing climate change (adaptation). The report reflects a shift in this debate by focusing on both. Further, it places a sense of control and responsibility into the hands of the many instead of the few. The authors recommend that local businesses and communities lead the way rather than waiting for the international community to agree on policies. The report also notes that many collective efforts are already under way to adapt to climate changes. There are people who will never accept the science of climate change, but responding to current disasters by developing community resources to prepare for the worst just makes good sense. Key risks and adaptation prospects are presented for public-private partnerships to consider (Friedman and Narula, 2014).

INTERNATIONAL PROGRESS

As climate change is a global problem, the need for mitigation is critical. To date, nation-state policies have been focused on reducing carbon dioxide and other greenhouse gas emissions. The Global Legislators Organization (GLOBE) completed a recent study tracking climate legislation across the 66 countries (accounting for almost 90% of global emissions). The study finds that 64 countries have put in place or are putting in place strong legislation to reduce fossil fuel use. In addition, 61 countries have laws to promote clean energy sources within their borders and 54 have mandated strengthened energy efficiency standards (Biron, 2014). The number of national climate laws around the world has increased from 40 in 1997 to nearly 500 (Friedman and Narula, 2014).

Unfortunately, the United States is lagging far behind other nations in these legislative efforts. None of the bills currently in Congress includes targets for reducing greenhouse gas emissions. Aside from modest legislation aimed at increasing clean energy sources, the United States does not have a comprehensive climate change law (Lefton, 2014).

ADAPTATION IS LOCAL

What does adapting to climate change look like in practice? Communities have long practiced climate-change adaptation, such as inner city rooftop gardens, planting trees to combat urban heat, and planting drought-tolerant crops. In many of these cases, people are not even thinking that they are adapting to climate change; they are just doing what needs to be done to make the environment healthier and to improve their quality of life. But people must do more.

Policy choices in local communities, such as those at the state and national levels, are shaped by the distribution of money, power, and resources. Nurses need to advocate with public health professionals, environmentalists, and other diverse stakeholders to promote healthy communities where they live. One way to do this is to engage in legislation that promotes what is called Health in All Policies (HiAP). HiAP (www.apha.org/hiap) uses a collaborative approach to improve population health by embedding health considerations into many areas of local and state government decision making. Policy decisions that affect the social determinants of health are often made outside of the local health department by other government agencies and by the private sector. Decisions made in a range of areas, such as education, workplace practices, transportation, and criminal justice procedures, all contribute to the social determinants of health. HiAP seeks to ensure that decision makers are informed about the health equity and sustainability consequences of various policy options, and to integrate these considerations of health with other areas throughout the policy process (National Association of County and City Health Officials [NACCHO], 2012).

EXAMPLES OF HEALTH IN ALL POLICIES

What are the questions policymakers need to ask (applying a HiAP lens) regarding how a policy might affect children, food, water, land, and air? For example, what will be the impact on the levels of toxins in the environment by placing a power plant in the community? What are the associated health outcomes? Another illustration might be related to the environmental impact of a proposal to develop a new light rail service versus expansion of a current state highway. Questions regarding the impact of these options on air pollution, associated asthma rates, and so on would be considered as part of the policy discussion (NACCHO, 2012).

Several best practice initiatives have been implemented recently. California has been an early adopter of HiAP at the state level. Local community initiatives that exemplify best practices in HiAP include King County's Equity and Social Justice Ordinance in Washington, DC and Denver's Environmental Public Policy in Colorado (NACCHO, 2012).

NURSING ACTION ORIENTED LEADERSHIP

At the community level nurses can lead efforts to ensure the health facilities they work in are prepared. In addition to preparing for disasters, staff can also be educated about local climate risks and how they could impact patient and community health. Nurses can promote green initiatives reducing the carbon footprint in communities and within hospitals and clinics. Serving on environmental health task forces, ensuring the use of recyclable products, and making purchasing decisions are examples of effective professional activities (Sayre et al., 2010).

Beyond the collective efforts noted, nurses can make a difference at the individual level. For one, we can use our knowledge of climate change and environmental health to make wiser choices in our daily lives. In mitigating the effects of climate change, nurses might want to consider reducing their personal carbon footprint. There are simple things people can do to reduce their carbon footprint. Examples include reducing energy use by turning down the heat, economizing on electricity use, eating locally sourced produce, and using a reusable water bottle instead of a plastic disposable one (Goodman, 2013). Nurses need to join forces with other health care professionals to help with mitigation, adaptation, and policy surrounding this issue.

CONCLUSION

The issues we face are increasingly complex and the political power within our country at the national, state, and local levels has become more decentralized and polarized. The ongoing tensions regarding the appropriate role of the government in the lives of its citizens continues to play out not only in determining the size of the government's budget but also what services it provides and to whom it provides services.

As the gap between rich and poor widens and climate change continues, the quality of life (and health) of the middle class and the poor will be disproportionately impacted. Political leaders must be held accountable through transparency in decision making and holding conversations that provide substance, not sound bites. Extreme political rhetoric and partisanship must be condemned, not condoned, on both sides.

As America's historic health care reform continues to unfold, nurses will be on the front lines. This makes us responsible for advocating quality health care for all, demanding action to address pervasive social problems, and using knowledge of issues impacting the health of our communities to engage effectively in the political and policy process for the betterment of all.

DISCUSSION QUESTIONS

1. What makes the Affordable Care Act such a divisive issue both politically and economically?
2. With the increase in the number of baby boomers reaching retirement age and holding strong political power, what are the economic issues that both federal and state governments will need to address?
3. Identify some of the social, ethical, and economic reasons for addressing immigration policy reform.

REFERENCES

Amadeo, K. (n.d.a). U.S. debt ceiling. What it is, and what happens if it's not raised? Retrieved from *useconomy.about.com/od/glossary/g/National-Debt-Ceiling.htm*.

Amadeo, K. (n.d.b). What was Obama's stimulus package? Retrieved from *useconomy.about.com/od/candidatesandtheeconomy/a/Obama_Stimulus.htm*.

Baicker, K., Taubman, S., Allen, H., Bernstein, M., Gruber, J., Newhouse, J., et al. (2013). The Oregon experiment—Effects of Medicaid on clinical outcomes for the Oregon Health Study Group. *New England Journal of Medicine, 368*, 1713–1722.

Barnes, R. (2014). Upcoming Supreme Court cases are weighty if not numerous. *The Washington Post*, Retrieved from *www.washingtonpost.com/politics/upcoming-supreme-court-cases-are-weighty-if-not-numerous/2014/01/12/0fa0ad0c-79f1-11e3-af7f-13bf0e9965f6_story.html*.

Benko, R. (2014). How the GOP can win the upcoming battle over income inequality. *Forbes*, Retrieved from *www.forbes.com/sites/ralphbenko/2014/01/20/how-the-gop-can-win-the-upcoming-battle-over-income-inequality/print/*.

Berlinger, N., & Gusmano, M. (2013). Undocumented patients: Undocumented immigrants and access to health care. Garrison, NY: The Hastings Center. Retrieved from *www.undocumentedpatients.org/wp-content/uploads/2013/03/Undocumented-Patients-Executive-Summary.pdf*.

Bernstein, D. (2013). The impact of inequality on growth. Washington, DC: Center for American Progress. Retrieved from *www.americanprogress.org/wpcontent/Uploads/2013/12/BerensteinInequality.pdf*.

Biron, C. (2014). Global study finds "impressive" wave of climate legislation. Rome: Inter Press Service. Retrieved from *www.ipsnews.net/2014/02/global-study-finds-impressive-wave-climate-legislation/*.

Blodget, H. (2014). Eric Schmidt just revealed a key truth about the economy that very few rich investors and executives want to admit. Retrieved from *www.businessinsider.com/eric-schmidt-on-inequality-2014-1*.

Camarota, S. (2011). Welfare use by immigrant households with children: A look at cash, Medicaid, housing, and food programs. Retrieved from *cis.org/immigrant-welfare-use-2011*.

Chetty, R., Hendren, N., Kline, P., & Saez, E. (2014). Where is the land of opportunity? The geography of intergenerational mobility in the United States. Retrieved from *obs.rc.fas.harvard.edu/chetty/mobility_geo.pdf*.

Cohn, N. (2013). Obama is wrong: Gerrymandering is not to blame for the GOP fever. *New Republic*, Retrieved from *www.newrepublic.com/article/112410/obama-blames-gerrymandering-gop-fever-hes-wrong*.

Congressional Budget Office. (2014a). Updated estimates of the effects of the insurance coverage provisions of the Affordable Care Act. Washington, DC: Congressional Budget Office. Retrieved from *www.cbo.gov/publication/45231*.

Congressional Budget Office. (2014b). The budget and economic outlook: 2014 to 2024. Washington, DC: Congressional Budget Office. Retrieved from *www.cbo.gov/sites/default/files/cbofiles/attachments/45010-Outlook2014_Feb.pdf*.

Corak, M. (2013). Income inequality, equality of opportunity, and intergenerational mobility. DP No. 7520. Ontario, Canada: University of Ottawa and Bonn, Germany: IZA. Retrieved from *ftp.iza.org/dp7520.pdf*.

Davenport, C. (2014). Rising seas. *New York Times*, Retrieved from *www.nytimes.com/interactive/2014/03/27/world/climate-rising-seas.html*.

Debate.org. (2014). History and debate of redistribution. Retrieved from *www.debate.org/redistribution/*.

DeSilver, D. (2013). Congress ends least-productive year in recent history. Washington, DC: Pew Research Center. Retrieved from *www.pewresearch.org/facttank/2013/12/23/congress-endsleast-productive-year-in-recent-history/*.

Drake, B. (2014). Polls show strong support for minimum wage hike. Washington, DC: Pew Research Center. Retrieved from *www.pewresearch.org/fact-tank/2014/03/04/polls-show-strong-support-for-minimum-wage-hike/*.

The Economist. (2011). The rich and the rest: What to do (and not do) about inequality. Retrieved from *www.economist.com/node/17959590*.

The Economist. (2012). For richer or poorer. Retrieved from *www.economist.com/node/21564414*.

The Economist. (2014). The Hobby Lobby hubbub. The Supreme Court ponders the contraceptive mandate. Retrieved from *www.economist.com/news/united-states/21599789-supreme-court-ponders-contraceptive-mandate-hobby-lobby-hubbub*.

Edsall, T. (2012). Separate and unequal. *New York Times*, Retrieved from *www.nytimes.com/2012/08/05/books/review/the-price-of-inequality-by-joseph-e-stiglitz.html?pagewanted=all&_r=0*.

Elmendorf, D. (2014). Testimony on the budget and economic outlook: 2014 to 2024. Washington, DC: Congressional Budget Office. Retrieved from *www.cbo.gov/publication/45087*.

Emanuel, E. (2013). Op-ed; How to fix the glitches. *New York Times*, Retrieved from *www.nytimes.com/2013/10/23/opinion/emanuel-how-to-fix-the-glitches.html?pagewanted=2*.

Fischl, J. (2013). Income inequality in America: What we should be doing about it? *Policy.Mic*. Retrieved from *www.policymic.com/articles/26805/income-inequality-in-america-what-we-should-be-doing-about-it*.

Fitz, M., Wolgin, P., & Oakford, P. (2013). Immigrants are makers, not takers. Washington, DC: Center for American Progress. Retrieved from *www.americanprogress.org/issues/immigration/news/2013/02/08/52377/immigrants-are-makers-not-takers/*.

Fox, A. (2014). Inequality: The defining challenge of our time. *The Huffington Post*, Retrieved from *www.huffingtonpost.com/arthur-fox/income-inequality-the-defining-c_b_4604230.html*.

Friedman, U., & Narula, S. K. (2014). The UN's new focus: Surviving, not stopping, climate change. *The Atlantic*, Retrieved from *www.theatlantic.com/international/archive/2014/04/the-uns-new-focus-surviving-not-stopping-climate-change/359929/*.

Galbraith, J. (2012). *Inequality and instability: A study of the world economy just before the great crisis*. New York: Oxford University Press.

Galea, S., Tracy, M., Hoggatt, K. J., Dimaggio, C., & Karpati, A. (2011). Estimated deaths attributable to social factors in the United States. *American Journal of Public Health, 101*(8), 1456–1465.

Gallup. (2014). Trust in government. Retrieved from *www.gallup.com/poll/5392/trust-government.aspx*.

Gillis, J. (2014). Climate change study finds U.S. is already widely affected. *New York Times*, Retrieved from *www.nytimes.com/2014/05/07/science/earth/climate-change-report.html?hp*.

Goldenburg, S. (2014). Climate change: The poor will suffer most. *The Guardian*, Retrieved from *www.theguardian.com/environment/2014/mar/31/climate-change-poor-suffer-most-un-report*.

Goodman, B. (2013). Role of the nurse in addressing the health effects of climate change. *Nursing Standard, 27*(35), 49–56.

Goss, S., Wade, A., Skirvin, P., Morris, M., Mark Bye, K., & Huston, D. (2013). Effects of unauthorized immigration on the actuarial status of the social security trust funds. Actuarial note. Number 151. Baltimore, MD: Social Security Administration. Retrieved from *www.socialsecurity.gov/oact/NOTES/pdf_notes/note151.pdf*.

Hamel, L., Firth, J., & Brodie, M. (2014). *Kaiser health tracking poll: March 2014*. Menlo Park, CA: Kaiser Family Foundation. Retrieved from *kff.org/health-reform/poll-finding/kaiser-health-tracking-poll-march-2014/*.

Hansen, J., Sato, M., & Ruedy, R. (2014). Global temperature update through 2013. Washington, DC: National Aeronautics and Space Administration. Retrieved from *www.columbia.edu/~jeh1/mailings/2014/20140121_Temperature2013.pdf*.

Hass, R. N. (2013). What is the effect of U.S. domestic political gridlock on international relations? Council on Foreign Relations. Retrieved from *www.cfr.org/united-states/effect-uzsz-domestic-political-gridlock-international-relations/p30725.*

Hinojosa-Ojeda, R. (2010). Raising the floor for American workers—The economic benefits of comprehensive immigration reform. Retrieved from *americanprogress.org/issues/immigration/report/2010/01/07/7187/raising-the-floor-for-american-workers/.*

Holland, J. (2014). Obamacare is widening the gap between "red" and "blue" America. *BillMoyers.com*, Retrieved from *billmoyers.com/2014/04/07/obamacare-is-widening-the-gap-between-red-and-blue-am.*

Institute on Taxation and Economic Policy. (2013). Undocumented immigrants' state and local tax contributions. Retrieved from *www.itep.org/pdf/undocumentedtaxes.pdf.*

Intergovernmental Panel on Climate Change (IPCC WGII AR5). (2014). Climate change 2014: Impacts, adaptation, and vulnerability. Summary for policymakers. Retrieved from *ipcc-wg2.gov/AR5/images/uploads/IPCC_WG2AR5_SPM_Approved.pdf.*

International Budget Partnership. (2014). Why are budgets important? Retrieved from *internationalbudget.org/getting-started/why-are-budgets-important/.*

Johnson, L. (2013). Government shutdown cost $24 billion, Standard & Poor's says. *The Huffington Post*, Retrieved from *www.huffingtonpost.com/2013/i0/16/government-shutdown-cost_n_4110818.html.*

Jones, S. (2014). CBO director: Important to give advance warning about coming changes to social security. *CNSNews.com.* Retrieved from *www.cnsnews.com/news/article/susan-jones/cbo-director-important-give-advance-warning-about-coming-changes-social.*

Kaiser Family Foundation. (2009). Medicaid: Timeline of key developments. Retrieved from *kaiserfamilyfoundation.files.wordpress.com/2008/04/5-02-13-medicaid-timeline.pdf.*

Kaiser Family Foundation. (2013a). Key facts on health coverage for low-income today and under the Affordable Care Act. Kaiser Commission on key facts. Medicaid and the uninsured. Retrieved from *kaiserfamilyfoundation.files.wordpress.com/2013/03/8279-02.pdf.*

Kaiser Family Foundation. (2013b). Immigration reform and access to health coverage: Key issues to consider. Kaiser Commission on key facts. Medicaid and the uninsured. Retrieved from *kaiserfamilyfoundation.files.wordpress.com/2013/02/8420.pdf.*

Kaiser Family Foundation. (2014). Status of state action on the Medicaid expansion decision, 2014. Retrieved from *kff.org/health-reform/state-indicator/state-activity-around-expanding-medicaid-under-the-affordable-care-act/.*

Khimm, S. (2012). The sequester explained. *Washington Post Wonkblog*, Retrieved from *www.washingtonpost.com/blogs/wonkblog/wp/2012/09/14/the-sequester-explained/.*

Klein, E. (2013a). This is what would happen if we breach the debt ceiling. *Washington Post Wonkblog*, Retrieved from *www.washingtonpost.com/blogs/wonkblog/wp/2013/01/07/this-is-what-would-happen-if-we-breach-the-debt-ceiling/.*

Klein, E. (2013b). Inequality isn't "the defining challenge of our time". *Washington Post Wonkblog*, Retrieved from *www.washingtonpost.com/blogs/wonkblog/wp/2013/12/13/inequality-isnt-the-defining-challenge-of-our-time/.*

Kliff, S. (2013a). Arkansas's unusual plan to expand Medicaid. *Washington Post Wonkblog*, Retrieved from *www.washingtonpost.com/blogs/wonkblog/wp/2013/02/28/arkansass-different-plan-to-expand-medicaid/.*

Kliff, S. (2013b). When Medicare launched, nobody had any clue whether it would work. *Washington Post Wonkblog*, Retrieved from *www.washingtonpost.com/blogs/wonkblog/wp/2013/05/17/when-medicare-launched-nobody-had-any-clue-whether-it-would-work/.*

Kogan, R. (2012). How the across-the-board cuts in the Budget Control Act will work. Budget and policy priorities. Retrieved from *www.cbpp.org/cms/?fa=view&id=3635.*

Koger, G. (2012). Congress: Partisan, not polarized. Blog posting. Retrieved from *www.transportationissuesdaily.com/four-explanations-for-congressional-gridlock-you-may-not-know-about/.*

Koh, H., Oppenhheimer, S., Massain-Short, S., Emmons, K., Geller, A., & Viswanath, K. (2010). Translating research evidence into practice to reduce health disparities: A social determinants approach. *American Journal of Public Health, 100*(S1), S72–S80.

Krasney, R. (2013). Obama signs bipartisan budget deal, annual defense bill. *Reuters.com*, Retrieved from *www.reuters.com/article/2013/12/26/us-usa-obama-idUSBRE9BP0HK20131226.*

Kraushaar, J. (2014). The most divided Congress ever, at least until next year. 2013 vote ratings. *National Journal*, Retrieved from *www.nationaljournal.com/2013-vote-ratings/the-most-divided-congress-ever-at-least-until-next-year-20140206.*

Kuhnhenn, J. (2014). Debts, deficits—Once a focus—Fade from agenda. New York: Associated Press. Retrieved from *http://bigstory.ap.org/article/fading-passion-debt-deficits-recede-view.*

Leflar, R. B. (2013). Reform of the United States health care system: An overview. *University of Tokyo Journal of Law and Politics, 10*, 44–59.

Lefton, R. (2014). U.S. falling behind as other countries pass climate legislation, new survey shows. *Climate Progress*, Retrieved from *thinkprogress.org/climate/2014/02/27/3338011/countries-climate-legislation/.*

Levey, N. (2014). Obamacare has led to health coverage for millions more people. *The Los Angeles Times*, Retrieved from *touch.latimes.com/#section/-1/article/p2p-79773450/.*

Longmire, S. (2013). Immigration reform shouldn't include taxpayer-funded health care. *Fox News Latino*, Retrieved from *latino.foxnews.com/latino/opinion/2013/04/22/immigration-reform-shouldnt-include-taxpayer-funded-health-care/.*

Mann, T., & Ornstein, N. (2012). *It's even worse than it looks: How the American constitution system collided with the new politics of extremism.* New York: Basic Books.

McCarthy, J. (2014). No improvement for Congress' job approval rating. *Gallop.com*, Retrieved from *www.gallup.com/poll/168428/no-improvement-congressional-approval.aspx.*

McNamara, R. (2014). Gerrymander: 19th century history. Retrieved from *history1800s.about.com/bio/Robert-McNamara-36749.htm.*

Melillo, J., Richmond, T. C., & Yohe, G. (Eds.) (2014). Climate change impacts in the United States: The Third National Climate Assessment. *U.S. Global Change Research Program*, Retrieved from *nca2014.globalchange.gov/.*

Morgan, D. (2014). Obamacare enrollment to surpass 7.5 million: U.S. official. *Rueters.com*, Retrieved from *www.reuters.com/article/2014/04/10/us-usa-healthcare-obama-idUSBREA3918920140410.*

National Association of County and City Health Officials. (2012). Health in all policies: Frequently asked questions. Retrieved from *www.naccho.org/topics/environmental/HiAP/upload/HiAP-FAQs-Finals-12.pdf.*

National Immigration Law Center. (2013). Summary and analysis: The Senate Bill (S.744). Retrieved from *www.nilc.org/s744summary1.html.*

National Oceanic and Atmosphere Association. (2014). Greenhouse gases. Asheville, NC: National Climatic Data Center. Retrieved from *www.ncdc.noaa.gov/monitoring-references/faq/greenhouse-gases.php.*

Nichols, J., & McChesney, R. (2013). Dollarocracy: How special interests undermine our democracy. *BillMoyers.com*, Retrieved from *billmoyers.com/2013/11/08/dollarocracy-how-special-interests-undermine-our-democracy/.*

Ohlemacher, S. (2014). GOP enjoys advantage of house control. *Associated Press*, Retrieved from *bigstory.ap.org/article/gop-redistricting-advantage.*

O'Keefe, E. (2014). The House has voted 54 times in four years on Obamacare. Here's the full list. *Washington Post*, Retrieved from *www.washingtonpost.com/blogs/the-fix/wp/2014/03/21/the-house-has-voted-54-times-in-four-years-on-obamacare-heres-the-full-list/*.

O'Neil, R. (2012). Inequality increases political influence of wealthiest. IMPACT: Research from Harvard Kennedy School. Retrieved from *www.hks.harvard.edu/news-events/publications/impact-newsletter/archives/spring-2012/inequality-increases-political-influence-of-wealthiest*.

Passel, J., & Cohn, D. (2012). Unauthorized immigrants: 11.1 million in 2011. Pew Research Hispanic Trends Project. Retrieved from *www.pewhispanic.org/2012/12/06/unauthorized-immigrants-11-1-million-in-2011/*.

Pew Research Center. (2013). Public trust in government: 1958-2013. Retrieved from *www.people-press.org/2013/10/18/trust-in-government-interactive/*.

Pew Research Center. (2014). Most see inequality growing, but partisans differ over solutions. Retrieved from *www.people-press.org/2014/01/23/most-see-inequality-growing-but-partisans-differ-over-solutions/*.

Piketty, T. (2014). *Capital in the twenty first century*. Translated by A. Goldhammer. Cambridge, MA: Harvard University Press.

Rampton, R. (2014). Health secretary resigns after Obamacare launch woes. *Rueters.com*, Retrieved from *www.reuters.com/article/2014/04/11/us-usa-healthcare-idUSBREA3926R20140411*.

Rector, R. (2007). Amnesty will cost U.S. taxpayers at least $2.6 trillion. Retrieved from *www.heritage.org/research/reports/2007/06/amnesty-will-cost-us-taxpayers-at-least-26-trillion*.

Reich, R. (2014). Why widening inequality is hobbling equal opportunity. Retrieved from *robertreich.org/post/75696787369*.

Richy, W. (2014). Hobby Lobby 101: Explaining the Supreme Court's birth control ruling. Retrieved from *http://www.csmonitor.com/USA/DC-Decoder/2014/0710/Hobby-Lobby-101-explaining-the-Supreme-Court-s-birth-control-ruling*.

Riffkin, R. (2014). In U.S., 67% dissatisfied with income, wealth distribution. *Gallup.com*, Retrieved from *www.gallup.com/poll/166904/dissatisfied-income-wealth-distribution.aspx*.

Roche, C. (2011). Buffet discusses the USA's plutocracy, lessons from the crisis & dabbles in mint. *Pragmatic Capitalism: Practical Views on Money and Finance*, Retrieved from *pragcap.com/buffett-on-the-usas-plutocracy-lessons-from-the-crisis-dabbles-in-mmt*.

Rome, E. (2013). Immigration bill shouldn't limit immigrants' access to health care. Press release. *Healthcare for America Now*, Retrieved from *healthcareforamericanow.org/2013/04/19/immigration-bill-shouldnt-limit-immigrants-access-to-health-care/*.

Ruffing, K., & Stone, C. (2013). Separating the debt limit from the deficit problem. Washington, DC: Center for Budget and Policy Priorities. Retrieved from *www.cbpp.org/cms/?fa=view&id=3888*.

Saez, E. (2013). Striking it richer: The evolution of top incomes in the United States. Retrieved from *elsa.berkeley.edu/users/saez/saez-UStopincomes-2012.pdf*.

Samuelson, R. (2014). The end of government. *Washington Post*, Retrieved from *www.washingtonpost.com/opinions/robert-j-samuelson-the-end-of-government/2014/02/09/94096a0c-9021-11e3-b46a-5a3d0d2130da_story.html*.

Sayre, L., Rhazi, N., Carpenter, H., & Hughes, N. (2010). Climate change and human health: The role of nurses in confronting the issue. *Nursing Administration Quarterly*, *34*(4), 334–342.

Schmitt, M. (2014). Here's how we should think about the inequality debate: We need a whole new framework. *NewRepublic.com*, Retrieved from *www.newrepublic.com/article/116285/problems-inequality-debate*.

Shapiro, T., Meschede, T., & Osoro, S. (2013). *The roots of the widening racial wealth gap: Explaining the black-white economic divide*. Waltham, MA: Institute on Assets and Social Policy. Retrieved from *iasp.brandeis.edu/pdfs/Author/shapiro-thomas-m/racialwealthgapbrief.pdf*.

Skopec, L., & Sommers, B. D. (2013). Seventy-one million additional Americans are receiving preventive services coverage without cost-sharing under the Affordable Care Act. Issue Brief. Washington, DC: Office of the Secretary of Planning and Evaluation (ASPE). Retrieved from *158.74.49.3/health/reports/2013/PreventiveServices/ib_prevention*.

Social Security Online. (2014). Frequently asked questions: Ratio of covered workers to beneficiaries. Retrieved from *www.ssa.gov/history/ratios.html*.

Sommers, B., Baicker, K., & Epstein, A. (2012). Mortality and access to care among adults after state Medicaid expansions. *New England Journal of Medicine*, *367*, 1025–1034.

Stiglitz, J. (2012). *The price of inequality: How today's divided society endangers our future*. New York: W. W. Norton.

Sullivan, S. (2013). The Republican Party's big state-level advantage, in one chart. *Washington Post: The Fix*, Retrieved from *www.washingtonpost.com/blogs/the-fix/wp/2013/02/04/the-republican-partys-big-state-level-advantage-in-one-chart/*.

Urban Institute. (2014). 10.3 Million poor uninsured Americans could be eligible for Medicaid if States opt for ACA expansion. Washington, DC: Health Policy Center, Urban Institute. Retrieved from *www.urban.org/health_policy/health_care_reform/map.cfm*.

U.S. Department of Health and Human Services. (2012). Press release. New health care law helps more than 3 million young adults get and keep health coverage. Retrieved from *www.hhs.gov/news/press/2012pres/06/20120619b.html*.

U.S. Department of the Treasury. (2013). The potential macroeconomic effect of debt ceiling brinkmanship. Retrieved from *www.treasury.gov/initiatives/Documents/POTENTIAL%20MACROECONOMIC%20IMPACT%20OF%20DEBT%20CEILING%20BRINKMANSHIP.pdf*.

Vanic, D. (2014). John Boehner believes income inequality is a problem. But the GOP doesn't have a solution. *NewRepublic.com*, Retrieved from *www.newrepublic.com/article/117748/boehner-admits-income-inequality-problem-offers-no-solution*.

Wade, L. (2014). Opinions on economic inequality driven by ideology, not income. Retrieved from *thesocietypages.org/socimages/2014/01/28/opinions-on-economic-inequality-driven-by-ideology-not-income/*.

Watts, A. (2014). Two scathing reviews by scholars working with the IPCC show why the organization is hopelessly corrupted by politics. Retrieved from *wattsupwiththat.com/2014/04/26/two-scathing-reviews-by-scholars-working-with-the-ipcc-show-why-the-organization-is-hopelessly-corrupted-by-politics/*.

Weatherford, K. (2014). President Obama's use of his executive power: Facts vs. hyperbole. Washington, DC: Center for Effective Government. Retrieved from *www.foreffectivegov.org/president-obamas-use-of-his-executive-power-facts-vs-hyperbole*.

Wessler, S. (2011). Thousands of kids lost from parents in U.S. deportation system. *News for Action*, Retrieved from *www.raceforward.org/research/reports/shattered-families?arc=1*.

The White House, Office of the Press Secretary. (2013). Remarks by the President on economic mobility. [Press release]. Retrieved from *www.whitehouse.gov/the-press-office/2013/12/04/remarks-president-economic-mobility*.

Wilkinson, R., & Pickett, K. (2009). *The spirit level: Why more equal societies almost always do better*. London: Allen Lane.

Ydstie, J. (2015). The ruling against Obamacare would have broad implications. *NPR.org*, Retrieved from *www.npr.org/2015/03/04/390694492/a-ruling-against-obamacare-would-have-broad-implications*.

CHAPTER 41

How Government Works: What You Need to Know to Influence the Process

Karrie Cummings Hendrickson   Christine Ceccarelli Schrauf[1]

"What government is the best? That which teaches us to govern ourselves."

Wolfgang von Goethe

Nurses need to know how government works so that they can convince public officials to create policies that improve access to quality and affordable health care for all. This chapter provides an overview of the federal, state, and local levels of government, how each level works, and the relationships among them in a federalist system. Such information is essential to affect policy and bring nurses' unique perspective to those who make the final decisions: legislators, regulators, and the staff who support them. Because budget policies underlie all health policy issues, this chapter also reviews the federal budget process and related state and local processes. All health programs require funding, and the budget process is the means by which the executive and legislative branches reconcile competing priorities and make budgetary decisions. In this chapter, we identify key access points for influencing policy at different levels and branches of government and throughout the federal budget process. We have used long-term care (LTC) to demonstrate how nurses can influence the government.

FEDERALISM: MULTIPLE LEVELS OF RESPONSIBILITY

The United States government is a federalist system. This means that the government consists of multiple levels, including a centralized, national tier and at least one decentralized, subnational tier, and that power is shared among them. In the case of the United States, tiers include the federal, state, and local levels of government. Unlike a unitary state, a federalist system constitutionally divides sovereignty among the different governmental levels so that the policymakers at each level have final authority in some areas and can act efficiently and independently of each other. The U.S. Constitution divides governmental authority by prescribing the duties and responsibilities of the federal government and withholding both specified and unspecified powers for the states. The Tenth Amendment to the Constitution (the States' Rights Amendment), helps to clarify how this authority is divided among the levels of government. It states, "The powers not delegated to the United States by the Constitution, nor prohibited by it to the States, are reserved to the States respectively, or to the people." This means that states have jurisdiction over issues that the Constitution does not explicitly grant to the federal government. This is a fundamental aspect of the Constitution; and state policymakers often interpret their constitutional states' rights liberally.

[1]The authors wish to acknowledge the mentorship and previous contributions in the development of this chapter to Sally S. Cohen, PhD, RN, FAAN. Sally was previously the Associate Professor and Director of the Robert Wood Johnson Foundation Nursing and Health Policy Collaborative at the University of New Mexico in Albuquerque. Currently she is the Distinguished Scholar-In-Residence at the Institute of Medicine of the National Academies in Washington, DC.

Because the U.S. government is one of divided powers, citizens are accountable to three levels of authority. In a federalist system, the allocation of authority among the levels may vary over time, and programs benefiting the public are implemented through the collaboration of local, state, and federal initiatives as part of the "marble cake federalism" of the United States (Grozdin, 2013). The federal government may participate in, and influence, local policy through government grants, incentives, and federal mandates (federal requirements for state, local, or tribal governments to expend their own resources to achieve certain goals) (O'Toole & Christensen, 2013). Many powers, such as taxation and law formation and enforcement, are shared equally among the levels of government and may be exercised in either conjunction or independently.

Because governmental powers and responsibilities laid out in the Constitution are imprecise and subject to interpretation, controversy and conflict have occurred among all the levels of government, particularly between federal and state authorities (Derthick, 2013). The U.S. Supreme Court works to interpret the Constitution and maintain the balance of power among the levels of government (O'Toole & Christensen, 2013). It is important to understand the Court's stand on federalism and states' rights when designing a federally administered program and planning its implementation.

THE FEDERAL GOVERNMENT

The U.S. federal government is centered in Washington, DC and has 10 regional offices (Figure 41-1). These regional offices are instrumental in policy implementation and enhance access to federal officials for issues concerning health. Like the three levels of government, the three branches of the federal government represent a separation of powers and work as a series of checks and balances on one another. These branches require policymakers to work together to formulate policy that is acceptable to as many people as possible, and they are designed to prevent any individual or small group from making sweeping changes.

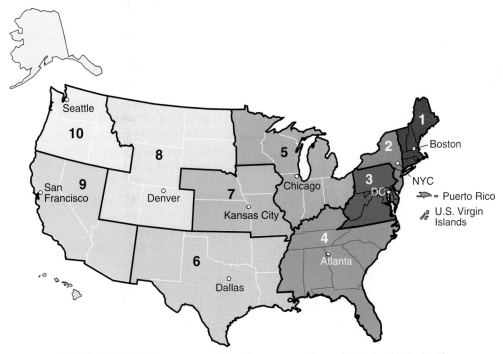

FIGURE 41-1 Federal government regions (*Source: www.hhs.gov/iea/regional/index.html.*).

THE EXECUTIVE BRANCH

The role of the executive branch is to implement laws and oversee enforcement. The executive branch is made up of the Executive Office of the President (EOP), the Executive Cabinet, and many independent agencies, boards, committees, and commissions, the staff of which advise the president and help to oversee the programs.

Executive Office of the President. The EOP consists of the president, the vice president, and related White House offices and agencies (Box 41-1) who develop and implement the policy and programs of the president. The Office of Management and Budget (OMB) is one of the most relevant to nursing. It prepares the president's budget for presentation to Congress on the first Monday of February. The budget reflects the president's national agenda and provides those seeking to influence policy a realistic picture of the likelihood of their project receiving funding. It also serves as a potential access point for policy change.

BOX 41-1 Obama Administration Offices and Agencies of the Executive Office of the President

Council of Economic Advisors: *www.whitehouse.gov/administration/eop/cea*

Council on Environmental Quality: *www.whitehouse.gov/administration/eop/ceq*

The National Security Council: *www.whitehouse.gov/administration/eop/nsc*

Office of Administration: *www.whitehouse.gov/administration/eop/oa*

Office of Science and Technology Policy: *www.whitehouse.gov/administration/eop/ostp*

Office of Management and Budget: *www.whitehouse.gov/omb*

Office of the U.S. Trade Representative: *www.ustr.gov*

Office of National Drug Control Policy: *www.whitehousedrugpolicy.gov*

Office of the Vice President: *www.whitehouse.gov/about/vp-residence*

The White House Office

The Executive Residence

The president is the highest ranking elected federal official and serves as the head of the executive branch. The president also serves as the commander-in-chief of all U.S. military forces, and with the approval of the Senate, grants pardons, makes treaties, and appoints high-ranking officials such as Supreme Court justices and Cabinet secretaries. One of the president's most notable domestic powers, however, is the veto, which effectively stops (or at least delays) a newly passed piece of legislation from becoming a law. This power is not to be taken lightly because, if the president invokes the veto, it can only be overridden by a two-thirds majority vote in both houses of Congress.

Of importance to those hoping to influence policy are the powers of the president not defined in the Constitution, including the power to set the national agenda. This is sometimes referred to as the power of the pulpit. Newly elected presidents bring their priority issues to the forefront of the American political agenda. Though this may not result in policy change, it does open the door for discussion and debate of some issues and closes the door on others. At the beginning of his presidency, President George W. Bush's proposals regarding Social Security, Medicare prescription drug coverage, and homeland security were high on the public and policy agendas. But the election of President Barack Obama in 2008 shifted emphasis away from those issues and onto discussions of revitalizing the domestic and worldwide economies, ending the war in Iraq, and providing universal health care. A savvy activist must be aware of policymakers' priorities and anticipate how changes in the political climate following an election may affect the politics of health policymaking.

White House staff are influential in setting national agendas and disseminating the president's priorities. These individuals are appointed by the president but are not confirmed by Congress. They usually hold views similar to those of the president and are instrumental in White House decision-making. One can determine White House staff perspectives on health policy through media reports.

The Cabinet. The Executive Cabinet is made up of the heads of 15 departments. After confirmation by Congress, cabinet members work with the president and oversee the enforcement and administration of federal law through regulation and the appropriation of funds. Although all cabinet departments may have jurisdiction over areas of interest to nurses, the ones most relevant to nursing practice are discussed in the following sections.

The U.S. Department of Health and Human Services. According to their website (*www.hhs.gov*), the U.S. Department of Health and Human Services (HHS) is "the United States government's principal agency for protecting the health of all Americans and providing essential human services, especially for those who are least able to help themselves." The HHS incorporates the Office of the Secretary and 11 agencies (Box 41-2) that oversee more than 300 programs such as Head Start, Vaccines for Children, Medicare, and Medicaid. The HHS is responsible for the distribution of the second largest portion of federal budget. New programs or changes to existing programs advocated by health professionals will probably be overseen by the HHS. It is vital to understand its structure and functions.

BOX 41-2 The 11 Agencies Included in the U.S. Department of Health and Human Services

Centers for Medicare and Medicaid Services: *www.cms.hhs.gov*

Centers for Disease Control and Prevention: *www.cdc.gov*

Food and Drug Administration: *www.fda.gov*

Indian Health Service: *www.ihs.gov*

Administration for Children and Families: *www.acf.hhs.gov*

Administration on Community Living: *www.acl.gov*

Agency on Toxic Substances and Disease Registry: *www.atsdr.cdc.gov*

Health Resources and Services Administration: *www.hrsa.gov*

Substance Abuse and Mental Health Service Administration: *www.samhsa.gov*

National Institutes of Health: *www.nih.gov*

Agency for Healthcare Research and Quality: *www.ahrq.gov*

The Social Security Administration. Economic security for most retired workers age 65 years or older in the United States is guaranteed through Social Security and funded through payroll contributions. The Social Security Administration (SSA) also provides monthly benefits to permanently disabled workers who have contributed to the program, as well as Supplemental Security Income (SSI) payments to needy older adults, blind individuals, and disabled individuals. Participation in the program also enables older adults and individuals who are disabled to qualify for Medicare health coverage, currently administered by the Centers for Medicare and Medicaid Services (CMS).

The Department of Defense. U.S. military spending makes up the largest portion of the federal budget, and a large part of that money goes to health care. The Department of Defense (DoD) provides care to all active duty military personnel, retirees, National Guard and Reserve members, and their families: approximately 9.6 million people stationed throughout the world (DoD, 2013). The military employs over 35,000 nurses, runs 65 military hospitals, oversees 413 medical and dental clinics, and provides funding for nursing research. Provision and coordination of health care for DoD members is provided by TRICARE, its health maintenance organization.

The Department of Veterans Affairs. Through the Veterans Health Administration (VHA), the U.S. Department of Veterans Affairs (VA) oversees programs to provide health care and other services to U.S. military veterans and their families. In 2012, approximately 6 million people received care at a VHA facility (VA, 2013a). The VA also manages the largest medical, nursing, and health professions training program in the U.S. Over 90,000 health professionals receive training in VA medical centers annually (VA, 2013b).

The U.S. Department of Education. The U.S. Department of Education, along with the Health Resources and Services Administration (HRSA) of the HHS, provides billions of dollars in grants and loans for students to attend college and professional schools, including nursing. This is relevant to nurses, particularly in times of nursing shortage, because the department works with hospitals and other government agencies to provide incentives such as loan repayment programs, which attract nurses to the most underserved areas (HRSA, 2013).

Regulatory Functions of the Executive Branch of Government. The executive branch of the government is responsible for implementing laws enacted by Congress. This falls to staff of the relevant departments and agencies, with input from the agencies of the EOP. Once a law is enacted, the federal agency staff develops regulations for implementation of the program, which specify definitions, authority, eligibility, benefits, and standards. This is necessary because although the laws passed by Congress or a state's legislative body express the legislators' intentions, they do not specify the details of the new program (Smith & Greenblatt, 2013).

Federal regulations (or rules) are published in the *Federal Register*, giving interested individuals and organizations a limited opportunity to review and comment. This is an important access point for nurses interested in shaping health policy. Agency staff review all of the comments and then issue final regulations in the Federal Register. These regulations govern how agencies and individuals in states and localities are to implement the law.

THE LEGISLATIVE BRANCH

The legislative branch of the federal government consists of the Congress, which is divided into two chambers: the Senate and the House of Representatives. Members of Congress are elected by their constituents. The Senate, with two members from each state, has 100 seats. The House of Representatives has 435 voting seats and 6 nonvoting seats, with each state's number of representatives based on its population. The number of members in each state's delegation may change every 10 years based on the results of the national decennial census. Members of the Senate and House are elected for 6-year and 2-year terms, respectively.

The primary role of the legislative branch is the formulation of laws for recommendation to the president. The process of creating such laws can be long and arduous, requiring much discussion and compromise. However, once a new topic or bill is introduced into a congressional chamber, it is often assigned to one of the committees or subcommittees for further discussion and hearings. In 2013, the Senate had 16 standing committees and four select committees, while the House of Representatives had 20 standing committees and one select committee. Select committees do not have the legislative jurisdiction of standing committees, but facilitate agenda setting by focusing on a specific issue. Between them, the House and Senate share four joint committees. The committee stage is a critical step for the nurse activist to recognize because it provides one of the primary points of entry into the policy arena. The assignment of a bill to a committee signals to those who care about the issue that it is time to act. Although this point of entry is not without roadblocks, measures can be taken to help keep the issue salient. Successful entry requires that the policy advocate be knowledgeable about the committee with jurisdiction, its members, and their priorities. It also requires that they be prepared with both a primary and backup policy plan, be willing and able to educate committee members and their staff, and be capable of providing persuasive testimony before committee members. For a complete list of committees and their health-related jurisdictions, see Tables 41-1 and 41-2. By following the link to each committee, one can obtain information about committee and subcommittee membership, complete jurisdiction, hearings, recent bills, and other timely health policy information. The status of all federal bills can be obtained at one of the most important websites for congressional information: *www.congress.gov*. It is also important to recognize that members of the congressional staff are accessible by telephone and the Internet. Nurses should be familiar with not only representatives from their home state but also other legislators who either support their issue or sit on a committee with jurisdiction over it.

Congressional caucuses are another way that congressional members provide a forum for issues or legislative agendas. Caucuses generally exist in the House of Representatives and can consist of both Representatives and Senators interested in diverse topics including individual disease conditions and health professions. The 113th

TABLE 41-1 Standing Committees of the U.S. Senate with Jurisdiction over Health Policy Issues

Committee	Jurisdiction
Agriculture, Nutrition, and Forestry *www.agriculture.senate.gov/*	Agricultural economics and research Food Stamp programs Human nutrition School nutrition programs
Appropriations *www.appropriations.senate.gov/*	Appropriation of revenue
Armed Services *www.armed-services.senate.gov/*	Issues relating to national (common) defense
Banking, Housing, and Urban Development *www.banking.senate.gov/public/*	Insurance Construction of nursing homes Public and private housing
Budget *www.budget.senate.gov/*	Congress's annual budget plan
Commerce, Science, and Transportation *www.commerce.senate.gov/public/*	Science, engineering, and technology research and development and policy
Energy and Natural Resources *www.energy.senate.gov/public/*	Emergency preparedness Nuclear waste policy
Environment and Public Works *www.epw.senate.gov/public*	Air pollution and environmental policy Solid waste disposal and recycling
Finance *www.finance.senate.gov*	Public monies and customs Health programs under Social Security Act Health programs financed by a specific tax or trust fund
Homeland Security and Government Affairs *www.hsgac.senate.gov/*	Census and collection of statistics Studying the efficiency of government departments Evaluating the effects of enacted laws National security
Health, Education, Labor, and Pensions *www.help.senate.gov*	Aging Biomedical research and development Domestic activities of the Red Cross Individuals with disabilities Public health Student loans Wages and hours of labor
Indian Affairs *indian.senate.gov/public*	Indian Health Service
Veterans Affairs *veterans.senate.gov*	Life insurance for members of the armed forces Veterans hospitals and medical care

Congressional Nursing Caucus is currently co-chaired by Lois Capps, RN (D-CA) and David Joyce (R-OH). Nurses interested in a specific area of health care can identify whether a caucus exists for that area and its congressional members by searching on the House of Representatives website: *www.house.gov/representatives.*

THE FEDERAL BUDGET

Anyone involved with national health policymaking follows the federal budget process closely. The federal budget is the end result of collaboration between the executive and legislative branches. The executive branch sets the national agenda as

UNIT 3

TABLE 41-2 Standing Committees of the U.S. House of Representatives with Jurisdiction over Health Policy Issues

Committee	Jurisdiction
Agriculture *agriculture.house.gov/*	Human nutrition and home economics Special Supplemental Nutrition Program for Women, Infants and Children, Food Stamps Licensing of animal research facilities Rural development Bioterrorism
Appropriations *appropriations.house.gov*	Appropriation of revenue
Armed Services *armedservices.house.gov*	Common defense National security Benefits of members of the armed forces (including health care) Scientific research and development support of the armed services
Budget *budget.house.gov*	Budget resolutions and budget process
Education and the Workforce *edworkforce.house.gov/*	Child labor Head Start and other early childhood education Child abuse prevention and adoption Food programs for schools Education and labor generally Worker's compensation
Energy and Commerce *energycommerce.house.gov*	Biomedical research and development Health and health facilities (except health care supported by payroll deductions) Public health and quarantine
Financial Service *financialservices.house.gov/*	Public and private housing Insurance
Homeland Security *homeland.house.gov*	National security Science and technology Emergency preparedness
Natural Resources *naturalresources.house.gov/*	Water and power Native American affairs
Science, Space, and Technology *science.house.gov*	Environmental research National Science Foundation Science Scholarships
Veterans Affairs *veterans.house.gov*	Veterans hospitals, medical care, and treatment
Ways and Means *waysandmeans.house.gov*	Customs Tax exempt foundations National Social Security Health programs under the Social Security Act and those financed by a specific tax

outlined in the presidential budget, and the legislative branch, with the help of the Congressional Budget Office (CBO), reevaluates the budget and divides and allocates the available monies among the programs seeking funding.

Policy advocates need to be very familiar with the federal budget process because it sets the structure and timeline for important policy work. Its appropriation process provides key access points for nurses to educate staff members and provide testimony. The federal government's fiscal year runs from October 1 through September 30. For example, the fiscal year 2014 runs from October 1, 2013 to September 30, 2014. The budget process officially begins each year in early February when, after months of analysis by the OMB, the president presents his budget to Congress.

The House and Senate budget committees work with the CBO to create budget resolutions for their respective chambers. According to congressional rules, these are supposed to be passed during March, but as a result of conflicts over budget priorities, consensus is not always easily reached. Once passed, a conference committee composed of both Senators and Representatives works to resolve the differences between the two budget resolutions and combine them into a single resolution that should pass both houses by April 15, but again, may be delayed. Once passed, the final budget resolution lacks the power of law, but is important as a blueprint for subsequent budget legislation.

After passage of the resolution, the next steps are enacting budget reconciliation legislation and enacting appropriation bills. A reconciliation bill is a piece of legislation that reconciles the amount of money coming into the government (taxes) with the amount of money the government is spending. Figure 41-2 depicts the data used to calculate the reconciliation each year and shows how tax revenues compare to government spending. An appropriations bill is a piece of legislation that prescribes how much money will go to each program in the federal budget. Figure 41-3 depicts early appropriations for President Obama's 2014 budget.

Both reconciliation and appropriation deliberations entail hearings and opportunities for nurses to present testimonies as the legislators try to determine how best to allocate the funds for the upcoming fiscal year. Many programs such as Social Security and Medicaid receive nondiscretionary funds as laid out by their authorizing legislation. These programs are entitlements, meaning Congress is required to fund all individuals and programs that are eligible under law. The only way entitlement funding can be decreased is by changing eligibility or diminishing services through revisions in law. Such highly contentious discussions may be part of reconciliation or budget deliberations in an effort to reduce federal spending.

Programs such as the National Institutes of Health and AIDS funding are discretionary,

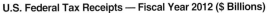

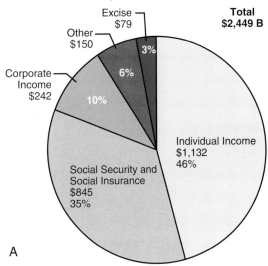

A

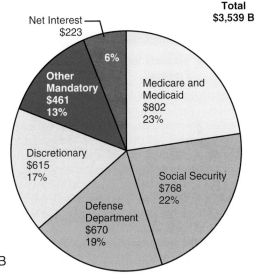

B

FIGURE 41-2 Federal revenues (**A**) and government spending (**B**) and for fiscal year 2012. (*Source:* Congressional Budget Office, Washington, DC, Historical tables, *www.cbo.gov/.*)

meaning that their funding is determined annually under the appropriations process. Figure 41-4 depicts discretionary spending and major expenditures of the HHS. Representatives of the constituent organizations involved with these programs must, with the help of advocates, provide testimony and

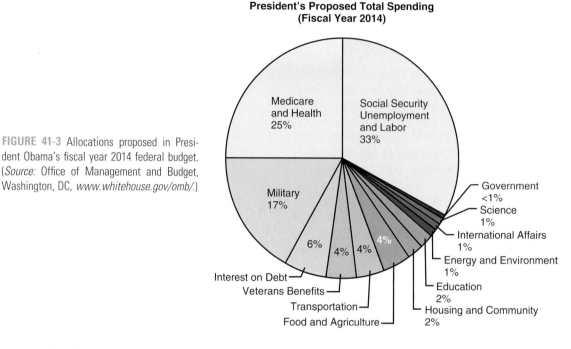

**President's Proposed Total Spending
(Fiscal Year 2014)**

FIGURE 41-3 Allocations proposed in President Obama's fiscal year 2014 federal budget. (*Source:* Office of Management and Budget, Washington, DC, *www.whitehouse.gov/omb/.*)

BOX 41-3 Glossary for the Federal Budget Process

Reconciliation Bill: A piece of legislation that balances the amount of money coming into the federal government (taxes) with the amount of money the government intends to spend in the coming year.

Appropriations Bill: A piece of legislation that prescribes how much money will go to each program named in the federal budget.

Entitlement (Mandatory) Spending: Money for programs that, by law, Congress must fund in full each year. For example, Medicare.

Discretionary Spending: Money for programs, the funding for which is debated annually during the appropriations process.

---

lobby to request annual funding from the government. (For budget terminology, see Box 41-3.)

The Senate and House Committees on Appropriations. The role of the appropriations committees is described in the U.S. Constitution, which states that before the federal government may spend any money, it must be reviewed by Congress and

appropriated by law. This power is sometimes referred to as the power of the purse. Appropriations bills must be enacted by September 30 for the ensuing fiscal year, which begins on October 1. Failure to do so may result in a government shutdown, as occurred in fiscal year 2014. The appropriations access point is important because Congress has money ready to spend and is weighing its options as how best to spend it. Successful testimony at this point can result in money being dispersed to your program.

More information on the federal budget is available from the Office of Management and Budget at *www.whitehouse.gov/omb/budget.*

STATE GOVERNMENTS

Each state government has its own constitution, which, similar to that of the federal constitution, defines the roles of each of the three branches of government at the state level. Each state's constitution is unique and is based on the state's history, population, philosophy, and geography. State constitutions and individual state laws cannot conflict with federal law or with the U.S. Constitution.

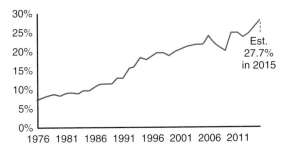

Medicare and Health as a Percent
of Total Federal Spending
(Fiscal Years 1976–2015)

Est.
27.7%
in 2015

Examples of proposed Department of Health and Human Services expenditures FY 2014 budget ($80.1 billion requested to support the HHS mandate):

- o $31 billion for the National Institutes of Health
- o $4.6 billion for the FDA
- o $4.4 billion for the Indian Health Service
- o $3.8 billion to enable health centers to provide affordable high-quality primary and preventive services to underserved populations, including the uninsured
- o $327 million for Title X family planning
- o $130 million to improve mental health services for students and to train teachers and professionals in mental health
- o $30 million to the CDC for gun violence prevention and research
- o $26 million to the Office of Health IT to support the advance of electronic health records technology and standards

FIGURE 41-4 Federal health spending: Medicare and health as a percentage of total federal spending (FY 1976-2015) and discretionary budget authority in billions of dollars (FY 2014). (*Source:* From National Priorities Project: Federal budget tip sheet: health care spending. September 2014. Available at *media.nationalpriorities.org/uploads/publications/health .tipsheet.9_16_14.pdf.*)

Although there is much variation in the structure and day-to-day functioning of state governments, there are enough similarities for comparison. Only the basics of the state executive and legislative branches will be discussed in this chapter. For complete information on each state, visit your state government's website, available through links on the federal government web portal at *www.usa.gov/ Agencies/State-and-Territories.shtml.*

EXECUTIVE BRANCH

Similar to the president at the federal level is the governor at the state level. All but three states also have lieutenant governors, whose roles are comparable to that of the vice president. The powers of these officials vary widely among the states, but they all have some common duties: the preparation of the state budget for presentation to the legislature, and management of the approved budget. Also, like the president, the governors have the power to veto or approve state-level legislation along with the power to make appointments to influential positions such as the state board of health. Most states also have lieutenant governors who often have a leadership position in the legislature (National Lieutenant Governors Association, 2013).

The governor's veto power, however, is slightly different from that of the president. Known as the line item veto, it allows the governor to cross out or delete sections of a bill before signing it into law. This is helpful for combating riders, legislators' favorite programs, which may be attached to bills. President Bill Clinton sought a line item veto on the federal level, but it was ultimately struck down by the Supreme Court. Attempts by Presidents Bush and Obama to enact an alternate way for the president to exert pressure on Congress to rescind portions of legislation have also been unsuccessful. Some believe it would give the President too much power and upset the system of checks and balances existing among the three branches of government (Brown, 2012). Therefore, the president must still sign a bill in total or veto it.

Regulatory Function of State Governments

Translating Laws into Regulations. The 50 states employ about 3.5 million people in state agencies who work to translate the intentions of state legislatures, outlined in new laws, into sets of rules and regulations, which define how those intentions will become reality (Smith & Greenblatt, 2013; U.S. Census Bureau, 2013). The crafting of regulation language is a process as important as the law itself, because it determines how it will be implemented. Once a set of rules is approved, within 30 days, it has the force of law and becomes a part of the state's administrative code. Laws and regulations work together to determine how public policy is implemented (Donovan, Smith, & Mooney, 2013).

The leaders of state agencies also work to influence policy. Many are elected officials, who attempt to keep campaign promises through the rules and

UNIT 3

regulations outlined in the agency (Smith & Greenblatt, 2013). The regulatory role of the executive branch makes it a prime target for the nurse activist. Creating and maintaining relationships with both appointed and elected officials helps to ensure that once the bill is enacted, its implementation matches the law's intent and the original vision. Agency personnel responsible for writing new regulations often benefit from the input of practicing health professionals, especially in specialty practice areas. Nursing input in these situations can be critically important to ensure that rules governing professional practice are realistic and meet patient needs adequately.

Regulation of Health Professionals. One of the most visible roles of the state executive branch with respect to health care is the licensing and regulation of professionals, including nurses. Each state sets both the educational and testing requirements for licensure and limits the scope of nursing practice through the state's nurse practice act. Even though some states have entered into compacts allowing nurses to practice in multiple states, the practice regulations continue to vary widely among states, particularly with regard to the scope of advanced nursing practice. Questions or disputes related to interpretation of state regulations are typically referred to the state's office of the Attorney General. Complete information on the regulations in your area, a list of states in the licensure compact, and links to all 50 state boards of nursing are available on the website of the National Council of State Boards of Nursing at *www.ncsbn.org*. Familiarity with state licensing boards, as well as with state agencies such as departments of public health or social services, can be very beneficial to nurses in their quest to influence policy. These agencies also serve as consultants on issues pertaining to health care to both executive and legislative branches of government. Working with staff of these agencies can help enhance your policy efforts.

LEGISLATIVE BRANCH

All 50 states have state legislatures with roles similar to that of the U.S. Congress. These groups create and pass new laws and serve as a check and balance to the executive branch by evaluating the governor's budget and appointments. Beyond this basic structure, aspects of the state legislatures may differ. Nebraska has a legislature with a single house, whereas the other 49 states have bicameral (two-house) legislatures. Although most state legislatures meet every year, 4 states have legislatures that meet every other year: Montana, Nevada, North Dakota, and Texas. Just as at the federal level, it is important to get to know not only the representatives from your home district but also those who support your issue and members of committees with jurisdiction over your area of interest.

LOCAL GOVERNMENT

There are many types of local governments in the United States, including counties, cities, towns, villages, and school districts. Local governments often have elected executive leaders. They may be referred to as mayors, in a county, city, or town, or as superintendents in school districts. The legislative branch at the local level is often composed of an elected council or board, which works to create the laws governing the locality. These laws cannot conflict with state or national laws.

Although the structure and function of local-level governments vary more widely than the governments at the state level, they serve as vital links between the local citizens and the state and nation (Donovan, Smith, & Mooney, 2013). Federal health policy can influence local health initiatives through transfer of billions of dollars in grant money to local entities, which disperse funds to community health agencies. These grants are often accompanied by defined health goals such as improved child immunization (Metzenbaum, 2008). As a result of rising health care costs of municipal employees and retirees, local governments often elect to institute their own health care reforms without waiting for federal or state initiatives. These programs can take the form of health screenings, wellness programs, and environmental control (Korfmacher, 2012; Wagner, 2010).

As local government responsibility for the health care of citizens has increased, it offers nurses increasing opportunities to influence policy. Getting to know and maintain a relationship with local officials is often much more feasible than it is with officials at the state or federal levels. Addressing issues and testing proposals at the local level will allow evaluation and improvement before moving to the state or federal level.

The nurse's strategies for influence at the local level are the same as those at the state and national levels, with one possible exception. Because of the nature of localities, policy advocates and policymakers may also be neighbors, friends, or colleagues. Such informal relationships must be carefully balanced, but they may also aid the advocate in gaining access to influence change.

TARGET THE APPROPRIATE LEVEL OF GOVERNMENT

The principle of divided powers is a cornerstone of our government (federal, state, and local) and the branches (executive, legislative, and judicial). The founding fathers saw this system of checks and balances as key to preventing the accumulation of power by any one group, thereby helping to maintain a democratic nation. Although this organizational structure may present challenges to nurses aiming to influence policy, it is important to understand which issues fall under the jurisdiction of each level of government, and the tasks that are shared responsibilities among the levels.

When it comes to the health and health care of U.S. citizens, the preamble to the Constitution addresses the government's responsibility by stating that one of the government's purposes is to promote the general welfare. At the time of the writing in 1787, the term, welfare, referred to the health, happiness, prosperity, and well-being of the people, and should not be confused with the social programs it may be associated with today (Mount, 2013).

The federal government is broadly responsible for many health policies regarding the organization, financing, and delivery of health care. Federal issues typically include programs enacted by Congress and the president, such as Medicare, Medicaid, and Veterans Affairs, as well as the administration of programs that fall under federal jurisdiction, including National Institutes of Health, the Centers for Disease Control and Prevention, the Food and Drug Administration, and the HHS.

At the state level, governments protect the public and affect the delivery of health care through policies within their jurisdiction, such as licensing of health care professionals and developing Long-Term Care (LTC) policy options (Brous, 2012; Harrington, 2012). States also control expansion of Medicaid health insurance to low-income individuals through Affordable Care Act provisions. Local governments oversee the provision of health care through administration and funding of safety-net programs and public hospitals and, more broadly, by addressing the public's general health by providing public education, waste management, fire and police protection, and public health initiatives (Donovan, Smith, & Mooney, 2013).

Over time, the powers associated with the implementation of programs have shifted from the federal level to the state and local governments, a process called devolution. Each state and locality implements federal programs, such as those funded by block grants and those that are shared federal-state responsibilities (e.g., Medicaid), in very different ways. Despite the fact that this may or may not result in better outcomes for the program, it definitely creates challenges for the nurse activist trying to understand the policies that affect patient care. Remember that the system is murky, and any issue may require attention at all three levels of government. Federal laws often provide funding and overarching direction, states are often the lead funding agencies under block grants or matching federal-state programs, and local agencies may receive funding from state or federal authorities to administer programs. Each level of government operates programs that are independent of the others.

Many health care initiatives fall to multiple levels of government for both funding and administration. For example, covering the uninsured falls under all three domains, depending on the proposal under debate. Medicaid, which provides insurance for the poorest Americans, is administered by federal and state authorities. Similarly, many education programs, although administered by local education agencies, entail some federal involvement. Laws such as the Elementary and Secondary Education Act (reauthorized as the No Child Left Behind

Act) are federal initiatives with grants to states, which in turn allocate funds to local agencies.

Some public health issues, such as emergency preparedness, which is overseen by the U.S. Department of Homeland Security and executed by the Federal Emergency Management Agency, involve all three levels of government. Implementation of disaster response and security of mass transit has become primarily a local responsibility, resting with local public health, hospital, and crime enforcement authorities. The federal and state governments retain a great deal of administrative control and responsibility for security of air traffic.

PULLING IT ALL TOGETHER: COVERING LONG-TERM CARE

This example will demonstrate how an issue can span multiple levels (federal, state, and local) of government, with each level developing and implementing policy to reach the best workable solution for the public welfare. Meeting the LTC needs of older adults and Americans who are disabled is too complex and costly for one government level. This issue is addressed through a federal/state partnership, with each state deciding the combination of LTC services available and the eligibility criteria required for persons to access them. According to the Centers for Medicare and Medicaid Services, the United States spent $136.2 billion for LTC services in 2011 (Eiken et al., 2013). The responsibility for this cost is shared between the federal government and the states, occupying an increasingly larger share of state Medicaid budgets. Efforts to include a voluntary government LTC insurance program within the Affordable Care Act were unsuccessful because the program was judged to be actuarially unsound (Frank, 2013). Current systems for reimbursement of LTC services do not expect to change for the foreseeable future.

Millions of older adults and Americans who are disabled currently require help with activities of daily living to ensure their safety and health, and this population is expected to grow rapidly. According to the U.S. Census Bureau (2010), the population 65 years or older is projected to grow to 88.5 million in 2050, more than double its population

in 2010 (Vincent & Velkoff, 2010). Most help is given by family and friends, but when this is not available, personal resources are usually used to pay for needed care. Medicaid is the safety-net program available to Americans when they exhaust personal resources to pay for their LTC needs.

Federal Medicaid funds available to states to help cover LTC costs are supplemented by matching state funds, and states must conform to federal rules and regulations, including the right of every eligible beneficiary to benefit from the program. Each state develops its own policies governing Medicaid eligibility, benefits provided, and reimbursement levels. This enables states to respond to the needs of its citizens as well as the limits of its budget. Because institutional care must be a covered Medicaid LTC service, all those eligible to receive services can be cared for in a nursing home. Local governments participate by ensuring that these facilities meet all local fire and safety requirements.

The majority of Americans wish to remain in their homes as long as they can, receiving in-home LTC services. To accommodate public preference and reduce institutional Medicaid costs, many states have sought Medicaid waivers from the federal government to offer alternate home and community LTC services. Federal Real Choice System Change grants are available to assist states to address barriers to provision of more home- and community-based LTC. Both federal and state LTC policy continues to evolve, responding to public demand for changes in services and the need to control escalating costs. Nurses can help to advocate for choice in patients' LTC settings by lobbying state legislators to pass enabling legislation and testifying at public hearings on these issues. States and localities assist older adults and persons who are disabled in additional ways, recognizing that their resources may be limited. These efforts indirectly help defray LTC costs and can include reductions in property taxes, grants to cover energy costs, and sliding-scale fees for home care services.

The nurse interested in improving LTC choices, or any other health policy issue, needs to know how the government works to plan appropriate strategies.

DISCUSSION QUESTIONS

1. How can a nurse who is interested in a specific health care issue learn about current government policies and funding that affects it?
2. During which parts of the lawmaking process does a nurse have an opportunity to influence final bill language?
3. How do the executive and legislative branches of government work together to create and regulate laws benefiting the public?

REFERENCES

Brous, E. (2012). Nursing licensure and regulation. In D. Mason, J. Leavitt, & M. Chaffee (Eds.), *Policy and politics in nursing and health care* (6th ed., pp. 506–513). St. Louis, MO: Saunders.

Brown, A. R. (2012). The item veto's sting. *State Politics & Policy Quarterly, 12*(2), 183–203.

Derthick, M. (2013). Ways of achieving federal objectives. In L. J. O'Toole & R. K. Christensen (Eds.), *American intergovernmental relations* (5th ed., pp. 148–1459). Los Angeles, CA: CQ Press.

Donovan, T., Smith, D. A., & Mooney, C. Z. (2013). *State and local politics. Institutions and reform* (3rd ed.). Boston, MA: Cengage Learning Wadsworth.

Eiken, S., Sredl, K., Gold, L., Kasten, J., Burwell, B., & Saucier, P. (2013). Medicaid expenditures for long term services and supports in 2011. Retrieved from *www.medicaid.gov/Medicaid-CHIP-Program-Information/By-Topics/Long-Term-Services-and-Support/Downloads/LTSS-Expenditure-Narr-2011.pdf.*

Frank, J. A. (2013). W(h)ither Medicaid? *National Academy of Elder Law Attorneys Journal, 9*(1), 67–89.

Grozdin, M. (2013). The federal system. In L. J. O'Toole & R. K. Christensen (Eds.), *American intergovernmental relations* (5th ed., pp. 37–46). Los Angeles, CA: CQ Press.

Harrington, C. (2012). Long-term care policy issues. In D. Mason, J. Leavitt, & M. Chaffee (Eds.), *Policy & politics in nursing and health care* (6th ed., pp. 206–213). St. Louis, MO: Saunders.

Korfmacher, K. S. (2012). Rochester's lead law: Evaluation of a local environmental health policy innovation. *Environmental Health Perspectives, 120*(2), 309–315.

Metzenbaum, S. H. (2008). From oversight to insight: Federal agencies as learning leaders in the information age. In T. J. Conlan & P. L. Posner (Eds.), *Intergovernmental management for the twenty-first century* (pp. 209–242). Washington, DC: The Brookings Institution.

Mount, S. (2013). The U.S. Constitution online. Retrieved from *www.usconstitution.net/glossary.html.2006-09-02-updating_theories_of_american_federalism.pdf.*

National Lieutenant Governors Association. (2013). Roster of lieutenant governors. Retrieved from *www.nlga.us/lt-governors/roster/.*

O'Toole, L. J., Jr., & Christensen, R. K. (2013). American intergovernmental relations: An overview. In L. J. O'Toole & R. K. Christensen (Eds.), *American intergovernmental relations* (5th ed., pp. 1–32). Los Angeles, CA: CQ Press.

Smith, K. B., & Greenblatt, A. (2013). *Governing states and localities* (4th ed.). Washington, DC: CQ Press.

U.S. Census Bureau. (2010). The next four decades. The older population in the United States: 2010 to 2050. Suitland, MD: U.S. Census Bureau. Retrieved from *www.census.gov/prod/2010pubs/p25-1138.pdf.*

U.S. Census Bureau. (2013). 2011 Public employment and payroll data, state governments, United States total. Suitland, MD: U.S. Census Bureau. Retrieved from *www2.census.gov/govs/apes/11stus.txt.*

U.S. Department of Defense. (2013). TRICARE. Arlington County, VA: U.S. Department of Defense. Retrieved from *www.tricare.mil/Welcome/AboutUs/Facts/BeneNumbers.aspx.*

U.S. Department of Veterans Affairs. (2013a). 2012 Highlights for the citizen. Washington, DC: U.S. Department of Veterans Affairs. Retrieved from *www.va.gov/budget/docs/report/2012-VAPAR_Highlights.pdf.*

U.S. Department of Veterans Affairs. (2013b). Department of Veterans Affairs: Students/trainees. Washington, DC: U.S. Department of Veterans Affairs. Retrieved from *www.vacareers.va.gov/students-trainees/.*

U.S. Health Resources and Services Administration. (2013). NurseCorp loan repayment program. Rockville, MD: U.S. Health Resources and Services Administration. Retrieved from *www.hrsa.gov/loanscholarships/repayment/nursing/.*

Vincent, G. K., & Velkoff, V. A. (2010). The next four decades, the older population in the United States: 2010 to 2050. U.S. Census Bureau Publication P25-1138. Suitland, MD: U.S. Census Bureau. Retrieved from *www.census.gov/prod/2010pubs/p25-1138.pdf.*

Wagner, D. M. (2010). Local government leaders initiate health care reforms. *Public Management, 92*(1), 11–12.

ONLINE RESOURCES

The National Council of State Boards of Nursing
www.ncsbn.org
U.S. Bills and Resolutions
www.congress.gov
U.S. Government Official Web Portal
www.usa.gov

CHAPTER 42

Is There a Nurse in the House? The Nurses in the U.S. Congress

C. Christine Delnat

"The members of the legislative department …. are numerous. They are distributed and dwell among the people at large. Their connections of blood, of friendship, and of acquaintance embrace a great proportion of the most influential part of the society … they are more immediately the confidential guardians of their rights and liberties."

James Madison

The U.S. Congress is elected to represent the people of the United States in regularly held democratic elections. There are two houses, the House of Representatives which has 435 voting members serving 2-year terms, and the Senate which has 100 voting members serving 6-year terms. The 113th Congress, elected in November 2012, includes members of many professions, predominantly business, law, public service and politics, and education. However, there are also a number of health care professionals: 19 physicians, 2 dentists, 1 psychiatrist, and 6 nurses (Manning, 2014). The first U.S. Congress met in 1789. In 1992, 203 years later, Eddie Bernice Johnson (Figure 42-1) became the first nurse elected to serve in the U.S. Congress. Congresswoman Johnson (D-TX-30) continues to serve, now joined by Karen Bass (D-CA-33) (Figure 42-2), Diane Black (R-TN-06) (Figure 42-3), Lois Capps (D-CA-23) (Figure 42-4), Renee Ellmers (R-NC-02) (Figure 42-5), and Carolyn McCarthy (D-NY-04) (Figure 42-6).

Although elected to represent their constituents, Congress as a whole does not always reflect the population characteristics of the nation (Heineman, Peterson, & Rasmussen, 1995). For example, 51% of the 2010 U.S. population was female (U.S. Census Bureau, 2010). However, only 18.7% of the 113th Congress was female (Manning, 2014). Fortunately, nursing is well represented in Congress. With 3.1 million nurses in the U.S. (American Nurses Association, 2011), at least 4 nurses would have been expected in the 113th Congress and 6 were elected.

THE NURSES IN CONGRESS

Nursing is diverse, and the six nurses who served in the 113th Congress reflect that diversity. Rep. Johnson's background is in psychiatry, Representatives Elmer and McCarthy were intensive care nurses, Rep. Black's background is emergency nursing, Rep. Capps was a school and community nurse, and Rep. Bass was a nurse before becoming a physician's assistant. The six nurses who served in the 113th Congress arrived at their positions through uniquely different paths. One replaced a spouse who died while serving in Congress, another ran for office after the incumbent refused to take a stand on gun control following an act of gun violence that killed her husband, several ran for Congress after serving at the state level, and one ran for office because of deeply held opinions on patient rights and access to health care.

THE HONORABLE KAREN BASS

Congressmember Bass is a former nurse, physician's assistant, and nonprofit community activism organization founder who was elected to her second term in the House of Representatives in 2012. She serves California's 37th Congressional District which includes parts of Central, West, and South Los Angeles. Before Rep. Bass was elected to Congress, she served in the California Assembly, where

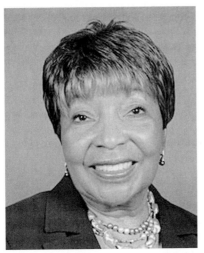

FIGURE 42-1 Congresswoman Eddie Bernice Johnson.

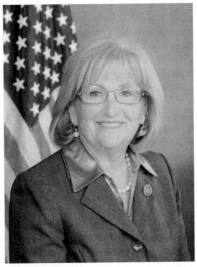

FIGURE 42-3 Congresswoman Diane Black.

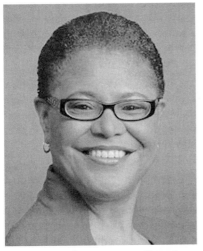

FIGURE 42-2 Congresswoman Karen Bass.

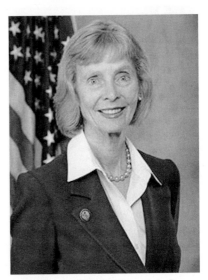

FIGURE 42-4 Congresswoman Lois Capps.

she earned the distinction of being the first African-American woman in U.S. history to be elected to the powerful role of state Speaker. She serves on the Steering and Policy Committee, which sets policy for the Democratic Caucus and also serves in the Congressional Black Caucus as the Whip for the 113th Congress (Bass, 2014a).

Rep. Bass has taken a strong stand on health care with consistent support of the Affordable Care Act (ACA), the introduction of legislation to increase health care technology in underserved communities, and cosponsoring legislation to improve education on sexually transmitted infections and unintended pregnancies. A life-long advocate for foster children, she founded the Congressional Caucus on Foster Youth, a bipartisan effort with the goals of overhauling the nation's foster system and providing advocacy for the needs of the nation's foster children (Bass, 2014b).

UNIT 3

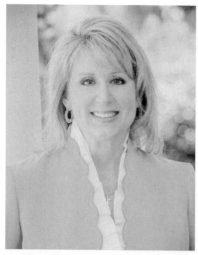

FIGURE 42-5 Congresswoman Renee Ellmers.

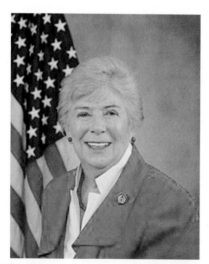

FIGURE 42-6 Congresswoman Carolyn McCarthy.

THE HONORABLE DIANE BLACK

Diane Black was elected to the Tennessee 6th Congressional District in 2010, on a platform of small government and limited taxes (Black, 2014a). Rep. Black is one of three female U.S. Representatives that use the term title Congressman instead of Congresswoman. Rep. Black has been a registered nurse for over 40 years. She began her career in the emergency department in 1971 and worked as a nurse until 1998, when she was elected to the Tennessee

House of Representatives. Rep. Black is a member of the House Committee on Ways and Means and its Subcommittee on Oversight, as well as the Committee on Budget (GOP.gov, 2013).

Rep. Black represents a constituency that believes that the ACA should be repealed and replaced by market-based health care reform (GOP.gov, 2013). Health care legislation that she has sponsored includes Title X Abortion Provider Prohibition, which would prohibit agencies performing abortions from receiving federal family planning assistance; the Health Care Conscience Rights Act, which would prohibit requiring people to purchase health insurance covering abortions; and the Safety Net Abuse Prevention Act of 2013, to terminate the Partnership for Nutrition Assistance Initiative between the United States and Mexico (Black, 2014b).

THE HONORABLE LOIS CAPPS

Congresswoman Lois Capps was a school nurse in Santa Barbara, California, a nursing instructor in Portland, Oregon, holds an MA in Religion from Yale University, and maintains her registered nurse license. She won her seat in the House of Representatives in a special election resulting from the death of her husband, Walter Capps. She holds influential seats on the Committee on Energy and Commerce and the Health, Energy and Power, and Environment and the Economy subcommittees. Rep. Capps maintains that her health care background is very influential in informing her work in Congress. She is also the cochair of the House Cancer Caucus, the Congressional Heart and Stroke Coalition, as well as a founding member of the Congressional Nursing Caucus, the Infant Health and Safety Caucus, and the School Health and Safety Caucus (Capps, 2014a).

Lois Capps's legislative priorities include better schools, quality health care, and a cleaner environment. Through her leadership in public health, she has sponsored legislation to reduce the nation's nursing shortage, protect victims of domestic violence, decrease underage drinking, improve mental health services, and improve Medicare coverage for people with Lou Gehrig's disease. Rep. Capps states that she is committed to increasing access to affordable health coverage and working toward quality health care availability for everyone. According to Rep. Capps, "Our nation's health care system is broken, but through health care reform we are now taking critical steps to repair it." (Capps, 2014b)

THE HONORABLE RENEE ELLMERS

Congresswoman Ellmers was elected in 2010 to serve the constituents of North Carolina's second District in the U.S. House of Representatives. Rep. Ellmers worked as a nurse for 21 years, first in surgical intensive care, and then with her husband in their general surgery practice. She became interested in politics as a result of health care reform and ran for office on a platform that included repealing the ACA, lowering health care costs, increasing health care access, protecting the physician-patient relationship, and reducing government spending. She serves on the House Energy and Commerce Committee, the Health, Communications, and Technology Subcommittee, and the Oversight and Investigations Subcommittee (Ellmers, 2014a).

Like fellow Congressman Black, Rep. Ellmers believes that health care reform should be based on the free market and that government involvement takes away individuals' control over their benefits and health care decisions. Rep. Ellmers' health care related legislative efforts in the 113th Congress included cosponsoring legislation to repeal the ACA, to prohibit abortion after 20 weeks' gestation, and to allocate money for pediatric research (Ellmers, 2014b).

THE HONORABLE EDDIE BERNICE JOHNSON

Congresswoman Eddie Bernice Johnson was the chief psychiatric nurse at the Dallas Veterans Administration Hospital until 1972, when she became the first African-American woman from Dallas, Texas to win an elected office. Elected to the Texas House of Representatives, she then became the first woman in Texas history to lead a major committee, and in 1977 she was tapped by President Jimmy Carter to serve as Regional Director of the U.S. Department of Health, Education, and Welfare. In 1986, she became the first African

American to hold the office of Texas State Senator since Reconstruction, and she became known for spearheading measures to improve neighborhoods, health, and childcare. In 1992, Johnson was elected to the U.S. House of Representatives and has become a leader in science, technology, transportation, election reform, and civil rights issues. In December 2010, Congresswoman Johnson was elected as the first African-American female Ranking Member of the House Committee on Science, Space, and Technology (Johnson, 2014a).

A former nurse in the Veterans Administration, Rep. Johnson has a long history of advocating for veterans' access to mental health services. She has recently sponsored bills to improve community assistance for persons with mental illness, as well as assistance for family caretakers caring for a family member with Alzheimer's disease (Johnson, 2014b). These bills are currently under legislative review. Rep. Johnson believes that laws need to change for citizens with severe mental illness to have access to nondiscriminatory health care (Johnson, 2013).

THE HONORABLE CAROLYN MCCARTHY

In 1993, Carolyn McCarthy was a New York wife, mother, and nurse. McCarthy's life changed course on December 7, 1993, when her husband Dennis and son Kevin were shot by a gunman aboard the Long Island Railroad. Her husband died and her son was critically injured. McCarthy, fueled by the senseless tragedy, began to advocate for stiffer gun control. In 1996, the Congressman in her home district voted to repeal a ban on assault weapons causing her to reshape her activism to a campaign, and she won her seat that year to serve in the House of Representatives (WP Politics, 2014).

Although much of her legislative focus has remained on controlling gun violence, Rep. McCarthy has also worked to help shape health care reform. She is a member of the Committee on Education and the Workforce, which is one of the committees responsible for drafting health care reform plans. She believes that reform is necessary and supported the passage of the ACA during the 111th Congress. Other health-related efforts include sponsoring the Children's Access to Reconstructive

Evaluation and Surgery Act in the 110th and 112th Congress, as well as the Student-to-Nurse Ratio Improvement Act in the 112th and 113th Congress, both of which have stalled in committee. Rep. McCarthy has also introduced legislation to help address senior citizen needs through Medicare legislation, and a tax credit for hearing aid assistance. She has been a strong supporter of women's issues, including breast cancer education and women veterans' health care (McCarthy, 2014. Rep. McCarthy announced her retirement in January, 2014, after 17 years in Congress.

EVALUATING THE WORK OF THE NURSES SERVING IN CONGRESS

The performance of members of Congress has been in the limelight during the 113th Congress. Major partisan differences centering on the ACA and economic policies are blamed for increasing dissatisfaction with members of Congress. Overall approval ratings are reported to be very low by many organizations conducting polls. PollingReport.com provides a compilation of polls related to politics and current political events and is useful in getting an overall picture of how Congress is doing.

The public is increasingly involved in evaluative political dialogue through the steady adoption of new technology. Social media, including Facebook and Twitter, have provided constituents with immediate, up-to-the-moment, unfiltered communication from politicians and are arguably changing the face of political media strategy. Congressmen post to their Twitter accounts, engaging directly with their followers providing direct access to personal thoughts and opinions (Peterson, 2012). Within minutes of a statement being made by a political leader, the public can, and does, begin discussing and analyzing. Regardless of the results of polls, opinions of analysts, or social media judgments, the ultimate evaluation of a Congressman's success is measured by their reelection.

POLITICAL PERSPECTIVE

There are several tools available for evaluating political perspective. PolitiFact.com is a Pulitzer Prize winning Tampa Bay Times fact-checking project designed to find the truth in American politics. Reporters and editors of *The Times* evaluate and rate the factuality of comments made by politicians (PolitiFact.com, 2014). A search of PolitiFact can rapidly confirm or debunk statements and helps constituents evaluate their Representatives. Every year, the nonpartisan *National Journal* uses voting records to compare lawmakers on an ideologic, liberal/conservative scale based on controversial economic, foreign, or social issues (National Journal, 2013). The most recent National Journal ratings of the six nurses in Congress are listed in Table 42-1.

TABLE 42-1 *National Journal's* Ratings of the Nurses in the 112th U.S. Congress (2013)

	LIBERAL RATINGS			CONSERVATIVE RATINGS			COMPOSITE SCORE Liberal	COMPOSITE SCORE Conservative
	E	S	F	E	S	F		
Eddie Bernice Johnson, D-TX	68	80	76	32	0	24	78.0	22.0
Carolyn McCarthy, D-NY	68	77	78	31	30	39	66.5	33.5
Lois Capps, D-CA	74	80	78	25	0	18	81.5	18.5
Karen Bass, D-CA	87	80	88	12	0	0	90.5	9.5
Diane Black, R-TN	0	0	0	90	83	91	6.0	94.0
Renee Ellmers, R-TN	10	0	0	83	83	91	8.8	91.2

How to read the ratings: A score of 68 on economic issues in the liberal column, for example, means that the Representative was more liberal than 68% of her House colleagues on key economic votes in 2011. The designations *E, S,* and *F* refer to the economic, social, and foreign policy votes used to determine overall ratings (*National Journal*, 2013).

INTEREST GROUP RATINGS

Some interest groups grade, rate, or rank members of Congress on issues of interest to the group. For example, the Cato Institute, a libertarian public policy research organization, evaluates the support that members of Congress provide for open trade. They host an interactive website that allows the user to see how individual Congressmen have voted on legislation affecting free trade (Cato Institute, 2014). The National Rifle Association (2014) graded the 113th Congress on their voting record on gun rights, and The New York Times mapped their ratings in an interactive website (New York Times, 2012). Project Vote Smart is a political website devoted to providing the public with factual, timely, accurate information on politics in the United States. In addition to keeping a searchable database on performance evaluations of politicians from an extensive list of special interest groups, they provide interactive tools that allow comparing elected officials and potential candidates according to issue areas (Project Vote Smart, 2014).

CAMPAIGN FINANCING

There is big money in politics. In 2012, the cost of winning the office of U.S. Representative averaged $1,689,580, and the average cost of a Senate seat was $10,476,451 (Costa, 2013). Candidate's campaign funds come from a variety of sources, including interest groups, lobbyists, political action committees, organizations, and individuals. The Center for Responsive Politics is a nonpartisan organization dedicated to tracking money and analyzing the effects of money on U.S. politics and public policy. Their website, OpenSecrets.org, houses unbiased information on campaign contributions and lobbying that anyone interested can easily access (Center for Responsive Politics, 2014). Table 42-2 demonstrates overall fund-raising and expenditures of each nurse in Congress during the 2012 congressional election cycle.

SOURCES OF CAMPAIGN FUNDS

As of 2014, for the first time in history, more than half of the elected Representatives in Congress

TABLE 42-2 Nurses in the 113th Congress: 2012 Election Cycle Fund-Raising

	Raised	Spent
Karen Bass, D-CA	$812,448	$933,375
Diane Black, R-TN	$2,497,751	$2,207,350
Lois Capps, D-CA	$3,325,296	$3,289,188
Renee Ellmers, R-NC	$1,136,890	$1,238,946
Eddie Bernice Johnson, D-TX	$779,237	$882,303
Carolyn McCarthy D-NY	$2,278,000	$1,860,331

	Small Individual	Large Individual	Political Action Committees	Candidate Self-Financing	Other
Karen Bass, D-CA	$21,423 (3%)	$215,672 (31%)	$442,998 (64%)	$0	$12,896 (2%)
Diane Black, R-TN	$50,410 (2%)	$862,880 (35%)	$1,178,331 (48%)	$304,523 (12%)	$41,086 (2%)
Lois Capps, D-CA	$419,388 (13%)	$1,697,422 (51%)	$1,132,703 (34%)	$0	$70,557 (2%)
Renee Ellmers, R-NC	$106,653 (10%)	$349,274 (32%)	$597,024 (55%)	$0	$33,919 (3%)
Eddie Bernice Johnson, D-TX	$23,390 (3%)	$236,340 (30%)	$518,496 (67%)	$1000 (0%)	$12 (0%)
Carolyn McCarthy, D-NY	$718,316 (32%)	$730,072 (32%)	$823,663 (36%)	$0 (0%)	$5950 (0%)

From Center for Responsive Politics (*www.OpenSecrets.org*).

were millionaires (Center for Responsive Politics, 2014). This has sparked increased public discussion about how well Congress represents the actual population and the increasing wealth inequality. In the United States, 75.4% of all wealth is held by the richest 10% of the people. This is among the highest in the developed nations and has been steadily increasing (Credit Suisse Research Institute, 2013). Two nurses in Congress are in the multimillionaire category: Diane Black with an average net worth of $69.6 million, and Carolyn McCarthy with $4.3 million. With campaigns becoming increasingly expensive, the field of prospective legislators has narrowed. Table 42-2 outlines the campaign financing for the nurses serving in the 113th Congress.

Evaluating members of Congress is difficult. The reader may recall the Hindu fable where six sightless men touching an elephant came to six different conclusions about what an elephant was like. The six men touched six different parts and came to six different conclusions about the elephant. Although each man may have been telling a truth, each man was wrong about his conclusion. This also applies in Congress. A true picture of a Congressperson's effectiveness will necessarily include a variety of measures from a variety of perspectives.

REFERENCES

American Nurses Association. (2011). Fact sheet: Registered nurses in the U.S. Retrieved from *nursingworld.org/NursingbytheNumbersFactSheet*.

Bass, K. (2014a). About me: Full biography. Retrieved from *bass.house.gov/about-me/full-biography*.

Bass, K. (2014b). Issues. Retrieved from *bass.house.gov/issues*.

Black, D. (2014a). About me: Biography. Retrieved from *black.house.gov/about-me/full-biography*.

Black, D. (2014b). Legislative work. Retrieved from *black.house.gov/legislative-work*.

Capps, L. (2014a). About me: Full biography. Retrieved from *capps.house.gov/about-me/full-biography*.

Capps, L. (2014b). Legislative work: Issues. Retrieved from *capps.house.gov/issues*.

Cato Institute. (2014). Free trade, free markets: Rating the Congress. Retrieved from *www.cato.org/research/trade-immigration/congress*.

Center for Responsive Politics. (2014). About us. Retrieved from *www.opensecrets.org/pfds/*.

Costa, J. (2013). What's the cost of a seat in Congress. MapLight. Retrieved from *maplight.org/content/73190*.

Credit Suisse Research Institute. (2013). Global wealth databook, 2013. Retrieved from *www.international-adviser.com/ia/media/Media/Credit-Suisse-Global-Wealth-Databook-2013.pdf*.

Ellmers, R. (2014a). About Renee: Biography. Retrieved from *ellmers.house.gov/biography/*.

Ellmers, R. (2014b). Legislation: Issues. Retrieved from *ellmers.house.gov/issues/*.

GOP.gov (2013). Republicans in Tennessee: Diane Black. Retrieved from *www.gop.gov/republicans/dianeblack/bio*.

Heineman, R., Peterson, S., & Rasmussen, T. (1995). *American government* (2nd ed.). New York: McGraw-Hill.

Johnson, E. B. (2013). Press release: Congresswoman Eddie Bernice Johnson introduces legislation to expand access to mental health care. Retrieved from *ebjohnson.house.gov/media-center/press-releases/congresswoman-eddie-bernice-johnson-introduces-legislation-to-expand*.

Johnson, E. B. (2014a). About Eddie Bernice Johnson. Congresswoman Eddie Bernice Johnson. Retrieved from *ebjohnson.house.gov/meet-ebj/*.

Johnson, E. B. (2014b). Health care. Congresswoman Eddie Bernice Johnson. Retrieved from *ebjohnson.house.gov/health-care1/*.

Manning, J. (2014). *Membership of the 113th Congress: A profile*. Washington, DC: Congressional Research Service. Retrieved from *www.fas.org/sgp/crs/misc/R42964.pdf*.

McCarthy, C. (2014). Legislation. Retrieved from *carolynmccarthy.house.gov/legislation/*.

National Journal. (2013). National Journal's 2012 vote ratings. Retrieved from *www.nationaljournal.com/2012-vote-ratings*.

National Rifle Association. (2014). NRA Digital Network. Retrieved from *home.nra.org/home/list/cpac-2014*.

Peterson, R. (2012). To tweet or not to tweet: Exploring the determinants of early adoption of Twitter by House members in the 111th Congress. *Social Science Journal, 49*, 430–438.

PolitiFact.com. (2014). About Politifact.com. Retrieved from *www.politifact.com/*.

Project Vote Smart. (2014). National special interest groups. Retrieved from *votesmart.org/interest-groups#.UtNsPbT6dD0*.

New York Times. (2012). How the N.R.A. rates lawmakers. Retrieved from *www.nytimes.com/interactive/2012/12/19/us/politics/nra.html*.

U.S. Census Bureau. (2010). *Age and sex composition: 2010*. Suitland, MD: U.S. Census Bureau. Retrieved from *www.census.gov/prod/cen2010/briefs/c2010br-03.pdf*.

WP Politics. (2014). Carolyn McCarthy (D-NY). *The Washington Post*. Retrieved from *www.washingtonpost.com/politics/carolyn-mccarthy-d-ny/glQAiZEKAP_topic.html*.

ONLINE RESOURCES

Find your elected officials and look at voting records and positions on key issues
votesmart.org
Track money in U.S. politics through this nonpartisan, independent, and nonprofit organization
www.opensecrets.org
Watch the U.S. House of Representatives live and follow floor proceedings, votes, bills, and reports
www.house.gov
Watch the U.S. Senate live and check bills, hearings, schedules, and voting
www.senate.gov

CHAPTER 43

An Overview of Legislation and Regulation

Nancy Ridenour

"Law is order, and good law is good order."

Aristotle

INFLUENCING THE LEGISLATIVE PROCESS

Public policy formation in the United States often appears to be indecisive and slow, and it can be difficult for the casual observer to distinguish the subtleties of the process. These nuances require that the observer select a conceptual model of policy-making to assist in understanding the specifics of policymaking process (that is, why a particular proposal is enacted or defeated). Chapter 7 sets forth several models for policy analysis. These can clarify how an issue is placed on the formal agenda for authoritative decision making. Nurses who understand this process can better influence the development of sound health policies for their patients, their patients' families, and the profession of nursing.

This chapter will describe the path by which a bill becomes a federal or state law in the United States, with primary emphasis on federal processes. The legislative path differs only slightly between the federal and state levels and from state to state.

INTRODUCTION OF A BILL

Only a member of the U.S. Congress (or of a state legislature) can introduce bills, although the idea for a bill can come from anyone. A legislator can introduce several types of bills and resolutions by simply giving the bill to the clerk of the house or,

in Congress, placing the bill in a box called the hopper. Legislation is often introduced simultaneously in the House of Representatives and the Senate as companion bills that will have different bill numbers and may differ in their details.

A legislator who understands the legislative process in depth can contribute more to either the passage or defeat of a bill than one who is an expert only on its substance. However, the numerous players involved (the executive branch, the legislature, constituents, and special interest groups) and the complexity of the legislative process make it far easier to defeat a bill than to pass one.

Every bill introduced in Congress faces a 2-year deadline; it must pass into law by then or die by default. Box 43-1 provides an overview of the types of bills that can be introduced by members of Congress. Legislators introduce bills for a variety of reasons: to declare a position on an issue, as a favor to a constituent or a special interest group, to obtain publicity, or for political self-preservation. Some legislators, having introduced a bill, claim that they have acted to solve a problem but do not continue to work toward enactment of the measure, blaming a committee or other members of the legislature if no further action is taken. Passage of a bill requires that, at critical points in the policymaking process, three streams come together, creating a window of opportunity. These streams include a problem for which a potential solution is identified and the political climate supports the proposed action (Kingdon, 2010). Although meeting these conditions helps a bill to rise on the decision agenda, nothing can guarantee enactment.

BOX 43-1 Types of Bills in the U.S. Congress

Bill: This is used for most legislation, whether general, public, or private (i.e., initiated by noncongressional sources). The bill number is prefixed with HR in the House and S in the Senate.

Joint resolution: This is subject to the same procedures as bills, with the exception of any joint resolution proposing an amendment to the U.S. Constitution. The latter must be approved by two thirds of both chambers, whereupon it is sent directly to the Administrator of General Services for submission to the states for ratification, rather than to the president. There is little difference between a bill and a joint resolution, and often the two forms are used interchangeably. One difference in form is that a joint resolution may include a preamble preceding the resolving clause. Statutes that have been initiated as bills have later been amended by a joint resolution and vice versa. The bill number is prefixed with HJ Res in the House and SJ Res in the Senate.

Concurrent resolution: This is used for matters affecting the operations of both houses. The bill number is prefixed with H Con Res in the House and S Con Res in the Senate.

Resolution: This is used when a matter concerns the operation of either chamber alone; adopted only by the chamber in which it originates. The bill number is prefixed with H Res in the House and S Res in the Senate.

From U.S. Government Printing Office. (2013). *About congressional bills.* Washington, DC: U.S. Government Printing Office. Retrieved from *www.gpo.gov/help/about_congressional_bills.htm.*

INFLUENCING THE INTRODUCTION OF A BILL

Nurses can influence the introduction of bills as constituents and as members of professional associations that lobby Congress. They can call attention to problems in funding health care, such as the need for expanded services for uninsured children or to increase reimbursement for nursing services. Legislators like to work with groups that have strong positions on a bill, such as the American Nurses Association, American Association of Colleges of Nursing, American Association of Nurse Anesthetists, or state nurses' associations.

Frequently, associations are asked to assist in drafting legislation and in lobbying members of the legislature. Coalitions of interested organizations are created to present a united front, a clear message, and a strong constituency to persuade legislators to support a particular bill. Enactment, if achieved at all, may take several legislative sessions.

Identifying the appropriate sponsor to introduce a bill is critical to its success. In selecting a primary bill sponsor, it is best to ask a member of a committee that has jurisdiction over the issue that needs to be addressed. For example, in the U.S. Senate, the Finance Committee has jurisdiction over the Medicare program and decides which Medicare-related legislation is sent to the full Senate for a vote (U.S. Senate, n.d.). Legislation that would address changes in direct reimbursement of nurse practitioners (NPs) or nurse anesthetists under Medicare would be less likely to be tabled (not acted upon) if a member of the Senate Finance Committee was a primary sponsor of the measure.

COMMITTEE ACTION

Committees are centers of policymaking at both federal and state levels. It is in committee that conflicting points of view are discussed and legislation is often refined and amended. Successful committee consideration of bills requires organization, consensus building, and time; only about 15% of all bills referred to committees are reported out for House and Senate consideration.

The Senate and House have separate committees with distinct rules and procedures. Committee procedure provides the means for members of the legislature to sift through an otherwise overwhelming number of bills, proposals, and complex issues. Within the respective guidelines of each chamber, committees adopt their own rules to address their organizational and procedural issues. Generally, committees operate independently of each other and of their respective parent chambers (Davis, 2012b; Schneider, 2008; U.S. Senate, 2013).

There are three types of committees at the federal level: standing, select, and joint. A standing committee has permanent jurisdiction over bills and issues in its content area. Some standing committees set authorizing funding levels, and others set appropriating funding levels for proposed laws. This two-step authorizing-appropriating process is designed to concentrate the policymaking decisions within the authorizing committee and decisions about precise funding levels within the appropriations committees.

A select committee cannot report out a bill and is often created by the leadership to address a special concern. A joint committee consists of members of both the House and Senate. One type of a joint committee is the conference committee, in which members of each chamber and party work together to address differences in their respective bills.

In congressional committees, leadership and authority is centered in the chair of the committee. The chair, always a member of the majority party, decides the committee's agenda, conducts its meetings, and controls the funds distributed by the chamber to the committee (Heitshusen, 2012). The senior minority party member of the committee is called the ranking minority member (or ranking member). The committee's subcommittees also have chairs and ranking members. Often, but not always, the ranking member assists the chair with some of the responsibilities of the committee or subcommittee. The committee chair usually refers a bill to the subcommittees for initial consideration, but only the full committee can report out a bill to the floor. For example, the House Ways and Means Committee refers most Medicare bills to the House Ways and Means Subcommittee on Health. If the subcommittee wishes to take action on the bill, it usually will schedule at least one hearing to discuss the substance of the bill.

In very unusual circumstances, a few bills will bypass the committee process. This can only happen if the leadership of the majority consents. Committees and subcommittees usually select the bills they want to consider and ignore the rest. Committees thus perform a gate-keeping function by selecting, from the thousands of measures introduced in each session, those that meet their party's leadership priorities and those that they consider to merit floor debate.

Consideration of bills whose content overlaps the jurisdictions of different committees falls to the leader of the chamber to decide. Health care issues can cut across the jurisdiction of more than one committee. When this occurs in the House, upon advice from the Parliamentarian, the Speaker of the House will base his or her referral decision on the chamber's rules and precedents for subject matter jurisdiction and identify the appropriate primary committee and other committees for the bill's referral. The Parliamentarians in both chambers have a key role in advising the member of Congress presiding over a bill on the floor. Although a member is free to take or ignore the Parliamentarian's advice, few have the knowledge of the chamber's procedures to preside on their own. The primary committee has primary responsibility for guiding the referred measure to final passage. Referrals to more than one committee can have a positive effect by providing opportunities for greater public discussion of the issue and multiple points of access for special interest groups, but this can also greatly slow down the legislative process (Davidson, Oleszek, & Lee, 2013). A committee can handle a bill in any of the following ways (U.S. Senate, 2013): (1) approve a bill with or without amendments; (2) rewrite or revise the bill, and report it out to the full House or Senate; (3) report it unfavorably (i.e., allow the bill to be considered by the full House but with a recommendation that it be rejected); or (4) take no action, which kills the bill.

AUTHORIZATION AND APPROPRIATION PROCESS

A considerable amount of congressional activity is concerned with decisions related to spending money, and much of this activity has a direct effect on health care and nursing programs. It is thus especially important for nurses to be familiar with the distinction between authorization and appropriation. Programs and agencies such as the Nurse Education Act, Scholarships for Disadvantaged Students, the National Health Service Corps, the National Institute of Nursing Research, the National Institutes of Health, and the Agency for Healthcare Research and Quality are all subject to the authorization-appropriation process.

Before any of these programs can receive or spend money from the U.S. Treasury, a two-step process must occur. First, an authorization bill allowing an agency or program to come into being or to continue to exist must be passed. The authorization bill is the substantive bill that establishes the purpose of, and guidelines for, the program, and usually sets limits on the amount that can be spent. It gives a federal agency or program the legal authority to operate. Authorizing legislation does not, however, provide the actual dollars for a program or enable an agency to spend funds in the future. Renewal or modification of existing authorization is called reauthorization.

Second, an appropriation bill must be passed to enable an agency or program to make spending commitments and actually spend money. In almost all cases, an appropriation bill for an activity is not supposed to be passed until the authorization for that activity is enacted. That is, no money can be spent on a program unless it first has been authorized to exist. Conversely, if a program has been authorized but no money is provided (appropriated) for its implementation, that program cannot be carried out (Schick, 2007). For example, the Affordable Care Act (ACA) authorized The National Health Care Workforce Commission, but no funds were appropriated. The commission was appointed with nurse Peter Buerhaus as chair, but, without funding, the commission has never met.

The authorization-appropriation process is determined by congressional rules that, like most congressional rules, can be waived, circumvented, or ignored on occasion. For example, failure to enact an authorization does not necessarily prevent the appropriations committee from acting. If an expired program (e.g., the Nursing Education Act) is deemed likely to be reauthorized, it may receive funds. These must be spent in accordance with the expired authorizing language.

Today, much of the federal government is funded through the annual enactment of 13 general appropriations bills. Whether agencies receive all the money they request depends, in part, on the recommendations of the authorizing and appropriating committees. Each chamber has authorizing and appropriating committees with differing responsibilities. For federal nursing education and research activities, the authorizing committees are the Senate Health, Education, Labor, and Pensions Committee and the House Energy and Commerce Committee.

The appropriating committees are the Senate and House appropriations committees and their subcommittees on Labor, Health and Human Services, Education, and Related Agencies (Figure 43-1).

COMMITTEE PROCEDURES

Committee consideration of a measure usually consists of three steps: hearings, markups, and reports.

Hearings. Hearings can be legislative, oversight, or investigative; each of these types of hearing may be either public or closed (Heitshusen, 2012). When the committee leadership decides to proceed with a measure, it will usually conduct hearings to receive testimony in support of a measure. From these hearings the committee will gather information and views, identify problems, gauge support for and opposition to the bill, and build a public record of committee action that addresses the measure. Although most hearings are held in Washington, DC, field hearings in the members' respective states are also held.

Most witnesses are invited to testify before the committee by the chair, who is a member of the majority party and who sets the agenda for the hearing proceedings. The ranking minority member may have an opportunity to request a witness, but it is up to the discretion of the chair to agree to the selection of the witness. Written testimony can also be submitted to the committee by persons who do not have the opportunity to speak their position on a measure in person.

Nurses can influence the policymaking process by testifying at bill hearings. Frequently, committees prefer to deal with large, organized groups that have a position on an issue rather than with private individuals. Professional nursing organizations testify on behalf of their members. Congressional hearings are listed in the official House and Senate websites at *www.house.gov* and *www.senate.gov*. C-SPAN provides live and recorded coverage of hearings at *www.c-span.org*.

Constituents can influence the committee process by meeting with and writing to members of the committee. Concerns expressed by constituents are given serious consideration.

HOW A BILL BECOMES A LAW

The Federal Level

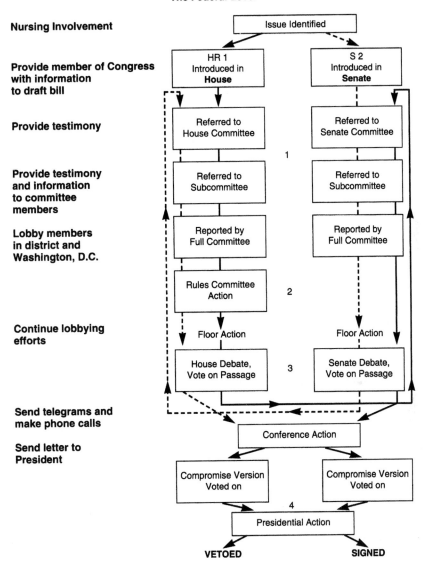

Nursing Involvement

Provide member of Congress with information to draft bill

Provide testimony

Provide testimony and information to committee members

Lobby members in district and Washington, D.C.

Continue lobbying efforts

Send telegrams and make phone calls

Send letter to President

Issue Identified

HR 1 Introduced in **House**

S 2 Introduced in **Senate**

Referred to House Committee

Referred to Senate Committee

Referred to Subcommittee

Referred to Subcommittee

Reported by Full Committee

Reported by Full Committee

Rules Committee Action

Floor Action

Floor Action

House Debate, Vote on Passage

Senate Debate, Vote on Passage

Conference Action

Compromise Version Voted on

Compromise Version Voted on

Presidential Action

VETOED   SIGNED

1, A bill goes to full committee first, then to special subcommittees for hearings, debate, revisions, and approval. The same process occurs when it goes to full committee. It either dies in committee or proceeds to the next step.

2, Only the House has a Rules Committee to set the "rule" for floor action and conditions for debate and amendments. In the Senate, the leadership schedules action.

3, The bill is debated, amended, and passed or defeated. If passed, it goes to the other chamber and follows the same path. If each chamber passes a similar bill, both versions go to conference.

4, The President may sign the bill into law, allow it to become law without his signature, or veto it and return it to Congress. To override the veto, both houses must approve the bill by a $2/3$ majority vote.

FIGURE 43-1 How a bill becomes a law.

UNIT 3

Lobbyists often meet with all members of the committee to express their client's position on a measure. Professional associations often activate a grassroots network of members, asking them to contact the committee members to request cosponsorship of, or opposition to, the measure.

The hearing process at the state level is similar, as is the importance of an organized approach to presenting testimony. When several representatives of nursing plan to testify on a bill, it is more efficient and effective for them to coordinate their testimony, raising different aspects of an issue rather than repeating the same points. It is also important for various nursing representatives to emphasize those issues where there is agreement; a unified message can strengthen the impression of a powerful coalition. And a hearing room packed with a supportive audience makes a powerful statement to legislators about support for an issue.

Markups. When legislative hearings are concluded, a subcommittee decides whether to attempt to report a measure. If the chair decides to proceed with the measure, she or he will generally choose to continue with the legislative process to mark up the bill. A markup is the committee meeting where a measure is modified through amendments to clean up problems or errors within the measure. A quorum of one third of the committee is required in both chambers to hold a markup session (Heitshusen, 2012). A markup session can weaken or strengthen a measure. Pressure from outside interest groups is often intense at this stage. Under congressional sunshine rules, markups are conducted in public, except on national-security or related issues.

After conducting hearings and markups, a subcommittee sends its recommendation to the full committee, which may conduct its own hearings and markups, ratify the subcommittee's decision, take no action, or return the bill to the subcommittee for further study.

Reports. The rules of both the Senate and the House dictate that a committee report accompany each bill to the floor. The report, written by committee staff, describes the intent of legislation (i.e.,

its purpose and scope). It explains any amendments to the bill and any changes made to current law by the bill, estimates the cost of the bill to the government, sets out documentation for the bill's legislative intent, and often contains dissenting views from the minority-party committee members.

A committee's description of the legislative intent of the bill is extremely important, especially for the government agency that will implement and enforce the law. Sometimes the report contains explicit instructions on how the agency should interpret the law in regulations, or the report may be written without great detail. Sometimes an agency will interpret the law narrowly, particularly if it is written vaguely. For example, when certified nurse midwives received reimbursement authority under the Medicare program, the agency chose to reimburse them only for gynecologic services, not for all the services covered by Medicare, which they are legally able to provide. This was a narrow interpretation of the law and was not the intent of Congress. It is important to provide comments on proposed regulations so that final regulations reflect legislative intent. In the event that a regulation narrowly interprets the law, additional legislative action may be needed.

The committee report is also important because it offers those interested in the bill an opportunity to promote or protect their interests. Committee staff frequently include the report language suggested by special interest groups if it is congruent with the bill.

FLOOR ACTION IN THE HOUSE AND SENATE

After a bill is reported out of committee, it can be placed on a calendar of chamber business and scheduled for floor action by the leadership of the majority party. Because the Speaker of the House is the leader of the majority party and the presiding officer of the House, the Speaker can influence floor debate. The Speaker has the discretion to recognize members to speak. The Speaker is considered a member of the House and can speak in the debate (Heitshusen, 2012). In the Senate, the Senate Pro Tempore as presiding officer is not a member of the body and does not have the same powers to control floor actions as does the Speaker of the House (Davis, 2012a). Although members of the House have time limits, Senators have no limits on how long they can speak. In the Senate, the presiding officer is required to recognize the first Senator who seeks recognition (Davis, 2012a; U.S. Senate, 2013).

The filibuster is used in the Senate to prevent a measure from coming to a vote (Beth & Heitshusen, 2013). (A vote of 60 members of the Senate is required to stop a filibuster of legislation or Supreme Court confirmations. See section on Senate Role in the Confirmation Process.) If the bill is not controversial, it may be dealt with expeditiously. Otherwise, it is placed on the chamber's calendar for future consideration. Both the rules governing the calendar on which a bill is placed, and the subsequent floor procedures, differ between the House and Senate and among state chambers. Box 43-2 compares the House and Senate procedures for scheduling and raising measures.

The influence of the committee chair and ranking member of the committee that reports out a measure is maintained throughout the floor proceedings. They continue to manage the measure by developing parliamentary strategy, controlling debate time, responding to colleague questions, deflecting unwanted amendments, and building coalitions to support their positions. Box 43-3 compares House and Senate rules for floor consideration of a measure. In the House, the Committee on Rules governs proceedings on the floor; there is no such committee in the Senate.

When a bill moves to the floor, special interest groups continue to lobby its opponents, its proponents, and particularly undecided legislators, attempting to influence the outcome of the vote. This process is usually begun after the introduction of the bill, when lobbyists meet with the members of the referring committee to gather support for the measure, and continues until the bill is signed into law. When a bill moves to the floor, constituents are activated to contact the members of the legislature from their own districts. Members listen attentively to their constituents, and so lobbying should continue until the moment of the vote, especially lobbying of undecided members. Lobbyists are known to wait outside the cloakroom in the

---

BOX 43-2 Scheduling and Raising Measures in the U.S. House and U.S. Senate

House

Four calendars (Union, House, Private, Discharge)

Speaker sets Calendar

Special days for raising measures*

Scheduling by Speaker and majority party leadership in consultation with selected representatives

No practice of "holds"

Powerful role for Rules Committee

Special rules (approved by majority vote) govern floor consideration of most major legislation

Noncontroversial measures usually approved under suspension of the rules procedure

Difficult to circumvent committee consideration of measures

Senate

Two calendars (Legislative and Executive)

No special days

Scheduling by majority party leadership in broad consultation with minority party leaders and interested senators

Individual senators can place "holds" on the raising measure, within limits

No committee with role equivalent to that of House Rules Committee

Complex unanimous consent agreements (approved by unanimous consent) govern floor consideration of major measures

Noncontroversial measures approved by unanimous consent procedure

Easier to circumvent committee consideration of measures

Adapted from Schneider, J. (2008). *House and Senate rules of procedures: A comparison.* Congressional Research Service order code RL30945, CRS-6. Washington, DC: Congressional Research Service. *There are special days for calling up bills under the suspension of the rules and Calendar Wednesday procedures, for raising measures from the Private Calendar, and for bringing up legislation involving the District of Columbia.

---

lobby to catch the attention of members as they move in and out of the chambers.

A vote is taken after the debate and amendment process is completed. There are three methods of voting: (1) voice vote, which calls for members to

---

BOX 43-3 Floor Procedures of the U.S. House and the U.S. Senate

House	Senate
Presiding officer has considerable discretion in recognizing members	Presiding officer (Senate Pro Tempore) has little discretion in recognizing senators
Rulings of presiding officer seldom challenged	Rulings of presiding officer frequently challenged
Debate time always restricted	Unlimited debate;* individual senators can filibuster
Debate ends by majority vote in the House and in the Committee of the Whole (i.e., the membership of the House)	Super-majority vote required to invoke cloture; up to 30 hours of postcloture debate allowed[†,‡]
Most major measures considered in Committee of the Whole	No Committee of the Whole
Number and type of amendments often limited by special rule; bills amended by section or title	Unlimited amendments; bills generally open to amendment at any point
Germaneness of amendments required (unless requirement is waived by special rule)	Germaneness of amendments not generally required
Quorum calls usually permitted only in connection with record votes	Quorum calls in order almost any time; often used for purposes of deliberate delay
Votes recorded by electronic device; electronic vote can be requested only after voice or division vote is completed	No electronic voting system; roll-call votes can be requested almost any time
House routinely adjourns at end of each legislative day	Senate often recesses instead of adjourning; legislative days can continue for several calendar days

Adapted from Schneider, J. (2008). *House and Senate rules of procedures: A comparison*. Congressional Research Service order code RL30945, CRS-6. Washington, DC: Congressional Research Service.

*Except when complex unanimous consent agreements or rule-making provisions in statutes impose time restrictions.

[†]Adoption of the motion to table by majority vote also ends Senate debate. Use of this motion, however, is generally reserved for cases when the Senate is prepared to reject the pending bill.

[‡]Simple majority vote for non-Supreme Court confirmations.

---

answer yea or nay (victory is judged by ear); (2) division vote, which requires a head count of those favoring and those opposing an amendment; and (3) recorded teller vote in the Senate and electronic voting system in the House that records each legislator's name and position taken on the vote. Recorded votes are the most valuable to lobbyists and constituents because they document how the member voted—helpful information in determining whether to continue to support a legislator and as a predictor of a legislator's future stand on issues.

CONFERENCE ACTION

Before a bill can be sent to the executive branch, identical bills must be passed in both chambers. Frequently, the bills originally considered by the House and Senate chambers are not identical, so members of each chamber must meet to resolve the differences. This is often where much of the hard bargaining and compromising takes place in the

passage of legislation. The leaders of each chamber appoint conferees, usually senior members of the committees with jurisdiction over the bill, to meet with the conferees of the other chamber.

A joint conference offers another opportunity for groups and individuals to persuade members to support positions on controversial aspects of the bill. Frequently, there is controversy over the amount of money allocated to a federal program. For example, House and Senate funding authorizations for nursing education programs can differ by millions of dollars. Supporters of a program would usually lobby for the version of the bill authorizing the largest amount of funding.

When agreement is reached on the controversial provisions of the measure, a conference report is written explaining the differences considered in resolving the issue. Both chambers must then approve the conference version of the bill for the bill to become law.

SENATE ROLE IN THE CONFIRMATION PROCESS

The Senate gives advice and consent to presidential appointments, Supreme Court nominees, and other high-level positions in the cabinet departments and independent agencies of the government. The Senate also confirms appointments of members of regulatory commissions, ambassadors, federal judges, U.S. attorneys, and U.S. marshals. Appointees named to be Supreme Court Justices and Cabinet Secretaries receive close scrutiny by the full Senate and Senate committees.

There are several steps in the confirmation process. First, the president submits a nomination in writing and forwards it to the Senate. The nomination is read on the floor of the Senate and is given a number. Second, the Senate Parliamentarian, acting on behalf of the presiding officer, refers each nomination to the committee or committees of jurisdiction. Confirmation hearings, generally open to the public, can be held, but they are not held on all nominations. Supreme Court nominees and senior administration officials or controversial nominees are given the closest scrutiny in hearings. Senators can use the committee hearings as a forum to advance their own policy and political agenda, to determine or challenge the administration's positions on policy issues, and to receive commitments from a nominee. The committee has the option to report the nomination favorable, unfavorable, or without recommendation, or take no action at all. If the committee moves to report the nomination, it is filed with the Senate's executive clerk, who assigns a calendar number and places the nomination on the Executive Calendar.

The third step in the confirmation process involves floor consideration of the nomination. During this step, the Senate will meet in an executive session to consider the nomination. Nominations are subject to unlimited debate, except when cloture, the only way the Senate can vote to place a time limit on debate, and thereby overcome a filibuster, is invoked. Because of frustration with the increased use of the filibuster, Democrats in the 113th Senate used parliamentary procedure to change the filibuster rules for Senate confirmations so that a simple majority, rather than the previous 60-vote majority, is now required (Bolton, 2013; Klein, 2013). The Supreme Court nominations were excluded from this rule change, still requiring the 60-vote majority. This new rule does not apply to legislative action. (The 60-vote majority is still required for a cloture vote on legislation.) The Senate has three options in its advice and consent role: confirm, reject, or take no action on the nomination. Confirmation requires a simple majority vote. Once the Senate has acted on a nomination, the Secretary of the Senate transmits the results of the nomination to the White House. In some instances, one or more senators can place a hold on a nomination, which can delay or prevent the nomination from reaching the floor for further action. Senate rules require any pending nominations to be returned to the president when the Senate is in recess for more than 30 days or adjourns between sessions. Presidents have made recess appointments, without consent of the Senate, when the Senate was in recess. These appointments are temporary, with the nominee's term expiring at the end of the next session of the Senate.

EXECUTIVE ACTION

After both chambers have passed identical versions of a bill, it is ready to go to the executive branch. The executive (president or governor) has the power to sign a bill into law, veto it, or return it to the legislature with no signature and a message stating his or her objections. If no further action is taken, the bill dies, or the legislature may decide to call for another floor vote to overturn the executive's veto. A two-thirds vote is required to override an executive veto in Congress and in many states. Under the U.S. Constitution, a bill becomes law if the president does not sign it within 10 days of the time she or he receives it, provided Congress is in session. Presidents occasionally permit enactment of legislation in this manner when they want to make a political statement of disapproval of the legislation but do not believe that their objections warrant a veto. If Congress adjourns before the 10-day period expires, the unsigned bill does not become law. In this case, the bill has been defeated by the pocket veto (U.S. Senate, 2013).

UNIT 3

REGULATORY PROCESS

Legislation is only the first phase of the process. As important as it is to become skilled at influencing the legislative process, it is equally important to influence the regulatory process (see Chapter 43). Regulations are written to guide the implementation of the laws that are passed. The implementation of the ACA, for example, requires the Centers for Medicare and Medicaid Services (CMS) to promulgate rules and regulations covering new aspects proposed in the law. Some of these topics include value-based payments, accountable care organizations, and meaningful use of electronic health records. Regulations such as these have a direct impact on a nurse's work and professional life. As changes in health care financing and delivery structures are driving changes in the current health care provider licensing system, many states are considering changes in the regulation of nursing, from amending the Nurse Practice Act to accomplishing a major overhaul of the entire licensing system. Many of these changes will take place in the regulatory arena within a nurse's state. Other health care related regulations that can impact nursing practice may also take place within the federal domain.

Although some regulations may be developed or amended without legislation, other regulations are created by the details of new or amended laws. The development of such regulations takes months or years. It is this important step, the development of regulations, which may be overlooked by those working to influence policy and the political process (Figure 43-2).

One of the largest federal agencies having primary responsibility for health care programs is the U.S. Department of Health and Human Services (HHS). The CMS is the administrative agency in the HHS that directs the Medicare and Medicaid programs. A major role of government regulation is to interpret the laws. The laws that Congress and state legislatures pass rarely contain enough explicit language to closely guide their implementation. It is the responsibility of administrative agencies to promulgate the rules and regulations that fill in the details. The health policy positions of the executive or legislative branches will

THE REGULATORY PROCESS

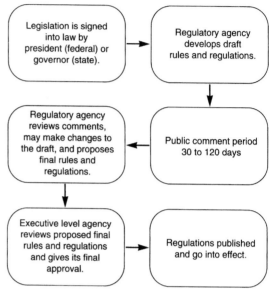

FIGURE 43-2 The regulatory process.

determine the laws that are passed, but once enacted, laws and their accompanying regulations shape the way the law is translated into programs and services.

Regulations specify definitions, authority, eligibility, benefits, and standards. Their development is shaped by the law and by the ongoing involvement and input of professional associations, providers, third-party payers, consumers, and other special interest groups (Box 43-4).

The administrative agencies, usually part of the executive branch of government, may enact, enforce, and adjudicate their own rules and regulations, thus assuming (in this context) the functions of all three branches of government (legislative, executive, and judicial). For example, some administrative agencies can sit in judgment of previously enforced agency regulations that are now in dispute and judge whether to uphold or overturn them. Agencies are created through legislation that broadly defines their structure and function. They must develop their own regulations that set policy to govern the behavior of agency officials and regulated parties; spell out their procedural requirements, such as rules governing notices of intent,

---

BOX 43-4 How to Influence Legislative and Regulatory Processes

- Become informed about the public policy and health policy issues that are currently under consideration at the local, state, and federal levels of government.
- Become acquainted with the elected officials that represent you at the local, state, and federal levels of government. Communicate with them regularly to share your expertise and perspective on health care and nursing issues.
- Call, write, or send a fax or e-mail message to your legislator, stating briefly the position you wish him or her to take on a particular issue. Always remember to mention that you are a registered nurse and that you live and vote in the legislator's district.
- Request that legislation be introduced or a regulatory change made. Offer your expertise to assist in developing new legislation or in modifying existing legislation and rules.
- Become active in your professional association and work to activate a strong grassroots network of members who

- are prepared to contact their elected representatives on key health care issues.
- Attend a public hearing on a bill or regulation to show support for an issue, or actually testify yourself.
- Build your own political résumé by becoming active in local politics in your area.
- Volunteer to work on the campaigns of candidates who are knowledgeable and supportive of nursing's perspective on health care issues.
- Seek appointment to a government task force or commission to have the opportunity to make legislative, regulatory, and public policy changes.
- Seek election to public office or employment in an administrative or executive agency.
- Explore opportunities to be involved with the policy and legislative process through internships, fellowships, and volunteer experiences at the local, state, and federal levels.
- Provide comments on proposed regulations

---

comment periods, and hearings; and develop enforcement procedures. For example, the Food and Drug Administration sets and monitors standards for foods and tests drugs for purity, safety, and effectiveness, although the Environmental Protection Agency, among other activities, controls health risks from water-borne microbes in drinking water through the development and implementation of regulations.

The promulgation of regulations is guided by certain rules. Key among these, at the federal level, is the requirement that the agency responsible for implementing a law publish a draft of any proposed regulations in the *Federal Register*. The *Federal Register* is the official daily publication for administrative regulations, including rules, proposed rules, and notices of federal agencies and organizations, as well as executive orders and other presidential documents. The publication of proposed regulations offers an opportunity for interested parties to react to the draft before it becomes final. Following the regulatory process and providing comments on proposed regulations is an important aspect of nursing advocacy (Centers for Medicare and

Medicaid Services, 2009; Office of the Federal Register, 2013b). States follow similar procedures.

A REGULATORY EXAMPLE: NURSE PRACTITIONERS AS ESSENTIAL COMMUNITY PROVIDERS

Insurance industry practices can restrict NPs expansion of primary care access. Some insurers do not permit NPs into credentialed networks as primary care providers, even in states that have independent practice laws covering NPs. To bill insurers directly for services, NPs must be credentialed in the insurer's network (Appleby, 2013). The Patient Protection and Affordable Care Act (2010) directs the Secretary of Health and Human Services to develop rules related to the requirement to include essential community providers in qualified health plans (QHPs) that are listed on the Health Insurance Exchanges (Patient Protection and Affordable Care Act, 2010, Section 1311). Proposed rules allow a QHP to be decertified if it fails to meet requirements related to inclusion of essential community providers (Office of the Federal Register, 2013a).

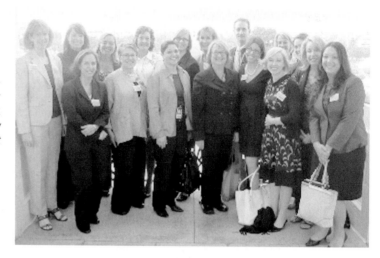

FIGURE 43-3 Nursing policy and organizational leaders on the Capitol balcony. Nancy Ridenour, first row, center. They met to work on the document *Commitment to quality health care reform: A consensus statement from the nursing community.* (Photo published with permission of Nancy Ridenour.)

The American Nurses Association submitted comments to proposed rules related to essential community providers (Weston, 2013). Documenting the expanded numbers of NPs, the quality of care provided by NPs, and citing publications by the Institute of Medicine (2011) and the National Governors Association (2012), the American Nurses Association requested that the regulations include NPs in QHPs. Despite significant evidence of quality outcomes and increased access to primary care, many insurers continue to refuse to credential NPs (Hansen-Turton, Ritter, & Torgan, 2008). The American Nurses Association has asked the CMS, through comments to the proposed regulations, to ensure that State Exchanges verify that potential insurers have secured access to NP services to be authorized as a QHP (Weston, 2013). It is important for nurses to monitor and suggest changes to proposed regulations to ensure access to health care and support for health providers working at the top of their expertise and license. The issue of credentialing by insurance providers and QHPs has not been resolved. Nurse advocates will continue to scrutinize this issue.

DISCUSSION QUESTIONS

1. What are the state and federal regulations applicable to an issue of importance to you that is affected by the ACA?

2. What impact has the 113th Senate change in the cloture rules had on Senate confirmations?

3. What advocacy actions might you take to improve health care through legislation at the state or federal level?

REFERENCES

Appleby, J. (2013). Nurse practitioners try new tack to expand foothold in primary care. *Kaiser Health News*, Retrieved from *www.kaiserhealthnews.org/Stories/2013/September/09/nurse-primary-care-slowed-by-insurer-credentialing.aspx.*

Beth, R., & Heitshusen, V. (2013). *Filibuster and cloture in the Senate.* Congressional Research Service, RL30360. Washington, DC: Congressional Research Service.

Bolton, A. (2013). Senate guts filibuster power. *The Hill*, Retrieved from *thehill.com/homenews/senate/191042-dems-reid-may-go-nuclear-thursday.*

Centers for Medicare and Medicaid Services. (2009). *E-rulemaking overview.* Baltimore, MD: Centers for Medicare and Medicaid Services. Retrieved from *http://cms.hhs.gov/eRulemaking.*

Davidson, R. H., Oleszek, W. J., & Lee, F. E. (2013). *Congress and its members* (14th ed.). Washington, DC: Congressional Quarterly.

Davis, C. (2012a). *The president pro tempore of the Senate: History and authority of the office.* Congressional Research Service, RL30960. Washington, DC: Congressional Research Service. Retrieved from *www.senate.gov/CRSReports/crs-publish.cfm?pid='0E%2C*PL%3F%3D%22P%20%20%0A.*

Davis, C. (2012b). *The legislative process on the house floor: An introduction.* Congressional Research Service (pp. 95–563). Washington, DC: Congressional Research Service. Retrieved from *www.senate.gov/CRSReports/crs-publish.cfm?pid=%26*2H4Q%5CC8%0A.*

Hansen-Turton, T., Ritter, A., & Torgan, R. (2008). Insurers' contracting policies on nurse practitioners as primary care providers: two years later. *Policy, Politics & Nursing Practice, 9*(4), 241–248.

Heitshusen, V. (2012). *Introduction to the Legislative Process in the U.S. Congress.* Congressional Research Service, R42843. Washington, DC:

Congressional Research Service. Retrieved from *www.fas.org/sgp/crs/misc/R42843.pdf*.

Institute of Medicine. (2011). *The future of nursing: Leading change, advancing health*. Washington, DC: National Academies Press.

Kingdon, J. (2010). *Agendas, alternatives, and public polices update edition, with an epilogue on health care* (2nd ed.). New York: Longman Classics in Political Science.

Klein, E. (2013). Nine reasons the filibuster change is a huge deal. *The Washington Post*, Retrieved from *www.washingtonpost.com/blogs/wonkblog/wp/2013/11/21/9-reasons-the-filibuster-change-is-a-huge-deal/*.

National Governors Association. (2012). *The role of nurse practitioners in meeting increasing demand for primary care*. Washington, DC: National Governors Association. Retrieved from *www.nga.org/files/live/sites/NGA/files/pdf/1212NursePractitionersPaper.pdf*.

Office of the Federal Register. (2013a, June 19). Patient Protection and Affordable Care Act; Program Integrity: Exchange, SHOP, Premium Stabilization Programs, and Market Standards. Retrieved from *www.gpo.gov/fdsys/pkg/FR-2013-06-19/pdf/2013-14540.pdf*.

Office of the Federal Register. (2013b). A guide to the rulemaking process. Retrieved from *www.federalregister.gov/uploads/2011/01/the_rulemaking_process.pdf*.

Patient Protection and Affordable Care Act. (2010). Retrieved from *beta.congress.gov/bill/111th-congress/house-bill/3590?q={%22search%22%3A[%22110+th+Congress+Affordable+Care+Act%22]}*.

Schick, A. (2007). *The federal budget: Politics, policy, process* (3rd ed.). Washington, DC: Brookings Institution.

Schneider, J. (2008). *House and Senate rules of procedure: A comparison*. Congressional Research Service, RL30945. Washington, DC: Congressional Research Service.

U.S. Government Printing Office. (2013). *About congressional bills*. Washington, DC: U.S. Government Printing Office. Retrieved from *www.gpo.gov/help/about_congressional_bills.htm*.

U.S. Senate. (2013). Legislative process: How a Senate bill becomes a law. Retrieved from *www.senate.gov/reference/resources/pdf/legprocessflowchart.pdf*.

U.S. Senate. (n.d.). Glossary. Retrieved from *www.senate.gov/reference/glossary_term/pocket_veto.htm*.

Weston, M. (2013). Re: PPACA; Program Integrity: Exchange, SHOP, Premium Stabilization Programs, and Market Standards. 78 Fed Reg/37032 (June 19, 2013). Retrieved from *www.nursingworld.org/cms71913*.

ONLINE RESOURCES

Congress.gov
beta.congress.gov
Federal Register
www.federalregister.gov
House Committee on Ways and Means
waysandmeans.house.gov
Senate Committee on Finance
www.finance.senate.gov
Senate Committee on Health, Education, Labor, and Pensions
www.help.senate.gov

UNIT 3

CHAPTER 44

Lobbying Policymakers: Individual and Collective Strategies

Kenya V. Beard[1]

"Our lives begin to end the day we become silent about things that matter."

Martin Luther King Jr.

For some, the word lobbying may conjure up images of elite salaried individuals who are well versed in evoking a persuasive discourse, poised in navigating the halls of Congress, and artistically skilled at setting the stage for change. This contextual view of the lobbying experience may sound daunting. However, simply stated, lobbying is described as an attempt to shape policy and influence government by ensuring that key policymakers are aware of and understand the concerns of their constituents (Zetter, 2011). Although lobbying should not engender silence, it sometimes does. For example, when I suggested to graduate level nursing students that they speak to their legislators about what advanced practice nurses do and the barriers to care that exist, they were eagerly receptive. Yet, when lobbying was used to describe the encounter, a look of trepidation washed over some of their optimistic faces and it was perceived as an insurmountable task. When I asked the students who wanted to sign up, many became silent.

Lobbying should not strike fear in individuals and need not be a formidable endeavor. Conversely, it should germinate from a space that is empowering so that individuals are willing to voice their opinions. Sometimes it is simply from a place that matters. Still, with the right combination of passion, knowledge, and commitment, individual citizens can and do have access to and accountability from elected officials, and you do not have to be a paid lobbyist to make a difference.

Many citizens lobby Congress, as well as state and local officials. Nurses have some significant advantages when it comes to working to influence an elected official. They are ranked first in trustworthiness in the Gallup most recent poll on honesty and ethics in professions (Gallup, 2013) and in each Gallup poll ranking since nursing was added in 1999, except for 2001, when firefighters topped the list after their heroic acts on September 11. Nursing is 3.1 million individuals strong, composing the largest group of health care professionals in the United States. The combination of credibility and numbers is important to legislators.

LOBBYISTS, ADVOCATES, AND THE POLICYMAKING PROCESS

Lobbying is a form of advocacy (Jacobs & Skocpol, 2012). Both paid, professional lobbyists and unpaid advocates may lobby a specific issue with the intention of influencing policymakers. However, the Internal Revenue Service (IRS) makes a clear distinction between lobbying and advocacy. The IRS defines a lobbyist as "a person who represents the concerns or special interests of a particular group or organization in meetings with lawmakers" (Internal Revenue Service, 2010). Most have experience in some aspect of the political or policy process, often as former elected officials or their staff, and have expertise in the legislative process or a specific policy area. Professional lobbyists are

---

[1]This chapter is an adaptation of earlier versions authored by Melinda Mercer Ray, Shelagh Roberts, Mary Foley, Catherine Dodd, Ellen-Marie Whelan, and Michael P. Woody.

employed by trade associations (such as the American Nurses Association), law firms, companies, public interest groups, and nonprofit agencies. Traditionally, lobbying regulations were lax. Today, there are limits on the lobbying activities of non-profit agencies as determined by the IRS. Typically, 501(c)(3) organizations are restricted from political campaign activities and risk losing their tax exemption status if lobbying is found to be excessive (Kupfer, 2011). However, depending on whether the 501(c)(3) is a public charity or private foundation, different rules may apply. For example, Section 501(h) of the Internal Revenue Code provides that 501(c)(3) organizations *not* classified as "supporting organizations" with an opportunity to make an "election" and are thus restricted in what they can do. Supporting organizations are viewed as electors and have more flexibility with regard to what constitutes lobbying activities.

LOBBYIST OR ADVOCATE?

Citizen advocates are not paid and spend most of their time doing something else. Although both lobbyists and advocates may lobby Congress, there is an important legal distinction between the two. The Lobbying Disclosure Act of 1995 made federal lobbying activities and some contributions and expenses more transparent. In 2007, the act was amended by the Honest Leadership and Open Government Act. A lobbyist who spends more than 20% of his or her time on lobbying activities is required to register with Congress, report what he or she is working on, and report political contributions above a certain limit. Requirements may differ at the state and local levels. Indeed, organizations are required to disclose lobbying activities once certain thresholds are met. Lobbying continues to be a politically charged word, with professional lobbyists often being blamed for policy failures, corruption in the political process, and symbols of what is wrong with Washington, DC. Antilobbyist sentiment was a prominent part of President Barack Obama's campaign narrative, but has been central to the political dialogue for years. Politicians often decry special interests and purport to favor the public interest even though the terms are subjective.

Indeed, the Jack Abramoff scandal[2] and other high-profile cases help solidify the view of lobbyist as villain in the public's mind. However, antilobbyist rhetoric undermines the profession's legitimate place in the policy process and denigrates the essential work lobbyists and advocates do to communicate policy ideas to Congress and the executive branch. In reality, legislation, the regulation of human activity, can be blindingly complicated (Nelson & Yackee, 2012). Members of Congress and state legislators write the laws, presidents and governors execute the laws, but all have precious little experience with every aspect of the complex society they are elected to govern. Oftentimes minute details that could have disastrous effects may go unnoticed. Providing information to elected officials is essential to the coherence of policymaking through law and regulation, its function in the real world, on professions, and on real people. Without lobbying, policy would have more unintended consequences than it already does. Between 2009 and 2010, pharmaceutical companies spent over $500 million lobbying lawmakers (Blumenthal, 2012). Smaller companies are finding it increasingly difficult to compete with well-funded corporations to get their voices heard. Many are turning to grassroots lobbying and using the influence of communities to help educate and influence legislators.

WHY LOBBY?

The most common reason people get involved with lobbying is because they see something that needs to be changed. For example, The Future of Nursing: Leading Change, Advancing Health (Institute of Medicine, 2011), calls for nurses to practice to the full extent of their education and training. However, in some states, nurse practitioners are not able to

---

[2]Jack Abramoff was a powerful lobbyist who was convicted in 2006 for conspiracy and fraud. He owned several nonprofit organizations and received millions of dollars in donations which went to bribe congressional leaders into supporting his clientele's positions. In an interview, at a Georgetown University Lecture Fund event, he admitted to spending $1.5 million a year on sports tickets alone so he could entertain policymakers and influence their decisions.

practice without having a physician supervise or collaborate with them. These barriers to care oftentimes impact the quality, timeliness, and cost of care that patients received. Nursing organizations may hire lobbying firms, or individual nurses may meet with their legislators to apprise them of the ramifications of current policies and suggest alternatives. Another example is the mandate in the Affordable Care Act that went into effect on October 1, 2013, requiring providers and suppliers to comply with face-to-face encounter requirements. This has impacted the way practitioners are able to obtain durable medical equipment and imposed unintended consequences for the patient. Knowledgeable nurses, nursing groups, and lobbyists explained the benefits and potential harm of this policy and, although the policy was not amended, more time was given to establish proper protocols surrounding this requirement. Unless a nurse represents their professional association as a paid lobbyist or serves as an appointed or elected representative, they often lobby because of their beliefs and values.

STEPS IN EFFECTIVE LOBBYING

RESEARCH

The first step in the lobbying process is to find out as much as you can about the issue that concerns you. Become a kind of detective. Uncover the legislative history, stakeholders, important elected officials, and policy particulars of bills related to your issue of interest. Your job is to learn as much as you can about the issue so that you can decide what your best lobbying approach will be.

Nearly all professional nursing associations, health care associations, and think tanks post political position statements on their websites. Many have legislative affairs sections that display sample letters or issue briefs to help you frame your arguments in favor of, or in opposition to, a particular bill or policy. If you have expertise to offer, contact someone in the government affairs department. For additional guidance, most government agencies make detailed documents, including bill texts and summaries, federal agency reports and studies, and countless sources of federal data available online.

The website of the Library of Congress (formerly *www.thomas.loc.gov*, this service has been transitioned to *www.Congress.gov*) offers complete listings of bills that can be searched by subject, keyword, cosponsor, date of introduction, and bill title or number. In addition, every state has a webpage with detailed information regarding elected officials and legislative activity. Although the websites of the states vary in the degree of detail they provide, almost every one includes the names of, and contact information for, state senators and representatives, as well as a search function to identify your legislator according to zip code or city name. These searches will identify bills on your issue of interest in great detail and can help you gain knowledge of the legislative histories behind a given subject. Tracking a bill is also very important, as the legislative process is, by design, one of compromise. Knowing where a bill is in the process, and what has changed or remained the same, will enable you to speak accurately about your support for, or opposition to, a bill at the right time.

IDENTIFYING SUPPORTERS

First, identify members of Congress or state legislatures who have been leaders on the particular issue. For example, if you search a site using the keyword, breastfeeding, you can identify legislators with a long history of introducing or cosponsoring breastfeeding legislation. When approaching the legislator for support, you will be able to build on his or her previous knowledge and initiatives to craft a workable legislative strategy. Remember to thank the legislator for their previous support. Once you identify the issue that you want to lobby on, and you have educated yourself as to its legislative history and the current status of bills related to it, the next step is to determine (1) whom you need to contact to bring about change and (2) the best mode of communication to accomplish that change.

CONTACTING POLICYMAKERS

At the federal level, your primary contacts are the congressional staff members in the offices of your representatives and senators. They work with other congressional offices and interest groups to craft provisions in legislation. Your first step at the federal level is to identify the person in your legislator's office who is responsible for your issue. For nursing and health-related issues, this will likely be the legislative assistant who works on health care policy. Sometimes, though, responsibility for health care issues can be divided among several staff, particularly if the member of Congress serves on a committee that has jurisdiction over health. Therefore, it is best to obtain specific information about who covers your particular issue of interest, not just who covers health care issues. Usually, the easiest way to identify the correct person on your issue is to telephone your member's Capitol Hill office and ask for the name of the individual who handles that issue. Once you have identified the proper staff member, you should address all correspondence or requests for meetings to that person.

Types of Congressional Staff. At the federal level, there are two types of staff who work on policy: those in the members' personal offices and those who work at the committee level. Some members of Congress are leaders on an issue because they have a personal or constituent-related connection to it, whereas others serve on committees that have jurisdiction over significant health care matters, such as the committees that oversee federal health programs or appropriations. Although there are also district offices for both representatives and senators in the members' home states, these offices generally handle constituent services rather than policymaking responsibilities. However, this might be a good place to start if your issue has implications for your state or district.

Political staff often experience high turnover rates, so you should confirm that the contact information you have is current, particularly if you are relying on a published directory. Staff usually rely on experts in the field to help them understand the background of certain legislative issues. A staff member would need input from experts who actually work in nursing to get a firm grasp on what might be short-term and long-term strategies to promote workforce diversity. Some members of professional nursing organizations have the insight and the credibility to explain how a diverse workforce contributes to a healthier nation.

At both state and federal levels, it is important to recognize the critical role the staff plays in crafting legislation and helping to determine legislative priorities for the member of Congress for whom they work. With the broad range of issues that members of Congress must address, they rely on staff to brief them on issues. Members also look to staff to craft legislation and make recommendations about what issues to champion. It is unrealistic to expect a meeting with a member of Congress in most circumstances, and you can accomplish a great deal by meeting with a staff member who will be involved in writing legislative language. Additional avenues of access may result from your participation in an association or coalition that has broad appeal to the member.

Building Relationships. Opportunities to build personal relationships are often easier at the local and state levels than at the federal level, for the simple reason that there are more occasions for networking and building personal relationships with policymakers where you both live. In your community, you can invite an official or his or her staff to meetings of your professional organization, or you can invite the policymaker to address the group at a meeting or luncheon. You should also regularly attend local and state meetings or committee hearings on issues in the home district. Additional opportunities for networking and visibility occur when you volunteer to serve on a task force in your community, take part in a political campaign, become involved in the political party structure, or run for office yourself. Through the informal exchanges with legislators and policymakers these activities provide, you can build the foundations for lasting relationships.

HOW SHOULD YOU LOBBY?

PERSONAL VISITS

Face-to-face lobbying is generally perceived as the most effective strategy. If you have arranged a personal visit with a legislative assistant or other staff member, or with a member of Congress or state or local official, you can apply many of the same guidelines for crafting your message that you would employ in letter-writing. Know the current status of legislation; keep the visit brief, as time is usually short; keep your points succinct and germane to the topic; illustrate your expertise or concern with personal examples; and identify your practice setting. Finally, do not forget to ask for a specific action or request to close the meeting. This is your "ask" and the reason for the visit. For example, "We hope we can count on you to vote next Wednesday to increase funding for nursing education." Box 44-1 contains tips for effective visits to policymakers.

It is recommended that you provide a one-page fact sheet to staff in advance of the meeting, and have a copy available to leave with whomever you meet as well. For example, if you are demonstrating the need for increased funding for nursing scholarships, you could provide a graphic representation, a chart or table, which illustrates the low rate of increase for nursing scholarships since they were initiated, particularly compared with grants or scholarships for other health professions. Make sure your name and contact information is on this document. Any resource that provides data or illustrates points in the form of easily digestible tidbits (talking points) can be useful to the staff member when he or she briefs the elected official, writes speeches, or drafts press materials. Be sure to bring business cards to distribute.

TELEPHONE CALLS

Telephone calls are not ideal for introducing yourself to a legislative assistant. It is better to write a letter or make a personal introduction at an appropriate forum, such as a legislative briefing, to make the initial point of contact. After a letter has been received, it is perfectly acceptable to call the legislative assistant to whom you have written to confirm that the letter was received or to ask if he or she would like any further information. Telephone calls are, of course, expected if you are actively working with a legislative assistant or other staff member on a particular piece of legislation or if you have an ongoing relationship with that person. Placing numerous telephone calls to someone with whom you have no established relationship, however, can

identify you as a nuisance. With written communication, the person can respond according to his or her own timetable, whereas a phone call is sometimes an interruption.

A pitfall of communicating by telephone is that there is no written record of the call. Additionally, when you communicate with staff via telephone, you have no way of guaranteeing that either your message or your personal information (e.g., your name, telephone number, or address) is recorded correctly. If they are recorded correctly, you have no assurance that they will be forwarded to the correct person. A telephone call may be worthwhile simply to express your support for, or opposition to, a legislative issue that is currently on the floor of the House or Senate for debate and will be coming up for a vote. Most congressional offices keep a running tally of yes or no votes from constituents who call the office during a contentious debate. Telephone calls can also be a good means of obtaining brief information or following up with someone with whom you have already established a relationship.

LETTER-WRITING

Written communication to Congress has changed dramatically after the anthrax attack in 2001, where letters containing anthrax spores were mailed to several news media offices and two U.S. Senators. Since that time, all mail delivered to Congress must go through an irradiation process. This process creates new compounds, which results in a different look, feel, and even smell. In many cases, it ruins the mail, rendering it virtually unreadable. Because of this, electronic correspondences have become the norm for communicating with Congress. Although letters are still a critical way of communicating with Congress, they should be put into the body of an e-mail when possible. Note that using the correct address and salutation makes your letter more effective.

When you write a letter to a member of Congress or a state or local official, there are some general guidelines to follow. First, identify who you are. For example, you might state that you are a constituent, a registered nurse, and a member of the

---

BOX 44-1 8 Tips for a Successful Legislative Visit

1. **Make the appointment.** Make an appointment with the policymaker or his or her staff member. Arrive on time and be ready to wait because often schedules change at the last minute. Reconfirm the appointment a day before the meeting. Remember that often staff members know more about specific issues than the legislator. If you meet with a staff person, find out what you can do to help them stay informed, and in turn inform your legislator.

2. **Plan the meeting.** Create an agenda. Time is limited. Develop a policy brief (one page) to leave behind. Agree on who will open and close the meeting and who will speak to each agenda item and ensure that everyone generally knows what will be said before the meeting. Meetings are often cut short, so be prepared with an essential message. Meetings should generally follow these steps: (1) have each person introduce himself or herself (e.g., name, whether or not you're a constituent, position with the organization); (2) state the purpose of the meeting, along with bill number(s) if appropriate, and provide relevant materials; (3) tell your story (making a clear and simple ask of the legislator); (4) ask for a response; (5) and follow up as necessary.

3. **Do your homework.** Credibility is everything. Know your facts. You only get one chance to make a first impression, so express your talking points accurately and succinctly. Know your issue as well as your legislator's background and priorities. What committees does he or she serve on? Learn all you can about the legislator you plan to visit. If you can connect your interests to those of the legislator, then do so. It is imperative that if there is opposition to your issue you make your legislator aware of this to avoid any surprises. Prepare for what the opposition's points of contention will be and what your responses are to those points.

4. **Build rapport.** Legislators are just people. They are members of a community, a home town; if your organization does work in that home town or district, let

the legislator know. Don't expect your legislator to understand your issue. Provide a one-page issue brief, then begin with a general explanation of the topic and the necessary background. Give good eye contact; if he or she appears distracted, inquire if this is a good time to speak because you think your message is very important and the legislator's support critical. Time is always limited, so getting to the point efficiently is important. Present your views with conviction, but don't give a speech.

5. **Know your "ask."** What do you want from the legislator? It is important to know and to be clear what it is before the meeting. Is it is a vote on a specific bill? Are you asking them to hold a hearing or to persuade others? Ask directly for your legislator's support. If he or she is not willing to support your cause, ask what would be needed (e.g., more data, other supporters) to consider changing his or her mind. Don't conclude the meeting until you have agreed upon the next steps and are clear on the position and direction the legislator is heading on your issue.

6. **Present specific examples.** On many issues, legislative representatives are not experts. Personal stories as well as facts are important to present.

7. **Agree to disagree.** Be respectful that legislators may not be ready to decide on the spot. Actively listen and respond to questions and concerns with facts and clarity. If you don't know, state that you will find out the answer. Never "fake" an answer. Never threaten, and don't burn bridges because you will probably need to work together in the future.

8. **Follow up after the visit.** It is very important to say thank you at the end of the meeting and to send a personal handwritten thank-you note to the legislator. Personal notes are appreciated and stand out, as this practice has become less common. It demonstrates to the legislator how important the issue is to you.

Adapted by Deborah Gardner from the experiences of nurses who have lobbied and the specific resources that follow: American Nurses Association. (2010). Hill basics: Lobbying. Retrieved from *nursingworld.org/HillBasics-Lobbying.aspx;* Friends Committee on National Legislation. Eight tips for a successful lobby visit. Retrieved from *fcnl.org/assets/flyer/lobby_flyer1105.pdf;* and Tips for effective grassroots lobbying. Retrieved from *www.hsd.k12.or.us/Portals/0/District/Budget_Matters12-2010/Stand_Lobbying%20tips%202013.pdf.*

National Hispanic Nurses. Next, direct your letter according to the legislator's responsibility. For example, do not write a letter regarding problems with your state's nurse practice act to a federal legislator, who has no authority on that issue. In most cases, your correspondence will be considered only if you write to the elected official who represents you. If you have a reputation as an expert or you have a personal relationship with an elected official, your letter may have impact. Personal letters still carry more weight than form letters, petitions, or phone calls. If the elected official has a history of support of the issue, it is always important to start each communication with a thank you for his or her support.

A further clarification of who to write pertains to an issue you may want to influence at the committee level, but your elected official is not on that committee. At the federal level, if your member of Congress is not on the committee, you can still communicate your opinion by addressing your letter to the chair of the committee at the committee address (not at the chair's congressional personal office address). Committee information, such as chair names, committee members, and committee address, is available on the Internet. State practices may vary, so again, check with your local guidelines. In crafting the message of your letter, identify yourself as a nurse, particularly if the legislation has anything to do with health care. Include hospital or other practice setting information as well as professional credentials, and make sure to include a return address, telephone number, and e-mail address if appropriate. See Box 44-2 for an example of a letter to a policymaker.

Include information about how proposed legislation would influence your personal experiences, or provide personal anecdotes that demonstrate your firsthand knowledge of, and experience with, a certain issue. State clearly what your position is, what your major concern about the proposal is, and whether you want the official to support, or oppose, the proposal. Again, tracking the legislation throughout the process will require that you include relevant committee or hearing information and bill numbers in your correspondence. Keep your letter brief and to the point.

BOX 44-2 Sample Letter/E-Mail to a Policymaker

Lisa Dunner, RN
2500 Wingate Street
New York, NY 10010
The Honorable Brad Hoylman
Room 413, Legislative Office Building
Albany, NY 12247

Dear Senator Hoylman,

I am a certified adult/geriatric nurse practitioner, a member of the Nurse Practitioners of New York, and one of your constituents. I am writing to urge your support for Senator Velmanette Montgomery's bill, S04611-A, which will amend the education law and allow nurse practitioners to either collaborate with a nurse practitioner in the event that a collaborating physician has to terminate the practice agreement or if the nurse practitioner has been practicing for more than 3600 hours, provide documentation to support that he or she has collaborative relationships with one or more licensed physicians. This bill will allow nurse practitioners to expand access to low-cost, effective, safe care for all who wish to use our services.

I have practiced as a nurse practitioner for the past 10 years and can vouch for the professional relationship I have with my collaborating physician. In most instances, she never sees my patients, nor is she required to do so, although under current law she is required to review a sample of my charts quarterly. We both agree that this as an unnecessary step that bears no relationship to patient care or safety. In fact when my last collaborator became ill and suddenly died, I had to refer all of my patients to different providers. The delay in care and treatment for some of these patients impacted the quality of care they received and generated a great deal of stress for them. Barriers, such as the requirement to collaborate with a physician, only add an additional expense and may delay or prevent access to care. I urge you to support S04611-A, and I would appreciate knowing your position on the bill.

Sincerely,
Lisa Dunner, DNP, RN, GNP-BC, NP-C
ldun@myemail.com
212.345.3333

E-MAIL

For many members of Congress and their staff, e-mail is a preferred means of communication because it has these advantages:

- *Directness:* The information is sent directly to the person you identify.
- *Timeliness:* Correspondence is immediate, in most cases.
- *Flexibility:* Legislative staff can open e-mail in their own time frame, unlike telephone calls, which are often unscheduled interruptions.
- *Attachments:* Important articles, reports, or other information that support your ideas can be attached with e-mail.

When sending e-mail, include your name, address, telephone number, and e-mail address. Observe the usual rules for written correspondence.

PROVIDING HEARING TESTIMONY

Providing testimony at a government hearing is an important way to go on the record about an issue on behalf of an organization or as a constituent. Hearings are increasingly designed by committee staff to highlight an issue, but they are not, in fact, where most of the key information is shared or decisions are made. As an individual, or on behalf of an association, you may request to testify on a particular issue. It is more likely that your coalition or organization will receive a call from a legislative office requesting that testimony be given from your group. Federal testimony is accepted in two forms for most committees: as oral remarks (those who are asked to testify) or as written testimony. Written testimony can be provided to the committee by the witness as a supplement to the oral remarks, or it can be provided by any association or individual choosing to submit it for the record. This testimony and the transcript of the hearing will eventually be published as a permanent record of the hearing.

Although there is limited opportunity to testify at hearings, it is important that you know how to prepare and conduct yourself in the event that you do testify. All committees and their subcommittees have a format they use to conduct the hearing; formats differ not only from state to federal committees, but also from one committee to the next.

Generally, there is a time limit placed on the length of an individual's remarks. You will use this time to present your position on the legislation or issue in an interesting and informative way. Frequently, this is not your last word on the subject, as the committee will often engage in a question-and-answer period with a witness following the presentation of testimony.

A senior legislator chairs committee hearings. The hearing is called to order, and then the chair often begins with remarks. Following the chair's remarks, any other legislators on the committee that choose to provide opening remarks will be given the opportunity to do so. Do not be surprised if the elected officials come and go during the meeting. The staff are always present and, in fact, will be responsible for the key messages you bring, and they will also rely on the written materials.

If you are asked to testify, it is important that you learn all you can about the politics and the issue before your testimony. This is where association representatives are invaluable. Typically, they will be the ones who call and ask if you would be willing to testify. If you receive the call from them, rely on them for the drafting of remarks, briefing on the issue, the politics and rules of the hearing, and other matters. Request that they attend the hearing with you and support you through the process. If you receive a request directly from a legislator's office, you may choose to call your association representative to see if he or she is willing to provide support for your testimony. Review your remarks; practice them before friends, family, and colleagues, even a mirror. Make sure you personalize your testimony and use phrases that are comfortable for you. Identify some of the questions you might be asked, and think through your responses.

COLLECTIVE STRATEGIES

Although the potential power of the individual nurse-constituent is great, the power base grows when nurses come together with a unified voice to advocate for change. Nursing groups can be influential with policymakers at all levels of government, from local boards to Congress. Elected officials often welcome opportunities to address the core constituencies in their districts to show that they care about the issues back home, and the possibility of good coverage in local newspapers can also be an incentive to those representatives with an eye toward reelection. Local nursing groups can sponsor legislative luncheons or celebrate National Nursing Week by inviting a policymaker to either join them at a meeting or address the group. Groups can award legislators with annual leadership or advocate recognition. Such grassroots activities are excellent ways to increase awareness of nursing issues and to make sure that nurses are represented when health care policy is being developed. The other model for grassroots action works in a reverse organizational pattern. Many national nursing organizations have local or statewide chapters. The headquarters of an association might be in Washington, DC, whereas the local chapters, sections, or branches can be spread out nationwide. This model is effective because the local or regional branch of the organization has the name recognition, resources, and prestige of the national association on their side as they pursue activities at the local level. In this way, local chapters enjoy the added strategic benefit of integrating their grassroots activities with the overall strategic lobbying goals of the national organization. The local group can then look to the national organization for position papers, copies of testimony, briefing documents, or other data on a given issue for use at the local level. Coordination of activities at the local and national levels of the same organizations is critical to ensure that all members are spreading consistent messages and positions with policymakers and to avoid any conflicts that might undermine the overall lobbying strategy.

In terms of collective lobbying strategies, one of the most common, and increasingly most effective, options for bringing about change is to create or join a coalition. As the number of interest groups has increased, with almost every niche group having its own association or group, it has become more important to reach consensus and refine priorities with groups that share your interests before approaching federal policymakers with priorities or legislative remedies. Coalitions simplify the workload of legislators and their staff by saving them time. A meeting with one coalition representing 25 groups will take much less time than 25 meetings with representatives from each group.

DISCUSSION QUESTIONS

1. Your school is planning an advocacy day to educate students on the salient aspects of the legislative process. How would you prepare students for this experience?
2. Identify a practice issue and describe the steps you would take to influence a local politician to draft a bill in favor of your concern.
3. Lobbyists have been rated at the bottom of the Gallup poll list on ethics and honesty. Why do you believe this occurs and what needs to happen to change the public's view of this essential role?

REFERENCES

Blumenthal, P. (2012). Auction 2012: How drug companies game Washington. *Huffington Post*. Retrieved from *www.huffingtonpost.com/2012/02/01/auction-2012-drug-companies-lobby_n_1245543.html*.

Gallup. (2013). Honesty/ethics in professions. Retrieved from *www.gallup.com/poll/1654/honesty-ethics-professions.aspx*.

Institute of Medicine. (2011). *The future of nursing: Leading change, advancing health*. Washington, DC: National Academies Press.

Internal Revenue Service. (2010). Glossary. Retrieved from *www.irs.gov/app/understandingTaxes/student/glossary.jsp#L*.

Jacobs, L. R., & Skocpol, T. (2012). *Health care reform and American politics: What everyone needs to know*. New York: Oxford University Press.

Kupfer, J. I. (2011). Restrictions on lobbying by exempt organizations: How much advocacy is too much? *NPQ: Nonprofit Quarterly*. Retrieved from *www.nonprofitquarterly.org/index.php?option=com_content&view=article&id=16636:restrictions-on-lobbying-by-exempt-organizations-how-much-advocacy-is-too-much&Itemid=336*.

Nelson, D., & Yackee, S. W. (2012). Lobbying coalitions and government policy change: An analysis of agency rulemaking. *The Journal of Politics, 74*(2), 339–353.

Zetter, L. (2011). *Lobbying: The art of political persuasion* (2nd ed.). Hampshire, UK: Harriman House Ltd.

ONLINE RESOURCES

Congress.gov
beta.congress.gov
GovTrack
www.govtrack.us

CHAPTER 45

TAKING ACTION:
An Insider's View of Lobbying

Betty R. Dickson

"There are two things you don't want to see being made—sausage and legislation."
Attributed to Otto von Bismarck

"So, what do you do?" is a question I am frequently asked. To which I reply, "I am a lobbyist." The looks that follow are either scornful, surprised, quizzical, astonished, or thoughtful. I wonder if the questioner associates all lobbyists with those who have been involved with high-profile scandals. Most likely the question is a reflection of not knowing what I do and a curiosity about the job.

The reality is that few people know what really happens in the halls and offices of government. To be a successful lobbyist includes attending plenty of committee meetings, knowing the bill-writing process, watching and understanding political maneuvering, sitting through innumerable working meals and receptions, developing different friendships, watching and working in elections, and imparting reams of information. Although nurses are excellent caregivers and the backbone of the health care system, few understand the influence that laws and regulations have on their practice; fewer are skilled at the long process of creating positive outcomes. My role as a lobbyist parallels advice from my mother: "Don't cross the street without looking both ways." In other words, "don't approach a legislative body without a professional lobbyist, one who knows the ins and outs of the system."

I watch hundreds of schoolchildren, parents, teachers, and single-issue citizens converge on the Mississippi state capitol during the annual 3-month legislative session. I watch as they wander the halls of what is probably one of the most beautiful capitol buildings in the United States. They come to observe, speak out about their issue, be recognized from the visitor gallery, and tour the magnificent capitol building. Then they go home.

For 20-plus years, I mentored nursing students and practicing nurses as they came to observe and be publicly recognized by legislators in the chambers. A few spent the entire day with me, following closely as I attended committee meetings, listening to testimony and debates, and conducting personal visits with legislators. They left with a new respect for the role of a lobbyist and the importance of having someone represent nursing during the legislative session.

GETTING STARTED

I started working as a lobbyist in 1989 when I began a long journey learning the ropes of lobbying in a small state rich with tradition and history, some bad, some notorious. In 1988, I became Executive Director of the Mississippi Nurses Association (MNA) and began my career as a lobbyist. Thankfully, my background as a journalist and newspaper editor, and my experience in government and public relations was a perfect combination for the responsibility of lobbying.

Until 2012, the MNA had 95% of its legislation passed, some of which includes the following:
- Securing significant annual funding for nursing education
- Obtaining additional pay for school nurses who become certified
- Increasing the number of school nurses
- Creating a $12,000 per year stipend for nurses to obtain a master's or doctoral degree if they teach in a school of nursing

- Securing inclusion of nurse practitioners (NPs) in most health care networks and getting reimbursed at the same rate as physicians
- Obtaining controlled substance authority for NPs
- Establishing the Office of Nursing Workforce

WINDS OF CHANGE COMING IN STATE LEGISLATURES

In recent years especially in the South, many state legislatures have seen a change in the power structure. During my career, I have seen the structure change from both Houses controlled by Democrats, to a Senate with a Republican majority and the House with a Democratic majority, to both chambers controlled by Republicans. Many states are experiencing the same change in leadership.

It is complicated when a new regime enters the picture and the entire system is changed: a new speaker of the House, new committee chairs, many of whom never chaired a committee before, and staff changes. Here lobbyists perform an important task of educating the new committee chairs, working with staff changes, and helping clients adjust to the change. It is like starting all over again after years of working with many of the same faces.

But nursing's messages haven't changed. We still must provide adequate nursing staff to care for the state's citizens in every health care arena; more Americans support giving NPs full authority to provide health care services; more school nurses are needed in the ever-complex educational system; there must be adequate funding for nursing schools; nurses are the largest number of health care providers in the health care arena, and the list goes on. Take your message to those in control.

MONEY! MONEY! MONEY!

Today's lobbyists and their clients are many times the go-to people to help with fund-raising for various candidates. When I started lobbying in 1988, rarely was I approached about fund-raising activities. Today, prior to and following the election cycle, I receive monthly invitations to attend events for the various elected officials. It's almost as if the first thing on many agendas following swearing in is to begin a fund-raising cycle to build a hope chest for the next election. Much of what is driving the financing of campaigns is the high cost of television advertising, direct mailing, and competition between political action committees (PACs).

Nurses are not noted as big contributors to political campaigns. But they must become more involved financially through the various nursing PACs at either the state or federal levels.

Consider this simple math: There are 3.1 million nurses in the United States. If every nurse gave only $1 to the American Nurses Association PAC, that PAC would be pretty formidable. Make that $5 and we talking serious money. In a state with 50,000 nurses who each contributed only $10 to their state association PAC, that would create a very competitive sum to help elect candidates who are open to nursing issues.

POLITICAL STRATEGIES

GETTING NURSES ON EVERY HEALTH-RELATED STATE AGENCY

My lobbying career got off to a big start. Innocently, I took the MNA leadership seriously when they told me their major objective was to have nurses at the seat of every table where health care decisions were made. During my first year at the MNA, our lobbyist was a nurse-attorney. During Desert Storm, the nurse/lobbyist went to work full-time for a law firm to fill a vacancy created by an attorney/guardsman who was called to active duty. I became MNA's only lobbyist.

However, while she was still working, we developed a strategy to access every code section in the law for every health care agency. We planned to try to amend the law to mandate that a nurse be on every governing board of any health-related agency, including the Department of Education. Although the legislation would define my career and reputation, I was totally unaware of the enormous opposition to touching any regulatory board's composition. That first legislative session turned out to be one of getting acquainted with division and department heads, getting a comprehensive education about government agencies, and getting a ton of teasing from other lobbyists who thought this was a pretty gutsy move for a newcomer.

Of course, the bill had little chance of passage, but once we searched the Mississippi code, drafted the bill's language, asked a legislator to introduce the bill, and attempted to get a committee hearing on the bill, I learned the legislative process from the bottom up. To this day, those agency heads who are still around ask me at the beginning of each session if I have any surprises up my sleeve. It's good to keep them guessing. As a result of that initiative and even without passage of the bill, the Mississippi Department of Mental Health and the Department of Health, to this day, has a registered nurse (RN) on the Boards, including one who served as chair. As nurses serve on various boards, their value increases. Today, nurses serve on numerous boards and committees in state government. Every time a piece of legislation comes forward in the Mississippi legislature, I am there as a lobbyist to ensure the insertion of the words nurse, school nurse, and NP where appropriate in health-related legislation and regulation.

NUMBERS CONNOTE STRENGTH

Lobbying is about counting. I can count, nursing leadership can count, and legislators know the value of numbers. In the early 1990s, there were over 40,000 RNs and licensed practical nurses practicing in Mississippi, and we had to establish a mechanism to bring representatives from all those nurses together. We created the MNA's Nursing Organizations Liaison Committee (NOLC) to bring 25 nursing organizations together to plan and agree on a legislative agenda. Representatives from each group worked collaboratively on a statewide nursing summit that 700 to 800 RNs and students attend annually. We invited key legislators to join the summit, and they could count the numbers for themselves. It was through this coalition that nursing began to be recognized as a significant force at the state capitol. That same coalition continues to work today in a collaborative effort to maintain a strong legislative presence.

LONG-TERM STRATEGIES FOR LONG-TERM SOLUTIONS: TACKLING THE NURSING SHORTAGE

When the NOLC was formed, I told the group, "MNA is furnishing the lobbying for all of you. There's a way for you to participate and to provide support for this effort", and they have. This group was involved in passing the law creating the Office of Nursing Workforce. My role as a lobbyist is to ensure that this office is adequately funded.

The group developed long-range plans. The first step was to retain nursing faculty, and the best way to do so was to provide faculty with a competitive salary. In 2007, we worked with the legislature to obtain a $6000 pay raise for all nursing faculty. In 2008, the second installment of the pay raise of $6000 for nursing faculty was enacted. Many of those considering retiring changed their minds, while others decided to become teachers. In 2008, the next step was to add one additional faculty in all schools of nursing. That too was successfully enacted.

In 2008, I lobbied to fund a study about simulation labs and how they could increase enrollment. The legislature appropriated $75,000 for this initiative. In 2009, they funded the next step, allocating $500,000 to the Office of Nursing Workforce to coordinate where, when, and how to implement a simulation lab program. A million here, a million there, and the next thing you know, Mississippi has invested millions of dollars to resolve the nursing shortage. As a result, faculty numbers have stabilized and enrollment in schools of nursing has increased.

CALL IN THE NURSES

It helps to have a successful political action committee behind you (which the MNA has), and it helps to have a plan to call in the nurses when the need arises. I know that legislators really fear having large droves of citizens come to the capitol, whether it's truckers, physicians, loggers, hair braiders—or nurses. I remember one issue in the early 1990s when an attempt was made to establish medication technicians in nursing homes. Nurses were strongly opposed to this new provider whose only requirement was a high school education and a few weeks of training. The vice chair of the House of Representatives Public Health and Welfare Committee was assigned the bill and scheduled a public hearing. The MNA arranged for over 100 nurses, in uniform, to attend the hearing. When the committee chair couldn't get everyone in the regular conference room on the first floor because there were so many nurses, he moved us to a larger room on the second floor. It became apparent that the second room was too small, so he moved us to an even larger room back again on the first floor. Imagine 100 nurses marching from floor to floor, room to room. It created a lot of excitement, stares, and curiosity, and made several points about the nursing community: there are a lot of us, we're well organized, and we'll make lots of calls to our legislators.

When the chair finally got the hearing under way, the nurses were breathing pretty heavily; but when testimony began, the breathing became a little more pronounced. And when one of the opponents, during testimony, said something disparaging about nurses, all 100 gasped in unison. It even scared me, and I was on their side. Needless to say, the chair ended the hearing without a vote on the bill. Mississippi still does not have medication technicians.

BE IN THE RIGHT PLACE AT THE RIGHT TIME

Successful lobbying often depends on being in the right place at the right time. Once a state senator called me to review an immunization bill he wanted to introduce. After reading through the bill, I told him that I thought we were already doing what he wanted to do with the legislation. His reply was that he wanted an immunization bill! I told him I would get back with a suggestion. I was the MNA's representative on the Mississippi State Health Department's Immunization Task Force, so I called the chief of staff at the health department, a nurse. She suggested that we convince him to introduce a bill for a statewide immunization registry, one of the goals of the task force. I did. He loved the idea. He introduced a bill, and we worked very hard for passage. Today there is a statewide registry for tracking immunization. The result is that Mississippi has one of the highest immunization rates in the United States.

The same nurse and I were in the capitol during a legislative session when we were called by the chair of the Public Health and Welfare Committee, who wanted to implement a school-based clinic pilot for the state. We were given the assignment to come up with language for an amendment to an education bill that would authorize the pilot project. She grabbed an envelope, and we crafted the language on the back. Reading it over carefully, we went back into the meeting where she handed the chair the envelope. He passed it to the bill writer. It became law.

PUTTING FROGS IN A WHEELBARROW: USE HUMOR AS A TOOL

Sometimes humor can disarm even the most stoic adversary. After we were successful in getting the bill passed to create the Office of Nursing Workforce through the House and the Senate and then back to the House for final approval, a community college president appeared at the weekly committee meeting and told the chair that the community colleges were opposed to the bill. We were completely blown away by this opposition at the final hour. The chair gave us 1 day to work out the problem. Luckily, the community college presidents were meeting the next day, so I arranged an audience with them by convincing an old friend, who was a president, to get a group of us on the agenda. Several of us appeared the next day but were getting nowhere. The head of the community college board kept saying we didn't need the Office of Nursing Workforce. We tried to reason with him: "We have no accurate data on nursing in Mississippi; we need better communication between the schools of nursing and hospital nursing administration; we need to develop workforce strategies." Nothing was working with the all-male audience. Finally, I placed both hands on the table and asked: "Mr. Chairman, have you ever tried to put frogs in a wheelbarrow?" A slight smile appeared on his face. "Where are you going with this?" he asked. I explained, "We have been trying to get these folks working together. First, we get the community college nursing programs in the wheelbarrow. Then we turn around and try to pick up the baccalaureate programs and put them in the wheelbarrow. Then we try to get hospital administration in the wheelbarrow. Then we turn around, and the other two have jumped out. We need a way to get them all in the wheelbarrow at the same time." They all laughed and, with further discussion, agreed to support the bill.

USE YOUR BEST ASSETS

When Mississippi's first Republican governor since reconstruction, Kirk Fordice, created the state's Health Care Commission, I was appointed to represent nursing. When it came time for nursing to make a presentation on nursing's role in health care and how we could improve the status of health care in Mississippi, the MNA chose three outstanding leaders to make our case. The first was a diminutive, perky nurse president of the MNA who could spit out data in rapid fire delivery; the second was our impressive Board of Nursing (BON) executive director, whose ability to think on her feet and whose sense of humor were incredible; and finally, a tall blond dean of a school of nursing and former Alabama Maid of Cotton, whose intelligence was only exceeded by her good looks. When the nurses finished their presentation and walked back to their chairs, the president of the hospital association whispered to me, "You don't play fair!" As a result of our "unfair play, the commission recommended, and the legislature passed, legislation to increase funding to three existing NP programs and to add two new programs, all to increase the numbers of NPs so that rural Mississippi could experience better access to care.

USE PROVEN STRATEGIES

Learning from past experiences was important when NPs asked the MNA to help with regulations about signing forms that, by law, required a physician signature. Once again, we did a code search of the rules, found every law requiring a physician signature, and drafted a bill to change the language to say "or nurse practitioner" (see Chapter 66). The process was the same as the one we used to get nurses on state agency boards: finding a simple word or phrase that could be added to an existing law and thus expanding NP practice. It involved

numerous forms, one of which was an authorization for handicapped parking. The addition of "nurse practitioner" affected many agencies, thus creating a lot of attention. We explained that the NP was the provider and that the physician was not always on site. To get a physician signature, the patient had to schedule an appointment with the physician, thus creating additional cost and additional paperwork. The bill passed, and the result was that all agencies changed all their forms to include NP signatures.

BE PATIENT: DO NOT GIVE UP

My job as a lobbyist has been to shepherd legislation to expand NP practice. In the early 1980s, there was only a handful of NPs practicing in the state. In the early 1990s, there were about 400. By 2009, there were almost 2000, not including certified registered nurse anesthetists. Some NPs opened their own practices. The Mississippi State Board of Medical Licensure and the Mississippi Medical Association saw this as a threat.

Under the old law, the BON was required to jointly promulgate any regulation affecting the NP. The MNA was successful in getting a law passed in 1994 that required the Board of Medical Licensure (BOML) to also jointly promulgate any regulations affecting NPs, meaning that meant that both boards had to jointly promulgate. This set up a scenario in which we spent 15 years arguing back and forth between the two professions whenever any regulatory changes were suggested by one of the boards. We were able to gain ground by introducing bill after bill to remove the restrictions, and, through legislative support, we actually forced the BOML to compromise on many of the restrictions. But keeping the regulatory process effective and timely was impossible, much like walking through molasses. It took 2 to 3 years to get anything done.

When the NPs approached the MNA regarding prescriptive authority for controlled substances, we went to the BOML asking to jointly promulgate regulations to make it happen. They refused. We went to the legislature and asked for a bill to give the NPs controlled substance prescriptive authority. We also told the legislators that it could be done through the regulatory process, but the BOML would not cooperate. The chairman of Public Health and Welfare called all stakeholders to his office and gave strong directions for the two parties to work together through the regulatory process, or else he would look at a change in the law. It took another year, but regulations were passed to give controlled substance prescriptive authority to NPs.

In 2009, the MNA went back to the legislature with a bill to completely remove joint promulgation of rules. Once again, the chairman of the Public Health and Welfare Committee forced the parties to work together, and, after many negotiations, all parties came to agreement and the bill became law on July 1, 2010. Now the BON could regulate NPs without joint promulgation with the BOML. But it took 20 years!

What made the difference? First was the fatigue factor; after all those years, key legislators were tired of trying to resolve issues between the BON and the BOML. Secondly, there was a vast increase in the number of NPs. More and more legislative families were using NPs as their primary provider. Many had daughters and sons who were NPs. And the MNA pounded the legislators with the outcome data about NP practice. Thirdly, we figured out some fancy political maneuvering. When the BOML opposed our legislation, we suggested that we take the regulations under which the NPs had been successfully practicing for years and move them into legislation. This was a strategy I had considered for 20 years. It actually was suggested by a physician who supported NPs and encouraged us to consider legislation instead of regulation. The legislators thought the logic was sound, because NPs were already practicing successfully under the regulations, and moving them into legislation did not change any of their practices. Today, NPs continue to work in a collaborative arrangement with physicians.

Eliminating joint promulgation has greatly shortened the process of rule-making. For example, practice guidelines for NP hospitalists and NPs in pain management were developed quickly but thoroughly. The process is simple: Bring together interested NPs, look at national guidelines, study the research, create appropriate practice guidelines, present them to the BON, seek public and medical input, and present final proposals to the BON. Instead of taking 2 years under joint promulgation, it took from 1 to 3 months to implement. This new seamless, timely process would not have been possible without years of work by a seasoned lobbyist.

THERE REALLY IS A NEED FOR LOBBYISTS

There are no secret ingredients to lobbying. Legislators, especially in states where staff are limited, depend on lobbyists to provide information about issues, to muster support for pet projects, and to help with their campaigns. There is so much legislation that can affect nursing practice. From issues such as Medicaid to the State Department of Health, from the nursing shortage to mandatory overtime, there must be nursing representation in state and federal policy arenas. It requires expertise in the intricacies of the legislative and regulatory process, in knowing the implications of suggested legislation or regulation, knowing who is your ally and who is your obstacle, developing trust among policymakers and other stakeholders, and knowing when the right people are in the right places to implement change. It requires seeing the process like a puzzle or poker game: Know when to hold and when to fold. It helps to be creative and look at surprise approaches to problems. Lobbyists keep their fingers on the pulse of health care legislation and regulations. They are skilled communicators, who know when to call out the nurses. Organizational success in policy arenas is often directly related to the effectiveness of the lobbying effort. Unless nurses do this as a full-time job, they rarely have the time to assume the lobbying function. My advice to nursing: Don't be caught without one.

CHAPTER 46

The American Voter and the Electoral Process

Karen O'Connor   Alixandra B. Yanus

"Suffrage is the pivotal right."

Susan B. Anthony

American democracy requires elected officials in the legislative and executive branch to create public policy. Legislation is created in state legislatures and Congress and signed into law by the governor or president. Consequently, it is critical who those legislators and chief executives are because they determine whose interests are represented in the policy arena.

Citizens exercise a key political act when they vote for candidates who support particular policy positions. In the United States, opportunities to vote abound. Elected officials range from local party leaders to the U.S. President and members of Congress. Thus, the 3.1 million registered nurses in the United States have significant potential to affect health policy through both the ballot and direct lobbying activity. As the ongoing debates over the implementation of the 2010 health care reform legislation (Obamacare) have revealed, it is crucial to have elected officials who support the interests of the health care community.

Yet U.S. voter turnout for elections remains low compared with other industrialized nations, perhaps attributable to the sheer number of elections and lack of clarity on the issues or stakes of any contest. This chapter examines basic election law, voting behavior, how campaigns work, and how lobbying. In so doing, it optimizes the potential for nurses and voters more generally to affect the policy process.

VOTING LAW: GETTING THE VOTERS TO THE POLLS

The framers of the U.S. Constitution initially granted voting rights to all property-owning, white men. But, as our notions of equality expanded, so did voting opportunities for additional groups. Over time, the Constitution has been amended to grant suffrage first to free men regardless of "race, color … [or] previous condition of servitude," (Fifteenth Amendment, 1870), then women (Nineteenth Amendment, 1920), and, most recently, those age 18 years and older (Twenty-Sixth Amendment, 1971). The U.S. Constitution also prohibits poll taxes (Twenty-Fourth Amendment, 1964), which were passed largely by southern lawmakers with the intent to disenfranchise largely poor African Americans.

Federal legislation has also eliminated literacy tests and property ownership as qualifications to vote. The Voting Rights Act (VRA) of 1965 was enacted with support from President Lyndon B. Johnson. The Act targeted all of the southern states and others with high concentrations of minority voters, particularly blacks, whose voter turnout lagged behind their percentage of the voting-age population.[1] Recognizing that voter repression and intimidation was happening, the Act introduced national standards (and compliance measures)

---

[1]The Voting Rights Act was also applicable in states in the North with high concentrations of Hispanic voters. District lines were also audited in some areas of New York City with high concentrations of Puerto Rican voters, for example.

designed to promote electoral equality. Where necessary, it also authorized the U.S. Attorney General to replace local voting registrars with federal registrars, and procedures to register voters were standardized in specific states. The immediate consequence was to enfranchise large blocks of African-American voters, particularly in the South. It also caused formerly conservative Democrats to join the Republican Party. A more recent Supreme Court decision, however, has limited the Act's application in most states covered by the law. This decision has led some states, such as Texas, to enact voter identification laws, which may have a disproportionate impact on poor and minority voters.

CALLS FOR REFORM

Voter registration of minorities and the poor continued to lag behind that of white voters until the early 1990s. Grassroots civil rights and good government organizations around the country pushed for voter registration reform, citing much higher registration and turnout rates in other nations. In many locales, registration was difficult. Before the passage of the National Voter Registration Act of 1993 (known hereafter as the "Motor Voter Act"), modes of registration varied widely from state to state. Some states made registration easy at shopping malls and post offices, other states required citizens to go to more isolated board of elections offices, removed from public transportation. Behind the push for the Motor Voter Act was the argument that increased accessibility of voting registration would increase voter turnout. When President Bill Clinton signed the Motor Voter Act, voter registration sites were expanded specifically to include social services and motor vehicle registry offices, hence the designation. Although the Motor Voter Act was effective in increasing registration dramatically, its effects on actual turnout were less notable (Brown & Wedecking, 2006).

In 2000, the hotly disputed presidential election between Vice President Al Gore and Texas Governor George W. Bush produced a second, albeit brief, public outcry for reforms of voting methods. Across the nation, especially in Florida, voting technology was revealed to be outdated, malfunctioning, or still inaccessible for certain voters, especially African Americans and Hispanic people who repeatedly found their names wrongfully purged from lists of eligible voters. With visions of hanging chads dancing in their heads, members of Congress passed the Help America Vote Act (HAVA) in 2002. It provided federal funding to states and localities to replace old voting technologies. It also mandated that at least one voting device at each precinct be accessible to voters with disabilities. In addition, HAVA allows voters whose names do not appear on registration lists to vote with provisional ballots, which can later be verified, and if proven legal, counted. This measure allows all citizens who are properly registered to have their votes counted. Although these reforms sought to expand not only the number of Americans registered to vote but also the percentage of those voting, overall turnout increased only moderately after the passage of HAVA (Kropf & Kimball, 2012).

Still, many new technologies sought to streamline the voting process as well as improve its ease and accuracy. The efforts were not without controversy. For example, many voters argued that some digitized ballots that leave no paper trail for verification could be manipulated easily or sabotaged. Steps have been taken to ameliorate these concerns, but the reforms have been gradual and have not yet yielded immediate, tamper-free, accurate results across localities and states (Alvarez & Hall, 2010). Congress has considered a variety of bills to modify current HAVA verification standards, such as requiring all states to have voter-verifiable paper audit trails, but these efforts have failed and have lost their sense of immediacy as the tainted 2000 election has faded from memory and been replaced by concerns about the economy, health care, and international security.

Unless a requirement is specified in the Constitution or by federal law, states have the power to define and change election laws. Despite the Voting Rights Act of 1965, the Motor Voter Act, and HAVA, voting laws still vary considerably from state to state. All states allow some sort of early or absentee voting with mail-in ballots if individuals are unable to vote in their designated precincts on Election Day.

Modes of voting are different from jurisdiction to jurisdiction. Oregon residents, for example, vote by mail-in ballot only, making voting booths obsolete. As of 2013, 10 states and the District of Columbia allow same-day voter registration, and several states do not require any voter registration at all. In the 2008 and 2012 general elections, many states opened polling places days or even weeks before Election Day in a process called early voting; in these states, a significant number of voters opted to vote early. Early voting, however, does not appear to increase overall voter turnout (Giammo & Brox, 2010). Hence, voting is among the simplest ways for nurses to influence public policy.

VOTING BEHAVIOR

Research on voting behavior seeks primarily to explain two phenomena: voter turnout (i.e., what factors contribute to an individual's decision to vote or not to vote) and voter choice (once the decision to vote has been made, what leads voters to choose one candidate over another).

VOTER TURNOUT

Turnout is the proportion of the voting-age public that votes. Those eligible to vote include all citizens of the United States who are age 18 years or older. States regulate voting eligibility in a number of ways, from preventing felons from voting to having strict single-day, limited voting hours.

Turnout is especially important in American elections because most candidates are elected in winner-take-all systems, where an election's outcome can be influenced by a single voter. (A few states still require candidates to receive 50%+1 of the vote; without it, runoff elections are necessary.)

In spite of the reforms, the United States continues to lag well behind many other constitutional democracies in terms of voter turnout. Many industrialized societies report that upwards of 90% of all eligible voters do so. In contrast, only about 58% of eligible voters went to the polls during the 2012 presidential election. This was a significant decline from the 2008 presidential election, when the historic candidacy of Barack Obama energized many Americans; however, even in this election, only 63% of eligible voters turned out to the polls (Gans, 2008). Turnout is of great concern, especially if nonvoting is seen as a sign of political alienation, dissatisfaction with the status quo, anger at negative campaigns, and/or voter cynicism.

Why such low voter turnout rates? According to one 2012 U.S. Census Bureau study, 18% of Americans say that school or work conflicts made them too busy to vote. Approximately 15% cite illness or personal emergencies in explaining why they did not vote. Other explanations include apathy, being out of town, not knowing or not liking the candidates, registration problems, or forgetfulness (U.S. Census Bureau, 2012). A breakdown of turnout rates by demographic categories reveals dramatically different turnout rates among different groups (Table 46-1). Among eligible voters, turnout was

TABLE 46-1 Voter Turnout by Age, Race/Ethnicity, and Gender, 2012 Presidential Election

	Reported Registered (%)	Reported Voted (%)
Age		
18 to 24 years	49.4	38.0
25 to 44 years	59.4	49.5
45 to 64 years	70.5	63.4
65 to 74 years	77.0	71.0
75 years and over	76.7	67.8
Race/Ethnicity		
White, non-Hispanic	72.4	63
Black	68.4	61.8
Asian	37.2	31.3
Hispanic	38.9	31.8
Gender		
Male	63.1	54.4
Female	67.0	58.5

From U.S. Census Bureau. (2012). Voting and registration in the election of November 2012. Retrieved from *www.census.gov/hhes/www/socdemo/voting/publications/p20/2012/tables.html.*

lowest among Asian and Hispanic[2] Americans, two groups with large noncitizen populations, and highest among white, non-Hispanic people.[3] Turnout rates increase with age, and a higher percentage of women than men voted in the 2012 presidential election.

PATTERNS IN VOTER CHOICE

Getting voters to the polls and providing fair and dependable mechanisms is one issue; how people vote is another. Deep divisions exist within the electorate across different social and demographic factors. Understanding the habits of American voters is important as nurses seek allies for their policy agendas.

From the earliest days of the U.S. democracy, most political power has been vested in two political parties. Although some third parties are powerful at the local level, no third-party candidate has won a presidential election. Political scientists have long sought to discover why people vote the way they do. Research reveals that several demographic characteristics correlate with voting behavior. Factors known to influence voter turnout include political party, religion, race and ethnicity, gender, and age.

Political Party. Party identification is the most powerful predictor of voting behavior. Rather obviously, self-described Democrats tend to vote for Democratic candidates, and self-described Republicans often vote for Republican candidates. Although intense partisanship has increased over the past electoral cycles, many voters now identify as independents, in addition to those who register for either party. Voting for candidates from other parties, especially in state presidential primaries where independents may choose a party at the poll, or if the state allows voters of either party to vote in the primary of another, can affect electoral outcomes drastically. Independents who make up as much as one third of the voters in a general election are a focus of partisan candidates trying to sway them to their side (O'Connor, Sabato, & Yanus, 2015).

Religion. Since the 1980s, religion has become the second most common predictor of voting. Religious groups also vote in distinct patterns. Fundamentalist or Evangelical Christians are most likely to vote for conservative, Republican candidates. Jewish voters are also a politically cohesive group; the vast majority align with Democrats and have done so for decades. In 2013, for example, 69% of all Jewish-American voters cast their ballots for President Barack Obama in the general election (CNN, 2012).

Catholics are a somewhat politically divided group. For years, they tended to be Democrats. However, many support Republican candidates when issues of gay rights or abortion are major issues in an election. The Roman Catholic Church, too, often makes voter recommendations largely based on candidates' positions on abortion. The Church hierarchy has threatened high-profile legislators such as House Democratic Leader Nancy Pelosi. Rep. Patrick Kennedy (D-RI) even cited pressure from the Church as one of the reasons he chose not to seek reelection in 2010. In 2012, 50% of the Catholic voters chose Barack Obama for President in the general election in spite of his pro-choice views (CNN, 2012).

Race and Ethnicity. Democrats have long enjoyed the support of the black[4] community. Single, black women are the most supportive of Democratic Party candidates. In the 2012 presidential election, 93% of African Americans voted for Barack Obama, whereas only 6% supported Mitt Romney (Table 46-2).

Although African Americans tend to have consistent voting patterns, other racial groups are less consistent. In California, Texas, Florida, Illinois,

---

[2]The authors acknowledge the controversy over the proper terminology of this group, ranging from *Hispanic* to *Latino* and/or other terms; the term *Hispanic* is that which is used in the U.S. Census and is thus used in this work.
[3]However, when we only look at eligible voters, blacks outvoted whites for the first time in American history.

---

[4]The authors use the term *black* rather than *African American* to be consistent with the language employed by the U.S. Census Bureau.

TABLE 46-2 Voter Choice by Age, Race/Ethnicity, and Gender, 2012 Presidential Election

	Obama (%)	Romney (%)
Age		
18 to 29 years	60	37
30 to 44 years	52	45
45 to 64 years	47	51
65 years and older	44	56
Race/Ethnicity		
White, non-Hispanic	39	59
Black	93	6
Asian	73	26
Hispanic	71	27
Gender		
Male	45	52
Female	55	44

From CNN. (2012). President: Full results. Retrieved from *www.cnn.com/election/2012/results/race/president.*

and New York, five key electoral states, Hispanic voters have emerged as powerful allies for candidates seeking office, and, no doubt, were among the major reasons for President Barack Obama's selection of the self-proclaimed wise Latina woman, Judge Sonia Sotomayor, to be his first appointment to the U.S. Supreme Court. Hispanics tend to align with the Democratic Party except for those of Cuban descent, who overwhelmingly vote for Republicans. In 2012, approximately 71% of Hispanic voters cast their ballots for Barack Obama. Asian Americans are even more heterogeneous than their ethnic counterparts. In 2012, for example, Indian and Cambodian Americans were comparatively more supportive of President Obama, whereas Vietnamese and Samoan Americans were comparatively less supportive (Asian Americans Advancing Justice, 2012). Citizens who identify as Asian/Pacific Islanders are diverse in terms of political leanings, so generalizing for this broad minority group can be misleading.

Gender. In general, women are more Democratic than white men. Unmarried women are even more likely to vote for a Democrat. The Democratic Party tends to support more liberal policies of concern to women, such as health care, contraceptive and reproductive rights, and equal pay. Women also are more likely than men to align with the Democratic Party's positions on social welfare and military issues (Box-Steffensmeier, De Boef, & Lin, 2004). In every election since 1980, women have supported Democratic candidates, especially at the presidential level, at statistically significant higher rates than men. Furthermore, women are far more likely to support female candidates than are men. Studies on representation suggest that women and minority groups tend to vote for candidates who match their demographic characteristics because they believe that the candidates can understand their life experiences and will thus promote policies that are friendly to them.

Age. Age has long been associated with party identification, as most voters develop their partisan affiliations based on formative political experiences. Today, generally the youngest voters—many of whom are moderate but socially progressive—tend to prefer the Democratic Party. Middle-aged voters, in contrast, disproportionately favor the Republican Party (CNN, 2012). These voters, often at the height of their careers and consequently at the height of their earning potential, tend to favor the low taxes championed by Republicans (Flanigan & Zingale, 2006).

ANSWERING TO THE CONSTITUENCY

Does it make a difference if the members of Congress come from or are members of a particular group? Are they bound to vote the way their constituents expect them to vote even if they favor another policy? In the 18th century, British political theorist Edmund Burke and members of Parliament posited that the answers to these questions depend on a person's philosophy of representation. One perspective argues that a representative is a trustee who listens to the opinions of constituents and then can be trusted to use his or her own best judgment to make final decisions. In contrast, delegate representation contends that representatives should vote exactly how their constituents would, regardless of the representatives' own views. Clearly, these two modes of representation are not exclusive, nor do representatives subscribe to one view entirely. Therefore, a third theory exists: legislators act as politicos, alternately donning the hat of trustees or delegates, depending on the issue or the environment (O'Connor, Sabato, & Yanus, 2015).

Of course, how representatives view their roles does not completely explain whether it makes a difference if a representative is young or old; male or female; white, black, or Hispanic; or gay or straight. Can a man, for example, represent interests of women as well as women can?

CONGRESSIONAL DISTRICTS

According to the Constitution, the U.S. Senate is composed of 100 senators: two from each state, and two shadow senators who have nonvoting status from the District of Columbia. Representation in the U.S. House of Representatives is based on the population of each of the states. There are 435 seats in the House of Representatives (plus 5 nonvoting delegates representing the District of Columbia, the U.S. Virgin Islands, Guam, American Samoa, and the Northern Mariana Islands, and a resident commissioner representing Puerto Rico). The Congress determines the number of seats in the House, and each state is apportioned seats based on a census taken decennially by U.S. constitutional mandate. How those seats are allotted within the states is up to the states and is a process referred to as redistricting. In most states, state legislators, who want to optimize the majority party's political power, are responsible for redistricting. When legislators redraw district lines, they often engage in a practice called gerrymandering, or drawing lines most advantageous to their political party. Two common tactics used when redrawing district lines are packing and cracking. Packing concentrates voters of one type into a single electoral district to reduce their influence in other districts. They may also break up the districts of prominent representatives of the opposite party (cracking), which weakens the

chances of a member of the opposition from winning in the redrawn district.

In the past few decades, Northern and Mid-Atlantic states have lost congressional seats to the South and West, particularly California, which has one seventh of the members of Congress. Thus, state lawmakers have ended up drawing oddly shaped districts to achieve their goals. Although insisting that districts facilitate the election of minorities, the U.S. Supreme Court has ruled that racially gerrymandered districts do not serve a compelling government interest and are thus unconstitutional (O'Connor, Sabato, & Yanus, 2015).

Redistricting is an extremely contentious process that has tremendous potential to affect the outcome of elections and the types of lawmakers elected. Many states hold hearings as new district maps are drawn, providing citizens and groups of citizens, such as nurses, input into a process that is critical to the outcome of public policy.

INVOLVEMENT IN CAMPAIGNS

CHOOSING YOUR CANDIDATE

Political parties and interest groups recruit candidates and can tap into resources of time, money, and volunteers to execute a successful campaign. Interest groups, such as the American Nurses Association, provide invaluable information on national and state candidates. (See Chapters 72 and 74.) Interest groups also publish materials such as voter guides or scorecards to direct potential voters toward or away from candidates. Tracking which groups give money to a particular candidate is also an indication of how a candidate might be influenced to vote.

Researching candidates via the Internet is another effective way to determine a candidate's positions on issues of concern to nurses and patients. Websites of candidates and political parties present their policy positions. Reputable media sources may profile and endorse candidates. But, ultimately, it is up to the individual to consider questions such as those posed in Box 46-1 to make a decision about which candidates to support.

BOX 46-1 Questions to Ask When Considering Candidates

- What kinds of experiences would the candidate bring to office?
- Are the candidate's political skills and knowledge sufficient and respected by his or her peers?
- If the candidate is an incumbent (already holding the office and seeking reelection) or held another office previously, what is his or her voting record in terms of nursing or comparable policies?
- Has the candidate established positions on issues pertaining to health care and nursing policy, and, if so, what are they?
- What positions of leadership could enable this candidate to be more effective if elected?
- Is the candidate's campaign well organized and relatively straightforward in its message?
- Can the candidate raise money well and keep an organized and transparent budget?
- Can the candidate actually be elected by the population at large? Is his or her name recognizable by the general public?
- What does public opinion indicate about the potential of this candidate to be victorious?
- Who supports this candidate's campaign, both through fund-raising and endorsements?
- How has the media covered the candidate?
- Is there any damaging evidence—whether it be a policy stance or personal shortcoming—that would be exploited by opposition or would prevent you or the general public from voting for the candidate?

Adapted from Dato, C. (2006). The American voter and electoral politics. In D. Mason, J. Leavitt, & M. Chaffee (Eds.), *Policy & politics in nursing and health care* (5th ed.). St. Louis, MO: Elsevier.

CAMPAIGNING

One opportunity for nurses to get their voices heard is by participating in political campaigns as a group. Nurses have participated in political workshops offered by numerous national women's groups, unions, and the American Nurses Association. Nurses have unique skills that enable them to be both consultants on policy as well as orga-

nizers, negotiators, and communicators on behalf of candidates they support. Even making small monetary donations or distributing campaign materials can make an impact on the outcome of elections.

Of course, nurses can seek elective office, and they often do. Service on town councils, school or advisory boards, as well as in state legislatures and Congress, are essential in increasing the visibility of nurses as political players.

GETTING THE BEST CANDIDATE

Women's rights groups have been vital to the political success of nurses, especially as the majority of nurses are women. Six nurses (two Republicans and four Democrats) served in the 113th Congress. The Susan B. Anthony List, a political action committee (PAC) formed in 1992 to support prolife women candidates, supported both Republican nurses. Likewise, EMILY's List supported all four Democratic nurses. EMILY's List was founded in 1985 to support prochoice Democratic women candidates. Now one of the largest and most influential PACs, it dwarfs all other women's PACs in size of contributions to candidates. Both organizations bundle contributions for endorsed candidates and provide candidate training, consultants, and get-out-the-vote efforts to increase the number of women in Congress, as well as create more public awareness of important issues and those candidates' stances on issues.

PACs are the fund-raising arm of organizations. Although the Bipartisan Campaign Reform Act of 2002 (also known as BCRA or the McCain-Feingold Act in honor of its sponsors) places a limit on the amount of money PACs may give directly to candidates in national elections, no such limit exists on uncoordinated expenditures on behalf of candidates. Other types of groups, such as Super PACs, 527s, and 501(c) groups, may also raise and spend money in the electoral environment. Nurses and others must be aware of these changes when dealing with campaign contributions, because the broader health insurance industry has more money than nurses or physicians to spend on elections.

CAMPAIGN FINANCE LAW

Campaign finance laws were created in the 1970s amid public concerns about transparency in campaign spending. Although the original 1971 Federal Election Campaign Act (FECA) was largely ineffective and vague, amendments to FECA in 1974 had more ambitious goals, including the following:

- Contribution limits for individuals, interest groups, and political parties in national elections
- Spending limits for individuals, interest groups, political parties, and candidates in national elections
- Mandatory disclosure of campaign contributions and spending
- Establishment of a nonpartisan Federal Election Commission to oversee and enforce campaign laws

PACs were established to channel money to candidates, but since these spending limits were put in place, nearly 4000 PACs have been established (Francia, Joe, & Wilcox, 2008). The stringent spending requirements were loosened after the Supreme Court's ruling in *Buckley v. Valeo* in 1976, which found that spending money was a right of free speech. Only if presidential candidates waived their First Amendment rights by accepting public funds, could they be subjected to campaign spending limits. Every presidential candidate who was eligible for public funding accepted it and waived their free speech rights until Barack Obama in 2008. His decision not to accept public financing allowed him unlimited fund-raising power. He was still subject to contribution limits, but he had no limits on how much he could spend, so he was able to raise and spend over $750 million. Spending in the 2012 presidential contest topped $1 billion on behalf of each of the candidates.

During the 1990s, soft money contributions, unreported and unlimited, could legally be provided to political organizations but not individual candidates. This reflected loopholes within FECA and led to the passage of BCRA. This law banned large soft money contributions and enacted limits on campaign advertising, timing, and spending. The provisions of this law, however, were greatly weakened by a 2010 Supreme Court decision that declared many of these limits unconstitutional on the grounds that money is a form of speech, and restricting spending, thus, amounts to a violation of the First Amendment.

TYPES OF ELECTIONS

There are three types of elections: primary, general, and presidential.

PRIMARY ELECTIONS

In the primary election, voters decide which candidate will represent the party in the general election. In some states, there are closed primaries, meaning only a party's registered voters may cast a ballot to determine the candidate for the general election. In contrast, open primaries allow independents and members of other parties to participate. Closed primaries are generally considered healthier for the two-party system because they prevent members of one party from influencing the elections of another party. In some states, if none of the candidates in the primary secures a majority of votes, a runoff primary occurs, where the top two candidates vie in a second contest for at least 50%+1 of the votes.

GENERAL ELECTIONS

Once candidates from the primary election are decided, each state holds its general election. (States often hold elections for state and local office on off- and odd-numbered years.) In general elections, voters decide which candidates from opposite parties will hold elective public office. Many local elections, especially for judges, are nonpartisan.

PRESIDENTIAL ELECTIONS: A SPECIAL CASE

In all elections except for the presidential election, people vote directly for the candidate. In the case of presidential elections, most voters actually vote for electors instead of the candidates themselves. Electors are representatives from each state who convene at the Electoral College to elect a president. Although the Electoral College itself has been a contentious issue recently, it remains intact.

THE MORNING AFTER: KEEPING CONNECTED TO POLITICIANS

After a candidate wins the election, it is vital to advance one's interests even if the person who won was not the preferred candidate. Just as their roles in campaigns are crucial, nurses can continue to act as champions of policy and sources of information to influence the politicians while in office. Nurses can join the staff of or volunteer for the elected official and be involved with policy issues more directly. In whatever way possible, nurses must develop relationships with policymakers, perhaps through the newly formed Congressional Nursing Caucus, if they expect to influence policy.

DISCUSSION QUESTIONS

1. Are you registered to vote? How do you register to vote in your state? What are the absentee and early voting requirements in your jurisdiction? How do these laws affect turnout among groups (such as nurses) that may not have a traditional work schedule?

2. On what policy issues might nurses lobby Congress? What strategies might nurses use to have their voices heard?

3. How might nurses get involved in campaign politics? What strategies might nurses use to have their voices heard?

REFERENCES

Alvarez, M., & Hall, T. E. (2010). *Electronic elections: The perils and promises of digital democracy*. Princeton, NJ: Princeton University Press.

Asian Americans Advancing Justice. (2012). Strength in numbers: Infographics from the 2010 AAPI post-election survey. Retrieved from *www.advancingjustice-aajc.org/sites/aajc/files/sin_final.pdf*.

Box-Steffensmeier, J., De Boef, S., & Lin, T. (2004). The dynamics of the partisan gender gap. *American Political Science Review, 98*(3), 515–528.

Brown, R. D., & Wedecking, J. (2006). People who have their tickets but do not use them. *American Politics Research, 34*(4), 479–504.

CNN. (2012). President: Full results. Retrieved from *www.cnn.com/election/2012/results/race/president*.

Dato, C. (2006). The American voter and electoral politics. In D. Mason, J. Leavitt, & M. Chaffee (Eds.), *Policy & politics in nursing and health care* (5th ed.). St. Louis, MO: Elsevier.

Flanigan, W., & Zingale, N. (2006). *Political behavior of the American electorate* (11th ed.). Washington, DC: CQ Press.

Francia, P., Joe, W., & Wilcox, C. (2008). Campaign finance reform—Present and future. In R. J. Semiatin (Ed.), *Campaigns on the cutting edge*. Washington, DC: CQ Press.

Gans, C. (2008). Much-hyped turnout record fails to materialize: Convenience voting fails to boost balloting. Press release. *AU News*. Retrieved from *www1.media.american.edu/electionexperts/election_turnout_08.pdf*.

Giammo, J. D., & Brox, B. (2010). Reducing the costs of participation: Are states getting a return on early voting? *Political Research Quarterly, 63*(2), 295–303.

Kropf, M., & Kimball, D. (2012). *Helping America vote: The limits of election reform*. New York: Routledge.

O'Connor, K., Sabato, L., & Yanus, A. (2015). *American government: Roots and reform* (2014 election ed.). New York: Pearson.

U.S. Census Bureau. (2012). Voting and registration in the election of November 2012. Retrieved from *www.census.gov/hhes/www/socdemo/voting/publications/p20/2012/tables.html*.

ONLINE RESOURCES

American Nurses Association
www.nursingworld.org
United States Election Assistance Commission
www.eac.gov
United States legislative information
www.congress.gov

UNIT 3

CHAPTER 47

Political Activity: Different Rules for Government-Employed Nurses

Shanita D. Williams   Josepha E. Burnley[1]

"Government of the people, by the people, for the people, shall not perish from the Earth."

Abraham Lincoln

The 2008 Presidential election was historic in many ways. The election was the first in which an African American was elected to the Presidency, and the first time the Republican Party nominated a woman for Vice President. With the highest voter turnout in at least 40 years, more Americans were mobilized than ever before to be politically active. Although the voter turnout in the 2012 election was lower than 2008 (Bipartisan Policy Center, 2012), more Americans continued to stay politically engaged and active.

U.S. citizens and legal residents celebrate many political freedoms such as speaking out on radio call-in shows, participating in public demonstrations, and campaigning for political candidates. It seems paradoxical, then, that the U.S. government restricts the type of political activity in which government-employed nurses, as well as other public employees, may participate. Political activity is defined as any activity that is directed toward the success or failure of a political party, candidate for partisan political office, or partisan political group. U.S. government restrictions on certain political activities may appear to be a violation of one's political freedom and the right to free speech, but the limits serve as a means of protecting government employees from coercion. Nearly 60,000 nurses nationwide are subject to these political activity restrictions.

The Hatch Act of 1939, officially An Act to Prevent Pernicious Political Activities, is a U.S. federal law whose main provision prohibits employees in the executive branch of the federal government, except the President, Vice President, and certain designated high-level officials of that branch, from engaging in partisan political activity (U.S. Office of Special Counsel, 2014). The law was named for Senator Carl Hatch of New Mexico (Box 47-1). The Hatch Act was amended in 1993 and again in 2012. It is the regulatory aspects of the Hatch Act that limit the political activity of civilian nurses and other health professionals serving in a variety of government agencies including the U.S. Department of Veterans Affairs and U.S. Veterans Health Administration, the U.S. Department of State, the U.S. Public Health Service, and the federal civil service. In addition, the political activities of members of the Armed Forces are governed by the U.S. Department of Defense (DoD) Directive 1344.10 titled Political Activities by Members of the Armed Forces on Active Duty (DoD, 2008). The DoD regulatory directive limits the political activity of nurses who serve on active duty in all branches of the U.S. Armed Forces.

WHY WAS THE HATCH ACT NECESSARY?

The political activity of government employees is restricted to protect employees from coercion by

---

[1]This is a revision of a chapter in the 6th edition that was authored by Tracy A. Malone and Mary W. Chaffee.

BOX 47-1 The Hatch Act (1939)

The Act to Prevent Pernicious Political Activities, more commonly known as the Hatch Act, was passed in 1939. The Hatch Act restricts the political activity of executive branch employees of the federal government, the District of Columbia (DC) government, and certain state and local agencies. Nurses employed by the federal government in any status (i.e., full-time, part-time, permanent, temporary) are subject to restrictions on political activity. Nurses covered by the Hatch Act include federal employees, DC employees, employees of state or local agencies funded by the federal government, and commissioned officers in the U.S. Public Health Service.

Because the original Hatch Act was extremely restrictive, multiple attempts have been made to amend the legislation and loosen restrictions. In 1993, Congress passed legislation that substantially amended the Hatch Act, allowing most federal and DC employees to engage in many types of political activity. Although these amendments did not change the provisions applying to state and local employees, they do allow most federal and DC government employees to take part in political management or in political campaigns. The Office of Personnel Management (OPM) published the translation of the amendment into specific regulations in the Federal Register on July 5, 1996.

On December 19, 2012, the U.S. House of Representatives passed S. 2170, the Hatch Act Modernization Act of 2012. The Hatch Act Modernization Act removes the federal prohibition on most state and local government employees who want to run for partisan political office. Under current law, state and local government employees may not run for partisan office if their job is connected to federal funding, a prohibition that prevents well-qualified candidates from serving their local communities. S. 2170 will strike this prohibition unless the employee's salary is fully funded by federal dollars. The Hatch Act will continue to restrict state and local government employees from engaging in coercive conduct, or otherwise using their government positions to advance partisan political ends (U.S. Office of Special Counsel, 2014).

---

corrupt politicians and political organizations. In the 1930s, a Senate panel discovered that certain federal employees had been coerced to support specific political candidates to keep their jobs. Senator Carl Hatch of New Mexico introduced legislation that was enacted in 1939 to end this practice.

Senator Hatch also feared the development of a national political machine made up of federal employees following the directions of their employers. In addition, the Hatch Act maintains the political neutrality of government offices. See Box 47-2 for the do's and dont's on political participation for federal employees, including nurses.

HATCH ACT ENFORCEMENT

The U.S. Office of Special Counsel (OSC) is an independent federal agency charged with enforcing the Hatch Act and several other federal laws. Headquartered in Washington, DC, the OSC investigates and, when warranted, prosecutes violations before the Merit Systems Protection Board. The OSC serves a dual role under the Hatch Act. Its mission includes preventing Hatch Act violations through the use of advisory opinions, and enforcing and prosecuting violations of the act when they do occur. Each year the OSC issues approximately 2000 advisory opinions, enabling individuals to determine whether and how they are covered by the act and whether their contemplated activities are permitted under the act. The OSC also enforces compliance with the act, receiving and investigating complaints alleging Hatch Act violations (OSC, 2014).

The OSC reports increased requests for advisory opinions on political activity during Presidential election periods. During the 2008 election period, the OSC saw a considerable increase in both the number of complaints (the highest on record) and the seriousness of Hatch Act violations by federal employees (OSC, 2009). With a rise in political advocacy by federal employees, there are more possibilities for violations.

Today, the most common way federal employees run afoul of the Hatch Act is through misuse of e-mail. When federal employees send e-mails that advocate support or opposition of a partisan candidate running for office and do so from government computers, in a government building, or while on duty in a federal job, they violate the Hatch Act. Most state employee violations involve members who were unclear as to their ability to run for public office while serving in state government.

BOX 47-2 Civilian Federally Employed Nurses Do's and Dont's Under the Hatch Act

For nurses covered by the Hatch Act, a wider range of political activities is now permitted because of Hatch Act reform (1993), with the following specific restrictions:

Nurses covered by the Hatch *Act* **may**:

- Register and vote as they choose and assist in voter registration drives
- Express opinions about candidates and issues
- Participate in campaigns in which none of the candidates represents a political party
- Contribute money to political organizations
- Attend political fund-raising functions, political rallies, and meetings
- Join and be active members of a political party or club
- Sign nominating petitions
- Campaign for or against referendum questions, constitutional amendments, or municipal ordinances
- Campaign for or against candidates in partisan (political party–affiliated) elections
- Be candidates for public office in nonpartisan elections
- Make campaign speeches for candidates in partisan elections, as long as the speech does not contain an appeal for political contributions
- Distribute campaign literature in partisan elections
- Help organize a fund-raising event, as long as they do not solicit or accept political contributions
- Display a partisan bumper sticker on a private automobile used occasionally for official business

- Contribute to a political action committee through a payroll deduction plan

Nurses covered by the Hatch Act **may not:**

- Solicit or receive political contributions from the general public
- Coerce other employees into making a political contribution
- Become personally identified with a fund-raising activity
- Participate, even anonymously, in phone-bank solicitations for political contributions or solicit political contributions in campaign speeches
- Display partisan buttons, posters, or similar items on federal premises, on duty, or in uniform
- Participate in partisan political activity while on duty, when wearing an official uniform, using a government vehicle, or in a government office
- Sign a campaign letter that solicits political contributions
- Use official authority or influence to interfere with an election
- Solicit or discourage political activity of anyone with business before their agency
- Be candidates for public office in a partisan election
- Wear political buttons on duty

Although Hatch Act reform has resulted in greater opportunity for political participation, handling political contributions remains off-limits. Personally accepting, soliciting, or receiving political contributions is not permitted under current regulations.

With the wave of new political appointees who entered government service as a result of the 2008 and 2012 Presidential election, the OSC stepped up efforts to get the message out that federal employees, political and career, must use the many opportunities available to them to learn about Hatch Act regulations.

PENALTIES FOR HATCH ACT VIOLATIONS

Nurses and other health professionals who engage in political activities that violate the Hatch Act or DoD Directive are subject to a range of penalties and disciplinary actions. Penalties and disciplinary actions may include removal from federal service, reduction in grade, debarment from federal employment for a period not to exceed 5 years, suspension, reprimand, or a civil penalty not to exceed $1000.

For example, under a settlement with the OSC in August 2012, two federal employees agreed to serve suspensions for violating the Hatch Act's prohibitions against engaging in political activity while on duty or in the federal workplace or soliciting political contributions (OSC, 2012). One employee was found guilty of coordinating volunteer efforts for a gubernatorial candidate's 2010 campaign while on duty in his federal office. The second employee organized an Obama fundraiser and distributed campaign materials in the workplace.

In matters not sufficiently serious to warrant prosecution, the OSC will issue a warning letter to the employee. Although the OSC will prosecute violations of the Hatch Act, it views its primary role as helping federal employees avoid such violations in the first place.

U.S. DEPARTMENT OF DEFENSE REGULATIONS ON POLITICAL ACTIVITY

Restrictions similar to those in the Hatch Act regulate the political behavior of nurses in the U.S. Army, Navy, and Air Force, including those in the National Guard and/or in Reserve status. The spirit and intent of DoD Directive 1344.10 (DoD, 2008) prohibits any activity that may be viewed as associating the DoD with a partisan political cause or candidate. See Box 47-3 on Regulations on Political Activity of Military Personnel for the full directive. This directive is a lawful general regulation and violations by persons subject to the Uniform Code of Military Justice are punishable under Article 92, which is Failure to Obey Order or Regulation, Chapter 47 of Reference (b). Violators shall be punished as a court martial may direct.

INTERNET AND SOCIAL MEDIA INFLUENCE

Internet communication and social media have become the most efficient and effective means of information transfer and have significantly shaped

UNIT 3

BOX 47-3 Restrictions on Political Activity of Military Personnel

The following restrictions on political activity apply to military personnel, including nurses:

Nurses in the armed forces **may**:
- Register, vote, and express their personal opinions on political candidates and issues, but not as representatives of the uniformed services
- Encourage other military members to vote, without attempting to influence or interfere with the outcome of an election
- Contribute money to political organizations, parties, or committees favoring a particular candidate
- Attend partisan and nonpartisan political meetings or rallies as spectators when not in uniform or on duty
- Join a political club, and attend meetings when not in uniform
- Serve as nonpartisan election officials, if they are not in uniform, if it does not interfere with military duties, and approval is provided by the commanding officer
- Sign a petition for legislative action or for placing a candidate's name on a ballot, but in the service member's personal capacity
- Make personal visits to legislators, but not in uniform or as official representatives of their branch of service
- Write a letter to the editor of a newspaper or other periodical expressing personal views on public issues or political candidates
- Display a political bumper sticker on a private vehicle
- If an officer, seek and hold nonpartisan civil office on an independent school board that is located on a military reservation

Nurses in the armed forces **may not:**
- Use their official authority to influence or interfere with an election
- Solicit votes for a particular candidate or issue
- Require or solicit political contributions from others
- Participate in partisan political management, campaigns, or conventions
- Write or publish partisan articles that solicit votes for or against a party or candidate
- Participate in partisan radio or television shows
- Distribute partisan political literature or participate in partisan political parades
- Display large political signs, banners, or posters on a private vehicle
- Use contemptuous words against the president; the vice president; Congress; the secretaries of defense or transportation or the military departments; or the governors or legislators of any state or territory where the service member is on duty
- Engage in fund-raising activities for partisan political causes on military property or in federal offices
- Attend partisan political events as official representatives of the uniformed services
- Campaign for or hold elective civil office in the federal government, or the government of a state, a territory, DC, or any political division in those areas
- Nurses serving in the military are encouraged to obtain an official opinion from a military lawyer if they are unsure about participating in a specific political activity

political participation. They are the now preferred methods of communication and messaging in partisan political activities. Federally employed nurses can easily (and often unintentionally) break the rules regarding partisan political communication. John Mitchell, Communications Director for the OSC, has cautioned federal employees about accessing the Internet through computers on the job, including if remotely accessed. Easy access to the Internet at work "makes it easier for people to make a mistake." He added, "Now people can step into trouble very easily just by forwarding a message that someone else sent to them" (Federaltimes.com, 2008). The increased popularity of social media has also posed problems for government employees and has led to many questions to the OSC for clarification, resulting in the Frequently Asked Questions Regarding Social Media and the Hatch Act guidance issued in April of 2012 by the OSC (U.S. OSC, 2012).

CONCLUSION

American nurses have created new horizons in policy and politics by becoming increasingly sophisticated in their political knowledge and by becoming actively involved in influencing health care in many environments. Many have translated professional nursing skills into effective political skills. Government-employed nurses should have their voices heard, as all other nurses have the opportunity to do, and participate actively in the political process. However, it is critical that they be aware of and abide by the laws and regulations designed to offer them a nonpartisan workplace and protection from coercion. Although the availability of information and educational materials on political activity and government employment is abundant, it is the nurse's responsibility to review

and understand the provisions of the Hatch Act and U.S. Department of Defense regulations to avoid any unnecessary violations or misuse of their key positions in the U.S. government.

DISCUSSION QUESTIONS

1. Should there be different rules and regulations that guide the political activities of civilian nurses in the federal workforce as compared with nurses in the U.S. armed forces? Discuss pros and cons.
2. Do you believe the Hatch Act violates U.S. citizens' and/or legal residents' right of free speech? Why or why not?
3. Will knowledge of the Hatch Act and DoD Directive 1344.10 impact your employment decisions in the future?

REFERENCES

Bipartisan Policy Center. (2012). 2012 Voter turnout. Retrieved from *bipartisanpolicy.org/library/report/2012-voter-turnout.*

Federaltimes.com. (2008). What to know about Hatch Act. Retrieved from *www.federaltimes.com/index.php.*

U.S. Department of Defense. (2008). DoD Directive 1344.10, Political activities by members of the armed forces. Retrieved from *www.dtic.mil/whs/directives/corres/pdf/134410p.pdf.*

U.S. Office of Special Counsel [OSC]. (2009). *U.S. Office of Special Counsel fiscal year 2009 annual report to Congress.* Washington, DC: U.S. Office of Special Counsel. Retrieved from *osc.gov/Resources/ar-2009.pdf.*

U.S. Office of Special Counsel [OSC]. (2012). *Frequently asked questions regarding social media and the Hatch Act.* Washington, DC: U.S. Office of Special Counsel. Retrieved from *osc.gov/Resources/Social%20Media%20and%20the%20Hatch%20Act%202012.pdf.*

U.S. Office of Special Counsel [OSC]. (2014). *How does the Hatch Act affect me: Federal employees.* Washington, DC: U.S. Office of Special Counsel. Retrieved from *osc.gov/pages/hatchact-affectsme.aspx.*

ONLINE RESOURCES

U.S. Office of Special Counsel: The Hatch Act
www.osc.gov/hatchact.htm

CHAPTER 48

TAKING ACTION:
Anatomy of a Political Campaign

Greer Glazer   Charles R. Alexandre   Angela K. Clark

"Every election is determined by the people who show up."

Larry J. Sabato

Is it hard to imagine why anyone would stand in the rain or snow from 6:00 AM to 6:00 PM on Election Day handing out information about a political candidate? How about someone driving a candidate to eight events in one long 14-hour day covering 250 miles? Or a group of volunteers battling against the clock to create 250 new polling stations the week of the presidential election in response to the fury of Hurricane Sandy (Rowley, 2012)? People work on political campaigns for a variety of reasons, and understanding their motivation is critical to building a strong volunteer program.

WHY PEOPLE WORK ON CAMPAIGNS

People's motivations for working on campaigns fall into four general categories: (1) belief in an issue or a candidate, (2) network building, (3) party loyalty, and (4) personal payback. These four categories are not mutually exclusive and often closely overlap. For example, unpaid volunteers donate their time and/or resources because they believe strongly in an individual or an issue. They tend to be party loyalists who build networks at the grassroots level to create change that may, in the end, dually advance the party's agenda and result in personal gain.

BELIEF IN AN ISSUE OR CANDIDATE

There are traditionally two types of paid staff on a campaign—those who 'believe in the man and the mission' and those who do it for personal gain. (Chris Burger, Romney Presidential Campaign, 2012)

Some people work for a candidate because they feel strongly about issues they support and champion or conversely want to defeat the opponent because of where he or she stands on the issues. For example, in 2008, Democratic presidential candidate Barack Obama preached a message of change that resonated with voters, and the presidential election resulted in a higher voter turnout than had been seen in many years (Pew Research Center, 2008). The 2012 presidential election turned out fewer voters overall than the two previous elections, but a shift in voter demographics gave Obama his second term. The turnout of white voters dropped to 71.1% of eligible voters from 75.5% and 73.4% in 2004 and 2008, respectively (Frey, 2013). During the same period, minority voting rates rose to a quarter of eligible voters. The presidential election of 2012 was the first time in history that the rate of African-American voter turnout was higher than for whites. It may be that the high turnout of African Americans can be attributed to support for the first African-American president, whereas the drop in white voters may be the result of a lack of commitment to either candidate (Frey, 2013).

NETWORK BUILDING

Some people are drawn to campaigns to advance their own social or professional network. Professional network building may include paid campaign staff that start at a basic level and by mobilizing all lines of networking move up in the organization (Democratic Gain, 2013). For volunteers, getting them involved in social activities will

419

keep them involved in campaign activities, thus propelling the campaign agenda.

PARTY LOYALTY

Many individuals work for the candidate because they are loyal to the political party. Candidates target close races in which they believe an infusion of financial and human resources can change the outcome of the election. Party loyalists will travel to different states to work on campaigns in which they can make a difference. In 2012, nurses traveled to a variety of states to attend rallies and events to support presidential candidates and help their candidate gain visibility to garner press coverage. The American Nurses Association dedicated October 17, 2012 as Nurses Campaign Activity Night (Nurses CAN). This movement was about getting nurses involved in the campaign of their choice to advance nursing's core issues across all political parties (American Nurses Association, 2012).

PAYBACK

Tangible paybacks include paid work for the campaign, course credit for students, and, if the candidate is elected, appointment to staff, appointment to key commissions or boards or other political appointments, and support for specific legislation. In fall 2013, President Obama nominated Jeh Johnson, a long-time Obama supporter and prominent campaign fund-raiser, to run the U.S. Department of Homeland Security (Delreal, 2013; Sullivan, 2013). Understanding why people work on campaigns enables the campaign to successfully recruit volunteers. However, understanding why people work on campaigns does not necessarily help to retain them. You must also be aware of why people stop working on campaigns.

WHY PEOPLE STOP WORKING ON CAMPAIGNS

The major reason why people stop working on campaigns is that their roles and campaign activities are not aligned with their motivation for working on the campaign. People leave campaigns because they lose interest, are not given enough positive feedback and recognition, do not feel part of the larger whole, lose faith that the candidate can win the election, feel that the work is boring, have competing outside interests such as family and work obligations, and are not enjoying themselves. The following describes campaign activities that either engage or disengage campaign workers.

THE INTERNET AND THE 2012 ELECTION CAMPAIGN

The Internet has been a tool in presidential elections since Howard Dean's extraordinary Internet-based fund-raising in 2004. Obama expanded on Dean's success, raising a record amount of money and mobilizing supporters nationwide. Since then, the growth of technology and the impact of social media have revolutionized the electoral process (Pew Research, 2012). Hong and Nadler (2012) note that in a 2-year span from 2010 to 2012 "politicians in modern democracies across the world have eagerly adopted social networking tools, such as Facebook and Twitter, seeing in them powerful new mediums for engaging their constituents" (Hong & Nadler, 2012, p. 456). Another example of new uses of the Internet was that, with the support of Governor Chris Christie, New Jersey residents were able to submit online ballots in the 2012 presidential election. This decision was instrumental in supporting the voting rights of Americans recovering from the aftermath of Hurricane Sandy (State of New Jersey, 2012).

Use of the Internet during an election campaign is based purely on demographics (gender, race, and geography), and users are similar in makeup to the adult population as a whole, although the political Internet user tends to have a higher level of income and education than the total U.S. population (Pew Research Center, 2009). In the 2010 midterm elections, 24% of American adults stated they received the majority of their campaign information from the Internet, a threefold increase from the 2002 midterm elections (Smith, 2011). Although news from in-press sources such as newspapers has decreased, the proportion of Americans who log on to get their campaign news has increased by 60% in just 4 years (Smith, 2011). As a result of the increase in Internet use among voters, it is no surprise that the 2012 Obama for America presidential campaign was very strategic about how to connect with voters. The Obama for America data and technology operations staff comprised 30% to 40% of headquarters staff. Staff members were recruited from Silicon Valley, Fortune 500 companies, and various other technologically savvy corporations such as Microsoft, Twitter, and Pixar (Engage Research, 2013).

This presence gave the Obama campaign the ability to fully utilize predictive analytics that are driven by the net, allowing the campaign to develop strategies and direct campaign resources to where they are needed the most (WPA Opinion Research, n.d.). Winston Churchill was quoted as saying "However beautiful the strategy, you should occasionally look at the results." Predictive analytics offers a statistically calculated prediction of current results based on responses to campaign activities and voter demographics. In the 2012 presidential election, President Obama's Campaign Manager, Jim Messina, stated, "We were going to put an analytics team inside of us to study us the entire time to make sure we were being smart about things" (Engage Research, 2013, p. 18). True to Messina's statement, the Obama for America analytics team ran 66,000 simulations each night to project the victor in each of the battleground states to guide strategy and allocate real-time resources (Engage Research, 2013).

SOCIAL NETWORKING WEBSITES

The changing landscape of presidential elections has long been molded by the advent of technology. The televising of presidential debates during the 1960 election between Nixon and Kennedy increased visual accessibility of the candidates to the voters. Voters could put a face to the message and, perhaps most importantly, identify with the candidates. Since the 1960s the use of technology has continued to grow. Phenomena not readily available during the previous campaigns but used extensively during the 2008 campaign were social networking websites (e.g., MySpace and Facebook) and video-sharing websites (e.g., YouTube). By the 2012 election, Twitter, Tumblr, Instagram, and Storify were capturing all aspects of the election. Candidates were using Twitter to deliver their messages right up until the closing of the polls. At 2:57 PM on November 6, 2012 @MittRomney tweeted, "I am asking for your vote because I want to keep America the hope of the earth" (Romney Presidential Campaign, 2012). Barack Obama himself (as signified by his Twitter signature "@bo") tweeted, "We're coming to the end of a long campaign, all that's left to do is get out the vote. Let's win this." At the same time, campaign supporters and celebrities were retweeting pro-voting tweets. The Pew Research Center, in 2012, reported that 38% of those who use social networking sites promote material related to politics and 35% have used social networking sites to encourage people to get out and vote (Duggan, 2012) (Box 48-1).

CAMPAIGN ACTIVITIES

Campaign activities can be divided into basic-level campaign activities and advanced-level campaign

---

BOX 48-1 Social Media and Voting in the 2012 Presidential Election

- 30% have heard from family and friends via postings on social networking sites or Twitter in the past 30 days that they should vote for either candidate.
- 29% have heard from family and friends in phone conversations in the past 30 days that they should vote for either candidate.
- 21% have heard from family and friends in e-mails in the past 30 days that they should vote for either candidate.
- 20% have posted voting messages to others on a social networking site or Twitter, encouraging them to vote for one of the candidates.
- 22% of registered voters have announced on a social networking site or Twitter how they voted or planned to vote.
- The "social vote" cohort included anyone who related messages about voting, or posted messages about their presidential choice on social media, and accounted for 74% of registered voters.

Adapted from Rainie, L. (2012). Social media and political engagement. Pew Internet and American Life Project. Washington, DC: Pew Research Center. Retrieved from *pewinternet.org/Reports/2012/Social-Vote-2012.aspx*.

activities. Basic-level campaign activities include organizing phone banks and literature drops, office work, poll watching, organizing house parties, driving candidates, fund raising, serving as a health policy advisor, organizing voter registration, and providing Internet communication about a candidate. Advanced-level campaign activities and roles usually require full-time involvement and include the campaign manager, finance director, political director, operations director, communications director, and new-media or Internet director.

BASIC-LEVEL CAMPAIGN ACTIVITIES

Basic-level campaign activities are easily undertaken by nurses because they are used to working on teams and in groups, have good communication skills, and are well organized.

Although there are no limitations on your involvement in a campaign as a private individual, in some cases it may be inappropriate for you to work on a political campaign as a representative of a particular organization. Some organizations are prohibited from engaging in political activity or candidate endorsements based on federal election law and their tax status. Political involvement on behalf of that organization may cause problems for the organization as well as the campaign. Be sure that your participation in a campaign is approved by the organization that you represent.

Once you have the green light, do not be shy about making sure the campaign is aware of your affiliation. If you want an organization to get credit for your participation, you need to identify yourself as a representative of that organization. It would be best to have a group of individuals from your organization take responsibility for a specific campaign activity or project.

The second issue to consider is how much time you have to volunteer. Campaigns count on their volunteers, and if you sign up to do something, it is important that you follow through. Obviously the more time and involvement you have, the greater will be the payback. For those who have more time, decide whether you want to be involved in many activities or stay focused on one activity. Keep in mind that it is easier to quantify one's contribution and get credit for the work when you can

be identified as filling a specific role such as driver, house party coordinator, or heath policy advisor.

TYPES OF CAMPAIGN ACTIVITIES

Phone Banks. Phone banks are frequently used to contact voters for voter identification, to communicate the candidate's message, to determine support or nonsupport of a specific candidate or issue, and to ensure turnout on Election Day. They are also used to recruit volunteers, raise money, and ensure turnout at campaign events. Nurses are usually experienced at phone banking because of their excellent communication skills.

Literature Drops. Volunteers often go door to door to drop off campaign literature. Leafleting is a form of literature distribution that is limited to public places. Literature drops and leafleting are low-impact voter contacts with low cost and little ability to target voters. Other low-impact activities include buttons and bumper stickers, lawn signs, billboards, and human billboards.

Door-to-Door Canvassing. Door-to-door canvassing is a traditional type of voter contact in which the volunteer knocks on the door and speaks with the voter. Your goal may be to share the candidate's message or to determine the voting preference of the residents of the house.

House Parties. House parties are given by a volunteer in a targeted area where neighbors, friends, and colleagues are invited to the volunteer's house to meet the candidate. Greer Glazer served as house party coordinator for Lee Fisher during his campaign for Ohio State Senate. When Fisher was elected State Senator, Greer served in an advisory capacity on nursing and health issues. He subsequently ran for and was elected to the Office of Ohio Attorney General. Fisher is currently CEO of CEOs for Cities, whose mission is "to be a strong, deep, and broad global, cross-sector, cross-generational, inter-connected network that serves as a cutting edge online and face to face platform and collaborative infrastructure for making American cities more vibrant, sustainable, and economically competitive and successful, with a focus on investing in the distinctive assets of cities." The relationship that had been developed by working on all of his campaigns was very helpful when Greer was able to have access to discuss Medicaid payments for advanced practice nurses.

Created Events. Created events are the best way to create the environment for the candidate's message and target it to a specific group. Senator Sherrod Brown of Ohio (D-OH) routinely holds such events. These include meetings with nurses to discuss health care issues, meetings with senior citizens to discuss prescription drug coverage, or town hall meetings to discuss larger policy issues such as Social Security. Every detail is planned in advance. Nurses participated in a variety of created events during the 2012 presidential campaign. For example, President Obama launched a national coalition, Nurses for Obama. Their role was to promote a campaign report on how the Affordable Care Act had benefited Pennsylvanians (Griffiths, 2012). The campaign used these events to elaborate on the candidate's position and to provide visual images, using the public's trust in nurses, to enhance support for his candidacy.

Timing for media events can be created by the campaign or dictated by opportunities that arise to highlight a candidate's position. Examples of events created by the campaign might include staging a worker rally, holding a press conference in front of a hospital to discuss the need for enhanced medical insurance for children, or interviewing senior citizens about Medicare. For added exposure, clips from rallies or interviews might also be posted as a video on the candidate's website.

Unplanned media opportunities use news events to highlight a candidate's position with regard to a current event. It can provide an opportunity to differentiate the candidate from the opposition candidate or to highlight one's leadership. Unplanned media opportunities may also derail the focus of a campaign. While speaking to a group of wealthy donors in the Republican Party, Romney, captured on a smartphone video, described supporters of Obama as "freeloaders who pay no taxes, who don't assume responsibility for their lives, and who think the government should take care of them" (Corn, 2013). He was quoted saying that it was not his job to worry about these people. Arguably, the quote could have been taken out of context; however, the Obama campaign was able to successfully use this as an example of Romney being out of touch with the average American citizen. Media coverage of such events creates powerful messages for the public.

Political Action Committees. In addition to candidate media events, supportive organizations and individuals may use their own resources to generate media coverage for a particular issue. Political action committees (PACs) are groups that are organized to engage in political activity, although they are not endorsed by a particular candidate or political party (Law Library, n.d.). PACs may be sponsored by businesses, labor unions, or special-interest groups for the purpose of raising and spending money to support or denounce legislative initiatives. For example, Emily's List *(www.emilyslist.org)* is a PAC that supports prochoice women running for governor or Congress. The American Nurses Association's (ANA's) political action committee, ANA-PAC, has actively taken out newspaper ads, made radio spots, and purchased political paraphernalia to advocate for nurse-friendly candidates.

Get-Out-the-Vote Activities. The candidate can have the most campaign funds, best message, and most efficient operation, but if the campaign is

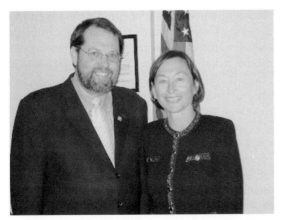

FIGURE 48-1 Dr. Greer Glazer with Congressman Steven LaTourette (R-OH) at the American Association of Colleges of Nursing congressional reception.

unable to get supporters out to vote on Election Day, the candidate will not win. Phone banks, e-mail, and door-to-door canvasing are all effective strategies for getting out the vote, yet 2012 saw a significant rise in the use of social media to encourage people to vote. A total of 30% of registered voters were encouraged to vote for either Obama or Romney by family and friends via social media platforms such as Facebook and Twitter, while 20% of registered voters used these platforms to encourage others to vote (Rainie, 2012).

ADVANCED-LEVEL CAMPAIGN ACTIVITIES

The campaign manager has overall responsibility for the strategic and technical decisions of the entire campaign and creates the campaign and business plans. The campaign manager sets the tone to motivate staff and volunteers, who work long hours for little or no payment. For example, the 2012 campaign did not have the resounding theme of hope and change as it did 4 years earlier, but it did have an all-encompassing focus on operational technology. Despite being evenly matched financially, the Obama campaign built an operation four times the size of Romney's (Engage Research, 2013).

The finance director has overall responsibility for campaign finances. This individual manages fund-raising and oversees a finance committee and fund-raising events and how the money is spent. This is the person who determines, with the political director and the communications director, how much to spend on media, special events, travel, staff, and so on. By the 2008 election cycle, all candidates used the Internet to enhance fund-raising for their campaigns. No one was more effective than the Obama campaign, which raised nearly $750 million while establishing a database of 13 million donors (Brooks, 2009). In the 2012 cycle, the Obama campaign, using the donor lists created in 2008, greatly exceeded previous fund-raising, reporting $1.1 billion in fund-raising efforts with $525 million brought in through online means (Tau, 2012).

The political director has overall responsibility for campaign strategy to determine how to position the candidate as the person to win. A major responsibility is developing an opposition strategy. In the 2008 election, the Internet not only became an effective medium for fund-raising, but it also provided extensive constituent outreach that resulted in a very large online constituency. The Obama campaign did an outstanding job of recruiting and developing an online constituency by having people register on the campaign's website; sending routine e-mail messages with consistent and compelling messages; creating online polls, surveys, and discussions (blogs); asking those visiting the website to forward messages to friends and relatives (viral marketing); and creating urgency. Importantly, every contact from the Obama campaign included a request for a campaign donation with an active credit card link. During the 2012 campaign both candidates worked to maintain and expand their online constituencies; however, it was the Obama campaign that more effectively used direct digital messaging by targeting specific voter groups such as African Americans; the lesbian, gay, bisexual, and transgender (LGBT) community; Latinos; and veterans/military families (Journalism.org, 2012).

The communications director has overall responsibility for the campaign theme. A campaign message is the basis for a successful communication plan. Joe Rospars, former new media director for the Obama 2008 presidential campaign, defined the prerequisite for a successful campaign as "a candidate and a message that resonates with people and a staff of dedicated people that believe in the candidate and the message in order for it to work" (Rospars, 2009, p. 9). Rospars went on to state that "building of networks among the supporters within the context of your organization and the campaign where people can step up and become owners of the campaign and owners of the organization and recognize the collective power to come together in small groups, and also in a big way, together create change" (Rospars, 2009, p. 10).

Throughout a campaign, candidates seek as much control as possible over how they and their opponents are perceived by the media and the electorate. Communications directors carefully craft messages about their candidate as well as about the opponent, often based on research and polling. The goal is to ensure that their campaign defines the candidate and, to the greatest extent possible, the opponent, on their own terms.

Involvement in political campaigns provides nurses with a wonderful opportunity for influencing candidates about health issues, for meeting people, and for bringing a nursing perspective to the political process. Campaigns are ultimately very local and grassroots-oriented, requiring a solid ground game to reach the voter. The final step requires convincing the electorate to vote for your candidate or issue and then make sure each voter goes to vote on Election Day.

DISCUSSION QUESTIONS

1. Identify a political issue or agenda in health care. How would you formalize support to advance this agenda?
2. Discuss the role and potential impact of predictive analytics in advancing your agenda. Who would your target population be?
3. How will you mobilize the Internet to reach this population?

REFERENCES

American Nurses Association. (2012). Nurses campaign activity night. Retrieved from *www.rnaction.org/site/PageServer?pagename=nstat_take_action_nursescan_home&ct=1*.

Brooks, M. A. (2009). Challenges ahead for new White House Web team. Retrieved from *www.america.gov/st/usg-english/2009/January/20090123153511hmnietsua0.1627008.html*.

Corn, D. (2013). Secret video: Romney tells millionaire donors what he really thinks of Obama voters. Retrieved from *www.motherjones.com/politics/2012/09/secret-video-romney-private-fundraiser*.

Delreal, J. (2013). 10 things to know about Jeh Johnson. Retrieved from *www.politico.com/story/2013/10/jeh-johnson-facts-98531.html*.

Democratic Gain. (2013). How to get a political job. Retrieved from *www.democraticgain.org/?page=howtogetajob*.

Duggan, M. (2012). Pew Internet: Politics (11/14.12). Pew Internet and American Life Project. Retrieved from *pewinternet.org/Commentary/2012/November/Pew-Internet-Politics.aspx*.

Engage Research. (2013). Inside the cave. Retrieved from *engagedc.com/download/Inside%20the%20Cave.pdf?*.

Frey, W. H. (2013). Minority turnout determined the 2012 election. Retrieved from *www.brookings.edu/research/papers/2013/05/10-election-2012-minority-voter-turnout-frey*.

Griffiths, B. (2012). Obama campaign launches nurses coalition to defend health care law. Retrieved from *www.politicspa.com/obama-campaign-launches-nurses-coalition-to-defend-health-care-law/32765/*.

Hong, S., & Nadler, D. (2012). Which candidates do the public discuss online in an election campaign? The use of social media by 2012 presidential candidates and its impact on candidate salience. *Government Information Quarterly, 29*(4), 455–461.

Journalism.org. (2012). How the presidential candidates use the web and social media. Retrieved from *www.journalism.org/analysis_report/how_presidential_candidates_use_web_and_social_media*.

Law Library. (n.d). Political action committee—Further readings. Retrieved from *law.jrank.org/pages/9252/Political-action-Committee.html*.

Pew Research Center. (2008). Social networking and online videos take off: Internet's broader role in campaign 2008. Pew Internet and American Life Project. Washington, DC: Pew Research Center. Retrieved from *www.people-press.org/report/384*.

Pew Research Center. (2009). The Internet's role in campaign 2008. Pew Internet and American Life Project. Washington, DC: Pew Research Center. Retrieved from *www.pewinternet.org/Reports/2009/6-The-Internes-Role-in-Campaign-2008.aspx*.

Pew Research Internet Project. (2012). Politics fact sheet: Highlights of the Pew Internet Project's research related to politics. Retrieved from *www.pewinternet.org/fact-sheets/politics-fact-sheet/*.

Rainie, L. (2012). *Social media and voting*. Pew Internet and American Life Project. Washington, DC: Pew Research Center. Retrieved from *pewinternet.org/Reports/2012/Social-Vote-2012.aspx*.

Rospars, J. (2009). Joe Rospars discusses online outreach in political campaigns. Retrieved from *www.america.gov/st/washfile-english/2009/March/20090331113206xjsnommis0.5156214.html*.

Rowley, J. (2012). Business week. Some voting places being moved in storm-ravaged northeast. Retrieved from *www.businessweek.com/news/2012-11-05/some-voting-places-being-moved-in-new-york-new-jersey*.

Romney Presidential Campaign. (2012). Retrieved from *twitter.com/MittRomney*.

Smith, A. (2011). *The Internet and campaign 2010*. Pew Internet and American Life Project. Washington, DC: Pew Research Center. Retrieved from *www.pewinternet.org/Reports/2011/The-Internet-and-Campaign-2010/Section-2/The-internet-and-political-news-sources.aspx*.

State of New Jersey. (2012). Christie administration announces e-mail and fax voting available to New Jerseyans displaced by Hurricane Sandy. Trenton, NJ: Office of the Governor. Retrieved from *www.nj.gov/governor/news/news/552012/20121103d.html*.

Sullivan, E. (2013). What about Jeh Johnson? Jeh Johnson, Obama's DHS nominee, not well known by law enforcement associations. *The Huffington Post*. Retrieved from *www.huffingtonpost.com/2013/11/05/jeh-johnson-obama-dhs_n_4218025.html*.

Tau, B. (2012). Obama campaign final fundraising total: $1.1 billion. *Politico.com*. Retrieved from *www.politico.com/story/2013/01/obama-campaign-final-fundraising-total-1-billion-86445.html*.

WPA Opinion Research. (n.d). Predictive analytics. Retrieved from *www.wparesearch.com/our-tools/predictive-analytics/*.

ONLINE RESOURCES

Federal Election Commission
www.fec.gov
Gallup Poll
www.gallup.com
Open Secrets
www.opensecrets.com
Pew Research Center
www.pewinternet.org/topics/2014-election

UNIT 3

CHAPTER 49

TAKING ACTION:
Truth or Dare: One Nurse's Political Campaign

Barbara Hatfield   Brenda Isaac

"All serious daring starts from within."

Harriet Beecher Stowe

STEPPING INTO POLITICS

My dream (Barbara Hatfield) had always been to be a wife, mother, and nurse. Never in my wildest dreams did I envision a career in politics. Having graduated from a hospital-based diploma program, I was content to raise my family and work as a staff nurse in Charleston, West Virginia. As I became more experienced in my career, I began to be increasingly frustrated by the lack of power that nurses have in health care decisions. My colleagues and I saw the problems on a daily basis but felt powerless to make needed changes. Taking a leap of faith, I decided to run for the House of Delegates, with the support of nurses throughout my district.

My campaign staff consisted of volunteer nurses who took pictures, researched key issues, designed brochures and flyers, and formed phone banks. We found out that if you are not one of the "good ole boys," you get very little help or advice from the party. There was no money to buy mailing lists, so we had to be creative. Much of my funding came from nurses giving $10, $25, or whatever they could. After a while we got a few endorsements from the nurses' groups and the teachers' associations. Even the Medical Association and the Hospital Association endorsed me the first time because of my nursing background. They never really expected me to win and quickly dropped me after my first victory.

No one was more surprised than I was when we won our first campaign. With name recognition and a positive voting record, I continued to win elections. We still struggled to raise money, and I depend heavily on the dedicated nurses and other friends who volunteer to help me. Over the years we broadened our base to include social workers, teachers, labor unions, and others who fight for the little guys. The nurses, however, were always my mainstay. As the battles got tough, they kept me focused on our real objective: making life better for the people of West Virginia. In 2012, with some clever redistricting on the part of the opposition, I was defeated, losing my seat by 41 votes.

ETHICAL LEADERSHIP

Twenty-two years as a Delegate in the West Virginia House of Delegates has been a learning experience of monumental proportions. Although experience can mean power, it does not always turn out that way for members of governmental bodies, especially for women. A legislator can serve for many years, and if he or she is not in the majority party or in a leadership position, it is very difficult to get issues noticed and bills passed. This is where my nursing background paid off. As a nurse, I knew how to work with people and how to get people to work with me. Accomplishing anything in the legislature requires the ability to compromise, but it also requires knowing when to refuse to compromise and stick to what you know is right, even when some powerful people might get mad at you. In a

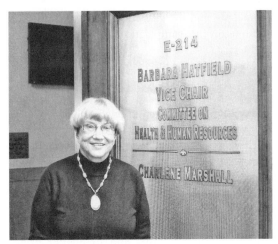

FIGURE 49-1 Barbara Hatfield.

couple of situations, I refused to compromise on bills that were just plain bad for the health of our constituents. I was able to use my health care expertise to speak against these bills, and because it was well known that I was a nurse, others listened, and I prevailed.

One of these issues involved tobacco. The tobacco industry is powerful and going against them was scary. I knew they could hurt me in future elections but this was just too important to back down on. Other more civic-minded lobbying groups got behind my cause and I was able to get enough delegates on my side to defeat the tobacco legislation. Although I did alienate a powerful lobbying group, I was seen by others as someone who knew what she was talking about and would not back down when it came to the health of my constituents.

In 2007, Delegate Richard Thompson was elected Speaker of the West Virginia House. He in turn put a record number of women legislators in positions of power. Because of my health care background, he felt I was the ideal person to serve as Vice Chairperson of the Health and Human Resources Committee. Of even greater significance, I was also awarded a position on the powerful House Rules Committee. The Speaker of the House chairs the Rules Committee and the members of this committee decide which bills are going to be brought to the floor of the House for a vote. As a member of this powerful committee, I was able to be a true voice for women, children, and health care. During my tenure I also served on the Government Organization Committee, Homeland Security Committee, Committee on Veterans Affairs, and a Special Committee on Senior Citizens.

MAKING A DIFFERENCE

After several sessions and a lot of hard work, I was able to get a bill passed to create a Commission on Behavioral Health, dealing with mental health issues for both adults and children. Specifically, I also took the lead in developing legislation to ensure early intervention for young children, 4 to 11 years old, whose mental health needs were not being adequately met. Many of these children had been abused and ended up in the foster care system without receiving appropriate mental health counseling and treatment. As a mother and a nurse, I understood the importance of treating children early and preventing more serious problems later on, perhaps even preventing these children from becoming status offenders and ending up in juvenile facilities or worse. This law requires specialized training for certain foster families before these children are placed in homes. This training helps to decrease multiple foster care placements for troubled children and provides the necessary continuity and ongoing treatment. The law has been dubbed Jacob's Law, after a little boy who from the age of 4 years had been in and out of foster homes and even mental health facilities, never receiving the continuous intensive care that he needed. The West Virginia Alliance for Children honored me for my work on this bill, and my advocacy for children's issues in general.

LESSONS LEARNED

Throughout my 22 years as a Delegate, I have fought tirelessly to improve the lives of our citizens, especially women and children. My reputation as an expert in health care has grown owing to my work in the Legislature. My time in the West Virginia Legislature has come to an end. However, I continue to further the causes that are important to

UNIT 3

me through service on various boards and commissions, such as the Board of Directors for a community federally qualified health care center, a state Supreme Court Commission on the rehabilitation of adjudicated juvenile offenders, and the Behavioral Health Commission. With my experience and connections through my years of service, I hope to continue making a difference.

I am sorry to say that I have not fulfilled my wish of having more nurses as West Virginia Delegates and Senators. Currently there is only one nurse in the House and none in the Senate. I continue to educate and mentor younger nurses in the political process, hoping that perhaps the dream of more nurses in government will become a reality. Grassroots campaigning is harder now, though, and it takes a lot more money to run a successful campaign. It is almost always harder for women to raise the necessary money to overcome the big boys and the big money. The media, through television and the Internet, plays a much bigger role in today's campaigns, and the grassroots idea of handshakes and one-on-one campaigning is becoming a thing of the past.

My last campaign, sadly, even involved some false-negative advertisements against me from outside groups that I had never worked with and knew little about. Even though the fights were tougher, my loyal group of friends, mostly nurses, stuck by me and together we fought the good fight. Other supporters I got to know along the way, such as members of women's groups, labor unions, and children's advocates, were there for me, too, and still are as we continue to advocate for those issues that we all believe in. I will continue to fight for those issues close to my heart and to mentor bright younger nurses who want to enter the political arena to make a difference. As Eleanor Roosevelt once said, "We [women] are half the people, we should be half the Congress," and nurses can help to make it happen.

CHAPTER 50

Political Appointments

Judith K. Leavitt   Andréa Sonenberg[1]

"Ask not what your country can do for you. Ask what you can do for your country."

John F. Kennedy

The wheels of the U.S. government and state governments are powered by three groups of employees: those elected to office, those who are career employees, and those appointed to serve. Each group offers an opportunity to influence public policy, and for nurses a political appointment is an outstanding chance to influence health policy. It addresses findings of the Robert Wood Johnson Foundation survey that, "while nurses are knowledgeable sources of information, they are not perceived as leaders" in the development of health care delivery systems (Mund, 2012, p. 423). Influencing public policy through a seat at the table fulfills one of the recommendations of the Institute of Medicine (IOM) (2011) in its report *The Future of Nursing: Leading Change, Advancing Health* that nursing should become instrumental in the transformation of health care delivery by assuming more leadership and policymaking roles (Mund, 2012). Seeking political appointments allows nurses to apply skills expertly demonstrated in clinical practice, translating clinical evidence to support policy reform (Armstrong, 2005; Clarke, Swider, & Bigley, 2013; Feetham, 2011; Mund, 2012). To attain a political appointment, nurses need to be familiar with the requirements for the position, how the appointment process works, and how to prepare for the process.

WHAT DOES IT TAKE TO BE A POLITICAL APPOINTEE?

Richard Nathan (2009), an authority on political appointments, states:

The politics of getting appointed and then being in the public service are intense. One appeal of appointive office is that, unlike elective offices, most people in these jobs are not constantly caught up in political fundraising and campaigning. Still, one cannot succeed in government without being political. A thick skin, the courage to take a stand, and the quickness of wit to defend it are essential qualities for appointive public service. It is exhilarating at the top, but it can also be nerve-racking too. Successful appointed leaders need a keen intuitive feel for the constant bargaining that the American political process requires. Most appointees are qualified and willing to serve when asked. (p. 11)

Then why seek a political appointment and the resulting political pressures? Nathan (2009) identified the following reasons why individuals seek political appointments:

- Public service can produce a gratifying sense of accomplishment.
- Public service can lead to recognition and prestige.
- Successful leadership in public service can enhance the chances of landing a well-paid job after exiting government service.

---

[1]The authors would like to thank Mary Chaffee for her work on the previous version of this chapter.

There is a large demand for appointees. Nathan (2009) estimates that 400,000 individuals serve in appointed positions in the federal, state, and local governments. In addition to recognizing their extensive numbers, Nathan tips his hat to their influence: These (appointed) officials "do the heavy lifting of policymaking and management inside America's governments and play a significant role as change agents in the nation's political system. Yet books about American government tend to ignore them and focus instead on elected office holders" (Nathan, 2009, p. 10). David Lewis (2008), a political scientist at Vanderbilt University, examined 600 government programs and the 234 managers that ran them. He found that the political appointees were better educated and had excellent records before their appointments. However, Vedantam (2008) found it was the career employees who were better at getting the work done through strategic planning, program design, and financial oversight. Yet the political appointees may bring fresh ideas, enthusiasm, and a closer connection with the public to the government workplace. Lyttle (2011) stresses that "nurses in particular are being called upon to parlay their expertise and experience into careers in politics" (p. 19), citing that they offer something that non-nurse candidates cannot offer: the personal and accurate reporting of what happens at point of service, whether it be in the hospital, in ambulatory settings, or in the community. Nurses are uniquely positioned to serve in this capacity; having the experience of directly witnessing the effects of policies on population health outcomes is a perspective not many other potential appointees can offer. In appointee roles, nurses are "likely to do exactly what they've been doing in health care settings … adjust and adapt to ever-changing situations; listen carefully; gather facts; and discern, decide, and deal thoughtfully with unexpected outcomes and turns of events" (Lyttle, 2011, p. 19).

GETTING READY

Once you decide you are interested in a political appointment, how do you get started? Determine where your interests and experience lie. Is there something you wish to change or a service needed

---

> **BOX 50-1** Government Political Appointment Resources
>
> **State Government**
> Contact the offices of individual secretaries of state or check their websites for appointment opportunities at the state level. For example, search online for "California Secretary of State." Employment sites and professional organizations update postings for appointment opportunities on a regular basis.
>
> **Federal Government**
> The federal government provides many public resources. One of the most important is the official *Plum Book*. Every 4 years, just after the Presidential election, Congress publishes U.S. Government Policy and Supporting Positions, more commonly known as the *Plum Book*. (The *Plum Book* is so called because of the color of the book.) The electronic version of the *Plum Book* is located at the Government Printing Office's website at *www.gpoaccess.gov/plumbook/*.

in your community or state? Do you have the expertise to be competitive for a federal appointment? Is your goal to seek political office? Will serving in a political or public role enhance advancement in your career? See Boxes 50-1 and 50-2 for resources.

IDENTIFY OPPORTUNITIES

How does a nurse determine where the opportunities are? The types of political appointments run the gamut. For instance, a position on a state board of health affords an opportunity to develop policy, whereas an appointment to an election commission is a mechanism for carrying out state law. If a nurse is interested in being considered for such a nomination, he or she should be visibly involved in service within the community and organization and make it known that he or she would be willing to serve. State and federal health-related coalitions may support nurses for particular positions, and political parties may offer support. For example, MassGAP is a bipartisan coalition of Massachusetts women's groups that works to increase the number of women appointed by the governor to senior-level cabinet

---

BOX 50-2 Non-Government Political Appointment Resources

- American Nurses Association (ANA) *(www.nursingworld .org)*. The ANA is the national professional nurses' association that represents nurses on many national nursing and multidisciplinary health care coalitions, as well as federal governmental committees and task forces. The ANA assists in the identification, recruitment, and support of nurses for elected and appointed representation or office at various levels of government.
- State Nurses Associations (locate your state association through the ANA website at *www.nursingworld.org/ FunctionalMenuCategories/AboutANA/WhoWeAre/ CMA.aspx*). State Nurses Associations, in response to solicitation of nominations of qualified candidates for consideration for appointment as a member of an advisory committee or other governmental position, submit a nomination package for nurses identified as qualified and willing to serve.
- National League for Nursing (NLN) *(www.nln.org)* and myriad nursing specialty organizations, in response to calls for nominations for appointment to advisory committees and other federal government positions, identifies qualified nurses who are able and willing to serve and then submits appropriate nomination packages.
- The National Women's Political Caucus (NWPC) *(www.nwpc.org)*. The NWPC is a grassroots membership organization that assists in the identification, recruiting, training, and support of women for elected and appointed office at all levels of government. The NWPC is also the chair of the Coalition for Women's

Appointment, a 60-member organization that assists women who seek Presidential and gubernatorial appointments.
- The National Council of Women's Organizations (NCWO) *(www.womensorganizations.org)*. The NCWO is an organizing council of more than 200 women's organizations representing more than 10 million members. Their goal is to advocate change on many issues of importance to women, including equal employment opportunity, economic equity, media equality, education, job training, women's health, and reproductive health, as well as the specific concerns of mid-life and older women, girls and young women, women of color, business and professional women, homemakers, and retired women.
- The Brookings Institution *(www.brookings.edu)*. The Brookings Institution provides information for those interested in pursuing a presidential nomination. They have done a number of studies about the appointment process and making government processes more effective.
- The Rutgers Center for American Women and Politics (CAWP) *(www.cawp.rutgers.edu)*. The CAWP is a unit of the Eagleton Institute of Politics at Rutgers University, the state university of New Jersey. It is nationally recognized as the leading source of scholarly research and current data about American women's political participation. It is an excellent source for learning about campaigns, elections, and appointments and provides a state-by-state guide to learning how to run for office.

---

positions, as agency heads, and to state-selected authorities and commissions (MassGAP, 2010).

Nurses interested in impacting population health can seek positions at the community level: on county health boards, task forces on redevelopment, or a local recreation committee to address policies that expand walking paths and bike trails. Community and county appointments could include the zoning commission, planning commission, hospital boards, boards of education, or councils on aging or economic development. State appointments could be as a public university trustee, a department head, or to a state board or commission. Federal opportunities exist in all federal agencies, both in Washington, DC and in regional offices around the nation (Box 50-3).

MAKING A DECISION TO SEEK AN APPOINTMENT

Seeking a political appointment is not a decision to be taken lightly. Consider the following questions to determine whether or not this path is right for you. Some questions will be more important if you are considering a full-time federal assignment rather than a part-time community role (Box 50-4).

PLAN YOUR STRATEGY

When you have identified the appointment you are interested in, the next step is being nominated. Determine the process used for nomination and identify who will make the appointment. Having

---

BOX 50-3 Finding Opportunities to Serve in an Appointed Status

Although health and health care services appointments may be attractive to nurses, there are many types of appointments, not directly related to health, where nursing expertise can benefit constituents. These include the following:

- Commerce and economic development: Tourism and industrial development appointments could benefit from nursing expertise. A nurse's knowledge of the health care system could provide industries considering relocation with valuable information about what they can expect for their employees' health care. In many states, health care is one of the top three industries.
- Conservation: Environmental issues affect the health care of every community. For example, a nurse could provide expertise regarding hazardous waste, the value of clean water systems, or preserving green space.
- Corrections: Nurses' expert health care knowledge could play a valuable role in policy decisions regarding the health care and education of incarcerated persons. Nurse practitioners provide much of the health care in many of today's correctional facilities (both public and private).
- Education: Nurses could offer valuable insight on policy decisions regarding school-based health care services and health curricula. A nurse's knowledge of budgeting

and cost-effective management could assist in the budget process.
- Health and human services: A wide variety of appointments exist at the local, state, and federal levels.
- Higher education: Policy decisions are made by state agencies and boards that have authority over colleges and universities.
- Licensure and regulatory boards: State boards of health determine policy regarding the health of the public, including drinking water, restaurant inspections, and health care provider licensure. State boards of nursing regulate the practice of nursing and offer the opportunity to nurses to serve on their governing boards. Some state boards of medicine make decisions regarding the practice of nurse practitioners and may have seats available for a nurse appointee.
- Public safety: Nurses can bring important perspectives to agencies and boards involved in public safety related to domestic violence, gun laws, and motor vehicle safety.
- Transportation: Nurses have seen firsthand the effect of motor vehicle accidents and can be valuable partners in improving safety through political appointments to transportation and highway safety organizations.

---

the support of more than one organization strengthens your chance. A number of factors should be considered when a plan is developed.

THE VETTING PROCESS

The scrutiny of an appointee's past is called the vetting process and serves as a quality check before appointment. Vetting involves the review of financial history, personal history and relationships, tax records, business transactions and ventures, family history, and other personal credentials. Vetting can also involve the process of preparing a candidate for the nomination hearing process. Vetting can result in the withdrawal of a nomination when unfavorable information is uncovered. In 2009, the vetting of former Senator Tom Daschle, nominated by President Barack Obama to serve as Secretary of Health and Human Services, resulted in his withdrawal following a revelation of unpaid taxes from consulting fees and unreported gifts of a car and driver services. Bernard Kerik, nominated by President George Bush, abruptly withdrew his name

from nomination for Secretary of Homeland Security when multiple issues were uncovered during his vetting. At the state level, scrutiny is less intense but will include a thorough review of a candidate's personal and public life. Now that so much information is available on social media sites, it becomes critical to use caution about personal posts.

POLITICAL PARTY AFFILIATION

Political party affiliation is an important factor in securing support for a political appointment. Most appointments are made as rewards for loyal support. The support could be as simple as volunteering in a local or state party office, organizing a fundraising event for your party, writing letters, or making contributions to a candidate or the party. It can also involve becoming recognized for expertise in the appointment domain. For example, Virginia Trotter Betts identified her political affiliation as key to her appointment as Senior Advisor on Nursing and Policy to the Secretary and Assistant Secretary of Health of the U.S. Department of

UNIT 3

BOX 50-4 Questions to Consider When Seeking a Political Appointment

If you are considering a political appointment, ask yourself these questions:

- Can you take time away from your job or your family to meet the demands of the position?
- How often will meetings be held? What will your time obligation be? Is this a full-time position or a group that meets occasionally?
- Will your employer support you? Will you have family support?
- Will your employer provide the time for you to serve, or will you be required to take vacation time?
- Why do you want to serve in this position? Can you articulate why you are qualified?
- What are the strengths and weaknesses you would bring to the position?
- What is your connection to your community? Do you know your neighbors? Have you served in volunteer organizations? Having a solid base of support from your neighbors, your friends, and your fellow volunteers in local organizations will enhance your chances of success.
- Where do you fit in the political spectrum? Are you registered to vote as a Democrat, Republican, or Independent? Party affiliation provides important linkages to support from individuals and groups.
- How will your education, background, and experience serve you in the desired appointment? Candidates should

be able to identify aspects of each that will qualify them for the position.

- How are your health and your family's financial situation? Careful analysis should be given to each.
- Who makes the appointment? Is it the governor, the lieutenant governor, or the Speaker of the House of Representatives?
- Are there educational or geographic requirements? In Mississippi, the Nurse Practice Act requires a baccalaureate degree as the basic qualification for one board of nursing position and an associate degree as the basic qualification for another. One position is designated for an advanced practice nurse and another is designated for a nurse educator. Some appointments require certain credentials (e.g., being a physician or a nurse).
- Which stakeholders care about who gets this position? Do you have influence with them? Are there other nominees under consideration?
- Is there a match between your qualifications and the requirements of the position? Carefully review local, state, or federal laws applicable to the appointment.
- Do you have a chance of getting the position? What connections do you have with individuals and organizations that will make the decision?

Health and Human Services (HHS) under President Bill Clinton. She credited a long-standing relationship with the Clinton-Gore administration after the American Nurses Association (ANA) became the first health care group to endorse the candidates in 1992. Betts had been a Robert Woods Johnson fellow in the office of then-Senator Al Gore. When he ran for Vice President, she worked on his campaign. After her federal appointment, Betts was appointed by Tennessee Governor Phil Bredesen as Commissioner of Mental Health and Developmental Disabilities because of her federal experience and her expertise in mental health.

GETTING SUPPORT

Federal appointee Shirley Chater, PhD, RN, FAAN, served as U.S. Commissioner of the Social Security Administration during the Clinton administration from 1993 to 1997. Dr. Chater's appointment was

unusual because she did not seek it. Rather, it evolved from her leadership, her health care knowledge, and her experiences with Ann Richards, former Governor of Texas, when she chaired a commission on health reform in Texas. Governor Richards had urged President Clinton to consider her for a senior position in government. Her appointment was supported and promoted by former colleagues in education (she had been President of Texas Woman's University as well as Vice Chancellor for Academic Affairs at the University of California, San Francisco), as well as in nursing, through the ANA. It is a story of unexpected opportunity that resulted in the most senior appointment of a nurse in the Clinton administration. She advises that it is most important to develop a strategy with supporters who provide different perspectives of the candidate's expertise and experience (S. Chater, personal communication, December 2010).

USING THE POWER OF NETWORKS

Few people have the clout or power to be appointed without broad support. Networks are important in serving as early-information systems (Jansson, 2011), providing opportunities and contacts who can lend insight into issues, problems, and trends relevant to developing strategies for policy reform. It must also be "[recognized] that an opponent in one circumstance may be an essential ally in another" (Milstead, 2011, p. 75). The executive responsible for making an appointment needs to be certain that the appointee is respected and approved by many constituents. For nurses, this means mobilizing groups or individuals outside of nursing, such as members of Congress if one is seeking a federal position. At the state level, it might mean other health professionals, such as physicians, social workers, or the hospital association, as well as consumer groups such as the AARP. The benefit and outcomes of networking can be likened to the success of the women's suffrage movement, as Trivedi (2003) envisioned it: "Opportunity creation is defined as strategic action taken by a social movement to reshape those norms and established power alignments by modifying institutional constraints to its own advantage" and therefore "forming alliances within the existing power structure and attempting to function within the institutional constraints instead of challenging them as political outsiders." Although the suffrage movement was a concerted coalition effort, individual opportunities can be fostered through similar networking strategies. In this electronic age and climate of social networking, it is politically savvy, and relatively easy, to connect with professionals in a variety of health and policy-related fields.

CONFIRMATION OR INTERVIEW?

Depending on the type of appointment you desire, you may need to participate in confirmation hearings or interviews. It is vital to be familiar with the position and the organizational hierarchy in which it falls, as well as current issues facing the organization. Such interviews can be intense and require careful preparation.

When preparing for either a hearing or interview, consider the following questions:
- What do I need to bring?
- Who will be conducting the hearing or interview?
- What questions will I be asked?
- Will I have the opportunity to ask questions?
- Should I have representation or sponsorship at the confirmation hearing?

Be honest about personal and family finances and anything in the past that could be damaging, such as public records, media reports, and postings on social media sites. Be prepared to respond to questions; it helps to practice for the interview with someone who is familiar with the issue, can be tough, and can give honest feedback.

COMPENSATION

Federal appointments follow published compensation schedules. State appointees may have compensation set by statute. Potential appointees should request information in advance of an appointment about compensation (both direct compensation and reimbursement for expenses incurred) before accepting an appointment. Pay alone generally does not motivate appointees; some high-level appointees may actually receive less compensation than they could receive in the private sector.

AFTER THE APPOINTMENT

RELATIONSHIPS WITH SUPPORTERS

Once you have passed the background checks, survived the interviews, and have been appointed to a position, there is nothing more important than thanking those who supported your appointment. Send letters of appreciation to recognize their efforts in helping you attain your appointment.

Once you are appointed, consider whom it is your duty to serve. If yours is a public appointment, your allegiance must be to your constituents. If it is to a health care organization's board of directors, your responsibility is to the patients and community. It is important that you retain your autonomy if the appointment is of a regulatory nature. If an association or other group was instrumental in your nomination and subsequent appointment, maintain open communication to keep them informed and to listen to their concerns. If your appointment is to represent a specific group on a task force or other group, close communication is necessary to convey their viewpoints.

EXPERIENCES OF NURSE APPOINTEES

DR. MARY WAKEFIELD

Dr. Mary Wakefield was appointed by President Obama as Administrator of the Health Resources and Service Administration (HRSA) in the HHS. She is former Chief of Staff to two North Dakota Senators and was an appointee to several major federal health care commissions, including the Medicare Payment Advisory Commission (MedPac), and chair of the National Advisory Council for the Agency for Healthcare Research and Quality. She was appointed to the HRSA by President Obama very early in his first term, one of the first positions filled in the HHS.

Dr. Wakefield had an extensive network of support from physicians and other health providers (she had been Associate Dean for Rural Health at the School of Medicine and Health Services at the University of North Dakota) and was elected as a fellow at the IOM where she worked on landmark reports on quality, health professional education, and rural health. She had a breadth of experience in nursing and public and rural health but also in higher education and quality issues.

She advises that expertise alone may not be enough to get a position; it requires becoming known to the decision makers. She always had the support from the nursing community in all her work in Congress, in higher education, and on advisory commissions and committees. She emphasizes the need to have other major non-nursing organizations and influential individuals advocate for you. The more broad-based support you have, the better your chances of being recognized. Wakefield says that to successfully obtain an appointment, you must have a two-pronged approach: You need to have the expertise required by the position and a network of relationships with policymakers and other influential stakeholders that has been nurtured over time. She laughingly states that there is only six degrees of separation among policy folks, so if one is trying to get an appointment, it is essential to use those networks to provide access. In Dr. Wakefield's case, former Senator Tom Daschle, who was chair of President Obama's health transition team and knew her well, made the recommendation for her appointment to the HRSA.

Her advice to those seeking appointments is to expand one's expertise and networks beyond nursing. Volunteer on policy committees in health or community organizations (e.g., American Health Association, American Heart Association), take classes or audit courses in political science and business, read policy articles, serve in political party positions, and get to know local political leaders. Most importantly, learn the connections between the provision of health services and policy, such as government regulations, proposed legislation, and institutional policy.

Wakefield highlights the importance of making it easy for people to help you. She recommends that nurses not just ask someone to write a letter of support but that the potential nominee write the letter and give it to the person providing the recommendation or that person's staff. If you desire, a phone call can be made on your behalf; provide the person making the call with a brief memo about your qualifications and why you would make a great candidate. In her position at the HRSA, Dr. Wakefield has made a significant improvement in funding for nursing higher education, expanding opportunities for the health care workforce, and provision of services to underserved populations (M. Wakefield, personal communication, November 2013).

MARILYN TAVENNER

Marilyn Tavenner served as Virginia Secretary of Health and Human Services from 2006 to 2009. In 2010, President Obama appointed her as Principal Deputy Administrator for the Centers for Medicare and Medicaid Services (CMS), an agency within the HHS. She served as Acting Director for 2 years, and in 2013 she was appointed as Administrator.

UNIT 3

Tavenner oversees the $800 billion federal agency, which ensures health care coverage for 100 million Americans, with 10 regional offices and more than 4000 employees nationwide. The CMS administers Medicare, Medicaid, and the Children's Health Insurance Program (CHIP). Most importantly, she is responsible for the implementation of the Affordable Care Act.

She started her career as a staff nurse, moved to chief nursing officer, and eventually moved to chief executive officer (CEO) of two hospitals in the Hospital Corporation of American (HCA) system in Virginia. She then moved to a more senior position in the HCA, as Group President of Outpatient Services in their corporate office in Tennessee. During that time, she served as chair of the Virginia Hospital Association and was a member of the Board of Trustees of the American Hospital Association.

Tavenner became acquainted with Tim Kaine before his election as Virginia's governor. As a hospital CEO, she worked on projects with Mr. Kaine as well as serving as head of his campaign's policy working group. After his election, she called to congratulate him, and he asked her to interview for a position in his administration. It was the broad support of groups she had worked with that moved her nomination forward. These included the Virginia Nurses Association, the Virginia Hospital Association, the Virginia Medical Association, the American Organization of Nurse Executives, insurance firms, long-term care organizations, and other nursing groups close to the governor. That multidisciplinary network was glad to rally support when she asked for help.

In the state position, she created one of the first state health reform commissions during a time of extreme budget challenges. Tavenner was able to introduce nursing representation in many agencies by creating nursing positions in them, including the nurse directorship of the Department of Health Professions. She established a health workforce center that instituted nursing scholarships for graduate education and resulted in a major increase in nursing faculty in the state. It also resulted in a 50% increase in nursing school enrollment. In addition, she expanded medical school enrollment to meet the projected shortfall of physicians.

Her nomination for Administrator of the CMS was facilitated by support from Congressman Eric Cantor, the leader of the House of Representatives. She was supported by both parties, particularly because of her extensive business, as well as health, expertise.

Ms. Tavenner's advice for others seeking an appointment is threefold:
- Get involved in your community and develop a broad network of support.
- Get involved in political campaigns and party organizations, and in developing policy platforms.
- Give financial contributions to candidates whom you support. (M. Tavenner, personal communication, December 5, 2009 and November 2013).

RITA WRAY

Rita Wray, Deputy Executive Director of the Mississippi Department of Finance and Administration, got her start through a neighbor's invitation to a County Republican Women's Club meeting. She was drawn to the party because she agreed with the values that the party espoused: personal responsibility, free markets, low taxes, and fiscal conservatism. Wray was a nurse executive with a consulting business focused on regulatory compliance, risk management, corporate communication, and professional practice issues. She was active in leadership positions with the ANA, the Susan G. Komen Breast Cancer Foundation, and the National Coalition of 100 Black Women, Inc. She serves as co-chair of the Mississippi coalition for implementing recommendations for The Future of Nursing report (IOM, 2011). But her political connections, made through running for a seat in the Mississippi legislature (unsuccessfully) and working for the successful election of Governor Haley Barbour, made her a candidate for an appointment on his election. In 2008, she became the sixteenth President of the Mississippi Federation of Republican Women (MFRW) and the first African American. She has remained in her state position at the Department of Finance and Administration under Governor Phil Bryant.

Wray credits her selection for the political appointment as the result of her business acumen, her work with the party, her leadership ability, and her interpersonal and communication skills, in addition to her race and gender. She advises others to use the steps of the nursing process: Assess strengths and abilities, develop a plan to demonstrate how those match the ones needed for the appointment, implement the plan, and evaluate outcomes. Above all, she recommends, use the power of connections (R. Wray, personal communication, March 2010).

DEBRA A. TONEY

Dr. Toney, Director of Nursing for Nevada Health Centers, has had several appointed positions in Nevada. One of the most significant was Chair of the Nevada State Office of Minority Health Advisory Committee. Because of her work around health issues of underserved communities, including women, African Americans, and Native Americans, she worked with a cross-section of health advocates, and when the former governor, Jim Gibbons, was looking for a chair of the new Office of Minority Health, her name was offered and she received the appointment. She credits her appointment to her ability to work with diverse communities and her knowledge of health policy issues across the state. To enable others to recognize your ability to be knowledgeable, her advice is: Become involved in community issues, volunteer for boards and commissions, meet a cross-section of individuals, and develop speaking and communication skills. Dr. Toney said it takes courage to jump in and realize one does not have to know all the answers, but one does need to know where to find answers and experts (D. A. Toney, personal communication, October 2013).

CONCLUSION

Getting appointed to policy positions provides the opportunity for nurses to be at the table where decisions about health are made. Whether in the public arena, in a paid appointed position, or a volunteer appointed post, the guidelines are the same: take a risk, make yourself known as knowledgeable about health issues, volunteer for leadership positions, use your networks, and use the communication, business, research, and policy skills that make one successful as a nursing leader.

DISCUSSION QUESTIONS

1. Why would a nurse want to seek an appointed position in government?
2. How would you prepare for consideration to an appointed position?
3. Give examples of how nurses can affect public policy in various appointed positions.

REFERENCES

Armstrong, F. (2005). With knowledge comes innovation, and with innovation: POWER. (Cover story.). *Australian Nursing Journal, 13*(1), 14–17.

Clarke, P. N., Swider, S., & Bigley, M. (2013). Nursing leadership and health policy: A dialogue with nurse leaders. *Nursing Science Quarterly, 26*(2), 136–142. doi:10.1177/0894318413477146.

Feetham, S. L. (2011). The role of science policy in programs of research and scholarship. In A. S. Hinshaw & P. A. Grady (Eds.), *Shaping health policy through nursing research.* New York: Springer.

Institute of Medicine. (2011). *The future of nursing: Leading change, advancing health.* Washington, DC: National Academies Press.

Jansson, B. S. (2011). *Improving healthcare through advocacy: A guide for the health and helping professions.* Hoboken, NJ: John Wiley & Sons, Inc.

Lewis, D. (2008). *The politics of presidential appointments: Political control and bureaucratic performance.* Princeton, NJ: Princeton University Press.

Lyttle, B. (2011). Politics: A natural next step for nurses. *American Journal of Nursing, 111*(5), 19–20.

MassGAP (2010). MassGAP: Moving women ahead in Massachusetts. Retrieved from *www.massgap.org.*

Milstead, J. A. (2011). *Health policy and politics: A nurse's guide.* Boston, MA: Jones and Bartlett.

Mund, A. R. (2012). Policy, practice, and education. *AANA Journal, 80*(6), 423–426.

Nathan, R. P. (2009). *Handbook for appointed officials in America's governments.* New York: Rockefeller Institute Press.

Trivedi, R. (2003). *Marketing ideology: The role of framing and opportunity in the American Woman Suffrage Movement, 1850 to 1919.* Paper presented to American Political Science Association, annual conference 2003 (pp. 1–56). Philadelphia, PA. Retrieved from *citation.allacademic .com//meta/p_mla_apa_research_citation/0/6/3/0/7/pages63071/ p63071-2.php.*

Vedantam, S. (2008, November). Who are the better managers—Political appointees or career bureaucrats? *The Washington Post.* Retrieved from *www.washingtonpost.com/wp-dyn/content/article/2008/11/23/ AR2008112302485.html? sub=AR.*

ONLINE RESOURCES

American Nurses Association
www.nursingworld.org
American Nurses Association Activist Toolkit
www.rnaction.org
Health Resources and Services Administration
www.hrsa.gov
National League for Nursing
www.nln.org

CHAPTER 51

TAKING ACTION:
Influencing Policy Through an Appointment to the San Francisco Health Commission

Catherine M. Waters

"The only politics I am willing to devote myself to ... is simply a matter of serving those around us: serving the community and serving those who will come after us. Its deepest roots are moral because it is a responsibility expressed through action, to and for the whole."

Vaclav Havel

In this chapter, I reflect on my journey, experiences, and postanalysis of 5 years of public service as a Health Commissioner on the San Francisco Health Commission. The amount of data and reports that require reading, absorbing, and understanding in a relatively short time, usually 3 days and often instantaneously, to make policy and budget decisions about the lives of people who are vulnerable and in critical need of health, social, and housing services was daunting and challenged my ethical and moral compasses, values, and philosophical beliefs. I was able to maintain and uphold uncompromisingly my integrity and the art, science, and caring practice of nursing with honor and dignity.

DEMOCRACY AND SERVICE TO THE HEALTH COMMISSION

I served as a member, and during my final year, as Vice President of the Health Commission. My colleagues' vote of confidence was a testament to their respect for my style as an evidence-based thought leader, who was fair and democratic, who facilitated discussion with diplomacy, and who listened first,

then spoke. This style of leadership baffled a few critics who queried about my commitment and dedication. A government appointment is not carte blanche for disseminating a personal agenda without consideration of other perspectives. As the governing and policymaking body of the Department of Public Health, the City and County Charter mandates the San Francisco Health Commission to manage its hospitals, monitor and regulate emergency medical services, and oversee matters pertaining to the health preservation, promotion, and protection of its citizens (Health Commission, 2008).

I took a stand with courage and fortitude for the health and well-being of San Francisco residents. When I spoke about health issues on behalf of the people, I spoke in the spirit of inquiry with conviction, precision, and data. I applied the principles of diplomacy and democracy even when the newly elected Mayor was considering reappointing me for an additional 4-year term. The Mayor's Chief of Staff for Commission Boards was concerned that the Health Commission did not represent all of San Francisco's citizenry. My reappointment would have been a redundant representation of San Francisco's constituency. I reminded the Chief of Staff that we live in a democracy where a person does not hold a position for eternity. When a term expires, an appointed or elected official peacefully vacates the position in a democratic society (Magstadt, 2013).

As one of the Charter Commissions, the Health Commission is structured such that there is a majority of nonhealth-related Commissioners, an indication that the Health Commission is accountable to the public; its intent is not to serve as a health care expert committee. Moreover, the Health Commission was created with fixed terms so that it would transcend any mayoral administration (Health Commission, 2008). When Gavin Newsom, the former Mayor of San Francisco, appointed me as a Commissioner to the San Francisco Health Commission in 2008, I replaced a nurse, Dr. Catherine Dodd, who had 1 year left in her term when she was appointed as the Mayor's Deputy Chief of Staff for Health. Commissioner Dodd recommended me to the Mayor's Office to complete her term. I, too, recommended a nurse as my replacement because I believe wholeheartedly that a nurse provides a unique perspective to the mission of the Health Commission and to the importance of protecting the health and human rights of all citizens, in particular vulnerable individuals, populations, and communities. Supporting my belief, the newly elected Mayor appointed a nurse to the Health Commission when my term expired in 2013.

CHECKS AND BALANCES OF HEALTH COMMISSION ACTIVITIES

The balance of power in San Francisco's local government is similar to the balance of power in the U.S. federal government. The Health Commission falls under the executive branch because the Mayor

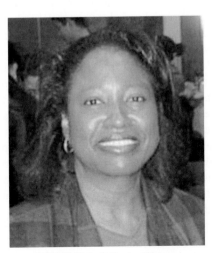

FIGURE 51-1 Catherine Waters.

appoints its members. The powers and duties of the Health Commission are in accordance with the City and County Charter (Health Commission, 2008). The Board of Supervisors composes the legislative branch and approves the Mayor's Health Commission appointments. Serving as the judicial branch, the City Attorney Office provides legal services to the Mayor, the Board of Supervisors, and the Health Commission. This balance of power is in perpetual action. When the Health Commission recommends funding, elimination, or reduction of programs, the Board of Supervisors determines expenditures for those programs and sometimes (because of scrutiny by the public) restores the Health Commission's cuts to or elimination of programs. At other times, the Board of Supervisors approves the Health Commission's cuts regardless of the public's scrutiny.

SCOPE OF WORK OF THE HEALTH COMMISSION

The Health Commission considers issues including budget approval of the San Francisco Department of Public Health, estimates of revenues and expenditures, budget modifications, fund transfers and reappropriations, accepting and expending grants, receiving gifts, entering contractual agreements, and reviewing hospital proposed rates, fees, and other charges. The Health Commission considers policy matters relating to the public's health needs, including program additions, deletions, and modifications, and closing and building of hospitals in San Francisco. All policy declarations are in the form of a resolution, and, if approved, the Health Commission forwards the resolution to the Mayor for submission to the Board of Supervisors.

INFRASTRUCTURE OF THE HEALTH COMMISSION

The Health Commission, facilitated by the president and vice president, is composed of seven members from diverse backgrounds, who serve a 4-year term. The Health Commission conducts all of its business in a public forum; however, it may meet in closed sessions. Members of the public are encouraged to attend meetings and address the

Health Commission. The Health Commission hears public comments before voting on action items. Four Joint Conference Committees compose the Health Commission. One committee reviews financial reports and approves contracting services for the Department of Public Health. Another committee provides oversight for the Department of Public Health programs and its citywide contractors that deliver services on its behalf. The remaining two committees provide oversight of health care delivery for the City and County of San Francisco's two hospitals: Laguna Honda Hospital and Rehabilitation Center, and San Francisco General Hospital and Trauma Center. In addition to the Joint Conference Committees, the president and vice president of the Health Commission appoint commissioners to serve as liaisons to three governing bodies needing Health Commission representation.

BALANCING HEALTH COMMISSION SERVICE WITH ACADEMIA

Balancing my primary responsibility as a tenured full professor in a School of Nursing at a research-intensive university with being a member and Vice President of the Health Commission was challenging; however, it was a rich and rewarding experience. Of my many responsibilities as a Health Commissioner, serving as a Board Member of the San Francisco Health Plan enriched my perspective as a clinician and scientist. The San Francisco Health Plan provides quality affordable health care coverage to low- and moderate-income San Franciscans. My leadership skills and understanding of the health care insurance industry, affordable quality care, and health outcomes as a result of safe health and nursing care were enhanced by this experience.

Reflecting on this exciting journey as a Health Commissioner, I wish I had more time to delve deeply into issues before making instantaneous budgetary and policy-related decisions, as the Health Commission often had to do. I wish I had asked for more time-off compensation from teaching, service, research, and clinical residency responsibilities from the School of Nursing as my Health Commission experiences informed my

teaching, service, practice, and research. My community-based participatory research in collaboration with public and private sector partnerships and public health nursing expertise informed my policy work and decision making on the Health Commission. On occasion, study findings of colleagues' research would receive attention by the Health Commission. I wish I had encouraged more nurse scientists to highlight the influence of their work on public health policy to the Health Commission. Because of my experience as a Health Commissioner, I realize the importance of bridging academic and public service endeavors.

INTROSPECTION: RE-EXPERIENCING DECISION MAKING ON THE HEALTH COMMISSION

I developed grace and humility that comes with collaborating with a diverse mix of individuals from different backgrounds with whom I had little or nothing in common. The Health Commission hears arguments from disparate sides. I listened with diligence and in earnest from a nursing perspective. I tried to give voice to stakeholders who often could not speak for themselves. Making decisions and having debates about the multifaceted issues that came before the Health Commission required the application of diplomacy, democracy, politics, and the art and science of nursing. Diplomacy and democracy are about differences, which are bound to diverge when different viewpoints and demands are expressed freely by interest groups and individuals competing for limited funds and resources. My nursing expertise in public health nursing guided my decision making in the context of mutual respect, fairness, and justice (American Nurses Association, 2013).

During the economic downturn, some people would question my use of morality and dismiss it as naïve, but morality has a place in policymaking and decision making, especially when it involves the safety of the public's health. Ideology may not be a prudent course of action during economic strife, but making sure that every person has a fair chance for a healthy life and an equal opportunity for quality health care is not about ideology. The inalienable right to life, liberty, and the pursuit of happiness is not possible without good health. It is a Fata Morgana, a mirage, to believe budget cuts will not have a negative impact on the health of vulnerable people. In a decent, democratic society, there are certain obligations that are not subject to trade-offs or negotiations. Health care should be one of those obligations. The public values and trusts nurses (Newport, 2012), a trust that is an honor that brings with it responsibility and commitment to serve the public with mindful vigilance and discriminate decision making.

I spent a majority of my tenure on the Health Commission participating in decision making about the transitioning of Healthy San Francisco and planning for the implementation of the Affordable Care Act (ACA). Healthy San Francisco is a health access, not health insurance, program that uses the medical home concept to subsidize universal health care for certain uninsured residents. Even though health reform is law now, Healthy San Francisco will continue to fill the gap for certain uninsured and undocumented residents. The Health Commission decisions included voting on which programs are redundant with health reform and need to be eliminated and which programs are unique and will meet health reform requirements. Understanding the impact of health reform on Healthy San Francisco is essential because certain health care services costs now incurred by the General Fund will be funded under the ACA.

Looming and ever-present was the vote on which mid- and end-of-year program budget cuts had to be made in order to deal with San Francisco and the Department of Public Health's fiscal reality. As a nurse, how do I, in good conscience, vote for the reduction and elimination of programs that I know may prove to be detrimental to the public's health, particularly to vulnerable populations? The vote often was a choice either to eliminate or reduce patient services or fund-mandated cost-of-living allowances for health care personnel. These patient services included ophthalmologic services for persons with diabetes, weekday and weekend urgent

care, and integrated behavioral and medical services for persons with human immunodeficiency virus (HIV) infection, and were implemented to prevent complications, such as blindness, emergency department overuse, and HIV stigmatization. Why would the Health Commission dismantle services that were designed to save lives, improve quality of life, and decrease health care costs?

Many health needs exist in San Francisco, but there are limited funds and resources available to address them. The Health Commission cannot do everything that would eliminate health disparities. Budget cuts to programs that serve as the safety net for vulnerable populations are difficult to prioritize, and there is no magical formula to determine budget cuts. The Health Commission cannot spend money that it does not have. The Health Commission's budget principles dictate that it will develop a budget to maximize revenues, minimize the impact on vulnerable populations, and preserve its core functions. Using these budget principles, I voted initially in favor of a wait-and-see approach before approving cuts in services that might harm the most vulnerable populations. After waiting for a thorough assessment of the fiscal impact and because of the fiscal reality, I voted to both reduce and eliminate, as well as preserve, programs that serve as the safety net for vulnerable populations.

Despite it being difficult to prioritize resources among people who are all at risk, I have learned to articulate my viewpoint, defend my position, face controversy, build a consensus, compromise with trade-offs, and debate issues with diplomacy, skills that are essential when making difficult and controversial decisions.

REFERENCES

American Nurses Association. (2013). *Public health nursing: Scope and standards of practice* (2nd ed.). Washington, DC: American Nurses Association.

Health Commission. (2008). *Rules and regulations.* San Francisco, CA: Health Commission.

Magstadt, T. M. (2013). *Understanding politics: Ideas, institutions, and issues* (10th ed.). Belmont, CA: Wadsworth Cengage Learning.

Newport, F. (2012). Congress retains low honest rating. Nurses have highest honesty rating; car salespeople, lowest. Retrieved from *www.gallup .com/poll/159035/congress-retains-low-honesty-rating.aspx.*

CHAPTER 52

TAKING ACTION:
A Nurse in the Boardroom

Marilyn Waugh Bouldin

"What I want in my life is compassion, a flow between myself and others based on a mutual giving from the heart."

Marshall B. Rosenberg

One evening in February 2012, I sat in the audience at a hospital board meeting in rural Colorado wondering how I could convince five board members to support the local clinic for uninsured patients. As president of the independent nonprofit clinic board of directors and a past public health director and nurse, I was concerned about meeting this population's needs. When the discussion began about the election of new hospital board members, a light bulb came on. I thought, "I could do that!"

This is the story of my campaign to become a member of the Board of Directors of the hospital in my community, the factors leading to my decision to run for the board, the campaign I launched, its success and challenges, and my experience serving as a board member.

I have always believed nurses should be full partners with other health care professionals in designing health care systems, as the Institute of Medicine's (IOM) report on *The Future of Nursing* recommended (IOM, 2011). Here was my opportunity! I knew it would be a challenge, and I would be stretching my comfort zone. Historically, nurses have not been welcomed into the boardroom (Hassmiller & Combes, 2012); nor have many sought out board membership. However, with nurses' broad holistic perspective of patient care, knowledge of quality and safety issues, and understanding of concepts such as team leadership, accountability, professionalism and relationship building, nurses are, in fact, perfect for the job.

At a very young age, as I helped my mother care for younger siblings, I decided to become a nurse. Raising a family, returning to school, and becoming aware of the feminist movement, I enjoyed learning new things, meeting new people, and accepting challenges. Sometimes I failed. The infant-toddler childcare center I started went bankrupt, and once I was fired for insubordination. But I learned that failure wasn't the end of the world, and I always maintained my passion for taking care of people and my community.

I have been a risk taker ever since I left my promising career at a major urban hospital and moved by myself to a small town in Colorado. When I began developing a new Associate Degree nursing program at our local community college, I was not afraid to ask for help. Fellow nursing directors across the state were a tremendous source of information and support as I tackled this major project. I learned that positive relationships and collaborations were critical to any accomplishment.

MY POLITICAL CAREER

Friends have been key assets on my journey. I met a friend in my rural community (where everyone knows everyone!) who was extremely politically active. One day, she told me about an opening on the state board of health and encouraged me to apply, as they needed representation from my geographic area. I still remember a comment made during my interview with the State Senate Confirmation Committee almost 40 years ago: I was "good looking enough to be appointed." I felt humiliated

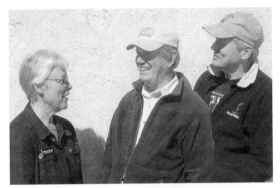

FIGURE 52-1 Hospital Board candidate Marilyn Bouldin talking to two constituents during her campaign.

but was too intimidated to reply. My term in office was a time of tremendous learning and growth, as I was young and very inexperienced. My fellow board members treated me with respect, and I enjoyed discussing state health issues.

Throughout my public health career I learned the importance of developing positive and diverse relationships through my involvement with many community projects. I participated in assessing my community's health needs and developing new programs to meet those needs. I served on several not-for-profit boards and learned how to be an effective board member. Professionalism and respectful communication were key characteristics being an effective board member. My job required I make periodic presentations to the county commissioners about our work, so I learned how to speak clearly, concisely, and in a politically correct manner, speaking within my time allotment and answering questions truthfully but sensitively.

MY CAMPAIGN

When I became aware of the upcoming election for hospital board members, I decided this would be an interesting and valuable board to serve on. I had something to offer, and I could influence the board's direction; also I was retired and had the time to serve. Because of our hospital's quasi-governmental designation as a "special hospital district," the board members must be elected by the voters who reside within the hospital district. (Special districts are

described in Box 52-1.) However, I had no experience in running a campaign or giving political speeches. I thought I did not have much to lose by trying. Over the years I had developed a tough skin and had learned I could never please all the people all the time. Many professionals in the community assured me that I was very competent to do the job and supported me.

My friends volunteered to help. A nurse friend who was a retired Lt. Colonel decided to be my informal campaign manager. Another friend who was a graphic designer developed the campaign materials. Others offered to support me financially and introduce me to their friends.

The relationships I developed were extensive and varied, even though I had only lived in this community for 5 years. My membership in Rotary International, a service club with weekly meetings, provided me with many networking opportunities. I also belonged to a quilt guild, a church group, and a hiking group for women, all of which provided me with access to people who could be mobilized to support my candidacy and vote in the election.

CAMPAIGN PREPARATION

My campaign was 2 months long. There were nine candidates, two women and seven men, running for two seats. I decided to commit time, energy, and money to run an active, high-profile campaign.

My first job was to learn about the hospital so I could speak knowledgeably. I studied its website, read the bylaws, learned about the services offered, reviewed the latest strategic plan and interviewed existing board members. I also met with people in the C-Suite, a term I learned referred to all the executive chiefs: the Chief Executive Officer (CEO), Chief Operating Officer (COO), Chief Nursing Officer (CNO), and Chief Financial Officer (CFO). Understanding the management of a multimillion-dollar budget was one of my biggest challenges. I had to be willing to ask a lot of questions.

I became familiar with the characteristics of my hospital district (three rural counties with a population of 20,000) to learn about the demographics, the health issues, and other characteristics. I talked

UNIT 3

BOX 52-1 Special Hospital Districts of Colorado

Special Districts in Colorado are local governments (political subdivisions of the state). Local governments include counties, municipalities (cities and towns), school districts, and other types of government entities such as authorities and special districts.

Colorado law limits the types of services that county governments can provide to residents. Districts are created to fill the gaps that may exist in the services that counties provide and the services that the residents may want. Examples include ambulance, fire, water, sanitation, park and recreation, libraries, and health services.

Upon incorporation as a special district, bylaws are written which describe the election process for the board of directors in accordance with state statutes.

to health professionals to learn about their concerns, and to people in the district about their experiences and perceptions of the hospital.

Next, I learned about the Secretary of State's office and campaign laws and regulations. I sought advice from friends who had run campaigns and stayed in close communication with the designated election official at the hospital. She kept me informed about campaign law, election timelines, and report deadlines.

Then I determined my campaign platform. I felt strongly that the hospital (the second largest employer in the region) was essential to having a healthy and economically viable community. I believed the hospital should also be a community health partner and should extend services beyond their walls. The Affordable Care Act (ACA) had recently passed and I decided to use my campaign to increase awareness of this significant legislation. I am a firm believer in an integrated approach to health care using the triple aim model, and wanted to explain this concept to the community. This model promotes a three-pronged approach to developing an effective health care delivery system for the future: improving the experience of care by providing effective, safe, and reliable care; improving the health of the population by focusing on prevention, wellness, and managing chronic

conditions; and decreasing per capita health care costs (Bisognano, 2012). I thought there should be more diversity on the board as most of the directors had a financial or business background and all had limited health care experience.

Developing campaign materials was critical. Wherever I went, I wore a nametag that read "Marilyn Bouldin, RN, Hospital Board Candidate." I had business cards printed and used my personal phone number and e-mail address, as I believed accessibility was important. I developed fliers and newspaper ads, and a friend created a website about me, at the urging of my marketer sister.

LAUNCHING THE CAMPAIGN

I believe that most people are interested in their local hospital. If they haven't used it themselves, they know someone who has. Many people had stories to tell me about their experiences and I made a point to listen. If someone had a complaint I helped them contact the appropriate person. I empathized with them and sometimes gave health advice. I invited them to contact me anytime if they had concerns about the hospital and told them I hoped to represent them on the board.

I contacted community leaders to identify opportunities to speak to groups. One night I drove 30 miles out into the countryside to attend a community potluck dinner. Another time I drove to the other end of the district to speak at a women's luncheon. I was a guest speaker at a local political party meeting and a radio talk show, to discuss the ACA and the hospital board election process. I went to my favorite coffee shop and hung out all morning to engage people in informal conversations. I went to Business After Hours where local businesses network over appetizers, and attended Chamber of Commerce events. I talked with my friends as we hiked in the Rocky Mountains, and they in turn talked to their friends.

One effective strategy was having a letter-to-the-editor writing party. A friend hosted this in her home, complete with wine and cheese. We helped people compose letters of support and submit them to the newspapers. (See Box 52-2 for one of the letters that was submitted.) We had fun doing it! I

BOX 52-2 Letter to the Editor

April 26, 2012

Dear Editor,

I want to recommend Marilyn Bouldin to your community. It is logical and fortunate that she has offered herself to serve as an elected member of your HRRMC Hospital Board. As my clinical colleague, former boss, and years-long friend, I am familiar with her broad knowledge of health care, her respect for those who work in this field and of her advocacy for consumers who present for its services.

Marilyn is known for her fairness and ability to listen and intelligently weigh out multiple sides of the issues she tackles. Her enthusiasm and commitment to follow-up is legendary. Should I ever require such health-care decisions in my own behalf, Marilyn heads my list of go-to consultants. Though not a member of your community, I would confidently cast my vote for her in your upcoming election for HRRMC Hospital Board membership. It is my opinion that your community could do no better.

Sincerely,

Marilyn Russell, RN, MSN

had an extensive e-mail list and composed a message about who I was, what I believed and why I wanted to be on the hospital board. I then sent this out to everyone I knew asking for their vote.

One of my most nerve-racking experiences was participating in the League of Women Voters candidate forum. Each candidate was given 3 minutes to talk, followed by questions from the audience. The forum was videotaped to play in the library, and the a newspaper reporter was there to cover the story (the editor did not endorse me because he thought other candidates had a better financial background). I was worried I would make mistakes or not know all the answers, and had a sleepless night before the event, which, of course went fine!

I decided that, regardless of the outcome on election night, I wanted to celebrate with all the people who had helped me. We had a pizza party at a local restaurant and it was a truly wonderful time, especially when I got the news that, not only had I won a seat, but I had also received the most votes!

The following week I wrote by hand many personal thank-you notes to people who had helped

me. I also sent flowers to my informal campaign manager and graphic designer. I put one last ad in the paper expressing my appreciation to the people who had voted for me and invited them to contact me with any comments or concerns.

LESSONS LEARNED

Although I have had many professional successes and received many awards over the years, what mattered most in my election were my relationships with people. My ability to listen, to be genuinely interested and compassionate, and to follow through with people's questions and concerns served me well. Once people found out I was a nurse they trusted and confided in me.

I was pleased overall with my campaign strategies. I decided early on not to accept monetary donations for my expenses. I was intimidated by the additional requirements and documentation required by the Secretary of State's office for campaign donations. I was also bothered by the thought that I might be beholden to the people who contributed. Next time I will accept contributions! I did not develop a budget at the start and did not realize how much it would cost me to run a campaign, which turned out to be over $600.

I did have one negative experience. After going around town on a windy day to place fliers on windshields, a stranger came to my house to tell me he did not appreciate me polluting the streets with my papers. In hindsight, I think he had a good point!

During my first year on the board I spent a lot of time listening, reading, learning about the culture of the board, and building trust with my fellow board members. Even though I had served on many boards in the past and had spent decades working in health care, I was surprised at the steep learning curve necessary for me to understand how a hospital functions. Being the new kid on the block gave me permission to ask lots of questions. I had several one-on-one sessions with the board chair to learn more. I met with key nurses in the organization to hear their concerns and learn how I could be supportive. I read my board packet thoroughly in preparation for meetings. I was appointed to the performance improvement committee as the board representative and actively participated. Refreshing my knowledge of good communication skills was also helpful to me, and I attempted to use nonviolent communication (NVC) as much as possible. The objective of NVC is to establish relationships based on honesty and empathy that will fulfill everyone's needs (Rosenberg, 2003). I attended a national hospital conference, which I found enlightening and informative. I have also tried to take the initiative when appropriate. For example, I worked on developing a new board member orientation manual, compiling all the information that would have been helpful to me during my first month in office (such as an explanation of the bylaws of the foundation board to which I was automatically appointed when I was elected to the hospital board).

I learned quickly that serving on the board requires much more time than just attending monthly meetings! Although being a board member is a volunteer position, as an elected official I felt obligated to do the best job I could and to represent the hospital's interests and those of our constituents, the taxpayers in the district who legally own the hospital. Consequently, I committed a significant amount of time to reviewing policies, attending hospital-sponsored events and employee-recognition ceremonies, meeting physician candidates, supporting the volunteer auxiliary, serving on the hospital foundation board, and responding to feedback from community members. I also spent time reading publications related to hospital administration.

I have learned to pick my battles and to ask myself "How important is it?" There are times when I choose to remain silent. There are times when significant informal communication happens outside of board meetings, and I make sure to participate in hallway talks. I learned that maintaining positive relationships is of the utmost importance. Nothing happens through divisiveness. I try hard to keep an open mind and to be willing to compromise.

Even after 2 years, I continue to ask a lot of questions, which I find is very helpful to everyone during a meeting. The responsibilities I have in my position continue to be daunting to me and I take them very seriously, especially in the areas of credentialing physicians, overseeing a very large budget, and evaluating the CEO.

I have become skilled at answering the question I get from community members, "How's it going on the board?" Some people are just making polite conversation and don't need an in depth answer. I try to be honest yet tactful and am careful not to undermine anyone or gossip. I constantly need to determine what I can share and what I cannot, and am always aware of the language I use. Once the board has made a decision, we must all present a united opinion, whether we agreed personally with the decision or not. This is sometimes challenging.

THE FUTURE

The way we deliver health care and medical services is changing rapidly and represents a paradigm shift. Leaders need to have vision, health care knowledge, critical thinking skills, and collaborative expertise, all of which nurses possess. I look forward to a time when nurses are seen as essential participants in every boardroom in every hospital, and they see themselves that same way.

REFERENCES

Bisognano, M., & Kenney, C. (2012). *Pursuing the triple aim: seven innovators show the way to better care, better health, and lower costs* (1st ed.). San Francisco: John Wiley and Sons Inc.

Hassmiller, S., & Combes, J. (2012). Nurse leaders in the board room: A fitting choice. *Journal of Healthcare Management, 57*(1), 8–11.

Institute of Medicine [IOM]. (2011). The future of nursing: leading change, advancing health. Washington, DC: National Academies Press. Retrieved from *www.iom.edu/nursing*.

Rosenberg, M. B. (2003). *Nonviolent communication—A language of life* (2nd ed.). Encinitas, CA: PuddleDancer Press.

CHAPTER 53

Nursing and the Courts

David M. Keepnews   Virginia Trotter Betts

"Power concedes nothing without a demand. It never did and it never will."

Frederick Douglass

The courts are an important source of health policy. Their decisions hold significant implications for nurses and for the patients, families, communities, and populations they serve. Nurses and other health professionals who seek to understand policy need at least a basic knowledge not just of the impact of court decisions, but also of how advocates can respond to and even influence the outcomes of those decisions. This chapter provides an overview of the legal and judicial systems and the role of the courts in shaping policy. It is not a comprehensive overview; rather, it aims to provide the reader with a general understanding of this policy arena and its critical importance for nursing.

THE JUDICIAL SYSTEM

The United States has two parallel court systems: federal and state. The federal courts have jurisdiction over matters that involve federal law (generally speaking, those that pertain to the U.S. Constitution, federal statutes, and/or the actions of federal agencies). Federal courts can also hear complaints that arise between parties in different states if a sufficient monetary amount is in dispute. The trial courts for the federal system (the entry point for most federal cases) are called district courts; there are 94 federal district courts located throughout the United States and its territories. Federal courts of appeal, also referred to as Circuit Courts, are organized into 12 geographic circuits plus the Federal Circuit Court (Administrative Office of the U.S.

Courts, n.d.). The U.S. Supreme Court is the federal court of last resort; there is no higher court to which its decisions can be appealed.

Each state has its own court system. State courts generally rule on issues arising under the state's constitution and laws. State courts may also hear some claims that arise under federal law or the U.S. Constitution. The state court systems include trial-level and appellate courts, with a high court as the court of last resort. The high court is known as the Supreme Court in most states, but not all; in New York State, for example, its highest court is known as the Court of Appeal.

JUDICIAL REVIEW

In *Marbury v. Madison* (1803), the U.S. Supreme Court first asserted its power to declare a law unenforceable if it is found to violate the Constitution. This power of judicial review has given the courts a significant role in public policy since they have the power to affirm or strike down laws or other government action.

A significant recent illustration of this power was the U.S. Supreme Court's decision in *National Federation of Independent Business v. Sebelius* (2012). In this case, the Court heard challenges to provisions of the Affordable Care Act and upheld the law's minimum coverage provision (often referred to as the individual mandate), that is, the requirement that most people who are not covered through their employer or through a government program such as Medicare or Medicaid must purchase health insurance. Opponents argued that Congress does not have the authority to compel people to purchase something. This case was closely watched by opponents and supporters of the ACA since the outcome would determine whether a key component of the ACA could go into effect.

Most legal experts expected the outcome of the case to hinge on the Court's determination of the reach of the Commerce Clause, a provision in the U.S. Constitution that says Congress has the power to regulate interstate commerce. Instead, although finding that the Commerce Clause does not permit Congress to require people to purchase insurance, the Court narrowly (by a 5-4 majority) upheld the law on entirely different grounds. It found that the individual mandate, which is enforced by requiring people without insurance to pay a financial penalty that will be levied by the Internal Revenue Service, was within Congress' power to lay and collect taxes.

The Court also struck down another important part of the ACA. The ACA included an expansion of the Medicaid program. Medicaid, which provides health insurance to many poor people, is administered by the states with joint federal and state funding. States are not required to participate in the Medicaid program although all states currently do. The ACA called for making everyone with incomes below 133% of the Federal Poverty Level eligible for Medicaid. States that failed to comply with this provision could be excluded from federal Medicaid funding altogether.

The Court, by a 7-2 majority, found that this penalty was too severe and over-reaching and that it would coerce states into implementing the ACA's Medicaid expansion. Justices Ginsberg and Sotomayor wrote a strong dissent from the majority opinion, arguing that the penalty was within Congress's power, especially since state participation in the Medicaid program itself is voluntary. The impact of this ruling was to make states' implementation of the Medicaid expansion voluntary. Several states have so far opted not to implement it, thus excluding millions of potential Medicaid recipients.

Subsequently, the Supreme Court ruled in the case of *Burwell v. Hobby Lobby* (2014) that corporations could opt for a religious exemption to the ACA's requirement that employers cover women's contraception. (See Box 53-1.)

THE ROLE OF PRECEDENT

An important legal doctrine, *stare decisis* (let the decision stand), sets the course for judicial precedents by adhering to previous findings in cases with substantially comparable facts and circumstances. Thus courts grant deference to their prior rulings. Courts are not completely bound by precedent; they sometimes overrule prior decisions, but they are expected to depart from precedent based only on compelling and clearly articulated reasons. Lower courts are expected to follow the rulings of a higher court (Administrative Office of the U.S. Courts, 2010). Thus, for example, a federal district court in California or Oregon would look to rulings of the Ninth Circuit Court of Appeals (which includes those states) for guidance; the Ninth Circuit would look to the U.S. Supreme Court as well as the Ninth Circuit's own prior rulings.

THE CONSTITUTION AND BRANCHES OF GOVERNMENT

The U.S. Constitution sets out the basic structure of the federal government. State constitutions do the same for each state government. A key element of this structure is a system of checks and balances between the three branches of government: legislative branch (Congress, state legislatures, local legislative bodies), executive branch (President, governors, and the government agencies they administer), and judicial branch (federal and state courts). Each branch carries out specific functions, but no branch is completely autonomous. For example, Congress passes legislation but the President can either sign or veto it, and Congress can override a presidential veto by a two-thirds majority. Federal executive agencies such as the U.S. Department of Health and Human Services are accountable to the President, but their budgets depend on actions by Congress. The federal courts act independently of the President and Congress, but judges are nominated by the President, subject to confirmation by the U.S. Senate.

The Constitution is the fundamental source of U.S. law. All government action must be consistent with it. This is true of the U.S. Constitution (which

BOX 53-1 Contraceptive Services and the *Hobby Lobby* Decision

The Affordable Care Act (ACA) of 2010 requires health plans to cover a number of services including women's preventive services, without cost-sharing. Federal rules defined the scope of those services to include all FDA-approved contraceptive methods, sterilization procedures, and patient education and counseling for all women with reproductive capacity.

Religious organizations were exempt from this mandate. The rules also allowed an accommodation for nonprofit, religious-affiliated employers (such as faith-based universities and health care institutions): They could exclude contraceptive devices and services from their health plans, and the health plans would be required to cover these directly.

However, the contraceptive mandate was challenged in court by some private, for-profit employers, who claimed that being required to cover four types of contraception (two types of morning-after pills and two types of intrauterine devices) was contrary to their religious beliefs. They charged that the mandate thus violated the Religious Freedom Restoration Act (RFRA), which bars the federal government from taking action that substantially burdens the exercise of religion unless that action constitutes the least restrictive means of serving a compelling government interest.

In *Burwell v. Hobby Lobby*, the Supreme Court ruled by a 5-4 majority in favor of these employers. The Court found that the RFRA applies to religious expression by corporations, that the contraceptive mandate had placed a substantial burden on

the employers' exercise of religion, and that the Obama Administration had failed to show that this mandate was the least restrictive available means of assuring access to contraception.

Writing for the majority, Justice Alito characterized the court's decision as narrowly tailored, that it invalidated only the mandate to cover the four specific contraceptive methods that had been challenged and that it applied specifically to closely held private corporations (those for whom at least 50% of stock is owned by five or fewer owners).

In her dissent, Justice Ginsburg noted that this was the first time that the Court had ruled that the religious-expression protections of the RFRA apply to for-profit corporations. She also cautioned that the ruling could have broad implications, that other employers might raise religious objections to a broad range of health care services, including blood transfusions, antidepressants, and vaccinations.

As of this writing, it is too soon to know what the long-range implications of the *Hobby Lobby* decision will be and whether and how the administration will seek other options to ensure access to contraceptive devices and services, and if some employers will successfully resist other insurance mandates on religious grounds.

Reference
Burwell v. Hobby Lobby (2014). U.S. Supreme Court, No. 13–354.

---

applies to the actions of the federal and state governments) and each state constitution (which apply to the actions of each state).

Although much of the Constitution is concerned with the structure and functions of the federal government, the first 10 amendments to the Constitution, known as the Bill of Rights, define the basic rights of all people in the United States, including: freedom of speech; freedom of assembly; freedom of religion; freedom from unlawful searches and seizures; and protection against being deprived of life, liberty, or property without due process. In the United States, the rights outlined by the Bill of Rights are defined primarily as limitations on government's power to restrict or deny them. Thus, for example, the First Amendment reads as follows:

Congress shall make no law respecting an establishment of religion, or prohibiting the free exercise thereof; or abridging the freedom of speech, or of the press; or the right of the people peaceably to assemble, and to petition the Government for a redress of grievances.

Although the language of the Bill of Rights specifically focuses on the federal government, the 14th Amendment has had the effect of applying these rights to actions by state governments.

Because the Bill of Rights applies to government action, it does not directly limit the behavior of private individuals (including employers). Other laws may apply to actions by employers and individuals, for example, civil rights laws, which protect people from discrimination based on race, gender, national origin, or other factors, and whistleblower laws that protect employees' rights to report illegal conduct or unsafe practices.

Laws passed by Congress must be consistent with the U.S. Constitution. Laws passed by a state legislature must be consistent with both the U.S. Constitution and the state constitution.

Rules or regulations issued by the executive branch must be consistent with the Constitution. There must also be some statutory (legislative) source of authority for them to act. For example, the U.S. Secretary of Health and Human Services is authorized by federal law to issue rules and regulations to carry out the functions of her department, including the administration of the Medicare program (see, for example, Home Health Services Act, 42 U.S. Code, Section 1302, 2011); this is the basis for that agency to adopt regulations spelling out Conditions of Participation that hospitals and other health care organizations must meet to participate in the Medicare and Medicaid programs (Medicare Conditions of Participation, 2014.) The federal Administrative Procedure Act (5 U.S. Code, Chapter 5, 2011) and parallel state laws also spell out the procedures that government agencies must follow in issuing regulations, such as how much notice must be provided to the public and how members of the public can provide comments on any proposed regulations. The actions of an executive agency may be challenged on the basis that it has allegedly acted without legal authority or fails to comply with procedural requirements.

In *Spine Diagnostics Center of Baton Rouge, Inc. v. Louisiana State Board of Nursing* (2008), a Louisiana appellate court considered a challenge to a Board of Nursing advisory opinion that interventional pain management is within the scope of practice of Certified Registered Nurse Anesthetists (CRNAs). The court upheld a trial court finding that this Advisory Opinion constituted a rule (regulation) expanding the CRNA scope of practice into an area in which they had not traditionally practiced. The court agreed that interventional pain management is "solely the practice of medicine." Since this rule expanding (according to the court) CRNAs' scope of practice had not been issued in accordance with the state's Administrative Procedures Act (including advance notice and an opportunity for public comment), it was found to be an improper attempt at rule making. The state supreme court subsequently declined to hear an appeal of the decision (Louisiana Supreme Court, 2009), thus allowing it to stand.

Another example helps to illustrate the court's power to review agency actions. In 1999, California enacted Assembly Bill (AB) 394, which requires hospitals to abide by mandatory nurse staffing ratios. AB 394 directed the California Department of Health Services (CDHS) to issue regulations implementing the ratios. When the CDHS issued its ratios regulations in 2002, they included a proviso that the ratios be in effect "at all times." The state hospital association argued that this requirement was too rigid and that applying it during meal and bathroom breaks would be costly and impractical. They sued the CDHS, seeking to have that provision overturned. A California Superior Court ruled against them, finding that the "at all times" language accurately reflected the legislature's intent in passing AB 394 and that eliminating it would render the law "meaningless" (Egelko, 2004).

IMPACT LITIGATION

Advocates have developed a tradition of using the courts strategically to establish, affirm, or clarify rights. Litigation that is pursued with a goal of achieving a broad social affect that sets a significant precedent or benefits a class of people is often referred to as *impact litigation*. It "is most commonly understood to mean litigation that is expected to have far-reaching results" (Churchill, 2009).

An important example of such litigation is *Brown v. Board of Education,* the 1954 case in which the U.S. Supreme Court struck down school segregation and mandated that states begin a process of desegregating their public schools. The Court unanimously found that segregated public school education constituted a state policy of inferior education, that "separate educational facilities are inherently unequal," and that it thus violated the Equal Protection Clause of the Fourteenth Amendment to the U.S. Constitution. This case had been pursued by civil rights advocates as part of their broad efforts to end racial segregation.

EXPANDING LEGAL RIGHTS

Laws passed at the federal or state level often create rights or remedies that can be legally enforced through the courts. The Americans with Disabilities Act, 1990 (ADA) provides for equal treatment for disabled Americans and bars discrimination in a number of areas including employment and public accommodations. For example, a person with a disability who is able to perform the essential aspects of a job with reasonable accommodation cannot be fired or denied a promotion on the basis of a disability. The ADA applies principles of equality and fair play that are basic to American law and public life, but it also created specific rights that can be enforced through government action and litigation.

In *Citizens United v. Federal Election Commission* (2010), the Supreme Court ruled that restricting corporate or union campaign donations was a violation of the First Amendment. This ruling, described in Box 53-2, gave corporations the same protections to free speech as individuals have.

ENFORCING LEGAL AND REGULATORY REQUIREMENTS

The courts are often used as a means to seek enforcement of existing regulatory requirements. Nursing organizations sometimes turn to the courts to challenge practices they believe violate state nurse practice acts. For example, the California School Nurses Organization, the American Nurses Association (ANA), and ANA/California sued the California Department of Education (CDE) challenging a CDE directive authorizing insulin injection in public schools by unlicensed personnel. The CDE had issued this directive in connection with its settlement of a suit by parents of diabetic students who, the parents had charged, were being denied needed care by the lack of school personnel qualified to administer insulin (CDE, 2007). The nursing groups challenged this practice as a violation of California's Nursing Practice Act and questioned the authority of the CDE to issue a directive on nursing practice. The trial court and appellate court ruled in favor of the nurses but the state supreme court later ruled that the CDE directive

---

BOX 53-2 Citizens United

The influence of money in the political process has long been a contentious policy and legal issue. The Bipartisan Campaign Reform Act of 2002 (BCRA, also known as the McCain-Feingold Act) had imposed restrictions on how much money corporations and unions could spend on broadcast advertisement supporting or opposing political candidates shortly before an election. In 2010, the Supreme Court lifted these restrictions. In *Citizens United v. Federal Election Commission*, the Court—by a 5-4 majority—ruled that limiting the amount of money corporations and unions could spend to support or oppose a political candidate violated the First Amendment's guarantee of freedom of speech. In so ruling, the Court emphasized that corporations, and not just individuals, are entitled to protection of free speech rights. One result of *Citizens United* has been a significant growth in campaign advertising by "outside" groups—i.e., groups not directly associated with a candidate. Although the decision contemplates that these organizations are independent of candidates and their political campaigns, critics of the decision argue that, in practice, weak regulation has allowed for coordination between these "outside" groups and campaigns, leading to growing influence by wealthy donors in political campaigns, and thus in public policy.

Reference

Citizens United v. Federal Election Commission (2010), 558 U.S. 310.

---

did not violate the Nursing Practice Act, and allowed it to stand (*American Nurses Association v. Torlakson*, 2013). Nonnurses are thus permitted to administer insulin to students in schools.

ANTITRUST LAWS AND ANTICOMPETITIVE PRACTICES

Federal and state antitrust laws are designed to protect consumers by prohibiting anticompetitive business practices. These laws have their roots in the end of the 19th century when large and powerful businesses combined into alliances and colluded on prices, distribution, and other practices. Such collusion effectively eliminated competition among these businesses and blocked newer companies from entering the market, to the detriment of the consumer. Antitrust protections have been a legal area which nurses and others have sometimes looked to for relief from practices that block their full participation in the health care marketplace.

Although federal antitrust laws are enforced through two federal agencies, the Federal Trade Commission (FTC) and the Antitrust Division of the Department of Justice (DOJ), private parties can also bring antitrust suits directly to federal court. In June 2006, class action antitrust suits[1] were filed on behalf of nurses in Detroit, San Antonio, Albany, Chicago, and Memphis. These suits alleged that hospitals and health systems in each of those metropolitan areas had secretly shared nurses' pay and planned raises, agreeing not to compete with each other on compensation. This collusion between erstwhile competitors, the suits alleged, violated federal antitrust laws (Evans, 2007; Miles, 2007). Some hospitals opted to settle without going to trial. An Albany, New York, health system reached a $1.25 million settlement (Greenhouse, 2009); a Detroit health system agreed to a $13.6 million settlement (Greene, 2009). One Detroit hospital, however, did not participate in this settlement; as of the time this chapter was written, the class action suit against that hospital is continuing.

Professional associations can also be subject to antitrust scrutiny. For example, in a prominent case, the U.S. Supreme Court found that an agreement by a county medical society to establish maximum fees for medical procedures constituted illegal price-fixing (*Arizona v. Maricopa County Medical Society*, 1982). In *Wilk v. American Medical Association* (1990), the AMA was found to have violated antitrust laws by engaging in anticompetitive activities. The AMA had advised that physicians were guilty of unethical conduct if they referred patients to chiropractors or accepted referrals from them, since one of the AMA's ethical principles barred cooperation with "unscientific practitioners." A group of chiropractors filed suit against the AMA and prevailed in the Seventh Circuit Court of Appeals, which found that this was

an attempt to conduct an illegal group boycott of the chiropractic profession.

The FTC, in keeping with its charge "[t]o prevent business practices that are anticompetitive or deceptive or unfair to consumers…" (Federal Trade Commission Act of 1914; FTC, n.d.), has issued a series of opinions on state health care laws and regulations, analyzing their potential impact on competition. It has reviewed several existing and proposed state policies that restrict or expand the practice of different groups of health professionals, including Advanced Practice Registered Nurses (APRNs). For example, in March 2013, the FTC, in response to a request by a Connecticut legislator, issued a letter citing the procompetitive effect of proposed legislation to remove state requirements that APRNs must practice underwritten collaborative agreements with physicians (Federal Trade Commission [FTC], 2013).

In its 2011 report on *The Future of Nursing*, the Institute of Medicine (IOM) noted that the FTC "has a long history of targeting anticompetitive conduct in health care markets, including restrictions on the business practices of health care providers, as well as policies that could act as a barrier to entry for new competitors in the market." (p. 5). The IOM called on the FTC and the Antitrust Division of the Justice Department to "[r]eview existing and proposed state regulations concerning advanced practice registered nurses to identify those that have anticompetitive effects without contributing to the health and safety of the public" (p. 279).

CRIMINAL COURTS

Many of the court decisions that have an impact on health policy and nursing practice are civil actions. In some prominent instances, however, actions in criminal courts have resulted in significant policy implications for nursing as well. For example, although negligent acts or omissions that lead to patient injury or death are usually addressed in civil suits, on occasion they have led to criminal prosecution. In 2006, a Wisconsin nurse faced criminal charges for negligence leading to the tragic death of a teenage mother in labor. She was charged with Neglect of a Patient Causing Great Bodily Harm,

---

[1]Class action suits seek to vindicate the rights of an entire class of individuals who share a common interest giving rise to the suit and who seek a common outcome.

which is a felony. This case drew national attention because of concern that criminalizing medical errors was overreaching and excessive and that emphasizing individual blame rather than system-level accountability for errors and their prevention could actually impede efforts to improve patient safety. The Wisconsin nurse eventually accepted a plea bargain, agreeing to plead "no contest" to two misdemeanor charges and accepting 2 years' probation and restrictions on her work hours; in addition, the Wisconsin Board of Nursing suspended her license for 9 months (Treleven, 2006).

In 2006, 10 nurses simultaneously resigned their positions at a Long Island nursing home. These nurses were among a larger group, all of whom were recruited from the Philippines, working in facilities owned by the Sentosa Care nursing home chain. These nurses had complained that many of the promises made to them when they were first hired regarding wages and working and living conditions had been broken. The nurses, fearing retaliation by their employer, resigned with minimal notice. The facility, whose patients included ventilator-dependent children, covered their shifts with other nurses. After receiving a complaint from the nursing home, the state's board of nursing found no basis to proceed with a patient abandonment complaint. An investigation by the state Department of Health later yielded a conclusion that no patients had been put at risk. Nonetheless, the local county District Attorney filed criminal charges against the nurses, indicting them for conspiracy and for putting children and disabled patients at risk.

The case raised significant concerns not only about mistreatment of immigrant nurses but also about the rights of all nurses (Keepnews, 2009). Nursing organizations, including the ANA, the New York State Nurses Association, and the Philippine Nurses Association of America, supported the nurses' call for charges to be dropped. The trial court judge refused to drop the charges; however, the nurses filed an appeal of this decision. A state appellate court issued an order that the trial be stopped. The court found that "criminalizing [the nurses'] resignations" would have the effect of unjustifiably "abridging the nurses' Thirteenth Amendment rights," referring to that constitutional amendment's prohibition on involuntary servitude (*Vinluan v. Doyle*, 2009).

INFLUENCING AND RESPONDING TO COURT DECISIONS

Although judges are expected to rule based on facts and law, several other factors may influence the outcome of court decisions. Judges often take changing social attitudes and standards into account in their rulings. Judges also differ in their own judicial philosophies. The views of federal judicial appointees and their judicial records are factors in a president's judicial nominations and in the Senate's decision whether or not to confirm the nominations. Thus, the outcomes of presidential and senate elections can have an important impact in the composition of the federal courts, including the Supreme Court. Judges' views may shift over time and cannot always be reliably predicted or neatly categorized. Supreme Court Justice Harry Blackmun, often characterized as a liberal Court member, and who wrote the majority opinion in *Roe v. Wade*, had been nominated to the Supreme Court by President Richard Nixon.

PERSUADING THE COURTS: *AMICUS CURIAE* BRIEFS

An important route for influencing courts' decisions is through filing *amicus curiae* (friend of the court) briefs. Amicus briefs provide an important tool for advocacy groups to make their views known on a relevant case. When (with the court's permission) groups and/or individuals file an amicus brief, they bring their perspectives, data, and beliefs about the issues before the court to persuade it on how to rule.

Examples of cases in which nursing organizations have filed amicus briefs include:

- *National Federation of Independent Business v. Sebelius* (2012). The ANA, joined by five other health professional groups, filed an amicus brief in support of the Affordable Care Act's minimum coverage provision. The ANA filed amicus briefs in other federal cases regarding the ACA.
- *Lark v. Montgomery Hospice* (2008). The ANA, the Maryland Nurses Association, the American

College of Nurse-Midwives, and the Public Justice Center filed an amicus brief in Maryland's high court in support of a nurse who had accused her employer of violating that state's health care whistleblower law by firing her after she had reported safety concerns.

- *Olmstead v. L.C.* (1999). The American Psychiatric Nurses Association joined other organizations in an amicus brief before the U.S. Supreme Court to support the right of disabled persons to receive care in noninstitutional settings.
- *Sullivan v. Edward Hospital* (2004). The American Association of Nurse Attorneys filed an amicus brief with the Illinois Supreme Court, arguing that only nurses are qualified to provide expert testimony on nurses' standard of care.
- *Commonwealth Brands Inc. v. U.S.* (2010). The Oncology Nursing Society joined with 10 other organizations in support of FDA regulation of tobacco manufacturing, sales, and advertising.

RESPONDING TO COURT DECISIONS

Appealing an Unfavorable Decision. When faced with an unsatisfactory court ruling, a party may be able to appeal the decision to a higher court. Generally, there must be grounds to appeal beyond simply not being satisfied with the outcome. For example, the losing party may argue that the court made an error in how it applied the law or in refusing to consider relevant evidence. There is no guarantee that an appellate or higher court will agree to hear an appeal.

Repudiating the Court. When a court's decision is based on its interpretation of a statute, another option is to seek a change in that statute. Of course, this requires a political strategy to secure passage of new legislation, which may or may not be a viable option.

For example, in *Ledbetter v. Goodyear Tire & Rubber Co., Inc.* (2007), the U.S. Supreme Court interpreted the equal-pay provisions of Title VII of the Civil Rights Act of 1964 as meaning that a violation occurs only at the time that a biased pay scale is instituted, not each time workers are paid unequally as a result of that policy. This had the effect of sharply limiting an employee's ability to file a discrimination claim, even if an employee learned of this unequal pay policy only sometime after it had been implemented. In response, Congress passed and President Obama signed the Lilly Ledbetter Fair Pay Act of 2009. The preamble to the bill explicitly criticizes the Court's *Ledbetter* decision, stating that "[t]he limitation imposed by the Court ... ignores the reality of wage discrimination and is at odds with the robust application of the civil rights laws that Congress intended" (Lily Ledbetter Fair Pay Act of 2009).

Amending the Constitution. Another potential means of responding to an unsatisfactory court decision, particularly if the decision is based on an interpretation of the Constitution, is to amend the Constitution. This is much easier said than done. Amending the U.S. Constitution requires approval by not only a two-thirds majority of both houses of Congress but also by three-quarters of the states.

Amending state constitutions, however, is often a different story. States differ in their procedures for amending their constitutions: a vote of the legislature, a constitutional convention, popular referendum, and/or a combination of methods. One example that captured national attention occurred in California. In 2008, the California Supreme Court ruled that denying same-sex couples the right to marry was a violation of the equal protection clause of the California State Constitution (*In re Marriage Cases*, 2008). Opponents of same-sex marriage gathered enough signatures to place Proposition 8, a state constitutional amendment, on the ballot. That amendment, which California voters narrowly approved in November 2008, declared that only marriage between a man and a woman is valid or recognized in California, thereby repudiating the court's interpretation by changing the state constitution.

Subsequently, a federal district court ruled that Proposition 8 violated the Equal Protection Clause of the U.S. Constitution (*Perry v. Schwarzenegger*, 2010). Supporters of Proposition 8 appealed this ruling to the Ninth Circuit Court of Appeals, which affirmed the district court's decision. Supporters then appealed to the U.S. Supreme Court. The Court ruled that Proposition 8 supporters lacked standing to challenge the ruling. This had the effect of reinstating the ruling against Proposition 8, thereby allowing same-sex marriages to resume in California but without the Court addressing whether the U.S. Constitution requires all states to recognize a right of same-sex couples to marry (*Hollingsworth v. Perry*, 2013). That issue continues to be debated in the federal court system.

NURSING'S POLICY AGENDA

Health care practice and health policy continue to change rapidly in often chaotic and unpredictable ways. Successful policy strategies must include being knowledgeable about the role of the courts in health policy and being prepared to respond to and, when possible, seek to influence the outcome of court decisions.

DISCUSSION QUESTIONS

1. What impact do court decisions have on policy issues related to nursing and health care?
2. How can nurses have an impact on the outcome of legal issues related to nursing and health care?

REFERENCES

Administrative Office of the U.S. Courts (n.d.). The federal court system in the U.S. Retrieved from *www.uscourts.gov/uscourts/FederalCourts/Publications/English.pdf.*

Administrative Office of the U.S. Courts. (2010). Understanding the federal courts. Retrieved from *www.uscourts.gov/uscourts/educational-resources/get-informed/understanding-federal-courts.pdf.*

Administrative Procedure Act, 5 U.S. Code, Chapter 5 (2011).

American Nurses Association v. Torlakson, 57 Cal.4th 570 (2013).

Americans with Disabilities Act of 1990, P.L. 101-336, 42 U.S.C. § 12101 et seq.

Arizona v. Maricopa County Medical Society, 457 U.S. 332 (1982).

California Department of Education [CDE] (2007). Children with diabetes win assurance of legally required services at school. Retrieved from *www.cde.ca.gov/nr/ne/yr07/yr07rel97.asp.*

Churchill, S. (2009). Making employment civil rights real. Amicus (Harvard Civil Rights-Civil Liberties Law Review online supplement). Retrieved from *harvardcrcl.org/amicus/2009/10/22/employment-civil-rights.*

Commonwealth Brands Inc. v. U.S., 2010 U.S. Dist. LEXIS 6316, USDC W.D.Ky (2010).

Egelko, B. (2004). Judge upholds nurse rules/Hospitals must continue to maintain staffing ratios at all times San Francisco Chronicle. Retrieved from *articles.sfgate.com/2004-05-27/business/17427543_1_california-nurses-association-nursing-shortage-ratios.*

Evans, M. (2007). Nurses' wage war. *Modern Healthcare.* Retrieved from *www.modernhealthcare.com/article/20071217/REG/71213005.*

Federal Trade Commission [FTC] (n.d.). About the FTC. Retrieved from *www.ftc.gov/about-ftc.*

Federal Trade Commission Act of 1914, (15 U.S.C §§ 41-58, as amended.

Federal Trade Commission [FTC]. (2013). FTC Staff Letter to the Honorable Theresa W. Conroy, Connecticut House of Representatives, Concerning the Likely Competitive Impact of Connecticut House Bill 6391 on Advance Practice Registered Nurses. Retrieved from *www.ftc.gov/policy/policy-actions/advocacy-filings/2013/03/ftc-staff-letter-honorable-theresa-w-conroy.*

Greene, J. (2009). "St. John Health agrees to $13.6 million settlement with nurses." *Crains Detroit Business,* Retrieved from *www.crainsdetroit.com/article/20090330/FREE/903309950.*

Greenhouse. (2009). "Settlement in nurses' antitrust suit.". *New York Times.* Retrieved from *www.nytimes.com/ 2009/03/10/nyregion/10settle.html?_r=3.*

Hollingsworth v. Perry (2013). 570 U.S. ___ , 133 S.Ct. 2652.

Home Health Services, 42 U.S. Code, Sections 1302 and 1395 (2011).

In re Marriage Cases (2008). 43 Cal.4th 757.

Institute of Medicine. (2011). *The future of nursing: Leading change, advancing health.* Washington, DC: National Academies Press.

Keepnews, D. M. (2009). Welcome news in the Sentosa nurses case. *Policy, Politics, & Nursing Practice, 10*(1), 4–5.

Lark v. Montgomery Hospice, 414 Md. 215 (2008).

Ledbetter v. Goodyear Tire & Rubber Co., Inc. 127 S, Ct. 2162 (2007).

Lily Ledbetter Fair Pay Act of 2009, Pub.L. 111–2, S. 181.

Louisiana Supreme Court. (2009). News Release #019. Retrieved from *www.lasc.org/news_releases/2009/2009-019.asp.*

Marbury v. Madison, 5 U.S. 137 (1803).

Medicare Conditions of Participation, 42 CFR Chapter IV, Subchapter G (2014).

Miles, J. (2007). The nursing shortage, wage information sharing among competing hospitals, and the antitrust laws: The nurse wages antitrust litigation. *Houston Journal of Health Law & Policy, 7,* 305–378.

National Federation of Independent Business v. Sebelius, 567 U.S. ___ , 132 S.Ct 2566 (2012).

Olmstead v. L.C., 527 U.S. 581 (1999).

Perry v. Schwarzenegger, 591 F.3d 1147 (2010).

Spine Diagnostics Center of Baton Rouge, Inc. v. Louisiana State Board of Nursing, Louisiana Court of Appeal (First Circuit). No. 2008 CA 0813, December 23, 2008.

Sullivan v. Edward Hospital, 806 NE 645 (Ill. 2004).

Treleven, E. (2006). "I'd give my life to bring her back"; Nurse gets probation in pregnant teen's death. *Wisconsin State Journal*, A1. December 16, 2006.

Vinluan v. Doyle. (2009). 2009 NY Slip Op. 219.New York State Supreme Court, Appellate Division, Second Department. Retrieved from *www.courts.state.ny.us/courts/ad2/calendar/webcal/decisions/2009/D20723.pdf.*

Wilk v. American Medical Association, 895 F. 2d 352 (7th Cir. 1990; cert. denied, 498 US 982) (1990).

ONLINE RESOURCES

The American Association of Nurse Attorneys
www.taana.org
CDC Public Health Law Program
www.cdc.gov/phlp
Public Health Law Research
publichealthlawresearch.org
Network for Public Health Law
www.networkforphl.org

CHAPTER 54

Nursing Licensure and Regulation

Edie Brous

"[T]he liberty component of the Fourteenth Amendment's Due Process Clause includes some generalized due process right to choose one's field of private employment, but a right which is nevertheless subject to reasonable government regulation."

United States Supreme Court, *Conn v. Gabbert,*

The application process for nursing educational programs has become progressively more competitive. In fact, professional nursing programs turned away more than 75,587 qualified applicants in 2011 (American Association of Colleges of Nursing [AACN], 2012). Any accepted student must meet the stringent academic rigors of a challenging curriculum, followed by successful completion of state board examinations, before being licensed to practice. The extensive ordeals in qualifying for licensure have led some to believe they have earned the right to practice professional nursing. The practice of nursing, however, is not an unqualified right. It is also a privilege, and privileges must be preserved. To maintain one's license in good standing and continue practicing, nurses must understand that rights are always accompanied by responsibilities.

This chapter will provide an overview of the regulatory processes, both those that are internal to nursing and those that impose obligations from outside of the profession. Although external regulatory schemes impact all health care providers, it is the internal process of self-regulation that greatly influences nursing practice and defines nursing as an autonomous profession.

HISTORICAL PERSPECTIVE

Before 1903, nursing regulation in the United States was limited to lists or registries of those who had been trained as nurses. In 1903, North Carolina

created the first Board of Nursing (BON) and enacted a Nurse Practice Act (NPA). Within 20 years, this had been followed by all other states. As nursing boards developed standards to define nursing practice and prevent unqualified persons from practicing, licensure became mandatory and each state developed an examination process toward that end (Damgaard, Hohman, & Karpiuk, 2000). Members of each state BON met collectively with members of the American Nurses Association (ANA) Council on State Boards of Nursing. This gave way to the National Council of State Boards of Nursing (NCSBN) in 1978. Today there are 60 constituent member boards (including all 50 states and some U.S. territories). Educational requirements have been standardized and modernized, as has the examination process, and NCSBN has published a model NPA.

The scope of nursing practice has greatly expanded but remains state-specific at all levels of practice. Advanced practice nursing, as with registered nurse (RN), licensed practical nurse (LPN)/licensed vocational nurse (LVN), or nursing attendant practice, remains within the regulatory purview of each state or territory. The composition and authority of each board, the methodology for addressing complaints, the definition of professional misconduct, and the qualifications for remaining in good standing are examples of state-specific regulation. For this reason, nurses at all levels of practice must understand and abide by the NPAs or nursing statues and regulations of each state in which they practice.

THE PURPOSE OF PROFESSIONAL REGULATION

The government has an obligation to protect its most vulnerable citizens. This social contract with the public is the reason that nursing is a regulated profession. Those who are sick, infirm, young, elderly, disabled, or in any manner unable to advocate for themselves may be endangered by unqualified practitioners. Nursing regulation provides public accountability. A member of the lay public may not have the ability to recognize and protect himself or herself from incompetent providers. Government oversight of licensed nurses by a body of nursing experts is intended to keep patients safe by ensuring competence.

SOURCES OF REGULATION

NURSING BOARDS

The initial qualifications for licensure, continuing educational requirements, disciplinary procedures, complaint resolution processes, professional misconduct or unprofessional conduct definitions, mandatory reporting requirements, and specific scopes of practice are determined at the state level. Some states have separate licensing boards for RNs and LPNs/LVNs, although other states have unified boards for regulating all nurses. Boards of nursing (BONs) are given their authority through state laws or administrative procedure acts.

HEALTH AND HUMAN SERVICES

As stated on the HHS website, "[T]he Department of Health and Human Services (HHS) is the United States government's principal agency for protecting the health of all Americans and providing essential human services, especially for those who are least able to help themselves" (U.S. Department of Health and Human Services [HHS], 2013). Through various administrative agencies, HHS regulates issues such as civil rights, privacy, food and drug safety, the Medicaid and Medicare programs, health care fraud, medical research, technology standards, and tribal matters. It serves as the umbrella organization for such agencies as the Centers for Medicare and Medicaid (CMS), the Food and Drug Administration, the Centers for Disease Control and Prevention, and the Office for Civil Rights, among others. The integrity of all HHS programs is protected by the Office of the Inspector General (OIG)

through audits and exclusion lists, as discussed in the following paragraphs.

CENTERS FOR MEDICARE AND MEDICAID SERVICES

Medicare and Medicaid are government health insurance programs for qualifying individuals. Medicare is a federally administered program available to persons 65 or older, persons under 65 with certain disabilities, and persons of all ages with end-stage renal disease. Medicaid is a state-administered program available to low-income individuals and families meeting federal and state eligibility criteria. Health care providers must be compliant with regulations and criteria called Conditions of Participations (CoPs) and Conditions for Coverage (CfC) to be eligible for Medicare or Medicaid reimbursement. The OIG may place a provider on a List of Excluded Individuals/Entities. The exclusion program is designed to protect the health and welfare of the nation's older adults and poor individuals by preventing certain providers from participating in the Medicaid or Medicare programs. Nurses placed on the exclusion list may not be employed by any employers receiving state or federal funding.

THE JOINT COMMISSION

Compliance with the Medicare and Medicaid CoPs may be demonstrated by Joint Commission accreditation (United States Code, 2013). The CMS will deem an organization as meeting certification requirements by virtue of having met The Joint Commission's standards. Those standards include nursing performance elements such as policies and procedures, safety initiatives, reporting mechanisms, communication systems, sentinel events, quality improvement practices, staffing effectiveness, credentialing, and other performance indicators. The goal of The Joint Commission survey and accreditation process is to improve patient outcomes.

FEDERAL, STATE, AND LOCAL LAW

Public health codes are laws enacted to promote community health and safety. They address emergency preparedness, communicable diseases, environmental controls, use of health care facilities, staff credentials and competency, policies and procedures, sanitation, housing, childhood nutrition, mental health issues, food safety, and many other elements related to nursing care. Public health laws exist at the local, state, and federal level and may be enforced by civil or criminal penalties.

ORGANIZATIONAL POLICY

Nurses are responsible for being familiar with their employer's policies and procedures and to adhere to them. An organization's protocols may be used to establish the practice standards to which the nurse will be held. They exist to provide standardization and consistency. Failure to abide by an institution's rules may endanger patients and expose the nurse and the employer to liability.

LICENSURE BOARD RESPONSIBILITIES

PROTECT THE PUBLIC

The primary function of a BON is to protect the health, safety, and welfare of the public and to maintain the public's trust in the profession by ensuring that those individuals who engage in the conduct described in the Nurse Practice Act or nursing statutes are properly trained and licensed. The state in which an applicant seeks licensure (by reciprocity or endorsement) must confirm that the applicant is in fact a licensee in good standing in another jurisdiction. To confirm that this is the case, state boards will perform licensure verification. Approximately 38 states participate in NURSYS, an online process for providing immediate verification information to the requesting board.

ISSUE AND RENEW LICENSES

An initial professional license issued by a nursing board is valid for the licensee's lifetime but the licensee must periodically register that license to continue practicing. The licensee must meet the board's registration requirements to be issued a registration certificate. Such requirements typically include continuing education, clinical practice, the

absence of a criminal record, and continued good moral character. The cyclical process of reregistering a license is commonly referred to as a renewal process.

To comply with their legislative mandate to protect the public, BONs define the required elements of nursing education. Graduation from a school that is accredited in one state may not meet the requirements for licensure in another state.

INVESTIGATION AND PROSECUTION OF COMPLAINTS

BONs are statutorily mandated to investigate all complaints against health care providers covered by the state's administrative procedure act or NPA. Some cases may be resolved through informal procedures, although others require formal hearings. Licensees against whom a complaint has been lodged should be advised of the allegations and of their rights. Although nurses may represent themselves, it is strongly advised that they seek legal counsel when responding to Board inquiries, even when the allegations appear baseless.

LICENSURE REQUIREMENTS

EXAMINATION

A candidate for entry into nursing practice as an RN or LPN/LVN must apply for licensure to a board of nursing and receive an Authorization to Test (ATT). He or she then may be allowed to schedule an appointment to take the National Council Licensure Exam (NCLEX-RN or NCLEX-PN). Successful completion of the examination is required to be granted an initial licensure.

ENDORSEMENT

A nurse licensed in one jurisdiction may be granted a license in another jurisdiction without retaking the NCLEX upon meeting certain conditions. Typically the requirements include graduation from an accredited program, English proficiency, clinical practice experience or a refresher course, and good moral character. Additionally, the nurse may be required to explain criminal activity or any disciplinary actions in the home state. Interstate compact agreements may also allow multistate licensure.

NURSING LICENSURE COMPACT

A multistate compact, referred to by the NCSBN as a "mutual recognition model," allows RNs or LPN/LVNs to work across state lines in certain circumstances. Nurses residing in compact member states, known as residency or home states, may practice in other compact member states, known as remote states. Nursing practice must be compliant with the NPA and the nursing licensure compact administrative rules of each state. Nurses must remain within the specific scope of practice in the state in which they are practicing (the state in which the patient is located). Home states and remote states communicate through a coordinated database and both may take disciplinary action against a licensee when indicated. A separate licensure compact for advanced practice nurses has not been implemented, but three states, namely Texas, Iowa, and Utah, have passed laws authorizing their participation (National Council of State Boards of Nursing [NCSBN], 2012).

NURSE PRACTICE ACTS

The state regulation of nursing occurs within the context of statutory mandates. Sets of laws enacted to protect the public specify the scope of practice for nursing attendants, LPN/LVNs, RNs, and advanced practice registered nurses (APRNs); outline the authority of the Board; define professional misconduct; and detail the investigation and disciplinary processes for resolving complaints. Although most states have a specific statute called the Nurse Practice Act, some states embed nursing laws and regulations in other statutes.

SCOPE OF PRACTICE

The scope of practice for all levels of nursing has evolved and expanded considerably since the first NPA was enacted. Medical societies frequently react to advancements in nursing practice by challenging BON authority to define expanded roles, particularly regarding advanced practice roles. Medical societies have made arguments that advanced nursing practice encroaches upon the practice of medicine, specifically regarding nurse practitioners (NPs), nurse midwives, and clinical nurse specialists. The American Medical Association (AMA) for example has proposed or adopted resolutions opposing the creation of a board of midwifery and proposing greater physician oversight of midwifery practice (American Medical Association [AMA] House of Delegates, 2008, Res. 204), requiring Doctors of Nursing Practice to function under the supervision and authority of physicians (AMA, 2008, Res. 214) and protecting the terms doctor, resident, and residency by restricting their use to physicians, dentists, and podiatrists (AMA, 2008, Res. 232). Such actions by the AMA consistently oppose the independent practice of other practitioners and declare the need for physician supervision and authority over all other providers. In 2005, the AMA's Resolution 814 went so far as to suggest that physicians should usurp the legislatively granted authority of other licensing boards. Nursing organizations, such as the ANA, view these efforts as a divisive attempt to restrict the practice of other providers and presume authority over all professions. The use of terms such as limited licensure health care provider, mid-level professional, or non-physician reflects the AMA's anachronistic view of all health care providers as physician extenders (American Academy of Nurse Practitioners, 2006) and inaccurately suggests that nursing boards do not keep patients safe.

ADVISORY OPINIONS AND PRACTICE ALERTS

Many nursing boards publish opinions regarding scope of practice, professional misconduct definitions, or delegation questions to clarify the board's position. These advisory opinions may be published independently or in conjunction with other organizations. Practice alerts may also be published advising the nursing community and the public at large of any rule changes or urgent issues. Nurses should go to their BON's website periodically to monitor such communications.

THE SOURCE OF LICENSING BOARD AUTHORITY

Nursing is regulated at the state level. Laws referred to as Administrative Procedure Acts or Civil Procedure Codes vary by state and determine the structure and authority of the BON. In some states the BON is an independent agency, although in others the BON operates under a larger state agency. Typically the BONs that are consolidated under larger agencies are functionaries of the Secretary of State, the Department of Health, the Division of Consumer Affairs, Education Departments, or other regulatory and licensing agencies. BONs may also be hybrid organizations, functioning as institutions that are partially independent and partially affiliated with other agencies. Rules and regulations for nursing practice may also be found in public health and general business laws. The court system generally supports the exclusive authority of the BON but will consider conflicts between employment practices and BON directions.

Courts may also hear conflicts between the BON and other agencies, as exemplified in *American Nurses Association et al. v. Jack O'Connell et al.* (2008). The American Diabetes Association (ADA) and the parents of several diabetic students brought a class-action lawsuit claiming that the California Department of Education (CDE) violated the educational rights of diabetic students. In the absence of adequate numbers of school nurses, the parents claimed they had to remove their children from the school or leave their jobs to administer insulin. The CDE settled with the parents and issued a Legal Advisory on the Rights of Students with Diabetes in California's K-12 Public Schools in which local education agencies were required to train nonlicensed volunteers to administer insulin.

The ANA, the California Nurses Association (CNA), and the California School Nurses Association (CSNA) challenged this legal advisory in court, arguing that the directive could not be followed as it violated the California NPA. The NPA specifically restricted medication administration to licensed nurses. While the matter was pending, the California Board of Registered Nursing issued a public statement (California Board of Registered Nursing [CBRN], 2009) in which nurses were advised to adhere to the NPA and practice in accordance with the Board's standards.

The ADA intervened in the lawsuit arguing that federal disability laws entitled diabetic students to insulin administration as a component of their educational rights. As such, in the absence of sufficient school nurses, schools were required to train unlicensed employees in insulin administration. The court ruled that the CDE legal advisory was unenforceable as the CDE had exceeded its authority. The ruling stated that the CDE's legal advisory conflicted with state law because the NPA clearly defined the administration of medications as a nursing practice. Although the decision should imply that school funding decisions must include adequate nursing staffing, the case was appealed. Legislation and public hearings were conducted regarding the issue, and on August 12, 2013, the California Supreme Court sided with the ADA, finding that "California law permits unlicensed school personnel to administer insulin" (American Nurses Association et al., 2013). Many BONs are considering this issue in home care as well as school settings.

DISCIPLINARY OFFENSES

BONs investigate all complaints they receive. Although gross negligence and unsafe practice are obvious sources of disciplinary action, many actions not directly related to patient care may fall within the definition of professional misconduct and result in disciplinary action. Failure to advise the BON of name or address changes, failure to repay student loans, failure to pay child support, driving under the influence, failure to file or pay taxes, dishonesty in licensure or job applications, falsified or deficient documentation and record-keeping, improper delegation, diversion of controlled substances, or criminal convictions are some examples of actions that may result in BON disciplinary action.

COMPLAINT RESOLUTION

The BON may offer the nurse an opportunity to settle the matter informally rather than conducting a full hearing. A settlement called a Consent Order may be reached in which the nurse stipulates to certain findings and agrees to a disciplinary action that has been negotiated. Informal settlement conferences offer the advantage of lower legal costs and more rapid resolution of the complaint. The nurse may elect to attend a formal hearing rather than agree to a Consent Order if the settlement agreement offers a disciplinary action the nurse considers too harsh. A formal hearing may also be preferred when the disciplinary action of a proposed Consent Order would trigger an OIG exclusion.

DISCIPLINARY ACTIONS

The BON may close the file if its investigation finds no violations. The complainant will be advised that the investigation is complete and the matter is resolved. No action is taken against the nurse. Alternatively, the BON may find violations that can be addressed by issuing a letter of reprimand, but no other action. Letters of reprimand may be publicly posted as disciplinary actions. Nurses may also be fined and/or ordered to attend corrective education.

For more serious practice or ethical issues, the BON may impose practice restrictions and place the nurse on probation. During the probationary period, the nurse may be required to submit periodic employer reports, demonstrate attendance in an impaired provider program, and comply with other terms. Licenses may also be suspended. The period of suspension may be actual suspension, during which time the nurse is not permitted to work, or stayed (temporarily set aside), during which time the nurse is permitted to work while remaining on probation.

The most severe penalty, revocation, is reserved for cases in which the BON believes the nurse presents a serious danger to the public and cannot be rehabilitated to practice safely. A revocation permanently terminates a nurse's license, prohibiting practice and the use of nursing titles. The individual may no longer represent himself or herself as a nurse. The BON may entertain a petition for reinstatement after revocation in certain cases where the individual can demonstrate rehabilitation and competence. Mandatory waiting periods may be

imposed before requests for restoration will be entertained, and formal restoration hearings may be required.

When faced with formal disciplinary hearings, some nurses may agree to voluntarily surrender their nursing licenses. In doing so, the nurse must understand that the forfeiture of the license is permanent. Such surrender still constitutes a disciplinary action tantamount to revocation. The surrender process, sometimes referred to as Discipline by Consent, is an application that the BON may or may not accept. Temporary surrenders may be negotiated for nurses who agree to enter professional assistance programs for impaired providers. Entry into such programs may provide immunity from further disciplinary action if the licensee meets all other required criteria.

Nonpunitive peer assistance programs may provide an alternative to discipline but have not been uniformly adopted in all jurisdictions. Those states and territories that have adopted such alternatives to discipline programs may require the absence of patient harm for nurses to qualify for participation. The ANA endorses these programs stating, in part, that "alternative approaches have been demonstrated to be at least as effective in protecting the public safety as more antiquated punitive methods. The ANA has resolved to work with these few states to pursue the legislative and regulatory modifications necessary to implement an 'alternative to discipline' model for impaired nurses" (ANA, 2011).

Alternatives to discipline programs may address impairment from mental illness as well as from chemical addiction. The use of a medical model, as opposed to a punitive model, in addressing mental illness and/or chemical addiction is preferable because it is more consistent with the board's stated goal of protecting the public. Additionally, such diversion programs allow the nurse to be rehabilitated and support reporting systems. Nurses working in states without such programs should become active in lobbying for their adoption. Some states have an additional category of license surrender called Voluntary Relinquishment. This is a form of surrender unrelated to disciplinary action, in which the licensee is retiring, moving out of state, or for other reasons choosing not to practice nursing in the state.

Appealing board decisions is a difficult, expensive, and frequently unsuccessful process. All internal administrative steps must be completed before seeking redress in the courts. The court will only reverse BON decisions under narrowly defined circumstances. A licensee appealing a BON decision must prove that the BON has violated the constitution or the law and has exceeded its authority under the statute, that it took actions that were an abuse of discretion or arbitrary and capricious, or that the actions taken by the BON were unsupported by the evidence.

COLLATERAL IMPACT

The emotional, financial, legal, and professional impact of BON disciplinary action can be profound. Evidence of board disciplinary action may be admissible in medical malpractice lawsuits or in criminal prosecution. OIG exclusions and data bank listings may render a nurse unable to work, even when holding a license in good standing. Subsequent licensure in another profession or jurisdiction may be difficult or impossible to obtain. Reputation damage is very difficult to overcome. The emotional distress can be considerable, even disabling. Long after the BON has resolved the complaint the licensee may continue to experience sequelae.

REGULATION'S SHORTCOMINGS

Although professional licensing boards are entrusted with keeping the public safe, there is no evidence that the current regulatory system for BONs is effective in improving nursing practice. Some BON practices may in fact be antithetical to patient safety goals. Punitive cultures undermine patient safety by deterring essential reporting of errors. BONs that fail to distinguish between intentional misconduct and inevitable human error perpetuate an ineffective response to adverse events by blaming the end-user or direct provider for the error. This sharp-end focus fails to account for the dangerous systems in which nurses practice and compromises the error-analysis process necessary

to prevent recurrence. In opposition to a latent-error focus (a focus on less apparent failures of organization or design that contributed to the occurrence of errors or allowed them to cause harm to patients), which positively impacts patient safety, such active-error focus has a paradoxical and perverse effect on patient safety initiatives.

The level of penalty imposed may be determined by the level of injury to the patient, which is both inequitable and counterproductive. Outcome-oriented discipline results in inconsistency from one licensee to another for the same infraction. Safety experts recommend evaluating processes, not outcomes. The public is not kept safe by imposing a harsher penalty on a nurse because the patient was injured. The nurse whose patient is not injured by the identical error may be a less cautious provider and actually pose a greater risk to patients but would receive a lighter penalty with this approach.

Lengthy suspensions create rusty practice skills. The technical competence and knowledge required for safe practice are not enhanced by removing a clinician from the workforce. Practice deficiencies are not corrected by levying fines or publishing disciplinary actions on the Internet. Without addressing the underlying root causes and contributing factors of nursing errors they will persist and endanger patients.

Public safety cannot be attained in the absence of nursing advocacy. Patients cannot be kept safe unless their providers are adequately supported. BON advisory opinions are often unavailable or inadequate. Statements such as "Nurses should work collaboratively with their employers" or "Until the matter is resolved nurses are advised to use their best judgment" offer no direction to the practitioner faced with questionable work situations. Although the NCSBN could provide significant guidance, much of the Council's published materials are restricted to board members and are unavailable to the practicing nurse. Many NPAs use generic language when addressing "professional misconduct" or "unprofessional conduct" and do not provide definitions to guide practice or educate nurses regarding potential violations.

The defense of a licensee may be compromised when the BON has information which the licensee is unable to access. Privacy and confidentiality provisions of the administrative statutes are sometimes written or interpreted in such a manner as to prevent even the target of the investigation from obtaining all evidentiary materials. The discovery rights to which a criminal or civil defendant would be entitled may not be afforded to licensees in an administrative action. Disciplinary actions taken against licensees can destroy reputations and careers, and, as such, there should be an adequate appeal mechanism. Courts tend to defer to the expertise of the BON and to uphold BON decisions. This deference is based upon a rationale that the BON's unique nursing expertise distinguishes it as the most qualified body to render decisions. Disciplinary hearings in some states, however, may be conducted by nonnurse administrative personnel with absolutely no expertise in nursing.

The collateral impact of disciplinary action may be ultimately more destructive than the actual disciplinary action itself, even serving as a constructive revocation. Onerous practice restrictions compromise employment opportunities. A temporary suspension may be all that is required for OIG exclusion. The inability to practice for several years may make an eventual return to practice logistically impossible, regardless of licensure status. This undermines efforts to rehabilitate motivated professionals. Such constructive revocations contribute to the nursing shortage by accelerating the exodus of providers from the workforce. The consequent reductions in staffing levels endanger, rather than protect, patients.

Board members may not be selected by members of the nursing profession. They are frequently appointed by the governor or some other state-based selection method. As such, appointees may be selected more by political motivations than qualifications the regulated community would find essential. BONs are bureaucratic structures, many of which are underfunded and understaffed. Levels of efficiency vary. Due process rights in agencies differ substantially from due process rights in a court of law. The right to a speedy trial in the criminal system, as well as the standards and goals that move civil suits forward on mandated schedules, do not exist in the administrative setting. The investigative and hearing process can take months or even years from initial complaint to final resolution. This lengthy process is traumatizing even to those nurses who are ultimately vindicated.

Most people understand the need for legal representation to protect their freedom and physical possessions in criminal or civil lawsuits, yet many nurses try to represent themselves with the BON. A professional license is a valuable asset that requires protection and skilled advocacy. Some BONs make telephone calls to licensees. In these circumstances, nurses may unknowingly make statements against their interest. Nurses may also sign agreements with the BON not understanding the long-term collateral impact of doing so. BONs do not always advise licensees that they can and should seek legal representation at all stages of the process. Nursing board investigators and prosecutors may discourage nurses from being represented by counsel or not inform them that their professional liability insurance may provide for licensure defense.

CONCLUSION

It is critical that nurses read and understand their NPAs. Although all nurses make human mistakes, they should not unexpectedly find themselves defending their license for failure to educate themselves regarding the rules. Nurses must study and adhere to their state's continuing education requirements, scope of practice, definitions of professional misconduct, reporting requirements, and standards of practice. Nebulous areas of practice should be identified to the BON, and advisory opinions should be requested. Clinical practice can only be evidence-based if nurses belong to professional organizations and regularly read the literature. Physical limitations must be respected to reduce the clinical error associated with sleep-deprivation impairment. If contacted by telephone, nurses should advise the BON that they wish to speak with counsel before making any statements or signing any papers. All nurses should independently maintain professional liability insurance rather than relying on employer coverage. Personal policies may provide the coverage for disciplinary actions and licensure defense that employer policies do not.

UNIT 3

A professional license is a valuable asset that may be considered a property right. It is not a right that can be taken for granted, however, and nurses can only protect their licenses by fully understanding the responsibilities that accompany them.

DISCUSSION QUESTIONS

1. Do you consider your license to practice nursing a right or a privilege? What is the difference?
2. Why is nursing a regulated profession? How is it regulated in your state(s)?
3. What are the strengths and weaknesses of the current regulatory scheme for licensed professions?

REFERENCES

American Association of Colleges of Nursing [AACN]. (2012). New AACN data show an enrollment surge in baccalaureate and graduate programs amid calls for more highly educated nurses. Retrieved from *www.aacn .nche.edu/news/articles/2012/enrollment-data*.

American Academy of Nurse Practitioners. (2006). Health professionals urge cooperative care; Oppose SOPP & AMA Resolution 814. Retrieved from *www.apta.org/AM/Template.cfm?Section=Home&TEMPLATE=/CM/ ContentDisplay.cfm&CONTENTID=31550*.

American Medical Association House of Delegates. (2005). Resolution 814: Limited licensure health care provide training and certification standards. Retrieved from *www.google.com/url?sa=t&rct=j&q=&esrc =s&source=web&cd=1&cad=rja&uact=8&ved=0CCAQFjAA&url=http %3A%2F%2Fwww.ama-assn.org%2Fmeetings%2Fpublic%2Finterim05 %2Frefcomkannotateda05.doc&ei=0ZJWVJK0EI_4yQSRpYKQDg&usg =AFQjCNHC8DHAH7Wcsfqj03Ar45VVtUoP6w&sig2=DRfHHYUfSiwh PVwpsjtzbw&bvm=bv.78677474,d.aWw*.

American Medical Association House of Delegates. (2008). Resolution 204: Midwifery scope of practice and licensure. Retrieved from *www.google .com/url?sa=t&rct=j&q=&esrc=s&source=web&cd=1&cad=rja&uact =8&ved=0CCkQFjAA&url=http%3A%2F%2Fwww.mamasonbedrest .com%2Fwp-content%2Fuploads%2F2010%2F11%2FAMA-Resolution -204-Midwifery.doc&ei=zJJWVITWF8mgyASJv4GYAQ&usg=AFQjCNH 6u9QRGLPOkpTwI3L1WitYk-eEOg&sig2=Tau4kwiKM1vMRORFulYa _A&bvm=bv.78677474,d.aWw*.

American Medical Association House of Delegates. (2008). Resolution 214: Doctor of nursing practice. Retrieved from *svnnet.org/uploads/File/ AMAResolution214.doc*.

American Medical Association House of Delegates. (2008). Resolution 232 (formerly 303): Protection of the terms "doctor" "resident" and "residency." Retrieved from *www.healthy.net/Health/Essay/AMA_Escalates _Campaign_Against_Nurses_Chiropractors_Naturopaths_Midwives _and_Others/1001*.

American Nurses Association. (2011). Impaired nurse resource center. Retrieved from *www.nursingworld.org/MainMenuCategories/ WorkplaceSafety/Healthy-Work-Environment/Work-Environment/ ImpairedNurse*.

American Nurses Association, et al. v. Jack O'Connell, State Superintendent of Public Instruction, et al., (2008). California Superior Court, Judge Lloyd Connelly, No. 07AS04631.

American Nurses Association, et al. v. Tom Torlakson, 2013 Super. Ct. No. 07AS04631 filed August 12, 2013. Retrieved from *dredf.org/2013 -documents/S184583-ANA-decision.pdf*.

California Board of Registered Nursing. (2009). Insulin administration in public schools. Retrieved from *www.rn.ca.gov/pdfs/regulations/npr-i -38.pdf*.

Damgaard, G., Hohman, M., & Karpiuk, K. (2000). History of nursing regulation. Retrieved from *doh.sd.gov/boards/nursing/Documents/White PaperHistory2000.pdf*.

National Council of State Boards of Nursing [NCSBN]. (2012). APRN compact. Retrieved from *www.ncsbn.org/APRN_Compact_hx_timeline _April_2012_(2).pdf*.

United States Code. (2013). Title 42, chapter 7, subchapter XVIII, Part E, § 1395(bb): Effect of accreditation. Retrieved from *www.law.cornell.edu/ uscode/text/42/1395bb*.

U.S. Department of Health and Human Services [HSS]. (2013). About HHS. Retrieved from *www.hhs.gov/about*.

ONLINE RESOURCES

American Nurses Association
www.nursingworld.org
The National Council of State Boards of Nursing
www.ncsbn.org/index.htm
Nurses Service Organization
www.nso.com

CHAPTER 55

TAKING ACTION:

Nurse, Educator, and Legislator: My Journey to the Delaware General Assembly

Bethany Hall-Long

"I have come to the conclusion that politics are too serious a matter to be left to the politicians."

General Charles de Gaulle

MY POLITICAL ROOTS

I am a nurse and I became the first health care professional elected into the Delaware General Assembly, as well as the first registered nurse elected. The roots of my public service began in a farming community where I volunteered to help others in my church and at neighborhood organizations. At the age of 12, I was a candy-striper in a local hospital and continued my civic work during my teen years. When I entered college I joined a political party. Though my parents were not politically active, my great-grandfather was a member of the Delaware House of Representatives in the 1920s and I am a descendent of Delaware's 16th governor.

My interest in politics began while working with underserved residents at the same time I was completing my master's degree in community health nursing in the late 1980s. I used an earlier edition of this book in my graduate program and vividly recall reading the chapters about becoming involved in politics. I began working with my local city government, the League of Women Voters, and a federal health clinic that served the homeless. Before these experiences, I had thought that public policy was remote to nursing and somewhat dry. These experiences changed my perspective.

VOLUNTEERING AND CAMPAIGNING

I went on to volunteer with nonprofit and civic organizations, join professional associations, and to complete my doctoral degree in nursing administration and public policy. During this time, I served as a United States Senate Fellow and as a U.S. Department of Health and Human Services policy analyst for the Secretary's Commission on Nursing. These experiences exposed me to national policy work, federal officials, leaders in the nation's health associations, and international researchers. I became actively involved with veteran's organizations because my husband was on active duty in the military. I also became a volunteer on political campaigns with the Democratic Party. I had excellent mentors to assist me with both my nursing and political career paths. All of these experiences helped me to understand the policy process and the importance of building relationships.

I began my work in politics to make a difference in the lives of many citizens who lack life's necessary resources. As a public health nurse, I had an interest in improving the services available to vulnerable populations. I continue to work to advance issues important to the residents I represent. These include health care, the environment, land preservation, education, and economic development.

THERE'S A REASON IT IS CALLED "RUNNING" FOR OFFICE

A number of factors influenced my decision to run for public office in 2000, including my desire to make a significant contribution to the public's health. As a university faculty member, I assigned students to various public health and health policy assignments. During these experiences, I witnessed the need for expert health knowledge in the Delaware General Assembly. The time was ripe within the political party and within my district to run for the Delaware legislature. I ran for office for the first time in 2000 and lost by a mere 1%. I had run against a long-term, male incumbent and learned some important political lessons. In 2002, political redistricting left a vacant seat and I ran again. This time I won in a tough election against the president of the local school board. After serving 6 years in the House, I campaigned for, and won, a state senate race in 2008 (Figure 55-1).

A DAY IN THE LIFE OF A NURSE-LEGISLATOR

No two days in politics are alike. Each elected official's experiences and perceptions are linked to his or her beliefs, the district's beliefs, the state's legislative rules, and external economic or social pressures. In Delaware, serving as a legislator is a part-time job. Delaware's bicameral legislative session is active for a total of 45 days per year. Session convenes each January, and the legislature must pass the budget bill and recess by July 1. We meet three days a week: Tuesday, Wednesday, and Thursday. I spend the remaining days on

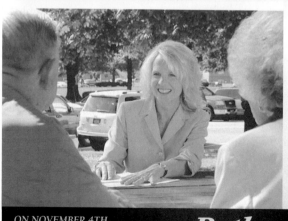

Homegrown leadership **with a real plan for** *change.*

Born and raised on a Delaware farm, Bethany Hall-Long's roots run deep in our state. As a nurse, a UD professor and a mother, Bethany understands the challenges facing Delaware's families. As our next State Senator, Bethany has a plan to improve the lives of Delaware's citizens – and the experience with proven results to make it happen.

ON NOVEMBER 4TH, give Delaware's families a strong voice in the State Senate.

www.hall-longforsenate.com

Bethany **HALL-LONG** **DEMOCRAT FOR STATE SENATE**

Paid for by the Committee to Re-Elect Bethany Hall-Long

FIGURE 55-1 Dr. Hall-Long's campaign literature identifies her as a nurse and educator.

constituent work, in meetings, delivering speeches, and conducting my job as a nursing faculty member. Between July and January, my days are filled with at least 8 to 12 hours of meetings, community work, and, in election years, campaign activities. On occasion, there are Special Sessions in the fall when the senate convenes.

Much of a state legislator's time is spent on the capital and operating budgets of the state, as well as handling senate confirmations. These activities need to be completed by the end of the state's fiscal year: July 1. My most important role is to represent my constituents at committee meetings, public hearings, on task forces, and as a sponsor or cosponsor of relevant bills. My district is both rural and suburban and has numerous policy needs: smart growth, transportation, education, health care, and economic development.

I juggle caring for my family, legislative work, and nursing education. I'm up at 5 AM to exercise and then I have breakfast meetings with constituents or campaign committee members. Following the meetings, I usually put on my other hat and spend time with my nursing students. I return phone calls in my car as I head into the state capital. When I arrive in my office, I'm greeted with phone messages, e-mail, and the pressing issues of the day. I share one staff member with another senator. Session begins around 2 PM when we enter caucus for 30 to 45 minutes to discuss the legislative agenda and bills to be voted upon. One day a week there are committee hearings. In the afternoons, I squeeze in more phone calls, RSVPs, research with the lawyers, and then head back to the floor for votes.

After each legislative day, there are usually receptions sponsored by interest groups. These provide time for lobbyists and members to review issues and concerns and highlight state funding efforts or programs. Typically, I attend several civic or association meetings each evening after the session in my district (I balance these with my son's sporting and school events.). These meetings are important for gathering community input, staying current on issues, and letting my constituents know that I am concerned about their issues. It all takes a lot of time, energy, and a few cups of coffee.

WHAT I'VE BEEN ABLE TO ACCOMPLISH AS A NURSE-LEGISLATOR

I have sponsored or cosponsored a range of legislation as a member of the house and senate: health, education, transportation, veteran's affairs, agriculture, natural resources and the environment, homeland security, community and county affairs, and insurance committees. As the only health care professional in the Delaware General Assembly, I have been the prime sponsor of some important health bills and on task forces such as the necessary code changes for the state's Health Exchange as a result of the federal Affordable Care Act *(www. heatlthcare.gov),* Governor's Cancer Council, and the Health Fund Advisory (Master Tobacco Settlement Committee). I have worked on many licensure/scope of practice and public health and environmental policies. These policy issues have included occupational health, substance abuse prevention and treatment, cancer, minority health, dental care access, health professions, environmental justice, chronic illness, mercury removal from the environment, school health, early childhood education, prescription assistance, and end-of-life care decisions. I have found that having a nursing background is extremely valuable in influencing a wide variety of policy issues.

I have worked very closely with the farmers in my district. I myself was raised on a farm, and my knowledge of farming has proved vital. I was pleased to sponsor, as my first piece of legislation, the farmland preservation license tag. In addition, I have sponsored land use legislation that helps with county, municipal, and state communication. Only 1% of the U.S. population consumes more than 20% of all health care expenditures, and 5% of the population accounts for more than 50% of the total expenditure (The National Institute for Health Care Management [NIHCM] Research and Educational Foundation Data Brief, 2012). Chronic illness is a major issue for Delaware, as it is for the nation. I sponsored legislation to establish a blue ribbon task force to analyze the problem of chronic illness in Delaware and to develop policy recommendations. The task force identified strategies including disease standards of care for health professions, improved communication between insurers and providers, outreach to the at-risk, and the use of a disease management approach with Medicaid patients and among the business community.

I was the prime sponsor of legislation creating a cancer consortium for Delaware. This group has completed a comprehensive assessment and plans to tackle our high cancer mortality rates. I am pleased to say that the cancer incidence and cancer rates have dropped since the creation of this body. The state has implemented the consortium's many recommendations, including establishing a free treatment program for cancer patients who lack insurance, adding statewide caseworkers, and creating screening programs. Recently, I was pleased to update the state's Indoor Tanning Laws to prohibit children under age 14 years from using tanning beds and for those aged 14 to 18 years to require parental consent.

HIV infection rates in Delaware are among the highest in the nation. Several years ago I cosponsored needle exchange legislation, and it has shown a positive impact on HIV infection rates. I was pleased to sponsor the legislation to create a state Office of Health and Safety for public programs. All these examples of sponsored legislation involve a team effort with other officials, individuals, lobbyists, and organizations or advocates.

TIPS FOR INFLUENCING ELECTED OFFICIALS' HEALTH POLICY DECISIONS

What have I learned as a legislator who can help other nurses who are seeking to influence policy? You must communicate well to influence policy, and nurses are naturally gifted communicators and problem solvers. In a study of nurse leaders in federal politics, I found that the political strategies used most frequently by nursing organizations are direct contacts, grassroots efforts, and coalition formation (Hall-Long, 1995). Nurses should not be intimidated by the need to call, write, or visit their elected officials. It is important when meeting with elected officials that you are prepared. Have a one-page fact sheet to leave behind (as opposed to a binder of information), and be prepared to summarize your issue and offer solutions in less than 5 minutes.

If nurses don't speak up on health care issues, who will? Physicians? Hospital associations? Insurers? If nurses don't speak up, legislators will only hear from other groups. Given health reform and a push for a nursing consensus model, advanced practice nurses are expected to take on a broader scope of practice and must be engaged in state-level policy discussions. You have heard the expression, "It's not whether you win or lose but how you play the game." Well, in politics, how you play the game can determine whether you win or lose an issue. Increasing your influence by working in a group or coalition is an extremely effective strategy.

IS IT WORTH IT?

Life as an elected official has been better than I could have imagined. Though it has taken some time away from my family and my scholarship, it has been worthwhile. I encourage other nurses to consider how they might serve the public, including running for elected office.

REFERENCES

Hall-Long, B. (1995). Nursing education at political crossroads. *Journal of Professional Nursing, 11*(3), 139–146.

The National Institute for Health Care Management [NIHCM] Research and Educational Foundation Data Brief. (2012). The concentration of health care spending. Retrieved from *www.nihcm.org/pdf/DataBrief3%20 Final.pdf.*

CHAPTER 56

Policy and Politics in Health Care Organizations

Sharon Pappas   Karren Kowalski   Erin M. Denholm

"We keep moving forward, opening new doors, and doing things because we're curious and curiosity keeps leading to new paths."

Walt Disney

New doors are opening for opportunities in health care. Incredible pressures are coming to bear on the traditional system as it fights off change. Some of these pressures are financial and are focused on payment or lack of payment for such things as readmission in less than 30 days or decreased payment for events that are sensitive to nursing care such as infections, falls, and readmissions. Other financial pressures come from bundled payments where a fixed payment must reimburse multiple providers for care across the continuum including acute, ambulatory, and postacute services. These all create an incredible opportunity for nursing to influence how health care organizations are being reshaped and redesigned. Much of the care is moving into the community, and mandates are focused on the engagement of patients and families in their own health promotion and chronic disease management. With the advent of Accountable Care Organizations (ACOs) the focus is on the continuum of care rather than acute episodes. The change in focus

demands that the traditional systems change, and change radically.

FINANCIAL PRESSURES FROM CHANGING PAYMENT MODELS

Some of the most immediate and visible changes seen are the intense financial pressures and their impact on providers. The financial pressures on hospitals and health care systems brought about by the Accountable Care Act (ACA) are significant. Although implementation of the ACA is expected to provide health coverage for an additional 36 million Americans, it would seem providers would be expanding services. However, multiple providers are responding to the financial pressures with major cost-reduction efforts, signifying the realities brought on by falling insurance payments and inpatient visits. Davidson and Hansen (2013) highlight the multiple reasons behind the declining revenue streams to hospitals including cuts in payment, shifts from inpatient to outpatient services, and movement of a large number of the baby boomer population into federal reimbursement programs and away from commercial insurance.

The federal budget cuts in Medicare and Medicaid can be classified into two categories: changes in payment rates and in payment methodology. Since

469

2010, Medicare and Medicaid payments for hospital services have been reduced by more than $121.9 billion (American Hospital Association, 2014). In addition to the rate changes, hospitals were faced with methodology changes that were implemented in 2008. The method changed from calculating reimbursement the same for all hospitals to reducing payment to hospitals that have lower quality, lower patient satisfaction, or high readmission rates. In 2013, Medicare cut payments to hospitals by 1.25% (The Medicare Payment Advisory Commission, 2013). They then redistributed the savings based on how hospitals performed on three measures: clinical standards, patient satisfaction, and mortality. It is estimated that around 1500 hospitals received reduced payments in this second year of Medicare's quality incentive program, called the Hospital Value-Based Purchasing (VBP) Program administered by the Centers for Medicare and Medicaid Services (CMS) (The Advisory Board Company, 2013).

In addition to changes in reimbursement rates, there is a shift from reimbursement for inpatient care to holding patients in observation and categorizing them as outpatients for 48 hours so a physician can decide if an individual is sick enough to be admitted. Although this designated observation status reduces reimbursement, no corresponding change in patient care requirements accompanies the reduced payment. Therefore, the cost of providing care is not reduced. Baugh and Schuur (2013) reported that the annual number of observation hours for Medicare beneficiaries nationally increased from 2006 to 2010 by almost 70%. Responses to these changes are acute and visible to health care providers, and, across the United States, many are activating major cost-cutting initiatives in response to the changes in revenue streams.

POLICY IMPLICATIONS FOR NURSING PRACTICE

Hospitals and health care systems are in a conundrum. In most hospitals, nursing labor costs are at least half of the overall labor budget, making nursing labor an appealing target for cost reduction. Clearly, nurses must optimize their economic relationship to hospitals by reporting the financial impact of effective nursing practice or nursing budgets will be subject to budget cuts. In a systematic review and meta-analysis, Kane and colleagues (2007) subsequently provided strong, consistent evidence that nurse staffing in hospitals plays a significant role in achieving improvements in quality and safety outcomes and in patient satisfaction. McHugh, Berez, and Small (2013) established that hospitals with higher nurse staffing had 25% fewer admission penalties. These data provided additional rationales for proceeding cautiously when considering nursing labor cost reduction as a solution to reduced revenue streams. Even with extensive research, it is difficult to set fixed standard registered nurse (RN) ratios. Every hospital and patient population is different. Establishing a standardized core staffing structure plus a mechanism to apply additional nursing resources that correspond to patient risk for adverse events or mortality could serve as a solution for improving outcomes. For example, hospitals with recurring central line-associated blood stream infections could put one third of the 1.25% withheld Medicare revenue at risk. Under a VBP approach (payment based on outcomes), nurses effectively managing these high-risk patients would prevent infections and thus capture full revenue.

Many nursing leaders support the fact that the ability to sustain good quality of care, and thus lowering costs, extends far beyond numbers of nurses. National and state efforts to legislate nurse staffing numbers only address one aspect of the prescription for achieving desired outcomes. These outcomes depend on adequate numbers of nurses and on work environments where better foundations for quality of care exist that emphasize professionalism and accountability. These foundations include nurse manager ability and support, collegial nurse-physician relationships, and the presence of RNs with BSN degrees, as summarized in the meta-analysis by Kane and colleagues (2007). The convergence of these health care changes amid a national shift from using patient value (good quality and lower costs) instead of volume as determinants of success stimulates the opportunity for policy and regulatory change. Successful hospitals have adequate staffing and high-quality work environments, as found in magnet facilities. McHugh Berez, and Small (2013) summarize this nicely when they call for policy that rewards care environments that are sufficiently staffed and resourced to allow clinicians to do their work most effectively.

BEYOND ACUTE CARE

Advancing health care system accountability beyond the acute phase is also a significant adjustment that requires change. The growing popularity of single payments for services across acute and postacute settings implicates and depends on nurses to achieve patient activation and engagement in ways that yield better patient outcomes through adherence to mutually agreed-upon treatment regimens. Porter and Lee (2013) outline a multitier hierarchy for achieving successful management of patient value. Figure 56-1 displays these tiers. Tier 1 outcomes describe health status achieved or retained in the immediate phase of recovery. Tier 2 outcomes capture the continuing process of

recovery. Tier 3 outcomes address the sustainability of health and the nature of recurrences of problem or disease and long-term consequences of therapy. The first tier is the historical focus of acute care, with tiers 2 and 3 addressing new territories that are essential for providing patient value and are a significant tenet of nursing practice. Achievement of tier 1 outcomes is the priority and basis of measurement of effective nurse staffing through hours per patient day (HPPD). To branch into tier 2, acute care registered nurse (RN) roles must encompass care coordination functions, which require more RNs. Regulators such as The Joint Commission and the CMS must expand their regulatory descriptions of acute inpatient nursing to assure that there is adequate RN staffing to assume a greater role in care coordination.

Similar to the importance of evaluating the long-term effects of acute care, the school health programs deserve similar analysis. The cost cuts in school nurse program support cannot be celebrated

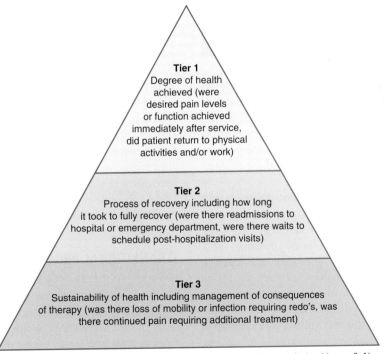

FIGURE 56-1 Outcomes that matter to patients. (From Porter, M. [2010]. What is value in health care? *New England Journal of Medicine, 363*[26], 2477-2481.)

as a short-term gain, but must be supported by policy to analyze the downstream impact of staff reductions. It is estimated that at least one third of school-age children have developed risk factors for heart disease and diabetes that could be modified by focused health education from an on-site school nurse. From an interview with a school nurse leader from a southeastern state (G. H. Chambers, personal communication, December 27, 2013), there are around 1.5 million school-age children; at least 13% are without health care insurance coverage; and one third have chronic health conditions. The state has funded a ratio of 1690 regular education students to only one school nurse for the entire state. The national ratio is 750:1. This exhibits a significant missed opportunity that likely exists in many states across the nation.

A common theme across multiple settings of patient care is the reduction of providers to achieve a desired financial impact. This myopic approach must be guided by political efforts to require robust measurement of the impact of these structural changes on consumers.

THE BROADENING INFLUENCE OF OUTCOME ACCOUNTABILITY

The very nature of health care provision is changing with the disruptive forces of the ACA. The ACA has spurred three foci: reduced payments, accountability and quality, and new models of care. These disruptions are creating space for innovation and improved health. Payment models, as the incisive driver of disruption, have catapulted these changes into clinical practice.

Methods of reduced payment such as no reimbursement for hospital-acquired conditions (HACs) and VBP have driven new, more rigorous compliance with evidence-based practices and standardization. The accountability and quality focus have rendered penalties for such things as 30-day readmissions for key diagnoses, HACs, and lack of meaningful use (automated documentation). Remarkably, this has ignited care coordination activities across the traditional silos of care in unprecedented ways. The new models of care, including the patient-centered medical home, have

been adopted in the ambulatory setting. At the same time, ACOs and bundling of care across the continuum have notably influenced the scope of nursing practice. The Office of the Surgeon General's National Prevention Strategy (2011) describes new models using prevention science more applicably to improve the health of individuals and populations in pursuit of decreasing total cost of care. This type of national focus and influence begins to shift our traditional focus on sick care to wellness and preventative care.

In addition to patient-centered care and prevention science, consumer engagement has become an essential element of effective care that has increased the availability and accessibility of resources for patients who are demanding different approaches to patient education (motivational interviewing, use of social media, portals, and gameology). Consumer-driven demands as well as evolving science have accelerated the disruption, also causing major change. Hospital centrism no longer works with these new influences in play. ACA requirements for nonprofit hospitals to conduct community health needs assessments with an accompanying improvement plan calls for expanded competency in consumer engagement, measurement, and improvement. Outcome metrics that transcend sites of care and focus more fully on the overall health status of the patient and the community in which they reside, and the most efficient use of resources, are driving changes in regulation and policy. The use of telemonitoring equipment is a prime example whereby state and federal regulations have had to change to guide remote/virtual providers in supporting people living with chronic illness to achieve their active engagement in maintaining their optimal level of wellness in their home setting.

TRANSITIONAL PROGRAMMING— SUCCESSES AND OPPORTUNITIES

Historically, there have been three domains of care that have acted independently and in isolation of each other. Ambulatory, acute, and postacute care arenas have had separate and unique standards of care, regulations, and metrics that have been developed and audited from both public and private sectors. As a result, an evidence base for a cross-continuum best practice is lacking. There is an increasing focus on delivering high-quality care at the lowest cost, and in some payment models, such as bundling, singular reimbursement is provided for preacute, acute, and postacute episodic care. It is in this context that transitional programming has become a popular solution. Multiple studies have shown that specific handoffs and transition activities produce improved patient compliance and decreased readmissions.

Regulatory bodies, including the CMS, The Joint Commission, and others, have developed targeted transitional care standards and regulations that all sites of care now must address. The Transitions of Care Portal (The Joint Commission, 2014) is a good source of education for this advancement. With penalties for 30-day readmissions for the top chronic illnesses, the proliferation of care models that address these transitions has been growing. The future position of the National Quality Forum (NQF) is to enable, through health care technology, the use of care plan data communicated during transitions of care (e.g., problems/diagnoses, interventions/orders, and expected outcomes/goals) for quality measurement (National Quality Forum, 2012b).

An example of cross-setting management is the seminal work of Mary Naylor, PhD, RN (Naylor et al., 1994) and Eric Coleman, MD (Coleman, 2007) on care transitions. Although there is no standardized definition of transitions of care, many studies are galvanizing best practice with documented benefits of interventions that occur at the time of acute care discharge to other sites of care. The simple processes of establishing a follow-up primary care office visit, performing medication reconciliation, and making sure patients have filled their prescriptions has provided compelling data regarding the importance these efforts have on readmissions. Additionally, communicating directly with primary care providers regarding acute care stays as part of effective transition activities has enabled the providers in the ambulatory setting to reconcile the care plan.

Optimizing postacute care (home care, skilled nursing facilities, palliative care, and long-term acute care services) is paramount in ultimately supporting improved quality at the lowest cost. Home care profoundly impacts the efficacy of transitions as they receive referrals from other sites of care and often are responsible for conveying information among and between other providers. Supporting patients discharged from the hospital with a high risk for readmissions has challenged all providers, acute and postacute care, to innovate services for these patients that prevent readmission. The services that have been found to reduce readmissions include standardized discharge planning, home visits, coaching, and remote monitoring (Naylor et al., 2011). Acute care providers and physicians in the ambulatory setting are looking to partner with centers of excellence that can provide the clinical acumen and competency that address patient complexity to prevent penalties. Thus, they produce success under reimbursement models that cover a spectrum of care across the continuum.

EMERGING NEW MODELS

New models of care have developed within the postacute settings, such as telemonitoring. The home care setting has eagerly adopted this innovation with increasing frequency, as evidence is showing outcomes that include decreased 30-day hospital readmissions and improved health habits for those living with chronic illness. Telephonic monitoring provides the ability to collect objective clinical findings remotely and to respond immediately with appropriate nursing interventions without patients leaving their homes. The use of risk assessment tools enables acute care providers to identify who would best be served by this technology. Skilled nursing facilities that do not have 24-hour medical coverage can also use telemonitoring to strengthen their clinical competence through remote access to more skilled providers.

With more organizations participating in ACOs, population health is a term that has been coined for supporting individuals in a specific group that employs prevention science as its care model. This is a manifestation of moving from sick care to well care. With the financial incentives aligned to share cost savings for the defined population, well care strategies are now frequently employed to prevent hospital admissions and high cost interventions. With the use of risk stratification tools, ambulatory and postacute providers intervene with patients who have high predictive scores for hospitalization. The National Quality Forum (2012b) has established these measures. Acute care providers also conduct screenings. As an example, emergency room providers are changing to more fully address patients' long-term needs beyond the emergent chief complaint. This evolving paradigm expands the knowledge of this continuum of care and provides for the opportunity for research focused on the new standards and metrics. Research funding is essential to test and ensure effectiveness of these innovations.

In 2011, one in four nursing home residents was hospitalized, costing the Medicare program $14.3 billion. As an agent of the Office for Inspector General (OIG), Levinson (2013) published the rates of hospitalization and recommended new measures to track acute care admissions from nursing homes. The nursing home that provides postacute care will be forced to use these same risk assessment tools and proactive interventions to decrease their readmission rates. A 2013 Medicare Payment Advisory Commission (MedPAC) report noted a 5% annual growth in expenditures for postacute care (The Medicare Payment Advisory Commission, 2013). This prompted the CMS to test new payment methods that reimburse hospitals and postacute care in a lump sum instead of paying separately.

The NQF has undertaken the task of providing multistakeholder guidance on priorities for performance measurement under contract with the U.S. Department of Health and Human Services. Consistent with the Triple Aim (Institute for Healthcare Improvement, 2012), these measures are in support of quality improvement and better health at lower cost. The areas that have been identified for performance measurement include: adult immunization, Alzheimer's disease and dementia care, and care coordination. In 2012, the NQF published outcome measures for cross-continuum care coordination that compelled all sites of care to participate in transitional care programming (National Quality Forum, 2012a). Connecting patients functionally within the health care system without redundancy and with sharp communication among and between providers is essential to these measures.

As wellness care takes on greater significance in the coming years, policy and standards will continue to evolve. The implications for nurses' academic preparation and scope of practice are vast and require nursing leaders to take charge in imagining future possibilities.

A DOOR OPENS—POLICY TO SUPPORT THE ROLE OF THE NURSE PRACTITIONER

One of the opportunities from the ACA implementation has evolved in both the acute care setting and the patient continuum. In both situations, access to care is a key factor in addressing the issues presented in the significant increase in the numbers of insured patients. Consequently, new opportunities have opened for advanced practice nurses as a result of the cost restructuring, the changes in medical practice, and physician employment by hospitals. Not only is the need for nurse practitioners (NPs) increasing in primary care, the need for NPs working in acute care with hospitalists and in specialty services such as cardiology and cardiac surgery is also increasing. NPs are working in the emergency department screening patients and providing care for those who do not really need to see the physician. They are responsible for both quality and value to the patients. Some NPs who work in a specialty service may follow patients in clinics or the physician's office as well as in acute care and postacute care. NPs are employed by insurance companies to follow residents in long-term care, and reports indicate that NPs work in conjunction with the nursing personnel in these facilities more closely than physicians can.

At the same time, the need for NPs has significantly increased in ambulatory settings. One aspect of disruptive innovations in health care, as described by Christensen, Flier, and Vijayaraghavan (2013), has led to NPs working in retail clinics where they see patients with complaints, such as respiratory infections and bladder infections, and they treat these patients, often under protocol. In addition, some of the retail clinics have collaborative agreements with major medical facilities in which they follow patients with chronic illnesses and refer back to physicians as needed. It is convenient to see the NP while shopping for groceries at the grocery store. Christensen, Flier, and Vijayaraghavan (2013), in a *Wall Street Journal* op-ed piece, described this innovation as low cost, whereas similar care in a hospital or major physician practice is high cost with no evidence that it is better care. In fact, the Federally Qualified Health Centers (FQHCs) employ NPs as they are more cost-effective than physicians, who are very difficult to recruit and retain. The quality of the care delivered has been thoroughly researched and found to be equal or in some cases exceed that which is delivered by physicians (Newhouse et al., 2011). Although all health care sectors respond to these disruptions, Pappas (2014) encourages traditional nursing practice to reprogram our "professional DNA" to migrate to an accountability for consumer requirements across all health care settings. For example, in an ACO, one nurse might be responsible for the patient's care before acute care admission, following discharge, and for ongoing health maintenance. Historically, nursing is practiced in silos addressing patient needs whether patients are seeking solutions, interventions, or long-term management. Evolving nursing practice to universally adopt competencies and accountabilities across ambulatory, acute, and postacute settings will require innovation, increased use of technology, and designs that best meet consumer and community needs.

In addition, productivity and patient satisfaction increase when wait times are decreased. It has become clear that clinics can employ two NPs for the cost of one physician, thus increasing the ratio of providers to patients. NPs also understand working in interprofessional teams, and these teams have been strongly emphasized in the new ACOs. Many doctors have discovered that NPs are, in fact, a bargain as they support the practice by seeing patients but also take a nursing perspective on prevention and care coordination with many patients. Added to this broader scope of practice, nurse-managed clinics are gaining in popularity because

they are well run and have very good outcomes (Auerbach et al., 2013).

One concern is the differences in the scope of practice of NPs from state to state. States vary significantly in what is allowed in NP practice. A major focus of the Institute of Medicine's (IOM's) *The Future of Nursing* report (2011) is that all nurses be able to practice at the full scope of their education and training; however, the current emphasis is on allowing NPs to practice to the full scope of their education and preparation. This effort was identified nationally by the National Council of State Boards of Nursing (NCSBN). In 2008, the NCSBN created a consensus model for advanced practice registered nurses (APRN) regulation (Cahill, Alexander, & Gross, 2014; Madler, Kalanek, & Rising, 2012; Phillips, 2014). The key elements of the consensus model for APRN practice are outlined in Box 56-1. The goal was that all states would enact these principles and would consequently be similar across state settings by 2015. That does not seem

---

BOX 56-1 Consensus Model Elements

- Title: Advanced practice registered nurse (APRN).
- Roles of APRNs and recognition of each: CNP, CNS, CRNA, CNM.
- Licensure: APRNs hold both an RN and APRN license.
- Education: Graduate education is required for APRNs regardless of role.
- Certification: Every APRN is required to meet advanced certification requirements.
- Independent practice: The APRN shall be granted full authority to practice independently without physician oversight or a written collaborative agreement.
- Full prescriptive authority: The APRN shall be granted full prescriptive authority without physician oversight or a written collaborative agreement.

CNM, Certified nurse midwife; *CNP,* certified nurse practitioner; *CNS,* clinical nurse specialist; *CRNA,* certified registered nurse anesthetist.
From Cahill, M., Alexander, M., & Gross, L. (2014). The 2014 NCSBN consensus report on APRN regulation. *Journal of Nursing Regulation, 4*(4), 5-12.

likely. However, progress is being made. North Dakota changed the state regulation in 2011. Other states are attempting to follow the consensus model. For those interested in the health policy and legislative aspects of changing such laws, Madler, Kalanek, & Rising (2012) have outlined a process that works in the political arena. The state nurse practitioner association began this process with support from the state board of nursing (BON). The next step was to select the right legislator to sponsor the bill, and the one chosen had a history of work on health-related legislation and was well respected. Then, this group chose a well-respected lobbyist, an attorney who had worked with the BON and had vast experience in governmental regulation, health law, and professional issues. The NP group and the lobbyists dedicated extensive time at the legislature talking to representatives, answering questions, and building coalitions. They had strong data from the BON describing the scarcity of disciplinary issues and the national data supporting this same trend (Miller, 2013). Testimony for the bill was prepared and delivered by four NPs and representatives from the BON. With this careful planning and execution of a sound strategy, the bill passed. Furthermore, Madler, Kalanek, and Rising (2012) provided several recommendations regarding changing the laws (Box 56-2). These changes are essential to ensuring transformation of the health care system to facilitate access to care for the patient populations.

BOX 56-2 Recommendations for Changing Nurse Practitioner Law

1. Be patient. Be resilient and committed to the project; occasionally incremental change is required versus radical change.
2. Promote and maintain transparency. Professional associations and advocacy groups must be open and educate all stakeholders including the opposition. Meet with adversaries and stakeholders throughout the process.
3. Create partnerships. Potential partners are not only nursing organizations but other organizations interested in such issues as access to care. Some of these possible partners include organizations such as AARP, federally qualified health centers, groups interested in the underserved, and rural health care associations.
4. Form alliances between nursing organizations and these other groups who are interested in access to care.
5. Cultivate relationships. Be mindful of respectful approaches with groups having opposing points of view.
6. Focus the message. The message must be clear and consistent in all communications. Communication professionals can help with this effort. What is the elevator speech that can convey the message?

From Madler, B., Kalanek, C., & Rising, C. (2012). An incremental regulatory approach to implementing the APRN consensus model. *Journal of Nursing Regulation, 3*(3), 11-15.

CONCLUSION

Nurses at all levels must have the ability to articulate the clinical and financial impact they bring to patients and consumers. In nursing practice settings, nurses must focus beyond the activities they perform to demonstrate the impact of nursing care on patient outcomes. Nurses must also be open to innovations in the delivery of care especially across traditional silos. Professional nurses need to be open to the impact of technology, such as telehealth, on the health maintenance of patients. Each year, more nurses express interest in advance practice roles and how these roles improve patient outcomes. Innovations in the use of these advanced practice nurses will significantly increase the effectiveness of the care provided.

DISCUSSION QUESTIONS

1. What competencies and capabilities do nurses need to optimize their economic relationship with health care organizations?
2. How do transition models impact acute care nursing processes and mental models?
3. What role do professional organizations play in developing these new models?
4. How should nurses assure policy change for advanced practice registered nurses?

REFERENCES

The Advisory Board Company. (2013). The daily briefing: Nearly 1,500 hospitals get penalties based on quality. Retrieved from *www.advisory.com/Daily-Briefing/2013/11/18/Nearly-1500-hospitals-get-penalties-based-on-quality*.

American Hospital Association. (2014). The financial state of U.S. hospitals. Retrieved from *www.aha.org/content/14/fs-financialstate.pdf*.

Auerbach, D., Chen, P. G., Friedberg, M. W., Reid, R., Lau, C., Buerhaus P. I., et al. (2013). Nurse-managed health centers and patient-centered medical homes could mitigate expected primary care physician shortage. *Health Affairs, 32*(11), 1933–1941.

Baugh, C., & Schuur, J. (2013). Observation care—High-value care or a cost-shifting loophole? *New England Journal of Medicine, 369*(4), 302–305.

Cahill, M., Alexander, M., & Gross, L. (2014). The 2014 NCSBN consensus report on APRN regulation. *Journal of Nursing Regulation, 4*(4), 5–12.

Christensen, C., Flier, J., & Vijayaraghavan, V. (2013, February 18). Opinion: The coming failure of 'accountable care.' *Wall Street Journal.* Retrieved from *online.wsj.com/news/articles/SB10001424127887324880504578296902005944398*.

Coleman, E. (2007). The care transitions program. Retrieved from *www.caretransitions.org*.

Davidson, P., & Hansen, B. (2013, October 13). A job engine sputters as hospitals cut staff. *USA Today,* Retrieved from *www.usatoday.com/story/money/business/2013/10/13/hospital-job-cuts/2947929/*.

Institute for Healthcare Improvement. (2012). The IHI Triple Aim. Retrieved from *www.ihi.org/Engage/Initiatives/TripleAim/Pages/default.aspx*.

Institute of Medicine. (2011). *The future of nursing: Leading change, advancing health.* Washington, DC: National Academy of Sciences. Retreived from *www.iom.edu/nursing*.

The Joint Commission. (2014). Transitions of care portal. Retrieved from *www.jointcommission.org/toc.aspx*.

Kane, R. L., Shamliyan, T. A., Mueller, C., Duval, S., & Wilt, T. J. (2007). The associate of registered nurse staffing levels and patient outcomes systematic review and meta-analysis. *Medical Care, 45*(12), 1195–1204.

Levinson, D. (2013). Medicare nursing home resident hospitalization rates merit additional monitoring. Retrieved from *oig.hhs.gov/reports-and-publications/archives/semiannual/2014/sar-s14-web-final.pdf*.

Madler, B., Kalanek, C., & Rising, C. (2012). An incremental regulatory approach to implementing the APRN consensus model. *Journal of Nursing Regulation, 3*(3), 11–15.

McHugh, M., Berez, J., & Small, D. (2013). Hospitals with higher nurse staffing had lower odds of readmissions penalties that hospitals with lower staffing. *Health Affairs, 32*(10), 1740–1747.

The Medicare Payment Advisory Commission. (2013). Testimony: Medicare post-acute care reforms. Retrieved from *www.medpac.gov/documents/congressional-testimony/20130614_wandm_testimony_pac.pdf?sfvrsn=0*.

Miller, K. (2013). The National Practitioner Data Bank: An annual update. *The Journal of Nurse Practitioners, 9*(9), 576–580.

National Prevention Strategy. (2011). Economic benefits of preventing disease. Retrieved from *www.surgeongeneral.gov/initiatives/prevention/strategy/appendix1.pdf*.

National Quality Forum. (2012a). Endorsement summary care coordination measures. Retrieved from *www.qualityforum.org/News_And_Resources/Endorsement_Summaries/Endorsement_Summaries.aspx*.

National Quality Forum. (2012b). Population health endorsement maintenance: Phase II technical report. Retrieved from *www.qualityforum.org/Publications/2012/12/Population_Health_Endorsement_Maintenance__Phase_II_Technical_Report.aspx*.

Naylor, M., Aiken, L., Kurtzman, E., Olds, D. M., & Hirschman, K. B. (2011). The importance of transitional care in achieving health reform. *Health Affairs, 30*(4), 746–754.

Naylor, M., Brooten, D., Jones, R., Lavizzo-Mourey, R., Mezey, M., & Pauly, M. (1994). Comprehensive discharge planning for the hospitalized elderly: A randomized clinical trial. *Annals of Internal Medicine, 120*(12), 999–1006.

Newhouse, R., Stanik-Hutt, J., White, K., Johantgen, M., Bass, E., Zangaro G., et al. (2011). Advanced practice nurse outcomes 1990-2008: A systematic review. *Nursing Economics, 29*(5), 230–251.

Pappas, S. (2014). Disruptive innovation and nursing. *VOICE of Nursing Leadership, 12*(1), 4–5.

Phillips, S. (2014). 26th annual legislative update: Progress for APRN authority to practice. *The Nurse Practitioner, 39*(1), 29–52.

Porter, M. (2010). What is value in health care? *New England Journal of Medicine, 363*(26), 2477–2481.

Porter, M., & Lee, T. (2013). The strategy that will fix health care. *Harvard Business Review, October 2013,* 50–70.

ONLINE RESOURCES

Centers for Medicare and Medicaid Services
www.cms.gov
Institute of Healthcare Improvement
www.ihi.org
The Joint Commission
www.jointcommission.org
National Association of School Nurses
www.nasn.org
National Council of State Boards of Nursing
www.ncsbn.org
National Quality Forum
www.qualityforum.org

UNIT 4

CHAPTER 57

TAKING ACTION:
Nurse Leaders in the Boardroom

Linda Burnes Bolton Catherine Alicia Georges Rita Wray

"Learn the craft of how to open your heart and to turn on your creativity. There's a light inside of you."

Judith Jamison

Nurses have always been amenable to opening their hearts to help others. Today it is important that they build on that willingness to be of use to humankind by turning on their creativity to lead the changes required to achieve a better life for all. The land-mark study from the Institute of Medicine (IOM) (2011) titled *The Future of Nursing* called for nurses to expand their contributions to improving our nation's health through leadership. Nurses have the knowledge and expertise regarding the demand for and resources needed to meet the health and human services needs of the United States. It is our legacy and one that we must commit to advancing if we are to achieve the recommendations from multiple reports on what will it take to improve the human condition.

Currently, only 0.8% of nurses in the United States serve on hospital boards and only 2.3% serve on community health system boards, compared with 5.1% and 22.61% of physicians, respectively (IOM, 2011). Stepping up to the challenges of today and the future requires us to be present when deci-sions are made about the allocation of resources, creation or closure of health and social services pro-grams, jobs, education, arts, music, business, and finance.

GETTING STARTED

There are many pathways to serving on govern-ing bodies, including appointments, winning an election, and volunteering. Regardless of the pathway, it is important that you let others know you are interested in a board position.

A first step that has proven successful for the authors is to volunteer to serve on local boards, including professional organizations. Leadership is a practiced art and the best way to prepare for a board position is to begin as a volunteer.

Second, you should follow your passion. Seek board positions around issues that are important to you. The more you care about an issue, the more likely you will be to seek opportunities that can enable you to make a difference on the issue. For example, our passion for seeking to eliminate health disparities, improve access to education for ethnic minorities, and provide access to information to improve health led us to pursue leadership roles in organizations with health and educational mis-sions. The types of organizations ranged from Part-nership for a Drug Free America to serving as trustees of universities.

Third, you should be prepared to lead. Programs such as Best on Board and the Robert Wood Johnson Foundation's Nurse Executive Fellows program provide necessary knowledge and skill acquisition. Serving on the American Hospital Association's Equity of Care Committee enabled one of the authors to promote nurse engagement in the hospital trustee program that prepares people to serve on hospital boards. Several nurses have been placed on hospital boards after completing this program. Many nursing and health care orga-nizations have programs to support nurses acquir-ing board positions.

Nurses can and must seek appointments outside of the health care facilities and organizations. City and county Chambers of Commerce, housing

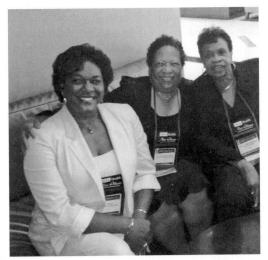

FIGURE 57-1 Leaders in action: authors Rita Wray, Linda Burnes-Bolton, and Catherine Alicia Georges.

programs, and neighborhood watch organizations play important roles in addressing the social determinants of health for communities. Nurses can influence the provision of services for individuals and communities by serving locally.

The following sections describe some of our individual experiences with serving in these leadership positions.

RITA'S JOURNEY

In my experience, nurses bring a unique perspective to board service, whether it is visioning, strategic planning, bringing nursing's values to policymaking, or attention to fiduciary matters. Nurses also make excellent leaders and decision makers, whether as executive leaders in health systems and hospitals, professional organizations, businesses, universities, or government, because of their academic preparation, work experience, and professional expertise. Nurses use a lens of human caring and patient-centeredness when making decisions, whether on behalf of an individual, population, or an organization.

The leadership skills learned in the classroom and honed in the clinical and academic settings are the same skills needed to serve effectively on

health care related and non-health care related boards and commissions; it is merely a transference and translation of core leader skills combined with a deep sense of commitment, experience, and expertise.

My professional clinical career track includes bedside nurse, nurse educator, nurse executive, nurse entrepreneur, and business owner with cumulative leadership skills that I have found highly transferrable in my role as a state government executive, as well as in-service on multiple boards and commissions. Many of those skills were cultivated, recognized, and used within nursing circles as the nursing process, the essential core of practice for registered nurses to deliver holistic patient-focused care. It requires each situation to be assessed by use of a systematic, dynamic way of collecting and analyzing data; creating a plan developed with critical thinking and crucial conversations; and implementing the plan with sound bridge building and evaluation. With demonstrated knowledge, ability, candor, and tact, I begin with acknowledging the value all bring to the table by actively listening and data gathering (assessing), solidifying the task (planning), engaging bridge builders, and getting the job done (implementing). After group engagement and buy-in is obtained, I close with my trademark charge: "Let's do this." For example, as president of the Greater Jackson Arts Council, the official cultural arm for both city and tourists, I led the board through a visioning exercise where we discerned the need for developing a signature sustainable event (assess). Through our grants program we chose to create new stories with neighborhood associations, emerging artists, community leaders, and major art providers such as museums, symphony, opera, ballet, and theater companies (plan). Begun in 2006, the Storytellers Ball invites all to be a part of the story. It is not only a successful annual fundraiser but is also a dynamic way of highlighting the importance of arts and culture in schools and communities within the capital city (implement).

Examples such as these were fundamental stepping stones to my passion for visioning and strategic planning, an essential need of boards and commissions whose charge is to take a concept

UNIT 4

to reality through the planning and implementation stages. These translatable core skills—data collection and analysis, communication, teamwork, planning, goal setting, and ascertaining effectiveness—honed early in my career prepared me to serve in board leadership positions and enriched my diverse career path.

A snapshot of my board and commission experience is varied and has included professional organizations (National Black Nurses Association, treasurer; and Mississippi Action Coalition, co-lead), private business entities (The Capital Club, president of a 1500-member private business club known for its social and cultural prominence in the capital city of Mississippi; treasurer of the Junior League of Jackson Sustainers Board, an organization of women committed to promoting volunteerism, developing the potential of women, and improving communities through the effective action and leadership of trained volunteers), political organizations (Mississippi Federation of Republican Women, president), religious organizations (National Advisory Council for the U.S. Catholic Bishops, vice chairperson; and Parish Pastoral Council, president), community organizations (Greater Jackson Arts Council, president; and Community Foundation of Greater Jackson, strategic planning committee chairperson), charitable organizations (Susan G. Komen Foundation, president of the Steel Magnolia Chapter; and the American Red Cross, chapter strategic development co-chairperson), and a gubernatorial appointee (Mississippi Commission on the Status of Women, commissioner).

The common thread for all of my board and commission service is an identified passion with the board's vision and mission; placement in a marketable pool for consideration when skills in communication, decision making, management, and leadership are sought; and investment in credible mentors or sponsors, all of whom were chosen because they were accomplished leaders with a track record of succeeding. These circumstances are then matched with my time, talent, and treasure (making financial contributions or otherwise raising money for the organization) to the board's mission-driven goals.

Health care reform is shaping board discussions about governance effectiveness and resource allocation based upon an understanding of patient and community needs. Additionally, non-health care boards are appointing highly respected and experienced nursing leaders to strengthen governance discussions. Skills and attributes such as broad-spectrum credibility, awareness of community needs, and an ability to identify and solve problems will not only bring nurses to the board table but also allow them to ascend as leaders.

If a seat at the boardroom table is your goal, start today to position yourself to be an effective board member and leader. I encourage you to use Rita Wray's Building Blocks of Board Service:

- Identify your passion.
- Network in health care and non-health care settings.
- Educate yourself on governance issues related to your targeted board or commission, as well as board roles and responsibilities often found in an organization's literature.
- Hone, master, and then market your transferable and translatable core leadership skills.
- Locate a sponsor—an influential current or previous board member, a member of the nominating committee, or an appointing authority—to facilitate your entry to board membership.
- Once the board seat is attained, tackle intriguing situations. For example, as a board member (from 2007 to 2013) and the appointed chairperson of the Strategic Planning Committee (from 2010 to 2013), I led a national search for the CEO of the Community Foundation of Greater Jackson, an organization which holds almost 200 charitable funds and endowments and invested more than $20 million in the community between 1998 and 2013.

Take the initiative and prepare yourself to become an effective leader on various boards and commissions. One initiative I found exceedingly beneficial for board development was through my community (and later state) Chamber of Commerce involvement. In 1987, as the first African-American Director of Nursing of a 500+ bed hospital in the state of Mississippi, I was one of 40 emerging and existing leaders selected in our metro area to participate in the Leadership Jackson inaugural program. The program is designed to educate participants about major community issues and alternate approaches to solutions to community problems. Participants sharpen their leadership skills while gaining a better understanding of various aspects of the community, including forums on politics, education, the legal system, health care, government, and economics.

Make a habit of succeeding; the benefits of board service will far outweigh the responsibilities!

ALICIA'S JOURNEY

Getting appointed or elected to a board is not an accident. My journey to being elected to the Board of Directors of the American Association of Retired Persons (AARP) in 2010 for a 6-year term started a number of years ago.

As a graduate student at New York University, I took an elective course in urban planning and development. One of the assignments was to attend a community meeting and to ascertain how decisions were made in such areas as infrastructure projects and zoning policies that would have a potential impact on community development. The first obstacle was to gain access to the community board meeting. After many barriers and challenges to my right to be present at such meetings, I finally got an invitation to attend the community board meeting in my district as a silent observer. What I observed was the vested interests of board members being politically played out during the meeting. Decisions about projects being considered were defined by political affiliations. There was no opportunity for community groups to have their voices heard. I left that meeting perplexed and disappointed in the process.

A few years later the New York City (NYC) charter was revised and gave communities an opportunity to influence the local governance process. There was a call for those interested in serving on boards to complete an application and submit it to the borough president in one's own borough. There are five boroughs in NYC and mine was the Bronx. My application was clearly delineated with my specific knowledge and skills. I had to undergo a series of interviews, culminating in a brief and final interview with the Bronx borough president. I was supported by my city councilperson and selected by the borough president for the appointment. I served on that board for 18 years and was reappointed by three borough presidents.

During my tenure on that board, I served as secretary, vice chair, and eventually chairperson. As a board member and an officer, I needed to be able to interact with diverse community groups, nongovernmental organizations, governmental agencies, and elected and appointed policymakers. Being aware of the issues and having data to support requests for capital and expensive projects were critical factors in being heard by the policymakers and getting projects funded. Understanding public budgets and being able to interact with the financial experts in the city agencies became a necessary skill. Problem solving, negotiation, and conflict resolution were paramount in being an effective community board member.

At the same time that I was participating as a member of the local community board, I also became very active in the local chapter of the National Black Nurses Association (NBNA). Using the experience and skills gained at the community board level, I was able to demonstrate to the members of the NBNA that I could serve as a board member, an officer, and eventually the president of the Association. During the periods of time that I served on the community board and the board of the NBNA, I attended various seminars and conferences to expand my knowledge of board governance, improve my performance as a board member, and network with board members from other organizations. These connections with other board nominating committees gave me the opportunity to serve on other boards, such as CGFNS International, a credentialing organization for internationally educated nurses and other selected health professionals, and in 2010 to be elected to the Board of Directors of the AARP.

As a member of a community board, a professional nursing organization, and the world's largest consumer organization, I have learned that being a board member requires:

- Being knowledgeable about the issues that the board will have to confront

UNIT 4

- Being committed to the mission and vision of the organization
- Thinking critically as a board member
- Acting strategically
- Understanding governance policies of the board
- Willingness to speak out on issues because they are socially just
- Always being prepared and having substantive information to share with board members when a contentious issue arises

My journey as a board member on these various boards has been challenging but exciting. I encourage nurses to undertake this journey to board service.

ARE YOU READY?

Ask yourself:

- What is my driving purpose for wanting to serve on a board?
- What am I willing to do to accomplish my purpose?
- What am I willing to give up so I will have the time and energy to fully engage in the work of the governing team?
- What knowledge must I acquire to be prepared for board service?
- What experiences must I have to prepare myself for the next level on boards outside of health care?
- Who can I seek out for mentoring and kitchen cabinet advice?
- What do I have to contribute and how do I maximize that contribution?

Nurses are valuable members of society with knowledge and experience about how to get things accomplished, motivate individuals, and engage diverse voices in efforts to design the best solutions for a variety of problems. On your leadership journey you should seek out progressive leadership positions with increasing responsibilities. Start by volunteering to chair a committee or task force.

Demonstrate your ability to make significant contributions. Let others know you are willing to serve. Board leadership requires a broad knowledge base about many topics beyond nursing. You must be willing to assume a role of posing questions that generate ideas for others to consider. You must have the ability to promote disruptive innovation while understanding the potential consequences of all board decisions.

Become a societal leader. Commit to leading on behalf of the larger public. Grow your leadership community by being responsive when others seek your assistance. The leadership network that you have assisted will remember you and help you on your journey to board positions.

DISCUSSION QUESTIONS

1. What are you passionate about in your personal and professional life?
2. What skills do you possess that might prepare you for a board role?
3. Which organizations are doing business in areas in which you have a passionate interest?
4. Who is currently involved on the board and how will you meet members to discuss your passion?

REFERENCES

Institute of Medicine. (2011). *The future of nursing: Leading change, advancing health.* Washington DC: The National Academies Press.

ONLINE RESOURCES

Best on Board
www.bestonboard.org
Integrated Nurse Leadership Program
www.futurehealth.ucsf.edu/Public/Leadership-Programs/Home.aspx?pid=35
Robert Wood Johnson Foundation Leadership Programs
www.rwjf.org
Robert Wood Johnson Foundation Executive Nurse Fellows
www.executivenursefellows.org

CHAPTER 58

Quality and Safety in Health Care: Policy Issues

Linda Hirota Hevenor   Ellen T. Kurtzman   Jean E. Johnson

"If a physician makes a large incision with an operating knife and cure it,…he shall receive ten shekels in money…. If a physician make a large incision with the operating knife, and kill him,…his hands shall be cut off."
Code of Hammurabi, Code of Laws, No. 215, 218; ca. 1760 BC

For nearly two decades, the United States and its policymakers have wrestled with three interrelated phenomenon that threaten the U.S. health care system: compromised patient safety and quality, escalating costs, and growing rates of uninsured and underinsured. To address each, Congress passed the Affordable Care Act (ACA) in 2010 (ACA, 42 U.S.C. § 18001, 2010). It increases access to health care for millions of Americans by expanding insurance coverage while creating incentives among providers, practitioners, and consumers to achieve higher levels of quality and efficiency. Defined by the Institute of Medicine (IOM) as "the best care for the patient, with the optimal result given the circumstances, delivered at the right price" (IOM, 2012, p. 25), high value health care is terminology that refers to the delicate balance among cost, quality, and access, which must be achieved under health care reform to ensure system sustainability. To achieve higher value, nurses must be knowledgeable about the factors that contribute to waste and suboptimal outcomes, and lead efforts to maximize quality and efficiency.

Provisions in the ACA establish programs and services that drive higher value health care, but expanding access, controlling costs, and enhancing quality are contingent on the law's implementation at the state, health system, practitioner, and consumer levels. Public policy at all levels, including the interpretation of the ACA through rule making and regulation, is critical. This chapter will review the past decade of federal policymaking including the expected impact of the ACA on health care delivery, with a particular focus on the implications of higher value health care for nurses and the nursing profession. It describes policy approaches intended to stimulate higher values that are most salient to nurses. Additionally, key organizations involved in quality are introduced and their contributions highlighted.

THE ENVIRONMENTAL CONTEXT

COST

The cost of health care has been and continues to be the main driver of health policies leading to high value approaches. Currently, the spending on health consumes about 17% of the U.S. gross domestic product (GDP) and is estimated to increase to 20% of the GDP by 2020 (Fuchs, 2013). In 2012, health care costs were estimated to be $2.8 trillion, or $8915 per person (Centers for Medicare and Medicaid Services [CMS], 2014).

Although the rate of increase in health care costs has slowed to between 3.7% and 3.9% since 2009 compared with growth rates of 10% and higher in the 1970s and 1980s, an average growth rate of 5.8% is projected through 2022 with total spending estimated to hit $5 trillion (Sommers, Kennedy, & Epstein, 2014).

The value, or lack of value, is underscored when comparing the United States with other developed countries. A landmark study conducted by the U.S. Burden of Disease Collaborators (2013) compared the 34 countries in the Organisation for Economic Co-operation and Development (OECD) and found that although the United States made improvements in population health over the 20-year period from 1990 to 2010, the United States fell behind other wealthy nations on key indicators: 27th for age-standardized mortality, 27th for life expectancy, and 26th for healthy life expectancy. Additionally, the United States lags significantly behind other OECD countries on infant mortality and premature mortality and holds the highest ranking for obesity among adults (OECD, 2011). Furthermore, when compared with the other OECD countries, the United States has higher prices for health care services and goods, higher use of expensive diagnostic equipment, and more elective surgery, all of which contribute to the high costs.

Whereas health care has been one of a few markets in which the cost of services is unknown to the consumer, more people are demanding information about price and quality (Yegian et al., 2013). As more costs are shifted to consumers in the form of consumer-borne insurance premiums (monthly fees paid for insurance coverage), deductibles (the amount during a benefit period that the insured pays before the insurers pays for covered services), and copayments (the insured person's share of cost of a covered service), a more informed purchaser has emerged and begun to demand cost information.

QUALITY

In 2000, it was estimated that 98,000 individuals die every year needlessly from health care errors (Kohn, Corrigan, & Donaldson, 2000). Although improvements have been demonstrated in some areas, safety and quality remain significant and unresolved issues. A study of three large teaching hospitals found adverse events occurred in one third of admitted patients (Classen et al., 2011). A new estimate of the number of needless deaths among hospitalized patients, using the Institute for Healthcare

Improvement's Global Trigger Tool, puts that number between 220,000 and 440,000 per year (James, 2013). Although there are questions around the different methods and calculations of these estimates, clearly harm and death from health care errors continue to plague the U.S. health care system.

Despite these estimates, the past decade has seen some successes in the area of patient safety and quality improvement. According to the 2012 National Healthcare Quality Report (NHQR) and the National Healthcare Disparities Report, 60% of all measures demonstrated improvement with a greater proportion of the improvement occurring in acute illness or injury as compared with preventive care and chronic disease management (Agency for Healthcare Research and Quality [AHRQ], 2012, 2013). Even with these improvements, however, the pace of improving care is lagging, particularly for minority and low-income groups (AHRQ, 2013).

The ACA, through demonstration projects and requirements for performance measurement and public reporting, is part of a broad array of efforts to spur improvements in quality. It complements the American Recovery and Reinvestment Act of 2009, which provided substantial funds for institutions and individual physician practices in implementing electronic health records and achieving meaningful use of the system to improve care and efficiency.

ACCESS

Access to health continues to be an unsolved problem that the ACA is intended to substantially address. The primary culprit behind the lack of health insurance coverage rests with the decline of employer-sponsored coverage (Kaiser Family Foundation [KFF], 2013). The major coverage provisions of the ACA are intended to reduce the number of uninsured by expanding Medicaid, establishing a health insurance marketplace, and providing subsidies for private coverage. The nonpartisan Congressional Budget Office (2014) estimates the ACA will result in an additional 25 million Americans who will have health insurance by 2020.

THE POLICY CONTEXT: VALUE-DRIVEN HEALTH CARE

Value-driven health care or high value health care are terms that typically refer to improving the quality of care while lowering its costs, thus linking affordable care and quality. In simple terms, value is obtaining higher quality for the same investment. Within the health care context, transparency and accountability are terms that typically refer to activities aimed at measuring and publicly disclosing provider performance along with a complementary set of tools that stimulate and reward (typically through financial payments) high performance (U.S. Department of Health and Human Services [HHS], 2009). And although the ACA is the current policy vehicle for driving higher value, the building blocks of transparency and accountability, performance measurement, public reporting, and value-based purchasing (VBP) have already been put in place.

PERFORMANCE MEASUREMENT

Performance measurement is foundational to high value health care. In fact, Florence Nightingale pioneered the systematic collection and analysis of hospital mortality rates that enabled comparative reporting and quality improvements in Great Britain's public health system (McDonald, 2001; Nightingale, 1863). Since recognizing its virtues and acknowledging its necessity, hundreds of quality measures have been developed by government agencies (e.g., CMS, AHRQ), accreditation organizations (e.g., The Joint Commission, National Committee for Quality Assurance [NCQA]), professional societies and certification boards (e.g., American Medical Association-Physician Consortium for Performance Improvement, American Board of Medical Specialties), quality improvement organizations, and private organizations (e.g., Leapfrog Group). Because public reporting and performance-based incentives cannot exist in the absence of cost and quality outcomes on which they are based, performance measurement is the central player in and precursor to public reporting and accountability.

It is important to note that nursing has made a significant investment in and contribution to the performance measurement landscape. Measures that portray the contributions of nurses to high quality inpatient care, typically referred to as nursing-sensitive indicators, have been developed, tested, and implemented by organizations such as the American Nurses Association (American Nurses Association [ANA], 2013), Veterans Health Administration, and Association of periOperative Registered Nurses (Kurtzman, Dawson, & Johnson, 2008). The largest regional nursing quality measurement network, the Collaborative Alliance for Nursing Outcomes (CalNOC), began in California as the first statewide initiative in the country. In 2004, the National Quality Forum (NQF) endorsed the National Voluntary Consensus Standards for Nursing-Sensitive Care, the first set of nationally standardized performance measures that assess the quality of hospital-based nursing care and include indicators such as patient falls, restraint prevalence, and nursing care hours per patient day (NQF, 2004). The ANA's National Database of Nursing Quality Indicators (NDNQI),[1] comprising structural, process, and outcome measures, is the largest repository of unit-level nursing-sensitive indicators in the United States, and is used by more than 2000 hospitals. These data have helped the nursing profession and organizations identify and address opportunities to improve the quality of care and patient safety. Furthermore, the value of measuring nursing's contribution to quality is evidenced by the inclusion of nursing-sensitive measures by the CMS and The Joint Commission.

The ACA has specific requirements to expand the value of health care related to performance measures; however, there is no requirement that specifically relates to measures of nursing care. The Secretary of the HHS is required by the ACA to identify areas where there are gaps in measures. The priority areas for creating measures include disparities, shared decision making, functional ability, care coordination, and efficiency. To comply with the

---

[1]The ANA sold the NDNQI to Press Gainey in 2014 and remains a co-brander of the dataset.

ACA, the 2012 NHQR included new measures of care coordination and health system efficiency. Several additional requirements in the law support the development of performance measures including the HHS convening the stakeholder group, the National Priorities Partnership, to advise the HHS on measures to be developed. The National Priorities Partnership is a group of 51 major national organizations convened by the NQF with the goal of achieving better health and a safe, equitable, and value-driven health care system (NQF, 2014).

Measures related to different populations are also required by the ACA. In 2012, measures referred to as the Medicaid Adult Core Set were defined by the CMS in collaboration with the AHRQ to measure care provided to Medicaid-eligible adults. The final core set includes 26 measures that are being collected under public or private auspices. Examples include flu shots for adults age 50 to 64 years, cervical cancer screening, breast cancer screening, blood pressure control, and annual monitoring for patients on persistent medications (Medicaid Program, 2012). New measures to evaluate hospice and palliative care were added in 2013.

The only valid and reliable way to assess quality of care is through measurement. Although providers intend to do no harm and are committed to providing safe and effective care, intending to do well is not sufficient.

PUBLIC REPORTING

Public reporting is part of the national strategy for improving quality. The purpose of public reporting is to: (1) provide information to consumers to make choices based on quality and therefore incentivize providers to do better and (2) give health care providers comparative information about their quality of care to improve care.

Within the HHS, AHRQ and CMS are primarily responsible for publicly reporting measures. The AHRQ has developed the Charter Value Exchanges as public reporting sites that currently include 17 states and 38 databases (AHRQ, 2013). The CMS has developed and maintains several public reporting websites including Hospital Compare

and Nursing Home Compare. Additional quality measures are publicly reported by states, regional collaboratives, managed care organizations, commercial health insurers, and professional organizations and societies.

In addition, several private entities also report measures. The 17 alliances within the Robert Wood Johnson Foundation's Aligning Forces for Quality make hospital and ambulatory care measures publicly available to a broad group of stakeholders in their communities (Aligning Forces for Quality, 2011). *U.S. News and World Report* ranks health plans and health insurance products. The NCQA produces performance reports on health plans and patient-centered medical homes (NCQA, 2013). The Leapfrog Group, in addition to other reports, provides a single composite letter grade ranking hospitals on safety (Leapfrog Group, 2013). All of the reports are intended to provide consumers with information about quality to make informed choices about health plans and care providers.

Even though there are many publicly reported measures, there are few reports that portray nursing care. Currently, only a few states publicly report hospital-level nursing-sensitive measures. According to state statute, both Maine (22 M.R.S.A. §8708-A, Chapter 270) and Colorado (Senate Bill 08-196) require uniform statewide reporting of data related to health care quality including nursing-sensitive measures. A voluntary initiative undertaken by the Massachusetts Hospital Association and Organization of Nurse Leaders of MA-RI and referred to as PatientCareLink led to the public disclosure of hospital-level nursing-sensitive measures in the state. Even though the CMS does not devote a dedicated public report to nursing care quality per se, several measures that address the quality of nursing care have been incorporated into Hospital Compare. In 2008, for example, performance results from the Hospital Consumer Assessment of Healthcare Providers and Systems (HCAHPS), which includes several measures related to nursing care, were posted to the website. In 2009, the CMS added failure-to-rescue (defined as the percentage of major surgical inpatients who experience a hospital-acquired complication and die) as a required measure under its pay for reporting program.

Because CMS typically selects pay for reporting measures to publish on Hospital Compare, failure to rescue is likely to be included in this CMS database at some point in the future.

Evidence that public reporting is associated with provider-driven improvements in quality of care is mounting. An extensive systematic review concluded that public reporting has a positive impact on hospital mortality, although the findings were not uniformly consistent and there were some concerns about the appropriateness of the comparison group in some of the studies (Totten et al., 2012). This review also found an association between quality improvement and public reporting among health plans and long-term care facilities. Qualitative research suggests that multidisciplinary clinician groups perceive the public disclosure of performance data to be a motivating factor for organizations to improve and maintain performance (Hafner et al., 2011). Although there is some evidence that public reporting is related to improvements in health care, an evidence-based review conducted by the AHRQ indicates there is little evidence that public reporting impacts patients' and purchasers' choices about providers (Totten et al., 2012). This report identified the following reasons for this finding: people were unaware that the quality measures were available; the publicly reported data were not what consumers needed or valued; the information was not available when needed; and it was presented in an incomprehensible way. With regard to nursing homes, public reporting resulted in a small increase in consumers choosing high-scoring facilities (Werner et al., 2012).

Research suggests consumers mistakenly conclude that high costs are associated with high quality and are unable to discern high value care unless cost is accompanied by a strong quality signal (Hibbard et al., 2012). Sofaer and Hibbard (2010) provide nine evidence-based recommendations, including the value of a framework and use of plain language, to accurately communicate health care data to consumers and motivate them to incorporate this information into their decision making. Despite the substantial efforts to standardize measurement and reporting, there is much work to be done to ensure the publicly reported measures are important and usable to consumers.

VALUE-BASED PAYMENT AND DELIVERY MODELS

PAYMENT REFORM

A central component of high value health care is the use of payment programs to reward health care plans and providers to improve clinical quality and resource utilization as opposed to traditional fee-for-service payment models that reward volume alone. These incentives typically take the form of private- and public-sector pay for performance (P4P) programs based on measures of structure, process, outcome, and patient experience. The CMS has taken the lead in pursuing performance-based payment with an overarching goal of fostering joint clinical and financial accountability. The Medicare Payment Advisory Commission (MedPAC) has recommended numerous payment changes, including those outlined in Table 58-1, in an effort to drive quality improvement and reduce costs (MedPAC, 2013).

The keen interest and swift adoption of performance-based payment programs in the public and private sectors is not yet matched with definitive results of its effectiveness. Two systematic reviews of hospital P4P and quality reported positive impacts (Christianson, Leatherman, & Sutherland, 2008; Mehrotra et al., 2009). The more rigorous studies examining the largest Medicare hospital VBP demonstration project, the Premier Hospital Quality Incentives Demonstration (PHQUID), found improved but unsustainable performance on composite process measures (Werner et al., 2011) and no impact on 30-day mortality (Jha et al., 2012). Using data from Medicare's flagship demonstration project, PHQUID, other reports on the impact of P4P on composite process measures have cast doubt on the ability of VBP to drive quality improvement and sustain those improvements, particularly among low-performing hospitals (Ryan & Blustein, 2011; Ryan, Blustein, & Casalino, 2012). Medicare's hospital VBP program is projected to alter payments by less

UNIT 4

TABLE 58-1 Characteristics of Payment Models Recommended by the Medicare Payment Advisory Commission (MedPAC)

Payment Model	Payment Details
Physician Quality Reporting System	Through 2014 incentive payments for reporting on specific quality measures. Payment adjustments will be applied for nonreporting beginning in 2015. Additional incentive for working with a Maintenance of Certification entity.
Hospital-acquired conditions and present on admission indicator reporting provision	Hospitals do not receive the higher payment for cases if one of the selected hospital-acquired conditions develops during admission.
Value-based purchasing	The Centers for Medicare and Medicaid Services will reduce all diagnosis-related group (DRG) payments to participating prospective payment system hospitals by 1% of base inpatient payments and redistribute through value-based incentive payments. The size of the redistribution pool is mandated to increase 0.25% per year up to 2% of DRG payments in fiscal year 2017.
Medicare Advantage plan bonus	Bonus based on quality scores (star rating), which comprises 53 performance measures.
Hospital readmissions reduction program	Penalty for higher than expected risk-adjusted readmissions for certain conditions. Penalty for individual hospitals is capped at 1% of base inpatient operating payments in 2013, 2% in 2014, and 3% in 2015 and beyond.

than 1% among only two thirds of acute care hospitals and has a limited impact on hospital income, thus raising questions about the ability of VBP to substantially affect the quality of care (Kruse et al., 2012; Werner & Dudley, 2012).

There is a need for research on the impact of P4P methodologies on both cost and quality across various settings. Given the potential for unintended, negative consequences related to gaming, limiting access to high-risk patients, and equitable care, careful monitoring is critical.

DELIVERY REFORM

Although restructuring payment is one approach to stimulating increased value, an alternative strategy is changing the way health care is delivered. The ACA designated an Innovation Center within the CMS (CMMI) to encourage experimentation and identify health care delivery models that are most effective at producing high value care. Innovative health care delivery models being explored under health reform, such as bundled payments, global payments or capitated care, patient-centered health or medical home (PCMH), and accountable care organizations (ACOs), are meant to stimulate the development of a more integrated and value-oriented health care system and are among the

models being examined and replicated by the CMMI. In 2013, the CMS began the bundled payments for care initiative, in which selected organizations enter into payment arrangements that include performance and financial accountability for certain episodes of care. Bundled payments provide a single payment that covers all services related to an episode of care, including physician visits, laboratory tests, hospitalizations, and any other services needed. They are intended to provide incentives to providers to eliminate care that has limited or no benefit. Early evidence found weak but consistent associations between bundled payments and reduced spending and use and inconsistent and small effects on quality (Hussey et al., 2012). Recently, Blue Cross Blue Shield of Massachusetts established the Alternative Quality Contract with seven provider groups. In this program, providers received a budget to care for their patients representing a global payment model. After the first year of the program, studies have found reduced spending and improved quality compared with a fee-for-services approach (Song et al., 2012).

Two alternative models, the PCMH and the ACO, are integrated service delivery models that incorporate a variety of payment methods and financial incentives, including but not limited to P4P. In theory, cost savings will be manifested through reduced hospitalizations, readmissions, and avoidable complications. The PCMH emphasizes care coordination and communication to transform primary care and meet the triple aim of high quality, reduced costs, and improved patient experience. Payment models vary but a common model consists of a traditional fee-for-service component, fixed supplemental payments based on per member per month calculation, and P4P bonus payments. Studies and systematic reviews of the PCMH model or elements of the model revealed mostly favorable results, although a few interventions were associated with higher costs and some yielded inconclusive findings (Gilfillan et al., 2010; Maeng et al., 2012; Nielsen et al., 2012; Peikes et al., 2012). Future research on PCMHs may be more conclusive based on a recently constructed core set of standardized measures (Rosenthal et al., 2012).

An ACO is a locally or regionally organized group of health care providers and suppliers of services that is responsible for the quality and cost delivered to a panel of patients across the continuum of care. ACOs are an effort to improve efficiency through better care coordination. The ACA authorized Medicare to contract with ACOs through the Medicare Shared Savings Program. Alternative ACO models are also being tested by the CMS, such as the Pioneer ACO Initiative. ACOs that deliver better care will receive financial bonuses. The CMS estimates net federal savings of $940 million in the first 4 years of the Shared Savings Program (Berenson & Burton, 2012). Given the recent introduction of the ACO model, research on the impact on quality and cost is limited. Although the details of these value-based care delivery models differ, they shift payment away from rewarding volume with the intention of stimulating greater value through more efficient use of resources and more coordination within and across providers.

IMPACT OF VALUE-DRIVEN HEALTH CARE ON NURSING

Nurses are exceedingly well positioned to deliver care that creates greater value. First, nurses are the single largest provider of health care in the United States (U.S. Bureau of Labor Statistics, 2013) with frequent points of patient contact in many care settings. Therefore, nurses represent a significant workforce that can alter the value equation. Although laws and regulations continue to unfold, they are not specifically designed to recognize nursing's contribution to the quality agenda. Nurses both impact and are impacted by the transformative policy initiatives. The following are major areas of opportunities and challenges for nurses to contribute to high value health care through: (1) cost reduction, (2) quality improvement, and (3) better access.

NURSES AND COST

The business case for nursing has not been well defined across settings and as a result nursing has been invisible to payers and the public. However, there is a growing body of literature related to advanced practice registered nurses (APRNs) and cost. The salary of nurse practitioners (NPs) on average is lower than physicians and NPs usually do not benefit from practice bonus plans. Most practices bill for NP services through a physician billing number to get reimbursed at the full physician rate rather than through an NP charge that would be at the 85% rate. This makes it difficult for consumers to benefit from lower NP costs. In addition, limits on scope of practice have produced barriers to the effective use of NPs. A recent study on retail clinics showed that states with a broad scope of NP practice reduce costs (Spetz et al., 2013). In addition, an NP-led inpatient care management model has been shown to reduce drug use and decrease costs (Chen et al., 2009). APRNs are demonstrating the potential for cost savings while maintaining a quality of care.

For hospital-based nurses, there is an opportunity to link nursing care to the financial state of the hospital because payment is now linked to several key quality measures that are sensitive to nursing care, such as readmission, patient satisfaction, and hospital-acquired conditions. Although executives generally view nursing as a cost center and not an income generator, researchers have begun to look at the effect of hospital nursing on economic indicators with signs of positive impact (Dall, Chen, Seifert, Maddox, & Hogan, 2013). A cost analysis of unit staffing levels and readmissions indicated that investing in additional non-overtime RN hours resulted in significant net savings for payers through reduced postdischarge use (Weiss, Yakusheva, & Bobay, 2011). Moreover, improved RN staffing has been linked with reduced turnover (Brennan, Daly, & Jones, 2013), a factor that can be cost saving for an organization. A synthesis of the literature on staffing levels and nursing-sensitive indicators highlights the potential impact of improved RN staffing in hospitals by demonstrating an association between higher staffing levels and lower medical costs, improved national productivity, and saved lives (Dall et al., 2009). In addition, nurses are taking a greater role in case management by coordinating care and improving transitions of care across settings and providers. This can translate into cost savings and is an important component of the ACA (Naylor et al., 2013).

Although no federal performance-based payment programs target nurses per se, incentives to improve inpatient care such as paying for performance, penalizing for readmissions, and withholding payment for hospital-acquired conditions represents opportunities to demonstrate the economic value of nursing care within hospitals. Strategies that nursing should pursue to further demonstrate nurses' contribution to cost savings include:

- Continue to demonstrate through research the costs associated with restricted scope of practice for APRNs and all nurses.
- Continue to work with the CMS to capture cost data related to APRN practice.
- Create a robust research agenda examining nurses' contributions to revenue generation and/or cost savings for hospitals vis-à-vis high quality nursing care and sufficient nurse staffing.
- Continue to build the business case for care coordination and care transitions with a particular focus on work done through PCMHs and ACOs.
- Create financial models of nursing care across settings that recognize nursing as a revenue generator and not solely as a cost center.
- Prepare more nurse researchers to use cost data and partner with health services researchers to explore ways of capturing the cost benefit of nursing care.

NURSES AND QUALITY OF CARE

Nurses are vital to providing high quality of care throughout the health care system. APRNs have led the charge in defining the level of quality of care provided. The evidence accumulated over decades has demonstrated that NPs, nurse midwives, and nurse anesthetists provide safe, high quality care that is comparable and, in some cases, better than physician care (Newhouse et al., 2011). Medicare demonstration projects are evaluating nurse-managed clinics, PCMHs, and ACO models dependent on nursing roles for care coordination and transitions of care and will be useful in continuing to document nursing's contribution to quality.

In addition to the literature on APRN quality of care, a maturing body of evidence is demonstrating the contribution of hospital nurses to quality of care including the positive impact the size, composition, and educational preparation of the nursing workforce has on patient outcomes such as hospital mortality and failure-to-rescue (Aiken et al., 2012; Kane et al., 2007; Kutney-Lee, Sloane, & Aiken, 2013; Needleman et al., 2011; Park et al., 2012; Shekelle, 2013).

To better understand nurses' contributions to quality across all settings of care, the following strategies are recommended:

- Further examine how the size, composition, and preparation of the nursing workforce contribute to improved quality care across settings.
- Continue to explore, evaluate, and disseminate nurse-led models of care that contribute to high quality of care.
- Work with the CMS to publically report nursing-sensitive quality measures.
- Conduct and disseminate research regarding consumers' understanding and use of performance results related to nursing in their decision making.
- Prepare more nurses at the doctoral level to develop and test performance measures that are relevant to nursing.
- Target influential quality organizations and work to have nurses appointed to committees and boards that will make decisions about quality of care issues.

- Build on the Quality and Safety Education for Nurses (Sherwood & Barnsteiner, 2012) to design nursing education curricula that can develop a critical mass of nurse leaders in patient safety and quality in both the academic and clinical areas.

NURSING AND ACCESS

Coverage aside, a major concern about access is focused on primary care. To this end, the growing number of APRNs continues to be instrumental in expanding access. The rate of medical graduates has plateaued over the recent decade (Jolly, Erikson, & Garrison, 2013), although the number of new APRNs and physician assistants over this same time period has nearly doubled (Robert Wood Johnson Foundation, 2013). Employment of APRNs is projected to grow 31% from 2012 to 2022 in response to three factors: the ACA, a shift in focus to preventive care, and a growing baby boomer population (U.S. Bureau of Labor Statistics, 2013). The Health Services Resources Administration (HRSA) estimates that as of 2012 more than 35 million individuals living in 5870 Health Professions Shortage Areas lacked adequate primary care services, yet physician assistants and APRNs are more likely to practice in underserved remote and rural areas than physicians, and constitute a greater proportion of the United States' safety net providers (Hing & Uddin, 2011). To enhance access further, the legal, regulatory, institutional, and cultural barriers that unnecessarily prevent APRNs from practicing to the full extent of their education and training need to be addressed (IOM, 2011; National Governors Association, 2012). To meet the current and future demands for high quality primary care as access expands, state-based barriers to full scope of APRN practice remain the most important issue for policymakers to address; however, a robust set of strategies are needed and include:

- All major nursing organizations commit to having a priority to eliminate barriers to full scope of practice.
- Establish coalitions of nurses, business leaders, and policymakers to address barriers to full scope of practice.

- Continue to assess the financial impact of limiting nursing full scope of practice across settings.
- Support policies that recognize the contribution of nurse-managed clinics to providing access.

CONCLUSION

Broad changes in organizational culture, information technology, payment and delivery models, and health care leadership are necessary to expand health care access, reduce costs, and improve quality. Nurses need to share their firsthand accounts, along with the evidentiary basis and business case, for nursing's role in the quality enterprise. Additionally, nurses need to intensify their involvement in policy development, as well as build leadership and advocacy capacity, to effectively participate in this discourse; collaborate with consumers, providers, other health care professionals, payers, and policymakers in novel ways; and hold themselves accountable for higher value care.

DISCUSSION QUESTIONS

1. Discuss the fundamental strategies of public reporting, performance measurement, and value-based payments that policymakers are leveraging to drive the high value health care agenda.
2. How can health care payment and delivery models be formulated to drive quality of care.
3. Discuss how nursing impacts, and is impacted by, the quality and safety agenda emphasized in the ACA.

REFERENCES

Affordable Care Act [ACA]. (2010). 42 U.S.C. § 18001.

Agency for Healthcare Research and Quality [AHRQ]. (2012). 2012 National healthcare quality report. Rockville, MD: U.S. Department of Health and Human Services, Agency for Healthcare Research and Quality. AHRQ publication no. 13-0002. Retrieved from *www.ahrq.gov/research/findings/nhqrdr/nhdr12/nhdr12_prov.pdf*.

Agency for Healthcare Research and Quality [AHRQ]. (2013). National healthcare disparities report 2012. Rockville, MD: U.S. Department of Health and Human Services, Agency for Healthcare Research and Quality. AHRQ publication no. 13-0003. Retrieved from *www.ahrq.gov/research/findings/nhqrdr/nhdr12/nhdr12_prov.pdf*.

Aiken, L. H., Cimiotti, J. P., Sloane, D. M., Smith, H. L., Fynn, L., & Neff, D. F. (2012). Effects of nurse staffing and nurse education on patient deaths in hospitals with different nurse work environments. *The Journal of Nursing Administration*, *42*(10 Suppl.), S10–S16.

Aligning Forces for Quality (2011). Lesson learned in public reporting: Deciding what to report. Washington, DC: Aligning Forces for Quality. Retrieved from *forces4quality.org/af4q/download-document/3014/633*.

American Nurses Association. (2013). Nursing alliance for quality care. Retrieved 2013, from: *www.naqc.org/*.

Berenson, R. A., & Burton, R. A. (2012, January 31). Health policy brief: Next steps for ACOs. *Health Affairs*. Retrieved from *healthaffairs.org/healthpolicybriefs/brief_pdfs/healthpolicybrief_61.pdf*.

Brennan, C. W., Daly, B. J., & Jones, K. R. (2013). State of the science: The relationship between nurse staffing and patient outcomes. *Western Journal of Nursing Research*, *35*(6), 760–794.

Centers for Medicare and Medicaid Services. [CMS] (2014). National health expenditure data–Historical. Baltimore, MD: Centers for Medicare and Medicaid Services. Retrieved from *www.cms.gov/Research-Statistics-Data-and-Systems/Statistics-Trends-and-Reports/NationalHealthExpendData/NationalHealthAccountsHistorical.html*.

Chen, C., McNeese-Smith, D., Cowan, M., Upenieks, V., & Afifi, A. (2009). Evaluation of a nurse practitioner-led care management model in reducing inpatient drug utilization and cost. *Nursing Economic$*, *27*(3), 160–168.

Christianson, J. B., Leatherman, S., & Sutherland, K. (2008). Lessons from evaluations of purchaser pay-for-performance programs: a review of the evidence. *Medical Care Research Review*, *65*, 5S–35S.

Classen, D. C., Resar, R., Griffin, F., Federico, F., Frankel, T., Kimmel, N., et al. (2011). "Global trigger tool" shows that adverse events in hospitals may be ten times greater than previously measured. *Health Affairs*, *30*(4), 581–589.

Congressional Budget Office. (2014). Effects of the Affordable Care Act on health insurance coverage–February 2014 baseline. Washington, DC: Congressional Budget Office. Retrieved from *www.cbo.gov/sites/default/files/cbofiles/attachments/43900-2014-02-ACAtables.pdf*.

Dall, T. M., Chen, Y. J., Seifert, R. F., Maddox, P. J., & Hogan, P. F. (2009). The economic value of professional nursing. *Medical Care*, *47*(1), 97–104.

Fuchs, V. R. (2013). The gross domestic product and health care spending. *New England Journal of Medicine*, *369*(2), 107–109.

Gilfillan, R. J., Tomcavage, J., Rosenthal, M. B., Davis, D. E., Graham, J., et al. (2010). Value and the medical home: Effects of transformed primary care. *American Journal of Managed Care*, *16*(8), 607–614.

Hafner, J. M., Williams, S. C., Koss, R. G., Schurtz, B. A., Schmaltz, S. P., & Loeb, J. M. (2011). The perceived impact of public reporting hospital performance data: Interviews with hospital staff. *International Journal for Quality in Health Care*, *23*(6), 697–704.

Hibbard, J. H., Greene, J., Sofaer, S., Firminger, K., & Hirh, J. (2012). An experiment shows that a well-designed report on costs and quality can help consumers choose high-value health care. *Health Affairs*, *31*(3), 560–568.

Hing, E., & Uddin, S. (2011). Physician assistant and advance practice nurse care in hospital outpatient departments: United States, 2008-2009. NCHS data brief, no. 77. Hyattsville, MD: National Center for Health Statistics. Retrieved from *www.cdc.gov/nchs/data/databriefs/db77.htm*.

Hussey, P. S., Mulcahy, A. W., Schnyer, C., & Schneider, E. C. (2012). Bundled payment: Effects on health care spending and quality. Closing the quality gap: Revisiting the state of the science. Evidence report/technology assessment no. 208. Prepared by the RAND Evidence-based Practice Center under contract no. 290-2007-10062-I. AHRQ publication no. 12-E007-EF. Rockville, MD: Agency for Healthcare Research and Quality. Retrieved from *www.effectivehealthcare.ahrq.gov/reports/final.cfm*.

Institute of Medicine [IOM]. (2011). *The future of nursing: Leading change, advancing health*. Washington, DC: The National Academies Press.

Institute of Medicine [IOM]. (2012). *Best care at lower cost: The path to continuously learning health care in America*. Washington, DC: The National Academies Press.

James, J. T. (2013). A new, evidence-based estimate of patient harms associated with hospital care. *Journal of Patient Safety*, *9*(3), 122–128.

Jha, A. K., Joynt, K. E., Orav, J., & Epstein, A. M. (2012). The long-term effect of premier pay for performance on patient outcomes. *New England Journal of Medicine*, *366*(17), 1606–1615.

Jolly, P., Erikson, C., & Garrison, G. (2013). U.S. Graduate medical education and physician specialty choice. *Academic Medicine*, *88*(4), 468–474.

Kaiser Family Foundation. (2013). The uninsured: A primer–Key facts about health insurance on the eve of coverage expansions. Menlo Park, CA: Kaiser Family Foundation. Retrieved from *kff.org/uninsured/report/the-uninsured-a-primer-key-facts-about-health-insurance-on-the-eve-of-coverage-expansions/*.

Kane, R. L., Shamliyan, T., Mueller, C., Duval, S., & Wilt, T. J. (2007). *Nursing staffing and quality of patient care*. Evidence report/technology assessment no. 151 (pp. 1–115). Rockville, MD: Agency for Healthcare Research and Quality.

Kohn, K. T., Corrigan, J. M., & Donaldson, M. S. (Eds.), (2000). *To err is human: Building a safer health system*. Washington, DC: National Academies Press.

Kruse, G. B., Polsky, D., Stuart, E. A., & Werner, R. M. (2012). The impact of hospital pay-for-performance on hospital and Medicare costs. *Health Services Research*, *47*(6), 2118–2136.

Kurtzman, E. T., Dawson, E. M., & Johnson, J. E. (2008). A current state of nursing performance measurement, public reporting, and value-based purchasing. *Policy, Politics, & Nursing Practice*, *9*(3), 181–191.

Kutney-Lee, A., Sloane, D. M., & Aiken, L. H. (2013). An increase in the number of nurses with baccalaureate degrees is linked to lower rates of postsurgery mortality. *Health Affairs*, *32*(3), 579–586.

Leapfrog Group. (2013). Current Leapfrog initiatives. Retrieved from *www.leapfroggroup.org/about_leapfrog/other_initiatives*.

Maeng, D. D., Graham, J., Graf, T. R., Liberman, J. N., Dermes, N. B., et al. (2012). Reducing long-term cost by transforming primary care: Evidence from Geisinger's medical home model. *American Journal of Managed Care*, *18*(3), 149–155.

McDonald, L. (2001). Florence Nightingale and the early origins of evidence-based nursing. *Evidence-Based Nursing*, *4*(3), 68–69.

Medicaid Program. (2012). Initial core set of health care quality measures for Medicaid-eligible adults, 1CMS-2420-FN. Retrieved from *medicaid.gov/Federal-Policy-Guidance/Downloads/CIB-01-04-12.pdf*.

The Medicare Payment Advisory Commission [MedPAC]. (2013). *Report to the Congress: Medicare payment policy*. Washington, DC: The Medicare Payment Advisory Commission (MedPAC).

Mehrotra, A., Damberg, C. L., Sorbero, M. E. S., & Teleki, S. S. (2009). Pay for performance in the hospital setting: What is the state of evidence? *American Journal of Medical Quality*, *24*, 19–28.

National Committee for Quality Assurance. (2013). NCQA patient-centered medical home. Retrieved from *www.ncqa.org/portals/0/PCMH%20brochure-web.pdf*.

National Governors Association. (2012). The role of nurse practitioners in meeting increasing demand for primary care. Washington, DC: National Governors Association. Retrieved from *www.nga.org/cms/home/news-room/news-releases/page_2012/col2-content/nurse-practitioners-have-potenti.html*.

National Quality Forum [NQF]. (2004). National voluntary consensus standards for nursing-sensitive care. Washington, DC: National Quality Forum. Retrieved from *www.qualityforum.org/pdf/nursing-quality/txNCFINALpublic.pdf*.

UNIT 4

National Quality Forum [NQF]. (2014). National Priorities Partnership. Retrieved from *www.qualityforum.org/Setting_Priorities/NPP/National_Priorities_Partnership.aspx*.

Naylor, M. D., Bowles, K. H., McCauley, K. M., Maccoy, M. C., Maislin, G., et al. (2013). High-value transitional care: Translation of research into practice. *Journal of Evaluation in Clinical Practice, 19*(5), 727–733.

Needleman, J., Buerhaus, P., Pankratz, V. S., Leibson, C. L., Stevens, S. R., & Harris, M. (2011). Nurse staffing and inpatient hospital mortality. *New England Journal of Medicine, 364*(11), 1037–1045.

Newhouse, R. P., Stanik-Hutt, J., White, K. M., Johantgen, M., Bass, E. B., et al. (2011). Advanced practice nurse outcomes 1990-2008: A systematic review. *Nursing Economics, 29*(5), 1–21.

Nielsen, M., Langner, B., Zema, C., Hacker, T., & Grundy, P. (2012). Benefits of implementing the primary care patient-centered medical home: A review of cost and quality results, 2012. Retrieved from *www.pcpcc.org/sites/default/files/media/benefits_of_implementing_the_primary_care_pcmh.pdf*.

Nightingale, F. (1863). *Notes on hospitals.* London: Longman, Green, Longman, Roberts, & Green.

Organisation for Economic Co-operation and Development. (2011). Health at a glance 2011: OECD indicators. OECD Publishing. Retrieved from *dx.doi.org/10.1787/health_glance-2011-en*.

Park, S. H., Blegen, M. A., Spetz, J., Chapman, S. A., & De Groot, H. (2012). Patient turnover and the relationship between nurse staffing and patient outcomes. *Research in Nursing & Health, 35*(3), 277–288.

Peikes, D., Zutshi, A., Genevro, J. L., Parchman, M. L., & Meyers, D. S. (2012). Early evaluation of the medical home: Building on a promising start. *American Journal of Managed Care, 18*(2), 105–116.

Robert Wood Johnson Foundation. (2013). Improving patient access to high quality care: How to fully utilize the skills, knowledge, and experience of advanced practice registered nurses. In Charting nursing's future: Reports on policies that can transform patient care. Princeton, NJ: Robert Wood Johnson Foundation. Retrieved from *www.rwjf.org/content/dam/farm/reports/issue_briefs/2013/rwjf405378*.

Rosenthal, M. B., Abrams, M. K., Bitton, A., & Patient-Centered Medical Home Evaluator's Collaborative. (2012). Recommended core measures for evaluating the patient-centered medical home: Cost, utilization, and clinical quality (report no. 1601). Retrieved from *www.commonwealthfund.org/~/media/Files/Publications/Data%20Brief/2012/1601_Rosenthal_recommended_core_measures_PCMH_v2.pdf*.

Ryan, A. M., & Blustein, J. (2011). The effect of MassHealth pay-for-performance program on quality. *Health Services Research, 46*(3), 712–728.

Ryan, A. M., Blustein, J., & Casalino, L. P. (2012). Medicare's flagship test of pay-for-performance did not spur more rapid quality improvement among low-performing hospitals. *Health Affairs, 31*(4), 797–805.

Shekelle, P. G. (2013). Nurse-patient ratios as a patient safety strategy: A systematic review. *Annals of Internal Medicine, 158*(5 pt 2), 404–409.

Sherwood, G., & Barnsteiner, J. (Eds.). (2012). *Quality and safety in nursing: A competency approach to improving outcomes.* West Sussex, UK: Wiley-Blackwell.

Sofaer, S., & Hibbard, J. (2010). Best practices in public reporting no. 2: Maximizing consumer understanding of public comparative quality reports: Effective use of explanatory information. AHRQ publication no. 10-0082-EF. Rockville, MD: Agency for Healthcare Research and Quality. Retrieved from *www.ahrq.gov/professionals/quality-patient-safety/quality-resources/tools/pubrptguide2/pubrptguide2.pdf*.

Sommers, B. D., Kennedy, G. M., & Epstein, A. M. (2014). National health spending in 2012: Rate of health spending growth remained low for the fourth consecutive year. *Health Affairs, 33*(1), 67–77.

Song, Z., Safran, D. G., Landon, B. E., Landrum, M. B., He, Y., et al. (2012). The "alternative quality contract," based on a global budget, lowered medical spending and improved quality. *Health Affairs, 31*(8), 1885–1894.

Spetz, J., Parente, S. T., Town, R. J., & Bazarko, D. (2013). Scope-of-practice laws for nurse practitioners limit cost savings that can be achieved in retail clinics. *Health Affairs, 32*(11), 1977–1984.

Totten, A. M., Wagner, J., Tiwari, A., O'Haire, C., Griffin, J., & Walker, M. (2012). Public reporting as a quality improvement strategy. Closing the quality gap: Revisiting the state of the science. Evidence report no. 208. (Prepared by the Oregon Evidence-based Practice Center under contract no. 290-2007-10057-I.) AHRQ publication no. 12-E011-EF. Rockville, MD: Agency for Healthcare Research and Quality. Retrieved from *www.effectivehealthcare.ahrq.gov/reports/final.cfm*.

U.S. Burden of Disease Collaborators. (2013). The state of U.S. health, 1990-2010: Burden of diseases, injuries, and risk factors. *Journal of the American Medical Association, 310*(6), 591–608.

U.S. Bureau of Labor Statistics. (2013). Occupational outlook handbook, 2012-13 edition–Registered nurses. Washington, DC: U.S. Department of Labor. Retrieved from *www.bls.gov/ooh/healthcare/registered-nurses.htm*.

U.S. Department of Health and Human Services [HHS]. (2009). Value-driven health care. Washington, DC: U.S. Department of Health and Human Services. Retrieved from *www.hhs.gov/valuedriven/*.

Weiss, M. E., Yakusheva, O., & Bobay, K. L. (2011). Quality and cost analysis of nurse staffing, discharge preparation, and postdischarge utilization. *Health Services Research, 46*(5), 1374–1494.

Werner, R. M., & Dudley, R. A. (2012). Medicare's new hospital value-based purchasing program is likely to have only a small impact on hospital payments. *Health Affairs, 31*(9), 1932–1940.

Werner, R. M., Kolstad, J. T., Stuart, E. A., & Polsky, D. (2011). The effect of pay-for-performance in hospitals: Lessons for quality improvement. *Health Affairs, 30*(4), 690–698.

Werner, R. M., Norton, E. C., Konetzka, R. T., & Polsky, D. (2012). Do consumers respond to publicly reported quality information? Evidence from nursing homes. *Journal of Health Economics, 31*(1), 50–61. doi:10.1016/j.jhealeco.2012.01.001.

Yegian, J., Dardess, P., Shannon, M., & Carman, K. (2013). Engaged patients will need comparative physician-level quality data and information about out-of-pocket costs. *Health Affairs, 32*(2), 328–337.

ONLINE RESOURCES

Agency for Healthcare Research and Quality
www.ahrq.gov
American Nurses Association: National Center for Nursing Quality
www.nursingworld.org/ncnq
Centers for Medicare and Medicaid Services
www.cms.hhs.gov
Institute for Healthcare Improvement
www.ihi.org/Pages/default.aspx
Leapfrog Group
www.leapfroggroup.org
Medicare Payment Advisory Commission
www.medpac.gov
National Quality Forum
www.qualityforum.org

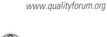

CHAPTER 59

Politics and Evidence-Based Practice and Policy

Sean P. Clarke

"The union of the political and scientific estates is not like a partnership, but a marriage. It will not be improved if the two become like each other, but only if they respect each other's quite different needs and purposes. No great harm is done if in the meantime they quarrel a bit."

Don K. Price

Health care has been a conservative field characterized by deep investments in tradition. Evolution of treatment approaches and facility and service management often has been very gradual, punctuated by occasional breakthroughs. For many years, it was said that nearly 2 decades could pass between the appearance of research findings and their uptake into practice. Although this statement bears revisiting in the era of evidence-based practice and in the Internet age, disconnects between evidence and care practices are still common, as are inconsistencies in practice and variations in patient outcomes across providers and institutions. It is clear that bringing research findings to real world settings remains a slow and uneven process.

Clinicians, researchers, and policymakers are aware of poor uptake of research evidence and lost opportunities to improve service, which has spurred an interest in clinical practice and, recently, health care policy, driven by high-quality scientific evidence. An often-cited definition of evidence-based practice is "the conscientious, explicit, and judicious use of current best evidence in making decisions about the care of individual patients" (Sackett et al., 1996). Evidence-based policy is an extension or extrapolation of the tenets of evidence-based practice to decisions about resource allocation and regulation by various governmental and regulatory bodies. Recognition of the scale of investments in health and social service programs and research around the world, the enormous stakes of providers and clients in the outcomes of policy decisions, and increasing demands for transparency and accountability influenced its rise.

Evidence-based policy has been defined as an approach that "helps people make well informed decisions about policies, programs, and projects by putting the best available evidence from research at the heart of policy development and implementation" (Davies, 1999).

This approach stands in contrast to opinion-based policy, which relies heavily on either the selective use of evidence (e.g., on single studies irrespective of quality) or on the untested views of individuals or groups, often inspired by ideological standpoints, prejudices, or speculative conjecture. (Davies, 2004, p. 3)

Controversies in clinical care and policy development are sometimes very intense. Political forces can influence the types of research evidence generated, how it is interpreted in the context of other data and values, and, most significantly, how it is used (if at all) in influencing practice. This chapter will review the politics of translating research into evidence-based practice and policy, from the generation of knowledge to its synthesis and translation.

THE PLAYERS AND THEIR STAKES

Translating research into practice involves many stakeholder groups. Health care professionals are often influenced by practice changes based on evidence. Many are invested in particular clinical methods or work practices and structures of practice or in the status quo of treatment approaches they use and the way care is organized. They often have preferences, pet projects, and passions and may have visions for health care and their profession's role that might be advanced or blocked by change. Health professionals may seek to protect their working conditions or defend turf from other professions, notably lucrative services or programs.

There are often direct financial consequences for industries connected with health care when research drives adoption, continued use, or rejection of specific products, such as pharmaceuticals and both consumable (e.g., dressings) and durable (e.g., hospital beds) medical supplies but also less visible (but equally expensive and important) products, such as consulting services.

Managers, administrators, and policymakers have stakes in delivering services in their facilities or organizations or jurisdictions in certain ways or within specific cost parameters. In general, administrators prefer to have as few constraints as possible in managing health care services and may be less enthusiastic about regulations as a method of controlling practice; however, changes that increase available resources may be better accepted.

For researchers, wide uptake of findings into practice is one of the most prestigious forms of external recognition, particularly if mandated by some sort of high-impact policy or legislation. This is especially the case for researchers working in policy-relevant fields where funding and public profile are mutually reinforcing. Researchers and academics involved in the larger evidence-based practice movement also have stakes in the enterprise. There are researchers, university faculty, and other experts who have become specialists in synthesizing and reporting outcomes and have interests in ensuring that distilled research in particular forms retains high status. Furthermore, funding

agency advisers and bureaucrats may also be very much invested in the legitimacy conferred by the use of evidence-based practice processes.

The general public, especially subgroups that have stakes in specific types of health care, wants safe, effective, and responsive health care. They want to think their personal risks, costs, and uncertainties are minimized, and they may or may not have insights or concerns about broader societal and economic consequences of treatments or models of care delivery. Expert opinions and research findings tend to carry authority, but for the public, these are filtered through the media, including Internet outlets.

Elected politicians and bureaucrats want to maintain appearances of being well informed and responsive to the needs of the public and interest groups, while conveying that their decisions balance risks, benefits, and the interests of various stakeholder groups. Elected politicians are usually concerned about voter satisfaction and their prospects for reelection. They, like the public, receive research evidence filtered through others, sometimes by the media but often by various types of civil servants. Nonelected bureaucrats inform politicians, manage specialized programs, and implement policies on a day-to-day basis. They may be highly trained and come to be very well informed about research evidence in particular fields. As top bureaucrats serve at the pleasure of elected officials, they are sensitive to public perceptions, opinions, and preferences.

THE ROLE OF POLITICS IN GENERATING EVIDENCE

Health care research is often a time- and cost-intensive activity involving competition for scarce resources and rewards. Much is on the line for many stakeholders. Which projects are attempted, what results are generated, and what is reported from completed studies are all very much affected by political factors at multiple levels.

Much research likely to influence practice or policy requires financial support from outside institutions. Researchers write applications to funders for grants to pay for the resources to carry out their work. Before agreeing to underwrite projects, external funders must believe that a topic being researched is important and relevant to the funding mission; the research approach is viable; and the proposed research team is able to carry out the project. Funders are often governmental or quasi-governmental agencies, but producers or marketers of specific products or services can subsidize research. When research is supported by suppliers of particular medications, products, or services, funders may have overtly stated or implicit interests in the results of the studies, and researchers may face pressures around the framing of questions, research approaches, and how, where, and when findings are disseminated. Only recently has the full extent of potential conflicts of interest related to industry-researcher partnerships come to light. However, not-for-profit and government agencies have stakes and preferences in what types of projects are funded and their decisions are also influenced by public relations and political considerations.

Researchers must please their employers with evidence of their productivity (e.g., successful research grants and high-profile publications). Not surprisingly, researchers choose to pursue certain types of projects over others and gravitate toward topics they believe will help them secure funding. They may defend or try to increase the profile of their approaches or topics through their influence as reviewers or members of editorial boards of journals or grant review committees and appointments to positions of real or symbolic power. There can be a great disincentive to move away from research approaches that have garnered support and recognition in the past. Nonetheless, research topics and approaches go in and out of style over time; subjects become relevant or capture the public's or professionals' imaginations and then often fade. As a result, academic departments, funding bodies, institutions, and dissemination venues become locales where specific tastes and priorities emerge or disappear. This also applies to methodologies within research fields.

Some subject matter areas or theoretical stances for framing subjects are so inherently controversial that securing funding and carrying out data collections are extremely challenging. Anything touching on reproductive health or sexual behavior tends to be potentially volatile, especially in a conservative political climate, and the questioning of the effectiveness or cost-benefit ratio of a health service much beloved by providers, the public, or both as potentially wasteful can encounter resistance.

COMPARATIVE EFFECTIVENESS STUDIES

Research that compares the effectiveness of different clinical approaches or different approaches to managing services is the most relevant for shaping practice and making policy. Comparative effectiveness research (CER) was defined by a federal coordination body established to guide $1.1 billion in earmarked funds under the American Recovery and Reinvestment Act (and later abolished under the Affordable Care Act [ACA]) as:

The conduct and synthesis of research comparing the benefits and harms of different interventions and strategies to prevent, diagnose, treat, and monitor health conditions in "real world" settings. The purpose of this research is to improve health outcomes by developing and disseminating evidence-based information to patients, clinicians, and other decision-makers, responding to their expressed needs, about which interventions are most effective for which patients under specific circumstances. (Federal Coordinating Council, 2009, p. 5)

Although important, comparative effectiveness research is difficult to carry out. Obtaining access to health care settings and to ethically conduct studies exposing patients or communities to different approaches requires a freely acknowledged state of uncertainty regarding the superiority of one approach over another. To conduct meaningful research, the interventions or approaches in question need to be sufficiently standardized and researchers must be able to rigorously measure harms and benefits across sufficient numbers of patients over enough clinical settings (Ashton & Wray, 2013). Comparative intervention research is complicated, demanding, and expensive work to carry out. It is also likely to plunge researchers into politically sensitive debates. It may not be surprising that, because of the practical challenges and political pitfalls involved in evaluating or testing interventions, many researchers in health care are engaged in research intended to inform understandings of health-related phenomena that will enable the design of potentially useful interventions. Unfortunately, when careful evaluations are carried out, history has shown that many widely accepted treatments are shown to be ineffective and needlessly increase both health care costs and risks to the public, suggesting that more rather than less of this difficult research is needed. Funding for comparative effectiveness research, which many hope will stimulate this essential type of inquiry, is included in the ACA of 2010.

THE POLITICS OF RESEARCH APPLICATION IN CLINICAL PRACTICE

INDIVIDUAL STUDIES

To stand any chance of influencing practice or policy, findings must be disseminated and read by those in a position to make or influence clinical or policy decisions. Individual research papers may or may not receive attention depending on timeliness of the topic, whether or not findings are novel, the profile of the researchers, and the prestige of a journal or conference where results are presented.

A key principle of evidence-based practice and policy is that one study alone never establishes anything as incontrovertible fact. In theory, single studies are given limited credence until their findings are replicated. Despite evidence that dramatic findings in landmark studies, especially using nonrandomized or observational research designs, are rarely replicated under more rigorous scrutiny (Ioannidis, 2005), there is often an appetite for novel findings and a drive to act on them. As a result, single studies, particularly ones with findings that resonate strongly with one or more interest groups, can receive a great deal of attention and even influence health policy, even though their findings are preliminary.

Journalists must find the most newsworthy of the findings in research reports and make them understandable and entertaining to their audiences. In contrast, for scientists, legitimacy hinges on integrity in reporting findings. Use of simplistic language or terminology or the reworking of complex scientific ideas into layman's terms in the popular press may result in broad statements unjustified by the data. Being seen as a media darling, especially one whose work is popularized without careful qualifiers, can be damaging to a researcher's scientific credibility. Furthermore, given that reactions and responses (and backlashes) can be very strong, researchers seeking media coverage of their research must be cautious. It is generally best to avoid popular press coverage of one's results before review by peers and publication in a venue aimed at research audiences. Avoiding avoiding overstating results and ensuring that key limitations of study findings are clearly described is essential, particularly if a treatment or approach has been studied in a narrow population or context or without controlling for important background variables.

SUMMARIZING LITERATURE AND THE POLITICS OF GUIDELINES AND SYNTHESES

Despite the appeal of single studies with intriguing results, the principles of evidence-based practice and policy dictate that before action is taken, synthesis of research results be carried out. Studies with larger representative samples and tighter designs are granted more weight in such syntheses.

Conducting and writing systematic reviews and practice guidelines are labor-intensive exercises requiring skill in literature searching, abstracting key elements of relevant research, and comparison of findings. The process is expensive and time-consuming, often requiring investments from stakeholder groups to ensure completion. Synthesis and guideline development are often conducted by teams to render the work involved manageable and increase the quality of the products and user perceptions of balance and fairness in the conclusions. Procedures used to identify relevant literature are now almost always described in detail to permit others to verify (and later update) the search strategy. It is worth noting that except in contexts such as the Cochrane Collaboration (where all procedures are extremely clearly laid out and designed to be as bias-free as possible), the grading of evidence and the drafting of syntheses can be somewhat subjective and reflect rating compromises.

Political forces will influence which topics, clienteles, or areas of science or practices are targeted for synthesis, often high-volume or high-cost services or services where clients are at high risk. Who compiles synthesis documents and under what circumstances reflects research and professional politics as well as influences from funders and policymakers. The credibility of syntheses hinges on the scientific reputation of those responsible for writing and reviewing them. There is debate regarding whether or not subject matter expertise is required of those conducting a synthesis and whether or not having conducted research in an area creates a vested interest that can jeopardize integrity of a review. Interestingly, different individuals tend to be involved in conducting research as opposed to carrying out reviews. Key investigators in the area may not want to take the time away from their research to work on reviews, but may feel a need to defend their studies or protect what they believe to be their interests. Often, recognized experts are brought in at the beginning or end of a search and synthesis exercise to ensure that relevant studies have not been omitted and that study results have been correctly interpreted.

Systematic reviews, disseminated by authoritative sources, can be especially influential for both clinical practice and health policy. When the usefulness of a treatment for recipients is brought into question or it is suggested that some diagnostic or treatment approaches are superior to others, it is very likely that the creators, manufacturers, or researchers involved with the losers will bring their resources together to fight. In 1995, the Agency for Health Care Policy and Research (AHCPR), the federal entity that was the precursor of the Agency for Healthcare Research and Quality (AHRQ), released a practice guideline dealing with the treatment of lower back pain that stated spinal fusion surgery produced poor results (Gray, Gusmano, & Collins, 2003). Lobbyists for spinal surgeons were able to garner sympathy from politicians averse to continued funding for the agency. In the face of other political enemies and threats to the AHCPR, the result was the threatened disbanding of the agency. The AHCPR was reborn in 1999 as the AHRQ, with a similar mandate to focus on "quality improvement and patient safety, outcomes and effectiveness of care, clinical practice and technology assessment, and health care organization and delivery systems" (www.ahrq.gov), but without practice guideline development in its portfolio.

Skepticism is warranted when reading literature syntheses involving the standing of a particular product or service that has either been directly funded by industry or interest groups or had close involvement by industry-sponsored researchers (Detsky, 2006). Guidelines and best practices to reduce bias in literature synthesis and guideline creation are being circulated (Institute of Medicine [IOM], 2009; Palda, Davis, & Goldman, 2007) in much the same way as parameters, checklists, and reporting requirements for randomized trials and observational research (e.g., the CONSORT guidelines at www.consort-statement.org) were first created and disseminated years ago.

THE POLITICS OF RESEARCH APPLIED TO POLICY FORMULATION

Distilling research findings and crafting messages to allow research evidence to influence policy can be even more complex and daunting than translating research related to particular health care technologies or treatments. Direct evidence about the consequences of different policy actions is often sparse, and much extrapolation is necessary to link available evidence with the questions at hand. Attempts have been made in the United States and elsewhere, often through nonprofit foundations such as the Robert Wood Johnson Foundation and the Canadian Foundation for Healthcare Improvement (formerly the Canadian Health Services Research Foundation) to educate the public and policymakers about health services research findings. The political challenges in implementing health policy change are considerable. The amounts of money are often higher, and symbolic significance of the decisions is even greater, which makes conflict across the same types of stakeholder interests discussed throughout this chapter even more dramatic. Box 59-1 shows pearls and pitfalls of using research in a policy context.

Glenn (2002) explores the role of scientific evidence in policymaking with regard to ultimate and derivative values and their relationships to each other. He frames ultimate values as those held without real justification (or need for justification) with facts. Notions that patient suffering is bad and is to be avoided at all costs, that health care is a right (and that society has a duty to help those in need), or that patients deserve care free of errors could all be considered as ultimate values. Ultimate values

---

BOX 59-1 Pearls and Pitfalls of Using Research in Policy Contexts

Pearls

- Before trying to link research with a policy issue, understand the underlying policy issue as well as possible to determine how results in question add to a debate.
- Consider the way opponents of a particular policy stance will interpret study findings, and consider adjusting messages accordingly.
- Be aware of major limitations in the study findings (e.g., weaknesses or Achilles' heels such as lack of randomization in an evaluation study or a failure to consider an important confounder), and be prepared to respond to them and explain why results are relevant anyway.
- Refer to bodies of similar or related research rather than individual studies, where possible, and acknowledge controversies.

Pitfalls

- Assuming policymakers and journalists are familiar with or interested in research method details.
- Writing research results with needlessly biased or strong language and/or citing such research in policy without reservations.
- Exaggerating the magnitude of effects and ignoring all weaknesses or inconsistencies, particularly those that are easily identified by educated nonspecialists.
- Citing research and/or researchers without checking credibility or verifying scientific quality of the results.
- Failing to recognize that research findings are only one component of wider policy debates.

---

are by nature ill-suited to scientific investigation, and in addition to value judgments, they may be fundamental political views about the role of government or religious beliefs. Derivative values result from (or are derived from) the combination of an ultimate value with a stance about the realities of the world. Some may argue that because low nurse staffing leads to higher error rates (an interpretation of research offering a testable insight about the clinical world) and their belief that patients should be exposed to as few errors as possible (an ultimate value), that low staffing should be avoided (or legislated against) through the use of minimum nurse staffing ratios (a derivative value).

In Glenn's words "...science can assess the validity of the beliefs about reality that link derivative to ultimate values" (Glenn, 2002, p. 69). Verifying statements about reality, not defending either ultimate or derivative values, is its role. Researchers are expected to remain objective and fair: to use the rules of evidence for scientific inquiry properly, clearly reporting facts that contradict their impressions or hypotheses, as well as ones consistent with their and others' ultimate and derivative values. However, several forces, namely, a tendency to resist admitting having drawn incorrect or overly simplified conclusions in the past, as well as social and political pressures from one's fan base (what Glenn calls the researcher's significant others) can create problems with keeping these boundaries clear. Researchers may be accused of bias or, worse, promulgating junk science. Journalists have commented on inflated estimates of prevalence or impacts of various diseases or conditions using research data (using loose definitions, questionable assumptions, or data with limited potential to be verified) (Barlett & Steele, 2004) to lobby for increased funding for research, treatment initiatives, or policy actions.

When research findings collide with the interests of stakeholder groups in a policy debate, the responses can be extreme. The ethical integrity, scientific competence, or motivations of the researchers involved can be called into question by stakeholders whose interests are in conflict with particular results. Late in 2009, controversy emerged when e-mail messages exchanged between prominent

United Kingdom climate researchers were made public. These scientists' work is often cited to document claims of global warming and to justify tighter vehicular, industrial emission, and environmental controls. The content of the e-mail messages was considered by some to show clear evidence of departures from objectivity, data massaging, and politicking to reduce the impact of conflicting findings from competing scientists (Booker, 2009; Sarewitz & Thernstrom, 2009). Equally high-profile and bitter arguments surround the potential health hazards associated with genetically modified crops and pit scientists, industry, and government stakeholders against each other. Within health care, as of this writing (winter 2014), controversy continues to simmer about public opinion on the ACA, the consequences of ACA for health insurance premiums, and the impact of the ACA's provisions penalizing employers who do not offer health insurance on unemployment rates and job creation (Bowman & Rugg, 2013; FactChecking "Pernicious" Obamacare Claims, 2013).

The culture of critique and a media appetite for sensationalism, fueled by rapid dissemination of news stories through the Internet, have undermined claims of complete objectivity in research and highlighted the political aspects of research. Whether or not the scientific claims or conclusions of any researchers are correct or even whether objectivity can ever exist in research is probably immaterial to the discussion here. Today, researchers, like politicians, are assumed to have vested interests unless proven otherwise. Good scientific practice is the best defense against claims of bias or worse, but it does not confer immunity from accusations. Nurse researchers aspiring to policy relevance and politically active nurses seeking to use research findings in their endeavors should be aware of the pitfalls and consequences. It is useful for researchers and activists to identify potential winners and losers under proposed policy changes and anticipate their likely interpretations of research findings. In making policy from the research literature tying outcomes to nurse staffing levels, opposing stakeholders at their extremes either cast managers and executives as untrustworthy when it comes to decisions where the bottom line and

patient safety might collide or frame nurses, their associations, and collective bargaining units as self-interested and prepared to see hospitals become insolvent by insisting on unnecessarily high staffing levels and/or expensive staffing models.

In the end, it is probably wise to avoid exaggerating the ultimate influence of research findings on shaping policy. Policy victories attributed to research evidence may be more about skill and luck in turning opinion than the research evidence itself and how it is spun in various forums. Furthermore, policy changes stimulated by or defended by research can be short lived. The balance between various political forces and interest groups can and often do influence the outcomes of many policy debates as much as, or more than, thoughtful application of research evidence. Resistance from organized medicine to expanded scope of practice for advanced practice nurses is one example of where a critical mass of evidence supports a change but political forces have conspired against it (Hughes et al., 2010).

The translation of evidence into clinical practice and policy is, by nature, a political process. Researchers are most likely to influence policy by designing studies that will yield the clearest possible answers to questions with policy relevance.

DISCUSSION QUESTIONS

1. Think about a specific area of clinical care you are familiar with where one or more interest groups are attempting to bring about a change in the nature of clinical care or systems of service delivery. Assume a new, potentially game changing research finding appears in the literature and receives wide attention. Using the list of types of stakeholders in translating research into practice in this chapter, identify the groups that might have an interest in these findings and hazard a guess about their likely reactions to new research.

2. Thinking about Glenn's explanation of the role of scientific evidence in policymaking and returning to the area of care or practice that you considered in connection with the preceding discussion question, what deeply held beliefs (ultimate values) and derivative values (conclusions

and values from interpretation of empirical data about the world in the light of ultimate values) do stakeholders claim in this area of clinical/policy controversy? Do you agree that the purpose of research is to add empirical data to policy debates rather than to support or refute ultimate or derivative value statements?

REFERENCES

Ashton, C. M., & Wray, N. P. (2013). *Comparative effectiveness research: Evidence, medicine and policy.* New York: Oxford University Press.

Barlett, D. L., & Steele, J. B. (2004). *Critical condition: How health care in America became big business—And bad medicine.* New York: Doubleday.

Booker, C. (2009). Climate change: This is the worst scientific scandal of our generation. *The Telegraph.* Retrieved from *www.telegraph.co.uk/comment/columnists/christopherbooker/6679082/Climate-change-this-is-the-worst-scientific-scandal-of-our-generation.html.*

Bowman, K., & Rugg, A. (2013). Top 10 takeaways: Public opinion on the Affordable Care Act. Retrieved from *www.american.com/archive/2013/october/top-10-takeaways-public-opinion-on-the-affordable-care-act.*

Davies, P. T. (1999). What is evidence-based education? *British Journal of Educational Studies, 47*(2), 108–121.

Davies, P. (2004). Is evidence-based government possible? Jerry Lee lecture, 2004. Presented at the 4th Annual Campbell Collaboration Colloquium, Washington, DC: National School of Government (UK). Retrieved from *www.nationalschool.gov.uk/policyhub/downloads/JerryLeeLecture1202041.pdf.*

Detsky, A. S. (2006). Sources of bias for authors of clinical practice guidelines. *Canadian Medical Association Journal, 175*(9), 1033.

FactChecking "Pernicious" Obamacare claims. (2013). Articles/featured posts. Retrieved from *www.factcheck.org/2013/09/factchecking-pernicious-obamacare-claims/.*

Federal Coordinating Council. (2009). Federal Coordinating Council for Comparative Effectiveness Research: Report to the President and the Congress. Washington, DC: Department of Health and Human Services. Retrieved from *books.google.com/books?id=DP9rLEEKjTgC&pg=PA133&lpg=PA133&dq=federal+coordinating+council+for+comparative+effectiveness+research+wray&source=bl&ots=SAoti-DzHz&sig=PfMicRVY_xSWuLQDWOuILbP9prl&hl=en&sa=X&ei=khpiVN7DHcukgwTaiYGIAQ&ved=0CB4Q6AEwAA#v=onepage&q=federal%20coordinating%20council%20for%20comparative%20effectiveness%20research%20wray&f=false.*

Glenn, N. (2002). Social science findings and the "family wars.". In J. B. Imber (Ed.), *Searching for science policy.* New Brunswick, NJ: Transaction.

Gray, B. H., Gusmano, M. K., & Collins, S. R. (2003). AHCPR and the changing politics of health services research. *Health Affairs,* Suppl Web Exclusives, W3-283-307.

Hughes, F., Clarke, S. P., Sampson, D. A., Fairman, J., & Sullivan-Marx, E. M. (2010). Research in support of nurse practitioners. In M. D. Mezey, D. O. McGivern, & E. M. Sullivan-Marx (Eds.), *Nurse practitioners: The evolution and future of advanced practice* (5th ed.). New York: Springer.

Institute of Medicine [IOM]. (2009). Conflicts of interest and development of clinical practice guidelines. In B. Lo & M. J. Field (Eds.), *Conflict of interest in medical research, education, and practice.* Washington, DC: National Academies Press. Retrieved from *www.ncbi.nlm.nih.gov/bookshelf/picrender.fcgi?book=nap12598&blobtype=pdf.*

Ioannidis, J. P. (2005). Contradicted and initially stronger effects in highly cited clinical research. *Journal of the American Medical Association, 294*(2), 218–228.

Palda, V. A., Davis, D., & Goldman, J. (2007). A guide to the Canadian Medical Association handbook on clinical practice guidelines. *Canadian Medical Association Journal, 177*(10), 1221–1226.

Sackett, D. L., Rosenberg, W. M. C., Gray, J. A. M., Haynes, R. B., & Richardson, W. S. (1996). Evidence based medicine: What it is and what it isn't. *British Medical Journal, 312*(7023), 71–72.

Sarewitz, D., & Thernstrom, S. (2009). Climate change e-mail scandal underscores myth of pure science. *The Los Angeles Times.* Retrieved from *articles.latimes.com/2009/dec/16/opinion/la-oe-sarewitzthernstrom16-2009dec16.*

ONLINE RESOURCES

Academy Health (professional association for health policy and health services research)
www.academyhealth.org
Canadian Foundation for Healthcare Improvement
www.cfhi-fcass.ca
Commonwealth Fund
www.commonwealthfund.org

UNIT 4

CHAPTER 60

The Nursing Workforce

Mary Lou Brunell   Angela Ross

"Producing a health care system that delivers the right care—quality care that is patient centered, accessible, evidence based, and sustainable—at the right time will require transforming the work environment, scope of practice, education, and numbers of America's nurses."

The Future of Nursing report
(Institute of Medicine [IOM], 2011)

The supply of nurses in the United States is made up of all licensed practical/vocational nurses (LPNs), registered nurses (RNs), and advanced practice nurses (APNs). Those with active licenses that are clear (without disciplinary or other limitation) are eligible for employment and represent the potential nurse employment pool. The actual nursing workforce is composed of those working in the practice of nursing or those whose job requires a license. To demonstrate the significance of these distinctions, Figure 60-1 illustrates the breakdown of licensed LPNs, RNs, and APNs in Florida, compared with those who define Florida's potential nursing workforce, and then with those who are actually working (Florida Center for Nursing [FCN], 2014b, 2014c, 2014d).

Successful planning requires knowing the real workforce supply numbers. As shown in Figure 60-1, there is a difference of more than 91,500 RNs (34%) between licensees and working nurses. Using the wrong base number could make it appear that a shortage does not exist, on paper, when reality says otherwise. A shortage or surplus exists when the supply does not meet the demand. If there is a need for 220,000 RNs, a supply of 269,760 implies a surplus, although a supply of 178,232 indicates a shortage of more than 40,000 nurses. Identifying the workforce supply can be achieved by collecting

information from nurses or employers. A weakness in seeking the information from employers is their tendency to think in terms of jobs as opposed to people; two full-time jobs could be filled by four part-time nurses. As is the case in Florida, many nurse workforce centers have partnered with their board of nursing to collect supply data during the license renewal process.

The greater difficulty is the collection of demand data. The demand for any profession is based on the willingness of employers to hire and pay for their services. Although several national sources of demand data exist—U.S. Bureau of Labor Statistics, Occupational Employment Statistics, Current Employment Statistics—each has limitations and the ideal source is through employer survey (Spetz & Kovner, 2013). The challenges in conducting a nurse employer survey include high cost, low return rates, and inconsistent definitions of terms. Since 2007, the FCN has been collecting and reporting nurse demand by surveying six nurse employing industries that represent approximately 72% of LPNs, 79% of RNs, and 53% of APNs in Florida. The industries surveyed are hospitals, psychiatric hospitals, hospices, public health departments, home health agencies, and skilled nursing facilities. The wealth of information obtained provides turnover rates, vacancy numbers, skill mix information, and projected growth (FCN, 2014a). Being able to compare supply to demand at the national, state, and local level is critical for strategic health workforce planning, policy development, and funding decisions.

However, demand is not the same as need. How many nurses are needed to meet the population's health care needs (Spetz & Kovner, 2013)? Forecasting models project future need based on the supply of nurses and the anticipated demand

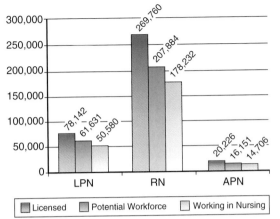

(employment) for nurses. They factor in changes in supply, such as retirements or expanded nursing education programs, and changes in demand, such as population aging or in-migration. Although several sources of forecasts and methods to project need exist, they are not without their limitations and challenges, leaving the door open for the development of a tool that can be adapted at the state level.

CHARACTERISTICS OF THE WORKFORCE

Nurses are the front-line providers of care for most health care consumers. The U.S. nursing workforce is the largest potential nursing workforce in the world and is still predominately female and white/non-Hispanic, with only 9.1% of surveyed respondents reporting as male and 24.6% reporting as a race other than white (U.S. Department of Health and Human Services[HHS], Health Resources and Services Administration [HRSA], 2013).

Although there is a lack of nationally collected and analyzed data on the nursing workforce, researchers have predicted a nursing shortage of between 300,000 to nearly 1 million nurses by 2030 (Jurasheck et al., 2012). A nursing shortage exists because demand, or need, exceeds the supply. Demand is expected to increase more rapidly than the supply as the baby boomer cohort of the U.S. population reaches retirement age. In 2007, the United States entered a severe economic recession. Buerhaus, Auerbach, and Staiger (2009) evaluated the impact of this economic recession on the projected nursing shortage. The authors found that in 2007 and 2008 combined, hospital RN employment increased by 243,000 full-time equivalent RNs; the largest 2-year increase in their 30-year dataset. The U.S. Bureau of Labor Statistics estimated that registered nursing will create 581,500 jobs by 2018, representing the largest absolute projected increase in any occupation (Benson, 2012). According to the Health Resources and Services Administration (HRSA), growth in the nursing workforce has surpassed that of the general population. Comparing census 2000 long form data to the American Community Survey 08-10 showed a 24.1% growth in the RN population to 2,824,641, representing a nearly 14% increase in supply per capita (HRSA 2013). In addition to representing increased education capacity over the previous 9 years, this influx and high employment rate is probably attributable to delayed retirements by older nurses, increases in hours worked, and reentry of younger nurses to the workforce following spouse layoffs or reduction in work. Thus, even with record-setting growth in the nursing workforce, the increase in supply is not necessarily adequate to keep up with increasing demand. In addition to increased demand created by an aging U.S. population that may be living longer with more chronic conditions, the passage of the Affordable Care Act in 2010 will lead to increased demand for RNs and APNs. New models of care delivery as well as an emphasis on prevention require greater care coordination and underscore the importance of an adequate supply of nurses (Auerbach et al., 2013). In addition, it is critical to not just ensure the right number of nurses but also the correct skillset needed to manage the increasingly complex health care needs of the U.S. population.

It is no surprise that the current nursing shortage is not the first. During the 1980s, the United States faced two marked nursing labor shortages, caused primarily by wage controls and cost-cutting approaches. They were essentially resolved through wage increases and increased funding for nursing education. What makes the current shortage different is that it is not driven by the cyclic nature of the economy. Over the next 10 to 15 years, one million nurses—nearly one third of the entire RN workforce—will approach retirement age. The average age of the RN population was 44.6 years in 2010. The majority of growth has occurred in the older and younger populations of nurses such that there are actually fewer RNs aged 36 to 45 working today. This influx of novice nurses and exodus of experienced nurses has grave implications for patients, nurses, and employers (HRSA 2013).

Studies have corroborated the intuitive idea that when nurses are understaffed, patient safety suffers and medical errors increase (Aiken et al, 2002; Diya et al., 2012; Needleman et al., 2002; Needleman et al., 2011). Understaffing also leads to nurse burnout (Aiken et al., 2002; Aiken et al., 2009), which, of course, causes increased turnover. The demand for nurses is expected to dramatically increase as consumers are living longer with more chronic diseases and a significant proportion of the population is approaching retirement age, creating increased need for health care services. As patients, these consumers will require a level of care that is best provided by an appropriate balance of nurses: those with years of hands-on experience and knowledge along with new nurses fresh from the education system.

Although it is difficult to accurately calculate the full cost of nurse turnover as a result of varying methods (Li & Jones, 2013), estimates range from between $22,000 to over $64,000 per turnover (Jones & Gates, 2007) and up to $2 billion in turnover costs to the U.S. health care system based on 2006 salary figures (Brewer et al., 2012). The costs associated with turnover and understaffing have a powerful impact on the economy. In an article analyzing the economic value of RNs, Dall and colleagues (2009) found significant economic value when even a single RN was added to an understaffed unit. The authors calculated the costs of patient mortality resulting from understaffing and evaluated the benefits of adding 133,000 full-time equivalent RNs to the acute care hospital workforce, the number needed to improve staffing at hospitals with low to medium staffing levels. Adding these nurses could save 5900 patient lives each year, with a productivity value of $1.3 billion annually. They also found that this increase in workforce would reduce hospital stays by 3.6 million days and thus generate additional productivity value of $231 million annually and $6.1 billion in annual medical savings. In Florida alone, the FCN found that the cost of turnover for LPNs and RNs exceeded $1.6 billion in fiscal year 2010 to 2011 (FCN, 2013a).

This research makes a compelling case to address nurse supply needs not only by expanding the workforce but also by retaining current nurses. Although continuing to expand education capacity and produce new nurses is important, it is not the only answer. As with the nursing workforce in general, the educator workforce is also aging and a mass wave of faculty retirements is anticipated within the next decade. There is already a faculty shortage, making it impossible for nursing education programs to accept the number of students needed to meet the demand. More than 75,587 qualified applicants were turned away from baccalaureate and graduate nursing programs in 2011 as a result of limited funding for faculty, lack of clinical sites, and lack of qualified faculty applicants (American Association of Colleges of Nursing [AACN], 2012). Even if education capacity could be expanded to meet demand, there will still be a lapse before an adequately experienced workforce is operational. Policy initiatives must take a multipronged approach by focusing on expanding both the general nursing and faculty education capacity, retaining the current nurse workforce, and increasing the diversity of nurses.

EXPANDING THE WORKFORCE

Nursing education programs must be expanded to facilitate growth in the nursing workforce. Successful expansion should be measured not just by increased admissions but also by increased graduations and successful passage of the National Council Licensure Examination for Registered Nurses. Lack of funding to hire additional faculty members and lack of qualified faculty applicants are consistently identified as reasons why programs turn away qualified applicants (AACN, 2012). Increased funding for graduate education is an essential first step toward increasing capacity. Funding for graduate education could help expand the faculty pipeline while also expanding the pool of candidates for other hard-to-fill nursing positions. Through the HRSA, the federal government has a variety of grant programs that offer loan repayment for nurses (HHS, 2009).

A key reason for lack of faculty applicants is the wide discrepancy between industry and academic salaries. Nurses can often earn significantly more in clinical practice than in teaching (Evans, 2013). The National League for Nursing (2010) suggests that this salary difference is a significant issue in recruiting new faculty. Funding aimed at increasing salaries for nurse faculty in entry-level programs would have considerable impact on reducing the faculty shortage. Many employers partner with local colleges to develop faculty-sharing programs; employers pay for salary and benefits and then donate 50% to 100% of the nurse's time to the school. These programs have been very successful, enabling educational institutions to expand admissions while providing faculty who are familiar with the clinical sites and policies. Employers may also offer tuition reimbursement for nurses seeking an advanced degree; this not only serves as a retention strategy for the employer but may also expand the pool of potential nurse educators. Private donations are another source of funding for educational programs.

Strategic use of scarce resources is a critical component of effectively expanding education capacity. Lack of access to clinical sites ranks as a barrier to expansion for all levels of nursing education. In Florida, Deans and Directors within all types of prelicensure nursing programs reported that "limited clinical sites" was the most common barrier to admitting more students (70% of Bachelor of Science in Nursing, 49% of Associate Degree Nursing programs) (FCN, 2013b). As a result, simulation is being implemented as an educational process or strategy designed to imitate the workplace or clinical environment. The National Council of State Boards of Nursing (NCSBN) is conducting a national, multisite, longitudinal study of simulation use in prelicensure nursing programs. Collaborating with learning institutions across the United States, the NCSBN is exploring the role and outcomes of simulation in prelicensure clinical nursing education. The results of such studies will provide the evidence needed to guide its use in nursing education. Although the cost of simulation technology is still high, collaboration among educational programs may be beneficial. Examples of collaboration include the following:

- *Oregon Simulation Alliance (OSA):* An innovative public-private partnership in health care education, the OSA Governing Council includes representation from the state's community colleges, public and independent 4-year colleges and universities, health care provider organizations, and simulation users. Their goal is to increase the health system's simulation capacity, using high-fidelity simulators and virtual reality software, in all regions of the state for multisector, multidisciplinary, and interdisciplinary use for health care workforce development, including both pre- and post-service, reentry and refresher, and career ladder programs (*OregonSimulation.com*).
- *Florida Healthcare Simulation Alliance (FHSA):* Inspiring a culture of innovation in health care simulation, the FHSA was established in 2012 by the FCN to coordinate and expand the use of all forms of simulation in academic settings, health care institutions, and agencies across the state to advance health care education and to foster patient safety. It serves as a resource to facilitate collaboration, networking, and the development and integration of best practices into health

workforce education and the delivery of patient care (*www.FloridaHealthSimAlliance.org*).

Critical to expanding the nursing workforce is the successful entry of new graduates into work settings. The Future of Nursing report recommends the implementation of nurse residency programs in support of nurses' transition to practice after completion of a prelicensure or advanced practice degree program or when they are transitioning into new clinical practice areas (IOM, 2011). Residency programs help ease the transition from education to clinical practice, strengthen commitment to the profession, and improve retention for newly licensed nurses. Development of experience and practical knowledge improves the quality of care and patient outcomes. As demand increases for APNs, the expectation that applicants enter graduate education with years of experience as an RN is no longer present. The resulting need for intense practical experience before a recent APN graduate assumes responsibilities of the new role should be met through a residency program. At the same time, the nurse workforce must respond to changing health industry demands as hospital admissions and lengths of stay decline, resulting in increased levels of care required in long-term care settings and home health. As such, a nurse residency program should be implemented to transition nurses from acute care to the community setting. Increasing the availability of specialized training for experienced nurses may also help produce a workforce with qualified applicants to enter hard-to-fill positions such as critical care and front-line management.

INCREASING DIVERSITY

As the U.S. population continues to grow and increase in diversity, it is important that the nursing workforce reflect these changes to effectively meet patient care needs and ensure cultural competency. Nursing is a predominately female profession; only 9.1% of the national nursing workforce is composed of men, although men make up nearly 50% of the population. Increasing the visibility of men in nursing is a crucial first step toward attracting more male applicants. The same is true for improving the appeal of nursing to ethnic and racial minorities. Stereotypical views of nurses as white women may be limiting their entry. Buerhaus, Auerbach, and Staiger (2009) project that increasing the numbers of men and Hispanics could add enough RNs to the workforce to resolve the projected shortage. The American Assembly for Men in Nursing, with the IOM, has set a goal of 20% male enrollment in U.S. nursing programs by the year 2020 (MacWilliams, Schmidt, & Bleich, 2013). Several state nursing workforce centers and nursing associations have also led diversity efforts. The New Mexico Institute for Nursing Diversity and the Oregon Center for Nursing's Nurturing Cultural Competence in Nursing program are examples.

Increasing diversity in the nursing workforce also requires increasing diversity in the education pipeline. Diverse nursing education faculty is also key to attracting and maintaining a diverse student population. Currently, only about 12.6% of nursing faculty members are from minority backgrounds compared with 37% for the national population (AACN, 2013). The AACN has also worked with several foundations and stakeholders to spearhead efforts to improve diversity in the nursing student pipeline, including scholarships, fellowship programs, and workforce grants (AACN, 2013).

RETAINING WORKERS

Policy efforts to address the shortage must include a focus on retention in both the public and private sectors. At the national level, grants have been given by the HRSA for demonstration programs that can be evaluated and replicated. Foundations have given grants to pilot regional initiatives, and employers have used different types of retention approaches. The Partners Investing in Nursing's Future (PIN) grants, sponsored by the Robert Wood Johnson Foundation (RWJF) and the Northwest Health Foundation, provide funding for localized initiatives and encourage regional collaboration. By requiring a dollar-for-dollar commitment from a local funder, the PIN program, which ran from 2006 to 2011, awarding 61 grants, also sought to encourage a framework for collaborative efforts addressing the shortage. The RWJF has also commissioned numerous reports, including *Wisdom at Work: Retaining Experienced Nurses* and *Wisdom at Work: The Importance of Older and Experienced Nurses in the Workplace.* To retain experienced nurses, health care leaders must focus on creating a healthy work environment for nurses. Negative work cultures within nursing impact both nurse retention and quality of care (McHugh & Ma, 2013). The American Association of Critical-Care Nurses has developed six standards for establishing a healthy work environment with the goal of improving nurse retention and patient outcomes (AACN, 2005).

Understanding that meeting workforce demand cannot be accomplished through a single effort of expanding the education of new nurses, state workforce centers and professional organizations offer nursing leadership development programs to not only enhance the professional image of nursing and promote nurses into policy setting positions but also to improve training for front-line managers. The American Organization of Nurse Executives provides a variety of programs, such as the Emerging Nurse Leader Institute, Nurse Manager Institute, and Essentials of Nurse Manager Orientation (American Organization of Nurse Executives, 2013).

With research showing that job satisfaction is an indicator of turnover (Hayes et al., 2006), improving the work environment at the facility level is perhaps the most effective strategy for improving the retention of both new and experienced nurses. An important and effective first step toward improving nurse retention is ensuring that the organization's leadership clearly values nurses. The Magnet Recognition Program administered by the American Nurses Credentialing Center is one example of a process that supports nursing work (see Chapter 64). It provides a focus on improved collaboration, increased autonomy/accountability for nurses, improved decision-making abilities, safe staffing levels, effective leadership, and improved access to professional development opportunities. Another highly successful initiative was Transforming Care at the Bedside (TCAB), a quality improvement program initiated by the RWJF and the

Institute for Healthcare Improvement that ran from 2003 through 2008. One TCAB goal was to increase the amount of time nurses spent in direct care, thereby improving the work environment and reducing turnover. Successful pilot projects in 10 facilities have facilitated the model being implemented in more than 100 hospitals across the country (RWJF, 2011).

In addition to visible leadership at the organizational level, effective nurse managers can have a significant impact on turnover. To ensure that front-line managers are both a good fit and adequately trained, some organizations have divided the traditional role into two: one focused on clinical activities and the other on administrative and management functions. Separating the roles not only helps reduce what was previously an overwhelming workload for one person but also enables nurses with strong clinical skills to lead without being responsible for management. Identifying new roles is an important step in developing career pathways, which may improve retention. Lack of clear opportunities for professional advancement can also increase turnover (Hayes et al., 2006). Developing new roles, such as patient liaison or admissions counselor, is an important step toward retaining older nurses while also reducing the workload for staff nurses (RWJF, 2006). To date, little is known if such roles have been designed and/or implemented.

To keep a safe mix of new and experienced nurses, nurse employers must implement strategies specifically aimed at retaining older nurses. In addition to the improved benefit to patients, the expertise that older and experienced nurses bring to the workplace is invaluable. This expertise is particularly beneficial when older nurses are paired with new nurses in mentorship programs. Not only do experienced nurses possess extensive clinical knowledge from years of hands-on experience but they also possess a strong knowledge of the organizational culture. Mentorship initiatives help organizations facilitate the transfer of the institutional knowledge to new nurses. New graduates in particular benefit from mentorships, to help ease the transition from school to real-life clinical work. Strategies aimed at retaining older nurses may also serve to improve retention among other groups, including working mothers or inactive nurses. These strategies include implementing tools to reduce the physical demands of the job, offering alternative shorter shifts and reduced workweeks, enhancing retirement benefits, and rewarding loyalty by creating incentives for longevity (Armstrong-Stassen & Stassen, 2013).

ADDRESSING THE NURSING WORKFORCE ISSUES

To address the nursing shortage on a local level, many states have established nursing workforce centers. Although the activities of centers vary, in general they focus on collecting, analyzing, and reporting state-level nursing workforce data while also serving as a source of information related to the shortage and identifying strategies for resolution. Because these centers collect data at a state level, they are typically able to produce more accurate information than previously published by national groups. The 2013 FCN survey of primary nurse employers (hospitals, skilled nursing facilities, home health agencies, hospices, and public health departments) asked responders to identify the top five most difficult-to-fill positions (FCN, 2014a). As was the case with past surveys, the majority of the most difficult-to-fill positions identified required advanced experience, advanced education, or both (e.g., adult critical care, emergency department, unit manager, nurse practitioners). The surprising result in 2013 was the inclusion of positions that would be open to certified nursing assistants, LPNs, and RNs, potentially as new graduates (e.g., inpatient staff nurse, home hospice staff RN, nurse aide, LPN). The only industry that did not indicate a need for entry-level positions was hospitals, sending a clear message to nurse educators: It is time to stop emphasizing hospital settings as the favored location for new graduate entry into practice. Nursing's academic partners must adjust to change and meet future demands, which indicate decreasing acute care bed use and increasing home health and long-term care needs. Nursing workforce centers also focus on workforce planning within the state, and they serve a key role in

presenting recommendations and educating legislators and policymakers.

Leaders of state nursing workforce centers came together in 2004 to establish the National Forum of State Nursing Workforce Centers (the Forum). With 33 participating states (as of 2014), the Forum seeks to create a unique dialogue that serves as a medium for wisdom sharing and strategy development in promoting the development of an optimal nursing workforce to meet the health care needs of the population. Many of these centers have established data-collection methods and are producing extremely accurate state-level information. However, there can be substantial differences in both the methods and metrics used for collecting nursing workforce data, making it difficult to produce an accurate national picture of the nursing shortage. After evaluating data-collection practices, the Forum established three datasets—Minimum Nurse Supply, Minimum Nurse Demand, and Minimum Nurse Education Program—to standardize the collection of state-level nursing workforce data and to create a national repository of data. The goal is to enable state and national workforce planners to identify and implement accurate and timely approaches to resolve the shortage. Planners and policy analysts will be able to benchmark progress and improve accuracy in forecasting the future workforce supply and demand. For more information on the Forum, visit *www.nursingwork forcecenters.org*.

In addition to state nursing workforce centers, private foundations, consumer groups, and professional practice associations have collected information and made recommendations for policy changes in the public arena as well as in the workplace. One major funder, the RWJF, has provided millions of dollars in funding for a broad range of nursing research and nursing workforce retention initiatives. The RWJF partnered with the AARP Foundation to create the Center to Champion Nursing in America (CCNA), which focuses on developing nurse leaders, expanding nursing education capacity, and retaining the existing nursing workforce. The CCNA provides leadership and technical support for the Future of Nursing: Campaign for Action (see Chapter 79). Numerous professional practice associations have initiated efforts to address the shortage, particularly efforts to improve the work environment and enhance the image of nursing. The American Nurses Association, the American Association of Colleges of Nursing, the American Hospital Association, and the National League for Nursing have made the shortage a priority issue. The Joint Commission has a Nursing Advisory Council on initiatives to resolve the nursing shortage.

At the federal level, the HRSA distributes funding for Nursing Workforce Development Programs through Title VIII of the Public Health Service Act; in fiscal year 2012, funding for these programs totaled nearly $148 million. Through the American Recovery and Reinvestment Act (ARRA) of 2009, the HRSA dedicated $200 million to provide grants, loans, loan repayments, and scholarships to expand training within the health care profession; $39 million of these funds were specifically for nurses and nurse faculty. The U.S. Department of Labor (DOL) provided funding for workforce initiatives, dedicating ARRA funds to the health care profession, including $220 million for high-growth industries with a priority on training workers within the health care sector. The DOL actively sought projects in nursing that facilitated progression along the nursing career pathway. In 2003, the Congressional Caucus on Nursing was founded by a nurse member of Congress, Lois Capps (D-CA), to better educate members of Congress about nursing (see Chapter 42). The Caucus has focused specifically on the shortage and workforce issues. It also serves as a clearing house for information and a sounding board for ideas brought forth by the nursing community.

CONCLUSION

The uniqueness of the nursing shortage is related to a variety of factors that require new solutions. It is not a simple issue of supply and demand. It is time to consider what changes and enhancements must be implemented to assure an adequate, qualified nurse workforce to meet the health care needs of the U.S. population. Increasing salaries and expanding education capacity alone will not assure an adequate, qualified workforce for the coming decades. Strategic resolution must include strategies that will (1) increase education capacity by addressing the nurse faculty shortage and clinical space limitations; (2) retain the current nursing workforce by improving the work environment, addressing age-related challenges, and valuing nurses' contributions; and (3) collect necessary data as the base for accurate forecasting, evaluation of interventions, sound health policy development, and allocation of scarce resources. The National Forum of State Nursing Workforce Centers provides a vehicle to bring state-level data and resolution strategies to the national level. Good policy requires good data, and this is particularly evident in developing policy surrounding the nursing shortage in the United States. Continued sharing of information, collaboration to successfully implement programs, and funding to support the work are critical to effectively address nurse workforce issues.

DISCUSSION QUESTIONS

1. Why do you think the issues presented in this chapter persist in today's workforce culture?
2. What steps can be instituted at the management level that might help to curb these problems?
3. In your opinion, who are the biggest stakeholders for this chapter? Why?

REFERENCES

Aiken, L., Clarke, S., Sloane, D., Lake, E., & Cheney, T. (2009). Effects of hospital care environment on patient mortality and nurse outcomes. *Journal of Nursing Administration, 39*(7–8), S45–S51.

Aiken, L. H., Clarke, S. P., Sloane, D. M., Sochalski, J., & Silber, J. H. (2002). Hospital nurse staffing and patient mortality, nurse burnout, and job dissatisfaction. *Journal of the American Medical Association, 288*(16), 1987–1993.

American Association of Colleges of Nursing. (2012). Fact sheet: Nursing faculty shortage. Washington, DC: American Association of Colleges of Nursing. Retrieved from *www.aacn.nche.edu/Media/FactSheets/FacultyShortage.htm.*

American Association of Colleges of Nurses. (2013). Fact sheet: Enhancing diversity in the nursing workforce. Washington, DC: American Association of Colleges of Nursing. Retrieved from *www.aacn.nche.edu/Media/FactSheets/diversity.htcm.*

American Association of Critical-Care Nurses. (2005). AACN standards for establishing and sustaining healthy work environments: A journey to excellence. Viejo, CA: American Association of Critical-Care

Nurses. Retrieved from *www.aacn.org/wd/hwe/content/hwehome.pcms?menu=*.

American Organization of Nurse Executives. (2013). Programs. Retrieved from *www.aone.org/education/programs/shtml*.

Armstrong-Stassen, M., & Stassen, K. (2013). Professional development, target-specific satisfaction, and older nurse retention. *Career Development International, 18*(7), 673–693.

Auerbach, D. I., Staiger, D. O., Muench, U., & Buerhaus, P. I. (2013). The nursing workforce in an era of health care reform. *The New England Journal of Medicine, 368*, 1470–1472.

Benson, A. (2012). Labor market trends among registered nurses. *Policy Politics Nursing Practice, 13*(4), 205–213.

Brewer, C., Kovner, C., Greene, W., Tukov-Shuser, M., & Djukic, M. (2012). Predictors of actual turnover in a national sample of newly licensed registered nurses employed in hospitals. *Journal of Advanced Nursing, 68*(3), 521–538.

Buerhaus, P. I., Auerbach, D. I., & Staiger, D. O. (2009). The recent surge in nurse employment: Causes and implications. *Health Affairs, 28*(4), w657–w668.

Dall, T. M., Chen, Y. J., Seifert, R. F., Maddox, P. J., & Hogan, P. F. (2009). The economic value of professional nursing. *Medical Care, 47*(1), 97–104.

Diya, L., Van den Heede, K., Sermeus, W., & Lesaffre, E. (2012). The relationship between in-hospital mortality, readmission into the intensive care nursing unit and/or operating theatre and nurse staffing levels. *Journal of Advanced Nursing, 68*(5), 1073–1081.

Evans, J. (2013). Factors influencing recruitment and retention of nurse educators reported by current nurse faculty. *Journal of Professional Nursing, 2013*(1), 11–20.

Florida Center for Nursing. (2013a). The economic impact of Florida's nursing workforce. Orlando, FL: Florida Center for Nursing. Retrieved from *www.flcenterfornursing.org/ForecastsStrategies/EvidenceRationale.aspx*.

Florida Center for Nursing. (2013b). Florida pre-licensure registered nurse education: Academic year 2011–2012. Orlando, FL: Florida Center for Nursing. Retrieved from *www.flcenterfornursing.org/StatewideData/NurseEducationReports.aspx*.

Florida Center for Nursing. (2014a). Demand for nurses in Florida: The 2013 survey of Florida's nurse employers. Orlando, FL: Florida Center for Nursing. Retrieved from *www.flcenterfornursing.org/StatewideData/NurseDemandReports.aspx*.

Florida Center for Nursing. (2014b). Florida's advanced practice nurse practitioner supply: 2012–2013 demographics, workforce characteristics and trends. Orlando, FL: Florida Center for Nursing. Retrieved from *www.flcenterfornursing.org/StatewideData/NurseSupplyReports.aspx*.

Florida Center for Nursing. (2014c). Florida's licensed practical nurse supply: 2012–2013 demographics, employment characteristics and trends. Orlando, FL: Florida Center for Nursing. Retrieved from *www.flcenterfornursing.org/StatewideData/NurseSupplyReports.aspx*.

Florida Center for Nursing. (2014d). Florida's registered nurse supply: 2012–2013 workforce characteristics and trends. Orlando, FL: Florida Center for Nursing. Retrieved from *www.flcenterfornursing.org/StatewideData/NurseSupplyReports.aspx*.

Hayes, L. J., O'Brien-Pallas, L., Duffield, C., Shamian, J., Buchan, J., Hughes, F., et al. (2006). Nurse turnover: A literature review. *International Journal of Nursing Studies, 43*(2), 237–263.

Institute of Medicine [IOM]. (2011). *The future of nursing: Leading change, advancing health.* Washington, DC: National Academies Press.

Jones, C., & Gates, M. (2007). The costs and benefits of nurse turnover: A business case for nurse retention. *The Online Journal of Issues in Nursing, 12*(3), manuscript 4.

Jurasheck, S. P., Zhang, X., Ranganathan, V. K., & Lin, V. W. (2012). United States registered nurse workforce report card and shortage forecast. *American Journal of Medical Quality, 27*(3), 241–249. doi:10.1177/1062860611416634.

Li, Y., & Jones, C. B. (2013). A literature review of nursing turnover costs. *Journal of Nursing Management, 21*, 405–418.

MacWilliams, B. R., Schmidt, B., & Bleich, M. (2013). Men in nursing. *American Journal of Nursing, 113*(1), 38–44.

McHugh, M. D., & Ma, C. (2013). Hospital nursing and 30-day readmissions among Medicare patients with heart failure, acute myocardial infarction, and pneumonia. *Medical Care, 51*(1), 52–59.

National League for Nursing. (2010). 2010 NLN nurse educator shortage fact sheet. Retrieved from *www.nln.org/governmentaffairs/pdf/NurseFacultyShortage.pdf*.

Needleman, J., Buerhaus, P., Mattke, S., Stewart, M., & Zelevinsky, K. (2002). Nurse staffing levels and the quality of care in hospitals. *The New England Journal of Medicine, 346*(22), 1715–1722.

Needleman, J., Buerhaus, P., Pankratz, V., Leibson, C., Stevens, S., & Harris, M. (2011). Nurse staffing and inpatient hospital mortality. *New England Journal of Medicine, 364*(11), 1037–1045.

Robert Wood Johnson Foundation. (2006). *Wisdom at work: The importance of the older and experienced nurse in the workplace.* Princeton, NJ: Robert Wood Johnson Foundation.

Robert Wood Johnson Foundation. (2011). Transforming care at the bedside: An RWJF national program. Retrieved from *www.rwjf.org/en/research-publications/find-rwjf-research/2011/07/transforming-care-at-the-bedside.html*.

Spetz, J., & Kovner, C. T. (2013). How can we obtain data on the demand for nurses? *Nursing Economic$, 31*(4), 203–207.

U.S. Department of Health and Human Services. (2009). News release: Secretary Sebelius makes Recovery Act funding available to expand health professions training. Washington, DC: U.S. Department of Health and Human Services. Retrieved from *www.hhs.gov/news/press/2009pres/07/20090728c.html*.

U.S. Department of Health and Human Services, Health Resources and Services Administration. (2013). The U.S. nursing workforce: Trends in supply and education. Washington, DC: U.S. Department of Health and Human Services. Retrieved from *bhpr.hrsa.gov/healthworkforce/supplydemand/nursing/nursingworkforce/nursingworkforcefullreport.pdf*.

ONLINE RESOURCES

Florida Center for Nursing
www.flcenterfornursing.org
The National Forum of State Nursing Workforce Centers
nursingworkforcecenters.org
The Robert Wood Johnson Foundation
www.rwjf.org

CHAPTER 61

Rural Health Care: Workforce Challenges and Opportunities

Alan Morgan

"Both the ideal and the reality of rural community are hard to define."

M. Troughton, 1999

Rural America is a vast, sparsely populated geographic location in which approximately 62 million people currently live. Currently 75% of the nation's geography is considered "rural and frontier" (Gamm & Hutchinson, 2005). The obstacles that health care providers and patients face in these rural areas are very different from those in urban areas. Rural Americans face a unique combination of factors that create significant disparities in health care when compared with urban areas. To understand the rural health care system, one must first understand that rural is not simply a small version of urban. Rural America has specific defining characteristics that represent a distinctive health care delivery environment.

Economic factors, cultural and social differences, educational shortcomings, lack of recognition by policymakers, and the sheer isolation of living in remote rural areas all conspire to impede rural Americans in their struggle to lead a normal, healthy life. This unique health care environment requires a specialized health care approach to delivering care. Since rural health care providers often struggle to provide care while maintaining fiscal viability, it is a fragile health care system, and much like the Arctic tundra, it can be easily damaged by unintended state and/or federal health care policy actions.

This chapter examines what distinguishes rural health care systems and discusses policy options to address these issues, which include the following three key characteristics:

- High health disparities within the patient population
- Geographic challenges that work to impede health
- Lack of health care resources

WHAT MAKES RURAL HEALTH CARE DIFFERENT?

Health care problems in rural areas are higher than urban or suburban locations. This is a unique aspect that is a result of many factors including education and poverty. On average, rural populations have higher proportions of elderly and child patients; unemployment and underemployment; and poor, uninsured, and underinsured residents than urban areas.

The fact that the private sector health insurance system is an employer-based system creates a financial barrier for many rural residents who do not access insurance through their employer. This is because many rural residents are either self-employed, work for small businesses that do not provide health insurance, or are unemployed. Rural residents are less likely to have private health coverage and the rural poor are less likely to be covered by Medicaid benefits than their urban counterparts. In addition, rural adults are more likely to be uninsured than urban adults, with uninsured rates among rural Hispanic adults greater than 50%. Rural adults are more likely than urban adults to report having deferred care because of cost. On average, per capita income is $7000 lower in rural than in urban areas, and rural Americans are more likely to live below the poverty level (Gamm & Hutchinson, 2005).

The challenges of health care provision among rural residents are significant and include the following:

- Rural adults are more likely to be obese than urban adults, with particularly high rates of obesity among rural African Americans (Gamm & Hutchinson, 2005).
- Rural residents are less likely to receive an annual dental exam.
- Rural women are less likely than urban women to be in compliance with mammogram screening guidelines.
- Rural adults are more likely to have diabetes than urban adults.
- The death rate for people between the ages of 1 and 24 years old is 25% higher in rural areas than in urban areas (Bennett, Olatosi & Probst, 2008).

Rural residents have a significantly greater distance to travel to access health care on average than their urban counterparts, a problem compounded by the lack of public transportation within small towns and communities. This has a direct impact on patient care, follow-up care, and long-term outcomes. Although the traditional goal of pre-hospital emergency medical services (EMS) has been to provide patients with immediate transportation to the nearest hospital, this role has greatly expanded in rural communities to serve in multiple patient transport roles. Very few small communities have paid EMS services. As of 2005, volunteer providers respond to medical emergencies for over 50% of the country (Gamm & Hutchinson, 2005).

Rural health care systems, with small numbers of providers and sparse resources, are tenuously balanced to meet the needs of residents while providing adequate income and quality of life to health care providers. Specialty care is delivered differently in rural areas, with a greater reliance on nontraditional staffing arrangements. The national shortage of nurses within the health care system has been well documented. In rural areas, nursing shortages are exacerbated by the rural employers' inability to compete with urban employers in terms of wages,

start-up bonuses, and benefits offered (Gamm & Hutchinson, 2005).

DEFINING RURAL

The need to define what is rural remains a deceptively complex policy issue and there is no single universally accepted definition. For the purposes of federal programs that target public resources toward rural communities, there are more than 15 program-specific rural designations that are currently used within various programs and more than 70 federal definitions. The definition of rural remains a key issue of rural health care policy. The most widely used definitions of rural are based on either the federal Office of Management and Budget (OMB) characterization of counties or the Census Bureau Urbanized Area categorization of census blocks and block groups.

The Census Bureau classifies rural as being all territory, population, and housing units located in nonurbanized areas and nonurban clusters. For the purposes of the Census Bureau, urbanized areas include populations of at least 50,000. Urban clusters include populations between 2500 and 50,000. The core locations of both urbanized areas and urban clusters are defined based on a population density of at least 1000 persons per square mile, and adjacent areas have at least 500 persons per square mile.

The Office of Management and Budget classifies nonmetropolitan or rural counties as those counties outside the boundaries of metropolitan areas (50,000 people or more). A metropolitan area must contain one or more central counties with urbanized areas. These nonmetropolitan counties are subdivided into two types; micropolitan areas and noncore counties. Micropolitan areas are urban clusters of at least 10,000 but fewer than 50,000 people.

By successfully defining rural, Medicare and Medicaid payment methodologies can be adjusted for the purpose of ensuring access to care in these geographic locations. Many rural communities have adverse economic conditions that limit a local health care provider's ability to furnish a broad array of necessary services. Therefore, payment policy interventions are often necessary to preserve rural patients' access to high-quality care.

Low volumes of patients present a challenge in delivering care in rural areas in an economical manner and the patients are often older and have significant underlying health care problems. This situation leads to a lack of volume purchasing power, greater transportation costs, and higher health care needs in many situations.

The National Rural Health Association (NRHA), a nonprofit membership association, strongly recommends that definitions of rural be specific to the programmatic purpose in which they are used. According to the NRHA, those programs targeting rural communities, rural providers, and rural residents do so for particular reasons, and those reasons should be the guide for selecting the criteria for a programmatic designation. This position ensures that any rural designation is appropriate for a specific situation and that it will best fit specific programs (National Rural Health Association [NRHA], 2005b).

Despite ongoing federal and state efforts to adequately address rural health, Medicare payments to rural hospitals and physicians remain less than those of their urban counterparts for equivalent services (Gamm & Hutchinson, 2005). The federal government has often responded to these rural financial realities by modifying the Medicare payment system by means of rural payment add-ons or other payment enhancement methodologies that provide additional payments for providers practicing in rural areas.

In addition, multiple federal grant programs have been established to target rural health. These grant programs are designed to assist the resource challenges faced by rural health care providers. Most often these grant programs target issues of workforce, infrastructure investment, and health care outreach.

RURAL POLICY, RURAL POLITICS

The political context for rural health policy is an ever-evolving process as politicians consider the political weight of the rural-voting demographic. Federal policymakers first recognized the political and policy need for targeted rural legislation to address rural health care in the late 1990s. Since the Balanced Budget Act of 1997, federal legislation has not only recognized the importance of sustaining the rural health care safety net but also using its unique characteristics as a learning lab for successful systems of care.

Targeted rural Medicare provisions included within the Balanced Budget Act of 1997, and again within the Medicare Modernization Act of 2003, provided members of Congress with the ability to present a successful rural policy agenda to their constituents. Among these provisions was the establishment of new payment demonstration programs for rural hospitals and rural clinics, as well as new payment enhancements for rural home health care and increased payments for clinicians practicing in rural underserved areas.

Equally important in these payment reforms was the recognition from policymakers that rural health care systems are fragile, as they operate on slim margins, and that they possess limited resources. A loss of health care access in rural communities can have a significant adverse impact on the sustainability of the rural community itself.

Rural health care providers are usually part of small health systems, where response to health problems is easier to accomplish, allowing rural health to innovate and evolve easily, and provide policymakers with opportunities to launch demonstration projects at a lower cost, with the potential for a meaningful and sustainable return on investment (Institute of Medicine [IOM], 2006).

This represents a contradiction in rural health service delivery: It is a geographically defined area where the system is fragile yet capable of innovation and adaptation, making it unique among our nation's health delivery settings. Inherent within this contradiction is why it is so appealing to many health care professionals to choose to practice in a rural setting, and there is no path forward without a fully functioning nurse workforce, one in which nurses are allowed to practice to the fullest extent of their education (Robert Wood Johnson Foundation 2013).

THE OPPORTUNITIES AND CHALLENGES OF RURAL HEALTH

Ultimately, a key issue for rural health care policy and practice is the issue of access to care. With limited resources, the ongoing policy debate continues to center on the question of the appropriate level of care provided in a timely manner and with the appropriate providers. This is particularly true for the recruitment and retention of nurses. Nurses in rural areas are expected to be familiar with performing the expert generalist role. They must understand how to interface hospital services with community-based services and programs and be comfortable with rural social structures that can influence practice patterns. Rural social structures can include threats to confidentiality, problems associated with traditional gender roles, and geographic and professional isolation (Bushy, 2004).

The rural practice experience can, however, be successful and rewarding for rural nurses through increased professional experience and autonomy, quality of life outside the clinical setting, and the potential for federal support through grants that promote innovative rural nursing models of care. The small organizational structures in rural areas create an environment for creative solutions to address these challenges, and to realize these opportunities, proper access to tools and information must be readily available.

Access to current and complete information to perform clinical responsibilities effectively is a serious issue for rural professionals. Because of rising printing costs, libraries of all types are providing fewer resources, and travel costs to attend continuing education courses are significant challenges. Online courses are an emerging solution, but the issue remains a concern for recruitment and retention of health care providers.

Because of the limited number of physicians and the need for primary care practitioners, rural communities make widespread use of physician assistants (PAs) and advanced practice nurses (APRNs). These practitioners are well qualified to improve access in rural locations.

From a national perspective, significant rural workforce proposals were included within the Affordable Care Act (ACA) of 2010. These provisions included a permanent reauthorization of the federal health centers program and also the National Health Service Corps (NHSC). The NHSC provides scholarships and student loan repayments to individuals who agree to a period of service as primary care providers in a federally designated Health Professional Shortage Area. Also included within the new law were provisions designed to reauthorize and expand existing health workforce education and training programs under Titles VII and VIII of the Public Health Service Act (PHSA). Title VII supports the education and training of physicians, dentists, physician assistants, and other public health workers through grants, scholarships, and loan repayment. The ACA creates several new programs designed to increase training experiences for primary care workers in rural areas as well as community-based settings and provides specific training opportunities to increase the supply of pediatric subspecialists and geriatricians. The ACA also expands the nursing workforce development programs authorized under PHSA Title VIII to bolster undergraduate and graduate nursing education and training.

However, although these workforce provisions were authorized within the ACA, many of these provisions have yet to be funded by Congress in the appropriations process, and therefore are not yet available.

The health care providers most likely to serve in rural areas come from rural areas. In addition many providers also often cite that climate, geographic features, and recreational facilities had a positive influence on their choice of practice location. Health care students and professionals who work and live in rural communities feel appreciated by the communities in which they serve and cite the benefit of knowing that what they do makes a difference in their community (NRHA, 2005a).

Rural communities provide wonderful opportunities as well as significant challenges to providing health care that best meets the needs of their people. A thorough understanding of the unique issues can enhance the quality of life for both providers and recipients of care. The federal government's role in supporting innovative systems of care is critical.

Because of the nature of rural practice and workforce shortages, federal and state health policies which support the independence of Nurse Practitioners is an emerging policy issue today. Although telemedicine is often viewed as a tool to address workforce shortages, practitioners in the field will remain a critical part of the rural health care system.

DISCUSSION QUESTIONS

1. How are rural definitions used to address population health care access needs?
2. Describe how health care access issues impact community health. What role can nurses play in addressing these community health needs, including policy actions?
3. What are unique attributes of rural practice that are appealing to providers?
4. What role does the ACA play in addressing workforce shortages in rural communities?

REFERENCES

Bennett, K., Olatosi, B., & Probst, J. C. (2008). Health disparities: A rural-urban chartbook. South Carolina Rural Health Research Center, 3. Retrieved from *rhr.sph.sc.edu/report/(7-3)%20Health%20Disparities %20A%20Rural%20Urban%20Chartbook%20-%20Distribution%20 Copy.pdf.*

Bushy, A. (2004). *Rural nursing: Practice and issues.* American Nurses Association continuing education module, American Nurses Association, 51.

Gamm, L. D., & Hutchinson, L. L. (Eds.), (2005). Healthy people 2010: A companion document for rural areas: Rural healthy people 2010 (vol. 3). College Station, Texas: Health, Southwest Rural Health Research Center. Retrieved from *www.srph.tamhsc.edu/centers/rhp2010/Volume _3/Vol3rhp2010.pdf.*

Institute of Medicine [IOM]. (2006). *Quality through collaboration: The future of rural health.* Washington, D.C.: Institute of Medicine.

National Rural Health Association [NRHA]. (2005a). Recruitment and retention of a quality health workforce in rural areas. Retrieved from *www .ruralhealthweb.org/go/left/policy-and-advocacy/policy-documents-and -statements/issue-papers-and-policy-briefs.*

National Rural Health Association [NRHA]. (2005b). Definition of rural. Retrieved from *www.ruralhealthweb.org/go/left/about-rural-health/ how-is-rural-defined.*

Robert Wood Johnson Foundation. (2013). RWJF scholars work to strengthen rural nursing. Retrieved from *www.rwjf.org/en/about-rwjf/newsroom/ newsroom-content/2013/02/rwjf-scholars-work-to-strengthen-rural -nursing.html?cid=xsh_rwjf_em.*

ONLINE RESOURCES

The National Rural Health Association
www.ruralhealthweb.org
The Federal Office of Rural Health Policy
www.hrsa.gov/ruralhealth
The Rural Assistance Center
www.raconline.org
The Rural Recruitment and Retention Network
www.3rnet.org

UNIT 4

CHAPTER 62

Nurse Staffing Ratios: Policy Options

Joanne Spetz

"The problems of the world cannot possibly be solved by skeptics or cynics whose horizons are limited by the obvious realities."

John F. Kennedy

The importance of nursing to the delivery of high-quality health care has been recognized since the inception of the practice of nursing. Various factors contribute to the quality of nursing care including the expertise of nursing staff, availability of supportive personnel and other health professionals, good communication among the care team, and the nurse/patient ratio. It was not until the early 2000s that high-quality empirical research found consistent relationships between licensed nurse staffing and the quality of patient care (Lang et al., 2004; Kane et al., 2007).

Concerns about the effects of changes in nurse staffing levels in the 1990s, combined with the increasing influence of nursing unions, resulted in the passage of California Assembly Bill (AB) 394 in 1999, the first comprehensive legislation in the United States to establish minimum staffing levels for registered nurses (RNs) and licensed vocational nurses (LVNs) in hospitals. This bill required that the California Department of Health Services (DHS) establish specific staffing ratios. These were announced in 2002 and implemented beginning in 2004. Since then, other states and the federal government have considered developing regulations for nurse staffing in hospitals. In 2014, for example, Massachusetts passed legislation mandating a ratio of one or two patients per nurse in intensive care units (Associated Press, 2014).

THE ESTABLISHMENT OF CALIFORNIA'S REGULATIONS

Throughout the late 1990s and early 2000s, there was substantial debate about the changes in hospital staffing that had occurred in the 1990s and the effects of such changes on the quality of care (Aiken, Sochalski, & Anderson, 1996; Spetz, 1998; Unruh & Fottler, 2006; Wunderlich, Sloan, & Davis, 1996). In some states, legislators and regulatory agencies considered staffing requirements with an aim to increase the numbers of nurses and other health care personnel working in hospitals and other settings. As the 1990s ended, a shortage of RNs emerged, and concern about poor staffing in hospitals continued (Kilborn, 1999). It was in this environment that AB 394 was passed by the California legislature. Previous Republican governors had vetoed similar legislation, but union-friendly Democratic Governor Gray Davis signed AB 394, satisfying union efforts to pass minimum-ratio legislation. AB 394 charged the California DHS with determining specific unit-by-unit nurse/patient ratios.

The DHS began an extensive effort to determine the new minimum nurse staffing ratios, with little research to guide them (Kravitz et al., 2002; Lang et al., 2004; Spetz et al., 2000). To help develop the proposed ratios, the DHS commissioned a study by researchers at the University of California, Davis (Kravitz et al., 2002). It also received recommendations about the ratios from stakeholders, ranging from the California Hospital Association (CHA) proposal of a ratio of 1 licensed nurse per 10 patients in medical-surgical units and the California Nurses Association recommendation of 1 licensed nurse per 3 patients in medical-surgical units. The ratios established by DHS were between those recommended by the CHA and the unions, with a 1:6 ratio in medical-surgical units starting January 1, 2004, and a 1:5 ratio in medical-surgical units commencing in January 2005. Other units have higher minimum-ratio requirements. The minimum ratios do not replace the requirement that hospitals staff according to a patient classification system (PCS); if a hospital's PCS indicates that higher staffing is needed, the hospital should staff accordingly.

WHAT HAS HAPPENED AS A RESULT OF THE RATIOS?

The implementation of California's minimum nurse staffing ratio legislation led to legal challenges and state government efforts to expand RN education. It also drove increases in hospital nurse staffing and wages in California. Several studies have found that the ratios are linked to higher nurse satisfaction, but there is little evidence that the regulations improved patient outcomes. Some research has found that there may have been negative impacts on hospitals' finances and ability to provide charity care.

LEGAL CHALLENGES

Two days before the ratios went into effect, the CHA filed a lawsuit arguing that the staffing ratios should not apply if a nurse takes a scheduled break or unscheduled restroom visit. The DHS contended that if the ratios were to have any meaning, they must be effective at all times. The judge hearing the case agreed with the DHS in a May 2004 ruling (Berestein, 2004). The second major legal challenge to the ratio regulations came from Governor Arnold Schwarzenegger, who sought to delay the implementation of the stricter ratio of one licensed nurse to five patients scheduled for January 2005 due to the severe shortage of licensed nurses (Rapaport, 2004). The CHA filed suit against the DHS in December 2004 alleging that the emergency order had illegally bypassed the legislature (LaMar, 2005). In early March, a Superior Court judge tentatively ruled that the DHS had indeed not followed the law when issuing the emergency regulation (Salladay &

Chong, 2005), and the judge's decision was finalized in May 2005 (Benson, 2005a, 2005b; Gledhill, 2005).

EXPANSION OF NURSING EDUCATION

To assist hospitals in meeting the staffing ratio rules, both former Governor Davis and Governor Schwarzenegger dedicated funds to expanding nursing education and reducing attrition from nursing programs. Between 2004 to 2005 and 2009 to 2010, nursing graduations in California increased by 72%, reaching over 11,500 new RN graduates per year (Spetz, 2013).

ARE HOSPITALS MEETING THE RATIOS?

The inspection and enforcement mechanisms of the DHS are relatively weak. The DHS does not have the authority to impose fines or monetary penalties on hospitals that are found to violate the ratios, but instead requests and monitors plans submitted by hospitals to remedy the problem. However, other mechanisms do exist to ensure that hospitals adhere to the ratios. First, government payers such as Medicare and Medi-Cal (the state Medicaid program) require that hospitals meet all state and federal regulations and can deny payment to violators. Second, California's cap on malpractice awards does not apply in cases of negligence, and a hospital could be deemed negligent if it consistently did not adhere to minimum nurse staffing regulations (Robertson, 2004). Third, unions draw public attention to hospitals that do not meet the staffing requirements, resulting in negative publicity for hospitals and increased scrutiny from DHS inspectors. Fourth, labor organizations that represent nurses have sought to incorporate staffing standards in their contract negotiations, with some success (Gordon, 2005; Osterman, 2005).

Several studies of all California hospitals have found that annual average numbers of RN productive hours and nurse staffing ratios in medical-surgical units increased markedly between 2001 and 2006 (Conway et al., 2008; Cook et al., 2012; Mark et al., 2012; Munnich, 2013; Spetz et al., 2009; Spetz et al., 2013). Spetz and colleagues (2009) found that statewide average RN hours per patient day increased 16.2% from 1999 through 2006, to an average of 6.9 hours per patient day. Interviews conducted with hospital leaders by a research team at the University of California, San Francisco (UCSF) revealed that many chief nursing officers and other managers said they had hired nurses to meet the ratios, and most noted that it is challenging to adhere to the ratios at all times, including during scheduled breaks (Chapman et al., 2009).

Aiken and colleagues (2010) surveyed nearly 80,000 RNs in California, New Jersey, and Pennsylvania to learn their experiences with staffing, the work environment, and patient care. They found that nurse workloads, measured according to the average number of patients per shift, were lower in California than in New Jersey and Pennsylvania and that over 80% of California nurses reported that their assigned workloads were in compliance with the state's regulation.

HAS THE MIX OF STAFF CHANGED?

There have been concerns that hospitals may have eliminated support staff positions because of the minimum licensed nurse staffing requirements (Spetz, 2001). Analyses of staffing data collected by the Collaborative Alliance for Nursing Outcomes (CALNOC) suggest that the substitution of licensed nurses for unlicensed staff may be widespread as the increase in RN staffing was much larger than the overall staffing increase among their hospitals (Bolton et al., 2007; Donaldson et al., 2005). In a series of qualitative interviews, some hospital leaders reported that they had laid off ancillary staff to use budgets to hire more RNs (Chapman et al., 2009), and the survey conducted by Aiken and colleagues found that nurses perceived reductions in LVN and aide use (Aiken et al., 2010). However, more recent analyses have measured only a slight decline in LVN staffing (Cook et al., 2012; Spetz et al., 2009; Spetz et al., 2013) and aide staffing (Cook et al., 2012; Spetz et al., 2009).

HAVE HOSPITALS REDUCED SERVICES AND CHARITY CARE?

The California Hospital Association warned that strict minimum nurse/patient ratio requirements would force hospitals to reduce their services. To maintain the minimum ratios, hospitals might reschedule procedures, close selected units and beds, or shut their doors entirely. However, there have been few verified reports of the minimum nurse/patient ratios causing permanent closures of inpatient hospital units or beds. There is some indication that there was lower growth in the provision of uncompensated care services among hospitals on which the regulations had the greatest impact on staffing levels (Reiter et al., 2011).

HAVE HOSPITALS SUFFERED FINANCIAL LOSSES?

Since 1999, California hospitals have been financially buffeted by numerous factors, including changes in Medicare and Medicaid payment policy and requirements that hospital facilities meet seismic standards through retrofitting or new construction (Spetz et al., 2009). Thus, it is difficult to determine whether the staffing regulations had any discernable effect on hospital finances. Qualitative evidence reported that hospital CEOs absorbed the costs of the ratios by reducing other budget areas, and some hospitals were able to obtain higher insurance reimbursement rates to cover additional staff expenses (Spetz et al., 2009). However, one analysis found that hospital prices rose even more between 1999 and 2005 than could be explained by labor cost increases that resulted from the nurse staffing ratios alone (Antwi, Gaynor, & Vogt, 2009).

In an analysis of hospital financial data, Cook (2009) found no significant change in total annual labor costs for licensed nurses, total annual hospital costs, or hospital prices. Reiter and colleagues (2012) used data from Medicare cost reports to explore whether changes in financial status differed between California hospitals that had higher versus lower preregulation staffing levels, and between California and other states. They found that relative to hospitals outside California, operating margins for California hospitals with lower preregulation staffing levels declined, and operating expenses increased significantly.

DID WAGES FOR NURSES INCREASE?

In theory, when the demand for workers rises more rapidly than the supply, wages should rise. Two studies have examined whether growth in the hiring of RNs caused by the staffing regulations is linked to more rapid growth in RN wages. One study found that wage growth among urban RNs in California was as much as 12% higher than in other states (Mark, Harless, & Spetz, 2009). A more recent analysis measured a 4.9% increase in RN wages between 2000 and 2007 with one dataset, and no increase at all with a different dataset (Munnich, 2013).

ARE NURSES MORE SATISFIED?

Advocates of staffing ratio regulations link improved staffing to nurse satisfaction and argue that greater nurse satisfaction will reduce nurse turnover and lead to better patient outcomes (California Nurses Association, 2009; Public Policy Associates, 2004). An analysis of statewide nurse survey data found that there were significant improvements in overall job satisfaction among hospital-employed RNs between 2004 and 2006 (Spetz, 2008). Nurse satisfaction also increased with respect to the adequacy of RN staff, time for patient education, benefits, and clerical support.

Aiken and colleagues (2010) also found in their survey of nurses in three states that RNs in California were more satisfied with their working conditions. Nurses in California were significantly more likely to report that their workload was reasonable and allowed them to spend adequate time with patients and that they were able to take breaks during the workday. Nurses with lower workloads were significantly less likely to report that they received complaints from families, faced verbal abuse, were burned out, were dissatisfied, felt quality of care was poor, or were looking for new jobs.

DID THE RATIOS IMPROVE THE QUALITY OF CARE?

One of the main purposes of California's minimum staffing legislation was to improve the quality of patient care. However, to date there is no convincing evidence that patient safety or the quality of care has improved. In the first paper published on this subject, rates of patient falls and hospital-acquired pressure ulcers reported to CALNOC

between 2002 and 2004 were analyzed for 68 hospitals, and it was found that there was no statistically significant change that could be attributed to the ratios (Donaldson et al., 2005). A follow-up study of data through 2006 confirmed these results (Bolton et al., 2007). These analyses had two main shortcomings: They included only a subset of California's hospitals and the two outcomes examined might not be very sensitive to changes in licensed nurse staffing. Studies that examine whether licensed nurse staffing affects rates of hospital-acquired pressure ulcers and postoperative hip fractures from a patient fall have produced mixed findings (Agency for Healthcare Research and Quality, 2005).

Aiken and colleagues linked their survey data to secondary data on patient outcomes collected by state government agencies (Aiken et al., 2010) and found that in all three states studied, higher nurse staffing levels were associated with lower rates of 30-day inpatient mortality and failure-to-rescue. These relationships were stronger in California than in other states. However, this analysis cannot confirm that the staffing regulations directly caused changes in patient outcomes. Research based on a single year of data does not measure the effect of changes in policy or practice on changes in patient outcomes. Although the responses of nurses regarding the patient safety environment suggest that the lower workloads in California are associated with more positive nurse perceptions of patient safety, these perceptions may not lead to actual improvements in patient outcomes. It's important to note that the analysis of patient outcomes in this study was limited to two outcomes.

Several newer studies have used multiple years of statewide data and examined a wider variety of outcomes. For example, Spetz and colleagues examined OSHPD patient discharge data for all nonfederal, general acute care California hospitals from 1999 through 2006 but could not associate improvements in outcomes to the implementation of the ratios (Spetz et al., 2009). In a more rigorous analysis of OSHPD data from 2001 to 2006, Cook and colleagues (2012) found no association between changes in nurse staffing and changes in pressure ulcer rates or failure-to-rescue a patient after a

UNIT 4

complication. Using similar methods, Spetz and colleagues (2013) examined six patient safety indicators using OSHPD data from 2000 to 2006 and found that growth in registered nurse staffing was associated with an improvement for only one outcome, mortality following a complication. They also analyzed whether the average length of stay declined among patients who experienced adverse events to explore the possibility that improved surveillance in better-staffed hospitals might reduce the severity of any complications. They found growth in staffing was significantly associated with reduced length of stay for only one patient safety indicator: select infections due to medical care.

The most comprehensive analysis of the impact of California's regulations on patient outcomes was published by Mark and colleagues (2012). Using patient discharge data from California and 12 comparison states they examined whether differences in staffing changes between California and other states were associated with different patient outcome trajectories. Their analysis also considered differences between hospitals with high preregulation staffing as compared with low preregulation staffing. They found that failure-to-rescue following a complication decreased significantly in some California hospitals, and infections caused by medical care increased significantly in some California hospitals as compared with comparable hospitals in other states. There were no statistically significant changes in either respiratory failure or postoperative sepsis.

Together, this research indicates that California's regulations did not systematically improve the quality of patient care, although there remains a need for more research on this topic. The outcomes examined thus far have been relatively limited, and it is possible that patient care improvements will be found in other areas such as medication safety. It also is possible that changes in patient outcomes caused by the staffing ratios occur over a longer period of time. However, examining and interpreting data over a longer period of time will be complicated by the fact that many health systems and hospitals have established quality improvement programs in response to increased public attention to medical errors and patient outcomes.

WHAT NEXT?

One remaining issue central to the debate about minimum nurse/patient ratios has yet to be addressed: What was the total cost of the ratio regulations?

COST OF THE RATIOS

Any positive impact of minimum staffing ratios should be weighed against their cost (Donaldson & Shapiro, 2011). As of 2014, these costs had not been accurately quantified. A careful accounting of the extent to which increases in nurse staffing were necessitated by the ratios, and the cost of any such increases, is necessary. Moreover, it is important to quantify the value of other investments hospitals might have made if they were not required to adhere to the staffing ratios. A hospital may have delayed implementation of a new infection-control system that would have reduced infection rates, and such opportunity costs should be included as part of the overall cost of the staffing regulations.

LEGISLATIVE OPTIONS

The only federal regulation that directly referred to nurse staffing levels in hospitals at the time of writing is the 42 Code of Federal Regulations (42CFR 482.23[b]), which requires hospitals that participate in Medicare to have "adequate numbers of licensed registered nurses, licensed practical (vocational) nurses, and other personnel to provide nursing care to all patients as needed" (American Nurses Association, 2009). In 2009, Sen. Barbara Boxer (D-CA) introduced S 1031, and Rep. Janice Schakowsky (D-IL) introduced H.R. 2273, both of which would have required that hospitals implement nurse-to-patient staffing plans and meet minimum RN nurse-to-patient ratios for specified patient care units. These bills did not pass, although the bills were reintroduced in 2011 and 2013.

Some states have pursued their own staffing regulations. State regulations generally take one or more of three approaches: a requirement that hospitals develop and implement nurse staffing plans with direct input from nurses, requiring public disclosure of staffing levels, and/or establishment of fixed minimum staffing ratios. California is the only state to have implemented a law using this third strategy, although similar legislation has been proposed in other states including Illinois, Kentucky, Maryland, New Jersey, New York, Vermont, and West Virginia.

Some states have opted to develop staffing regulations that offer hospitals more flexibility than fixed minimum staffing ratios. Connecticut, Illinois, Nevada, Ohio, Oregon, Texas, and Washington have signed into law requirements that hospitals implement and enforce a written nurse staffing policy. In most of these states, the staffing policy must be developed by a committee that includes staff nurses. Rhode Island requires that hospitals submit a "core staffing plan" to the state department of health annually, with specific staffing for each patient care unit and each shift (American Nurses Association, 2013).

The third, and least binding, approach to nurse staffing regulation is to mandate reporting of staffing ratios to the public or to a regulatory agency. In New York, for example, facilities must make available to the public information about nurse staffing and patient outcomes. Specific adverse events, such as medication errors and decubitus ulcers, are considered reportable information under this law. Other states with public reporting requirements are Illinois, New Jersey, Rhode Island, and Vermont. New Jersey's regulation mandates that hospitals post daily staffing information for each unit and shift and provide these data to state regulators, and in 2009, New York added a similar posting requirement to its regulations.

Even without new legislation, hospitals are likely to continue to focus on nurse staffing improvements as the evidence suggests that nurse staffing is a good financial investment in quality improvement (Rothberg et al., 2005). More research is needed, however, to determine whether the lack of measured benefit from California's regulation is caused by limitations of prior research or indicative of an actual lack of impact. If California's regulation can one day be shown to have improved patient outcomes at an acceptable cost, it will be easier for other states to follow in California's footsteps.

DISCUSSION QUESTIONS

1. It is not clear from the research conducted thus far whether California's staffing regulations have improved patient outcomes. However, several studies have found that nurse satisfaction has improved and that nurses perceive that they are providing better care. Is improving nurse satisfaction a sufficient reason to establish this type of regulation?

2. Several studies have suggested that hospitals responded to the staffing regulations by reducing staffing of non-RN personnel. What might be the benefits and consequences of reducing non-RN staffing?

3. Are regulations that require staffing committees likely to effectively address concerns about inadequate nurse staffing? What about laws that require public reporting of staffing levels?

REFERENCES

Agency for Healthcare Research and Quality. (2005). *AHRQ quality indicators —Guide to patient safety indicators, Version 2.1, Revision 3.* AHRQ Publication No. 03-R203. Rockville, MD: Agency for Healthcare Research and Quality.

Aiken, L. H., Sloane, D. M., Cimiotti, J. P., Clarke, S. P., Flynn, L., Seago, J.A., et al. (2010). Implications of the California nurse staffing mandate for other states. *Health Services Research, 45*(4), 904–921.

Aiken, L. H., Sochalski, J., & Anderson, G. F. (1996). Downsizing the hospital nursing workforce. *Health Affairs, 15*(4), 88–92.

American Nurses Association. (2009). Nurse staffing plans and ratios. Retrieved from *www.nursingworld.org/MainMenuCategories/Policy -Advocacy/State/Legislative-Agenda-Reports/State-StaffingPlansRatios.*

American Nurses Association. (2013). Nurse staffing plans and ratios. Retrieved from *www.nursingworld.org/MainMenuCategories/Policy -Advocacy/State/Legislative-Agenda-Reports/State-StaffingPlansRatios.*

Antwi, Y. A., Gaynor, M., & Vogt, W. B. (2009). A bargain at twice the price? California hospital prices in the new millennium. National Bureau of Economic Research Working Paper 15134. Retrieved from *www.nber .org/papers/w15134.pdf.*

Associated Press. (2014). Massachusetts hospital staffing law takes effect. *Washington Times.* Retrieved from *www.washingtontimes.com/news/ 2014/oct/1/massachusetts-hospital-staffing-law-takes-effect/.*

Benson, C. (2005a). Final ruling backs higher nurse ratio. *Sacramento Bee,* A5.

Benson, C. (2005b). Judge orders launch of nurse staffing rule. *Sacramento Bee,* A4.

Berestein, L. (2004). Industry group contends measure may hurt patients. *San Diego Union-Tribune,* C3.

Bolton, L. B., Aydin, C. E., Donaldson, N., Brown, D. S., Sandhu, M., Fridman, M., et al. (2007). Mandated nurse staffing ratios in California: A comparison of staffing and nursing-sensitive outcomes pre- and post-regulation. *Policy, Politics, & Nursing Practice, 8*(4), 238–250.

California Nurses Association. (2009). *The ratio solution: CNA/NNOC's RN-to-patient ratios work—Better care, more nurses.* Oakland, CA: California Nurses Association.

Chapman, S., Spetz, J., Kaiser, J., Seago, J. A., & Dower, C. (2009). How have mandated nurse staffing ratios impacted hospitals? Perspectives from California hospital leaders. *Journal of Healthcare Management, 54*(5), 321–336.

Conway, P. H., Konetzka, R. T., Zhu, J., Volpp, K. G., & Sochalski, J. (2008). Nurse staffing ratios: Trends and policy implications for hospitalists and the safety net. *Journal of Hospital Medicine, 3*(3), 103–199.

Cook, A. (2009). *Is there a nurse in the house? The effect of nurse staffing increases on patient health outcomes.* Unpublished doctoral dissertation. Pittsburgh, PA: Carnegie Mellon University.

Cook, A., Gaynor, M., Stephens, M. Jr., & Taylor, L. (2012). The effect of a hospital nurse staffing mandate on patient health outcomes: Evidence from California's minimum staffing regulation. *Journal of Health Economics, 31*(2), 340–348.

Donaldson, N., Bolton, L. B., Aydin, C., Brown, D., Elashoff, J., & Sandhu, M. (2005). Impact of California's licensed nurse-patient ratios on unit-level nurse staffing and patient outcomes. *Policy, Politics & Nursing Practice, 6*(3), 1–12.

Donaldson, N., & Shapiro, S. (2011). Impact of California mandated acute care hospital nurse staffing ratios: A literature synthesis. *Policy, Politics and Nursing Practice, 11*(3), 184–201.

Gledhill, L. (2005). Governor loses to nurses in ruling: He illegally blocked law that set staffing ratios, judge says. *San Francisco Chronicle*, A1.

Gordon, R. (2005). Nurses pact ready for vote: Plan would raise pay, offer higher signing bonus. *San Francisco Chronicle*, B4.

Kane, R. L., Shamliyan, T., Mueller, C., Duval, S., & Wilt, T. J. (2007). Nursing staffing and quality of patient care. *Evidence Report/Technology Assessment (Full Rep), 151*, 1–115. Retrieved from *archive.ahrq.gov/downloads/pub/evidence/pdf/nursestaff/nursestaff.pdf*.

Kilborn, P. T. (1999). Current nursing shortage more serious than those of the past. *New York Times*, A14.

Kravitz, R., Sauve, M. J., Hodge, M., Romano, P. S., Maher, M., Samuels, S., et al. (2002). *Hospital nursing staff ratios and quality of care.* Davis, CA: University of California, Davis.

LaMar, A. (2005). Nurses protest delay of lower patient ratio, 1500 rally at Capitol to fight 3-year wait. *San Jose Mercury News*, B2.

Lang, T. A., Hodge, M., Olson, V., Romano, P. S., & Kravitz, R. L. (2004). Nurse-patient ratios: A systematic review on the effects of nurse staffing on patient, nurse employee, and hospital outcomes. *Journal of Nursing Administration, 34*(7–8), 326–337.

Mark, B., Harless, D. W., & Spetz, J. (2009). California's minimum nurse staffing legislation and nurses' wages. *Health Affairs, 28*(2), w326–w334.

Mark, B., Harless, D. W., Spetz, J., Reiter, K. L., & Pink, G. H. (2012). California's minimum nurse staffing legislation: Results from a natural experiment. *Health Services Research, 48*(2 pt1), 435–454.

Munnich, E. (2013). The labor market effects of California's minimum nurse staffing law. *Health Economics, 23*(8), 935–950.

Osterman, R. (2005). Hospitals accept nursing ratios. *Sacramento Bee*, D1.

Public Policy Associates. (2004). *The business case for reducing patient-to-nurse staff ratios and eliminating mandatory overtime for nurses.* Lansing, MI: Michigan Nurses Association.

Rapaport, L. (2004). State eases nurse-staffing law until 2008—Hospital closings and delays in patient care prompt move. *Sacramento Bee*, A1.

Reiter, K. L., Harless, D. W., Pink, G. H., & Mark, B. (2012). Minimum nurse staffing legislation and the financial performance of California hospitals. *Health Services Research, 47*(3 pt1), 1030–1050.

Reiter, K. L., Harless, D. W., Pink, G. H., Spetz, J., & Mark, B. (2011). The effect of minimum nurse staffing legislation on uncompensated care provided by California hospitals. *Medical Care Research and Review, 67*(6), 694–706.

Robertson, K. (2004). New nurse law fails to cause emergency. *Sacramento Business Journal, 21*(9), 1.

Rothberg, M. B., Abraham, I., Lindenauer, P. K., & Rose, D. N. (2005). Improving nurse-to-patient staffing ratios as a cost-effective safety intervention. *Medical Care, 43*(8), 785–791.

Salladay, R., & Chong, J.-R. (2005). Judge backs nurses over staffing. *The Los Angeles Times*, B1.

Spetz, J. (1998). Hospital use of nursing personnel: Has there really been a decline? *Journal of Nursing Administration, 28*(3), 20–27.

Spetz, J. (2001). What should we expect from California's minimum nurse staffing legislation? *Journal of Nursing Administration, 31*(3), 132–140.

Spetz, J. (2008). Nurse satisfaction and the implementation of minimum nurse staffing regulations. *Policy, Politics & Nursing Practice, 9*(1), 15–21.

Spetz, J. (2013). *Forecasts of the registered nurse workforce in California.* Sacramento, California: Board of Registered Nursing.

Spetz, J., Chapman, S., Herrera, C., Kaiser, J., Seago, J. A., & Dower, C. (2009). *Assessing the impact of California's nurse staffing ratios on hospitals and patient care.* Oakland, CA: California HealthCare Foundation.

Spetz, J., Harless, D. W., Herrera, C.-N., & Mark, B. A. (2013). Using minimum nurse staffing regulations to measure the relationship between nursing and hospital quality of care. *Medical Care Research and Review, 70*(4), 380–399.

Spetz, J., Seago, J. A., Coffman, J., Rosenoff, E., & O'Neil, E. (2000). *Minimum nurse staffing ratios in California acute care hospitals.* San Francisco: California HealthCare Foundation.

Unruh, L., & Fottler, M. (2006). Patient turnover and nursing staff adequacy. *Health Services Research, 41*(2), 599–612.

Wunderlich, G. S., Sloan, F. A., & Davis, C. K. (Eds.), (1996). *Nursing staff in hospitals and nursing homes: Is it adequate?* Washington, D.C.: National Academies Press.

ONLINE RESOURCES

American Nurses Association: Nurse Staffing Plans and Ratios
www.nursingworld.org/MainMenuCategories/Policy-Advocacy/State/Legislative-Agenda-Reports/State-StaffingPlansRatios
National Nurses United: National Campaign for Safe RN-to-Patient Staffing Ratios
www.nationalnursesunited.org/issues/entry/ratios
Robert Wood Johnson Foundation: The Impact of Nurse Staffing on Hospital Quality
thefutureofnursing.org/resource/detail/impact-nurse-staffing-hospital-quality

CHAPTER 63

The Contemporary Work Environment of Nursing

Susan R. Lacey   Karen S. Cox   Jeanette Ives Erickson   Victoria L. Rich[1]

"We are in a new place, not on the edge of an old place."
Sister Elizabeth Davis, Montreal, 2005

Why is it necessary to frame a chapter on the contemporary work environment of nursing with the financial structures now in place and moving forward? The answer is that it is fundamental to understanding how resources, including human capital, are used and decisions are made. Nurses' work environments are affected by any shift in how health care goods and services are reimbursed. In addition, other factors are creating a need to change the way health care organizations are managed. These include regulatory mandates for transparency, population-specific quality agendas, reimbursement, staffing, the continued rise in the volume of high acuity patients, and an expanded pool of patients who have insurance for the first time. We will address how these and other key factors impact the professional practice of nursing and the current work environment.

The health care system is in the midst of seismic changes that will continue to accelerate as the Affordable Care Act (ACA) is implemented. The way in which health care is delivered and the nature of the work environment are inextricably linked to health care financing. These large-scale changes are predicated on the move from fee-for-service through diagnostic-related groups (DRGs) to bundled payments and value based purchasing (VBP) (Sanford, 2013). This plurality in financing, reimbursement, and quality, coupled with a national quality agenda requiring greater transparency, has created a conundrum for administrators trying to balance current operational realities with what is anticipated to be the reimbursement framework of the future (Sanford, 2013). Uncertainties of this nature can cause decision-making paralysis as health care executives try to maximize current fee-for-service revenues while holding off on key strategic decisions that are consistent with the new realities forged by the ACA.

We have divided these environmental drivers of health care change that impact the work environment into primary and secondary factors. Primary and secondary represent not a hierarchy, but rather the proximity the factor has to the direct care nurse's environment. For instance, a primary factor such as the skill set of the leader impacts the staff nurse directly, while a secondary factor such as the ACA impacts the entire health care system that will change the environment of nurses over time.

PRIMARY FACTORS

Figure 63-1 demonstrates those factors that directly impact the contemporary work environment of nurses on a day-to-day, shift-to-shift basis. Each factor has a different degree of influence over time and, when combined with other factors, may exponentially alter the contemporary work environment. This is not meant to be an exhaustive list; however, these factors weigh most heavily on the contemporary work environment of nurses.

SKILL SET OF UNIT LEADERS

As with any department leaders may or may not have the right skill sets to effectively manage

[1]The authors would like to thank Ms. Adrienne Olney for her assistance with the preparation of this chapter.

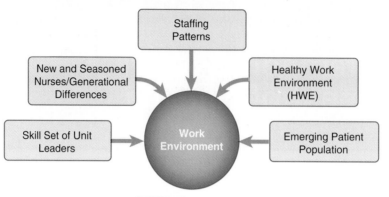

FIGURE 63-1 Primary factors.

resources and/or provide leadership for their staff. If the unit manager is not able to effectively provide timely feedback and constructive advice when needed, or advocate for patients, families, and staff, this can result in an adversarial dynamic between the staff and manager. Conversely, if the manager has the skills he or she needs to run the unit smoothly on all fronts, this creates a positive dynamic in an environment where nurses want to continue to practice (Heuston & Wolf, 2011).

Nurse managers must have both hard and soft skills to effectively manage their units. Hard skills include those appropriate to function in an appointed role in areas such as finance, organization, and human resources, while soft skills include good communication, professionalism, critical thinking, networking, teamwork, and enthusiasm (U.S. Department of Labor, 2014). One framework that has assisted managers in strengthening their soft skills is emotional intelligence. Conceived as a psychological theory by Mayer and Salovey (1997), emotional intelligence (EI) is defined as:

...the ability to perceive emotions, to access and generate emotions so as to assist thought, to understand emotions and emotional knowledge, and to reflectively regulate emotions so as to promote emotional and intellectual growth. (p. 5)

Bar-on (as cited in Goldman, 2005), who first attempted to understand emotional intelligence, asserts there are five characteristics of this concept. They are listed and defined in Table 63-1.

Clinical leaders are constantly faced with situations where emotional intelligence is key to successful change. For example, a nurse manager on a surgical unit was faced with higher-than-benchmarked central-line-associated bloodstream infections. Many staff were adamant their practices did not need to change. The leader could have simply issued an edict saying this is the change, without discussion or input. Instead, she sat with the critics and reviewed the unit data that provided evidence supporting the need for change. The loudest critic became the advocate, and their rates dropped below the benchmark.

Emotional intelligence is a dynamic and evolving skill set. Managers can strengthen their EI competence by informing themselves about current knowledge regarding generational differences that are emerging among staff in many workplaces.

GENERATIONAL DIFFERENCES

For the first time in the history of the United States, four generations are working side by side in the workplace. Table 63-2 shows some of the overarching characteristics of the four generations in the workplace today (Gronbach, 2008; Tolbize, 2008). While stereotypes can promote inaccurate assessment of individuals, there is a great deal of literature that examines how different generations approach both personal and professional issues. Some insight into the differences within this age-diverse workforce can help you to better understand the needs and expectations of your colleagues.

TABLE 63-1 The Five Components of Emotional Intelligence

Component	Definition	Hallmarks
Self-awareness	The ability to recognize and understand personal moods and emotions and their effect on others	Self-confidence, realistic self-assessment, self-deprecating sense of humor
Self-regulation	The ability to control or redirect disruptive impulses and moods; the propensity to think before acting	Trustworthiness and integrity, comfort with ambiguity, openness to change
Internal motivation	A passion to work for internal reasons beyond money and status; a propensity to pursue goals with energy	Strong drive to achieve, optimism, organizational commitment
Empathy	The ability to understand the emotional make-up of others; skill in treating people according to their emotional reactions	Expertise in building/retaining talent, cross-cultural sensitivity, service to clients/customers
Social skills	A proficiency in managing relationships and building networks; the ability to find common ground	Effectiveness in leading change, persuasiveness, expertise building/leading teams

Source: Goldman, D. (2005). *Emotional intelligence: Why it can matter more than IQ.* New York: Bantam Books

TABLE 63-2 Generational Characteristics

Generation	Year Born	Influences	Work Ethic
Matures/Traditionalists	1925-1944	Great Depression, WWII	Hardworking
Baby Boomers	1945-1964	Vietnam, civil rights	Live to work
Generation X	1965-1980	AIDS, latch-key kids	Work to live
Millennials (Y)	1981-2000	9/11, technology	Idealistic/Goal-oriented

Source: Gronbach, K.W. (2008). *The age curve: How to profit from the coming demographic storm.* New York: American Management Association; Tolbize, A. (2008). Generational difference in the workplace. Retrieved from *rtc.umn.edu/docs/2_18_Gen_diff_workplace.pdf.*

One key conclusion from the literature is that, generally, each generation has attributes that can be leveraged in work environments to achieve better outcomes. For nurse managers, this means identifying the different strengths in their staff and applying that knowledge to support the ongoing development of each staff member, and communicating the benefits such diversity brings to the team as well as to patients. A second finding of note is that within each generational cohort there will be a wide variability in characteristics and attributes among its members. Embracing each person as an individual, regardless of age or experience, will help create a culture of respect and can lead to better teamwork and patient outcomes.

NEW RNs AND EXPERIENCED RNS

Malcolm Gladwell (2008) described the point at which someone moves from a novice to an expert by looking at the careers and lives of professional athletes and other notable professionals. He found that the 10,000 Hour Rule seemed to apply in every instance. This rule says that the key to success in any field is in large part a matter of practicing for 10,000 hours. If you translate Gladwell's 10,000 Hour Rule to Benner's Novice to Expert framework, 10,000 hours of nursing practice is roughly five years of full-time experience. If this criterion were used when schedules are created for nursing units, there would be a sound mix of new and experienced nurses distributed across shifts. However, such a precise mix rarely occurs.

Although there are no hard and fast rules stating that all new RNs are less competent than experienced RNs, studies have shown that more experienced nurses are more likely to have developed the necessary critical thinking skills for better patient outcomes (Fero et al., 2008). In addition, researchers from Columbia University have found that more experienced nurses delivered better patient care and shortened the length of stay. The study, which examined 9000 patient records over 4 years from the VA health care system, found that a 1-year increase in RN tenure was associated with a 1.3% decrease in length of stay (Bartel et al., 2014).

It would be optimal if each unit and shift had a fairly even number of new and experienced nurses. By new, the authors employ Benner's model, Novice to Expert, which describes newer nurses as having less than 5 years' experience, while experienced nurses have more than 5 years of full-time practice in nursing (Benner, 2011).

REFRAMING STAFFING DISCUSSIONS

The literature on staffing and staff nurse ratios describes a plethora of findings that indicate nurse-to-patient ratios impact outcomes. However, we must not believe that simply creating a perceived ideal ratio keeps patients and nurses safe. To truly maximize and articulate what nurses individually and collectively bring to patient care, the debate about staffing ratios must be reframed. What if the new frame centered on nurses performing the most effective surveillance and therapeutic interventions? One might then ask, "On which unit would you want your loved one cared for—a unit where eight nurses perform 50% efficacious interventions or a unit where six or seven nurses perform 90% of the most efficacious interventions?" Answering this question moves the discussion from mandated ratios to achieving higher levels of professional practice. In addition, the new framework offers additional benefits, including: consistent use of evidence-based practice (EBP), accountability of the organization to support EBP, and decreased variation in nursing practice, making it less difficult to demonstrate what nurses do to keep patients safe.

The current national emphasis on quality outcomes, now tied to reimbursement, offers an opportunity to move the discussion from numbers to efficacy. Organizations will not receive payment for care if certain complications occur that are hospital acquired, many of which are nurse sensitive. Thus the next step is to have electronic medical record (EMR) systems record all individual nursing

actions and interventions. This idea and edict was described in *Modern Healthcare* in 2006 when the first of the Centers for Medicare and Medicaid (CMS) Never Events began, and yet we are no closer to this realization (Lacey, Cox, & O'Donnell, 2008).

It is important that nurses be able record and review nursing interventions related to specific patient level outcomes. Physicians have International Classification of Diseases (ICD)-9 codes for their interventions and it is clear to analysts which ones make a measurable difference. Nurses spend more time with the patient than any other provider, yet have no way of evaluating many of their care activities consistently and reliably. Until now there has been no real incentive to track every nursing action, but it is critical in determining the most efficacious care. Nurse executives and the entire profession must demand that information system vendors include this ability, as there is no other way to be certain that the nursing profession's contribution is realized. We must push for policies that require such systems to be part of the next generation of the electronic medical record.

HEALTHY WORK ENVIRONMENT

In 2005 the American Association of Critical-Care Nurses (AACN) embarked on a research-based program that outlined key components needed to create and maintain a healthy work environment (HWE). Those work environments deemed healthy foster a supportive milieu in which nurses can grow and learn. The fundamental tenets of HWE are found in Figure 63-2.

Everyone must be involved in the creation of healthy work environments, but the onus is on

- Skilled Communication
- True Collaboration
- Effective Decision Making
- Appropriate Staffing
- Meaningful Recognition
- Authentic Leadership

FIGURE 63-2 Healthy work environment tenets. (Source: American Association of Critical-Care Nurses [AACN]. [2013]. Healthy work environment resources. Retrieved from *www.aacn.org/wd/hwe/content/resources.content.*)

organizational, departmental, and unit leaders to ensure that it happens (AACN, 2013). When nurses perceive they are working within a healthy environment there is greater potential for reducing patient harm, increasing cost savings, and, most importantly, improving patient outcomes while the staff feels engaged and valued by the organization.

THE EMERGING PATIENT POPULATION

All of the aforementioned factors impact the contemporary work environment of nurses, but there has been little discussion of how the pool of newly insured patients will affect the complexity of nurses' work environments. This emerging patient population of individuals and families may have health insurance for the first time. How will they know what is expected of them, and how might this radically change the dynamic between the nurse and the patient, not only in terms of sheer increased volume, but also in teaching about use of preventative versus acute or emergency care?

The patients will need to learn how to use resources effectively for themselves and their families. Additionally, providers will need to learn to be more competent in the areas of culture, race and ethnicity, linguistics, socioeconomic status, religion, and sexual orientation. Nurses will need to be prepared to mentor, partner, and coach. This partnership between the nurse and patient must be built on mutual trust and care based on evidence that incorporates patient preferences. Nurses will need to be innovative and nimble while pursuing better outcomes and fiscal accountability, which are the key tenants of reform.

SECONDARY FACTORS

Figure 63-3 demonstrates the major secondary factors that impact the work environment.

THE AFFORDABLE CARE ACT AND ACCOUNTABLE CARE ORGANIZATIONS

The ACA is changing the landscape of the health care industry and how consumers access the system. One large system change driven by the ACA is

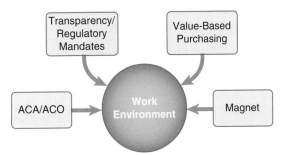

FIGURE 63-3 Secondary factors.

the development and testing of accountable care organizations (ACOs). Pioneer ACOs are a test bed of experienced organizations with the goal of increasing coordination of care and improving quality and savings. Nurses, with their inherent holistic approach to patient care, are well positioned to lead this coordination while ensuring safe practices (CMS, n.d.). While most nurses are accustomed to working in specialty or functional areas such as inpatient or outpatient settings, ACOs will expect nurses to provide care across the continuum.

REGULATORY MANDATES

Regulation plays a pivotal role in the health care industry and impacts the professional work environment of nurses. There are multiple regulatory agencies that seek to ensure the public's safety while encouraging best practices and cost effectiveness. Two of the largest and best known agencies are the Department of Health and Human Services (HHS) and The Joint Commission. HHS is the U.S. government's principal agency for protecting the health of all Americans and providing essential human services, especially for those who are least able to help themselves (HHS, 2014). The Joint Commission is the prevailing entity that sanctions the safety of a wide continuum of health care organizations. Their mission is to: "continuously improve health care for the public, in collaboration with other stakeholders, by evaluating health care organizations and inspiring them to excel in providing safe and effective care of the highest quality and value" (The Joint Commission, n.d.).

UNIT 4

KEEPING STAFF NURSES ENGAGED

There is no question that regulatory agencies and their regulations serve to promote the six quality aims of the Institute of Medicine (2001): to provide care which is safe, efficient, effective, timely, equitable, and patient-centered. How do organizations prepare themselves for regulatory reviews? Some health care organizations expend considerable effort gearing up for regulatory or accreditation reviews. The problem with cyclical preparedness is that it creates the impression organizations are not in compliance at other times and are only preparing to meet regulatory requirements.

One effective strategy to promote regulatory readiness is adopting the philosophy of Excellence Every Day. Excellence Every Day means striving to provide the best possible care to every patient and family in every moment of every day. It is both a philosophy and a commitment. Efforts to achieve Excellence Every Day include validation by external regulatory agencies such as on-site surveys, designation as a Magnet Hospital, or recognition in *U.S. News and World Report*.

Key to promoting the philosophy of Excellence Every Day is the engagement of staff champions selected from the professional teams and including staff nurses. Excellence Every Day Champions are charged with communicating key and timely quality and safety information to their colleagues. Another strategy is the use of tracers in inpatient, outpatient, and procedural areas. "Tracer methodology is an evaluation method in which surveyors select a patient, resident, or client and use that individual's record as a roadmap to move through an organization to assess and evaluate the organization's compliance with selected standards and the organization's systems of providing care and services" (The Joint Commission, 2014).

An additional strategy is the design and implementation of an Excellence Every Day portal (Massachusetts General Hospital, 2013). An Excellence Every Day portal provides easy-to-navigate access to internal and external information related to regulatory readiness. This up-to-date online resource includes potential dates for upcoming regulatory surveys, National Patient Safety Goals, policies and procedures, resource guides, and teaching materials. At a time when regulatory agencies are looking for staff to be able to articulate quality and safety efforts and speak knowledgeably about patient outcomes, this site could not be more relevant.

Providing the best possible care to every patient and family, every moment of every day, is a privilege and a responsibility. It requires teamwork and vigilance. It requires knowledge of current policies, procedures, and standards. That is the promise nurses make every time they enter a patient's room and that is the standard to which nurses should hold themselves accountable as they collaborate with the health care team to strive for nothing less than Excellence Every Day.

VALUE-BASED PURCHASING

The ACA is changing the health care paradigm to one based on the iron triangle of access, quality, and cost with preventative primary care as the cornerstone (Rich, 2013). This iron triangle was hardwired in 2013 by the CMS through the development of value-based purchasing (CMS, 2011).

Value-based purchasing is based on numerous evidence-based measures that improve patient outcomes and health status with the smallest outlay of money. It focuses on managing the use of the entire health care system to reduce unneeded, inappropriate care and to reward the best performing providers or penalize providers who are unable to meet the predetermined measures (Agency for Healthcare Research and Quality [AHRQ], 2002).

The first value-based purchasing measures, which began in 2013, involve 12 process measures and a patient satisfaction survey measure entitled Hospital Consumer Assessment of Healthcare Providers and Systems, better known as HCAHPS. These measures have different weights, and for each fiscal year the measures, weights, and financial incentives or penalties will be altered based on national comparative data. Hence value-based purchasing is predicated on the assumption that providers of health care will reduce medical errors, improve access to care, and decrease costs.

Nursing-sensitive outcomes are part of value-purchasing. Research has reported that acuity- and ratio-based nurse staffing, baccalaureate-prepared nurses, and teamwork are positively related to a decrease in adverse events and patient mortality (Kutney-Lee, Sloane, & Aiken, 2013; McHugh, Berez, & Small, 2013; Needleman et al., 2011). But more attention to measuring the impact of nursing care is needed. The National Database of Nursing Quality Indicators (NDNQI) is an example of a database that has demonstrated the importance of the professional nurse in decreasing hospital-acquired infections, pressure ulcers, falls, ventilated-related pneumonia, and failure-to-rescue patient outcomes. High patient satisfaction as reported by HCAHPS has been positively correlated with nurse communications (Kutney-Lee et al., 2009).

Regardless of recent evidence that clearly demonstrates the efficacy of professional nurses' impact on the metrics for value-purchasing, nurses remain the sleeping giant. We could create a voice for setting shared goals for accountability and offering exemplars that are reportable through leading nursing organizations and accessible to consumers and other stakeholders.

As value-based purchasing matures and reimbursement based on outcomes becomes the norm, the profession of nursing must assure that multiple stakeholders, including patients and families, understand the role professional nurses play in access, quality, and cost. It is imperative for nurse leaders to demonstrate the pivotal role professional nursing has in value-based purchasing. Strategies based on the Advisory Board Company 2011 Nurse Executive Center's Roundtable are shown in Figure 63-4. These seven strategies have the potential to awaken the sleeping giant (Rich, 2013).

VALUE-BASED STAFFING: MAGNET RECOGNITION PROGRAM

The Magnet Recognition Program, developed in the 1980s, recognizes organizations for quality patient care, nursing excellence, and innovations in professional nursing practice. To date, less than 7% of all hospitals have achieved this top designation that holds the professional practice of nursing to the highest standards (American Nurses Credentialing Center [ANCC], 2013). Central to Magnet is

1. Establish a nursing quality scorecard benchmarked with external, comparable agencies and strive for exceeding the target achievements.
2. Develop mechanisms for direct care nurses to become active members of interprofessional teams working on quality and process improvement outcomes.
3. Avoid preventable readmissions by actively enabling nurses to lead clinical rounds and function as a leader of the care team with advanced practice providers and pharmacists as partners; they actively role model the metaphor "a professional nurse sets the table for care."
4. Support the professional nurse and advance practice registered nurses (APRNs) to practice to the full scope of their license. Establish nurse staffing patterns based on acuity, evidence, outcomes, and cost so that senior leaders embrace and champion the impact of professional nurses on quality outcomes, patient satisfaction, and reduced rates of preventable readmissions.
5. Communicate to internal and external stakeholders and the public the Institute of Medicine (2011) recommendations as outlined in *The Future of Nursing.*
6. Provide leadership to activate patients and families in self-directed care and seek feedback from patients on how to improve care.
7. Provide tutelage and competence assessments in skills for all professional caregivers that include teach back or return demonstrations by patients and family members, therapeutic listening, and post-discharge phone calls.

FIGURE 63-4 Value-based purchasing strategies. (Source: Rich, V. [2013]. Affordable Care Act: Accountable care, and nurse leaders. *Nursing Administration Quarterly, 37*[2], 169-170.)

that direct care nurses be empowered to have control over their practice (ANCC, 2013). The most compelling aspect of Magnet is the growing evidence that shows these hospitals to have better clinical and organizational outcomes, and much higher staff nurse satisfaction, which is key for any hospital (Jayawardhana, Welton, & Lindrooth, 2012; Kalisch & Lee, 2012; Kelly, McHugh, & Aiken, 2011; Lake et al., 2010; McHugh et al., 2013).

Even if hospitals cannot allocate resources to pursue and maintain Magnet designation, they should look to this literature to determine what makes a measurable difference in performance and move forward with similar agendas.

UNIT 4

AMERICAN HOSPITAL ASSOCIATION (AHA) REPORT

In November 2013 the AHA published a new white paper, Reconfiguring the Model for a Bedside Care Team, to address the evolving health care system (AHA, 2013). Members of the panel were distinguished nurses and physicians from both the service and academic sectors. This report encouraged hospitals forging new bedside care models to do so by first assessing current resources and trends, and then determining where improvements can be made. It remains to be seen how hospitals will chose to adopt these recommendations. However, if adopted, these measures would significantly change the dynamic of health care and its delivery between providers and patients. Specific recommendations to reconfigure the bedside team include interprofessional education and teamwork, configuring the team that can best achieve established goals, limiting data in the electronic patient record to that which brings value to care, considering the clinical and psycho-social needs of the patient and family, and understanding that smooth transitions of care must exist (AHA, 2013).

CRUCIAL COMMUNICATION

Research indicates that ineffective communication among health care professionals is one of the leading causes of medical errors and patient harm (Dingley et al., 2008). Additionally, The Joint Commission found that poor communication is one of the top three root causes of all sentinel events (Joint Commission, 2013). When working in a high stakes, fast paced, complex environment such as health care, where lives can often hang in the balance, it is imperative there be mutual respect between those who work in these environments and those for whom care is provided. When the initial Institute of Medicine (IOM) report, To Err Is Human, was published in 1999 explicating that as many as 98,000 patients die each year from preventable errors, it shocked the entire health care industry and the nation (IOM, 1999). The fiscal impact of these errors was estimated at between $17 and $29 billion per year, to say nothing of the intense sense of loss a family experiences when a loved one dies

unnecessarily or the moral conflict imposed on the staff who are involved in the errors. This became a call to action to build a safer, high reliability system of care to eliminate these types of errors.

In 2001, the IOM issued a follow-up report, Crossing the Quality Chasm, which outlined the six aims for building better systems and identified 10 rules for health care design (IOM, 2001) (see Table 63-3 and Figure 63-5). Embedded in each aim and rule is a clear and focused attention to strong and effective communication between caregivers, as well as with patients and families. While much has been learned and there have been improvements (handoffs, checklists), a 2013 study found the number of deaths (estimated at 440,000) attributed to medical errors would rank it as the third leading cause of death in the United States,

TABLE 63-3 Institute of Medicine's Six Aims

Aim	Definition
Safe	Avoid injuries to patients
Effective	Provide services based on science to those who benefit and avoid services to those who would not benefit
Patient-centered	Provide care that is respectful and responsive to the patient
Timely	Reduce waiting and harmful delays
Efficient	Avoid waste
Equitable	Provide care that does not vary in quality because of personal characteristics

Source: Institute of Medicine [IOM]. (2001). Crossing the quality chasm: A new health system for the 21st century. Washington, DC: National Academies Press.

1. Care based on continuous healing relationships.
2. Customization based on patient needs and values.
3. The patient as the source of control.
4. Shared knowledge and free flow of information.
5. Evidence-based decision making.
6. Safety as a system property.
7. The need for transparency.
8. Anticipation of needs.
9. Continuous decrease in waste.
10. Cooperation among clinicians.

FIGURE 63-5 Rules for health care design. (Source: Institute of Medicine [IOM]. [2001]. Crossing the quality chasm: A new health system for the 21st century. Washington, DC: National Academies Press.)

according to the CDC statistics. One industry watchdog has likened these deaths to "burying a population the size of Miami every year who die from preventable errors" (Leapfrog Group, 2013).

There remains a false sense of security and staunch resistance to radically changing a health care system that appears to serve providers, and, in the for-profit sector, shareholders. The industry has touted the transition to the electronic medical record as key to making improvements aimed at preventing medication errors and as a way for providers to access timely patient information, but this has not made the measurable difference needed. The radical change required would be the development of an environment of safety for effective risk-taking communications between providers and between patients and providers and the ability to be safe to speak up when things are not congruent with the care that should be provided.

Two key reports, *Silence Kills* (Maxfield et al., 2005) and *The Silent Treatment* (Maxfield et al., 2010), have described the state of the science regarding communications between providers and what can be done to change these egregious practices of omission and commission. In *Silence Kills*, seven crucial concerns are listed and are directly linked to the conversations that those in health care need to feel safe to instigate (Maxfield et al., 2005). These are listed in Table 63-4.

In *The Silent Treatment*, the authors listed three undiscussables: (1) dangerous shortcuts, (2) incompetence, and (3) disrespect. The report found these three concerns were common (greater than 80% of respondents had seen them) and dangerous, although they were generally not discussed. The report continued by describing that caregivers who were able to speak up regarding these issues were more satisfied with their workplace and had better patient outcomes (Maxfield et al., 2010).

Perhaps it is time that nursing organizations join forces to support this critical agenda of keeping patients safe. There are many causes that organizations will support if they are framed as supportive of their primary mission. If we all joined together to address the life and death dangers of poor communication and undiscussable behavior with policymakers and the public, significant traction could be gained. The heart of the matter is to ensure

TABLE 63-4 Silence Kills: Crucial Concerns

Concern	Example
Broken rules	Taking shortcuts that could be dangerous
Mistakes	Using poor clinical judgment during assessments
Lack of support	Complaining when asked to help
Incompetence	Making decisions beyond competency level
Poor teamwork	Gossiping
Disrespect	Being condescending or insulting
Micromanagement	Abusing authority by pulling rank

Source: Maxfield, D., Grenny, J., McMillan, R., Patterson, K., & Switzler, A. (2005). Silence kills: The seven crucial conversations for healthcare. Retrieved from *www.aacn.org/WD/Practice/Docs/Public Policy/SilenceKills.pdf.*

safe, ethical work environments for the patients whose lives are at stake and for all providers.

The Joint Commission (2014) has hardwired the importance of creating an environment where disruptive behavior is not the expected norm. Its 2014 Hospital Accreditation Standards reflect the understanding that environments where intimidation occurs and people are fearful to speak up leads to unsafe environments. Leaders are required to regularly assess the culture of safety and to develop a code of conduct that defines acceptable behavior for everyone, including nurses, surgeons, and the CEO. This level playing field is key to developing a high reliability organization.

DISCUSSION QUESTIONS

1. Are you in favor of federal legislation for staffing levels? Provide a rationale with evidence.
2. What new roles for nurses and others do you see developing in the age of the Affordable Care Act?
3. What can the health care industry do to give personnel the authority to have crucial conversations and find solutions to undiscussables?

REFERENCES

Agency for Healthcare Research and Quality [AHRQ]. (2002). Evaluating the impact of value-based purchasing: A guide for purchaser. Retrieved from *www.ahrq.gov/professionals/quality-patient-safety/quality-resources/value/valuebased/index.html.*

UNIT 4

American Association of Critical-Care Nurses [AACN]. (2013). Healthy work environment resources. Retrieved from *www.aacn.org/wd/hwe/content/resources.content.*

American Hospital Association [AHA]. (2013). Reconfiguring the bedside care team of the future. Retrieved from *www.aha.org/content/13/beds-whitepapergen.pdf.*

American Nurses Credentialing Center [ANCC]. (2013). ANCC Magnet Recognition Program®. Retrieved from *www.nursecredentialing.org/magnet.aspx.*

Bartel, A. P., Beaulieu, N. D., Phibbs, C. S., & Stone, P. W. (2014). Human capital and productivity in a team environment: Evidence from the healthcare sector. *American Economic Journal: Applied Economics, 6*(2), 231–259.

Benner, P. E. (2011). From novice to expert. Retrieved from *currentnursing.com/nursing_theory/Patricia_Benner_From_Novice_to_Expert.html.*

Centers for Medicare and Medicaid Services [CMS]. (2011). Medicare program: Hospital inpatient value—based purchasing program. Final Rule. *Federal Register, 76*(88), 26490–26547.

Centers for Medicare and Medicaid Services [CMS]. (n.d.). Pioneering ACO models. Retrieved from *innovation.cms.gov/initiatives/Pioneer-ACO-Model.*

Dingley, C., Daugherty, K., Derieg, M. K., & Persing, R. (2008). Improving patient safety through provider communication strategy enhancements. In K. Henriksen, J. B. Battles, M. A. Keyes, & M. L. Grady (Eds.), *Advances in patient safety: New directions and alternative approaches* (Vol. 3). Rockville, MD: Agency for Healthcare Research and Quality.

Fero, L. J., Witsberger, C. M., Wesmiller, S. W., Zullo, T. G., & Hoffman, L. A. (2008). Critical thinking ability of new graduate and experienced nurses. *Journal of Advanced Nursing, 65*(1), 139–148.

Gladwell, M. (2008). *Outliers: The story of success.* New York: Little, Brown and Company.

Goldman, D. (2005). *Emotional intelligence: Why it can matter more than IQ.* New York: Bantam Books.

Gronbach, K. W. (2008). *The age curve: How to profit from the coming demographic storm.* New York: American Management Association.

Heuston, M. M., & Wolf, G. A. (2011). Transformational leadership skills of successful nurse managers. *Journal of Nursing Administration, 41*(6), 248–251.

Institute of Medicine [IOM]. (1999). *To err is human: Building a safer health system.* Washington, DC: National Academies Press.

Institute of Medicine [IOM]. (2001). *Crossing the quality chasm: A new health system for the 21st century.* Washington, DC: National Academies Press.

Jayawardhana, J., Welton, J. M., & Lindrooth, R. (2012). Adoption of national quality forum safe practices by Magnet ® hospitals. *Journal of Nursing Administration, 42*(10 Suppl.), S27–S43.

Joint Commission. (2013). Sentinel event data—Root causes by event type. Retrieved from *www.jointcommission.org/Sentinel_Event_Statistics/.*

Joint Commission. (2014). Standards information for hospitals. Retrieved from *www.jointcommission.org/accreditation/hap_standards_information.aspx.*

Joint Commission. (n.d.). About The Joint Commission. Retrieved from *www.jointcommission.org/about_us/about_the_joint_commission_main.aspx.*

Kalisch, B. J., & Lee, K. H. (2012). Missed nursing care: Magnet versus non-Magnet hospitals. *Nursing Outlook, 60*(5), e32–e39.

Kelly, L. A., McHugh, M. D., & Aiken, L. H. (2011). Nurse outcomes in Magnet ® and non-Magnet hospitals. *Journal of Nursing Administration, 41*(10), 428–433.

Kutney-Lee, A., McHugh, M. D., Sloane, D. M., Cimiotti, J. P., Flynn, L., Neff, D., et al. (2009). Nursing: A key to patient satisfaction. *Health Affairs, 28*(4), 666–677.

Kutney-Lee, A., Sloane, D. M., & Aiken, L. H. (2013). An increase in the number of baccalaureate degrees is linked to lower rates of postsurgery mortality. *Health Affairs, 32*(3), 579–586.

Lacey, S., Cox, K., & O'Donnell, R. (2008). Flying the murky skies: The roles nurses can play in solving 'never events'. *Modern Healthcare, 38*(26), 26.

Lake, E. T., Shang, J., Klaus, S., & Dunton, N. E. (2010). Patient falls: Association with hospital Magnet status and nursing unit staffing. *Research in Nursing and Health, 33*(5), 413–425.

The Leapfrog Group. (2013). Hospital errors are now the third leading cause of death in U.S. and new hospital safety scores show improvements are too slow. Retrieved from *www.leapfroggroup.org/policy_leadership/leapfrog_news/5123987.*

Massachusetts General Hospital. (2013). Excellence Every Day Portal. Retrieved from *www.mghpcs.org/EED_Portal.*

Maxfield, D., Grenny, J., Lavandero, R., & Groah, L. (2010). The silent treatment: Why safety checklists aren't enough to save lives. Retrieved from *www.aacn.org/WD/hwe/docs/the-silent-treatment.pdf.*

Maxfield, D., Grenny, J., McMillan, R., Patterson, K., & Switzler, A. (2005). Silence kills: The seven crucial conversations for healthcare. Retrieved from *www.aacn.org/WD/Practice/Docs/PublicPolicy/SilenceKills.pdf.*

Mayer, J. D., & Salovey, P. (1997). What is emotional intelligence? In P. Salovey & D. J. Sluyter (Eds.), *Emotional development and emotional intelligence* (pp. 3–31). New York: Basic Books.

McHugh, M. D., Berez, J., & Small, D. S. (2013). Hospitals with higher nurse staffing had lower odds of readmission penalties than hospitals with lower staffing. *Health Affairs, 32*(10), 1740–1747.

McHugh, M. D., Kelly, L. A., Smith, H. L., Wu, E. S., Vanak, J. M., & Aiken, L. H. (2013). Lower mortality in magnet hospitals. *Medical Care, 51*(5), 382–388.

Needleman, J., Buerhaus, P., Pankratz, V. S., Leibson, C. L., Stevens, S. P., & Harris, M. (2011). Nurse staffing and inpatient hospital mortality. *New England Journal of Medicine, 364*(11), 1037–1045.

Rich, V. (2013). Affordable Care Act: Accountable care, and nurse leaders. *Nursing Administration Quarterly, 37*(2), 169–170.

Sanford, K. D. (2013). Into the next era: An interview with Susan Lacey, PhD, RN, FAAN, and Karen Cox, PhD, RN, FAAN. *Nursing Administration Quarterly, 37*(3), 179–183.

Tolbize, A. (2008). Generational difference in the workplace. Retrieved from *rtc.umn.edu/docs/2_18_Gen_diff_workplace.pdf.*

U.S. Department of Health and Human Services [HHS]. (2014). About HHS. Retrieved from *www.hhs.gov/about/.*

U.S. Department of Labor. (2014). Youth in transition. Retrieved from *www.dol.gov/odep/topics/youth/softskills/.*

ONLINE RESOURCES

ANCC Magnet Recognition Program
www.nursecredentialing.org/magnet.aspx
Center for Medicare and Medicaid Innovation
innovation.cms.gov
The Joint Commission
www.jointcommission.org
U.S. Department of Health and Human Services
www.hhs.gov

CHAPTER 64

Collective Strategies for Change in the Workplace

Lola M. Fehr

"The art of progress is to preserve order amid change, and to preserve change amid order."

Alfred North Whitehead

Change is inevitable, but never has it been more predictable than in the current health care environment. Hundreds of books have been written about managing change, but few adequately describe the rapid complexity and day-to-day impact it is having on our health care delivery systems. The challenge of managing these systems requires nimbleness and flexibility just to stay afloat, let alone steer an organization on a positive course. This chapter will address key factors and strategies that can influence successful change in different hospital cultures, including unionized, Magnet facilities, and hospitals that are neither.

BUILDING A CULTURE OF CHANGE

There is strong evidence suggesting that complex systems can be effectively managed with the adoption and implementation of a framework for change. A change framework endorsed by leaders can provide guidance for the development of a work environment with the internal capacity to respond proactively to change. The framework is used to create transparency within the organization and can result in greater employee commitment to the change. One such framework has been suggested by John Kotter (2012a), who is considered an expert on leadership and change, and is comprised of eight critical stages as summarized in the following list. It is Kotter's contention that failure to implement a change process without following the stages in order will ultimately result in either failure or unnecessary and costly delays.

KOTTER'S EIGHT STAGES OF CHANGE

1. Establish a sense of urgency. Framing change in terms of urgency infuses energy and reduces resistance.
2. Create a guiding coalition. Identify key stakeholders to help plan and guide the process.
3. Develop a vision and strategy. Clearly articulate the end goal and guiding steps.
4. Communicate the vision. Messaging must be clear and repeated many times and in different ways.
5. Empower broad-based action. Employees are empowered to take action to strengthen the change process and value the work.
6. Generate short-term wins. Steps toward the goal are celebrated to sustain momentum for the duration of the process.
7. Consolidate gains and produce more change. This is the time to reevaluate all strategies to ensure that actions are achieving the desired results.
8. Anchor new approaches in the culture. Following the eight steps in every change process can build for future change efforts. (Kotter, 2012b)

WORKPLACE CULTURES DIFFER

Professional nursing practice in the acute care delivery setting will be the contextual focus of this discussion. There are three workplace culture prototypes: union or collective bargaining organizations, organizations that have Magnet designation, and organizations that are neither unionized or Magnet.

THE UNION CULTURE

According to Moberg (2013), although the number of nurses belonging to a union has declined (18% in 2012, down from 20% in 2008), they are still significant. Blackard (2000) believes that management attitudes toward unions are changing with the realization that treating employees right and allowing them to contribute and grow in their jobs is necessary to further the interests of managers themselves. Unions representatives are chosen through a secret ballot, and the results of the election are certified by the National Labor Relations Board (NLRB). The success of a union election is usually reflective of distrust in management. Kotter's eight stages (2012b) cannot be successfully implemented without trust in those responsible for the process. Trust in the union relationship may be built over years of successful contract negotiations, and evidence that management and the union are working together needs to be visible. Management in a unionized workplace is governed by the NLRB, and knowledge of the laws that are different from a nonunion environment is critical. Managers must work with the union's elected officers and may not approach union members individually in the change process. "Management must face more sources of resistance, more reasons for resistance, and a greater ability to resist in a unionized than nonunion workplace" (Blackard, 2000, p. 2). Those sources of resistance include the represented employees, the union, and nonrepresented employees.

Unions have the right to bargain for benefits and conditions of employment, including an appeal process for decisions related to discipline and termination. Management in a union setting will not be able to make unilateral decisions on these key matters. Opportunities for communication with the union are facilitated through channels defined in the union contract. In addition to the usual contract provisions for conditions of employment there are often groups that provide for the members' input into practice issues. These groups can form the basis of communication and discussion of proposed changes.

THE MAGNET DESIGNATION CULTURE

There are 397 Magnet-designated organizations in the United States. Some of these are as small as 50 beds, most are larger. The American Nurses Credentialing Center (ANCC) does not keep statistics on how many Magnet hospitals are unionized; however, we know there are some (Moran, 2014). There are five Magnet model components, three of which directly relate to Kotter's stages of change described above. If an institution has been designated a Magnet facility, it is safe to assume that it has a flat organizational structure with decentralized and shared decision making to support empowerment. It also means there is transformational leadership for coalitions, developing vision and strategy, and communicating the vision. The third Magnet model component, new knowledge, innovation, and improvements, reflects the presence of a learning culture and the encouragement of the innovations required to design successful change.

NONDESIGNATED HOSPITAL CULTURE

There are 5723 hospitals in the United States according to the American Hospital Association (AHA). Of these, 3019 are classified as urban and 1980 as rural (AHA, 2014). The remaining 724 are specialized facilities including psychiatric hospitals, most of which are in urban areas. The definition of rural and urban is not provided in this resource, but we can surmise that the urban facilities are generally larger and more complex. The majority of these hospitals are not unionized nor have they received a Magnet designation. Administrative leadership in these facilities reflect the management philosophy of the CEOs and key executives who assess the needs of the individual institutions. Relationships in small rural hospitals will extend into the community where many individuals will know each other through churches, schools, and social activities. These relationships are generally supportive of a high level of trust that may make the change process less challenging.

IMPLEMENTING THE CHANGE DECISION

The first step of clearly stating the problem to be resolved is crucial or it will not be possible to establish the required sense of urgency. In an organization with a culture of change, problem identification can come from any level. Problems identified by management are clearly their prerogative to solve, ideally with inclusion of key stakeholders. Management should also support problem solving at any level in the organization when steps for successful change are followed and all key stakeholders included.

Who will be invited to join the guiding coalition when complex systemic problems are identified? Obviously those with background information on the issue should be present as well as managers who will have the responsibility of implementing the designated change. Kotter (2012a) emphasizes the need to ascertain commitment from executive-level positions. A change process can be interrupted in the later stages if there is not a commitment from the top. Representation from relevant employee groups that will be affected by the change should also be included. By creating a guiding coalition of thought leaders from different areas in the organization, there is a stronger ability to define the scope of the problem and to develop strategies for root cause interventions. The implementation of the selected strategies will have greater potential for success when a larger number of stakeholders have a shared understanding of the problem and the rationale for the change. This creates champions for change and increased ability for the problem and strategies to be consistently communicated throughout the organization.

When a union is involved there will always be an extra voice at the table or, if not present, alert to respond as necessary to any information that is available. The extra voice is that of the elected union leaders within the institution who could be considered ex officio participants in any discussion that may affect their members. They will want to be able to assure the members that they have paid close attention to the protection of their interests. If the issue is one affecting nursing practice, there will be nurses who are union members sitting at the table. The determination of their participation may be defined in the union contract specifying the process for addressing nursing practice issues. Their role is to focus on identifying a best solution to the problem within the union guidelines.

It is important for each working group to understand their level of authority. Does the group have authority to make the decision or are they generating recommendations for change? How will the values of the union and/or the Magnet environments be upheld as groups fulfill their assignments? Although management may feel a sense of urgency in obtaining a solution and/or recommendations for change to the problem, it is important that all possible options be explored. This will be important for union leadership as they communicate the need for the change to their members because they can then assure them that the best possible option was chosen. These steps provide the groundwork for greater acceptance when the change is announced to the entire organization.

Blanchard (2007) has identified several reasons why changes may fail, even when the steps of a framework are carefully followed. One reason may be a history of past change initiatives that fell by the wayside for lack of commitment or follow-through. Employees may just decide to wait it out if that tactic has previously been successful in thwarting the outcome. Another factor is trust in the organizational leadership. Trust determines how accurately the change message is perceived and accepted.

A lack of trust may be present among those who are resisting the change, and the leaders will need to respect the power of this group. In fact resistance is a normal part of change. The ability to address the concerns voiced can lead to improved thinking about the problem as well as the interventions. Forums held to discuss a large organizational change should encourage those doubtful of the need for the change or of the interventions to openly discuss their concerns in the hope of increasing buy-in to the change. Often resisters are thought to be leaders who anticipate problems others may have missed and their comments should be heard and evaluated.

UNIT 4

EXAMPLES OF CHANGE DECISIONS

HEALTH CARE BENEFITS

Changing the group health insurance carrier for the institution is one example of a change that is a management prerogative. In a nonunion setting, the appropriate executives and managers may search for a new carrier for a variety of reasons. They will review proposals from other companies, compare the benefits, and make a decision. There will likely be staff meetings to announce the decision and explain the rationale. The employees will be more accepting of the changes in their own health care if management has communicated the decision elements clearly.

In a union environment, there will be a separate conversation with the union leaders, who will want to ascertain that no contract violations occur with the change. The employment contract may define what health benefits must be offered to the employee and their family members. If the union believes contract provisions are violated, grievances may be filed, prolonging the decision-making process. It is therefore better to have the union at the table early in the process.

CHANGES IN CARE DELIVERY

New evidence-based findings are regularly published about health care delivery. When an organization determines that a change in care delivery would be beneficial, the key people at the table must include the caregivers affected. Almost all facilities, including those with union contracts, have established practice committees to address patient care issues, and these groups should be key members of the guiding coalition. The union contract may define the composition and qualifications for such committees, although policies and procedures will provide guidelines in nonunion practice environments. The union leaders will again be another voice at the table, assuring their members that their interests are being protected.

CONCLUSION

The reality is that the implementation of a successful change process is related more to the leadership of an organization than whether the organization is unionized, a Magnet facility, or, as most acute care facilities are, neither. A unionized workplace may add an element of complexity, but it need not be an impediment when there is a known framework for making organizational change that is consistently followed. The successful implementation of any change builds a foundation to support changes in the future. Organizations that fail to develop that culture will find it difficult to be successful in the evolving world of health care.

DISCUSSION QUESTIONS

1. What limits might management encounter when planning change involving a unionized staff?
2. What do you believe is the most important factor in a successful change initiative?
3. What is the value of using a framework for change in your workplace?

REFERENCES

American Hospital Association [AHA]. (2014). Fast facts on US hospitals. Retrieved from *www.aha.org*.
Blackard, K. (2000). *Managing change in a unionized workplace* (p. 2). Westport, Connecticut: Quorum Books.
Blanchard, K. (2007). *Leading at a higher level.* Upper Saddle River, NJ: Prentice Hall.
Kotter, J. (2012a). *Leading change.* Boston: Harvard Business Review Press.
Kotter, J. (2012b). The 8-step process for leading change. Kotter International. Retrieved from *www.kotterinternational.com/our-principles/changesteps*.
Moberg, D. (2013, February 20). Are mergers the answer for fractious nurses? *In These Times.* Retrieved from *inthesetimes.com/working/entry/14631/are_mergers_the_answer_for_nurses_unions*.
Moran, J. (2014, January). Assistant Director, Magnet Operations, American Nurses Credentialing Center. Telephone interview.

ONLINE RESOURCES

American Hospital Association
www.aha.org
American Nurses Credentialing Center (ANCC)
www.nursecredentialing.org

CHAPTER 65

TAKING ACTION:
Advocating for Nurses Injured in the Workplace

Anne Hudson

"If you ever think you're too small to be effective, you've never been in bed with a mosquito!"

Wendy Lesko

When I was a nursing student, I learned to lift and move patients with techniques such as the under-axilla drag lift, bear hug, pivot transfer, two-person cradle lift, two-person arm and leg lug, and others. I later learned that these techniques could be dangerous to the person performing them and were not approved for use in the United Kingdom.

One of my instructors warned about cumulative trauma back injury from lifting patients. She said, "Be careful with your back. Your job depends on your back." Initially startled, I dismissed this as impossible. Surely registered nurses (RNs) would not lose their job if they hurt their back lifting patients. After all, it was their back, not their brain! I was unaware of the scope of back injuries in nurses or that manual lifting had been described as "deplorable … inefficient, dangerous to the nurses, and often painful and brutal to the patient" (Owen, 1999, p. 15). Patients can suffer pain, bruising, skin tears, abrasions, tube dislodgement, dislocations, fractures, and being dropped during attempts at manual lifting.

LIFE LESSONS

As an RN on medical/surgical, telemetry, and intermediate care units, I kept my patients pulled up in bed, turned frequently, and well-positioned, as well as lifting them to assist them to their walker, chair, and commode. In 2000, I suffered herniated lumbar discs and "cumulative trauma degenerative disc disease" from lifting patients. After spinal fusion surgery for placement of cadaver bone grafts and hardware, I had permanent lifting restrictions. I had to get an attorney and fight two court battles to prove that my spinal injury was caused by lifting patients to receive workers' compensation. I could not return to my position with lifting patients and was not selected for other nursing positions that did not require lifting. As a result, I was terminated. I became aware that what happened to me was part of a larger problem, and I began educating myself. I was troubled by what I found. Although patient-lift equipment used by lift teams or nurses had proven since 1991 to prevent injury, nurses were still suffering severe injuries from performing manual patient lifting (Charney, Zimmerman, & Walara, 1991). I could not find any efforts to develop safe patient handling legislation.

My online research revealed nothing about back-injured nurses. I contacted nursing schools, my state nursing association, and college and public research librarians; still I found nothing. I contacted the American Nurses Association and learned that the search term for the problem I was exploring was patient handling. Using this term, I found that 38% of nurses require time away from work during their career because of back injuries, and 12% leave nursing permanently as a result of back injuries, and that the U.S. Bureau of Labor Statistics (BLS) continually ranks nurses in the top 10 for work-related musculoskeletal disorders (MSDs). Called high-profile occupation categories, in 2011 the BLS ranked nursing assistants first with 25,010 MSDs and registered nurses fifth with 11,880 MSDs, the majority to the back from overexertion in lifting patients. The BLS reports a median of 7 days for RNs with an MSD to the back to return to work, without specifying to the regular position, or for temporary light duty, which often culminates in termination if the nurse is unable to return to the regular position. Thus, the severity of the injuries and impact on nursing career are not apparent in available data (U.S. Bureau of Labor Statistics, 2012).

I learned about cumulative trauma microfractures from lifting hazardous amounts of weight and about spinal injury to nurses from lifting patients. Because there are no pain receptors in the disc nucleus and vertebral endplates where microfractures typically begin, much spinal damage can occur over time without pain, just as there is no pain with tooth decay until it reaches the nerve. Thus, extensive damage to the spine may have already resulted in degenerative disc disease before severe pain announces extension of the injury from the center to nerves in the outer ring of the disc. By then, a career-ending or career-changing injury may have already occurred.

BECOMING A VOICE FOR BACK-INJURED NURSES

I discovered that the hospital had a Back Injury Prevention Task Force and requested to speak with the group. I presented research on safe lifting limits (35 lbs maximum for patient handling), spinal injury from patient lifting, preventing injuries with lift equipment, and how hospitals can save money through injury prevention techniques (Waters, 2007). I did not receive an enthusiastic response.

The group indicated that they were aware of what could be done to prevent injuries but had not tried to introduce workplace policies in the organization to prevent nurses from being injured.

My speaking out about preventing back injury began during a chance encounter with a patient-lift equipment vendor who introduced me to William Charney, pioneer of lift teams and no-lift policies. In 2001, Mr. Charney asked me to speak at a workshop in Portland, Oregon, on preventing back injuries with safe patient handling. I was glad to have the opportunity to discuss how nurses can be disabled by preventable injuries, issues related to loss of health insurance, and problems with employability.

Next, I spoke at the Third Annual Safe Patient Handling and Movement Conference in Clearwater, Florida. By networking with new contacts, I went on to speak around the country at health and safety conferences, meetings of nursing organizations, hospitals, schools of nursing, labor unions, workers' compensation training programs, and others. In 2005, I keynoted a conference for the Australian Nursing Federation (ANF) Victorian Branch No Lifting Expo, the ANF Industrial Relations Organizers, and the Injured Nurses Support Group (INSG) (Figure 65-1).

In 2002, I published my first article about back injury issues in nursing. It was titled, "Oh! My Aching Back!" (Hudson, 2002). In 2003, William Charney and I collaborated to co-edit a book titled *Back Injury Among Healthcare Workers: Causes, Solutions, and Impacts,* which was about the epidemic of back injuries caused by dangerous manual patient-lifting practices (Charney & Hudson, 2004). We addressed preventive technology and made a

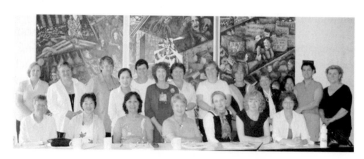

FIGURE 65-1 Author (standing, second row, sixth from left) with Injured Nurses Support Group and Coordinator Elizabeth Langford, AM, RN, RM, BN, Grad. Dip. (Adv. Nsg) (seated, front row, first on left) in Melbourne, Victoria, Australia. (Courtesy of Elizabeth Langford.)

case for eliminating manual patient lifting. We included personal stories of back-injured nurses, revealing the lasting, devastating impacts of severe injury caused by physically lifting patients. Mr. Charney and I were the first voices in America since 2001 calling for state and national safe patient handling-no manual lift legislation. I contacted my local television station to increase public awareness of injuries caused by patient lifting. As a guest on a television news program, I had the opportunity to raise awareness about the problem. I continued to write about the problem, collaborated on peer-reviewed articles, and served on the editorial board of the *Journal of Long-Term Effects of Medical Implants*. In 2007, my local newspaper published a full-page feature article about my efforts to address nurse injury from lifting patients. Despite all of these efforts to educate and raise awareness, action was still needed to address the problem.

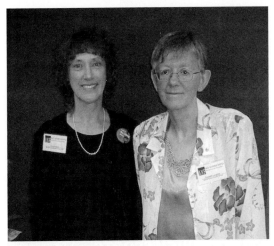

FIGURE 65-2 Author (left) with Elizabeth Langford, AM, RN, RM, BN, Grad. Dip. (Adv. Nsg), Australian Nursing Federation Victorian Branch, Coordinator Injured Nurses Support Group, author of *Buried but Not Dead: A Survey of Occupational Illness and Injury Incurred by Nurses in the Victorian Health Service Industry*.

ESTABLISHING THE WORK INJURED NURSES GROUP USA (WING USA)

I discovered that no-lifting policies had been in place for years in the United Kingdom, Australia, and other countries and that some foreign nursing organizations provided support services for injured and ill nurses. There appeared to be no such assistance, information, or support in place for back-injured nurses in the United States. I contacted nurses who were involved in back injury protection efforts in other countries. My first international contacts were Maria Bryson, RN, Royal College of Nursing Work Injured Nurses Group (RCN WING), Steward and Safety Representative in the United Kingdom, and Elizabeth Langford, RN, RM, BN, Grad. Dip. (Adv. Nsg), ANF Victorian Branch, and Coordinator of INSG in Melbourne, Victoria (Figure 65-2). Inspired by my new friends, who taught me about the services provided to injured nurses by RCN WING, and by ANF and INSG, I set out to work to develop similar services for U.S. nurses.

With the help of friends Teri Jennings and Marian Edmonds, we launched a website called

B.I.N. There—Back Injured Nurses, thus putting the phrase back-injured nurses into online search engines. In 2002, the name was changed to Work Injured Nurses Group USA (WING USA), and the website became *www.wingusa.org*. WING USA provides information about back injury in health care from manual patient lifting and serves as a meeting place for injured nurses from around the country. It includes a new attorney page with attorneys experienced in representing injured nurses, hopefully growing to cover every state. It is facilitated by an effort for leaders in each state to provide injured nurses with a contact in their area for mutual support and encouragement and for sharing experiences and information. Currently, 22 state leaders covering 36 states are active. State leaders may also be involved in a variety of activities including group meetings, writing for publication, media outreach, speaking events, and political involvement for safe patient handling/no manual lift legislation. We hope that national nurse organizations will initiate broad programs to help injured nurses, particularly advocacy programs to help work-injured nurses remain employed. There is only one known charity for nurses in the United States. Nurses House—A

UNIT 4

National Fund for Nurses in Need dates from 1922 and is a nurse-managed nonprofit "dedicated to helping registered nurses in need" *(www.nurses house.org)*.

More than 700 people receive WING USA's e-mail updates on legislation for safe patient handling. Legislative news posted at WING USA's website includes the Coalition for Healthcare Worker and Patient Safety (CHAPS) visit to Capitol Hill to meet with U.S. Representatives and their staff in support of HR 2381, the Nurse and Health Care Worker Protection Act of 2009.

LEGISLATIVE EFFORTS TO ADVANCE SAFE PATIENT HANDLING

Since 2001, I have worked to advance legislation for safe patient handling-no manual lift. This included working with labor unions, meeting with other back-injured nurses, meeting with legislators, and speaking out about the need for legislative efforts. I met with my U.S. Representative, Peter DeFazio (D-OR) (Figure 65-3) and his staff in the local district, in the state office, and in Washington, DC. Congressman DeFazio became cosponsor of HR 2381, the Nurse and Health Care Worker Protection Act of 2009. A companion bill, SB 1788, was introduced in the Senate. The legislation would have mandated use of mechanical lift equipment for patients and residents nationally, but both of these bills died in the 111th Congress.

We have, however, made progress on the state level. Texas became the first state to require hospitals and nursing homes to implement a safe patient handling program. WING USA's website identifies state legislative initiatives pertaining to safe patient or resident handling. Laws in the three states of Ohio, New York, and Hawaii lend support to efforts for safe patient and/or resident handling. Laws in the eight states of Texas, Washington, Rhode Island, Maryland, Minnesota, New Jersey, Illinois, and California require development of safe patient and/ or resident handling policies, and/or implementation of safe patient and/or resident handling programs, and/or use of specially trained lift teams,

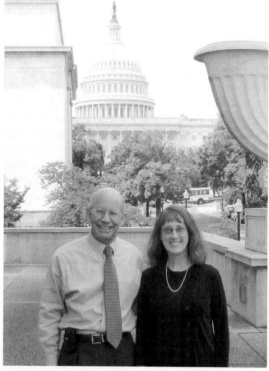

FIGURE 65-3 Author (right) with U.S. Representative Peter DeFazio (D-OR) in Washington, DC.

and/or use of mechanical patient-lift equipment, with variations in the scope and strength of requirements imposed by each state. With the above states, since 2004 a total of at least 20 states, 40% of the United States, have introduced or reintroduced bills to strengthen existing laws related to safe patient and/or resident handling including Florida, Hawaii, Iowa, Kansas, Maine, Massachusetts, Michigan, Missouri, Nevada, New York, Vermont, and possibly others.

I became a founding member of CHAPS to support passage of HR 2381/SB 1788, the Nurse and Health Care Worker Protection Act of 2009 (Figure 65-4). On July 23, 2009, 10 members of CHAPS met with members of Congress and their staff, including U.S. Representative John Conyers, Jr. (D-MI), author of HR 2381, which would have mandated safe patient-lift equipment to allow nurses and other health care workers to work without fear of being disabled and losing their

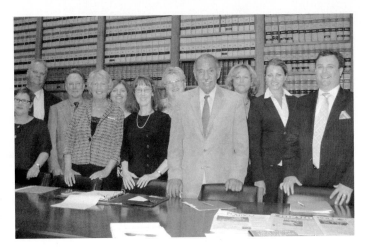

FIGURE 65-4 Coalition for Healthcare Worker and Patient Safety (CHAPS) members with U.S. Representative John Conyers, Jr. (D-MI) to support his sponsorship of HR 2381, the Nurse and Health Care Worker Protection Act of 2009. *Photo left to right:* Sara Markle-Elder, UAN, AFL-CIO; Walter Frederickson, UAN, AFL-CIO; Bill Borwegen, SEIU; Susan Epstein, WING USA Connecticut State Leader; Donna Zankowski, AAOHN; Anne Hudson, founder, WING USA; Elizabeth Shogren, Minnesota Nurses Association; Congressman John Conyers, Jr.; Marsha Medlin, founder, CHAPS; Erin Zrncic, senior nursing student, Indiana University of Pennsylvania; and Jay Witter, UAN, AFL-CIO.

position to back injury. After the first national bills for safe patient handling died in 2011, new legislation was introduced on June 25, 2013, HR 2480 Nurse and Health Care Worker Protection Act of 2013. At this writing, HR 2480 remains in committee (see *thomas.loc.gov/cgi-bin/query/z?c113:H.R .2480.IH:/*).

THE FUTURE

I look forward to the day when (1) losing nurses to disabling injuries caused by the dangerous nursing practice of manual patient lifting is recognized and addressed as a public health crisis, (2) legislation for safe patient handling forces the health care industry to protect all nurses and health care workers against life-altering injuries from lifting hazardous amounts of weight not permitted to be lifted by hand in other industries, (3) concern for the safety and well-being of nurses equals the concern for the patients in our care, and (4) nursing organizations lead national campaigns for retention of nurses back-injured in the line of duty so that nurses who have sacrificed their health and well-being caring for others are no longer treated as disposable.

REFERENCES

Charney, W., & Hudson, A. (Eds.). (2004). *Back injury among healthcare workers: Causes, solutions, and impacts.* Boca Raton, FL: CRC Press.

Charney, W., Zimmerman, K., & Walara, E. (1991). The lifting team: A design method to reduce lost time back injury in nursing. *Journal of American Association of Occupational Health Nurses, 39*(5), 231–234.

Hudson, A. (2002). Oh! My aching back! *Revolution: The Journal for RNs and Patient Advocacy, 3*(5), 31. Retrieved from *www.wingusa.org/aching.htm.*

Owen, B. (1999). Decreasing the back injury problem in nursing personnel. *Surgical Services Management, 5*(7), 15–21.

U.S. Bureau of Labor Statistics. (2012). Nonfatal occupational injuries and illnesses requiring days away from work, 2011. Table 18, Table A, Table B, Table C. Retrieved from *www.bls.gov/news.release/osh2.nr0.htm.*

Waters, T. (2007). When is it safe to manually lift a patient? *American Journal of Nursing, 107*(8), 53–58.

UNIT 4

CHAPTER 66

The Politics of Advanced Practice Nursing

Eileen T. O'Grady   Loretta C. Ford

"We shall be what we determine to be."
Margareta Madden Styles, legendary nurse leader
(1930-2005)

Since the 1960s, advanced practice nurses (APNs) have achieved unprecedented growth and recognition; political activism and social justice have always been at the heart of all four APN roles (nurse practitioner, nurse anesthetist, nurse midwife, and clinical nurse specialist). This chapter explores the political issues facing APNs with suggestions from the authors about ways to increase their political competence, visibility, and political power to impact the larger health policy context.

POLITICAL CONTEXT OF ADVANCED PRACTICE NURSING

THE ROLE OF POLITICS

Politics introduces divisive and self-interested agendas into the policymaking process. This resistance to APNs by some organized physician groups is a quintessential definition of politics: the struggle for ascendency or dominance among groups with different power relationships and agendas. The dominant group in any power struggle does all it can to maintain its role in the hierarchy, its status quo (Workforce Diversity Network, 2013). One strategy to level the playing field is for organizations to use the power of government to achieve what they cannot alone.

History informs the broader political forces currently in play around the politics of advanced practice nursing (Fairman & D'Antonio, 2013). Our past informs health policy because political issues resurface repeatedly but are framed differently with altered names and meanings. Nursing historians Fairman and D'Antonio (2013) use the examples of Social Security in the 1930s, Medicare in the 1960s, and the Affordable Care Act in 2010 as a resurfacing dialogue around those who are worthy and unworthy of entitlements. All three of these landmark programs are grounded in social justice, and what lay at the heart of the intense public dialogue on these programs is the concept of worthiness around class and socioeconomic status. As APNs mature and expand, our historical context bumps up against the overemphasized medical model on specialization. Fairman and D'Antonio (2013) describe nurses in the 1920s and 1930s who saw the need for pregnant women and children to receive care before illness took hold. They coined the term "periodic medical examination" and persuaded families to engage with the health system even without having symptoms. The early influence of these nurses and their ability to move their agenda and influence policy was transformative and to this day are still considered best practice. These nurses directly impacted decades of health policy around workforce, payment, and how the public interacts with the health care system (Fairman & D'Antonio, 2013). Historically, dating back to Florence Nightingale, nurses have had the knowledge and competency to carry out their political agenda and see it through to implementation.

The emphasis of medicine on specialization was not brought about by patient demand but by the rapid expansion of biologic and technologic discoveries, power, prestige, and tertiary care billing practices. In contrast, the nurse practitioner (NP) role was developed as a direct result of patient need. In the late 1960s, public health nurse Loretta Ford and pediatrician Henry Silver broke the traditional boundaries for nurses to provide care to the rural poor who had no access to health care in Colorado. This bold act, to broaden and deepen the scope and role of public health nurses, gave birth to the role of the pediatric NP. It is this innovative and entrepreneurial lens we will use to lay out a new APN politics, based on patient needs in this emerging health care reform era.

THE POLITICAL ISSUES

SCIENCE IS NOT VALUE FREE

If all scientific findings were value free, APNs would have no political resistance. The safety and quality of APN care is well documented and in no study did results suggest or even hint that APNs provided unsafe or poor quality care (Institute of Medicine [IOM], 2011; Mundinger et al., 2000; Newhouse et al., 2011; O'Grady, 2008). A systematic review by Newhouse and colleagues (2011) of APNs indicates that patient outcomes of care provided by NPs and certified nurse midwives are similar to and in some ways better than care provided by physicians alone. This extends what is already known about APN outcomes by reviewing APN studies over an 18-year period. These results strongly indicate that APNs provide high-quality care and play an increasingly important role in improving the quality of care in the United States, and could put to rest concerns about APN safety and quality. More compelling is that no studies suggest that care is better in states that have more restrictive APN regulations (IOM, 2011).

EXPANDING THE USE OF APN SKILLS

As health reform unfolds and millions of people obtain health insurance coverage, state payers and delivery systems will look for creative strategies to lower health care costs and improve quality, yet a considerable segment of the APN workforce remains underused because outdated state laws and regulations that govern APN practice are out of compliance with the U.S. national standards. The wide differences across the U.S. state practice acts reflect the lack of an evidence base in APN regulation, which categorically limits innovative care approaches and access to care. Although the regulation of health professions is intended to protect public safety, some of the restrictions on practice can have the opposite effect, not only impeding consumer access but also creating patient safety hazards. For example, West Virginia does not allow NPs to prescribe anticoagulants while Oklahoma requires certified registered nurse anesthetists to work under the supervision of podiatrists, dentists, or physicians, creating a potential for incomplete treatments, limited access to care, and poor quality as a result of unqualified professionals supervising certified registered nurse anesthetists (Phillips, 2013; Rudner et al., 2007).

MODERNIZING STATE NURSE PRACTICE ACTS

In 2008, APNs developed national standards (Consensus Document) for state licensing for APNs (National Council of State Boards of Nursing [NCSBN], 2008). This document contains the LACE framework; it aligns Licensing criteria for APNs, Accreditation of APN education programs, Certification of APNs once graduated, and Educational Standards (LACE) for all APNs. Although education, accreditation, and certification are necessary components to a cohesive and uniform approach to preparing APNs for practice, the state licensing boards are the final arbiters regarding who is recognized to practice within a given state. Each state independently determines the APN legal scope of practice, the roles that are recognized, the criteria for entry, and the certification examinations required.

The high degree of variability across the United States continues to create significant barriers for APNs and patients. The inability to have licensure recognized across states or to deploy innovative models of care not only decreases access to care but also creates confusion among patients and policymakers. Barriers to practice in many states include: requiring physician supervision, limiting reimbursement, and restricting prescriptive privileges (Brassard & Smolesky, 2011). APNs have built strong internal cohesion and thus political power

UNIT 4

by creating standards via the Consensus Document that unambiguously renders APNs to be self-regulating and self-determining. Licensing and credentialing is key to APN integrity and profession building, yet in more than half of the United States, national LACE standards for APNs are not in compliance because state legislatures have not modernized their state practice acts (American Association of Nurse Practitioners [AANP], 2013; IOM, 2011).

The LACE document establishes clear, professionally endorsed, national expectations for APN licensure, accreditation, certification, and education (Stanley, 2009). It has pointedly strengthened the position of APNs to confront resistance. It creates a pathway for state regulators to adapt a framework for modernizing their state nurse practice acts across the nation. One of the most pressing and urgent APN political issues is the implementation of LACE recommendations into each state nurse practice act. The APN community is challenged to modernize the nation's state practice act. All nursing organizations within a state, especially APN groups, must create a comprehensive plan to update their state nurse practice acts by addressing the issues of APN titling, standards, independent practice, and prescriptive authority so that they are consistent with the LACE framework. A gap analysis is a useful endeavor to list all of the changes that must be made in each state by creating an inventory of legislative and regulatory action that needs to take place in each state to accelerate the nurse practice act modernization process.

Many of the political issues confronting current APN practice are in some way addressed in the LACE framework. For example, as organized physician groups increase resistance to expanded scopes of practice, the LACE standard is for nursing to regulate itself, which will require APN unity. The degree of unity required to implement LACE is significant and necessary for APNs to become a far more effective and innovative force within health care.

APN UNITY AND INTERNAL COHESION

As internal cohesion strengthens among APNs, we learn to supply the APN movement with the validation that is not always provided by the larger health care environment. That is, as APN internal cohesion strengthens, so does its external validation. Exponential progress has been made by the merger of the American College of Nurse Practitioners into the American Association of Nurse Practitioners: Two of the United States' largest APN groups are significantly strengthened into one, so that power can be corralled. This merger represents a major step forward in unifying advanced practice nursing by significantly strengthening APN organizational internal cohesion (AANP, 2012).

PUBLIC TRUST

Based on Gallup polls (Gallup, 2012), the public strongly supports and trusts nurses, thereby creating a social covenant with the public. Having this consistent public trust, nurses, more than any other professional group, may need to be doing more on behalf of the pubic as it relates to high-level health care decision making. The public is solidly behind nurses and that sentiment has not been fully leveraged. There is no tension between public emotion and the evidence base deeming APN practice safe and of high quality.

THE SCLEROTIC OPPOSITION TO APNs AND WHY IT COULD BE IGNORED

The history of physician opposition to APNs is a long one, but was not present when the first NP program was developed, according to Loretta Ford. The early partnership between NPs and pediatricians was built on mutual respect, collaboration, and shared values and goals for patients. However, this relationship has deteriorated into turf battles as medical organizations seek to control the NP's expanding scope of practice. The belief by the physicians that they were and are captains of the ship has fueled a growing animosity between nursing and medical organizations.

Tensions around expansion of practice boundaries are not limited to APNs; there is an ever-increasing evolution of new technology and skill sets among dental hygienists and physical therapists, for example. In particular, some organized medical groups have consistently issued resolutions, petitions, and reports, which oppose state efforts to expand scope of practice for any group other than physicians. Resources from these oppositional organizations are directed at obstructing APN expansion by discrediting APNs as harmful to the public (IOM, 2011). As noted, these claims are not supported by five decades of research that have examined the safety, effectiveness, and efficiency of APN-delivered care. There are many opportunities for APNs embedded in this tired and sclerotic opposition. There are few innovative ideas or helpful solutions to the pervasive health care challenges in the United States. Physician opposition clings to the status quo and does not create a vision to move forward. By ignoring the overused and predicable opposition, which lacks any evidence base, APNs could more wisely focus their resources, considerable creativity, and pragmatism on innovations to fix what is broken.

States such as Arizona, Washington, and Wyoming that have fully modernized their nurse practice acts offer a powerful inoculation against these claims. In these modernized states, there is no economic collapse of the physician workforce, spikes in APN malpractice rates, or patient safety concerns. Yet there appears to be no research study or amount of credible resources that will change the opposition. In the wise words of historian, Joan Lynaugh, APNs should "Declare victory and move on!" (Lynaugh, 2013, personal communication).

Health care in the United States is fraught with fragmentation, persistent safety concerns, pervasive poor and uneven quality, workforce shortages, shocking health care disparities, and a chronic illness epidemic that appears to be deteriorating. In this context, to harken back to the nurses who created the periodic medical examination for preventive purposes, opportunities abound for APNs to improve the health of individuals and communities.

GENDER INEQUALITY AND ADVANCED PRACTICE NURSING PAYMENT ISSUES

It is impossible to discuss the tensions between medicine and nursing without recognizing the male-female dynamic. A key turning point in U.S. history was a Senate vote on June 4, 1920, approving the amendment granting women the right to vote by 56 to 25, which was then ratified by sufficient states in the same year. Thus, the Nineteenth Amendment was the law of the land prohibiting state or federal sex-based restrictions on voting. In 2013, women continue to be underrepresented in politics, in the Senate, in the House of Representatives, in State Houses, and in Governor's mansions. Women held only 18% of the seats of the 535 seats in the 113th Congress (Congressional Research Service, 2014). The Center for American Women and Politics (2013) attributes this to the ideologic political pull to the right, difficulty in recruiting candidates, and an overall lack of support once women are campaigning. Of the 98 women serving in the 113th Congress, six are nurses (American Nurses Association, 2013). However, the larger professional profile of those serving in the 113th Congress include 19 physicians, 173 lawyers, 51 teachers, and 130 business people (Congressional Research Service, 2014).

Comparable worth, also called pay equity, is the principle of equal pay for equal value. One of the very first laws that President Barack Obama signed during his first week in office was the Lilly Ledbetter Fair Pay Act of 2009, which protects those with wage discrimination attributable to race, sex, or national origin. This amendment to the Civil Rights Act addresses comparable worth and the Obama Administration's bold attempt to achieve pay equity across gender and race. For APNs, the difference in Medicare reimbursement can be considered such an issue. Current Medicare payment for NPs is set at 85% of the physician rate, a payment disparity that the APN community has quietly accepted. The Medicare Advisory Payment Commission (MedPAC) (2002), an independent advisory commission to Congress on Medicare, determined that there is no analytic foundation for these payment differentials. Medicare payment for treating otitis media by an NP, for example, is 15% less than when the same condition is treated by a physician.

APNs have not aggressively pursued 100% reimbursement or publicly marketed the reduced payments as a cost-saving measure to patients or insurers. There is a paradox in this payment differential. Providers must be paid the same rate for the same service, and APNs can provide high-quality care at a lower rate than physicians—both of which are true. In principle, Medicare could recommend equal pay if both physicians and APNs provide the same service and reimburse at the lowest cost, that is, to pay the provider who uses the fewest resources to provide the service (MedPAC, 2002). MedPAC recommends that Medicare pay for resources used, not provider type, regarding payment to physician specialists. MedPAC concluded that payment rates should adequately account for differences in resource costs among services and that "paying different amounts for services when they are provided by NPs may not be justified" (MedPAC, 2002, p. 8).

The influx of Doctor of Nursing Practice-prepared APNs into the workforce will strengthen and expand the role significantly. APNs have been ambivalent about using the argument of comparable worth. It does create problems when the emphasis in the policy arena is to seek lower costs. By contrast, adhering to an 85% payment standard limits income, especially for private practices, and communicates APNs as less than.

Instead, the best approach may be avoiding both polarizing positions. Placing emphasis on creating delivery systems that are patient-centered, longitudinal, and relationship-based is the type of care APNs can provide. They can also help develop systems that provide access 24/7 in person and online, that are designed around community and public health needs, looking at individuals within the context of their lives. This type of system must be provided by competent, innovative providers who use evidence-based care, like APNs. It is predicted that over time, more delivery systems will be integrated; care will be delivered by high-functioning teams of providers; and payments will be bundled (National Center for Interprofessional Practice and Education, 2013). Payment incentives are spurring innovative strategies for coordinated care to improve quality, outcomes, and satisfaction among patients and providers. APNs must position themselves at the forefront of new models of care delivery so that people can age in place, become their own providers, and maximize wellness in their lives.

OPPORTUNITIES IN HEALTH REFORM

The Patient Protection and Affordable Care Act (ACA) presents a number of astonishing opportunities and political shifts for APNs. The bill is full of provider-neutral language, opening up highly favorable circumstances for APNs to engage and fully participate in high-value health systems, such as accountable care organizations and health care homes. There are opportunities for nurse-managed health centers, school-based health centers, and faculty and nursing workforce centers to demonstrate how to measure and improve quality and reduce costs. If carried out with exceptional skill and unity, the APN community could position itself to be a sought-after and central component of redesigned systems of the future.

The Centers for Medicare and Medicaid (CMS) is the single largest payer of graduate medical education, contributing nearly $12 billion to teaching hospitals to pay for residency training, while the states add another $4 billion through their Medicaid programs (Health Affairs, 2012). MedPAC (1999, 2009) determined that payment for physician training (graduate medical education [GME]) is not aligned with Medicare's goals to ensure beneficiary access to care. They recommend delinking hospital payments based on the number of physician trainees, which creates a perverse incentive to increase the supply of physicians, rather than improve the quality of care. The ACA goes a step further and mandates increased flexibility in laws and regulations that govern GME funding to promote training in outpatient settings. The legislation mandates development of training programs that focus on primary care models such as medical homes, team management of chronic disease, and those that integrate physical and mental health services (Kaiser Family Foundation, 2010).

Bolder still, the ACA appropriated $50 million per year from 2012 through 2015 to establish a graduate nurse education demonstration program in Medicare. Five hospitals were selected to receive Medicare reimbursement for the educational costs attributable to the training of APNs to provide primary and preventive care, transitional care, chronic care management, and other care appropriate for the Medicare population (CMS, 2014). This demonstration, if carried out with methodological rigor, presents an enormous opportunity for APNs to demonstrate high-value care and gain a foothold on Medicare dollars for APN education for generations to come.

TOWARD NEW APN POLITICS: OVERCOMING APPEASEMENT AND APATHY

USING NURSING KNOWLEDGE

According to Chinn and Kramer (2008), "emancipatory knowing" is the capacity to notice social injustice and to explore why it is invisible. This type of knowing is grounded in power and gender dynamics and seeks to break free from institutional and political constraints that promote unjust practices. Emancipatory knowing seeks to challenge the forces that perpetuate advantage for a few and disadvantage for others. APNs have a long and strong history and are capable of creating a better vision for the future. The APN movement must stop appeasing opponents so that they can comfortably maintain their advantage and stop accepting the language of physician substitute, which diminishes both professions. A new nursing paradigm is needed centering around patient needs, as we still do not have a primary care delivery system that meets the needs of patients. Although there are pockets of excellence across the nation and many creative models, we are far from having a system that is designed to meet patient and population needs that makes or keeps them well. Such a visionary system would take into account social determinants, such as health literacy and access to wholesome food, which strongly predict one's health (Healthy People 2020, n.d.).

Health care has become a highly politicized topic and there is much that APNs can do to lower the temperature, politicization, and name-calling now common in health care policy. As a female-dominated workforce, APNs are masterful at consensus building and can do much to keep the focus on the triple aim: better journeys of care, higher quality care, and lower costs. Nurses' empathic approach must be used to promote more collegiality by negotiating, not appeasing. In states with polarizing politics, APNs could encourage more structured problem-solving approaches, for example, by bringing in respected, nonpartisan mediators who represent the public to help build consensus based on the best evidence.

REJECT THE TROJAN HORSE OF PHYSICIAN-LED COLLABORATION

As health care becomes increasingly measured by quality and outcomes, and care becomes more collaborative and interprofessional, it is critical that the care given by APNs is identified and evaluated. As more APNs earn doctorates and earn the terminal degree, we have a more balanced power gradient with other health care providers in care delivery settings. Being collaborative does not equate to supervision and must not hinge on a legal or regulatory definition of collaboration. Collaboration is a practice imperative for all health professionals and need not be put into a legal context. As the evidence base for interprofessional teams is created, APNs must not become invisible on the health team. Increasingly, opposition to APNs has called for physician-led teams in health care, which must be viewed as a Trojan horse. The story of the Trojan horse, according to the Merriam-Webster dictionary, comes from Greek mythology about the Trojan War, as told in the Odyssey by Homer. According to legend, the Greeks presented the citizens of Troy with a large wooden horse in which they had secretly hidden their warriors. During the night, the warriors emerged from the wooden horse and overran the city. This seemingly benign gesture is masqueraded and, at its core, is destructive to APNs. Forced, mandated, or legislated collaboration with the physician as the lead is in direct conflict the APN consensus standards (LACE).

The notion that physicians must lead health care teams should not be accepted and certainly not be legislated in any manner or form, as it is an unproductive gesture that sets APNs backward. According to the IOM (2011), the contribution of nurses must be fully realized and nurses must be full partners with physicians and other health professions to redesign health care in the United States. A physician as a team leader is not collaborative and thus must be seen as a disguise to maintain the status quo of those who oppose APNs.

There may be a perception among APNs of powerlessness in the face of opposition. Political strategies must be developed that do not center on appeasement. APN professional competency is established and the national standards must be implemented so that APNs are free to practice. Stakeholder coalitions must be broadened to include university presidents, citizen groups, health payers, and health insurers who cannot fully access the benefits that the APN workforce can offer. We must be more forceful in meeting the public covenant by engaging more fiercely on behalf of the public's health.

DISENGAGE FROM POWER STRUGGLES

Organizations engage in power struggles when they feel threatened; fear is at the core of all power struggles. Neither party has much to gain from engaging in a power struggle. When differences are perceived as being dangerous, dramatic amounts of organizational productivity are lost when groups operate from the win/lose perspective. This orientation buys into the belief that power is scarce and that there are only winners and losers. Engaging in a power struggle suppresses creativity and is a race to the bottom, so APNs must drop the notion of the power paradigm of survival, of eat or be eaten.

Power over is when leaders feel they can be safe if they control others. Power under stems from the belief that one can only get what one wants by pleasing others. It is easy to see the gender and power dynamics in the decades-old organized medicine/APN power struggle. The way out of a power struggle is to take full responsibility for one's actions and destiny and pursue a positive future independent of the opposition; that is, disengage from it (Berlinski, 2012). As pressure and opposition mount, it can feel overwhelming, but opposition can be faced and reduced or reversed by well-organized people who know how to play a better brand of defense, by creating a productive and creative offense. One example of a creative offense is Apple; although the Kodak company tried desperately to stay afloat in a digital age, it failed because it did not innovate.

HARNESSING NURSE INNOVATORS AND ENTREPRENEURS

Christensen, Bohmer, and Kenagy (2000) describe a disruptive innovation as an innovation that improves a product or service in ways that the market does not expect. Typically, this is done by creating a service for a new set of consumers and later by lowering prices in the existing market. A disproportionate amount of health care spending goes to caring for those with complex chronic illnesses and disabilities. In Boston, tech-savvy NPs are doing primary care house calls with the sole purpose of keeping people living as independently as possible in their homes. The program shows a 40% reduction in costs compared with those not receiving the home visits. The cost savings are attributable to team-delivered care, which assures continuous monitoring and management of all care needs, at all times, across all settings. The NP home visits are highly integrated and personalized and employ many technologically advanced interventions to meet those needs. APN home visits, with their potential to lower costs while improving health care quality, are more relevant than ever, and this is an exemplar of a disruptive innovation by reinvigorating home visits with a new twist and intention (CMS, 2013).

Blending technology fields with nurses to find new solutions to aging in place will be essential. Nurses have always found creative workarounds and crafted pragmatic solutions to patient problems. Pairing that clinical knowledge with the bioengineering field to create devices to age in place and manage disabilities seems to be an area rich with entrepreneurial opportunities.

There are other opportunities to leverage APN power. APN organizations must create opportunities for APNs to be appointed to public and private advisory commissions that develop quality-improvement measures. APN organizations must also identify key corporate boards and insurance companies and develop long-term strategies and political capital to get APNs appointed to these influential boards. These groups are increasingly influential as payers as well as consumers who seek to know more about what they are getting for their health care dollar. It is critical to broaden the base of stakeholders and policy communities knowledgeable about APNs. Certainly, the commitment of groups such as the American Association of Retired Persons and the positive response of the retail care industry will go a long way in leveraging support of the business community. Opportunities are available to APNs to innovate and drastically improve the health of the public.

DISCUSSION QUESTIONS

1. Think of an unmet health care/community need, taking into consideration the chronic illness epidemic. Describe an APN innovation that you think could address that need.
2. What do you think are some effective tactics for APN strategic positioning on comparable worth? Should APNs position themselves as lower-cost providers who do it better or push for comparable worth, same service, and same pay? Describe the pros and cons of each position.
3. Describe the most vexing political APN issue that you see persisting over the next decade. What are some ways to strategically corral APN political power and address it?

REFERENCES

American Association of Nurse Practitioners [AANP]. (2012). Press release: Nurse practitioners vote to form new national membership organization. Retrieved from *www.aanp.org/about-aanp/aanp-acnp-merger/28-press-room/2012-press-releases/1140-update-regarding-merger.*

American Association of Nurse Practitioners [AANP]. (2013). Issues at a glance: Full practice authority brief. Retrieved from *dhhs.ne.gov/publichealth/licensure/documents/FullPracticeAuthority.pdf.*

American Nurses Association. (2013). Policy advocacy brief: Nurses in congress. Retrieved from *www.nursingworld.org/MainMenuCategories/Policy-Advocacy/Federal/Nurses-in-Congress.*

Berlinski, C. (2012, December 1). Anatomy of a power struggle. *The Journal of International Security Affairs.* Retrieved from *afpc.org/publication_listings/viewArticle/1792.*

Brassard, A., & Smolensky, M. (2011). Removing barriers to advanced practice registered nurse care: Hospital privileges. Washington, DC: AARP Public Policy Institute. Retrieved from *campaignforaction.org/sites/default/files/RemovingBarriers-HospitalPrivileges.pdf.*

Center for American Women and Politics. (2013). Primary problems: Women candidates in U.S. House Primaries. Retrieved from *www.cawp.rutgers.edu/research/documents/Primary-Problems-10-1-13.pdf.*

Centers for Medicare and Medicaid [CMS]. (2013). Independence at home demonstration fact sheet. Baltimore, MD: Centers for Medicare and Medicaid. Retrieved from *innovation.cms.gov/Files/fact-sheet/IAH-Fact-Sheet.pdf.*

Centers for Medicare and Medicaid [CMS]. (2014). *CMS Center for Innovation, Graduate Nurse Education Demonstration.* Baltimore, MD: Centers for Medicare and Medicaid. Retrieved from *innovation.cms.gov/initiatives/gne/.*

Chinn, P., & Kramer, M. (2008). *Integrated theory and knowledge development in nursing* (7th ed.). St. Louis, MO: Mosby Elsevier.

Christensen, C., Bohmer, R., & Kenagy, J. (2000). Will disruptive innovations cure health care? *Harvard Business Review, 78*(5), 102–112, 199.

Congressional Research Service. (2014). Membership of the 113th Congress: A profile. Retrieved from *www.fas.org/sgp/crs/misc/R42964.pdf.*

Fairman, J., & D'Antonio, P. (2013). History counts: How history can shape our understanding of health policy. *Nursing Outlook, 61*(5), 346–352.

Gallup. (2012). Honesty/ethics in professions. Retrieved from *www.gallup.com/poll/1654/honesty-ethics-professions.aspx#4.*

Health Affairs. (2012). Health policy brief: Graduate medical education. Retrieved from *www.healthaffairs.org/healthpolicybriefs/brief.php?brief_id=75.*

Healthy People 2020. (n.d.). Overview on social determinants of health. Retrieved from *www.healthypeople.gov/2020/topicsobjectives2020/overview.aspx?topicid=39.*

Institute of Medicine [IOM]. (2011). *The future of nursing: Leading change, advancing health.* Washington, DC: National Academy Press.

Kaiser Family Foundation. (2010). Focus on health reform: Summary of health reform legislation. Menlo Park, CA: Kaiser Family Foundation. Retrieved from *www.kff.org/healthreform/upload/8061.pdf.*

Lynaugh, J. (2013). APNs should "Declare victory and move on!" (Personal communication with Dr. Loretta Ford).

Medicare Advisory Payment Commission [MedPAC]. (1999). Report to Congress: Rethinking Medicare's payment policy for graduate medical education and teaching hospitals. Washington, DC: MedPAC. Retrieved from *www.medpac.gov/publications/congressional_reports/august99.pdf.*

Medicare Advisory Payment Commission [MedPAC]. (2002). Report to Congress: Medicare payment to advanced practice nurses and physicians' assistants. Washington, DC: MedPAC. Retrieved from *www.medpac.gov/publications/congressional_reports/jun02_NonPhysPay.pdf.*

Medicare Advisory Payment Commission [MedPAC]. (2009). Report to Congress: Medical education in the United States: Supporting long-term delivery system reforms. Washington, DC: MedPAC. Retrieved from *www.medpac.gov/chapters/Jun09_Ch01.pdf.*

Mundinger, M., Lenz, E., Tottten, A., Ysai, W., Cleary, P., et al. (2000). Primary care outcomes in patients treated by nurse practitioners or physicians: A randomized trial. *JAMA: The Journal of the American Medical Association, 283*(1), 59–68.

National Center for Interprofessional Practice and Education. (2013). The Nexus. Retrieved from *nexusipe.org/about-nexus.*

National Council of State Boards of Nursing [NCSBN]. (2008). Consensus model for APRN regulation: Licensure, accreditation, certification & education. Retrieved from *www.ncsbn.org/Consensus_Model_for_APRN_Regulation_July_2008.pdf.*

Newhouse, R., Stanik-Hutt, J., White, K., Johantgen, M., Bass, E., et al. (2011). Advanced practice nurse outcomes 1990–2008: A systematic review. *Nursing Economics, 29*(5), 230–250.

O'Grady, E. T. (2008). Advanced practice registered nurses: The impact on patient safety and quality. In R. G. Hughes (Ed.), Patient safety and quality: An evidence-based handbook for nurses. Rockville, MD: Agency for Healthcare Research and Quality, U.S. Department of Health and Human Services. Retrieved from *www.ahrq.gov/qual/nurseshdbk/docs/O'GradyE_APRN.pdf.*

Phillips, S. (2013). 25th Annual legislative update: Evidence-based practice reforms improve access to APRN care. *Nurse Practitioner, 38*(1), 18–42.

Rudner, N., O'Grady, E. T., Hodnicki, D., & Hanson, C. (2007). Ranking state regulation: Practice environment and consumer health care choice. *The American Journal for Nurse Practitioners, 11*(4), 8–23.

Stanley, J. (2009). Reaching consensus on a regulatory model: What does this mean for APRNs? *The Journal for Nurse Practitioners, 5*(2), 99–104.

Workforce Diversity Network. (2013). Class: Power, privilege, and influence in the United States. Retrieved from *www.workforcediversitynetwork.com/docs/class_9.pdf.*

CHAPTER 67

TAKING ACTION:
Reimbursement Issues for Nurse Anesthetists: A Continuing Challenge

Frank Purcell[1]

"I was taught that the way of progress is neither swift nor easy."

Marie Curie

Since 1980 a number of federal initiatives have had a significant impact on the nurse anesthesia profession. Four federal reimbursement policies significantly affected the American Association of Nurse Anesthetists (AANA) and its 47,000 members. This chapter explores how federal policy can affect the economics of a profession, raise or lower barriers to practice, and cause or remediate inefficiencies in the delivery of anesthesia and pain management services. It also highlights that conflict can occur when two professional groups (in this case, certified registered nurse anesthetists [CRNAs] and anesthesiologists) have overlapping scopes of practice and major stakes in policy outcomes.

NURSE ANESTHESIA PRACTICE

CRNAs are educated in the specialty of anesthesia at the master's or doctoral level in an integrated program of academic and clinical study, and must pass a national certifying exam to practice anesthesia. In addition, they must meet recertification requirements. CRNAs are eligible to receive reimbursement for their services directly from Medicare, most Medicaid programs, TRICARE (the U.S. Department of Defense health program), and most private insurers and managed care organizations.

CRNAs, working with surgeons, anesthesiologists, and, where authorized, podiatrists, dentists, and other health care providers, administer 32 million anesthetics annually in the United States. CRNAs provide anesthesia for every age and type of patient using the full scope of anesthesia techniques, drugs, and technology that characterize contemporary anesthesia practice, as well as interventional pain management services. They work in every setting in which anesthesia is delivered: tertiary care centers, community hospitals, labor and delivery rooms, ambulatory surgical centers (ASCs), diagnostic suites, and outpatient settings. Predominant in rural America, CRNAs are the sole anesthesia providers in most rural hospitals, affording anesthesia and resuscitative services to these medical facilities for surgical, obstetric, and trauma care.

NURSE ANESTHESIA REIMBURSEMENT

Nurse anesthetists gained direct Medicare reimbursement in 1986. Medicare Part A establishes the regulations by which hospitals and ambulatory care facilities are reimbursed for services, supplies, drugs, and equipment used in the care of Medicare patients. Medicare Part B sets forth the payment regulations for health care professionals who are eligible to receive direct reimbursement through the Medicare program. With the advent of the Medicare program in 1965, payment for the anesthesia services provided by nurse anesthetists was provided through both Part A and Part B of the

---

[1]This updates a chapter originally developed by John Garde, CRNA, MS, FAAN and Rita Rupp, RN, MA and draws substantially upon their excellent work.

Medicare program. For the services provided by CRNAs who were hospital employed, the hospitals were reimbursed under Part A for reasonable costs of anesthesia services. For the services provided by CRNAs who were employed by anesthesiologists, the anesthesiologists who employed and supervised CRNAs could bill under Part B as if they personally had administered the anesthesia. These forms of payment were in effect until 1983, when Congress enacted the Prospective Payment System (PPS) legislation to control Medicare hospital costs, bundling all costs other than those reimbursable by Part B into a hospital diagnostic-related group (DRG) payment. The legislation created serious problems relative to the payment for nurse anesthesia services. Hospitals would have been required to pay for their CRNA employees from the fixed DRG payment, jeopardizing their ability to recoup actual costs and creating a disincentive for hospitals to employ CRNAs. Further, because the PPS precluded the unbundling of services, anesthesiologists who employed CRNAs would have been forced to contract with hospitals to get the CRNA portion of the DRG. Hospitals using more physicians for such services did not need to take the costs from the DRG payment; physician services were reimbursed from Medicare Part B. Further, for every $1 paid to CRNAs, anesthesiologists were being paid $3 to $4. If the substitution of anesthesiologists for CRNAs were to increase, the cost of anesthesia care to Medicare beneficiaries could be expected to escalate (Garde, 1988). Simply put, CRNA services were effectively nonreimbursable, and hospitals that accrued Medicare cost savings by using the services of CRNAs stood to be hurt the most by the move to a DRG payment system.

ADVOCACY ISSUES IN ANESTHESIA REIMBURSEMENT

Because of the potential negative effect of the PPS legislation on nurse anesthetists, the AANA advocated several legislative changes, most notably that the Omnibus Budget Reconciliation Act (OBRA) of 1986 should include direct reimbursement for CRNAs (to become effective January 1, 1989, with

extension of the two temporary provisions to the effective date of the legislation).

The mission of the AANA was to convince Congress and the Health Care Financing Administration (HCFA), renamed the Centers for Medicare and Medicaid Services (CMS) in 2001, that CRNAs were concerned about health care costs as well as equitable reimbursement for their services. Even though the American Society of Anesthesiologists (ASA) opposed the direct reimbursement legislation, AANA's message was understood because use of CRNAs in the provision of anesthesia services represents substantial cost savings from several standpoints. On average, the income of CRNAs is one third that of anesthesiologists. Also, for providing the same high quality of anesthesia care, the educational cost of preparing CRNAs is significantly less than that needed to prepare anesthesiologists. Congress passed the legislation granting CRNAs direct Medicare reimbursement, with two payment schedules incorporated in the law: one for CRNAs not medically directed by anesthesiologists and the other for CRNAs working under anesthesiologists' medical direction (Gunn, 1997). As a result of this legislation, all CRNAs, regardless of whether they are employed or are in independent practice, now have the ability to receive reimbursement from Medicare directly or to sign over their billing rights to their employers. In addition to Medicare direct reimbursement, CRNAs were reimbursed through many health plans.

TEFRA: DEFINING MEDICAL DIRECTION

Congress enacted the Tax Equity and Fiscal Responsibility Act (TEFRA) of 1982 to, among other provisions, control escalating Medicare costs for hospital-based services including anesthesiology, pathology, and radiology. Among the many cost concerns that TEFRA addressed was a need to ensure that an anesthesiologist provided specified services when billing Medicare for medical direction when a CRNA was administering the anesthesia. Before enactment of TEFRA, an anesthesiologist could bill for services in conjunction with supervision of hospital-employed CRNAs, without demonstrating that the anesthesiologist had provided specific services to qualify for such payment.

In 1983, the HCFA published the final rules implementing TEFRA relative to payment for anesthesiology physician services, limiting medical direction payment to an anesthesiologist to no more than four concurrent procedures administered by CRNAs. The rules implemented seven conditions that an anesthesiologist must satisfy in each case to obtain reimbursement for medical direction (U.S. Department of Health and Human Services [HHS], 1983). Interestingly, the TEFRA regulations also increased health care costs by providing incentives for the additional involvement of anesthesiologists in cases that could otherwise be provided by a CRNA as nonmedically directed. Medicare Part B did not require the involvement of anesthesiologists in CRNA services, except to the extent that an anesthesiologist submits a claim for medical direction.

In the early 1990s, the Physician Payment Review Commission (PPRC) study of anesthesia payments and individual research studies reported the need for changes in TEFRA. The 1992 Center for Health Economics Research (CHER) report to the PPRC recommended: "HCFA should consider whether to review the TEFRA requirements to see if modifications of the TEFRA rules would permit greater efficiencies without decreasing the quality of care" (PPRC, 1993). The PPRC concluded that "the use of the anesthesia care team seems to be determined by individual preferences for that practice arrangement. There appears to be no demonstrated quality of care differences between the care provided by the solo anesthesiologist, solo CRNA, and the team." No longer could anesthesiologists argue that medical direction of CRNAs by anesthesiologists and the TEFRA conditions under which medical direction is provided represent any safer or higher standard of care than the care provided by a CRNA practicing alone or an anesthesiologist practicing alone. The final conclusion reached by the PPRC on anesthesia payment represented a milestone in the recognition of anesthesia services provided by nurse anesthetists. A single payment methodology for anesthesia services was recommended by the PPRC and adopted by Congress, which resulted in a policy whereby the payment for anesthesia services would be the same, whether provided by a CRNA-anesthesiologist team, by a solo anesthesiologist, or by a solo CRNA providing nonmedically directed services. In the case of medically directed services, the payment would be split so that each practitioner receives 50% (PPRC, 1993).

In a joint meeting in 1998 with the ASA, AANA, and HCFA, proposals were advanced for revisions in the seven conditions of payment for physician medical direction. The ASA and AANA reached consensus on a revised recommended set of medical direction requirements. However, the ASA had second thoughts about the agreed-on revisions. The HCFA's response to the concerns posed by ASA membership and several state anesthesiologist societies was to retain the current requirements established in 1983 (HHS, 1998). The HCFA did decide that the physician who is responsible for medically directing must be present at induction and emergence for general anesthesia and present as indicated in anesthesia cases not involving general anesthesia and that the physician alone must attest in any claim for Medicare reimbursement of medical direction to having performed the seven medical direction tasks in each case (HHS, 1998). The AANA's influence on the development of medical direction policy helped secure the following:

- A published statement by the HCFA that medical direction should not be considered a quality-related standard, but a payment criterion.
- Adoption of a 50% split in payment by the anesthesiologist and CRNA for a case as long as the ratio of medical direction does not exceed 1:4.
- A 50% split in payment between the anesthesiologist and CRNA when the medical direction is 1:1. (Before this change, the physician received 100% of the payment.)

Nonmedically directed CRNA services represent an important value to patients, ensure a high quality of anesthesia service indistinguishable from more costly practice modalities, and create savings by comparison with medically directed services even though both are reimbursed identically under

BOX 67-1 Comparison of Cost of Four Types of Delivery of Anesthesia Services

Suppose that there are four identical cases: (a) has anesthesia delivered by a nonmedically directed CRNA; (b) has anesthesia delivered by a CRNA medically directed at a 4:1 ratio by a physician overseeing four simultaneous cases and attesting fulfillment of the seven conditions of medical direction in each; (c) has anesthesia delivered by a CRNA medically directed at a 2:1 ratio; and (d) has anesthesia delivered by a physician personally performing the anesthesia service. Further suppose that the annual pay of the anesthesia professionals approximate national market conditions in 2007, $145,000 for the CRNA and $380,000 for the anesthesiologist (American Society of Anesthesiologists, April 2007 newsletter). Under the Medicare program and most private payment systems, practice modalities (a), (b), (c), and (d) are reimbursed the same. Moreover, the literature indicates that the quality of medically directed versus nonmedically directed CRNA services is indistinguishable. However, the annualized labor costs (excluding benefits) for each modality vary widely. The annualized cost of (a) equals $145,000. For case (b), it is $145,000 + (0.25 × $380,000), or $240,000 per year. For case (c), it is $145,000 + (0.50 × $380,000), or $335,000 per year. Finally, for case (d), the annualized cost equals $380,000 per year.

Anesthesia Payment Model	FTEs/Case	Clinician Costs per Year/FTE
(a) CRNA nonmedically directed	1.00	$145,000
(b) Medical direction 1:4	1.25	$240,000
(c) Medical direction 1:2	1.50	$335,000
(d) Anesthesiologist only	1.00	$380,000

FTE, Full-time equivalent.

If Medicare and private plans pay the same rate whether the care is delivered according to modalities (a), (b), (c), or (d), some part of the health care system is bearing the additional cost of the medical direction service; most likely hospitals and other health care facilities, and, ultimately, patients, premium payers, and taxpayers. In the interest of patient safety and access to care, these additional costs imposed by medical direction modalities more than justify the public interest in continuing to recognize and reimburse fully for nonmedically directed CRNA services within Medicare, Medicaid, and private plans, in the same manner that physician services are reimbursed.

Medicare. Box 67-1 shows an example of this comparison.

PHYSICIAN SUPERVISION OF CRNAs: MEDICARE CONDITIONS OF PARTICIPATION

Medicare regulations in 2010 require physician supervision of CRNAs as a condition for hospitals, ASCs, and critical access hospitals (CAHs) to receive Medicare payment, except where the state has opted out of this requirement. These regulations do not require that a CRNA be supervised by an anesthesiologist.

During the 1990s, the AANA pursued a revision of these Medicare conditions of participation that would remove the physician supervision requirement for CRNAs. In December 1997, the HCFA released for comment the proposed revisions in the Medicare Conditions of Participation for Hospitals, ASCs, and CAHs, which would eliminate the requirement for physician supervision of CRNAs, deferring instead to state law. The HCFA's proposal to remove the physician supervision requirement was opposed by the ASA, whose main message was that if the rule was implemented, patients would die. To counter the claims, the AANA pointed to the extensive published literature documenting the safety of CRNA care, and commissioned a survey of Medicare beneficiaries in October 1999 by an independent research firm, Wirthlin Worldwide. The survey revealed that 88% of Medicare beneficiaries surveyed would be comfortable if their surgeon chose a nurse anesthetist to provide their anesthesia care; 81% surveyed preferred a nurse anesthetist or had no preference between a CRNA or an anesthesiologist when it came to their anesthesia care (American Association of Nurse Anesthetists [AANA], 2000). From the time that the proposed rule was announced, the AANA implemented a number of key activities to advocate its position on this supervision issue. Box 67-2 shows AANA strategies used in advocacy on this issue.

UNIT 4

BOX 67-2 American Association of Nurse Anesthetists (AANA) Strategies Used in Advocacy on the Supervision Issue

---

- AANA representatives met with key government personnel to advocate on behalf of CRNAs on the issue of supervision. Meetings were held with HCFA analysts, the Administrator of the HCFA (Nancy-Ann DeParle), members of Congress and their staff, the Secretary of Health and Human Services, staff members of the Clinton White House, the staff of the Office of Management and Budget, and others.
- As the ASA's opposition to the proposed rule increased, together with the delay in the HCFA's announcement of the final rule, the AANA called on Sen. Kent Conrad (D-ND) and Rep. Jim Nussle (R-IA) to introduce legislation requiring the HCFA to implement the proposed regulation related to deleting physician supervision of CRNAs in the hospital, ASC, and CAH as conditions for receiving Medicare payment.
- The AANA retained legislative consultants to assist in the promotion of its legislative initiatives.
- The AANA's public relations endeavors focused on increasing the public's awareness of the issues and advocating the position of the vital role that CRNAs play in anesthesia delivery in the United States. Efforts included advertising in many news publications, including Capitol Hill newspapers and *USA Today;* assisting with media training for AANA officers and staff to increase their effectiveness on radio programs and in interviews; and developing radio advertisements in Washington, DC to garner support for the AANA's position.
- The AANA retained grassroots political action consultants to assist in gaining letters of support for the new proposed regulations from key members of Congress.
- The AANA solicited a broad base of support from the nursing organization community, national hospital associations, related health professional associations, civic organizations, individual nurses, physicians, and the general public.

These advocacy efforts yielded an extensive base of support from all sectors. The AANA gained support for the proposed rule changes from the American Hospital Association; VHA, Inc.; Premier, Inc.; National Rural Health Association; Federation of American Health Systems; St. Paul Fire and Marine Insurance Company; Kaiser Permanente Central Office; California and Oregon Kaiser System; and numerous rural hospitals across the United States. On January 18, 2001, the HCFA published a final rule in the Federal Register, removing the federal physician supervision requirement for nurse anesthetists and deferring to state law on the issue. The HCFA refuted all major arguments advanced by the ASA opposition. Examples of several conclusions the HCFA reached in its study of the supervision issue are as follows:

- States have constitutionally and traditionally acted in matters of licensure and scope-of-practice and have not been found to be negligent in their exercise of this authority.
- There is no research that conclusively demonstrates a need for this federal requirement nor demonstrates that physician or anesthesiologist supervision makes a difference in anesthesia outcomes. The HCFA stated in the final rule that studies purported by the ASA to demonstrate such findings had serious limitations and did not support the ASA's conclusions. Furthermore, the HCFA stated that it cannot agree with the ASA's belief that anesthesia administration is the practice of medicine and therefore can be done only after medical school training.
- The HCFA's rule noted the safety of anesthesia as reported by the Institute of Medicine (IOM) (IOM Committee on Quality of Health Care in America, 2000).
- The flexibility resulting from the rule change would provide increased access to services in some areas and broaden the opportunity for providers to implement professional standards of practice that improve quality of care and promote more efficacious models of care delivery for anesthesia services.

However, on January 20, 2001, the incoming Bush administration placed a 60-day moratorium on all regulations published in the final days of the

Clinton administration. This action was not unexpected; every new administration takes the opportunity to review pending regulations that are not yet in effect.

The AANA took its case to HHS Secretary Tommy Thompson in 2001 and continued to urge the 107th Congress to leave the final regulation published by the HCFA on January 18, 2001, in place, although the ASA proposed legislation calling for continuation of the supervision requirements pending a study on supervision. Following extensions of the implementation moratorium, on July 5, 2001, the CMS published its new proposed rule (66 FR 35395-35399), which, if implemented, would replace the January 18 rule. The proposed rule would enable states to opt out of (or seek an exemption from) the federal supervision requirement for CRNAs. Hospitals, ASCs, and CAHs in a particular state would be exempted from the requirement if the governor submitted a letter to the CMS requesting the exemption. The letter would need to attest that the governor consulted with the boards of medicine and nursing about issues related to access to and quality of anesthesia services in the state; concluded that it is in the best interests of the state's citizens to opt out of the physician supervision requirement; and determined that opting out was consistent with state law. It would also have the Agency for Healthcare Research and Quality (AHRQ) design and conduct a prospective study to assess only CRNA practices with input from the CMS, anesthesiologists, and CRNAs or, alternatively, establish a registry to monitor only CRNA practice.

The AANA expressed concern that the proposed rule would potentially allow state medical boards to dictate how nurse anesthetists would be regulated on a state-by-state basis. In addition, the governors would be the targets of intense lobbying by organized medicine, and any exemption from supervision could be removed at any time because of this political pressure, creating a constant state of legal and professional limbo for CRNAs and the facilities they serve. The AANA's response to the CMS in response to the July 5 proposed rule urged the agency to revert to the January 18, 2001, final rule and defer to state law concerning anesthesia

services regarding the issue of physician supervision of CRNAs.

The CMS ultimately adopted a final rule on November 13, 2001 (66 FR 56762), closely mirroring the July 5 proposed rule. As of June 2014, 17 states had exercised the process authorized to opt out of the Medicare physician supervision requirement for nurse anesthetists: Alaska, California, Colorado, Idaho, Iowa, Kansas, Kentucky, Minnesota, Montana, Nebraska, New Hampshire, New Mexico, North Dakota, Oregon, South Dakota, Washington, and Wisconsin. To date, the AHRQ has not undertaken the study authorized by the final rule, which the agency already had authority to undertake. Anesthesia services continue to be delivered safely as the nurse anesthesia profession had promised, as measured by trends in nurse anesthetists' medical liability premiums to the extent that such premiums are a market proxy to measure relative risk (Fetcho, 2005) and as reported in the scholarly literature (Dulisse & Cromwell, 2010; Hogan et al., 2010).

MEDICARE COVERAGE OF CHRONIC PAIN MANAGEMENT SERVICES

Chronic intractable pain afflicts 100 million Americans at an annual economic cost exceeding $600 billion annually in the United States, and the country lacks a sufficient number of educated professionals to adequately diagnose and treat chronic pain (IOM, 2011). Thus, although such services are within CRNA's scope of practice, in 2011 a major Medicare administrative contractor acted to prohibit direct reimbursement of CRNA chronic pain management services in a dozen Western states, triggering another round of actions over Medicare coverage. Throughout a 20-month advocacy campaign in which the AANA called upon subject matter experts, members of Congress, and patient organizations to educate the Medicare agency, the CMS published a final rule (HHS, 2012) clarifying that CRNA "anesthesia and related care" services included chronic pain management and all other services within the CRNAs' scope of practice in the state where the service was provided. Taking effect

January 1, 2013, the final rule's initial impact was uneven at first, reflecting the variety of Medicare contractors as well as inconsistency in Medicare data reflecting CRNA services (Government Accountability Office, 2014).

CONCLUSION

The primary impetus for seeking direct reimbursement legislation was the problem created by a new Medicare payment system that had threatened the viability of the nurse anesthesia profession. However, the AANA saw a clear opportunity to seek this legislation to expand and secure patient access to care and to establish a more equitable market in which to promote CRNA services as fully qualified anesthesia providers. As of June 2013, 40 states do not have a physician supervision requirement for CRNAs in nursing or medical laws or regulations. Clearly, this is an indication that many states, as a matter of public policy, believe it is unnecessary to require physician supervision of CRNAs.

The AANA has learned from its experience in the political and legislative arena that politics is the use of power for change. Although politics may not always be nice or fair, health care professionals must engage in the political process. As has been illustrated in the federal policy initiatives discussed in this chapter, there are generally other forces at work to attempt to influence policy decisions that can have a detrimental impact on one's patients and profession. Therefore, the choice of whether or not to engage should be a simple one. The achievements won in the federal policy arena by the AANA would not have been possible without the commitment and dedication of its members.

However, it is very rare for a single group to be able to promote legislation or to effect major policy change. In the case of the federal supervision requirement for nurse anesthetists, networking with other groups, especially nursing organizations, has been critical to achieving support on Capitol Hill and in communications with the executive branch. The message to legislators has been loud and clear: Removing restrictive barriers to practice is in the public's interest and is sound health care policy.

REFERENCES

American Association of Nurse Anesthetists [AANA]. (2000). Nine out of 10 Medicare patients are comfortable with nurse anesthesia care. In *Roll Call*. Park Ridge, IL: American Association of Nurse Anesthetists.

Dulisse, B., & Cromwell, J. (2010). No harm found when nurse anesthetists work without supervision by physicians. *Health Affairs, 29*(8), 1469–1475.

Fetcho, J. (2005). CNA requests rate increases. *AANA News Bulletin, 59*(6), 34.

Garde, J. F. (1988). A case study involving prospective payment legislation, DRGs, and certified registered nurse anesthetists. *Nursing Clinics of North America, 23*(3), 521–530.

Government Accountability Office. (2014). Nurse anesthetists billed for few chronic pain procedures; implementation of CMS payment policy inconsistent. GAO-14-153. Washington, DC: Government Accountability Office. Retrieved from *www.gao.gov/products/GAO-14-153*.

Gunn, I. P. (1997). Nurse anesthesia. In J. J. Nagelhout & K. L. Zaglaniczny (Eds.), *Nurse anesthesia*. Philadelphia, PA: Saunders.

Hogan, P., Seifert, R. F., Moore, C. S., & Simonson, B. E. (2010). Cost-effectiveness analysis of anesthesia providers. *Nursing Economic$, 28*(3), 159–169.

Institute of Medicine Committee on Quality of Health Care in America. (2000). L. T. Kohn, J. Corrigan, & M. S. Donaldson (Eds.), *To err is human: Building a safer health system*. Washington, DC: National Academies Press.

Institute of Medicine [IOM]. (2011). *Relieving pain in America: A blueprint for transforming prevention, care, education, and research*. Washington, DC: National Academies Press.

Physician Payment Review Commission [PPRC]. (1993). *PPRC report to Congress. Payments for the anesthesia care team*. Washington, DC: PPRC.

U.S. Department of Health and Human Services [HHS]. (1983). *Federal Register, 48*, FR 8928.

U.S. Department of Health and Human Services [HHS]. (1998). *Federal Register, 63*, FR 58813.

U.S. Department of Health and Human Services [HHS]. (2012). *Federal Register, 77*(222), FR 68892.

CHAPTER 68

TAKING ACTION:

Overcoming Barriers to Full APRN Practice: The Idaho Story

Margaret Wainwright Henbest   Sandra Evans   Randall Steven Hudspeth

"There is nothing more difficult to take in hand, more perilous to conduct, or more certain in its success, than to take the lead in the introduction of a new order of things."

Niccolo Machiavelli

I (Margaret Henbest) was a licensed and practicing certified pediatric nurse practitioner (CPNP) when our family moved from Oregon to Idaho in 1986, 15 years after Idaho first began licensing nurse practitioners (NPs). When I came to Idaho, I experienced firsthand the restrictions that this early enabling legislation had created, then in 1996 became involved in changing them as a Representative in the Idaho State Legislature. It was only with the cooperation of other legislators, organizations, and leaders in nursing that ultimately an autonomous and full scope of practice was achieved in 2006. Sandy Evans, Executive Director of the Idaho Board of Nursing (IBN), played a significant leadership role on behalf of the IBN in 1998. Randy Hudspeth, Director of Patient Care at St. Alphonsus Regional Medical Center, followed by creating a vision, and then organizing and galvanizing the NP community to action in 2003.

Idaho has a long history of NP practice recognition beginning in 1971 when Idaho became the first state to license NPs. During the ensuing 40 years, the state circled from being an early adopter of the role to one of the most restrictive and then back to being one of the most progressive nationally. This story chronicles that work and highlights the critical importance of professional and legislative

leadership, perseverance, collaboration, compromise, and relationship building, all instrumental in achieving legislative success.

BACKGROUND

In the late 1960s and early 1970s, the emergence of the NP role in other states also received attention in Idaho as a means to improve rural access to health care. Supportive physicians, nurses, and citizens recruited two registered nurses (RNs) to complete the certificate NP program at Stanford University in 1971. The IBN and the Idaho Board of Medicine (BOM) came together as partners to design a mechanism to license and regulate this new professional entity, subsequently drafting a bill that created a dual regulatory framework for NP licensure. This meant the boards would jointly write the specific regulations that would apply to licensed NP practice. Regulations interpret the law and provide specificity that otherwise would be cumbersome in statute, and have the advantage of being much more adaptable to change. Regulations in most states are written and revised with the approval of the Governor and Attorney General. In Idaho, regulations must also be approved by the Legislature. This initial NP legislation was shepherded through the process by two legislators, one an RN and one a physician. Idaho was in the forefront nationally in the regulation of this new role with no experience to act as a guide. Controversy between the boards quickly emerged related to NP scope of practice and prescriptive authority.

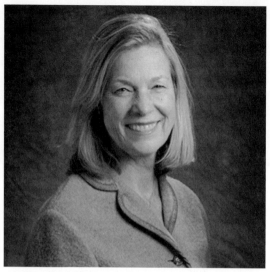

FIGURE 68-1 Margaret Henbest, MSN, APRN-CNP. (Photo courtesy of the author.)

NURTURING THE PASSION TO ACHIEVE STATUTORY CHANGE

After moving to Boise, I was readily granted an Idaho RN license, but I could not be licensed as an NP without the endorsement of a physician and the completion of an interview by the BOM, both requirements put in place through the joint rule-making process. In 1992, I joined with other NPs across Idaho who were frustrated by the stifling regulatory environment and recognized that access to health care for the underserved could be improved through a stronger and empowered NP workforce. As a group, we worked to introduce legislation to remove the dual regulation of NPs in Idaho, freeing the IBN alone to write rules for NP licensure and practice. Although the legislative effort was coordinated, and the NP community robustly engaged in lobbying legislators, the bill was defeated by a tie vote along partisan lines. Regrouping in the aftermath of defeat, a concerted effort was made to ensure that from that point forward, NPs were included in forums and discussions related to health care policy and that citizens and legislators had an accurate understanding of the role and preparation of NPs. This was accomplished over the ensuing years by putting ourselves in the room and at the table of health care discussions. We did not wait for invitations. In addition, a brochure and video was created and disseminated to all legislators explaining the preparation and role of the NP.

My growing immersion in Idaho health care politics made me realize the importance of getting personally involved in the political process to achieve change. I sought election to the Idaho House of Representatives in 1996 and won, defeating a three-term incumbent by seven votes, never to forget again that every vote counts. I served for 12 years.

BUILDING BROAD COALITIONS AND RELATIONSHIPS

Evolutionary changes to NP practice and general changes to nursing education curricula required the IBN to make major revisions to the act in 1998. The legislation, which was to become H445, removed the authority of the BOM to promulgate rules jointly with the IBN, defined the advanced practice professional nurse (APPN), and created a broad collaborative scope of practice for APPNs. (APPN was the first title used for the advanced practice registered nurse [APRN] in Idaho. When Idaho adopted the Consensus Model, it changed it to APRN.) In preparation for introducing the 1998 legislation, the IBN, led by Executive Director, Sandy Evans, worked with a broad coalition of interested nurses, physicians, health care organizations, citizens, and citizen organizations. The effort was funded by a grant from the American Nurses Association. The committee hosted a reception for legislators, distributed a press release, and published educational materials. As a legislator and finally a practicing NP, I was approached and agreed to be the House sponsor of H445. It was my opportunity to effect the changes that I sought so many years before.

Legislators have an aversion to interprofessional conflict. They label them "turf wars," recognizing them for what they often are: attempts to control trade and commerce, which may or may not be in the best interest of the public. H445 was referred to a subcommittee for further deliberations and negotiations, a strategic way to handle this conflict. Compromise was the inevitable and also desired outcome by legislators as it was the only means to save face and maintain relationships with both professions and constituents. The IBN entered negotiations focused on preserving four key points: (1) sole authority to promulgate rules; (2) APPN prescriptive authority for all classes of drugs consistent with nationally defined scope of practice for category and specialty; (3) requirement for a collaborative or consultative relationship with other providers; and (4) licensure based on established qualification, education, and demonstrated competence. The BOM and the Idaho Medicine Association (IMA) continued to demand dual promulgation of the rules for NPs and physician supervision. As a compromise, a new bill was written which removed the dual promulgation of rule making, but added language specifying that the APPN would practice with physician supervision, consultation, and collaborative management. This created a five-member Advanced Practice Advisory Committee to the IBN composed of two NPs, two physicians, and one pharmacist. The IBN had included physicians in the regulation of NPs in an advisory capacity only. With the assistance of three Senate sponsors, two of whom were nurses, the compromise legislation, H662, passed both houses unanimously and was signed into law by the Governor.

SUSTAINING THE EFFORT AND THE VISION

It seemed as if progress would be won or lost in the course of continuous skirmishes. After the legislation passed, the IBN began to promulgate new draft rules that for the first time it alone could write. The rules themselves were then opposed by the IMA because they did not require a specific supervising physician, a signed agreement with a physician, or direct physical supervision. Legislative leadership urged compromise on the rules, and during the following 1999 session, the amended rules were adopted over the continued objections of the IMA and BOM. It was becoming clear to me our early and continuous education of legislators was paying off. Policymakers understood what APPNs did,

who they were, and what it meant for improved access to care. Nursing had made significant political progress since 1992.

REMOVING BARRIERS TO AUTONOMOUS APRN PRACTICE

By 2003, however, it was apparent that there were unintended consequences from the passage of H662 in 1998. Both physicians and NPs had begun to question the strength and effectiveness of supervisory relationships that were separated in some cases by as much as 100 or more mountainous miles. Both physicians and NPs were concerned that supervision exposed them to increased liability. Clinical nurse specialists (CNSs), commonly employed by hospitals, were required to have supervision under the law, but in practice routinely did not. Finally, the departure of a supervising physician could result in a sudden interruption of APPN-delivered patient services. Legislation is written to solve problems, and it was now clear that there was a problem in need of a solution and that quality and access to care had not been compromised since 1998.

In an APPN practice meeting, Randy Hudspeth and others in attendance recognized that these problems had created an opportunity to remove the last barrier to autonomous practice: supervision. A workgroup was created, and the keys to success again would be leadership, coordination, communication, and leveraging of relationships and resources.

The NPs of Idaho assumed the lead. The IBN was supportive, as were physicians who worked with APPNs in the federally qualified health centers and hospitals, and citizens who appreciated the access and care that APPNs provided in their communities. A lobbyist with experience in health care was hired, and the representation of a well-respected and connected attorney secured. The attorney drafted the legislative language, which became H659, and I was one of two NP sponsors of the legislation. Together, the two of us represented both political parties and both houses of the Legislature. We recognized that nothing would be possible without compromise. However, the political environment was shifting; APPNs were significantly better known and valued than a decade and half before, and access to health care was becoming increasingly a critical issue as the uninsured rate in Idaho climbed to 16% to 20%.

THE STARS ALIGN

The legislative process from introduction, testimony, and floor debate to final passage lasted about 4 weeks. The committee heard about remote practices where NPs provided the only care available. They heard about physicians being paid $5000 to do monthly chart reviews. They heard about CNSs who were required to be supervised even though much of their practice was more nursing than medicine. They heard sometimes confusing and conflicting testimony from physicians. We were asked once again to meet and work out a compromise, a strategy that we were prepared for. I met with the IMA representative and the discussion centered around organized medicine's interest in ensuring a standard of APPN care in the absence of physician supervision. At the end of our meeting, we agreed that providing for collaboration with other health care providers and peer review in the statute would ensure professional standards of practice. It was a natural compromise from my perspective. As practitioners it was our responsibility to make sure we worked as a team with others as necessary to provide the wide array of services and expertise our patients needed, and if we could not subject ourselves to the transparent review of our peers, something was wrong. Compromise had been reached.

Again, grassroots lobbying was effective as NPs from each district personally contacted their legislators by e-mail, by phone, or in person. Votes were counted and legislators were personally lobbied. At the end of the 4 weeks, the bill to revise the Nurse Practice Act (NPA) and remove supervision was amended with the compromise wording. H659 passed both Houses by a large majority despite continued objections from the IMA. The rules created by the IBN in the interim, and which passed the following year, required that documentation of a peer-review process would be available to the IBN upon request, and a signed collaborative agreement with a physician would not be required.

THE 2012 NPA REVISION

After the Consensus Model was released by the National Council of State Boards of Nursing and the 2011 Institute of Medicine report *The Future of Nursing* called for nurses to work to the full extent of their education, Idaho was poised to adopt the model legislation. The foundation had been laid, and the Idaho Consensus Model Legislation, S1273, introduced in 2012, required only minor changes to the NPA. The IMA requested one change to the draft, that the make-up of the Advanced Practice Advisory Committee would remain equally representative of APRNs and physicians, and then took a neutral position on the legislation, paving the way for its smooth passage.

CONCLUSION

Although some would consider collaborative language and the creation of an advisory board related to APRN practice a dilution of independent NPA strength, I believe the path Idaho took was visionary. The redesign of health care in the United States places a priority on population health and paying for value, not volume. This can only be achieved effectively through enhanced interprofessional communication and coordination. Idaho has honored this by keeping our physician colleagues at the table of the APRN regulatory discussion and by acknowledging the need for us to collaborate with other health professionals to provide the best care for our patients.

For Idaho, an incremental approach contributed to our success. However, there is no doubt in my mind that the consistent, compelling, and truthful argument that APRNs could help to alleviate serious access to care issues in Idaho impressed legislators who had been intentionally and carefully educated about the role of the APRN. I believe that coordinated advocacy, citizen activism, leadership, nurses assuming key policymaking roles, compromise, and persistence can and will win the day.

CHAPTER 69

TAKING ACTION:
A Nurse Practitioner's Activist Efforts in Nevada

Elena Lopez-Bowlan

"Service is the rent we pay for being. It is the very purpose of life, and not something you do in your spare time."

Marion Wright Edelman

I have been a registered nurse for 30 years. In those 30 years, I have served on more than 30 community and state boards—four governor-appointed—and a presidential commission. I gained great experience in the area of communication, identification of leadership skills, and accessing funding for projects. I wrote about my experience as an activist in the last edition of this book. Some readers raised some good questions. Of importance was the question, "What are the leadership skills and behaviors that are useful to cultivate if you want to be an activist?" This question led me to examine the definition of a leader within the nursing profession. Some asked if there are communication strategies that work in certain situations but not others. Yet many felt that although community activism needed activists, these projects also needed funding; so if a nurse wants to be an activist, what are some strategies for locating resources that are useful? I hope that by answering these questions, I will inspire nurses across the United States to become leaders and advocates. Nurses can continue to better the lives of people across the world if they understand the importance of being a leader.

BEING A LEADER

Examining the leadership skills and behaviors required to be an activist, we need to understand there is some confusion in the health care system as to how a leader evolves. Although many ponder whether a leader is born or grown, I do not think that this is as important as being motivated to take a stand and make a difference. Many think that nurses are natural leaders and driven into leadership roles by their function as patient and family educators, their roles as liaisons between patient and physician, and by addressing the ever-changing needs in the health care system. However, the training provided to nurses in schools and in work settings may not prepare them to emerge as leaders. Often the development of nursing management skills focuses on staffing issues and planning for the immediate needs of patients. In contrast, leaders have the skill and ability to focus on a bigger picture that includes a vision for the future. Leaders can bring people together and inspire others to join them in their quest (McConnell, 2003, 2007; Pate, 2013).

The hierarchy of roles within the nursing profession such as the Chief Nursing Officer, House Supervisor, Director of Nursing Services, Nurse Manager, Staff Nurse, and Nursing Assistant does little to motivate or reward the development of leadership skills. Often nurses feel as though they must remain within their role. I have seen some supervisors use intimidation tactics to ensure that those who report to them stay within those boundaries. Although this system helps an organization run smoothly, it does not encourage the development of leaders within the nursing profession. I recently volunteered to serve on a nurse practitioner evaluation board, but an administrator told me that I needed to work at the facility for 2 years before I could join this board. Although I understand that the evaluation process is unique in every facility, if this person had read my curriculum vitae, she would have seen that I bring 30 years of nursing experience that is rich with knowledge from having served on many boards. This type of thinking by administrators must change if we are to encourage the development of leaders.

Although nurses are the largest subgroup in the health care system, they lack in representation on decision-making bodies. A Gallup survey conducted by the Robert Wood Johnson Foundation (RWJF), *Nursing Leadership from the Bedside to the Boardroom: A Gallup National Survey of Opinion Leaders,* reported that the individuals surveyed viewed government executives (75%) and health insurance executives (56%) as those who could exert more influence on health reform than nurses, which they ranked at a low of 14% (Khoury et al., 2011). These numbers demonstrate that nurses in positions of authority need to encourage the development of leaders within the profession.

ACTIVISM MEANS LEAVING YOUR COMFORT ZONE

In identifying leadership skills and behaviors, you must first step out of your comfort zone where you simply follow orders. Identify a compelling need in your community, state, or in the world. Before you take a stand, take a personal inventory and identify why you want to make a difference. Write down your vision for your project. For example, "I want to develop a clinic for homeless people so they will have a place to go to every Saturday." You must believe that you will make a difference, and above all do not allow others to stifle your passion. When you believe in yourself, you will behave in a way that is contagious, and inspire others to join you in your mission. In addition, to be a visionary you must have the communication skills to present your goals and requirements to others.

Communication strategies that are effective and those that hinder our process when moving toward a common goal can be limitless. I will touch on a few that have helped me in my advocacy role.

HONING YOUR VERBAL AND NONVERBAL MESSAGES

Some nursing books are worth keeping because of their important content. In the book *Interplay: The Process of Interpersonal Communication,* the authors explain the difference between hearing and listening (Adler, Rosenfeld, & Towne, 1992). Hearing occurs automatically when sound waves hit the eardrum and cause vibrations, which are transmitted to the brain. By contrast, listening is more purposeful, is not automatic, and requires that we interpret what is said and assign meaning to these sounds. Thus, at the start of any communication is active listening (Adler, Rosenfeld, & Towne, 1992). If your goal is to allow people to feel heard, use what some call "whole heart listening," which is listening without judgment (Fernandez & Baker, 2008). Once you get their attention, how you deliver the message is also important.

How many times have you heard a speaker who rambles, uses too many examples, and loses the crowd? I have always remembered a statement that one of my nurse practitioner professors, Dr. Alice Running, frequently used: "economy of words." As students, we wanted to show our great preparedness and our great enthusiasm, but this sometimes overshadowed our content. I have used Dr. Running's advice over the years, especially when addressing a large group. There are several components that will help keep the message organized and the delivery crisp: (1) Spend all the time you need to prepare what you are going to say, (2) choose a topic that you are familiar with and that is aimed at the right audience, and (3) define the purpose of your topic to aid in your research and your audience's understanding (Vollman, 2005). Lastly, if you must refer to bullet point notes, do so. There is nothing worse than addressing the legislature about an important issue and speaking without direction. Remember, economy of words is an essential component to the delivery of a message.

Examining your own body language and appearance is another critical step in communicating effectively. Dress in a way to project confidence. I remember taking a media training class through

TABLE 69-1 Body Language of the Audience That Signals Disinterest

Yawning	Person is tired or bored
Crossing arms	Defensive
Rolling eyes	Not accepting your point of view
Looking at watch	Lost interest
Bouncing feet go still	Stopped being interested
Side conversations	Stopped listening or agreeing

Developed by Elena Lopez-Bowlan. Adapted from Kelton, D., & Davis, C. (2013). Ask an expert: The art of effective communication. *Nursing Made Incredibly Easy, 11*(1), 55-56.

the Centers for Disease Control and Prevention (CDC) where they discouraged large pieces of jewelry (hub cap earrings), nonbusiness attire, or anything that would distract from your message. I became aware of what news people or politicians wore. Additionally, monitor your posture when speaking. Do not slouch; do not use your hands too much; and monitor any nervous ticks or sounds. One politician in Nevada would end every sentence or statement with "huh." After a while, his message was lost as we waited for the next "huh." After monitoring your body language, observe the posture of the audience to measure your effectiveness.

Watch your audience, as their body language is the best indicator of how they are receiving your message. Are people suddenly crossing their arms when you share a view? Are they checking their phone messages? It is very interesting to watch the group you are addressing. You will know if they are listening to your message. Your goal is to enlist the audience to support your cause (Table 69-1).

ACTIVISM REQUIRES FUNDING KNOWLEDGE

A question I am asked frequently by those interested in being an activist is, "Although community activism needed activists, these projects also needed funding; so if a nurse wants to be an activist, what are some strategies for locating resources that are useful?" Once you have chosen your project and delivered your message, locating funds for a project is probably the biggest challenge. Activists need to understand their responsibility when agreeing to serve on a committee or board or take on a cause, because you are also taking on the responsibility to raise funds for the development of the project. You may want to eliminate social inequalities, but if you cannot find the financial support needed to implement a project, you will not be able to deliver the service.

Many organizations have clear missions as to what types of issues they fund. The Rockefeller Foundation has had the same mission for 100 years, "to improve the well-being of humanity around the world." Your proposal must fit within their initiatives. They clearly state, "Your project should commit to nurturing innovation, pioneering new fields, expanding access to and distribution of resources, and ultimately generating sustainable impact on individuals, institutions, and communities within the context of our active initiatives" (Rockefeller Foundation, 2013). They also define what they do not fund. In addition to national foundations, many local organizations distribute funds in their state and communities.

Resources continue to get smaller. State divisions and county offices struggle to maintain their own funding. It is crucial for you to understand how your state and community distributes money. Several years ago, the CDC used to distribute money to states, which would then disseminate those funds to programs across the state. However, the CDC now allocates its HIV resources to High-Impact Prevention, which uses a combination of scientifically proven, cost-effective, and accessible interventions that can target the precise populations in the right geographic areas. Additionally, states are creating offices that can help procure funds for the needs of the state.

In 2011, the Nevada legislators passed Senate Bill 233, which led the way to the creation of the Office of Grant Procurement, Coordination, and Management (OGPCM). The office is to address the state's performance in the federal, corporate, and private grant arenas, increasing the value of grant funds to serve Nevadans. Before the creation of this office, Nevada ranked 50th in federal grant funding, and the money needed to provide much needed programs was dwindling. Many federal sources of funds require matching funds, which states struggle to produce. In its first fiscal year, the OGPCM identified and distributed $52.1 million in grant opportunities through established lists to 155 state internal contacts, 112 energy contacts, and 103 external grant contacts that included nonprofits (Office of Grant Procurement, Coordination, and Management, 2013).

One positive improvement in the world of fundraising has been the Internet and the ability to search for organizations that fund projects. There are sites that may charge a fee but they provide you with lists of grant makers from huge databases. For example, the Foundation Center offers online directories of funders and grants (Foundation Center, 2013). This organization houses databases on more than 108,000 foundations, corporate donors, and public charities that give out grants. They also provide training seminars to assist with proposals and grant writing. Some of these organizations assist with grant writing instructions as well. Some of the larger foundations who donate to health, arts, and other interests are:

- The Rockefeller Foundation *(www.rockefeller foundation.org/grants)*
- The Foundation Center *(www.foundationcenter .org)*
- The RWJF *(www.rwjf.org)*

If you have never written a grant proposal, it is worthwhile taking a class or researching books that can guide you in this process. Funders look for original ideas and have an understanding of projects that have succeeded and those that have failed. Advocacy work can include grant writing, knowledge of what funds are entering the state, and confidence that the program is a viable one. In addition to developing oral communication skills, you must have good writing skills.

Writing skills should be "clear, concise, and convincing" (Blum, 1996) when writing a proposal. Identify the problem that you will address. Establish and define a reasonable timeline that works with the granting source. Carefully read the requirements for submission of the grant and adhere to the specified length. Define a sensible budget for your project. Adhere to the established criteria for the grant, as this is how your grant will be reviewed (Linquist & Niloufar, 2013).

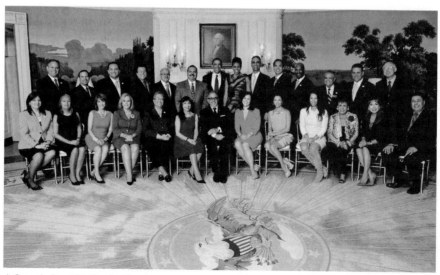

FIGURE 69-1 A Commissioner for the development of an American Latino Museum in Washington, DC, Elena Lopez-Bowlan (front row, second from right) in attendance at a White House reception celebrating the delivery of a report to the President and Congress.

DEVELOPING ACTIVIST SKILLS THROUGH EXPERIENCE

In concluding this chapter, I want to encourage nurses to continue to be activists in their own way. Find opportunities to serve on governing boards, to run for office, and to grow as leaders. In 2010, I ran for an Assembly seat for the Nevada Legislature. Although I did not win, I learned great lessons during the campaign and met wonderful people. On a national level, I continue the work as a Commissioner for the development of an American Latino Museum in Washington, DC. We presented our report to Congress and to President Obama. It awaits passage of legislation, which will make this vision a reality. As a Commissioner, I attended a reception at the White House with the President and the First Lady. I am now a nurse practitioner examiner and work with U.S. veterans in the Compensation and Pension section of the U.S. Veterans Health Administration. This division receives claims from injured soldiers who are seeking benefits. In the future, I hope to continue writing and my focus will be to examine the advocacy styles of nurses from around the world.

REFERENCES

Adler, B., Rosenfeld, L., & Towne, N. (1992). *Interplay: The process of interpersonal communication* (5th ed.). New York: Harcourt Brace Jovanovich College.

Blum, L. (1996). *The complete guide to getting a grant* (2nd ed.). New York: John Wiley & Sons, Inc.

Fernandez, C., & Baker, E. (2008). The management moment: Managing the difficult conversation. *Journal of Public Health Management and Practice, 14*(3), 317–319.

Foundation Center. (2013). Highlights of foundation funding. Retrieved from *www.foundationcenter.org/tour*.

Kelton, D., & Davis, C. (2013). Ask an expert: The art of effective communication. *Nursing Made Incredibly Easy, 11*(1), 55–56.

Khoury, C., Blizzard, R., Wright, M., & Hassimiller, S. (2011). Nursing leadership from the bedside to the boardroom: A Gallup national survey of opinion leaders. *Journal of Nursing Administration, 41*(7–8), 299–305.

Linquist, R., & Niloufar, H. (2013). Developing grant-writing skills to translate practice dreams into reality. *AACN Advanced Critical Care, 24*(2), 177–185.

McConnell, C. (2003). Accepting leadership responsibility preparing yourself to lead honestly, humanely, effectively. *The Health Care Manager, 22*(4), 361–374.

McConnell, C. (2007). The leadership contradictions: Examining leaderships' mixed motivations. *The Health Care Manager, 26*(3), 273–283.

Office of Grant Procurement, Coordination, and Management [OGPCM]. (2013). Highlights of the function of OGPCM. Retrieved from *grant.nv.gov*.

Pate, M. (2013). Nursing leadership from the bedside to the boardroom. *AACN Advanced Critical Care, 24*(2), 186–193.

Rockefeller Foundation. (2013). Highlights of the foundation's focus. Retrieved from *www.rockefellerfoundation.org/our-focus*.

Vollman, K. (2005). Enhancing presentation skills for the advanced practice nurse: Strategies for success. *AACN Advanced Critical Care, 16*(1), 67–77.

UNIT 4

Nursing Education Policy: The Unending Debate over Entry into Practice and the Continuing Debate over Doctoral Degrees

Elaine Tagliareni   Beverly Malone

"Great leaders are almost always great simplifiers, who can cut through argument, debate, and doubt to offer a solution everybody can understand."

Colin Powell

The educational entry level into nursing practice has been debated for decades. The old debate about entry into professional nursing at the prelicensure level and the latest debate about doctoral education and entry into advanced nursing practice inspire strong opinions from leaders in nursing education and practice. The early debate focused on entry at the prelicensure level, and more specifically, the movement of professional nursing practice into the academic setting. The current debate moves the dialogue to consideration of doctoral education, calling for acceptance of both the traditional research-focused doctorate and the rapidly increasing doctorate of nursing practice (DNP) as the profession's terminal degree. Both debates concern the transformation of nursing practice in the midst of changing health care systems and practice demands.

The belief that a nurse's educational entry point impacts the quality and competence of the nurse's work has fueled both debates. This notion, that entry affects practice, has resulted in numerous position statements from professional organizations describing the nature of education needed for the future. The first of these statements, the American Nurses Association (ANA) 1965, First Position on Education for Nursing (American Nurses Association [ANA], 1965) sought to change the trajectory of nursing education and move education out of the service sector and into academic settings. The paper's authors saw a future with two levels of nursing, technical and professional; two-year colleges would provide "minimum preparation for beginning technical nursing practice" (Committee on Nursing Education, 1965, p. 108) and four-year programs would prepare graduates for beginning professional practice. This document also called for practical nursing programs to eventually be replaced by technical programs. Its publication created controversy and debate in the nursing education and practice communities. Following the 1965 ANA position paper, colleges and university nursing programs created specialized master's programs (MSNs) that became the norm for credentialing and licensing of advanced practice roles. The 2004 position paper of the American Association of Colleges of Nursing (AACN), which called for the establishment of the DNP, proposed that study for the four advanced practice roles (midwives, nurse anesthetists, clinical nurse specialists, and nurse practitioners) should be elevated from the MSN to the DNP level by 2015. The DNP is viewed as the clinical path into specialized advanced practice (Donley & Flaherty, 2002). This was a radical departure from specialized master's programs and represented a new form of entry into advanced practice nursing.

THE ENTRY INTO PRACTICE DEBATE

HISTORICAL PERSPECTIVE

Following World War II, a shortage of nurses occurred because many nurses returning from military service did not re-enter the workforce. Also, changes in health care including hospital-based births, surgical procedures, and anesthesia necessitated more nurses working in hospitals (Haase, 1990). In 1948 the Carnegie Foundation commissioned a sociologist, Dr. Esther Lucille Brown, to study nursing education and to address the critical nursing shortage in the United States caused by a decreased supply of nurses and an increased demand following World War II. Brown's report, *Nursing for the Future*, called for nurses to be educated in colleges and universities instead of hospital-based programs (Brown, 1948). The ANA and the National League for Nursing (NLN) supported the Brown report and urged the profession to move nursing education into the college environment (Orsolini-Hahn & Waters, 2009). Simultaneously, President Harry Truman convened a National Commission on Higher Education which called for the expansion of community colleges. In response to both documents, the NLN representatives arranged a meeting with the Association of Community Junior Colleges (AAJC) (now known as the American Association of Community Colleges [AACC]), to explore teaching nursing in two-year community college programs (Haase, 1990).

While these events transpired on a national level, faculty at Teachers College, Columbia University, were engaged in the exploration of new models of nursing education. A doctoral student, Mildred Montag, proposed in her dissertation that nurses be educated at community colleges as nursing technicians (Montag & Gotkin, 1959). Based on Dr. Montag's dissertation, entitled *Education for Nursing Technicians*, she received funding to conduct research on this new model and in 1952, under her leadership, faculty from seven original associate degree programs created the 2-year technical program. Although the course of study was referred to as technical and terminal, a term used at the time to signify that the entire course of study could be accomplished in a set time-frame, faculty in the new programs viewed their mandate as more than the development of a shortened traditional program; they envisioned a program of learning that would revolutionize nursing education. The curriculum was no longer based on a "map of the hospital" (Waters, 2007). By 1980, associate degree programs were educating approximately 20% of new graduate nurses (Orsolini-Hahn & Waters, 2009). At the same time, professional nursing programs developed in baccalaureate programs, although not at the same pace as occurred in community college programs (Haase, 1990). The extraordinary growth of associate degree programs from the midpoint of the last century is compelling: in 2011 associate degree nursing graduates accounted for 60% of new Registered Nurse (RN) graduates from more than 900 associate nursing degree programs nationally (Human Resources Services Administration [HRSA], 2013).

UPHEAVAL WITHIN THE PROFESSION

Controversy followed the associate degree programs from their inception. The main reason for this was that the educational model was not consistent with the way associate degree graduates were used in practice. Dr. Montag had proposed this new model based on a two-level system of nursing care delivery. She intended that associate degree graduates would function in teams led by baccalaureate-prepared nurses due to the significant difference in technical and professional education. The practice environments, however, used the associate degree graduate in management and leadership positions where they performed satisfactorily (Orsolini-Hahn & Waters, 2009). For almost 50 years, nursing attempted to define the differences between graduates of the two types of nursing programs. Because these debates focused on practice in acute care both at the bedside and in management, where roles of both graduates were blurred and overlapped, they failed to clearly define the differences (Haase, 1990). In both education and practice, no clear distinctions between the two levels emerged and most employers never distinguished ADN and BSN nurses with regard to pay, function, or task.

UNIT 4

As early as 1965, organized nursing attempted to bring clarity to the differentiation debate. Due to the increasing complexity of health care and changes in practice, the ANA convened the Committee on Education to study nursing education, practice, and scope of responsibilities. The study group recommended that the minimum preparation for professional nursing practice should be the baccalaureate degree. The Committee on Education's statement became the ANA's position paper and contained a description of three levels of nursing education: baccalaureate education for beginning professional nursing practice, associate degree education for beginning technical nursing practice, and vocational education for assistants in the health service occupations (ANA, 1965). The authors of the position statement also recommended that associate degree programs replace practical nursing programs, further alienating vocational and practical nurses and faculty. That same year, the NLN published a document, Resolution 5, calling for examination of the differentiated functions of the two levels of nursing education (Haase, 1990). Subsequently, the 1965 ANA position paper was later reaffirmed by a 1978 ANA House of Delegates resolution which resulted in the recommendation that, by 1985, the minimum preparation for entry into professional practice would be the baccalaureate degree.

These actions divided the health and nursing community (Donley & Flaherty, 2002). Many associate degree nurse educators became disillusioned with the ANA and NLN, leaving both organizations to start a new organization in 1986, the National Organization for the Advancement of Associate Degree Nursing, which later became the National Organization for Associate Degree Nursing (NOADN). The NLN established separate councils for associate degree and baccalaureate educators; the councils rarely interacted. And strained relationships developed between faculty in both types of programs, resulting in little constructive dialogue on ways to differentiate between programs and build a more educated workforce, which had been the primary intent of the Brown report, the ANA 1965 position statement, and the NLN early documents. The central focus of the early debate

had been to improve educational preparation, elevate the status of nurses, and ultimately improve the quality and safety of patient care. Yet nursing had become mired in differentiation debates that served only to sidetrack the discussion. As a result, more than 50 years later, the need for a more educated workforce remained at the core of the entry into practice debate.

CURRENT CLIMATE: COLLABORATION WITH COMMON GOALS

The release of the Robert Wood Johnson Foundation (RWJF) and Institute of Medicine Report *The Future of Nursing: Leading Change, Advancing Health* (2011) was a pivotal event in the entry to practice debate. The report's wide dissemination and the positive response from the nursing community changed the national focus from differentiation debates to collaborative calls for an "action-oriented blueprint for the future of nursing" to advance the nation's health. Two of its recommendations related specifically to academic progression within nursing: (1) to support an increase in the proportion of nurses with a baccalaureate degree in nursing by 2020 from 50% to 80% and (2) to double the number of nurses with doctorates to add to the cadre of nurse faculty and researchers, with attention to diversity (Institute of Medicine [IOM], 2011). The report noted that nurses who enter the profession with either an associate or baccalaureate degree on average seek one more degree over the course of their careers and that approximately 60% of new nurses are associate degree graduates. Thus, having sufficient qualified faculty and advanced practice nurses to manage emerging models of care in a variety of settings would be unattainable with current articulation agreements. The report affirmed that in order to respond to increasing demands, nurses must achieve higher levels of education and training through an innovative education system that promotes seamless academic progression.

What factors influenced this change in thinking? What turned the dialogue away from differentiation to how academic progression could be accomplished to benefit the profession and advance the nation's health?

Factors Outside of Nursing. Numerous trends converged to coalesce around the need for a more educated workforce in the context of multiple entry points into the profession. The complexity of care and the predicted shortage of RNs in the mid-1990s to provide that care drove home the need for those RNs in the workforce to be better prepared to provide new models of care delivery, to manage the care of individuals with complex chronic care needs who require intervention in both institutional and home settings, and to teach future nurses in schools of nursing. Additionally, the calls for health care reform, which preceded the adoption of the Patient Protection and Affordable Care Act (2012), called for new approaches to delivering care to chronically ill individuals and a greater focus on health promotion and disease prevention. These approaches require nurses who are knowledgeable about research, care coordination, outcomes management, risk assessment, and quality improvement, skills that are core to the practices of professional nurses. New methods of care delivery required a systems approach to address the consequences of disparities in access to health care services that preclude quality care for all individuals. They also required that nurses have advanced study and practice experience.

Over time, the nursing community embraced the idea that the need for a highly educated workforce was the key issue, not the nurse's educational entry point. Academic progression would be the critical factor for the nursing profession to fully impact the quality and competence of a nurse's work, and the movement to embrace academic progression as essential to nursing's future gained new energy and momentum.

Factors Inside of Nursing. In 2011, the National League for Nursing released a statement promoting academic progression in nursing education. The statement made clear the NLN's conviction that transformation of nursing education is vital to the preparation of a nursing workforce prepared to tackle the demands of our ever-changing, dynamic 21st century health care system, with its advanced technologies, culturally diverse and aging patient population, and the shrinking of global borders.

The NLN reaffirmed its support of multiple entry points to the nursing profession and advocated for creating new opportunities for life-long learning and academic progression to advance the nation's health. Additionally, The Future of Nursing: Campaign for Action, was launched shortly after the release of the IOM report in 2010. The campaign, a national initiative to guide implementation of the report's recommendations, envisions a health care system where all Americans have access to high-quality care, with nurses practicing to the full extent of their capabilities. It is coordinated through the Center to Champion Nursing in America (CCNA), an initiative of the AARP (formerly the American Association of Retired Persons), the AARP Foundation, and the RWJF. As of 2014, the campaign included 51 state Action Coalitions and a wide range of health care providers, consumer advocates, and other leaders.

Internal Cohesion Comes to Nursing. In the wake of the IOM report's release, groups and organizations that were once viewed as adversarial developed joint position statements and programs. In 2012, The Joint Statement on Academic Progression for Nursing Students and Graduates brought together the NLN, AACN, American Association of Community Colleges, Association of Community College Trustees, and NOADN to declare that every nursing student and nurse needs to have access to additional nursing education (NLN, 2012).

The momentum generated by this report and the Campaign for Action resulted in dramatic changes in academic progression in nursing. The number of students enrolled in RN to BSN programs increased by 22% from 2011 to 2012 (American Association of Colleges of Nursing [AACN], 2012). By 2014, AACN data revealed a strong enrollment surge in baccalaureate nursing programs designed for practicing nurses looking to expand their education in response to employer demands and patient expectations. The number of students enrolled in RN to Bachelor of Science in Nursing (BSN) programs increased by 12.4% in 2013, the 11th year of enrollment increases in these programs (AACN, 2014a). These data reflect a trend in hospital employment that favors BSN graduates, and 59% of new BSN graduates had job offers at the time of graduation, which is substantially higher than the national average across all professions (29.3%) (AACN, 2013b). As employer demand has increased, more nurses from ADN and diploma programs recognize the need to advance their education to remain competitive in today's workforce.

Additionally, enrollment in master's and doctoral degree nursing programs also increased significantly. Nursing schools with master's programs reported an 8% jump in enrollments. In doctoral nursing programs, the greatest growth was seen in DNP programs where enrollment increased by 20% between 2011 and 2012. Enrollment in research-focused doctoral programs increased slightly by 1% (AACN, 2012).

At this time nursing students from minority backgrounds represented 28.3% of students in entry-level baccalaureate programs, 29.3% of master's students, and 27.7% of students in research-focused doctoral programs (AACN, 2014). RN-to-BSN programs exhibited the largest upturn, with minority enrollment gaining four percentage points to reach 26%. Although community college nursing programs are often the access point for entrance into nursing for individuals from minority backgrounds, there is much work to be done in nursing to have adequate representation reflective of the U.S. population.

The history of nursing progression in education includes years of debates about entry into practice at the prelicensure level, an exercise that proved to be divisive and counterproductive. For more than 50 years, from the time of the 1965 ANA position statement, the nursing community became sidetracked about how to achieve differentiation, and the ensuing debates diverted nursing's productive energy away from its fundamental vision to meet the needs of patients in changing practice environments. With the release of the IOM *Future of Nursing* report (2011) that energy is now channeled into productive dialogue about academic progression and creation of innovative programs to move new RN graduates more efficiently and effectively into advanced degrees. The next 50 years are poised to witness the transformation of nursing practice in the midst of changing health care systems and practice demands.

THE ENTRY INTO ADVANCED PRACTICE DEBATE

HISTORICAL PERSPECTIVE

Advanced practice nursing emerged as a response to the physician shortage in the late 1950s (Joelle, 2002). By the mid-1960s, nurse practitioner programs existed throughout the United States as post-baccalaureate certificate programs of varying length (O'Sullivan et al., 2005). In 1990 the National Organization of Nurse Practitioner Faculties (NONPF) published *Advanced Nursing Practice: Nurse Practitioner Curriculum Guidelines* and called for nurse practitioner education to be grounded in graduate level programs (National Organization of Nurse Practitioner Facilities [NONPF], 1990). Within the next decade, the shift away from certificated nurse practitioner (NP) programs was complete, with less than 1% of all NP programs representing non-master's education tracks (O'Sullivan et al., 2005).

Over time a growing movement evolved within nursing to reconsider nurse practitioner educational preparation in earnest. The practice doctorate was discussed as a means to meet the demand for increased knowledge and skills. The following societal changes and emerging health care trends sparked this movement:

- In the late 1990s, nurse-managed health centers emerged as safety net providers for underserved populations, extending the range of primary care services offered by nurse practitioners in autonomous practice settings (Hansen-Turton & Kinsey, 2001; O'Sullivan et al., 2005).
- The nursing community recognized that the demand for new models of care to manage complex chronic comorbidities, specifically of an aging population, required movement away from illness management to nontraditional approaches to case management involving multiple intersecting systems of care. Nurse faculty teaching in NP programs called for parity with other allied health professions. These disciplines,

for example, pharmacy, audiology, and physical therapy, had expanded their master's degree programs and created practice doctorates in response to the need for advanced practice professionals to work within complex systems, advocating for evidence-based quality care in an interdisciplinary environment. Nursing leaders argued that parity for nursing was not simply a matter of status but a necessary credential for credibility in leadership and policy positions (Lenz, 2005).

- The Institute of Medicine (2003) proposed changes in practice to reduce medical errors and increase the competencies needed to deliver quality care, including use of informatics, understanding of quality improvement, a focus on patient-centered care, wide acceptance of evidence-based practice, and movement to interdisciplinary care models. Changes in practice would require new approaches to the education of advanced practice health care professionals, including courses in health care finance and policy, process and outcomes measurement, and analysis and use of evidence-based methods to plan and implement care (O'Sullivan et al., 2005). These new educational demands resulted in increased clinical and classroom hours in NP programs; however, the credit allotment had not increased commensurately. It became apparent to faculty in NP programs that nursing may be under-credentialing its advanced practice graduates (Lenz, 2005).

EMERGENCE OF THE DNP: THE EARLY DEBATE

In 2004, AACN members endorsed a position statement on the Practice Doctorate in Nursing (AACN, 2004). This document was a response to calls for change in master's-level advanced practice nursing programs and advocated for moving entry from the master's to doctorate level by the year 2015. The DNP, as the new entry level would be termed, was viewed as a viable alternative to the research-focused doctorate in nursing for those nurses who desired to pursue excellence in nursing practice.

A collaboration between NONPF and the AACN created the publication of the AACN documents

(AACN, 2004, 2006). This generated considerable debate within the nursing community (Donley & Flaherty, 2002; Meleis & Dracup, 2005; NLN, 2007):

- What to do about schools in colleges or universities that are not authorized to offer doctorates or interested in offering a DNP?
- Was the AACN document released too soon, before adequate analysis and support from the nursing community could be garnered?
- Did the apparent separation of practice and research in the DNP program's curriculum lead to greater fragmentation in advanced nursing education?
- With the research-intensive environment of higher education, would the DNP undermine the scholarly productivity and funding advantage that schools of nursing receive from research grants?
- What was the impact on the need for well-qualified nursing faculty?

EXPONENTIAL GROWTH OF THE DNP: LESS DEBATE AND MORE DIALOGUE

Despite the initial concerns about the DNP, the growth of DNP programs across the United States has been unprecedented. From 2005 to 2011, DNP programs increased by 85%, with a 66% increase between 2009 and 2011 (Udlis & Mancuso, 2012). By 2014, almost 250 DNP programs existed and an additional 59 DNP programs were in the planning stages. From 2012 to 2013, the number of students enrolled in DNP programs increased from 11,575 to 14,699. During that same period, the number of DNP graduates doubled (AACN, 2014c).

Clearly the DNP program has addressed an unmet need for doctoral preparation in nursing as schools nationwide reported sizable and competitive student enrollment (AACN, 2013a). Although all DNP programs must adhere to the Essentials of Doctoral Education for Advanced Nursing Practice (AACN, 2006), numerous ways in which to organize and deliver programs currently exist (Udlis & Mancuso, 2012). The Essentials document called for moving the level of preparation necessary for advanced nursing practice from the master's degree to doctorate level by the year 2015, a deadline which has proved to be unrealistic. This variability in both intent and implementation of programs has led to a continuing debate about the purpose and value of the DNP. Three of the issues at the heart of the debate are: lack of standardization of the DNP program, uncertainty over nurse practitioner versus DNP practice, and lack of preparation of graduates for the faculty role.

Lack of Standardization. The DNP was viewed by proponents as a benefit to advanced practice nurses because it leveled the playing field in terms of status and authority between nursing and other health professions who have practice doctorates. Burns-Bolton and Mason (2012) argued that the DNP would distinguish advanced practice nurses as professionals that compare to other clinical doctorate health professionals but "has been undermined by the development, and now domination, of DNP programs that prepare administrators and educators" (p. 248). The DNP degree does not clearly represent the four roles of advanced clinical practice, and role definitions have been imprecise and unclear.

Lack of Preparation of Graduates for the Faculty Role. As more and more graduates of DNP programs begin or return to faculty roles in schools of nursing, the concern is that graduates will lack the complex and specialized knowledge intrinsic to the role of the nurse educator. In 2013, the NLN called for doctoral programs in nursing, including both research and practice doctorates, to prepare graduates with the knowledge and skills to teach, provide leadership for transforming education and health care systems, and conduct or translate research in nursing education. In practice disciplines such as nursing, it is especially important that educators and practitioners alike be able to evaluate and demonstrate links between educational outcomes and patient care quality, a particularly challenging task in a health system that is undergoing rapid change.

Calling for the doubling of the number of nurses with doctorates by 2020 to add to the number of nurse faculty, the IOM *Future of Nursing* report (2011) notes that at no time has there been a greater need for research on nursing education.

Consideration needs to be given to the urgent need to not only double the number of nurses with doctorates, whether DNP or PhD, but to prepare them to develop and incorporate evidence-based approaches to coordinated care within programs of learning and to expand graduates' views of patient-centered care, population-based care, and team-centered coordination during care transitions.

LESSONS LEARNED FROM NURSING'S JOURNEY

There are at least five major areas of learning from the profession's protracted journey in nursing education: vision, inclusion, diversity, the practice and education bridge, and the politics of connection: allies, partners, and champions (Box 70-1). To achieve transformation of a system, the nursing community must continually prioritize the essential components of the nursing education agenda and be sure they are consistently implemented across the country.

CONCLUSION

Donley and Flaherty (2002) have raised the question regarding the long-term achievements of the 1965 ANA position paper. The document called for all nursing education to take place in colleges and universities; today over 90% of prelicensure nursing programs exist in community colleges and bachelor's degree–granting institutions. In that sense, the position paper had a profound effect on changing the trajectory of nursing education. However if you consider the document to be a call for a more educated workforce, then the mandate has not yet been fully achieved. Similarly, if you consider that the major outcome of the DNP is parity for advanced practice nursing with other allied health disciplines, then the nursing profession is well on its way to establishing leadership and greater policy credibility. Moreover, if the intent is to advance excellence in nursing practice and nursing education to address the vision of a transformed health care system that is patient centered and community responsive, the outcome is, at present, unknown.

BOX 70-1 Lessons Learned from Nursing's Journey

There are at least five major areas of learning from the profession's protracted journey in nursing education: vision, inclusion, diversity, the practice and education bridge, and the politics of connection: allies, partners, and champions. These are not unknown areas of learning for nursing; however, they are frequently the forgotten and discounted priorities as change is pursued. As time moves us forward, to achieve not only change but transformation of a system, these priorities must be acknowledged and consistently implemented as essential components of the nursing education agenda.

Vision. By refusing to become distracted by old and new arguments related to entry, rather than focus on being responsive to a new vision for the nation's health care system, nursing/education today has the opportunity for leadership into a new era of lifelong learning and progression, claiming a stake in the vision without the perception of exclusive professional self-enhancement, sometimes referred to as tribalism. The vision is the overarching umbrella that allows space for dialogue, reflection, and debate that can exceed our individual or professional differences leading to creative pathways of collaboration and transformation. It is a vision that provides space for cocreation in alignment with the NLN definition of excellence: cocreating and implementing transformative strategies with daring ingenuity.

Inclusion. Nursing's history is replete with vivid examples describing the exclusion of nursing as a legitimate profession. It would seem that having been the recipient of a model of exclusion, we would be especially sensitive and proactive to dispel it within our ranks. Even at this time, however, the nursing profession still clearly disallows space for the licensed practical nurse (LPN) and the health care assistant (HCA). For nursing not to claim our relationship to our colleagues and exclude nurses from a variety of entry points for both prelicensure and postlicensure programs is shortsighted of the patient-centered, community-responsive care vision that a reformed health care system can offer.

Diversity. To focus on the vision for nursing, diversity has to be broader than race and ethnicity (NLN, 2012). Yet to be true to the vision for this nation with its multicultural people, race and ethnicity must also be a focus. Although the nursing workforce is still predominantly white, over time the proportion of racial/ethnic minorities has been increasing. Black/African Americans, Asians, and Hispanics/Latinos currently make up 25% of the RN population. Although this growth is notable, the RN workforce has a smaller percentage of Hispanics/Latinos and black/African Americans when compared with the total working-age population in the United States. The percentage difference for Hispanics/Latinos is particularly troubling: they compose 14% of the working-age population but only 5% percent of the RN workforce (HRSA, 2013). The old and new debates infrequently discuss these issues. Strategic efforts are still lacking in terms of making a difference in diversity. For a culture of diversity within the nursing/education workforce and workplace there must be the desire; the will to envision, create, plan, and implement; and to move to a culture of inclusiveness.

The Practice and Education Bridge. It would seem that the more recent debate on the DNP has learned from the earlier debate on entry for education and practice. This new learning involves an ongoing relationship between practice and education, and means a redesigning of both our nursing education and clinical organizations to be more inclusive of one another. The resounding question is "How can one think about a nursing education or clinical issue without practice and education playing primary roles in understanding the question and helping to determine the answer?"

The Politics of Connection: Allies, Partners, and Champions. From these nursing education debates of old and today, there is the message that nursing cannot stand alone or that even sectors of nursing cannot stand alone. Without allies, partners, and champions, we become so internally focused that we repeatedly lose sight of the vision. The vision of a transformed health care system that is patient centered and community responsive is the life line for the nursing profession. Nursing education with all of its twists and turns has consciously and unconsciously worked to create a strong diverse nursing workforce to heal the world.

DISCUSSION QUESTIONS

1. Is the current movement to produce a more educated workforce consistent with multiple entry points into the profession? Can these two realities exist in harmony?

2. How will the profession provide leadership to address the vision of a transformed health care system that is patient centered and community responsive? How will nurses with doctorates, whether DNP or PhD, lead the development and use of evidenced-based approaches to nursing

education? Will these two challenges be the next debate for the nursing profession?

3. How will the lessons learned from nursing's protracted journey in nursing education influence future debates about nursing's role in health care reform?

REFERENCES

American Association of Colleges of Nursing [AACN]. (2004). Position statement on the practice doctorate in nursing. Retrieved from *www .aacn.nche.edu/DNP/DNPPositionStatement.htm*.

American Association of Colleges of Nursing [AACN]. (2006). The essentials of doctoral education for advanced nursing practice. Retrieved from *www.aacn.nche.edu/DNP/pdf/Essentials.pdf*.

American Association of Colleges of Nursing [AACN]. (2012). AACN releases preliminary data from 2012 annual survey. Retrieved from *www .aacn.nche.edu/news/articles/2012/enrolldata*.

American Association of Colleges of Nursing [AACN]. (2013a). DNP fact sheet. Retrieved from *www.aacn.nche.edu/media-relations/fact-sheets/dnp*.

American Association of Colleges of Nursing [AACN]. (2013b). New AACN data confirm that baccalaureate-prepared nurses are more likely to secure jobs soon after graduation than other professionals. Retrieved from *www.aacn.nche.edu/news/articles/2013/new-data*.

American Association of Colleges of Nursing [AACN]. (2014a). Enrollment growth slows at U.S. nursing schools despite calls for a more highly educated nursing workforce. Retrieved from *www.aacn.nche.edu/news/ articles/2014/slow-enrollment*.

American Association of Colleges of Nursing [AACN]. (2014b). Enhancing diversity in the workforce. Retrieved from *www.aacn.nche.edu/media -relations/fact-sheets/enhancing-diversity*.

American Association of Colleges of Nursing [AACN]. (2014c). The Doctor of Nursing Practice (DNP). Retrieved from *www.aacn.nche.edu/media -relations/fact-sheets/dnp*.

American Nurses Association [ANA]. (1965). *A position paper.* New York: ANA.

Brown, E. L. (1948). *Nursing for the future: A report prepared for the National Nursing Council.* New York: Russell Sage Foundation.

Burns-Bolton, L., & Mason, D. J. (2012). Commentary on: Molding the future of advanced practice nursing. *Nursing Outlook, 60*(5), 248–249.

Committee on Nursing Education, American Nurses Association. (1965). American Nurses Association's first position on education for nursing. *American Journal of Nursing, 65*(12), 106–107.

Donley, R., & Flaherty, M. J. (2002). Revisiting the American Nurses Association's first position on education for nurses. *Online Journal of Issues in Nursing, 7*(2), 2.

Haase, P. T. (1990). *The origins and rise of associate degree nursing.* Durham, NC: Duke University Press.

Hansen-Turton, T., & Kinsey, K. (2001). The quest for self-sustainability: Nurse-managed health centers meeting the policy challenge. *Policy, Politics & Nursing Practice, 2*(4), 304–309.

Health Resources Services Administration [HRSA]. (2013). U.S. nursing workforce: Trends in supply and education. Retrieved from *bhpr.hrsa.gov/ healthworkforce/reports/nursingworkforce/nursingworkforcefullreport .pdf*.

Institute of Medicine [IOM]. (2003). *Health professions education: A bridge to quality.* Washington, DC: The National Academies Press.

Institute of Medicine [IOM]. (2011). *The future of nursing: Leading change, advancing health.* Washington, DC: Author.

Joelle, L. (2002). Education for entry into nursing practice: Revisited for the 21st century. *Online Journal of Issues in Nursing, 7*(2), Retrieved from *www.nursingworld.org/MainMenuCategories/ANAMarketplace/ANA Periodicals/OJIN/TableofContents/Volume72002/No2May2002/Entry intoNursingPractice.aspx*.

Lenz, E. R. (2005). The practice doctorate in nursing: An idea whose time has come. *Online Journal of Issues in Nursing, 10*(3), 2.

Meleis, A., & Dracup, K. (2005). The case against the DNP: History, timing, substance, and marginalization. *Online Journal of Issues in Nursing, 10*(3), 2.

Montag, M. L., & Gotkin, L. G. (1959). *Community college education for nursing: An experiment in technical education for nursing: Report of the cooperative research project in junior-community college education for nursing.* New York: McGraw-Hill.

National League for Nursing. (2007). Reflection and dialogue: Academic/ professional progression in nursing. Retrieved from *www.nln.org/ aboutnln/reflection_dialogue/refl_dial_2.htm*.

National League for Nursing. (2011). Academic progression for nursing education [NLN Vision Series]. Retrieved from *www.nln.org/aboutnln/ livingdocuments/pdf/nlnvision_1.pdf*.

National League for Nursing. (2012). *Joint statement on academic progressing for nursing students and graduates.* Retrieved from *www.nln.org/ aboutnln/academicprogression.htm*.

National League for Nursing. (2013). Doctoral preparation for nurse educators [NLN Vision Series]. Retrieved from *www.nln.org/aboutnln/ livingdocuments/pdf/nlnvision_6.pdf*.

National Organization of Nurse Practitioner Faculties [NONPF]. (1990). *Advanced nursing practice: Nurse practitioner curriculum guidelines.* NONPF.

O'Sullivan, A., Carter, M., Marion, L., Pohl, J., & Werner, K. (2005). Moving forward together: The practice doctorate in nursing. *Online Journal of Issues in Nursing, 10*(3), Retrieved from *www.nursingworld.org/Main MenuCategories/ANAMarketplace/ANAPeriodicals/OJIN/Tableof Contents/Volume102005/No3Sept05/tpc28_416028.aspx*.

Orsolini-Hahn, L., & Waters, V. (2009). Education evolution: A historical perspective of associate degree nursing. *Journal of Nursing Education, 48*(5), 266–271.

Udlis, K. A., & Mancusco, J. M. (2012). Doctor of nursing practice programs across the United States: A benchmark of information. Part I: Program Characteristics. *Journal of Professional Nursing, 28*(5), 265–273.

Waters, V. (2007). Reflecting on revolutions: A half-century in nursing education. In P. M. Ironside (Ed.), *On revolutions and revolutionaries: 25 years of reform and innovation in nursing education* (pp. 163–168). New York: National League for Nursing.

ONLINE RESOURCES

AACN Position Paper: The Baccalaureate Degree in Nursing as Minimal Preparation for Professional Practice
www.aacn.nche.edu/Publications/positions/baccmin.htm
Future of Nursing Campaign for Action
www.nln.org/aboutnln/livingdocuments/nln_vision.htm
NLN Vision Series
www.nln.org/aboutnln/livingdocuments/nln_vision.htm

CHAPTER 71

The Intersection of Technology and Health Care: Policy and Practice Implications

Carol A. Romano

"Technology is a useful servant but a dangerous master."

Christian Lous Lang

The invasion of information technology into the information-intensive area of health care has evolved together with the intent to improve access to care, enhance quality and safety, and reduce administrative and operational costs. Information technology holds great promise to improve a health care system in which patients cannot be assured they will receive the right care at the right time and in which coordination and communications related to care are lacking. Despite the introduction of information technology into the health care environment over half a century ago, in 2010 only 25% of physicians' offices and 15% of acute care hospitals took advantage of electronic records, and even fewer used remote monitoring and telehealth technologies (The National Ambulatory Medical Care Survey, 2010). Only in the past few years has a surge of national policies emerged to protect health information and facilitate and incentivize improved health outcomes and access to care through enhanced use of information technology. This chapter presents an overview of critical policies related to health information technology and addresses the implications that each poses to clinical practice. The chapter also presents considerations and concerns related to the unintended consequences of the technology–health care intersection.

The 1999 Institute of Medicine (IOM) report *To Err is Human: Building a Safer Health System* catalyzed a revolution to improve the quality of care and triggered the demand for a new direction and approach to health care. Health information technology (HIT) is viewed as a necessary tool to aid the health reform process (Berwick, Nolan, & Whittington 2008; Hebda & Czar, 2013). HIT encompasses a wide range of electronic tools that can help to access up-to-date evidence-based clinical guidelines and decision support and provide proactive health maintenance for patients. HIT can also facilitate better coordination of patient care with other providers through the secure and private sharing of clinical information. Given these benefits, concerns arise over the need to protect the privacy of personal health information in electronic form. There are also concerns about financial, technical, and social barriers to the implementation of HIT that may limit the benefits for improving care, access, and efficiency. In 2004, Executive Order 13335 by President George W. Bush initiated a more active role for government to address these concerns and spawned public policy that focused on HIT as a necessary tool to reform health and health care. Public sector involvement is critical if HIT is expected to protect patient safety. The federal government's official website for HIT is *www.healthit.gov*.

PUBLIC POLICY SUPPORT FOR HIT

Public policy can be generally defined as a system of laws, regulatory measures, courses of action, and funding priorities concerning a given topic promulgated by a governmental entity. A major aspect of public policy is laws that formalize funding and give statutory authority to initiatives (Kilpatrick, 2000). Several laws have formalized government support for HIT.

HEALTH INSURANCE PORTABILITY AND ACCOUNTABILITY ACT (HIPAA)

Patients and providers hold a long-standing concern over the privacy of and unprotected access to personal health information (Hebda & Czar, 2013). In 1996 HIPPA provided legal protection to individually identifiable health information and provisions for payments of care. It also mandated standard rules for the electronic exchange of health care data. The law named specific code sets for all Medicare related transactions, including the International Classification of Diseases (ICD) version 10 and the Clinical Modification component (ICD-10-CM), which provide more codes for the more detailed information available in electronic transactions. In 2009 the Department of Health and Human Services (HHS) released a Final Rule updating the standards for electronic transactions under HIPAA and set October 2014 as the deadline for compliance with version 10 and the Clinical Modification component (ICD-10-CM).

The new standards require conversion of the current alphanumeric designations given to every diagnosis, description of symptoms, and cause of death attributed to human beings. These codes are used by hospitals and other facilities to describe any health challenge a patient may suffer. As we move further toward electronic medical records, these codes will be increasingly used by medical and health professionals for documentation. The new coding system significantly increases the amount of data (by tenfold) to more accurately describe clinical conditions. However, the conversions to ICD-10-CM are expensive and expected to pose hardship to providers and institutions in meeting the standards (Hebda & Czar, 2013; Torrey, 2013). Federal policy was needed to help support nationwide implementation.

HEALTH INFORMATION TECHNOLOGY FOR THE ECONOMIC AND CLINICAL HEALTH ACT

Title XII of the American Recovery and Investment Act of 2009 (Pub. L. 111-5) is known as the Health Information Technology for Economic and Clinical Health Act or HITECH Act *(www.healthit.gov/policy-researchers-implementers/hitech-act-0)*. The provisions of this act are viewed not as investments in technology per se but as efforts to improve the health of Americans and the performance of their health care system (Blumenthal, 2010). The Act promotes the use of HIT to improve health care quality, safety, and efficiency (Subtitle A Part 1) by setting the "meaningful use" of interoperable electronic health record (EHR) adoption as a critical national goal and by financially incentivizing the meaningful use, not the adoption alone, of EHRs. The Act defined privacy and security provisions to protect electronic health information. Also, the HITECH Act funded programs to support the training and consulting needs of the many health care providers seeking to adopt EHRs by offering education, outreach, and technical assistance. To achieve the goal of EHR adoption, the Office of the National Coordinator (ONC) was formalized within the HHS and charged with coordination of national efforts to implement and use the most advanced HIT and the electronic exchange of health information. The ONC defined a 2011-2015 Strategic IT Plan *(www.healthit.gov/sites/default/files/utility/final-federal-health-it-strategic-plan-0911.pdf)* and certification processes to ensure EHR technologies meet standards to achieve certain quality and quantity goals to qualify for the financial incentive.

MEANINGFUL USE OF EHR

Section 4101 of the HITECH Act defines Meaningful Use as e-prescribing, engaging in health information exchange, and submission of information regarding quality measures. The goal is to change provider behavior by increasing the use and reporting of outcome measures and increasing the exchange of electronic patient information. The Centers for Medicare and Medicaid Services (CMS) sponsors the programs to incentivize the meaningful use of EHRs by defining objectives for EHR use *(www.healthit.gov/policy-researchers-implementers/meaningful-use)*. These objectives are categorized under five major policy initiatives: (1) improve quality, safety, and efficiencies and reduce health disparities; (2) engage patients and families;

(3) improve care coordination; (4) improve population and public health; and (5) ensure adequate privacy and security protections for personal health information. Requirements for EHRs include the entry of basic data such as vital signs, patient demographics, active medications, allergies, problem lists, clinical orders and medication prescriptions, reminders to patients for needed care, and identification and provision of patient-specific health education (Blumenthal & Tavenner, 2010). Eligible providers who do not participate in the use of EHRs by 2015 will have Medicare payments negatively adjusted. Criteria for meaningful use are being implemented in stages that address data capture and sharing first, followed by advanced clinical processes, and finally improved outcomes. Between 2009 and 2012, EHR adoption nearly doubled among physicians and more than tripled among hospitals. As of October 2013, progress on adoption of electronic records reported that 85% of eligible hospitals and greater than six in ten eligible providers had received federal EHR incentive payments (Reider & Tagalicod, 2013).

PRIVACY AND SECURITY PROVISIONS

It is recognized that electronic health information exchange cannot reach its potential benefit unless patients and providers are confident that patient data are private and secure. Thus the HITECH Act also provides new improved privacy and security provisions (Subtitle D Part 1) that have major implications for providers, hospitals, and health insurance plans. This act requires health care entities to report data breaches affecting 500 or more individuals to the HHS and to the media, as well as notifying the affected individuals within 60 days of any breach of unsecured health information. In addition, patients can restrict some disclosures in certain circumstances and can request an accounting of any disclosures made. Penalties for violation of these requirements can be as high as $1.5 million dollars.

THE PATIENT PROTECTION AND AFFORDABLE CARE ACT STRENGTHENS HIT ADOPTION

The Patient Protection and Affordable Care Act of 2010, as amended by the Health Care and Education Reconciliation Act of 2010, referred to collectively as the Affordable Care Act (ACA), builds on the HITECH Act and recognizes HIT as a critical enabler to broaden transformations in health care (*www.hhs.gov/healthcare/rights/law/index.html*).

Although the law includes a large number of insurance related provisions to be paid for by Medicare and other taxes and by fees on medical device and pharmaceutical companies, a number of provisions address the challenges facing the electronic health information exchange and the development of new methods to reimburse care expenses. The provisions can be organized into the general categories of quality health care, operating rules and standards, and supporting the HIT workforce (Healthcare Information and Management Systems Society [HIMSS], 2010). The first group of HIT provisions relate to quality and address areas such as increasing the accuracy of data collected by HIT, expanding the scope and type of data collected, creating new programs that involve HIT, and establishing and requiring reporting improvements (facilitated by HIT) in population health, health plans, service providers, and other clinical factors in the delivery of health care services. The second area of HIT provisions addresses operating rules and standards and attempts to simplify the administration of health care. These provisions establish a single set of consensus-based operating rules and establish federal grants to develop new or to adapt existing HIT to comply with the standards. The final group of HIT provisions relates to the HIT workforce and provides funding incentives for staff training in HIT and requires individuals with experience and skill in HIT to participate in working groups that address health quality. These policy provisions support the intersection of technology in the health care system.

POLITICAL AND CLINICAL IMPLICATIONS OF HIT POLICY FOR NURSING

HIPAA, HITECH, and the ACA policies are important to the clinical practice of nurses and affect the information handling practices of all clinicians. Standards for transmission of electronic information will allow for seamless exchange and communication of information across providers. The

ICD-10-CM requirements will foster continuity and coordination of care through detailed clinical documentation and accurate communications. The new standards and coding systems affect the documented information that reflects the practice and the care provided by nurses. The incentives for EHRs will increase the use of HIT and require all nurses to have knowledge and understanding of electronic information management. Skill in the effective use of EHRs is also required and affects how we prepare nurses in the academic and practice settings for such systems. Also, the advocacy role of nurses is critical to provide vigilance in advocating and monitoring privacy practices. The new requirements for meaningful use of technology also emphasize the need for informatics nurses to direct the development and implementation of EHR to meet the standards for certification. Hebda and Czar (2013) cite several political issues related to the implementation of these technology-related laws. Benefits of HIT are based on the assumption that health care practices and hospitals will have fully functioning, effective EHRs and supporting information systems in place. The reality is that many EHRs are not fully implemented; the technology infrastructures fall short of full support; and security measures are imperfect. Absent perfect systems, few hospitals or practices are paperless. Those with some EHR capacity need to expand their infrastructure, increase skilled personnel, and redesign their systems of care.

Critics of EHRs say they slow down providers, limit flexibility in care, and may increase opportunities for fraud. In addition there is a delicate balance between the free exchange of information and privacy protections; there are parties with vested interests in information access who pose potential problems for the protection of health information. Informed policy requires good information, and no perfect or complete information exists regarding outcomes or effectiveness of EHRs. In addition, the HITECH Act may trigger purchases without the due diligence of site visits, preparing staff, exploring decision support tools, and assessing compatibility with certification standards. It is also not clear which of these costs are covered by the HITECH Act or by the ACA. In addition,

controversy over the capacity to fund the ACA exists with many calling for the reduction, revision, or removal of the law. Initial technical difficulties and political communications related to the online health insurance marketplace have made initial realization of the tenets of ACA difficult, and while the nation has turned to widespread use of HIT to improve patient safety, there is a concern that poorly designed and implemented HIT can actually create new hazards in the complex care delivery system. Technology can only maximize safety and minimize harm if it is more usable, interoperable, and easier to implement and maintain than was previously the case. To address this concern, the IOM was asked by HHS to evaluate HIT safety concerns.

SAFETY AND UNINTENDED CONSEQUENCES OF HIT

HIT can improve patient safety in some areas such as medication safety; however, there are significant gaps in the literature regarding how HIT impacts patient safety overall. In 2011 the IOM report HIT and Patient Safety acknowledged that the information needed for an objective analysis and assessment of the safety of HIT and its use is not available. Little published evidence could be found quantifying the magnitude of the risk posed by HIT. Although specific types of HIT can improve patient safety under the right conditions, those conditions cannot be replicated easily and require continual effort to sustain. The report asserts that although some studies in the literature suggest improvements in patient safety, others have found either no effect or instances of harm. Examples of harm include medication dosing errors, failure to detect fatal illnesses, and treatment delays caused by poor human-computer interactions or loss of data. These have led to several reported patient deaths and injuries. The degree to which existing literature concerning the health care system can be generalized is limited, and the magnitude of harm is unknown because of the heterogeneous nature of HIT products, the diverse impact on different clinical environments and workflow, legal barriers and vendor contracts, and inadequate evidence in the literature. The absence of a central repository to collect and analyze information and the nondisclosure and confidentiality clauses that prevent users from sharing information about adverse events contribute to the lack of safety.

Many problems with HIT relate to usability, implementation, and how software fits with the clinical workflow. It is acknowledged that an EHR, or any software, is neither safe nor unsafe because safety is a function of how software is used by clinicians. The IOM report concluded that safety is the product of the larger sociotechnical system. The safe use of HIT is contingent on multiple factors that include the interplay of people, processes, and technology and the involvement of government, the private sector, and users and vendors of the technology. There is no single cause for safety problems or errors; however, poor user-interface design, poor workflow, and complex interfaces (or lack of interfaces) between systems threaten patient safety. Similarly, lack of system interoperability limits the availability of data and poses a barrier to improving clinical decisions and patient safety.

Creating safer systems begins with user-centered design principles and continues with quality assessments and adequate testing at each stage of design and implementation. Each of these areas should involve nurses, who are the largest users of HIT. A consistent commitment to safety is needed and all users of HIT bear the responsibility for diligent surveillance of any mismatches between user needs and system performance, unsafe conditions, adverse events, and unintended consequences. To build upon the recommendations made in the 2011 IOM safety report and to affirm the commitment to safety, HHS issued the Health IT Patient Safety Action and Surveillance Plan. This plan is available online along with evidence-based tools and interventions for various stakeholders and can be retrieved from *www.healthit.gov/policy-researchers-implementers/health-it-and-patient-safety*.

UNINTENDED CONSEQUENCES OF HIT

Although there are high expectations for HIT to achieve quality, safety, and cost benefits, studies have shown that unplanned and unexpected consequences have resulted from major policy and technology changes (Ash, Berg, & Coiera, 2004;

Bloomrosen et al., 2011). Bloomrosen and colleagues (2011) differentiate "unintended consequences," which implies lack of purposeful action or causation, from "unanticipated consequences," which implies an inability to forecast what actually occurred. These consequences can be positive, negative while achieving the desired effect, or negative without achieving what was originally intended. Ash and colleagues (2004) categorized two types of unintended consequences of patient care information systems related to silent errors: those occurring during the process of entering and retrieving information and those in the communication and coordination process that the HIT is supposed to support. Harrison, Koppel, and Bar-Lev (2007) view these unintended consequences from an interactive sociotechnical analysis (ISTA) perspective with recursive processes that effect second-level changes in social systems. The ISTA model refers to the influences of sociotechnical forces that shape work processes, the effects of work technologies and physical environments on individuals, the interactions among technology users, technology-in-practice as shaped by practitioners yet mediates practice, and social informatics that acknowledges the embedding of information technology in organizations and society.

The implementation of HIT and information systems results in changes to clinical practices and workflows and triggers emotions such as uncertainty and resentment. These can affect the clinician's ability to carry out complex physical and cognitive tasks. Patient safety is also impaired by the failure to quickly fix technology when it becomes counterproductive and when dangerous workarounds are developed to address unresolved problems. Safety is also compromised when health care information systems are not integrated or updated consistently. If not carefully planned and integrated into workflow processes, new technology can create new work and complicate or slow clinical care.

Front-line clinicians need to be involved in the HIT planning processes to consider best practices and the costs and resources needed for ongoing maintenance and to consult product safety reviews or alerts. Learning to use new technologies takes time and attention and places strain on demanding schedules yet needs to be addressed in HIT implementation to enhance safety in the longer term. Unintended consequences result from complex interactions between technology and the surrounding work environment even when HIT is well planned. The Joint Commission (2008) offers recommendations for safely implementing health information and converging technologies to avoid a range of adverse unintended consequences that can occur with daily use of HIT.

CONCLUSION

Policy can and does shape the intersection of technology in health and health care by removing barriers to the adoption and use of HIT, ensuring technology is designed and implemented to meet national standards for exchange through certifications, protecting the privacy and security of health information, and fostering new systems of care delivery to enhance coordination of care through the effective, interoperable exchange of information. As leaders in shaping health care reform and the policies that support it, nurses are critical to ensuring quality, safety, and cost-effective care and need to understand the role of technology as it intersects the health and health care systems as well as the power of policy to influence its use. Nurse involvement at the policy level is important so that issues related to care and reimbursement for advanced practice nurses can be included in the regulations.

DISCUSSION QUESTIONS

1. How can nurses inform and influence the development of health policy related to information technology?
2. How does the use of information technology in health care affect reimbursement for nursing care, evidence-based practice, and the use of data for population health?
3. What are some recommended practices for avoiding unintended consequences of electronic health record use?

REFERENCES

Ash, J. S., Berg, M., & Coiera, E. (2004). Some unintended consequences of information technology in health care: The nature of patient care information system-related error. *Journal of the American Medical Informatics Association, 11*(2), 104–112.

Berwick, D., Nolan, D., & Whittington, J. (2008). The triple aim: Care, health, and cost. *Health Affairs, 27*(3), 759–769. doi:10.1377/hlthaff.27.3.759.

Bloomrosen, M., Starren, J., Lorenzi, N. M., Ash, J. S., Patel, V. L., & Shortliffe, E. H. (2011). Anticipating and addressing the unintended consequences of health IT and policy: A report from the AMIA 2009 Health Policy Meeting. *Journal of the American Medical Informatics Association, 18*(1), 82–90. doi:10.1136/jamia.2010.007567.

Blumenthal, D., & Tavenner, M. (2010). The "meaningful use" regulation of electronic health records. *New England Journal of Medicine,* Retrieved from *www.nejm.org/doi/full/10.1056/NEJMp1006114*.

Blumenthal, D. (2010). Launching HITECH. *New England Journal of Medicine, 362,* 382–385. doi:10.1056/NEJMp0912825.

Harrison, M. I., Koppel, R., & Bar-Lev, S. (2007). Unintended consequences of information technologies in health care—An interactive sociotechnical analysis. *Journal of the American Medical Informatics Association, 14*(5), 542–549. doi:10.1197/jamia.M2384PMCID:PMC1975796.

Hebda, T., & Czar, P. (2013). *Handbook of informatics for nurses & health professionals* (5th ed., pp. 379–407). New Jersey: Pearson Education Inc.

Healthcare Information and Management Systems Society [HIMSS]. (2010). The Patient Protection and Affordable Care Act: Summary of key health information technology Provisions. Retrieved from *himss.files.cms-plus.com/himssorg/content/files/ppaca_summary.pdf*.

Institute of Medicine [IOM]. (1999). *To err is human: Building a safer health system.* Washington DC: National Academy Press.

Institute of Medicine [IOM]. (2011). *HIT and patient safety: Building safer systems for better care.* Washington DC: National Academy Press.

Joint Commission. (2008). Safely implementing health information and converging technologies. *Sentinel Event Alert,* (42), Retrieved from *www.jointcommission.org/assets/1/18/SEA_42.pdf*.

Kilpatrick, D. G. (2000). Definition of public policy and the law. Retrieved from *www.musc.edu/vawprevention/policy/definition.shtml*.

The National Ambulatory Medical Care Survey [NAMCS]. (2010). American Hospital Association IT supplement 2010. Retrieved from *www.hhs.gov/news/press/2011pres/01/20110113a.html*.

Reider, J., & Tagalicod, R. (2013). Progress on adoption of electronic health records. Retrieved from *www.healthit.gov/buzz-blog/electronic-health-and-medical-records/progress-adoption-electronic-health-records/*.

Torrey, T. (2013). What are ICD-9 or ICD-10 codes? How ICD codes affect your care. Retrieved from *patients.about.com/od/medicalcodes/a/icdcodes.htm*.

ONLINE RESOURCES

Federal Government's official website for Health InformationTechnology
www.healthit.gov
HHS Health IT Patient Safety Action and Surveillance Plan
www.healthit.gov/policy-researchers-implementers/health-it-and-patient-safety
Medicare and Medicaid Electronic Health Records (EHR) Incentive Programs
www.cms.gov/regulations-and-guidance/legislation/EHRincentivePrograms/index.html

CHAPTER 72

Interest Groups in Health Care Policy and Politics

Joanne R. Warner

"Politics isn't about big money or power games; it's about the improvement of people's lives."

Paul Wellstone

The ink from President Obama's pen was hardly dry as he signed the Patient Protection and Affordable Care Act (ACA) into law before interest groups were considering how to stall or prevent its implementation. In fact on that very day, March 23, 2010, a suit was filed declaring the law unconstitutional. Included in the suit's supporters were private interest groups such as Citizens United who objected to the law's mandate to buy insurance or pay a penalty. A legal conclusion to their questions came in a June 2012 Supreme Court ruling upholding the individual mandate, but striking down the requirement for states to expand Medicaid (Clemmitt, 2012). The legislative journey for the ACA presents many examples of interest group influence, including the citizen activists' organization Americans for Prosperity, who continue to cast doubts on the ACA's merits, warning that the implementation is "chaotic and frustrating" (Peters, 2013, paragraph 4). What promises to unfold for the ACA is the robust involvement of interest groups vociferously defending their preferences in the structure and financing of America's health care system.

Interest groups play a significant role in health care reform. However, they are a paradox within our governing system. We need and value them but at the same time they annoy and distract us. We embrace them as empowered citizen involvement, and we resent the perception of buying elections and votes. The love-hate ambivalence is born, in part, from the way a 1787 notion has translated into today's Washington-centric political era. Democracy within our individualistic society presents inherent tensions that are both our genius and our burden.

An interest group is a collection of people who pursue their common interests by influencing political processes. They are also known as factions, special interests, pressure groups, or organized interests. The original definition depicted them as "united and actuated by some common impulse of passion, or of interest, adverse to the rights of other citizens, or to the permanent and aggregate interests of the community" (Madison, 1787, paragraph 2). The mere act of organizing presupposes "some kind of political bias because organization is itself a mobilization of bias in preparation for action" (Schattschneider, 1960/2005, p. 279). Today, federal, state, and local political arenas experience the activity of organized groups who influence elections, votes, societal opinion, and the policy process itself.

581

This chapter gives context to the duality of distrust and appreciation for interest groups while also portraying them as a significant feature of our governing system. It traces the historical roots of interest groups, describes their functions and methods, and concludes that they embody the good, the bad, and the ugly of governance. It also describes the contemporary terrain of health care interest groups as well as a discernment framework for interest group involvement.

DEVELOPMENT OF INTEREST GROUPS

James Madison's *The Federalist No. 10* (1787) forms part of his treatise on the preferred structure of a republic. He proposes that rather than removing the causes of factions, the best wisdom is to control the effects of interest groups. To do otherwise is to undermine liberty. The legitimate roots of interest group organizing are therefore traced to the framers of the Constitution and the birth of the American version of democracy. Later, the French philosopher Alexis de Tocqueville observed the country from an outsider's view. His *Democracy in America* (1835) endures as a classic description of our inclination to form associations for common purpose and to create a vibrant political structure independent of the state (de Tocqueville, 1835/2010).

The impetus to organize exists not only within the American people but also within the political structure. Groups can influence policy through elections, lobbying the legislature, and pressuring the executive branch of any level of government. This diffusion of power presents many opportunities for persuasion. It also allows interest groups to shop for a different level of government if they are unhappy with policy; for example, federal versus state government (Anderson, 2011).

Historically, groups formed around interests such as slavery and alcohol prohibition. At the turn of the twentieth century, interest groups based in Washington blossomed. The social activism of the 1960s generated more groups focused on civil rights, the environment, and specific economic and humanitarian causes (Nownes, 2013). As the power and money of interest groups grew, Congress acted

to restrict their influence and limit direct contributions to candidates. However, the reforms that grew from the Watergate scandal of the 1970s inadvertently enhanced their power by promoting the formation of political action committees (PACs). The Bipartisan Campaign Reform Act of 2002 (the McCain-Feingold Act) revised the Federal Election Campaign Act of 1971 to control soft money contributions, that is, funds funneled through political parties to candidates, and the funding of issues ads (Federal Election Commission, 2013a). For good or ill, special interest money continues to grease electoral and political wheels.

From this historical perspective, several kinds of groups are in existence today: the trade unions and business associations that advance their economic interests, and the groups representing newer social movements (Fiorina et al., 2009). Within the latter group, there are interest groups that provide information and are active in the current health care reform debate. Examples include the U.S. Public Interest Research Groups (USPIRG), who "stands up to powerful interest when they threaten our health and safety" or when big money dominates the dialogue (U.S. Public Interest Research Groups, 2013); Essential Action, which wages campaigns on topics not visible in the mass media or on political agendas including access to medicines and the global effort to reduce tobacco use (Essential Information, 2013); and the Center for Science in the Public Interest (CSPI), whose consumer advocacy in health and nutrition involves novel research, providing information, and ensuring that science and technology serve the public good (Center for Science in the Public Interest [CSPI], 2012). These examples demonstrate the enduring nature of interest groups juxtaposed as an evolving list of groups and issues.

When is an interest group not what it appears? Astute citizens and policymakers need to be aware of front groups whose public persona is that of an unbiased group but whose funds and agendas are from an industry or political party. For example, the Center for Consumer Freedom, which has a message of individual choice but is a front group for the restaurant, alcohol, and tobacco industries. This group opposes public health messages of science, health, and environmental groups, calling them a "growing fraternity of food cops, health care enforcers, anti-meat activists, and meddling bureaucrats who 'know what's best for you'" (Source Watch, 2009). The popular Get Government Off Our Back (GGOOB) campaign was also exposed as a tobacco industry front group that rallied diverse groups to oppose policy. Analysis of GGOOB suggests that knowing the source of a group's funding can limit harmful misrepresentation and highlight how ideological arguments can diminish the power of solid science and research in policymaking (Apolionio & Bero, 2007). The presence of front groups calls each consumer to vigilance about the bias and intention of groups who advocate and provide information.

FUNCTIONS AND METHODS OF INFLUENCE

How do interest groups function within a complicated governance system? What methods can they use to advance their causes, and how do they determine which to use? Their methods are lobbying, grassroots mobilization, influencing elections, shaping public opinion, and litigation.

LOBBYING

Lobbying involves the direct influence of public officials and their decisions. Wolpe (1990) presented a concise description of lobbying as "the political management of information" (p. 9) because it involves educating, shaping opinions, and offering data and analyses. Lobbyists also often assist in bill drafting and revision. By hiring full-time Washington- or state-based lobbyists, groups have a more enduring presence; this also allows for ongoing relationships between staff, officials, and lobbyists to be the foundation of influence. Lobbyists become adept at the nuances of the legislative process and can provide nimble responses.

The largest number of registered federal lobbyists recorded to date is 14,842 in 2007 and the largest total lobbying expenditure was recorded at $3.55 billion in 2010. In 2012, 12,407 federal lobbyists were a part of $3.31 billion lobbying spending (Center for Responsive Politics, 2013a). Of the

top 8 lobbying industries in 2013, four are related to health: insurance, hospitals, pharmaceuticals, and physicians, in order of size (Center for Responsive Politics, 2013b). Lobbying is thus a substantial business.

GRASSROOTS MOBILIZATION

Grassroots mobilization involves indirectly influencing officials through constituency contact. More decentralized politics and expanded communication options make grassroots involvement effective. Pseudo-grassroots efforts that mobilize technology more than citizens are mockingly called AstroTurf lobbying; another version is grass-tops lobbying, when a prominent personality champions an issue. Most interest groups employ some version of grassroots mobilization (Bergan, 2009).

ELECTORAL INFLUENCE

Electoral influence can be considered the primary prevention of policymaking because it is an important activity that precedes policy work. It determines who is elected to shape future policies (Warner, 2002). Successful electoral campaigns need three resources: time, money, and people. Interest groups can provide the last two. Just as interest groups provide a collective voice, PACs provide the collective financial support. For example, the American Nurses Association (ANA) formed the ANA-PAC in 1974 to support federal candidates who are aligned with the ANA agenda and values, with the ultimate intent of improving the health care system (ANA, 2013). As a result of campaign reform efforts in 2002 the influence of PACs has been contained. During 2013 to 2014 PACs can only donate $5000 per election (primary, general, or special) and $15,000 annually to a national party, although individuals can give up to $2600 per year to each candidate (Federal Election Commission, 2013b).

SHAPING PUBLIC OPINION

Shaping public opinion overlaps with electoral influence and grassroots mobilization; it involves issue advocacy and public persuasion, similar to campaigning for an issue. It is similar to an infomercial that sells an issue or to direct mail blanketing an area with information promoting a particular perspective. The impression of societal consensus could, in turn, persuade policymakers as they create policy. These initiatives either cost money or are free media in the form of news coverage.

LITIGATION

Lastly, litigation can shape governance toward the goals of the group. The *Brown v. Board of Education of Topeka, Kansas* is a classic example of years of strategic effort culminating in a significant judicial ruling changing the landscape of society. The National Association for the Advancement of Colored People (NAACP) was the interest group championing social justice and the elimination of racial discrimination that organized 200 plaintiffs in five states to bring cases of racial segregation and discrimination in schools to the Supreme Court. This ruling affected racial discrimination through-out society and inspired interest groups to pursue their proposed change through the court system (Brown Foundation for Educational Equity, Excellence and Research, 2012).

To create their action plans, each interest group develops a distinct identity that originates in its methods, resources, and purpose. This discussion of function and method illustrates that their influence within the governance process, whether nuanced or bold, can span the entire process and can range from superficial to substantial.

Related to the scope of influence is the question of effectiveness. The critique ranges from the good to the bad and the ugly. Many maintain that they successfully enhance our democratic processes and actualize our early vision of democracy, as argued by James Madison. In doing so, they prevent violence and tyranny by engaging citizens in social change through other means. In theory, groups represent our pluralistic and transparent government. In practice, scholars believe that opposing groups' lobbying, media, or actions often cancel out their cumulative influence (Fiorina et al., 2009).

The bad and the ugly of their influence were termed demosclerosis, or the clogged vessels of our governmental body and subsequent policy gridlock. This acknowledges that the country's well-being cannot be achieved through the collective concerns of special interests and that the policy process grinds into inaction with too many special groups vying for their own advantage (Rauch, 1994). Quadagno (2005) presents a bold example of demosclerosis by concluding that health care reform has been thwarted over the years by special interests and that these groups are the "primary impediment to national health insurance" (p. 207). Even as the antireform coalition has changed over the years from primarily physicians to insurers, its goal of inertia and status quo has prevailed over the reformers' efforts. The chronicle of the ACA provides contemporary examples.

LANDSCAPE OF CONTEMPORARY HEALTH CARE INTEREST GROUPS

A *Pittsburgh Post-Gazette* editorial warned then President-Elect Obama against health care reform early in his presidency because "the field is a rat's nest of entrenched interests" (*Pittsburgh Post-Gazette*, 2008, p. 2). This unsavory reference underscores the complex nature of health care interests. Who are these players, what money is involved, and what is nursing's place and relative effectiveness in the context of federal lobbying groups?

Funds from interest groups are predominantly spent on lobbying and on campaign contributions, and the health industry is heavily involved in both. The Center for Responsive Politics (a nonpartisan research group that tracks money in politics) ranked the health sector as the sixth largest interest group contributor. During the 2012 election cycle, health professionals contributed a record $260.4 million to federal candidates; although Republicans received a larger proportion of those funds, nurses traditionally favor Democrats. Lobbying expenditures from the health care sector peaked in 2009 at $552 million as the ACA was being created. The pharmaceutical industry dominated the 2012 spending by contributing $235 million of the total $487 million of health spending (Center for Responsive Politics, 2013c). Stakeholders concerned with health care reform also include those outside the health industry (e.g., insurance corporations, labor unions, and myriad business and consumer groups). In fact, from an ecological perspective, most topics eventually trace back to health and the human potential it impacts.

Table 72-1 presents campaign contributions made by health professionals from 1996 to 2012, including both health professional PACs and individual contributions. It demonstrates dramatic increases in contributions and variation in the partisan allocations, usually related to whatever party is in power. Clearly, health professionals are engaged in electoral politics.

Nursing has experience and success with collective involvement in campaigns. The American Nurses Association (ANA) has provided a collective voice and presence in Washington from 1974 to the present. Their goal is the "improvement of the health care system in the United States" by contributing to candidates who support the ANA policy agendas (American Nurses Association [ANA], 2013a, p. 1). Decisions to endorse candidates are made by the Board of Trustees. It is important to realize that endorsement decisions are based on agreement with ANA's policy stands and not on the candidate's party. In the 2012 cycle, 82% of their $542,500 contributions went to Democrats and 16% to Republicans (Center for Responsive Politics, 2013d). Table 72-2 lists contributions of nursing PAC contributions to federal candidates in 2012.

TABLE 72-1 Health Professionals' PAC and Individual Contributions to Campaigns

Election Cycle	Total Contributions	% to Democrats	% to Republicans
2012	$152,275,788	43	57
2010	$77,614,465	48	52
2008	$101,791.889	53	47
2006	$56,758.918	38	62
2004	$75,280,121	37	63
2002	$42,738,790	38	62
2000	$48,042,286	42	58
1998	$31,587,151	41	59
1996	$37,811,666	36	64

Adapted from Center for Responsive Politics. (2012). Health professionals: Long-term contribution trends. Retrieved from *www.open secrets.org/industries/totals.php?cycle=2012&ind=H01*.

TABLE 72-2 Nursing PAC Contributions to Federal Candidates

Nursing Political Action Committee	Amount Contributed
American Association of Nurse Anesthetists	$683,800
American Nurses Association	$542,500
American College of Nurse Midwives	$70,500
American Academy of Nurse Practitioners	$63,050
American College of Nurse Practitioners	$26,500

Adapted from Center for Responsive Politics. (2012). PACS health: PAC contributions to federal candidates. Retrieved from *www.opensecrets.org/pacs/industry.php?txt=H01&cycle=2012.*

Trended data provide interesting information about the choices that nurses make for their collective electoral influence. The ANA PAC raised and spent over $1 million in one election cycle (1994) but has not reached that amount since. Contrast this to trended data about the American Association of Nurse Anesthetists whose PAC has exceeded $1 million in every election cycle since 2000, with a record high of $1.6 million in 2008 (Center for Responsive Politics, 2013d, 2013e). A simplistic assumption is that nurses donate closer to their specialty, yet the fuller explanation is likely more complex and not yet explained.

When the campaign dust settles and policymaking continues, lobbyists base their advocacy on the values and positions of the group. The ANA, for example, has a long history of supporting universal access to quality health care and advocating for a system that serves the interests of both patients and nurses (ANA, 2013b). The key elements of the 2008 Health System Reform Agenda continue to be relevant standards and values that infuse into ongoing reform efforts: access, quality, cost, and workforce. The ACA addresses most of these elements except health care as a human right for all and public funding through Medicaid expansion (ANA, 2010).

The landscape for health care reform therefore is populated with many interest groups, some in the health industry and many with vested interests in the cost and structure of the reform efforts. Significant money goes into elections and lobbying and nursing is involved in both. Although it may not be ranked as one of the most powerful groups, its political currency is trust, integrity, and a reputation for championing quality care for all within an equitable and accessible system.

ASSESSING VALUE AND CONSIDERING INVOLVEMENT

Most choices involve a "what's-in-it-for-me?" appraisal. In addition to that discernment, the robust ambivalence surrounding interest groups heightens the need for evaluation criteria. How can nurses and other health care providers assess the qualities of an interest group? Where should they allocate their finite resources of time, energy, money, and reputation?

Table 72-3 portrays queries that provide a framework for discernment to assess an interest group and determine the extent of involvement. The framework also provides language and justification for decisions. This approach matches the spirit, though not the rigor, of the scientific evidence-based nature of the health care profession. The nine queries are not listed by priority, as the weight of their importance will differ according to the individual. Nurses can engage in the discernment and defend their involvement in terms of the nine guiding principles, which may prove more thoughtful than replicating the behaviors of our parents or simply following the crowd.

CONCLUSION

In a democracy, interest groups are integral to the governing process. They are sanctioned by our Constitution and valued as a vehicle for citizen participation, but are also despised as an underhanded wielding of influence through money. Despite societal ambivalence, they are likely here to stay. Perhaps the best approach is to cleverly frame them. As Republican strategist Mary Matalin whimsically

TABLE 72-3 Framework for Assessing Interest Groups

Factor	Questions to Assess the Factor in an Interest Group
Efficiency	What portion of the group's budget supports advocacy, education, or the social interest represented, compared with the portion that supports the group's infrastructure, overhead, or administration?
Effectiveness	What is the track record of accomplishments related to education, awareness, legislation, or cultural change? What outcomes can be credited to the group, either individually or in coalition?
Values	Do the values of the group align with your personal, political, and professional values? Do your beliefs match the values that inspire the group's work? Does this work stir some passion in you?
Tactics	Do you support the methods used by the group? Do the tactics match your preferred approach to social change, including options such as violence, protesting, nonviolent resistance, media campaigns, or organized action?
Visibility and responsiveness	Does the group have the level of public visibility that you prefer? Do they employ the level of outreach to their members that you prefer? Do they communicate clearly and consistently with the constituency?
Social norms	Does the group match your local culture and the social norms of the people with whom you associate? Would your involvement in this group change the way people perceive you personally or professionally? Does that perception matter to you?
Perception	What is your perception of the leaders and key stakeholders of the interest group? Does that perception matter to you?
Costs	What would involvement require of you? Are there dues or voluntary financial commitments? Can you contribute the amount of time required? Will they ask to use your name, title, or reputation, and will any unintended implications involve professional cost? Does your employer prohibit or discourage involvement with this group?
Benefits	What's in it for you? Will you obtain any profit, professional advantage, or membership benefits? Do you value the social benefit of association? Are you willing to be involved for altruistic intentions? Are you willing to be involved if the benefits go to others, for example, an underrepresented population, the environment, or a cause beyond your immediate life?

noted, "They're stake-holders when they're with you, and they're interest groups when they're against you" (Espo, 2009, paragraph 8). Or perhaps the best advice is to intentionally discern our own involvement, know the rules of the game, and use interest group power to further the causes we treasure.

DISCUSSION QUESTIONS

1. In what ways is, or is not, the nursing profession a special interest group in American democracy?
2. What strategies would enhance the effective influence of nurses as a collective special interest group in policy advocacy and electoral politics?
3. What role does the nonpartisan stance of nursing PACs play in the broad engagement of nurses in electoral politics and policy advocacy?

REFERENCES

American Nurses Association [ANA]. (2010). ANA policy & provisions of health reform law. Retrieved from *www.nursingworld.org/MainMenu Categories/Policy-Advocacy/HealthSystemReform/Policy-and-Health -Reform-Law.pdf.*

American Nurses Association [ANA]. (2013a). ANA-PAC. Retrieved from *www.nursingworld.org/anapac.*

American Nurses Association [ANA]. (2013b). Policy & advocacy: Health care reform. Retrieved from *www.nursingworld.org/MainMenuCategories/ Policy-Advocacy/HealthSystemReform.*

Anderson, J. E. (2011). *Public policymaking: An introduction* (7th ed.). Boston: Wadsworth.

Apolionio, D. E., & Bero, L. A. (2007). The creation of industry front groups: The tobacco industry and "Get Government Off Our Back". *American Journal of Public Health, 97*(3), 419–427.

Bergan, D. E. (2009). Does grassroots lobbying work? A field experiment measuring the effects of an e-mail lobbying campaign on legislative behavior. *American Politics Research, 37*(2), 327–352.

Brown Foundation for Educational Equity, Excellence and Research. (2012). *Brown v. Board of Education*: Background, overview and summary. Retrieved from *brownvboard.org/content/background-overview -summary.*

Center for Responsive Politics. (2012). Health professionals: Long term contribution trends. Retrieved from *www.opensecrets.org/industries/totals .php?cycle=2012&ind=H01.*

Center for Responsive Politics. (2013a). Influence and lobbying: Lobbying database. Retrieved from *www.opensecrets.org/lobbyists/index.php.*

Center for Responsive Politics. (2013b). Lobbying: Top spenders. Retrieved from *www.opensecrets.org/lobby/top.php?indexType=s&show Year=2013.*

Center for Responsive Politics. (2013c). Influence and lobbying: Health. Retrieved from *www.opensecrets.org/industries/indus.php?ind=H.*

Center for Responsive Politics. (2013d). PACs: American Nurses Association. Retrieved from *www.opensecrets.org/pacs/lookup2.php?strID=C00017 525.&cycle=2012.*

Center for Responsive Politics. (2013e). PACs: American Association of Nurse Anesthetists. Retrieved from *www.opensecrets.org/pacs/lookup2 .php?strID=C00173153&cycle=2014.*

Center for Science in the Public Interest [CSPI]. (2012). Mission. Retrieved from *www.cspinet.org/about/mission.html.*

Clemmitt, M. (2012). Assessing the new health care law. *CQ Researcher, 22*(33), Retrieved from *library.cqpress.com/cqresearcher/document.php? id=cqresrre2012092100#.UkXBpz_ZWSo.*

Espo, D. (2009, August 19). "Special interests" on both sides in health fight. Associated Press. Retrieved from *www.newsday.com/special-interests -on-both-sides-in-health-fight-1.1380068.*

Essential Information. (2013). Essential action. Retrieved from *www .essentialinformation.org/about.html.*

Federal Election Commission. (2013a). Bipartisan campaign reform act. Retrieved from *www.fec.gov/pages/bcra/bcra_update.shtml.*

Federal Election Commission. (2013b). Contribution limits for (2013–2014). Retrieved from *www.fec.gov/ans/answers_general.shtml.*

Fiorina, M. P., Peterson, P. E., Johnson, B., & Mayer, W. G. (2009). *The new American democracy* (6th ed.). San Francisco: Pearson.

Madison, J. (1787, November 22). The Federalist No. 10: The utility of the union as a safeguard against domestic faction and insurrection. Retrieved from *constitution.org/fed/federa10.htm.*

Nownes, A. J. (2013). Interest groups in American politics: Pressure and power. New York: Routledge.

Peters, J. W. (2013, July 6). Conservatives' aggressive ad campaign seeks to cast doubt on health law. *New York Times*, Retrieved from *www .nytimes.com/2013/07/07/us/politics/conservatives-aggressive-ad -campaign-seeks-to-cast-doubt-on-health-law.html.*

Pittsburgh Post-Gazette. (2008, December 17). Road to reform: Daschle is well positioned to revamp health care [Editorial]. *Pittsburgh Post-Gazette*, Retrieved from *www.post-gazette.com/pg/08352/935535-192 .stm#ixzz OOz09rLM1.*

Quadagno, J. (2005). *One nation uninsured: Why the U.S. has no national health insurance.* New York: Oxford University Press.

Rauch, J. (1994). *Demosclerosis: The silent killer of American government.* New York: Random House.

Schattschneider, E. E. (1960/2005). The scope and bias of the pressure system. In G. M. Scott (Ed.), *Choices: An American government reader* (pp. 276–280). Boston: Pearson. (Reprinted from *The semisovereign people: A realist's view of democracy in America*, by E.E. Schattschneider, 1960, Austin, TX: Holt, Rinehart & Winston.).

Source Watch. (2009). Center for Consumer Freedom. Retrieved from *www .sourcewatch.org/index.php?title=Center_for_Consumer_Freedom.*

de Tocqueville, A. (1835/2010). *Democracy in America.* New York: Penguin Group.

U.S. Public Interest Research Groups. (2013). Mission statement. Retrieved from *www.uspirg.org/page/usp/about-us.*

Warner, J. R. (2002). Campaign management: Policy's primary prevention strategy. In D. J. Mason, J. K. Leavitt, & M. W. Chaffee (Eds.), *Policy & politics in nursing and health care* (4th ed., pp. 579–583). Philadelphia: W.B. Saunders.

Wolpe, B. C. (1990). *Lobbying Congress: How the system works.* Washington, DC: Congressional Quarterly.

ONLINE RESOURCES

Center for Responsive Politics
www.opensecrets.org

The Federalist Papers 10: The Utility of the Union as a Safeguard Against Domestic Faction and Insurrection (by James Madison)
constitution.org/fed/federa10.htm

UNIT 5

CHAPTER 73

Current Issues in Nursing Associations

Glenda Christiaens

"Associations are the hidden glue of our society and economy. Like the mortar that holds the bricks of a building in place, associations go largely unnoticed, yet they do much to hold the entire structure together."

Jim Collins

Associations are groups of people who have joined together to pursue a common purpose or goal. For registered nurses, the common purposes and goals can be summed up in the acronym CARE, representing Clinical practice, Advocacy, Research, and Education. Several associations have been established to create policies to promote the categories of CARE, such as evidence-based practice protocols, adequate compensation, hours of work that are safe for patient care and nurse well-being, practice according to educational preparation, engagement in lifelong learning, and research and professional development, among others. In addition, nursing specialty and subspecialty organizations create policies and education programs that promote their particular nursing domain. The work of professional nursing associations has the potential to benefit all nurses without regard to their membership in those organizations.

There are more than over 100 nursing organizations representing 3.1 million RNs licensed to practice in the United States (American Nurses Association [ANA], 2013a). Nurses have a wide choice of organizations to join, including a general organization such as the American Nurses Association (ANA), a specialty organization such as the American Psychiatric Nurses Association, or their own state nurses' association. Although each organization represents nurses, in fact only a small percentage of nurses belong to a nursing organization. Therefore, nurses are being represented by a wide variety of nursing associations even though they may not be familiar with those associations' policies or platforms.

NURSING'S PROFESSIONAL ORGANIZATIONS

Professional nurses are concerned about advocacy in three main areas: practice, research, and education. The interests of the nursing profession regarding leadership in these three areas are represented by the four autonomous nursing organizations that make up the Tri-Council for Nursing: the National League for Nursing (NLN), the American Association of Colleges of Nursing (AACN), the American Organization of Nurse Executives (AONE), and the American Nurses Association (ANA). Although not a decision-making body, the Tri-Council for Nursing comes together regularly "for the purpose of dialog and consensus-building, to provide stewardship within the profession of nursing" (Tri-Council for Nursing, 2013). When nursing organizations collaborate in this manner there is less potential for confusion by the public and legislators about exactly what the nursing profession represents. The Tri-Council concept is a step forward in unifying the voice of nursing. Unfortunately however, less than 10% of nurses are members of these organizations, a fact that weakens the position and credibility of the Tri-Council.

Two organizations in the Tri-Council for Nursing represent nursing education. The AACN is "the national voice for baccalaureate and graduate nursing education" (AACN, 2013). Its membership is made up of 725 schools of nursing. The NLN, with 33,000 individual and 1200 institutional members, is dedicated to excellence in all types of nursing education including associate degree and licensed practical nurse education (NLN, 2013).

The American Organization of Nurse Executives provides "leadership, professional development, advocacy, and research to advance nursing practice and patient care, promote nursing leadership excellence, and shape public policy for health care nationwide" (AONE, 2013). The organization focuses on the advancement of nursing leadership and has approximately 9000 members.

The American Nurses Association "advances the nursing profession by fostering high standards of nursing practice, promoting the rights of nurses in the workplace, projecting a positive and realistic view of nursing, and by lobbying the Congress and regulatory agencies on health care issues affecting nurses and the public" (ANA, 2013b). Individual registered nurses (RNs) are encouraged to join the ANA through their state nurses' associations. In response to the needs of members who cannot participate in their state organizations, ANA also offers ANA Only memberships.

Established in 1911, the American Nurses Association has generally been known as the organization that represents the profession across all education, practice, and demographic spectrums. However, more than 100 nursing specialty and subspecialty organizations have formed over the years. As with the ANA, many of these organizations engage in the following activities:

- Establishing standards of practice
- Creating specialty certification programs
- Offering continuing nursing education opportunities
- Educating nurses and the public
- Publishing professional journals
- Promoting nursing research
- Lobbying lawmakers and regulators on matters of public policy

See Box 73-1 for a list of all national nursing organizations. This list does not include the many international and state nursing associations.

Nursing organizations compete with each other for nurses' time, talent, and dues. There is often rivalry among organizations as to who will represent the profession in the halls of Congress, before state legislatures, or in the media. Because of this fractionation and dilution, nursing's voice is not being heard in public debates regarding access, cost, and quality of health care. As the largest group of health care providers and the most trusted profession, nurses in fact should be leading these discussions. Instead, other groups such as the American Medical Association, pharmaceutical companies, and insurance companies have been established by the public media as experts, thought leaders, change agents, and primary stakeholders in health care issues. Nurses and nursing organizations are generally absent in major media stories or serve to provide interesting background information only (Buresch & Gordon, 2013).

Individual nurses find it challenging to choose exactly which nursing organization is right for them. For example, if you are a nurse educator who teaches community health nursing and holistic nursing, which organization should you join? In addition to the ANA and your state nursing organization, you may want to join the NLN, which specifically represents nurse educators, or the American Holistic Nurses Association, the Association of Community Health Nursing Educators, the American Public Health Association, or the National School Nurses Association, along with a supporting membership in the National Student Nurses Association. It is easy to see how diluted the nursing profession's voice can be with so many organizations competing for membership. Florida alone has more than 27 nursing organizations. If nursing came together in one organization with one voice, the result would be a powerful force to influence the well-being and health of the profession and the nation.

The inability of the nursing profession to speak with one voice is an age-old predicament. The fragmentation stems from the many levels of education available such as an associate's degree, bachelor's degree, master's degree, doctor of nursing practice, or a PhD. In addition to several educational levels, nursing licenses may be classified as LVN, LPN, RN, or CNS as well as an assortment across the 50 states of advanced practice licensure requirements. This

BOX 73-1 Alliance Member Organizations

- Academy of Medical-Surgical Nurses
- Academy of Neonatal Nursing, LLC
- Air & Surface Transport Nurses Association
- American Academy of Ambulatory Care Nursing
- American Academy of Nurse Practitioners
- American Association of Colleges of Nursing
- American Association of Critical-Care Nurses
- American Association of Heart Failure Nurses
- American Association of Legal Nurse Consultants
- American Association of Neuroscience Nurses
- American Association of Nurse Anesthetists
- American Association of Occupational Health Nurses
- American College of Nurse Practitioners
- American Holistic Nurses' Association
- American Medical Informatics Association
- American Nephrology Nurses' Association
- American Nurses Association
- American Organization of Nurse Executives
- American Pediatric Surgical Nurses Association
- American Psychiatric Nurses Association
- American Society for Pain Management Nursing
- American Society of PeriAnesthesia Nurses
- American Society of Plastic Surgical Nurses
- Association for Radiologic and Imaging Nursing
- Association of Black Nursing Faculty, Inc.
- Association of Nurses in AIDS Care
- Association of Pediatric Hematology/Oncology Nurses (APHON)
- Association of periOperative Registered Nurses
- Association of Rehabilitation Nurses
- Association of Women's Health, Obstetric and Neonatal Nurses

- Commission on Graduates of Foreign Nursing Schools
- Dermatology Nurses' Association
- Developmental Disabilities Nurses Association
- Emergency Nurses Association
- Hospice and Palliative Nurses Association
- Infusion Nurses Society
- International Association of Forensic Nurses
- International Nurses Society on Addictions
- NATCO, The Organization for Transplant Professionals
- National Association of Neonatal Nurses
- National Association of Nurse Massage Therapists
- National Association of Orthopedic Nurses
- National Association of Pediatric Nurse Practitioners
- National Association of School Nurses
- National Council of State Boards of Nursing
- National Gerontological Nursing Association
- National League for Nursing
- National Nursing Staff Development Organization
- National Student Nurses' Association, Inc.
- Nutrition Support Nurses Practice Section of A.S.P.E.N.
- Oncology Nursing Society
- Pediatric Endocrinology Nursing Society
- Preventative Cardiovascular Nurses Association
- Rheumatology Nurses Society
- Sigma Theta Tau, International: Honor Society of Nursing
- Society of Gastroenterology Nurses and Associates, Inc.
- Society of Otorhinolaryngology and Head-Neck Nurses
- Society of Pediatric Nurses
- Society of Trauma Nurses
- Society of Urologic Nurses and Associates
- Wound Ostomy & Continence Nurses Society

Source: *www.nursing-alliance.org/content.cfm/id/members.*

large variance in education and licensing is reflected in the wide variety of nursing organizations to choose from, resulting in the lack of a cohesive and articulate nursing voice.

ORGANIZATIONAL LIFE CYCLE

Historically, organizations form around a particular issue. Some are formalized with bylaws, officers, dues, and staff, such as the National Nursing Staff Development Organization (NNSDO). Others, such as the International Academy of Nursing

Editors (INANE), convene but have no formal structure. Some organizations have dissolved over the years, such as the National Association of Colored Graduate Nurses, and others have been established, such as the National Black Nurses Association. If history is any guide, organizations will continue to be formed. Some will grow and prosper; others will languish, die, or refuse to die. As the nature of nursing practice and health care policy changes, so will its organizations.

Professional associations have a natural life cycle. According to Simon (2001), organizations travel through 5 stages of development. The first stage is visionary, when a motivated leader identifies a need and imagines an organization that could meet that need. The second stage is the start-up, when the organization is formally founded and operates with very little income and generally no paid staff. The third stage, also called the adolescent phase, is characterized by growth. The fourth or mature stage brings a focus on sustainability and relevance. This stage may last as long as 30 years (Speakman Management Consulting, 2013).

The fifth stage of professional association development is characterized by stagnation and renewal. It is here that nursing organizations may find themselves mired in an outdated structure, with programs that no longer fit the needs of members or the nursing profession and where interest, relevance, and volunteerism may be waning. There may be considerable internal conflict regarding the direction the organization is headed, further delaying progress. Strategic plans may be based on the nursing profession of the past, with many founding members feeling disaffected and alienated from the new leadership. Without change, the organization is headed for closure, which may be preceded by loss of credibility, negative press, and insufficient funding.

Familiarity with the natural lifespan of organizations is important in the wide arena of nursing professional organizations. Many nursing organizations were founded when nursing was a very different profession than it is today, with its emphasis on access to health care technology and evidence-based practice and research. Nursing can make a difference in quality of care and patient advocacy, but with so many organizations hanging on to old ways nurses are becoming less relevant in the health care discourse. It would serve the profession if organizations would align, uniting in a strong voice that truly represents the interests of nursing and public health. It is time for nursing organizations to honor the natural organizational life cycle and create something different, relevant, and powerful.

CURRENT ISSUES FOR NURSING ORGANIZATIONS

Although continuing to work on behalf of the profession, nursing associations are confronting issues such as shrinking resources, high member expectations, increasing competition for members' time from other groups, integration of cultures and generations, and rapid technological change. The issues can be broadly characterized as challenges in membership, advocacy, and leadership.

MEMBERSHIP

In their landmark book *Race for Relevance* (2011), authors Coerver and Byers outline the most common reasons people do not join professional organizations, including time, value expectations, technology, and generational differences. Many nurses are busy balancing work and family life. They just don't have the time to be involved in a professional organization unless they can gain a deep appreciation of the value of membership. Younger generations appeal to the Internet and hand-held devices for their information, entertainment, and sense of community. Each generation becomes less attracted to organizations that are still doing business based on face-to-face, hard copy models. Formidable competitors, including not-for-profit and for-profit groups that provide easy-to-access goods and services traditionally provided by professional organizations, increase the competition for membership. Organizations that do not use the latest technology are not appealing to upcoming generations and are unable to be nimble and up-to-date with the services they provide to members.

Nursing organizations are responding to today's challenges in a variety of ways. To increase productivity and efficiency, the ANA decreased the size of their board of directors in 2014 and changed from the cumbersome House of Delegates model to the Membership Assembly model (ANA, 2013b). Most organizations have websites that deliver information, continuing education, networking opportunities, resources, and online access to publications. Many offer webinars and podcasts in place of in-person conferences or hard copy guidebooks. To appeal to members who want to connect on their computers or hand-held devices, most organizations use social media outlets such as Facebook, Twitter, LinkedIn, and YouTube. In addition, the Internet brings members together instantaneously for opinion sharing and to vote on issues. Still, member participation is low. For example, a recent survey of 239 non-profit nursing and non-nursing associations found that voter turnout for association elections averaged just 20% to 26% for organizations with 500-10,000 members. Only 21% of the associations surveyed said they met the voter turnout goals they had established (Votenet, 2012).

Membership retention is another issue facing nursing organizations. A recent survey by Marketing General, Inc. (2013) revealed that the average renewal rate for individual nursing and non-nursing membership associations is 81%. Of 751 association representatives responding, the top reasons for non-renewal were company budget cuts, lack of engagement, and lack of significant return on investment of membership costs.

Although nursing organizations have worked hard to diversify membership across racial, ethnic, and gender lines with modest success, generational issues are now a central issue. Baby boomers (born between the mid-1940s and 1960s) and their parents, the silent generation (born between the mid-1930s and 1940s), have been loyal association supporters. Generation X (born between the mid-1960s and 1970s) has not joined associations in significant numbers. Generation Y (those born between the late 1970s and late 1990s) is perceived to be more involved and connected to others not only through the Internet but through the community volunteer experience required during their secondary education. The challenge is to get young people to join and older people to remain (Shinn, 2009). Interestingly, when asked about their biggest challenge to growth of membership, association representatives reported that membership was so diverse that they had trouble meeting the needs of the different segments. They also had difficulty attracting and/or maintaining younger members (Marketing General Inc., 2013).

Volunteering rates among Americans have increased dramatically in recent years, with 64.3 million Americans volunteering in formal organizations during 2011 (Corporation for National and Community Service, 2012). This may bode well for associations in the future, although current and future generations will want to make a meaningful contribution when volunteering their time. They to make a difference in their lives and the lives of others. Likewise, work-life balance has become a mantra for Generation Y, and association involvement is viewed as work. Volunteers are the lifeblood of organizations and provide countless hours in advancing the organizational mission.

According to Marketing General's (2013) report on association marketing, networking, access to specialized and current information, advocacy, and learning best practices in their profession are the top reasons people join and rejoin professional associations. The challenge for nursing associations is to give their members opportunities to network and access information in user friendly ways that are mindful of differences in age and culture, along with giving members a sufficient return on their investment of time and money.

ADVOCACY

Nursing organizations are concerned with causes or interests that advance their mission and promote and protect the health of the public. Advocacy includes activities such as:

- Developing and advancing public policy positions
- Creating political action committees
- Appearing before federal, state, and local agencies and courts of law
- Collaborating with other groups on matters of mutual concern
- Setting standards of practice
- Establishing a code of ethics
- Establishing credentialing mechanisms
- Working for the recognition and advancement of the profession
- Collectively bargaining

The work of advocacy is time-consuming, expensive, and resource-intensive. Often supported by member dues and contributions, advocacy efforts are threatened when membership or other sources of revenue decline. Although there are many national nursing organizations that lobby Congress, there are few at the state and local levels. The result is that other stronger groups have more influence. Physician groups, pharmaceutical organizations, hospital associations, and other provider groups can be counted on to fill any vacuum created by the lack of a strong voice for nursing.

One of the most controversial advocacy activities in the profession has been collective bargaining. Although some nurses have valued representation in the employment setting, others have found it foreign, labeling it unprofessional. Some nurses felt that the United American Nurses, the ANA's collective bargaining arm, was taking valuable resources away from more important areas of concern to all nurses. In 2008 the state nurses' associations of Montana, New Jersey, New York, Ohio, Oregon, and Washington came together to form the National Federation of Nurses labor union (National Federation of Nurses [NFN], 2013). In 2009, after a great deal of debate, United American Nurses merged with the California Nurses Association/National Nurses Organizing Committee and the Massachusetts Nurses Association to form National Nurses United (NNU), an AFL-CIO union. With 185,000 members NNU is currently the largest union and professional association of RNs in the United States (National Nurses United [NNU], 2013). The Service Employees International Union (SEIU) is another option for nurses, representing 1.1 million health care workers including but not limited to nurses (Service Employees International Union [SIEU], 2013). There are also many smaller, local unions nurses can join around the country. In 2012, nearly 20% of the 3.1 million RNs in the nation were represented by labor unions (Hirsch & Macpherson, 2013).

In response to nursing organizations' desire to have stronger voices in the ANA advocacy and policymaking process, in 2010, the ANA established the Organizational Affiliate program. Organizational representatives now have a voice and can vote on issues considered at the ANA annual Membership Assembly meeting. Organizational Affiliates, however, cannot vote in ANA elections or bylaws. More than 30 associations have joined the Organizational Affiliate program. Working together, the ANA and these organizations share information and collaborate in exploring solutions to issues that face the nursing profession, regardless of specialty (ANA, 2013b). For a list of ANA Affiliate Organizations, refer to the Online Resources section.

With so many nursing organizations advocating for important health and professional issues, it is remarkable how nursing has been generally unable to capture public media attention on a large scale. Organizations make statements about issues but do not put enough effort and funding into aggressive, effective lobbying efforts. Nursing organizations are good at identifying issues but have not been successful in leading or guiding public opinion or being recognized as health care leaders.

Because organizations are concerned with membership retention, they focus on internal communications such as publishing newsletters and journals and on advertising conferences. Their main audience is comprised of current and prospective association members who are usually nurses. Consistent outreach to the non-nursing public on pressing health care and nursing issues is missing, however (Buresch & Gordon, 2013). For nursing to gain relevancy and a strong voice in public debate, it is essential for organizations to turn their focus toward external communications including press releases, white papers, lobbying, and other ways to be heard and valued in the general media. They must urge their members to be involved in local and national politics regarding such issues as patient safety, safe workplace environments, and health care reform.

LEADERSHIP

Leaders may be elected or appointed to office and come from diverse practice, educational, experiential, and demographic backgrounds specific to a nursing specialty. Coerver and Byers (2011) refer to three reasons people will want to serve on a board of directors. The first is altruism, the unselfish desire to serve the organization for the good of the profession. The second is self-interest, the desire for personal or professional gain. The third reason is ego, or the opportunity to look good and enhance the resume. Although board members are motivated by all three factors, the more they are motivated by altruism, the better director they will be.

Motivation to serve is only one factor in making a good director. Experience and competency in leadership and governance are imperative. This creates a dilemma for nomination committees.

Although many volunteers are experts in nursing, they may not have experience in leadership or board membership. Many leaders are elected to office without any experience with leadership and lacking an understanding of association governance. With limited resources and few members desiring leadership positions, nursing associations have faced a challenge implementing the IOM recommendation that "nursing associations should provide leadership development, mentoring programs, and opportunities to lead for all their members" (Institute of Medicine [IOM], 2010).

A major issue in organizational leadership is succession planning, which is the identification, development, and engagement of future leaders. Younger nurses often work full-time and are unable to donate the large amount of time that board membership entails. Many boards appeal to retired nurses who are not currently practicing. However, as retirement ages continue to creep upward, it may be increasingly difficult to find leaders who have the time it takes to offer quality service to an organization. It is only recently that associations have paid attention to talent management, as volunteers are in short supply because of work demands, family commitments, and economic constraints. The answer may lie in putting board members on the payroll, although few organizations can afford this.

Many groups report the recycling of leaders, particularly at the local organizational level. Incumbents are often unopposed in elections and some board positions go unfilled caused by lack of candidates. In addition, those who aspire to leadership roles often report that there are social issue-related groups that are more worthy of the investment of time and energy. The lack of qualified, enthusiastic candidates causes a lack of diversity and forward thinking on boards that are populated by the same leaders year after year. With the onslaught of new information and new technology, it is imperative that nursing associations draw younger, technology savvy leaders with business skills and experience but without alienating long-term leaders and members. On the other hand, if associations are having trouble recruiting new leaders, it may be time to think about dissolving the organization and joining with another association with a similar mission.

Many associations that lack resources to orient and train incoming board members take advantage of the Nursing Alliance Leadership Academy (NALA), offered annually by the Nursing Organizations Alliance. NALA is an intensive program providing volunteer leadership education to officers, executive staff, and board members of nursing associations (Nursing Organizations Alliance [NOA], 2013). NOA also trains nurse leaders how to approach legislators through their annual Nurses in Washington Internship. Although NOA's programs provide a sound foundation to volunteer leaders, it is imperative that ongoing board development take place. Development plans often entail hiring expert consultants or purchasing training programs and can be cost prohibitive to some organizations.

Associations look to committee service as a way to groom future leaders. If people get burned out on the committee level, however, they are less likely to run for a board office. Some organizations are experimenting with virtual (online) volunteering to populate leadership ladders. Micro volunteering is also becoming popular, permitting people to do small jobs without making a long-term time commitment. Associations are also bringing people together for more time-limited, specific tasks. For example, the ANA eliminated the time-intensive Congress on Nursing Education and Practice, which required a 2-year time commitment from its members, replacing it with a Professional Issues Panels, where members can contribute meaningfully.

Organizations with a compelling purpose and those engaged in meaningful work have no shortage of volunteer leaders. Nursing organizations have to determine what these future leaders have a passion for and then determine how to match the jobs that need to be done to the interests of those in their ranks. It is time for nursing organizations to be creative and to encourage nurses to be invested in the association experience and motivated to lead.

CONCLUSION

The issues in contemporary organizations are complex and daunting. As the world becomes more technological and diverse, groups will be confronted with more and more challenges, especially in the areas of membership, advocacy, and leadership. Nurses are simply not joining organizations. Advocacy is expensive and time-consuming. Leaders are difficult to identify, train, and retain. The traditional association model is becoming less appealing and relevant to today's nurses who are working to balance personal and professional life while keeping their nursing skills and knowledge up to date.

More than 100 nursing organizations are competing for members and funding, resulting in fractionation and a dilution of nursing's voice on issues of health care access, cost, and quality. It is unclear who really speaks for nursing and no one group emerges as the single, strong, authoritative voice; a cacophony of disparate voices does the profession no good. It allows those outside the profession to fill the void by speaking for nursing. It dilutes the policy initiatives the profession undertakes on behalf of its members and the people for whom it cares. It is hoped that nursing associations will begin to address these problems in a way that unites and strengthens the profession and enables nursing to have a premier place in influencing health care.

DISCUSSION QUESTIONS

1. In what ways do nurses benefit from the work of professional organizations?
2. How do nursing associations work to promote policies that are patient-centered and lead the profession forward?
3. In what ways do nursing organizations compete with other organizations to maintain membership, generate and increase participation, and attract volunteers?
4. How can nursing organizations more effectively advocate for public policy?

REFERENCES

American Association of Colleges of Nursing [AACN]. (2013). About AACN. Retrieved from *www.aacn.nche.edu/about-aacn.*

American Nurses Association [ANA]. (2013a). Nursing by the numbers fact sheet. Retrieved from *nursingworld.org/nursingbythenumbersfactsheet.aspx.*

American Nurses Association [ANA]. (2013b). ANA 2012 annual report. Retrieved from *nursingworld.org/FunctionalMenuCategories/AboutANA/2012-AnnualReport.pdf.*

American Organization of Nurse Executives. (2013). About AONE. Retrieved from *www.aone.org/membership/about/welcome.shtml.*

Buresch, B., & Gordon, S. (2013). *From silence to voice: What nurses know and must communicate to the public* (3rd ed.). Ithaca, NY: ILR Press.

Coerver, H., & Byers, M. (2011). *Race for relevance: 5 radical changes for associations.* Washington, DC: ASAE.

Corporation for National and Community Service. (2012). Volunteering and civic life in America 2012. Retrieved from *www.volunteeringinamerica.gov/assets/resources/FactSheetFinal.pdf.*

Hirsch, B., & Macpherson, D. (2013). Union membership and coverage database from the CPS table V. occupation: Union membership, coverage, density, and employment by occupation, 1983-2012. Retrieved from *www.unionstats.com.*

Institute of Medicine [IOM]. (2010). Initiative on the future of nursing. Retrieved from *www.thefutureofnursing.org/about.*

Marketing General, Inc. (2013). 2013 Membership marketing benchmarking report. Retrieved from *www.marketinggeneral.com/resources/benchmark-report/.*

National Federation of Nurses [NFN]. (2013). Frequently asked questions. Retrieved from *www.nfn.org/about/faq.*

National League for Nursing [NLN]. (2013). About the NLN. Retrieved from *www.nln.org/aboutnln/index.htm.*

National Nurses United [NNU]. (2013). About us. Retrieved from *www.nationalnursesunited.org/pages/19.*

Nursing Organizations Alliance [NOA]. (2013). Nursing alliance leadership academy. Retrieved from *www.nursing-alliance.org/content.cfm/id/nala#objective.*

Service Employees International Union [SEIU]. (2013). SEIU healthcare. Retrieved from *www.seiu.org/seiuhealthcare/.*

Shinn, L. (2009). American Nephrology Nurses Association trends and considerations: Planning for the future: A report. Unpublished report.

Simon, J. S. (2001). *The five life stages of nonprofit organizations: Where you are, where you're going, and what to expect when you get there.* St. Paul, MN: Amherst H. Wilder Foundation.

Speakman Management Consulting. (2013). Nonprofit organizational life cycle. Retrieved from *www.speakmanconsulting.com/pdf_files/NonProfitLifeCyclesMatrix.pdf.*

Tri-Council for Nursing. (2013). Welcome. Retrieved from *http://tricouncilfornursing.org/.*

Votenet (2012). 2012 Votenet index of association and nonprofit voting and election trends. Retrieved from *www.votenet.com/whitepaper/2012-Index-of-Association-and-Non-Profit-Voting-and-Elections.pdf.*

ONLINE RESOURCES

American Association of Colleges of Nursing
www.aacn.nche.edu
American Nurses Association
www.nursingworld.org
American Organization of Nurse Executives
www.AONE.org
ANA Organizational Affiliates
nursingworld.org/FunctionalMenuCategories/AboutANA/WhoWeAre/AffiliatedOrganizations
National League for Nursing
www.nln.org
Nursing Organizations Alliance
www.nursing-alliance.org
Nursing Organization Links
www.nurse.org/orgs.shtml

CHAPTER 74

Professional Nursing Associations: Operationalizing Nursing Values

Pamela J. Haylock

"The profession of nursing, as represented by associations and their members, is responsible for articulating nursing values, for maintaining the integrity of the profession and its practice, and for shaping social policy."
Code of Ethics for Nurses with Interpretive Statements, Provision 9 (2001)

The tendency to form associations for common action characterizes American culture, something noted nearly 2 centuries ago by Alexis de Tocqueville during his 10-month stay in America (de Tocqueville, 1835/2000). Nursing associations facilitate and accomplish the work of the profession. Today, there are more than 120 nursing specialty associations in the United States (American Journal of Nursing, 2012). Other associations have international and multidisciplinary membership, and still more represent ethnic groups, specialties, and specific interests of nurses.

This chapter presents an overview of professional nursing associations, their critical roles in leadership development of members, and use of collective professional voices to shape policy, advocating for nursing and consumers of health care.

THE SIGNIFICANCE OF NURSING ORGANIZATIONS

Professional organizations and associations in nursing are critical for generating the energy, flow of ideas, and proactive work needed to maintain a healthy profession that advocates for the needs of its clients and nurses, and the trust of society (Matthews, 2012). Members can engage in discussions and advance solutions for issues of quality, access, and costs of care. In addition to advancing nursing

knowledge and clinical competencies, professional organizations build nurses' leadership skills and promote the advocacy component of nurse practice by (Schroeder, 2013):

- Providing networking and collaboration opportunities
- Facilitating discussion forums on issues
- Lending a collective voice to legislative and policy initiatives
- Providing leadership development opportunities

Active, engaged members feel more connected to the profession and tend to have broader perspectives beyond a particular community or practice setting (Cardillo, 2013). Personal and professional development occurs through volunteer activities, mentoring by more experienced members, and holding elected office. An association's publications, e-mail, and social media help members to be informed about clinical, employment, regulatory, and political issues affecting practice. Most importantly, professional associations allow nurses to speak in one voice, finding common ground and developing common messages, visions, and missions, reducing the fragmentation that hampers nurses' efficacy in shaping policy.

In 2010, the Institute of Medicine released the report *The Future of Nursing: Leading Change, Advancing Health* (Institute of Medicine [IOM], 2011). An underlying principle of the initiative is that "accessible, high-quality care cannot be achieved without exceptional nursing care." The report notes that realizing full economic value of nurses' contributions across health care settings can enable nurses to help bridge the gap between coverage and access, coordinate complex care, and meet the need for primary care. Four key messages structure the report's recommendations:

- Nurses should practice to the full extent of their education and training.
- Nurses should achieve higher levels of education and training through an improved education system.
- Nurses should be full partners, with physicians and other health professionals, in redesigning health care in the United States.
- Effective workforce planning and policymaking require better data collection and an improved information infrastructure.

The Future of Nursing Campaign for Action, an initiative of AARP (formerly the American Association of Retired Persons), the AARP Foundation, and the Robert Wood Johnson Foundation (RWJF), is rooted in pillars to drive and measure change (Campaign for Action, n.d.):

- Advancing education transformation
- Leveraging nursing leadership
- Removing barriers to practice and care
- Fostering interprofessional collaboration
- Promoting diversity
- Bolstering workforce data

There is uncertainty surrounding the profession's abilities to overcome major obstacles that prevent nurses from optimizing their impact in health policy. A Gallup poll of more than 1500 acknowledged national opinion leaders found that, although nurses were identified as the health professionals who should have greater influence in the areas of patient care quality and safety, major obstacles prevent such influence from becoming reality (RWJF, 2010). A crucial obstacle to maximizing nursing's influence is the fragmentation in the leadership of organized nursing (IOM, 2011). This dismal prophecy begs the question: How can nurses become full partners in America's health care redesign? The *Future of Nursing* report calls for nurses to assume leadership roles, provide mentorship for the next generations of nurses, and participate in policymaking processes (IOM, 2011). The IOM report has brought about significant unification among national nursing organizations around a policy agenda. Professional organizations offer nurses opportunities to be part of the answer to questions about promotion of health and well-being and providing safe and quality care to the diverse population of the United States.

EVOLUTION OF ORGANIZATIONS

Nursing organizations emerged as nursing became a social force. The first nursing organization, the Royal British Nurses' Association, was founded in 1887. In North America, nursing groups initially appeared as alumnae associations focused on nursing schools and alumnae groups. The need for a broader focus became apparent along with the recognition of the importance of nursing influence (Dolan, Fitzpatrick, & Herrmann, 1983). A meeting of superintendents of nurse training schools during the 1893 Chicago World's Fair resulted in the formation of the American Society of Superintendents of Training Schools (ASSTS). The ASSTS became the National League of Nursing Education and, later, the National League for Nursing. In 1896, 10 alumnae associations merged to become the Nurses' Associated Alumnae of the United States and Canada. The group's name changed in 1899 to the Nurses' Associated Alumnae (NAA) of the United States. The American Nurses Association (ANA) was formed in 1911 as the successor to the NAA. State nurses' associations were organized in 1901 to enhance nurses' influence in state legislative initiatives for the registration of nurses and to control nursing practice, including improving employment conditions, limiting duty hours, and advocating hospital employment of greater numbers of graduate nurses (Reverby, 1987).

The International Council of Nurses (ICN), founded in 1899, is the oldest international association of professional women (ICN, n.d.). The underlying philosophy of the ICN acknowledges nurses' four fundamental responsibilities: to promote health, to prevent illness, to restore health, and to alleviate suffering. Today, the ICN is a federation of more than 130 national nurses associations (NNAs) representing the world's 16 million nurses.

TODAY'S NURSE

Most nursing organizations are voluntary membership associations, requiring licensure as registered or vocational (or practical) nurses for access to full member benefits. Other levels of membership (honorary and corporate memberships, for example) are offered by some organizations to

UNIT 5

individuals and entities with expressed interest, commitment, and/or major contributions (financial or otherwise) to the mission of the organization. Elite organizations, exemplified by Sigma Theta Tau International (STTI) and the American Academy of Nursing (AAN) have restrictive member qualifications. Such entities are referred to as professional peak bodies (or peak professional bodies) (Middleton, Walker, & Leigh, 2009).

STTI was founded in 1922; founders chose the name from the Greek words *storgé*, *tharsos*, and *timé*, meaning love, courage, and honor. Its mission is to "support the learning, knowledge and professional development of nurses committed to making a difference in health worldwide" (STTI, n.d.). Membership is by "invitation to baccalaureate and graduate nursing students who demonstrate excellence in scholarship and to nurse leaders exhibiting exceptional achievements in nursing." Today, STTI has some 130,000 active members and 490 chapters in more than 85 countries. STTI supports its mission through products and services in education, leadership, career development, evidence-based nursing, research, and scholarship.

The AAN, affiliated with the ANA, held its inaugural meeting in 1973, welcoming the first 36 charter members, referred to as Fellows. Today, the AAN's more than 2300 Fellows are nursing's most accomplished leaders in education, management, practice, and research (AAN, 2014). Fellows are recognized for extraordinary contributions to nursing and health care, although invitation to the fellowship represents more than recognition of accomplishments: Fellows assume responsibility to contribute time and energies to the Academy and to engage with other leaders in transforming U.S. health care through a focus on health policy.

Nurses have historically been expected to join professional organizations, at least one, if not multiple organizations, as an obligation or duty of a professional (Felton & Van Slyck, 2008). However, this sense of professional obligation has dwindled over the past recent decades (Coerver & Byers, 2011). Organizations must adapt to changing circumstances to remain relevant and attend to potential and existing members' decisions to join. As a reflection of professional realities, the number of specialty nursing organizations continues to increase: today, most of the more than 120 nursing organizations are focused on specialty practice and offer means to get and maintain competencies, get information, find peer networks, and access other products and services that focus on their needs.

The IOM's *The Future of Nursing* contends that:

…nursing organizations must continue to collaborate and work hard to develop common messages, including visions and missions, with regard to their ability to offer evidence-based solutions for improvement in patient care. (IOM, 2011, pp. 239-240)

Establishment of common ground is an essential first step to eliminating fragmentation and maximizing nursing's leadership and influence. When common ground is established, organizations need to activate members and constituents to work together in support of shared goals. Only when confronted with the United States' largest group of health professionals acting in agreement on important issues, speaking with one voice, will policymakers listen and take action.

Quality and safety are practice areas in which nursing organizations can and do find common ground and provide needed leadership. For example, the Nursing Alliance for Quality Care (NAQC), now managed by the ANA, is a partnership of nursing organizations, consumers, and other stakeholders and is a model initiative designed to advance quality, safety, and value of patient-centered care (NAQC, 2013).

ORGANIZATIONAL PURPOSE

The Code of Ethics for Nurses (ANA, 2001) is an explicit statement of the primary goals, values, and obligations of those who enter the profession. Provisions 3 and 6 emphasize expectations of individuals and groups to advocate for social justice and the welfare of the sick, injured, and vulnerable, establishing a foundation for complementary roles of professional associations and association members. Provision 9 specifically articulates the complementary roles of the profession, associations, and individual members, as noted in the quotation that opens this chapter.

Nursing associations contribute to the work of the profession by means typically described in mission statements, bylaws, and charters of committees and other work groups. The existence of so many diverse nursing organizations has advantages and disadvantages for the profession. On one hand, the diversity and large number of organizations suggests that there is an organization to fit most, if not all of nurses' professional needs and interests. Conversely, the large number of diverse organizations creates competition for members, and resources, and, in general, complicates and weakens efforts of the profession to speak with a single and forceful voice.

Mission statements define organizational purpose—the reason to exist (Nanus, 1992). Organizational missions stipulate the "work" of the profession, sharing intentions to advance the profession and practice and enhance health-related outcomes. The ANA mission is "Nurses advancing our profession to improve health for all" (ANA, 2013). The ANA adds a more lengthy "statement of purpose" to claim a role in shaping health policy:

ANA advances the nursing profession by fostering high standards of nursing practice, promoting the economic and general welfare of nurses in the workplace, projecting a positive and realistic view of nursing, and by lobbying the Congress and regulatory agencies on health care issues affecting nurses and the general public. (ANA, 2013)

The mission of the American Organization of Nurse Executives (AONE), a subsidiary of the American Hospital Association, is "to shape the future of health care through innovation and expert nursing leadership" (AONE, 2013). The AAN's mission is to "serve the public and nursing profession by advancing health policy and practice through the generation, synthesis, and dissemination of nursing knowledge" (AAN, n.d.).

ASSOCIATIONS AND THEIR MEMBERS

Nursing associations need members, and nurses need associations. Benefits flow both ways: from the association to its members and from members back to the association. Traditional benefits of organizational involvement blend products and services that define the value of membership, including (Cardillo, 2013; Smith et al., 2008):

- Information and knowledge collection and dissemination
- Personal and professional development
- Chapter benefits (local, regional, and special interest networking and project participation)

Ultimately, products and services created and disseminated under the auspices of professional associations advance advocacy in the care of individuals, families, and populations. Guided by profession- and/or specialty-wide preparation, values, regulations, scope and standards of practice, and competencies, nurses are prepared to speak in one voice and assume advocacy as a fundamental aspect of nursing practice. The second edition of ANA's *Nursing: Scope and Standards of Practice* (ANA, 2010) identifies advocacy priorities, including health care evaluation and restructuring, reimbursement and value of nursing care, funding for nursing education, nursing roles in health and medical homes, and comparative effectiveness.

Benefits attributed to organizational engagement may contribute to career satisfaction among nurses. Societal expectations that nurses provide continual and compassionate care, even in the face of physical and emotional exhaustion, constant exposure to suffering, intense emotional experiences, limited budgets, diminished staffing levels, administrative demands, and workplace communication issues (a few of the challenges nurses face), can undermine career satisfaction among nurses, setting the stage for burnout, compassion stress, and compassion fatigue (Boyle, 2011; Lombardo & Eyre, 2011). Nurses who participate in association conferences or who use association-sponsored networking tools report feeling professionally supported and invigorated as an outcome of these collegial interactions (Sadovich, 2005).

LEADERSHIP DEVELOPMENT

The Future of Nursing (IOM, 2011) recommendations note that strong leadership is imperative for nurses to be full partners in redesigning health care systems. This transformation requires investment

UNIT 5

in nurse leadership development through experience and formal and/or informal education. Nursing organizations provide vital training grounds for personal and professional development, honing communication and writing skills, and enhancing big-picture awareness of nursing, political, and health care environments; in general, opportunities to learn and practice leadership skills (Maryland & Gonzalez, 2012). Table 74-1 lists examples of various nurse leadership training opportunities that have emerged in support of the IOM recommendations, many developed under the auspices of professional nursing associations. In addition to formal leadership training opportunities, associations offer members opportunities to develop and fine-tune critical leadership skills for nurses aspiring to influence within and outside of their professional organizations. Program and project development provides experience in group process, meeting facilitation, consensus building, negotiating, communication, and other essential leadership skills that will be useful throughout a lifetime, within and aside from nursing.

Many associations invest in tangible resources aimed at extending members' leadership skills. The Oncology Nursing Society outlines a leadership development pathway, describing competencies in five domains (personal mastery, vision, knowledge, interpersonal effectiveness, and systems thinking) that equip nurses to understand where and how they need to develop to lead at every level and in a variety of care settings (ONS, 2012).

The ICN identified three pillars crucial to enhancing nursing and health, each requiring an investment in leadership development, and focuses its activities in these areas: professional practice, regulation, and socioeconomic welfare (ICN, 2013). The Leadership for Change and the Global Nursing Leadership Institute (GNLI) projects fall under the professional practice pillar. The annual GNLI is an advanced leadership program for nurses and midwives at senior and executive level positions in developed and developing countries (ICN, 2014). Leadership for Change prepares nurses for leadership roles in nursing and the broader health sectors at country and organizational levels. Leadership in Negotiation, under the socioeconomic

welfare pillar, is operational in Africa, Asia, Caribbean, Latin America, the Middle East, and Russia.

OPPORTUNITIES TO SHAPE POLICY

Most nursing associations have missions that include advocacy around important nursing and health care issues. Often, the board or a legislative committee will set the policy agenda. The most sophisticated and well-resourced organizations have dedicated staff to organize the association's advocacy work, including engaging members to participate in lobby days and use of online tools for communicating with members' state and national policymakers around issues of importance to the association. In this way, local, state, and national organizations can provide a training ground for nurses to learn about policy and politics.

Often members get their first exposure to political advocacy work through participation in a lobby day, in which members go together to the state capitol or Washington, DC, to become oriented to the key policy issues of the association, learn the key messages to share with policymakers, and then meet with their individual representatives in to educate them about the issues and ask for their support. It is not uncommon for participants in lobby days to then volunteer to serve on a legislative or policy committee of the association or to get involved in its political action committee (PAC).

Membership in an organization that promotes interdisciplinary and interorganizational collaboration offers special opportunities to shape policy. Organizations whose members represent multiple disciplines connected to a specialty area, including nurses, physicians, industry, and administrators, expand the context of issues being considered.

Collaboration among the ANA, its affiliates, and specialty nursing associations is a way for nursing to speak with one voice with sufficient volume to achieve greater influence in health policy. In addition, the TriCouncil (ANA, American Association of Colleges of Nursing, the National League for Nursing, and the Organization of Nurse Executives) identifies important policy issues, seeks consensus

TABLE 74-1 Leadership Training Programs for Nursing Students and Nurses (partial list)

Program	Time/Location	Cost	Description	Link
AACN: Graduate Nursing Student Academy	Online	Free to AACN members	Websites and resources to advance leadership development in master's and doctoral degree students	www.aacn.nche.edu/ students/gnsa
AACN: Student Policy Summit	Washington, DC: 3 days	$199 registration fee, scholarships available	Focus on federal policy process and nursing's role in professional advocacy	www.aacn.nche.edu/ government-affairs/ student-policy-summit
NSNA: Leadership U	Online	Free to NSNA members	Provides opportunities for professional growth	www.nsna.org/ membership/leadership university.aspx
American Association of Critical-Care Nurses: Clinical Scene Investigator Academy	16 months at home institution	$10,000 to home institution to fund project	Teams of four nurses work with a leader and academy mentor	www.aacn.org/wd/csi/ content/csi-program -information,content? menu=csi&lastmenu=
ANA Leadership Institute	Live and recorded online seminars and self-paced courses	Costs vary by program	Programs sold as bundles, series, individually	www.ana-leadership institute.org
AONE: Emerging Leader Institute	3 days: multiple locations	$800 for AONE members; $900 nonmembers	For nurse managers with less than 6 months' experience	www.aone.org/aone _foundation/ENLI.shtml
Nursing Alliance Leadership Academy	2 days: Louisville, KY	$350 to $400	Board leadership development for newly elected or emerging leaders	www.nursing-alliance.org/ content.cfm/id/nala
American College of Health Care Administrators: Academy of Long-Term Care Leadership Development	Varies	1-year membership, $50; lifetime membership, $500	For health care and nursing home administrators and other professionals in long-term care	www.achca.org/index/php/ acacemy
National Hartford Centers of Gerontological Nursing Excellence Leadership Conference	2.5 days: location varies	$400	Leadership, management, and communication skills for experienced and aspiring gerontological nurses	www.geriatricnursing.org
STTI: Leadership Academies	18 months: leadership project at home institution— required travel to conferences and workshops	$500 to $625 registration for participant and mentor plus travel	Programs focus on maternal child health, geriatric nursing, nurse faculty, and board participation, using Kouzes and Posnner's (1995) *The Leadership Challenge* as the foundational element for several offerings	www.nursingsociety.org/ LeadershipInstitute/ Pages/default.aspx

AACN, American Association of Colleges of Nursing; *ANA,* American Nurses Association; *AONE,* American Organization of Nurse Executives; *NSNA,* National Student Nurses Association; *STTI,* Sigma Theta Tau International.
From Hassmiller, S. B., & Truelove, J. (2014). Are you the best leader you can be? Leadership resources for every nurse. *American Journal of Nursing, 114*(1), 61-67.

UNIT 5

on positions, and then mobilizes their membership to support this mutually agreed-upon agenda.

As interest groups, nursing associations provide an opportunity for nurses to bring a collective voice to the important nursing, health, and health care policy issues of the day. Clearly, however, an important issue is how members can influence the organization as it adopts a policy agenda.

INFLUENCING THE ORGANIZATION

Prospective members can gain understanding of an organization's mission, goals, priorities, political agenda, structure, and support resources, as well as a member's potential to be involved and heard. Attending local or national meetings, observing the levels of collegial exchange, and speaking with current members are useful ways to get a complete picture of an organization.

ORGANIZATIONAL STRUCTURE

It is important to understand an association's organizational structure and processes: why it exists, what it purports to do, how it runs, who runs it, and informal norms and expectations. Formal structure is determined by the organization's mission statement and bylaws, which are operationalized by governing policies and processes. These foundational documents are usually accessible to potential and current members and the general public. Procedural directions are most often available to members on request. The subtle, yet important, norms and expectations are discernible through formal and informal networking, collegial discussion, and astute observation.

BYLAWS

Bylaws, the organizational rule book, govern internal affairs, identify who has power and how that power works, and define purpose, membership criteria, financial and legal procedures, and governance operations (Tesdahl, 2003).

GOVERNANCE POLICIES

An organization's values and perspectives are blended into policy that codifies what staff can or cannot do and also the governing board's process and relationships (Carver, 1997).

PROCESSES AND PROCEDURES

Step-by-step how-to directions are offered in organizational policy and procedure manuals. Processes available to members who wish to influence organizational direction or agendas include:

- Drafting and presenting organizational resolutions and position statements;
- Suggesting organizationally branded projects, products, and services;
- Introducing issues for consideration by the governing board; and
- Presenting issues for discussion in forums offered during general business, town hall, or open meeting agendas.

Resolutions reflect organizational mission and goals and are used to inform members and other constituencies about an issue and to show support (or lack of support) for legislative initiatives.

Position statements or simply positions are issued under the auspices of a governing board to articulate an official stance on issues relevant to its mission and are intended as instruments of change to promote a common understanding and a collective response to issues of importance. Position statements succinctly define organizational stance and guide policy-shaping efforts.

GOVERNING BOARD, COMMITTEE, TASK FORCE, AND OTHER VOLUNTEER ROLES

Volunteer efforts are essential to an association's ability to survive and thrive. Governance roles relate to the elected leadership in the association: president, vice president, and/or president-elect, secretary, treasurer, and other members of the board of directors. The governing body is responsible for leading the organization in efforts consistent with stated values and mission, determining the priorities and goals, and providing stewardship and strategic planning efforts. In addition to governing board volunteer roles, nursing organizations use standing committees, task forces, and teams composed of volunteer members in functional areas to create programs, products, and services under the auspices of the organization. These structural elements differ primarily in the length of commitment involved and definition of function. Committees are likely to request longer-term commitments of committee members, although task force commitments are short term and last only for the duration of specific task-related efforts. Volunteer efforts allow the governing board to focus on "the big picture and critical decisions" (Lawrence & Flynn, 2006, p. 84). Any and all association work groups can influence the direction of the organization and health policy. The need for an organizational stance may be identified and suggested by general members and/or members in formal leadership roles. General members communicate this need via formal and informal member-leadership channels. Position statements are released only after the governing board gives final approval. Most nursing organizations post position statements on their websites so that perspectives are accessible to constituents and reach a broad audience.

Shepherding an idea from conception to completion and successful dissemination is probably one of the most rewarding aspects of membership. When the final product is perceived as valuable, it reflects well on the organization. This level of work is generally assigned to committees, teams, working groups, or task forces composed of appointed content-expert members. Through such involvement, nurses get to exercise creativity, use their skills and knowledge, and be part of a collaborative effort with opportunities to be mentored or to mentor others, to be exposed to new ideas and new ways of doing things, and to achieve success in a potentially complex process.

POLITICAL ACTION COMMITTEES

Some associations, particularly the ANA and state nurses' associations, create PACs to allow some engagement in political activities. It is illegal for incorporated nonprofit (designated 501[c][3] by the U.S. Internal Revenue Service) organizations to use funds to support candidates for federal elections, but association-related PACs can solicit funds and make contributions to candidates for federal office. PACs typically adopt bylaws and governing boards separate from the affiliated association, providing opportunities for members to focus on

issues of political influence. Since they were legitimized in 1971, PACs have become effective in channeling members' contributions to candidates who are sympathetic with organizational aims (Jacobs, 2007).

CONCLUSION

Nursing associations advocate, in one way or another, to advance the profession and promote the health and well-being of populations served. Opportunities to expand a nurse's level of influence beyond one-to-one direct care are the essence of association engagement for nurses. Volunteer contributions are essential for nursing associations to influence the well-being of individuals and the health of populations. Association involvement offers nurses opportunities to learn, practice, and polish the leadership skills that maximize their influence in associations, work, community, and health policy, and prepare the next generations of nurse leaders to continue the vital work of the profession.

DISCUSSION QUESTIONS

1. How do the nursing organizations with which you are familiar determine policymaking courses of action?
2. Identify and discuss a policy issue that merits use of organized nursing's resources.
3. How might you engage a nursing organization to influence a nursing or health policy issue of importance to you?

REFERENCES

American Academy of Nursing [AAN]. (n.d.). Strategic plan, 2014–2017. Retrieved from *www.aannet.org/strategic-plan-2014-2017*.

American Academy of Nursing [AAN]. (2014). Academy fellows. Retrieved from *www.aannet.org/fellows*.

American Journal of Nursing. (2012). Guide to nursing organizations: Lippincott's 2012 nursing career directory. *American Journal of Nursing, 112*(1), 39–42.

American Nurses Association [ANA]. (2001). *Code of ethics for nurses with interpretive statements*. Washington, DC: American Nurses Association.

American Nurses Association [ANA]. (2010). *Nursing: Scope and standards of practice* (2nd ed.). Silver Spring, MD: American Nurses Association.

American Nurses Association [ANA]. (2013). Mission statement. Retrieved from *nursingworld.org/aboutana*.

Association of Nurse Executives. (2013). About us. Retrieved from *www .aone.org/membership/about/welcome/shtml.*

Boyle, D. A. (2011). Countering compassion fatigue: A requisite nursing agenda. *OJIN: The Online Journal of Issues in Nursing, 16*(1), Manuscript 2.

Campaign for Action. (n.d.). Retrieved from *www.campaignforaction.org.*

Cardillo, D. (2013). Winning through associations. Retrieved from *donnacardillo.com/articles/associations.*

Carver, J. (1997). *Boards that make a difference* (2nd ed.). San Francisco, CA: Jossey-Bass.

Coerver, H., & Byers, M. (2011). *Race for relevance: 5 radical changes for associations.* Washington, DC: ASAE: The Center for Association Leadership.

Dolan, J. A., Fitzpatrick, M. L., & Herrmann, E. K. (1983). *Nursing in society: A historical perspective* (15th ed.). Philadelphia, PA: W.B. Saunders.

Felton, G., & Van Slyck, A. A. (2008). Self-examination: Giving, membership, and worth. *Nursing Outlook, 56*(4), 191–193.

Hassmiller, S. B., & Truelove, J. (2014). Are you the best leader you can be? Leadership resources for every nurse. *American Journal of Nursing, 114*(1), 61–67.

Institute of Medicine [IOM]. (2011). *The future of nursing: Leading change, advancing health.* Washington, DC: The National Academies Press.

International Council of Nurses [ICN]. (n.d.). About ICN. Retrieved from *www.icn.ch/about-icn/icns-mission/.*

International Council of Nurses [ICN]. (2013). Our mission. Retrieved from *www.icn.ch/about-icn/icns-mission/.*

International Council of Nurses [ICN]. (2014). Global Nursing Leadership Institute. Retrieved from *www.icn.ch/pillarsprograms/global-nursing -leadership-institute/.*

Jacobs, J. A. (2007). *Association law handbook: A practical guide for associations, societies, and charities.* Washington, DC: American Society for Association Executives and The Center for Association Leadership.

Kouzes, J. M., & Posner, B. Z. (1995). *The leadership challenge: How to keep getting extraordinary things done in organizations.* San Francisco, CA: Jossey-Bass.

Lawrence, B., & Flynn, O. (2006). *The nonprofit policy sampler* (2nd ed.). Washington, DC: BoardSource.

Lombardo, B., & Eyre, C. (2011). Compassion fatigue: A nurse's primer. *OJIN: The Online Journal of Issues in Nursing, 16*(1), Manuscript 3.

Maryland, M. A., & Gonzalez, R. I. (2012). Patient advocacy in the community and legislative arena. *OJIN: The Online Journal of Issues in Nursing, 17*(1), Manuscript 2.

Matthews, J. H. (2012). Role of professional organizations in advocating for the nursing profession. *OJIN: The Online Journal of Issues in Nursing, 17*(1), Manuscript 3.

Middleton, S., Walker, K., & Leigh, T. (2009). Why fellowship? Peak professional bodies, peer recognition and credentialing in Australia. *Collegian (Royal College of Nursing, Australia), 16*(4), 177–183.

Nanus, B. (1992). *Visionary leadership: Creating a compelling sense of direction for your organization.* San Francisco, CA: Jossey-Bass.

Nursing Alliance for Quality Care. (2013). About NAQC. Retrieved from *www.naqc.org/Functional/About-NAQC.*

Oncology Nursing Society. (2012). *Oncology Nursing Society leadership competencies.* Pittsburgh, PA: Oncology Nursing Society.

Reverby, S. M. (1987). *Ordered to care: The dilemma of American nursing, 1850–1945.* Cambridge, UK: Cambridge University Press.

Robert Wood Johnson Foundation. (2010). *Nursing leadership from bedside to boardroom: Opinion leaders' perceptions.* Princeton, NJ: Robert Wood Johnson Foundation. Retrieved from *www.rwjf.org/content/dam/web-assets/2010/01//nursing-leadership-from-bedside-to-boardroom.*

Sadovich, J. M. (2005). Work excitement in nursing: An examination of the relationship between work excitement and burnout. *Nursing Economic$, 23*(2), 91–96.

Schroeder, R. T. (2013). The value of belonging to a professional nursing organization. *AORN Journal, 98*(2), 99–101.

Sigma Theta Tau International. (n.d.). STTI organizational fact sheet. Retrieved from *www.nursingsociety.org/aboutus/mission/Pages/factsheet .aspx.*

Smith, B. G., Haas, J., Turner, M. M., Grant, M. N., Cleaver, S., et al. (2008). Member value proposition: ASAE Membership Associapedia Idea Swap. Retrieved from *www.asaecenter.org/wiki/indix.cfm?debug=false&page =Member%20Value%20Proposition.*

Tesdahl, D. B. (2003). *The nonprofit board's guide to bylaws: Creating a framework for effective governance.* Washington, DC: BoardSource.

de Tocqueville, A. (1835/2000). *Democracy in America.* New York: Bantam Classic Books.

ONLINE RESOURCES

American Nurses Association
www.nursingworld.org
American Society of Association Executives
www.asaecenter.org
BoardSource
www.boardsource.org

CHAPTER 75

Coalitions: A Powerful Political Strategy

Rebecca (Rice) Bowers-Lanier[1]

"When spider webs unite, they can tie up a lion."
Ethiopian proverb

The Affordable Care Act (ACA) and the resultant expansion of access to health care in the United States form the overriding context for health care policy at the federal and state levels. Key to expanding delivery of care is assuring that quality and timely health care can be delivered by all health care providers working within their educational capacity. In this context, the Institute of Medicine (IOM) delivered its report, *The Future of Nursing* (IOM, 2011), from which emerged the establishment of the Campaign for Action, an initiative to mobilize the development of State Action Coalitions (Center to Champion Nursing in America, 2011). The premise behind the emphasis on state action is that most of the policy and legislative resolutions to the IOM report would redound to the states. The ACA also provides the impetus for states to grapple with vexing policy options regarding access to health care, including whether or not to expand Medicaid. In 2013, in Virginia as in other states, expansion of Medicaid as a policy option was driven, in part, by the power of a coalition of health care providers, organizations, and patient advocacy groups working to overcome political opposition to Medicaid expansion. This chapter provides an overview of coalitions, from inception through evaluation, using as exemplars the action coalitions and the Healthcare for All Virginians (HAV) Coalition in Virginia.

The power of coalitions lies in their ability to bring people together from diverse perspectives around clearly defined purposes to achieve common goals. Strength lies in numbers, in working together and in strategizing for success. What factors contribute to success or failure of coalitions? How do we go about forming and maintaining coalitions? What are the ingredients? How do we know when or if coalitions achieve their goals? This chapter describes the ingredients for successful coalition building, maintenance, and success. The ingredients work in small sizes for local and regional coalitions and are equally effective in creating and sustaining larger coalitions at the local, state, national, and international levels.

BIRTH AND LIFE CYCLE OF COALITIONS

In simplest terms, coalitions are created to bring about collective action at the local, state, or national level. Rabinowitz (2010) defines a coalition as an alliance of individuals and organizations, sometimes referred to as an organization of organizations, that come together to address a specific problem or issue and reach a common goal. The League of Women Voters (2012) defines coalitions as groups of individuals and/or organizations with common interests that agree to work together toward mutually defined goals. When an individual or one association works on an issue, it, like the

[1]Personal thanks to contributions by the following State Action Coalition Leaders: Mary Foley (California), Mary Lou Brunell (Florida), Wanda Jones (Mississippi), Polly Johnson (North Carolina), Patricia Moulton (North Dakota), and Shirley Gibson (Virginia). Also thanks to Jill Hanken, Staff Attorney, Virginia Poverty Law Center, and co-lead of the Virginia Healthcare for All Virginians Coalition.

605

spider, creates a small web; working with others similarly minded creates a powerful network that can capture much more than an individual or association working alone. Coalitions create their effectiveness by empowering individual organizations to pool their resources and creativity to foster more strategic and effective action, enabling and enhancing communication and collaboration among members, increasing diversity by bringing together new and alternative voices, and increasing the impact through greater numbers.

Coalitions arise out of challenges or opportunities, and the key for all coalitions is to maintain their effectiveness until they achieve their goals. For some coalitions, the work may be completed within a matter of weeks; for others, the work may persist for years. The two coalitions discussed in this chapter have been in existence for several years and continue to press onward to achieve their goals.

BUILDING AND MAINTAINING A COALITION: THE PRIMER

ESSENTIAL INGREDIENTS

To build and maintain effective coalitions require four ingredients: leadership; membership; resources; and serendipity, or the ability to seize the moment. First and foremost is leadership. Coalitions cannot exist without outstanding leadership. Leaders may exist a priori or may emerge early from the membership of the coalition, but without leaders, coalitions will falter and fade away.

Two types of leaders are critical to coalition work: inspirational and organizational. Inspiring leaders use personal strengths and power to constructively and ethically influence others to an endpoint or goal. They motivate others to participate and meet their obligations; they encourage new ideas, problem solving, and risk taking. Inspiring leaders balance a personal inner drive to move forward while assisting coalition members to make decisions. They know when to steer forward, when to idle, and when to back up, if necessary. Organizational leaders possess the skills to keep members on track between meetings, ensure that

communication methods are in place, and follow through on coalition assignments. Inspiration and organization may coexist in one person, but frequently two leaders are needed to serve the coalition.

As important as leaders are, they are no more important than the coalition members, without whom the coalition would not exist. Members increase the productivity of the coalition. They also increase the visibility of the coalition, because they represent diverse constituencies and networks. Members must commit to the goals of the coalition, attend meetings, and communicate outcomes to their constituencies. Membership should be beneficial for the coalition and the individual (Berkowitz & Wolff, 2000; Coalitions Work, 2007a; Rabinowitz, 2010).

Coalitions need adequate resources to accomplish their work. Resources are the tools for the leaders and members to accomplish the coalitions' goals. They include money and in-kind donations from members and others, such as support for developing marketing materials, purchasing supplies, putting on educational sessions, and developing and maintaining websites. The use of social media is increasingly a means of communicating ideas and meetings and connecting members with one another.

The fourth ingredient for coalition success is serendipity, the happy occurrence of an opportunity not specifically sought, so long as coalition members take advantage of the opportunity by seizing the moment. To effectively seize the moment, leaders and members must obligate themselves to conduct continual environmental scans, such as tracking current events, connecting with many different types of people, and spending time thinking creatively (PolicyLink, n.d.a, n.d.b).

The 51 State Action Coalitions and the Virginia HAV Coalition illustrate these ingredients. Each action coalition is taking on one or more of the overall goals of the Campaign for Action: (1) remove scope of practice barriers, (2) expand opportunities for nurses to lead and diffuse collaborative improvement efforts, (3) implement nurse residency programs, (4) increase the proportion of nurses with a baccalaureate degree to 80%

by 2020, (5) double the number of nurses with a doctorate by 2020, (6) ensure that nurses engage in lifelong learning, (7) prepare and enable nurses to lead change to advance health, and (8) build an infrastructure for the collection and analysis of interprofessional health care workforce data (IOM, 2011). The HAV Coalition, formed in 2009, has been working over the past 4 years to increase access to health care for all Virginians, from enrolling pregnant legal immigrants through expanding Medicaid as part of the ACA (HAV Coalition, n.d.).

When the action coalitions were forming, the Center to Champion Nursing required coalition leadership to consist of one nursing organization and one non-nursing organization. The leadership of the action coalitions is thus relatively varied from state to state. All action coalitions adhere to this requirement; some have more than two leaders; one state has as many as 10 leaders. The HAV Coalition has two co-leads: one is a Staff Attorney at the Virginia Poverty Law Center, and the other heads a foundation that funds health initiatives in the Commonwealth of Virginia.

Membership of the action coalitions predominantly consists of nursing organizations (service, practitioners, and specialty groups), colleges and universities, and individual members. Most coalitions have work groups focused on one or more of the eight recommendations in the IOM *Future of Nursing* report. The HAV Coalition consists of 62 health care provider organizations, patient advocacy organizations, and related health policy organizations. Work is accomplished by calling together members around specific health policy initiatives, developing and disseminating information, and arranging for members to write letters for publication in newspapers.

Resources are invaluable for all coalitions and universally a source of frustration because of the need to raise funds to sustain coalition work. The action coalitions seek funds from foundations and members to accomplish their work. For example, some coalitions have initiated fundraising campaigns from organizational members. Others have been successful in securing grants to pursue one or more of their goals. Much of their work has been accomplished through in-kind contributions of members' time and talents. The HAV Coalition has obtained resources in a similar manner. In the early days of the HAV coalition, member organizations contributed nominal dues annually. Most recently, one or more organizations have contributed larger amounts to provide for some Web-based support and organizing for grassroots action. Very few coalitions of any stripe would report that they have sufficient funding to fully execute their work.

COALITION STRUCTURE

Structure refers to the organization of the coalition, and it defines the procedures by which the coalition operates. The structure serves the members, not the other way around. It also includes how members are accepted, how leadership is chosen, how decisions are made, and how differences are mediated. Effective coalitions operate using group process, meaning that they go through a life cycle that involves norming and storming (creating group behavioral norms and settling disagreements) before establishing group processes (Coalitions Work, 2007b).

Coalition structure, although necessary, is dynamic, depending upon the resources and the cause. Some coalitions are highly structured, with formal committees, task forces or work groups, and communication mechanisms; others are more loosely structured, with shared leadership and work done by ad hoc groups. Moreover, the structure may change over time, depending on the lifespan and work of the coalition. Highly structured coalitions may be necessary if the coalition work is complex and multifaceted, involving more than one goal. Committees and/or task forces may be established around the goals.

Coalition structure should make provisions for governance. This is especially true if the size exceeds 15 people. Beyond this number, the group becomes too large for effective, efficient decision making. The governance committee should, at the very least, include all committee and work group chairs to facilitate communication. The committee should represent the diversity of the members. Often the structure follows from coalition goals and/or complexity of the work. For example, the Pennsylvania

UNIT 5

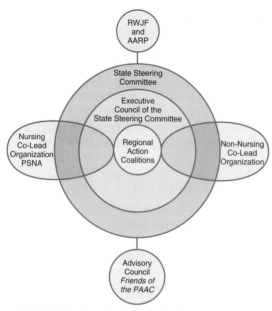

FIGURE 75-1 Pennsylvania Action Coalition organization.

Action Coalition (PAAC, n.d.) has published a schema that depicts the organizational structure of the coalition, including at its core nine Regional Action Coalitions and, in concentric circles, an Executive Council and the State Steering Committee (Figure 75-1). The two co-leads, nursing and non-nursing, intersect all concentric circles. The Virginia and North Carolina Action Coalitions have also formed regional coalitions around nursing education efforts (S. Gibson & P. Johnson, personal communication, October 25, 2013).

No matter what coalitions call themselves or how they structure themselves, an important factor to achieving goals is to engage appropriate support systems. Someone must agree to do a task, and have the means to get the task done. The work may be done by volunteers, as it is in many coalitions. However, there may be consequences to all-volunteer efforts; for example, a lack of accountability for achieving outcomes. Often, paid staff can deliver on the tasks and move the coalition along more effectively, especially when the work is complex and multifaceted (M.L. Brunell, W. Jones, and P. Moulton, personal communication, October 25, 2013).

DECISION MAKING

Decision making is a source of great concern, usually at the beginning of a coalition's life. Because members represent different constituencies and perspectives, they will often not trust one another, and conflict emerges. Everyone wants to protect his or her own interests. As the coalition decides on its mission and goals, it also has to figure out how it will make its decisions. Most often, decisions are made without voting by consensus; members simply agree or disagree. When decisions are controversial, coalition members enter into deeper dialogue. By operating on consensus, coalition members must come to a decision with which all are comfortable. What frequently happens is that alternative solutions are offered until one is made to which all can agree. Consensus building is by nature time-consuming, but it fosters involvement and buy-in from the members. The journey to consensus requires leadership skill and finesse (Berkowitz & Wolff, 2000).

Coalition work can be tricky. Member groups are bound to disagree on specific priorities or tactics. Moreover, participants' individual responsibilities will inevitably overtake their availability to support the coalition from time to time. When such challenges arise, coalition leaders should consider dialing back coalition expectations and/or shifting duties to other willing participants. Effective coalition leaders recognize the importance of creating a space for the disagreements to be discussed in an honest and forthright manner behind closed doors. In other words, what happens in Vegas, stays in Vegas. Divisions within coalitions should not become public, because advocacy requires a single message and a unified front (League of Women Voters, 2012).

MEETINGS

Coalitions must meet; otherwise, the work does not get done. Meetings take place in a variety of modes: face-to-face, conference call, and/or through Web-based connections. At least initially in the forming stage, face-to-face meetings are preferable because they facilitate conversation and getting to know one another. As coalitions mature, other types of communication may replace face-to-face venues. Coalition leaders should remember, however, that much of the cache and strength of coalitions comes from the interpersonal connections that members have with one another. Regardless of the venue, meetings must take place regularly and in an organized manner to keep members engaged.

The interval between meetings and the time of meetings are very important. The interval should be long enough for members to accomplish their assignments. Meetings should ideally consist of presenting alternatives for action and making decisions. If the interval between meetings is too long, little interim work will get done, as the human response is to wait until just prior to a meeting to complete an assignment. Leaders should confirm with members the amount of time each will need to get the work accomplished in the interim and then schedule the next meeting accordingly.

The content of the meeting should be focused on problem solving and decision making. There should be a sense among members that work is being done and decisions are being made; otherwise, results-oriented members will soon stop attending meetings. A good meeting has energy. If the meeting is primarily conducted to exchange information, some members will see this as a waste of their time, and they may drop out. Alternatives such as e-mail and electronic bulletin boards exist for disseminating information. Consequently, coalition leaders and members should regularly assess the content of the meetings to see what works and what does not and make necessary adjustments.

PROMOTING THE COALITION

What good is a coalition if no one knows it exists? Coalitions are formed to advance a common agenda, and communication is the vehicle with which that agenda is advanced. Early on in the coalition's life, members must develop and implement a communications plan aimed at getting the coalition's message out to the broader community of interest. The plan should include branding (i.e., logo and tag line), ways to reach intended audiences (i.e., website and social marketing venues, such as Facebook and Twitter), and assigning individuals to

keep the communication up-to-date and vibrant (Coalitions Work, 2007c).

FUNDING

Coalition work takes money. Some coalitions run on little or no money, using the time and talent of their members. In fact, many of the action coalitions began with little or no money, and fiscal resourcing continues to be a common challenge for these coalitions. Similarly, the HAV Coalition operates on little funding, depending upon the in-kind contributions of its members. Underfunded or unfunded coalitions may be unable to sustain their work over the long haul because of lack of resources. Generally speaking, coalitions will need to look for additional funds to stay solvent and accomplish their work. How much money is needed depends on several factors. First is the mission and aims of the coalition. Second, the strategic plan will define the resources needed; then members can decide how to best obtain the funds. Third, members should develop a fund-raising plan that includes tailoring the message to prospective funding sources, assigning people to make the contacts, communicating the mission and aims of the coalition, and seeking funding.

PITFALLS AND CHALLENGES

Coalitions usually start out with a flurry of excitement and activity. Action coalitions began in this manner, subsequent to the rollout of the IOM report. Sustaining the excitement and guiding the activity are ongoing challenges. Coalition work is difficult and complex. Following are some common pitfalls and challenges, with suggestions for overcoming them.

FAILURE TO GET THE RIGHT PEOPLE TO PARTICIPATE

Coalitions should attract those who are most interested in seeing that the work gets done, and these members will commit to participating in the coalition. At regular intervals, coalitions should assess who is at the table and who is not. The following three common membership errors exist: First is the error of exclusion of an entire group of stakeholders. In examining the purpose of the coalition, members should ask themselves these questions: "Who have we excluded?" "Whose expertise do we need?" "Who may work to derail the coalition's work if not invited to become a member?"

The second error in coalition membership is not achieving buy-in from major players, like the 800-pound gorillas. Coalition members should identify these individuals/organizations and seek their buy-in. For example, an action coalition that does not include the major leaders or associations, such as the hospital association, may have difficulty advancing its agenda. Action coalitions achieving some measure of success to date have diversified membership, but coalition leaders appreciate the need for increasing that diversity (M. Foley, W. Jones, & P. Moulton, personal communication, October 25, 2013).

The third error involves participation in the coalition by the wrong members. When organizations send representatives who do not have the authority to speak and represent the organization in coalition decision making, they hinder the work of the coalition. In reality, organizations sometimes use this approach as a passive aggressive way to derail the coalition.

CULTURAL AND LANGUAGE DIFFERENCES AMONG COALITION MEMBERS

Because coalition members represent different perspectives on the goals and mission of the coalition, all must learn the meaning of significant words used by coalition members. Sometimes simple words carry completely different connotations. For example, in nursing coalitions, the word time connotes entirely different interval spans for nurse administrators (who operate day-to-day) and nurse educators (who operate by semesters). In the HAV Coalition's earlier work, a legislative goal was to expand Medicaid to include pregnant immigrant women. In this case, immigrant by necessity was qualified to mean legal and within the United States for at least 5 years. Consequently, coalition leaders and members must continually be attuned to words that have different connotations, and they should agree on a common definition (if possible) or agree

to understand the differences in the meaning of words.

PERSISTENT DISTRUST AMONG COALITION MEMBERS

Distrust is perhaps one of the thorniest challenges that coalition leaders face, because much of the success of coalitions comes from the ongoing interaction among members that allays misperceptions and builds trust. When members become disengaged from coalition work, their absence can derail progress, especially if they fail to keep their own constituencies informed. To overcome distrust, leaders and members must work diligently on including potentially disenfranchised members such as nursing assistants. In the end, people must feel valued and treasured for their participation and contributions to the enterprise.

CONTROL FREAKS AND PROTECTING TURF

The tendency to control and protect turf can happen at the individual member level and at the coalition level. At the individual level, there are those in whom coalition success breeds a type of person: one who knows the truth and is always willing to share it. These individuals need to be gathered back into the fold and made to feel that their ideas are worthy, but at the same time, they must understand that they do not possess all the answers to the work at hand. At the coalition level, successful coalitions may easily rest on past achievement and ignore the need for retooling for ongoing challenges. Hence, competing coalitions may form, leading to turf protection and dysfunctional competing coalitions. One of the most unfortunate outcomes of competing coalitions aimed at the same outcome is that policymakers will disregard the petitions of both coalitions, and nothing will be gained.

POOR HANDLING OF DIFFERENT PERSPECTIVES

By their very nature, coalitions consist of individuals representing constituencies with differing perspectives on issues. For example, action coalitions' concerns relate to specific IOM recommendations such as removing barriers to scope of practice and increasing the numbers of nurses prepared at the baccalaureate level. As major employers of nurses, hospitals may or may not see it in their immediate best interest to aggressively support these recommendations. To engender buy-in from hospitals, some action coalitions might demonstrate that revising policies and procedures within hospitals that prohibit nurses from working to the full extent of their scope of practice might serve to improve patient care and increase nursing satisfaction. Both outcomes should contribute to hospitals' bottom lines. A similar potential conflict exists among educators and the increased pressure for the baccalaureate. Community college leaders must be able to identify the win-win in their participation in action coalitions, whether becoming full partners with baccalaureate education, enhancing their nursing workforce development initiatives, or other opportunities.

Coalition leaders and members have an obligation to recognize points of contention and determine how they will be handled. In fact, some worthy goals of a coalition might need to be postponed or shelved altogether if all of the members cannot agree on a selected outcome. That is not to say that the work will never be achieved, but that more time will be needed to come to consensus on strategies and goals.

FAILURE TO ACT

Coalitions begin with fire in their bellies. Going from words to action is sometimes more difficult than members had originally thought. Some coalitions formulate and reformulate action plans ad infinitum without getting to action. However, action is the coalition's currency. Without action, there will be no resources to support the work. At least two factors contribute to failure to act. One is lack of leadership and the other is the inability of the coalition to coalesce around solutions. To resolve the leadership issue, new leaders will have to emerge, and in this case, the coalition members may need to lead a quiet coup to replace leadership. Resolving the consensus issue requires a regrouping and reexamination of the purposes of the coalition and an analysis of whether or not any consensus can be achieved. Coalition members must adhere to working by consensus, as messy as the process is.

Coalitions are no vehicles for moving forward by majority rule.

LOSING BALANCE

Coalition leaders and members wear out. Managing, leading, and working in coalitions drain energy. Leaders of action coalitions, in particular, took on the IOM *Future of Nursing* recommendations with no promises of external funding, meaning that coalition work has been conducted, at times, by volunteers. Members are entitled to personal lives and must know that they do not have to keep their coalition jobs for life. Each person must assess his or her readiness to step aside and support the leadership and membership activities of new recruits. Therefore, coalitions should set in place a means for leadership succession planning at regular intervals (M.L. Brunell & P. Johnson, personal communication, October 25, 2013).

POLITICAL WORK OF COALITIONS

Should coalitions speak out on issues that matter to them? Should nursing coalitions speak out for nursing? Of course they should. But advocacy work has its downsides and upsides.

REASONS NOT TO ADVOCATE

When coalitions advocate for certain positions, they run into opposition from stakeholders who diverge from those positions. The further coalitions go out on the limb, the more people line up to saw off the limb. In fact, coalitions stand to lose their financial support if they go out too far. In addition, there are legal restrictions on advocacy by tax-exempt groups in lobbying, so coalitions whose members may be from tax-exempt organizations may be forced to pull back if they become too forcefully active in lobbying. Therefore, coalitions should choose their battles carefully, making certain that they are willing to accept the consequences of winning or losing (Bowers-Lanier, 2010).

REASONS TO ADVOCATE

Nursing and other health care coalitions that are established to advocate for particular legislative or policy initiatives will be successful if the initiatives are enacted into law or become established policies. When that happens, the coalition will have met its goal, and it may disband. Alternatively, it may envision another goal and begin work toward accomplishing that.

HOW TO ADVOCATE WITH GRACE

The solution, of course, is to proceed with care. By its very nature, advocacy involves risk. Coalition members should work out their differences and carefully select the words they will use when advocating for positions. Coalition members should agree in advance on the advocacy approaches they will take that will not jeopardize their legal status or disenfranchise funders and members.

EVALUATING COALITION EFFECTIVENESS

Coalitions should evaluate their effectiveness on a regular basis. Evaluation helps to keep members on track, determine strengths and areas for improvement, and in the final analysis, determine whether the coalitions' goals are met or if further work is needed. Evaluation should be both formative (assessing the progress of the coalition on a continual and regular basis such as after each meeting) and summative (assessing the status of coalition deliverables after a defined period of time such as annually) and should occur at regular intervals. Table 75-1 lists the questions governing formative and summative coalition evaluation.

Coalition work can be extremely exciting and fulfilling. By bringing together individuals who represent varying perspectives, coalitions can achieve their goals. Goal achievement occurs through active involvement of these diverse members and their constituencies. Leaders must emerge or be selected who are passionate about the cause and who can simultaneously attend to detail and create an organized structure for the coalition work. Coalitions must meet regularly and take action on their decisions. In the end, coalitions must determine how and when to advocate for their mission and evaluate their effectiveness to stay viable.

DISCUSSION QUESTION

1. As a direct-care provider with occasional unit management responsibilities, you and several of your colleagues identify a patient care issue that

TABLE 75-1 Coalition Formative Evaluation

Evaluation Type	Questions to Be Answered
Formative	Questions to be asked at a regular basis (by meeting, monthly, quarterly at maximum)
	Membership
	1. Are the right member organizations at the table? Who is missing?
	2. Are members fully engaged? If not, why not?
	3. Are all equal players? Why or why not?
	Coalition work
	1. Are goals realistic?
	2. How is the work being accomplished? By committees? By one person?
	3. Is there a better way to do the work?
	4. What are the barriers and facilitators to goal achievement?
	5. Are strategies in place for minimizing barriers? Maximizing facilitators?
	6. Is the work plan on schedule?
Summative	Semi-annually or annually: Goal achievement
	1. Have the goals been achieved? Why or why not? Should any strategies be changed?
	2. Are the goals still relevant to the mission of the coalition? Why or why not?
	3. Has the coalition achieved its stated goal? Should it be disbanded? Why or why not?
	4. Is there additional work to be done and the will to do it?

you believe needs to be resolved. When bringing up the issue with the clinical nurse specialist on your unit, she suggests that you form a coalition of individuals who could address the issue.

a. What other "stakeholder" groups should you consider asking to join in your work? Who are the 800-lb gorillas that need to be at the table?

b. Are you an inspirational or organizational leader? How would you go about seeking a co-lead who would complement your strengths?

c. As your coalition works to resolve the issue, coming to consensus on a solution may be the most difficult job of the coalition. Why is consensus important? What would likely occur if your coalition decides to vote on the resolution?

REFERENCES

Berkowitz, B., & Wolff, T. (2000). *The spirit of the coalition.* Washington, DC: American Public Health Association.

Bowers-Lanier, R. (2010). Advocacy in the public arena. In K. A. Polifko (Ed.), *The practice environment of nursing.* Clifton Park, NY: Delmar Cengage Learning.

Center to Champion Nursing in America. (2011). Campaign history. Retrieved from *campaignforaction.org.*

Coalitions Work. (2007a). Coalition membership. Retrieved from *coalitions work.com/resources/tools/.*

Coalitions Work. (2007b). Stages of team building. Retrieved from *coalitionswork.com/resources/tools/.*

Coalitions Work. (2007c). One-page organizational message for coalitions. Retrieved from *coalitionswork.com/resources/tools/.*

Healthcare for All Virginians (HAV) Coalition. (n.d.). Retrieved from *havcoalition.org/.*

Institute of Medicine [IOM]. (2011). *The future of nursing: Leading change, advancing health.* Washington, DC: The National Academies Press.

League of Women Voters. (2012). Coalition building strategies. Retrieved from *www.lwv.org/content/coalition-building-strategies.*

Pennsylvania Action Coalition [PAAC]. (n.d.). Organizational structure. Retrieved from *www.paactioncoalition.org.*

PolicyLink. (n.d.a). Advocating for change. Retrieved from *www.policylink.org.*

PolicyLink. (n.d.b). Seizing the moment. Retrieved from *www.policylink.org.*

Rabinowitz, P. (2010). Coalition building I: Starting a coalition. In T. Wolff (Ed.), *Community tool box.* Retrieved from *www.ctb.ku.edu/en/table-of-contents/assessment/promotion-strategies/start-a-coaltion/main.*

ONLINE RESOURCES

Center to Champion Nurses in America
campaignforaction.org
Coalitions Work
coalitionswork.com/resources/tools
Policy Link
www.policylink.org

CHAPTER 76

TAKING ACTION:
The Nursing Community Builds a Unified Voice

Suzanne Miyamoto   Lauren Inouye

Advocacy is a dish best served unified. No matter the issue, if more than one player in the process supports or opposes it, there is an increased potential that the final action will result in their favor. Although there are multiple factors that may impact this (i.e., the reputation of the players, their influence, or the political dynamics), the general rule is power in numbers. Legislators anticipate that their staff will thoughtfully investigate both sides of an issue and present them with sound options on how to proceed. The support of constituents, opinions of national or state organizations (depending on the legislative body), historical positions of the office, coalitions, and, of course, influence are major factors in the decision-making process. Of these, coalitions certainly make a sizable impression. If likeminded groups, particularly from diverse fields of expertise, join together for a common cause, it is noticed. There are many forms of coalitions, some more formal than others, but the question becomes, what makes a coalition effective? And, more importantly, why have they become increasingly necessary?

THE NECESSITY OF COALITIONS

Competition often necessitates coalition formation when political pressure to win is intense. Competition, in other words, is defined as the scenario when multiple parties have differing interests at stake, and the outcome of a particular policy favors one group's interests over another's (Holyoke, 2009). For example, in today's health care system, multiple parties, including health care professionals, hold interests and positions that do not always align and competition intensifies when the stakes are high. Essentially, the battle to advance a policy position focuses on who has the most presence on an issue, both the type that goes noticed and that which does not.

Consider any issue nurses would be passionate to promote. Does the profession have the resources to tip the odds in their favor (i.e., time, financial infrastructure, individual advocates)? The public assumes policy is formed on the basis of evidence, and this assumption is absolutely true. However, the wise citizen knows that evidence alone is not always the deciding factor. Take, for example, advanced practice registered nurses (APRNs) being able to practice to the full extent of their education and training. There are decades and mountains of evidence to show that APRNs are effective clinicians who can provide cost-effective, high-quality care. If evidence is all it took to create policy, then why is there not full practice authority for APRNs in all 50 states? There is much more to policy than evidence; there is politics. And politics is driven by competition. If competition is driven by those with the most resources to win, what are nursing's odds?

Time and time again we see advances made at the state level to amend practice acts that would allow APRNs to serve their patients to the level they were educated. Nursing organizations at the state level have made tremendous strides to find legislative champions, allies in the community, and partnerships among their associations, but when push comes to shove, the odds do not end up in their favor. It would appear that a perfect campaign was run, but the effort fell short. Ask any nurse who has endured this encounter and they will say their competition was intense.

Take, for example, a 2014 case in Nebraska. The efforts of the nurses in the state to pass Legislative Bill 916 were formidable. This bill would have eliminated the requirement that nurse practitioners must have a practice agreement with a collaborating physician. It passed the state legislature. However, when the bill was sent to the Governor's office, he notified the members of the legislature that he would not sign it, expressing the concern that the bill "goes too far too quickly" (Nebraska.gov, 2014, para 3), despite the fact that the legislation included a transition period in which new graduate nurse practitioners would have a 2-year transition into practice with a collaborating physician. In the Governor's official letter that vetoed the bill, he states,

... the Chief Medical Officer expressed concern that the "total independent practice for nurses practitioners ... without identifying an alternative means by which nurse practitioner can be included in viable practitioner referral networks creates potential safety issues for patients." The Chief Medical Officer also stated that "recent graduates of nurse practitioner programs ... lack sufficient clinical experience to practice independently"... (Nebraska.gov, 2014, para 4)

The Governor's letter does not mention the body of evidence supporting the APRN full practice authority or the Federal Trade Commission's (FTC) recent position that:

As explained herein and in prior FTC staff APRN advocacy comments, mandatory physician supervision and collaborative practice agreement requirements are likely to impede competition among health care providers and restrict APRNs' ability to practice independently, leading to decreased access to health care services, higher health care costs, reduced quality of care, and less innovation in health care delivery. For these reasons, we suggest that state legislators view APRN supervision requirements carefully.

Empirical research and on-the-ground experience demonstrate that APRNs provide safe and effective care within the scope of their training, certification, and licensure. (Federal Trade Commission, 2014, p. 38)

One of the glaring issues in this debate is always education and clinical hours, not necessarily the outcomes. In a letter written by the American Association of Colleges of Nursing, the rigor of APRN education was presented (American Association of Colleges of Nursing, 2014). Moreover, some health care disciplines are moving to a competency-based educational system over a prescriptive number of clinical hours. There are a host of factors that could have played a role in the Governor's decision, but he only cited one opinion in his veto letter: that of the Chief Medical Officer. One thing can be said in this case: there is competition in who helps inform the ultimate decision. Even the Institute of Medicine's (IOM's) *The Future of Nursing* report calls for nurses to assume more highly influential policy positions, stating, "Public, private, and governmental health care decision makers at every level should include representation from nursing on boards, on executive management teams, and in other key leadership positions" (IOM, 2011, p. 5).

In a competitive environment, as the number of players involved grows, the spectrum of positions becomes wider and the pot of resources needed to win becomes larger. Even within a larger group representing smaller, but similar interests, it is difficult to imagine that the positions and preferences of these smaller subgroups would be exactly the same (Moe, 1980). For example, the nursing profession is represented by more than 100 national organizations. Conceivably, one could assume that there are at least 100 policy positions that represent a segment of the nursing profession. Realistically, many of these nursing organizations have similar policy interests. Finding middle ground that appeals broadly helps to build the case for taking unified action (Holyoke, 2009). When multiple groups can convene around their common interests, the collective action of these groups helps promote competition and secure an outcome in their favor.

UNIT 5

COALITION FORMATION

In nursing school, many learn the Gestalt theory as an approach to patient care: the whole is greater than the sum of its parts. This is true in policy and politics and is at the core of coalition formation. Establishing a coalition for the purpose of advancing a shared interest allows individual parties to pool together resources and to amplify a unified voice. Say, for example, 10 health care associations are vying for their issue (a proposed solution that would increase access to primary care) to be placed on the federal agenda. Five of these 10 groups realize they have similar policy solutions and it would be in their interest to act collectively. As five, formerly separate groups now recognized as one unified entity, these groups have placed themselves in a higher position to leverage the policy's outcome. They can merge their collective resources to advance their policy solution. As a coalition, these groups represent one half of the political influence on this issue. Before this coalition formation, individually, they only represented one tenth (i.e., the whole is greater than the sum of its parts).

Moreover, the collaboration of multiple, vested stakeholders (individuals, groups, or established organizations) is intensified if coalition members provide diverse representation. Greater diversity among coalitions can increase the chances that the collaboration (and thus their interests) as a whole will appeal to legislators. If a health care coalition includes nurses, physicians, pharmacists, and physical therapists, legislators are less likely to see the issue as a provider issue, but rather as a health care issue. Knowing that coalitions are key in the policy process to overcome the competitive nature of the political process, what makes an effective coalition?

DEFINING A COALITION'S SUCCESS: THE IMPORTANCE OF LEADERSHIP AND GOAL SETTING

As discussed earlier, generally speaking, a coalition comprising numerous organizations will represent a spectrum of positions, perspectives, and values. It takes a highly skilled leader to draw together multiple organizations and channel the energy and resources of these groups toward a specific, common goal. A coalition leader must be able to clearly and concisely dialogue with all members involved so that each feels that they are being heard and recognized. Coalition leaders must be able to balance the individual perspectives of the organizations and consider how they will weight in when the coalition formulates a policy position on an issue, all the while making sure that the resulting message is one that the coalition as a whole can support.

A 2001 study interviewed coalition leaders on the complexities of coalition building. When asked how they defined their coalition's success, the highest ranked answer was "achieving our goals" (Mizrahi & Rosenthal, 2001). Although this may seem like an obvious response, it raises a very important point: it is not enough for interest groups to simply convene because they are likeminded; in addition to talking the talk, they must also walk the walk by channeling their collective support toward specific action. Setting goals helps coalitions to walk the walk. Goals may evolve over time, but it is important that they are communicated well among members of the coalition so that consensus and confidence in the coalition are maximized, and confusion, disappointment, and blame are minimized.

Goal setting is beneficial for a few reasons. First, the process of goal setting allows coalition members to create a clear plan of action and to divide up duties that are aimed at achieving that goal. This process creates commitment among the groups involved, which is essential for accountability. Second, goal setting ensures all members are on the same page regarding the desired result of the action plan. This is especially important because the end goal could realistically fall anywhere from raising awareness broadly about your issue of interest to a more concrete, long-term end goal, such as having a piece of legislation passed into law. Third, achieving goals builds a coalition's credibility. A coalition that can point to specific successes builds a reputation as being effective and collaborative. Within the nursing profession, the ability for nurses and nursing organizations to collaborate around common goals and present a unified front has not always been their strongest suit. This sentiment has been echoed by multiple parties, including Congressional staff (Begeny, 2009), and is a challenge that nursing continues to grapple with today (though it is making great strides forward).

A PERSPECTIVE ON NURSING'S UNIFIED VOICE

A 2010 Gallup study commissioned by the Robert Wood Johnson Foundation (RWJF) examined the perceived role of nurses in influencing health care reform, drawing on the opinions of 1500 leaders from several health-related industries (including insurance and health care services), as well as the government and academia. The survey unlocked perceptions about the degree to which nurses currently influence health care and to what extent nurses should influence the policies that dictate its delivery (RWJF, 2010). When respondents were asked which barriers prevent nurses' ability to contribute to improvements in policy development, 56% identified "Nursing lacks a single voice in speaking on national issues" as a major barrier, and 29% identified this barrier as a minor one (RWJF, 2010, p. 10). This was the fourth highest-ranking barrier out of 11 (RWJF, 2010). Furthermore, opinion leaders highlighted the importance of nurses taking accountability for elevating themselves into leadership roles. "In other words, respondents felt nurses should be held accountable for not only providing quality direct patient care, but also for health care leadership" (Khoury et al., 2011, p. 304).

What does this study tell the profession? Unite and take accountability for your own actions. The political process is fast moving and intense. Historically, nurses have been upheld in the public eye as among the most, if not the most, trusted profession in the United States (Swift, 2013). Nurses may believe it is not within their professional purview to be mingling in the political realm, or do not feel empowered to participate in the policy process as a result of feeling conflicted about what their role is when it comes to political leverage (Des Jardin, 2001).

However, if nursing wants a seat at the policy table, it is not simply awarded because nurses are trusted and well-respected publicly; it has to be earned. Earning that seat involves an empowered nurse to engage in the political process necessary to gain that seat. Ultimately, in every setting there is competition for relevance and if uniting is a way to be relevant in the political process, nursing must shed the perceptions of the opinion leaders in the RWJF study and be the leaders our patients need us to be.

NURSING UNITES: THE NURSING COMMUNITY

Comprising national nursing organizations, the Nursing Community (NC) coalition began as a forum of a handful of organizations with a shared interest in lobbying for federally funded nursing education programs. More specifically, the forum rallied around increasing federal support for the Nursing Workforce Development programs (Title VIII of the Public Health Service Act). Currently, the NC convenes 61-member organizations, and, over time, the expansion in its membership has brought with it an expanded portfolio of policy issues. Today, the NC is now a coalition representing more than 1 million registered nurses, APRNs, nurse executives, nursing students, faculty, and researchers who collaborate to improve the health of the nation by advancing the nursing profession (The Nursing Community, 2014). The NC's diverse nursing representation provides the coalition with expertise and insights into several aspects of the profession and adds to its political clout.

Earlier in this discussion, we addressed the importance of nurses being in influential roles to advance policy. After the Patient Protection and Affordable Care Act (ACA, Public Law 111-148) was passed into law, the NC met and evaluated opportunities for collective action. One identified goal was to ensure nursing leaders served on the commissions and boards newly established through the ACA. The traditional process for nursing organizations to nominate leaders onto commissions and boards was to look at their own membership and put forth one of their leaders. This resulted in

UNIT 5

multiple nurses being advanced for limited seats in a very competitive selection process. Two of the first calls for nominations into leadership positions from committees created through the ACA were the Patient-Centered Outcomes Research Institute (PCORI) and the National Health Care Workforce Commission. The NC realized that if nursing was to attain at least one representative within these policy bodies, the candidates must be supported on a unified front.

The mission of the PCORI is to "help people make informed health care decisions, and improved health care delivery and outcomes, by producing and promoting high integrity, evidence-based information that comes from research guided by patients, caregivers and the broader health care community" (PCORI, 2014, para 1). The NC engaged in creating a nomination process in which only a few, select nursing leaders would be nominated for these prestigious positions. Nursing organizations were able to submit candidates that would be collectively reviewed by all nursing organizations within the NC. The NC then established a vetting and voting process to select the top most-viable candidates from the names brought forth. The NC created a 168-page document outlining the strengths of each candidate. After nearly 2 months of thoughtful discussion among the organizations, four outstanding nursing candidates were put forth by the NC for the PCORI Board of Directors. The letter sent by the NC to the Comptroller General of the United States included the signatures of 33 organizations out of 55 national organizations belonging to the NC at the time.

The NC was pleased when one of the four candidates they put forth, Debra Barksdale, PhD, RN, FNP-BC, ANP-BC, CNE, FAANP, FAAN, was selected to serve on the PCORI Board of Governors (U.S. Government Accountability Office [GAO], 2010a) and another one of the candidates, Robin Newhouse, PhD, RN, NEA-BC, FAAN, was later selected to serve on PCORI's Methodology Committee (GAO, 2011).

The second policy body of interest, the National Health Care Workforce Commission, was established to "serve as a national resource for Congress, the President, and states and localities; to

communicate and coordinate with federal departments; to develop and commission evaluations of education and training activities; to identify barriers to improved coordination at the federal, state, and local levels and recommend ways to address them; and to encourage innovations that address population needs, changing technology, and other environmental factors" (GAO, 2010b). The NC put forth 5 candidates, with 32 NC member organizations supporting them. The Commission selected 15 leaders, and Peter Beurhaus, PhD, RN, FAAN, whom the NC supported as a nominee, was not only was selected onto the Commission but was also appointed as the Chairman by the Comptroller General.

Although the NC played a role in nominating these candidates, these nursing leaders engaged in the necessary process to gain a seat at the table. This example identifies the power of nursing unifying to meet goals set at the micro-level, which impacted the macro-level (i.e., the health care delivery system). As stated earlier, the IOM clearly calls for more nurses to serve in national leadership positions. The selection of Drs. Barksdale, Newhouse, and Beurhaus was a clear win in which the NC set goals and expectations, and delivered a successful outcome to meet this national agenda. Earlier in this chapter, we examined an example in Nebraska of how a few key individuals can significantly impact a policy dialogue. This story of the NC shows how it is imperative that our profession is represented in all policy and political circles, and this happens when we pool our resources. Since then, the NC has continued to collectively nominate nurse leaders such as Mary Naylor, PhD, RN, FAAN, who was appointed onto the Medicare Payment Advisory Commission, which is tasked with analyzing access to care, cost, and quality issues related to Medicare.

CONCLUSION

Effective coalitions can offer an amplified voice where the voice was once singular, marginal, or nonexistent. Leadership that can convene multiple perspectives is essential for setting the culture of the coalition and creating a unified voice. To use this voice effectively, clearly identifiable goals must be set so that coalition members understand their responsibility in the advocacy process and what constitutes a successful outcome. The NC has proven itself as an effective coalition for nursing when the profession needed unification most (i.e., when a seat at the policy table would give nursing political strength). However, the work is not done. The spectrum of issues continues to expand for nursing to pool its resources and elevate our public view as policy leaders, so that we can insert the expertise of nursing into the decisions that impact our patients. Now more than ever, the profession must be accountable for the outcomes we want to achieve for the national health care goals. United, we can achieve this.

REFERENCES

American Association of Colleges of Nursing. (2014). Letter to Nebraska, Chairperson Kathy Campbell, Health and Human Services Committee, Nebraska Unicameral Legislature. Retrieved from *www.aacn.nche.edu/government-affairs/SOP-in-Nebraska.pdf.*

Begeny, S. M. (2009). Lobbying strategies for federal appropriations: Nursing versus medical education. Retrieved from *hdl.handle.net/2027.42/64641.*

Des Jardin, K. E. (2001). Political involvement in nursing—Politics, ethics, and strategic action. *AORN Journal, 74*(5), 614–622.

Federal Trade Commission. (2014). Policy perspectives: Competition and the regulation of advanced practice nurses. Retrieved from *www.ftc.gov/system/files/documents/reports/policy-perspectives-competition-regulation-advanced-practice-nurses/140307aprnpolicypaper.pdf.*

Holyoke, T. (2009). Interest group competition and coalition formation. *American Journal of Political Science, 53*(2), 360–375.

Institute of Medicine [IOM]. (2011). *The future of nursing: Leading change, advancing health.* Washington, DC: National Academies Press.

Khoury, C. M., Blizzard, R., Wright Moore, L., & Hassmiller, S. (2011). Nursing leadership from bedside to boardroom: A Gallup national survey on opinion leaders. *Journal of Nursing Administration, 41*(7–8), 299–305.

Mizrahi, T., & Rosenthal, B. (2001). Complexities of coalition building: Leaders' successes, strategies, struggles, and solutions. *Social Work, 46*(1), 63–78.

Moe, T. (1980). *The organization of interests.* Chicago, IL: University of Chicago Press.

Nebraska.gov. (2014). Governor's veto letter on LB 916. Retrieved from *www.governor.nebraska.gov/news/2014/04/docs/0422_LB916_Veto_Message.pdf.*

Patient-Centered Outcomes Research Institute. (2014). Mission and vision. Retrieved from *www.pcori.org/about-us/mission-and-vision/.*

Robert Wood Johnson Foundation [RWJF]. (2010). Nursing leadership from bedside to boardroom: Opinion leaders' perceptions. Retrieved from *www.rwjf.org/content/dam/web-assets/2010/01/nursing-leadership-from-bedside-to-boardroom.*

Swift, A. (2013). *Honesty and ethics rating of clergy slides to new low.* Washington, DC: Gallup, Inc. Retrieved from *www.gallup.com/poll/166298/honesty-ethics-rating-clergy-slides-new-low.aspx.*

The Nursing Community. (2014). Members. Retrieved from *www.thenursingcommunity.org/#!members/cjg9.*

U.S. Government Accountability Office [GAO]. (2010a). Press release: GAO announces appointments to new Patient-Centered Outcomes Research Institute (PCORI) Board of Governors. Retrieved from *www.gao.gov/press/pcori2010sep23.html.*

U.S. Government Accountability Office [GAO]. (2010b). Press release: GAO announces appointments to new National Health Care Workforce Commission. Retrieved from *www.gao.gov/press/nhcwc_2010sep30.html.*

U.S. Government Accountability Office [GAO]. (2011). Press release: Appointments announced to Methodology Committee of Patient-Centered Outcomes Research Institute (PCORI). Retrieved from *www.gao.gov/press/pcori_2011jan21.html.*

CHAPTER 77

TAKING ACTION:

The Nursing Kitchen Cabinet: Policy and Politics in Action

Judith B. Collins   Rebecca (Rice) Bowers-Lanier

"Alone we can do so little; together we can do so much."

Helen Keller

THE CONTEXT

Raising the voice and visibility of nurses in Virginia is an ongoing challenge for Virginia nurse leaders. For the past three gubernatorial campaigns, 2005, 2009, and 2013, Virginia nurse leaders employed the Kitchen Cabinet as a strategy to influence and educate the gubernatorial candidates. This case example chronicles the journey focusing on the development and growth of the Kitchen Cabinet, from its inception in 2005 to the 2013 campaign. Through three gubernatorial campaigns and with varying degrees of success, we have employed strategies that increase nursing's influence. We will share those strategies and offer pointers for others wishing to influence political campaigns within their own states using the Kitchen Cabinet model.

Our journey began with nurse leaders' commitment to working together in the policy and political arenas. The mission of the Kitchen Cabinet was to educate the candidates about current nursing issues through a policy agenda, influence political campaigns, increase nurses' involvement, and ultimately change public policy and increase the visibility of nurses within the executive branch of government. The members were volunteer nurse opinion leaders who were passionate about the mission and were able to be dynamic and agile as the process unfolded. Throughout the campaigns, all nursing stakeholders were at the table: practice, education,

associations, and policy influencers. The methods required the Kitchen Cabinet to divide policy development from political action. Thus, the Kitchen Cabinet developed a common policy platform, although they differed on political persuasion.

POLICY DEVELOPMENT

The Kitchen Cabinet agreed on a plan to work together to develop a consensus, nonpartisan policy platform that has resulted in policy agendas that are nursing-centric and within the power of the Commonwealth's chief executive to implement (Box 77-1). These agenda items reflect the diverse perspectives of the nursing leaders and frame the issues that were (or continue to be) relevant in the campaign year.

POLITICAL ACTION

After completing the policy agenda, the Kitchen Cabinet focused its attention on the political work involved with communicating the message to the campaigns and working toward election of the candidates. In reality, the Kitchen Cabinet becomes two cabinets moving forward, Republican and Democrat.

The methods for achieving the political work have changed over the years. In 2005 and 2009, we were able to imbed nurses into the campaigns. In all three campaigns, meetings were held with the candidates themselves and/or their surrogates and Kitchen Cabinet members. The purpose of the meetings was to share with the candidates nursing's policy agenda, to educate about issues of importance to nurses, and to identify how they might assist the candidates toward successful election

---

BOX 77-1 Virginia Nurses' Kitchen Cabinet Policy Platforms 2005, 2009, and 2013

2005 Campaign	2009 Campaign	2013 Campaign
• A commitment to nursing workforce development with the creation of a statewide center for nursing. • A commitment from the Commonwealth to increase the educational capacity of the state's schools of nursing.	• A commitment from the Commonwealth to increase the educational capacity of the state's schools of nursing. • A commitment from the Commonwealth to allow full access to nurse practitioners. • A commitment for continued funding of the Department of Health Professions health care workforce data center.	• Enable advanced practice registered nurses to practice to their full scope of education and training. • Increase educational capacity and faculty salaries at the state's schools of nursing. • Ensure efficient regulatory process for the board of nursing. • Increase the number of nurses on public policy and regulatory boards.

---

campaigns. These nurses spearheaded efforts to hold nurses' fundraisers for the candidates and publicize their allegiances through bumper stickers and yard signs. In 2013, we scheduled meetings and looked for other opportunities to meet with the candidates and their campaign personnel. Increasingly, we are using social media to assist nurses in becoming politically active. This has involved posting candidate profiles on the Virginia Nurses Association's (VNA) website and information about campaign appearances through links to the candidates' websites.

RESULTS OF OUR WORK

In 2005, we met with huge success in our inaugural launch of the Kitchen Cabinet. Timothy Kaine was elected Governor, and he appointed two Kitchen Cabinet nurses to his health policy transition team. Both of these nurses then received gubernatorial appointments in the administration; one serving as the first nurse to head the Department of Health Professions (the umbrella health professions regulatory agency), and one as the Chair of the Virginia Council on Women.

The Governor also appointed other nurses in his administration and fostered the implementation of one of the long-term goals of the nursing community: he appointed a nurse, Marilyn Tavenner, as the Secretary of Health and Human Resources, a cabinet-level position (Tavenner is now the

Administrator for the Centers for Medicare and Medicaid Services). In 2006, he also appointed nurses to serve on his Health Reform Commission (HRC) and on Commission workgroups.

In addition to ensuring the presence of nurses in the executive branch and on gubernatorial appointed councils and commissions, we were incredibly successful in advancing our policy agenda. The primary overarching health workforce recommendation of the Governor's HRC was that the Commonwealth should invest in a health workforce data center. Although nursing's request and dream was a nursing workforce center, through the art of negotiation and compromise, we recognized the need for data on all health professions and thus supported this concept.

Our second policy platform request, to increase the educational capacity and faculty salaries in schools of nursing, was realized in 2007. The Governor submitted a budget request for a 10% increase in nurse faculty salary at all public colleges and universities. This request has been sustained throughout difficult economic realities.

In 2009, Virginia elected Bob McDonnell as Governor, who appointed Bill Hazel, MD, as his Secretary of Health and Human Resources. Secretary Hazel engaged all health care stakeholders around health reform and appointed VNA President Shirley Gibson to the Governor's Health Reform Initiative. Secretary Hazel ultimately recommended that nurses, especially advanced practice nurses, be used to the full extent of their scope of practice. To that end, the Virginia Council of Nurse Practitioners worked with the Medical Society of Virginia over a year-long process of negotiations to update the 1971 law, which required supervision of nurse practitioners by physicians. The result was a compromise bill that made incremental changes (dubbed the Virginia Way), removing some practice barriers. In particular, the language of physician supervision was replaced with consultation and collaboration. This relationship between the nurse practitioner organization and the physicians is ongoing, as nurse practitioners wish to fully implement the Institute of Medicine's (2011) *The Future of Nursing* recommendation on utilization of advanced practice nurses.

In 2013, Virginia elected Governor Terry McAuliffe and nurses were involved with developing questions for the gubernatorial candidates for a well-received and well-attended mental health forum. As Governor McAuliffe enters office at the time of this writing, he is informed about nursing issues and has key contacts who can advise him. These relationships are a direct result of nurses engaging early and throughout in the electoral process.

Through these years, Virginia nurses have grown in their ability to work collectively and collaboratively to achieve an agreed-upon set of common nursing policy goals. We also realize that our Kitchen Cabinet approach needs ongoing nurturing and rejuvenation with each election cycle. For the Kitchen Cabinet leaders, this process takes energy and commitment to advance the profession in a political environment. The goal continues to bring nursing leaders from both political party affiliation and all arenas of nursing to the table to develop a common public health policy agenda for nursing. Once the policy is established, political action is implemented to advocate/lobby/communicate/educate candidates based on the nurse leaders' party affiliation.

The major changes noted as the Kitchen Cabinet has evolved include:

- *Issues:* Policies needed reframing based on political realities and turbulence in the health care environment, such as passage and implementation of the Affordable Care Act (ACA) including Medicaid expansion and the health insurance exchange.
- *Communication styles:* Kitchen Cabinet members' face-to-face meetings have been replaced with conference calls, e-mails, and social media to increase political involvement.
- *Organizational dynamics:* Nursing organizations have a natural ebb and flow depending upon leadership. Kitchen Cabinet leaders must be attuned to these changes and inclusive of stakeholders.

DISCUSSION QUESTIONS

1. The Nursing Kitchen Cabinet members are meeting to develop the nurses' public/health policy agenda to present to the gubernatorial candidates in the upcoming statewide election. A serious concern for nursing is the lack of sufficient nursing faculty members for the student pipeline. The state is in financial difficulty. How would the Kitchen Cabinet proceed in developing a policy agenda?
2. The President of the State Nurses Association is invited to represent nursing at a fundraiser for a candidate for Governor. The President does not share the candidate's viewpoint. What are the President's options in responding to this request?
3. Describe three political actions nurses could take to strengthen their role in policymaking.

REFERENCES

Institute of Medicine. (2011). *The future of nursing: Leading change, advancing health.* Washington, DC: National Academies Press.

CHAPTER 78

TAKING ACTION:
Improving LGBTQ Health: Nursing Policy Can Make a Difference

Peggy L. Chinn   Michele J. Eliason   David M. Keepnews   Katie Oppenheim

"There are few moments in our lives that call for greater compassion and companionship than when a loved one is admitted to the hospital...Yet every day, all across America, patients are denied the kindnesses and caring of a loved one at their sides – whether in a sudden medical emergency or a prolonged hospital stay..."

Barack Obama, Presidential Memorandum,
Hospital Visitation, April 15, 2010

People with sexual and gender minority identities experience problems with access to quality health care and suffer physical and mental health disparities caused by societal stigma (Institute of Medicine [IOM], 2011), but their health care issues have not been sufficiently acknowledged in nursing education, research, policy, or practice (Eliason et al., 2009). In this chapter, we use both the acronyms LGBTQ (lesbian, gay, bisexual, transgender, and questioning/queer) and LGBTQI (lesbian, gay, bisexual, transgender, questioning/queer, and intersex), but there are a host of other identities that also comprise the larger population of sexual and gender minorities (Table 78-1). This chapter discusses nursing initiatives to address the needs of LGBTQ populations and outlines important steps that nursing organizations and individual nurses can consider to improve the quality of care to LGBTQ patients and their families.

LGBTQ RIGHTS IN THE UNITED STATES

Although organized advocacy for LGBTQ people in the United States dates back to at least the 1950s, the beginning of the current gay rights movement in the United States is most often attributed to the 1969 Stonewall riots in New York City in 1969. These riots erupted against a police raid, typical of the time, of gathering places for LGBTQ people. The riots also awakened widespread anger and frustration related to discrimination in housing, employment, health care, and other social institutions. The 1970s was a decade of progress for LGBTQ visibility. In the early 1980s, the advent of the HIV/AIDS epidemic initially sparked a backlash against LGBTQ rights, but by revealing widespread and damaging effects of stigma suffered by LGBTQ people it also raised their visibility. The epidemic was by no means limited to gay and bisexual men, the effect on these communities was devastating, and rallied many people to press for an end to health care practices that discriminated against or ignored the unique health challenges faced by LGBTQ people. The culture of silence that had shrouded the LGBTQ experience began to break open as more and more people came out to friends, family, and co-workers. Early in the twenty-first century, movements toward full equal rights for all LGBTQ individuals accelerated and scored significant successes in public policy and law. As of early 2015, 37 states and the District of Columbia had legalized same-sex marriage, and the U.S. Supreme Court had struck down legal prohibition of federal benefits for same-sex couples. In addition, research on health-related topics for LGBTQ people has broadened beyond HIV/AIDS and sexually transmitted infections to include issues of access to health care, quality of care, parenting, aging, and other topics.

623

TABLE 78-1 Definitions

Term	Definition
Lesbian	A woman who has romantic and sexual relationships primarily with other women and identifies as a lesbian.
Gay man	A man who has romantic and sexual relationships primarily with other men and identifies as gay.
Bisexual	Individuals whose romantic and sexual relationships are not dependent primarily on the sex of their partners.
Transgender	Individuals whose gender identification and/or expression differs from the sex assigned at birth. Trans men were born with female bodies; trans women with male bodies. Some have surgeries or use hormones to alter their bodies and some do not.
Queer	Some people do not identify with terms like lesbian, gay, or bisexual, but consider themselves to be outside of the mainstream heterosexual identity. Many youth use the term "gender queer" to indicate that they do not fit sexual or gender norms.
Questioning	Some individuals are not sure what sexual or gender identification best fits them and are in the process of exploring identities. This can happen at any age.
Intersex	A small subset of the population is born with genetic or endocrine differences that place their bodies somewhere on the spectrum between male and female. Because of the stigma often associated with a body that does not conform to societal norms, many people with intersex conditions have similar experiences of hiding their condition or experiencing shame and guilt about it as do LGBT people. Some people with an intersex condition identify as LGBTQ.
Allies	Many people who do not identify as LGBTQ are strong and active supporters of the struggle for LGBTQ equality.
LGBT, LGBTQ, LGBTQI, LGBTQIA, and so on	Organizations vary in how inclusive they are regarding the varieties of sexual and gender identifications. The most common acronym is LGBT, but if the organization serves many people with other identities, they may choose to include them all in their written materials. Every agency must make decisions about whom to include (and whom to exclude) when they issue policies or statements about cultural sensitivity. They may choose to use terms from specific populations they serve, such as Two Spirit (used by many indigenous people in the Americas) or Same Gender Loving (used by many African Americans).
Behavioral terms	Men who have Sex with Men (MSM) and Women who have Sex with Women (WSW) are terms often used by public health professionals to encompass individuals who have sex with others of the same sex but who may not identify as lesbian, gay, or bisexual.

NURSING AND LGBTQ ADVOCACY

Nurses were active in responding to the HIV/AIDS crisis. State and national nursing organizations advocated for HIV/AIDS care and funding and opposed discrimination against people with HIV/AIDS, including HIV-positive health professionals. The California Nurses Association played a leading role in initiating train-the-trainer programs to educate health professionals about the disease. Nurses helped to initiate specialized AIDS units in many hospitals to ensure compassionate, appropriate care for hospitalized patients with AIDS. They continue to be actively involved in HIV/AIDS care and research in the United States and globally.

However, the profession has been inconsistent in its willingness to advocate for LGBTQ issues in practice, education, research, or organizational policy (Keepnews, 2011). The American Nurses Association (ANA) adopted a statement in support of lesbian and gay rights in 1978, and in the 1990s opposed military discrimination against lesbian and gay people. The following sections summarize existing public policies and organizational initiatives that provide a foundation for LGBTQ advocacy in nursing.

ANTIDISCRIMINATION POLICIES

One of the most important steps that organizations and institutions can take is to create explicit non-discrimination policies related to LGBTQ people, including patients, employees, students, members, or participants. These examples of recent policy initiatives provide guidance in forming nursing antidiscrimination initiatives:

- In November, 2010, the U.S. Department of Health and Human Services issued a rule requiring hospitals to ensure equal visitation rights for same-sex partners (U.S. Department of Health and Human Services, 2010).
- The Joint Commission as of July 1, 2011 required that hospitals prohibit discrimination on the basis of sexual orientation and gender identity (Joint Commission, 2011).
- In 2011, the Institute of Medicine issued a landmark report that provided recommendations for an emphasis on LGBT populations in research, including improved methods for collecting and analyzing data to build a more solid evidence base for LGBT health care (IOM, 2011).

PUBLIC POLICY STATEMENTS ON LGBTQ HEALTH ISSUES

Adopting public policy statements representing a group's support for LGBTQ rights is a step that organizations can take. Recent policy statements provide examples that organizations can consider in making public policy statements.

- Two policy statements were initiated by the American Academy of Nursing (AAN) Expert Panel on LGBTQ Health in 2012: a statement in support of marriage equality and one on health care for sexual minority and gender-diverse individuals (American Academy of Nursing, 2012). The statement on marriage equality was also supported by the AAN Expert Panel on Cultural Competency and was subsequently endorsed by the Association of Nurses in AIDS Care. The ANA also adopted a position in support of marriage equality.

- The American College of Nurse Midwives issued a policy statement in December 2012 supporting access to safe, comprehensive, and culturally competent health care for transgender and gender-variant individuals and their families (American College of Nurse Midwives, 2012).
- The National Association of School Nurses adopted a revised statement entitled *Sexual Orientation and Gender Identity/Expression (Sexual Minority Students): School Nurse Practice* (National Association of School Nurses, 2012).
- The National Student Nurses Association (NSNA) adopted resolutions on LGBT health:
  - In 2010, the NSNA adopted a resolution submitted by Johns Hopkins University students calling for culturally competent education about LGBT individuals (National Student Nurses Association [NSNA], 2010).
  - In 2012, the NSNA adopted a resolution calling for implementation of The Joint Commission field guide (NSNA, 2012).

TAKING ACTION

It is time for nurses and nursing to take major steps to create policy changes and improve quality of care for all LGBTQ people and their families. Some of the changes require organizational actions and changes, but individual nurses can also take important steps to assure safe, culturally competent, and quality care for all LGBTQ people by being aware of their own beliefs and behaviors. All nurses can also refrain from engaging in any conversation that is derogatory or demeaning toward LGBTQ people, and interrupt such conversations by others.

In Table 78-2, we provide an LGBTQI Welcoming and Inclusive Services Checklist that nurses can use to assess the LGBTQI competency of an organization and to raise awareness of areas that need work. There are five sections on the Checklist. The first section, Institution or Agency Policies and Procedures, involves creating policies, procedures, and practices that assure LGBTQI patients, families, and employees are treated with respect and offered all the benefits and privileges afforded anyone else. The second section, Staff Training/Conduct, sets standards for educating providers about LGBTQI

TABLE 78-2 LGBTQI Welcoming and Inclusive Services Checklist

Yes	No	Institution or Agency Policies and Procedures
☐	☐	We have a nondiscrimination policy for staff members that includes sexual orientation and gender identity
☐	☐	We have a nondiscrimination policy for patients that includes sexual orientation and gender identity
☐	☐	Our mission statement is inclusive; it names LGBTQI people
☐	☐	We offer domestic partner benefits to LGBTQI employees
☐	☐	Patient confidentiality policies include how to deal with patients who do not want information about sexuality or gender on their records
☐	☐	Our sexual harassment policy includes LGBTQI issues
☐	☐	We have a procedure for staff or patients to grieve issues of discrimination based on sexuality and/or gender
☐	☐	Written notice is given to patients about when and for what reason information about them may be disclosed to a third party

Staff Training/Conduct

Yes	No	
☐	☐	All staff get basic training on LGBTQI people and issues at least once
☐	☐	Some staff get advanced training
☐	☐	At least one staff member has expertise in working with LGBTQI patients
☐	☐	All staff treat LGBTQI patients with respect and honor confidentiality
☐	☐	Staff members know how to intervene when patients act in a discriminatory manner to LGBTQI patients or their families

Inclusive Language: Forms/Assessments/Treatment

Yes	No	
☐	☐	Written forms have inclusive language and encourage disclosure
☐	☐	Assessments are inclusive and encourage discussion of whether gender or sexuality issues need to be addressed in treatment
☐	☐	Case management, treatment, and aftercare plans include issues related to sexuality and gender if appropriate
☐	☐	Staff members get a sexual history from all patients
☐	☐	Treatment groups, social activities, and all aspects of the institution are safe for LGBTQI patients (receptionists, laboratory technicians, housekeepers, ward clerks, kitchen staff, clergy)

Visibility of LGBTQI People and Issues

Yes	No	
☐	☐	We advertise employment opportunities in LGBTQI publications
☐	☐	We have openly LGBTQI people on staff
☐	☐	We have openly LGBTQI people on the board of directors, community advisory panels, agency task forces, and so on
☐	☐	We have openly LGBTQI people as volunteers, sponsors, mentors
☐	☐	Our nondiscrimination policy that includes LGBTQI is prominently displayed
☐	☐	Families of LGBTQI patients are included in visitation policies
☐	☐	LGBTQI issues are discussed in treatment groups, health education sessions, case management sessions, and other group settings when appropriate
☐	☐	Posters, pamphlets, magazines, and other materials reflect our LGBTQI patients
☐	☐	We do outreach/market our services to local LGBTQI communities

Resources and Linkages

Yes	No	
☐	☐	We have checked our referral sources to make sure that they are LGBTQI-sensitive (home care, clinics for follow-up care, community agencies, and so on)
☐	☐	We have linkages to our local LGBTQI community
☐	☐	We screen clergy, guest speakers, volunteers, mentors, sponsors, and so on, to make sure they know that we are welcoming and inclusive of LGBTQI people

appropriate care and assures that all patients and families have access to a provider who has sensitivity in caring for LGBTQI patients and families.

The section titled Inclusive Language: Forms/Assessments/Treatment is also part of a comprehensive program of staff training and conduct and involves changing both written and spoken language. This section and Visibility of LGBTQI People and Issues are essential to create a welcoming environment for any person or family who might identify as LGBTQI. If there is not a welcoming environment, the care that LGBTQI people receive is compromised because of fear of discrimination. The final section, Resources and Linkages, prompts an agency to become familiar with the groups, individuals, and organizations in the community that can provide additional care and support for LGBTQI employees, patients, and families. Achieving all of the points on the checklist is a formidable task, but well worth working toward!

CONCLUSION

Although nursing as a whole has been slow to respond to the needs of LGBTQ communities (Eliason, Dibble, & DeJoseph, 2010), as we have shown, significant policy initiatives have started to appear, and resources (see Online Resources) are beginning to appear in the nursing literature to guide institutions toward quality care for all patients in the communities that they serve (Eliason et al., 2009). The most important steps are for all nurses to be aware of biases and stereotypes that interfere with quality care for LGBTQ people and their families; to be sensitive to the perspectives, fears, and particular needs of LGBTQ people as they encounter a health care situation; and to be knowledgeable about LGBTQ health.

REFERENCES

American Academy of Nursing. (2012). Support for marriage equality. Retrieved from *www.aannet.org/assets/docs/marriage equality_7-26 12f.pdf*.

American College of Nurse Midwives. (2012). Transgender/transsexual/gender variant health care. Retrieved from *www.midwife.org/ACNM/files/ACNMLibraryData/UPLOADFILENAME/000000000278/Transgender%20Gender%20Variant%20Position%20Statement%20December%202012.pdf*.

Eliason, M., Dibble, S., & DeJoseph, J. (2010). Nursing's silence on lesbian, gay, bisexual and transgender issues: The need for emancipatory efforts. *ANS. Advances in Nursing Science, 33*(3), 1–13.

Eliason, M., Dibble, S., DeJoseph, J., & Chinn, P. L. (2009). *LGBTQ cultures: What health care professionals need to know about sexual and gender diversity*. Philadelphia, PA: Lippincott Williams & Wilkins.

Institute of Medicine [IOM]. (2011). *The health of lesbian, gay, bisexual, and transgender people: Building a foundation for better understanding*. Washington, DC: National Academies Press.

Joint Commission. (2011). Advancing effective communication, cultural competence, and patient- and family-centered care for the lesbian, gay, bisexual and transgender (LGBT) community: A field guide. Retrieved from *www.jointcommission.org/assets/1/18/LGBTFieldGuide.pdf*.

Keepnews, D. M. (2011). Lesbian, gay, bisexual and transgender (LGBT) health issues and nursing: Moving toward an agenda. *Advances in Nursing Science, 34*(2), 163–170.

National Association of School Nurses. (2012). Sexual orientation and gender identity/expression (sexual minority students): School nurse practice. Retrieved from *www.nasn.org/PolicyAdvocacy/PositionPapersandReports/NASNPositionStatementsFullView/tabid/462/ArticleId/47/Sexual-Orientation-and-Gender-Identity-Expression-Sexual-Minority-Students-School-Nurse-Practice-Rev*.

National Student Nurses Association [NSNA]. (2010). In support of increasing culturally competent education about gay, lesbian bisexual, transgender (LGBT) individuals. Retrieved from *www.nsna.org/Portals/0/Skins/NSNA/pdf/Final Resolutions 2010_11.pdf*.

National Student Nurses Association [NSNA]. (2012). In support of implementing practices suggested in the Joint Commission report "Advancing effective communication, cultural competence, and patient- and family-centered care for lesbian, gay, bisexual, transgender (LGBT) community: A field guide." Retrieved from *www.nsna.org/Portals/0/Skins/NSNA/pdf/20.pdf*.

U.S. Department of Health and Human Services. (2010). Medicare finalizes new rules to require equal visitation rights for all hospital patients. Retrieved from *www.whitehouse.gov/blog/2010/11/17/new-rules-require-equal-visitation-rights-all-patients*.

ONLINE RESOURCES

The Joint Commission: Advancing Effective Communication, Cultural Competence, and Patient- and Family-Centered Care for the Lesbian, Gay, Bisexual and Transgender (LGBT) Community
www.jointcommission.org/assets/1/18/LGBTFieldGuide_WEB_LINKED_VER.pdf

Fenway Health: Information for Providers
www.fenwayhealth.org/site/PageServer?pagename=FCHC_res_Provider Documents

Institute of Medicine: The Health of Lesbian, Gay, Bisexual, and Transgender People: Building a Foundation for Better Understanding
www.iom.edu/Reports/2011/The-Health-of-Lesbian-Gay-Bisexual-and-Transgender-People.aspx

UNIT 5

CHAPTER 79

TAKING ACTION:
Campaign for Action

Susan B. Hassmiller

"Commitment is an act, not a word."

Jean-Paul Sartre

There has long been a consensus across the political spectrum that the country's health care system is not doing all it can to improve patient and population health and that nurses are well positioned to be part of the solution to this problem. The Robert Wood Johnson Foundation (RWJF) has a proud history of supporting nurses, investing more than $600 million over its history in programs to support, grow and strengthen the nursing workforce. But change is never simple or easy, and persistent barriers to expanding nurses' roles exist.

To begin overcoming those barriers, identifying ways to address a debilitating nurse faculty shortage and to build an evidence base to support change, RWJF made what is arguably its most impactful nursing investment ever: a partnership with the esteemed Institute of Medicine (IOM) to support a major study on the future of nursing. The IOM brought together respected experts from diverse fields to define the health care challenges facing the United States and the role of nurses in meeting them. Chaired by Donna E. Shalala, president of the University of Miami and a former U.S. Secretary of Health and Human Services, the IOM committee spent two years reviewing scientific literature and talking to diverse experts about the nursing workforce.

THE FUTURE OF NURSING REPORT

The product of its work was *The Future of Nursing: Leading Change, Advancing Health* (2011), a report that envisioned new roles for nurses in the rapidly evolving U.S. health care system. The report noted the essential roles played by nurses, who are the providers who spend the most time directly caring for patients and, at 3.1 million in number, make up the largest segment of the health care workforce. The IOM report was a blueprint for action on nursing and it made a compelling case for a nursing workforce that is diverse, well educated, and prepared to practice to the full extent of its education and training to meet patient needs and become full partners in the implementation of health care reform.

The report recommended improving nurse education, fostering inter-professional education and collaboration, making nurses full partners in redesigning the health care system, creating an infrastructure to collect nursing workforce data, diversifying the nursing workforce, implementing nurse residency programs, and preparing and supporting nurses to lead change. It recommended increasing the number of nurses with bachelor's degrees to 80% by the year 2020 and removing barriers that prevent nurses from practicing to the full extent of their training and abilities. If implemented, these recommendations would be transformational for the nursing professional and the country's health care system.

A VISION FOR IMPLEMENTING THE FUTURE OF NURSING REPORT

RWJF put a plan in place to ensure that the IOM's *Future of Nursing* report did not simply sit on bookshelves. It created the Future of Nursing: Campaign for Action, a partnership between RWJF, the nation's largest health philanthropy, and AARP, the nation's largest consumer organization, to implement its recommendations. The ultimate test of the Campaign's

BOX 79-1 Join the Campaign for Action!

You can join the Future of Nursing: Campaign for Action by visiting its website (*www.CampaignForAction.org*) which contains a wealth of information on the Institute of Medicine report *The Future of Nursing: Leading Change, Advancing Health (CampaignforAction.org/evidence/iom -report)*, and the work to implement its recommendations. The Campaign website offers information about recent accomplishments, state activity, and upcoming events, as well as resources for those who want to support its work. In addition, you can follow the Campaign for Action on Facebook *(www.facebook.com/CampaignForAction)* or Twitter *(@Campaign4Action)*.

success would be whether or not the IOM's *Future of Nursing* became a catalyst for change (Box 79-1).

Launched in conjunction with the report's release, the Campaign moved quickly to mobilize the nursing community, sending the message that implementing the IOM recommendations was every nurse's responsibility. It also engaged a broad spectrum of partners from business, consumer organizations, government, health care, philanthropy, academia, and other sectors. The engagement strategy was successful, and the future of nursing became the IOM's most-read report in the years after its release, as well as the top reason people visited the IOM website.

Because much policy change happens at the state level, the Campaign created state Action Coalitions, each co-led by a nurse and a partner who is not a nurse. The focus on nurse leadership was designed both to harness enthusiasm in the nursing community and to help nurses see themselves as agents of change. In 2 years, Action Coalitions were active in all 50 states and the District of Columbia. All 51 chose to focus on the IOM's academic progression recommendation; many also opted to promote nurse leadership, seek to expand nurses' scope of practice, and support data collection on the nursing workforce. Most of the IOM recommendations were welcomed enthusiastically, but, as is often the case, there was some resistance also. At the federal level and for the Action Coalitions, progress came quickly on some fronts and barriers emerged on others.

Engagement with the Campaign for Action was impressive, with the nurse academic community

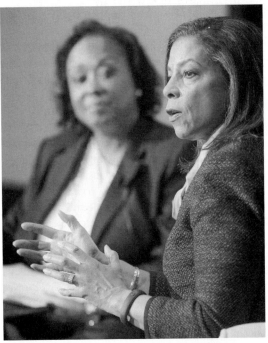

FIGURE 79-1 Risa Lavizzo-Mourey, MD MBA, President and CEO of the Robert Wood Johnson Foundation being interviewed at the 2013 Future of Nursing Campaign Summit. Interviewer is Linda Wright Moore, Senior Communications Officer, Robert Wood Johnson Foundation.

engaging nursing students, nursing associations, and highly educated nurses. Some nurses with associate degrees voiced concerns, however, regarding their ability to go back to school to get bachelor's degrees and that they would not be able to compete for jobs and promotions without them. Efforts to promote interprofessional education and collaboration picked up steam; nurse residency programs began springing up; and efforts to diversify the nursing workforce began to show slow but steady progress. However, efforts to remove barriers that restrict nurses' scope of practice faced opposition in Missouri, California, and several other states.

SUCCESS AT THE NATIONAL LEVEL

Progress has been tangible. Examples to date include: (1) For the first time in its history, Medicare announced it would pay to support training of advanced practice nurses through a $200 million demonstration project in five major hospital systems. (2) The late Sen. Daniel K. Inouye (D-HI) and Sen. Jay Rockefeller (D-WV) reached out to the Federal Trade Commission (FTC) regarding scope of practice restrictions in nursing. The FTC responded by challenging those limits in several states. (3) The Leapfrog Group reported that a hospital's Magnet status is an indicator of having an adequate and competent nursing staff and good nursing leadership in its 2011 Hospital Survey. The Magnet Recognition Program recognizes health care organizations for quality patient care, nursing excellence, and innovations in professional nursing practice. Before a hospital could apply or reapply for Magnet status, it would be required to adopt a plan that advances the goal of having 80% of its nurses holding baccalaureate degrees. (4) The National Organization for Associate Degree Nursing published a commentary expressing support for associate degree nurses to continue their education and urged employers to help them get higher degrees. A roundtable convened by RWJF found common ground between community colleges and nursing leaders on key issues, including the central role community colleges play in preparing and diversifying the nursing workforce and the need for all nurses to be lifelong learners. In several states, nursing and community college leaders began exploring ways to help both aspiring nurses and those already in the workforce to obtain higher degrees. At the state level, Action Coalitions made progress as well.

SUCCESS AT THE STATE LEVEL

ACADEMIC PROGRESSION

Texas, Idaho, and Washington were among the states to strengthen and standardize nursing education classes to create more seamless progression for associate degree nurses looking to continue their education. In 2013, New Mexico's governor announced a common curriculum between community college- and university-based nursing schools, and California implemented a groundbreaking effort to help nurses get advanced degrees.

CALIFORNIA: OPENING DOORS TO ACADEMIC PROGRESSION

An initiative designed to ease the transition between associate and baccalaureate degree nursing programs admitted its first students in the summer of 2013. Based at the School of Nursing at California State University, Los Angeles, the program enables students with associate degrees in nursing to earn baccalaureate degrees in nursing in just 12 months. Typically, this transition has taken students 2 years to complete and often involved redundant coursework because of inconsistent curricula across nursing schools. The new program allows students to get their bachelor's degrees in nursing with no repetition of courses. The program also enhances diversity in the nursing workforce and helps develop more nurse leaders.

SCOPE OF PRACTICE

In state after state, regulatory barriers to nurse practitioners' ability to practice to the full extent of their education and training were challenged, and some fell. Although some physicians groups opposed eliminating such barriers, many individual physicians spoke out in favor of doing so. In Colorado and Iowa, courts struck down barriers on nurses' scope of practice. In Nevada, the Action Coalition helped win a law eliminating them.

NEVADA: ACHIEVING POLITICAL CHANGE ON A CONTENTIOUS ISSUE

Nevada's governor signed a law in 2013 that gave advanced practice registered nurses full practice authority and expanded prescriptive authority. Enacting this law was a key priority of the Nevada Action Coalition because it frees advanced practice registered nurses from practice restrictions that required them to work under the supervision of a physician. The removal of that requirement is expected to increase access to care and to prescription medication in the heavily rural state, which has a low physician-to-population ratio, an aging population, and a shortage of primary care providers.

NURSE LEADERSHIP

Across the country, Action Coalitions have focused on preparing nurses to serve on boards of directors

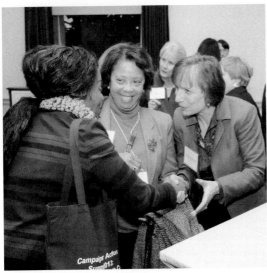

FIGURE 79-2 (From right to left) Susan Hassmiller, PhD, RN, FAAN, Director of the Future of Nursing: Campaign for Action, welcomes two new members of the District of Columbia Action Coalition, Pier Broadnax, PhD, RN, and Delores Clair Oliver, RN, MHA, CNAA, BC.

and on creating opportunities for them to do so. In Virginia, the Action Coalition created a statewide mentorship program to support emerging nurse leaders. The Texas and Montana Action Coalitions pioneered strategies to place nurses on boards of directors of health institutions. The New Jersey Action Coalition prioritized this work from the start.

NEW JERSEY PRIORITIZES PLACING NURSES ON BOARDS OF DIRECTORS

Shortly after it was formed, the New Jersey Action Coalition created a leadership workgroup that compiled a list of names of nurse leaders to recommend for appointments to various boards and other leadership positions. At the same time, the Action Coalition created a list of leadership opportunities to disseminate, so that nurses could prepare for becoming members of these boards and could develop leadership skills with these open positions in mind. Very quickly, nine nurses identified on the list assumed positions of influence, and the progress has continued.

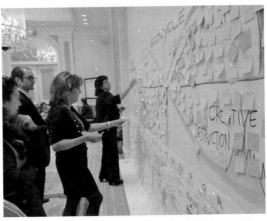

FIGURE 79-3 Future of Nursing: Campaign for Action members participating in a national summit.

CONCLUSION

By developing strategic partnerships, mobilizing a broad base of supporters, deploying resources wisely, and helping parties with different perspectives find common ground, the Future of Nursing: Campaign for Action has made progress in implementing the recommendations of the IOM's nursing report. However the work has really just begun. More challenges, and more progress, lie ahead in achieving the Campaign's goal: that everyone in America can live a healthier life, supported by a system in which nurses are essential partners in providing care and promoting health (Figs. 79-1 to 79-3).

REFERENCES

Institute of Medicine. (2011). *The future of nursing: Leading change, advancing health.* Washington, DC: National Academies Press. Retrieved from *www.iom.edu/nursing.*

ONLINE RESOURCES

Institute of Medicine: The Future of Nursing: Leading Change, Advancing Health
www.iom.edu/Reports/2010/The-future-of-nursing-leading-change -advancing-health.aspx
Future of Nursing: Campaign for Action
www.CampaignforAction.org
Robert Wood Johnson Foundation (nursing information)
www.RWJF.org/Nursing
Robert Wood Johnson Foundation: Charting Nursing's Future policy briefs
www.rwjf.org/en/search-results.html?cs=content_series%3Acharting -nursings-future

UNIT 5

CHAPTER 80

TAKING ACTION:
The Nightingales Take on Big Tobacco

Kelly Buettner-Schmidt   Ruth E. Malone

"Neglecting to discuss the industry's role as the disease vector in the tobacco epidemic is like refusing to discuss the role of mosquitoes in a malaria epidemic or rats in an outbreak of bubonic plague."

Rob Cushman, MD, Medical Officer of Health, Ottawa

TOBACCO KILLS

Tobacco use caused 100 million deaths in the twentieth century and kills about 6 million people worldwide annually (World Health Organization [WHO], 2013). Describing this in understandable numbers for laypeople should be among a nurse's roles. This translates into 1 out of every 10 adult deaths or one person every 6 seconds. In the United States, tobacco use and exposure remains the leading cause of preventable death, killing 480,000 people annually between 2005 and 2009, including more than 1000 infants (U.S. Department of Health and Human Services [HHS], 2014a). Since the first U.S. Surgeon General's Report in 1964, more than 20 million have died from tobacco use and exposure to secondhand smoke in the United States (HHS, 2014a).

Meanwhile, in the United States alone, in 2011 the tobacco industry spent $8.4 billion promoting cigarettes and another $450 million pushing smokeless tobacco products (Federal Trade Commission, 2013). Globally, tobacco companies are now aggressively targeting low- and middle-income countries, seeking new generations of young people and women who will develop tobacco addiction.

Electronic cigarettes (e-cigs) are the latest tobacco industry deception, with many tobacco control advocates concerned about the lack of regulation, misleading advertising, and the rapid uptake by youth.

RUTH'S STORY

"The latest news from me is that I died May 9, 1990, of lung cancer. Maybe my widower would like your free trip. Although I doubt it … You see, he has been mourning my death for 4 years. I was all he had left—me and my Benson & Hedges. Wish you were here" (Halpin, 1994). An elderly widower, perhaps sitting alone under the lamp at the kitchen table where he and his wife had eaten many meals together, wrote these words to the Philip Morris tobacco company in a trembling hand on the back of a glossy Benson & Hedges cigarette brand mailer.

I found his letter online, one of perhaps thousands written to tobacco companies by suffering customers and their families. Something about it would not let me rest. In many ways, he and the many others whose letters I found, were the founders of the Nightingales Nurses.

I smoked for years and felt guilty as I cared for patients suffering from emphysema, lung cancer, or heart disease. I tried to quit so many times but would slip back. I felt so alone. More than 20 years ago, I vividly remember reading about new studies showing that smoking was not really so bad, comparing it with eating chocolate or having a glass of wine. I never dreamed, then, that the tobacco industry was behind those phony studies (Smith, 2007).

What I didn't know then would fill a book, and several good ones have been written since by historians. Mainly, I didn't realize that the tobacco industry (TI) had set up front groups, hired scientists, organized massive campaigns to promote bogus ideas, and sponsored distracting scientific studies selected by industry lawyers to be sure they would result in findings favorable to the industry. They had promoted their intentionally deceptive ideas through an astonishingly large and varied assortment of paid consultants and front groups (Bero, 2003, 2005; Glantz, Slade et al., 1996). I had no idea that the TI had special marketing plans developed to reassure those, like me, who worried even as we lit up another cigarette (Brown and Williamson Tobacco Company, 1971; Cataldo & Malone, 2008) and that they were working on a global scale to fight tobacco control policies to ensure that smoking remained socially acceptable (Malone, 2009; McDaniel, Intinarelli, & Malone, 2008; McDaniel & Malone, 2009; Zeltner et al., 2000).

I didn't know that the cigarette had been carefully engineered to make it easy to start smoking and harder to quit and that in the process it had been made even more deadly (Proctor, 2011). I didn't realize then that tobacco companies had explicitly targeted their aggressive marketing and outreach efforts to the most vulnerable groups: the poor, less educated, and minority groups (Apollonio & Malone, 2005; Balbach, Gasior, & Barbeau, 2003; Cook et al., 2004; Landrine et al., 2005; McCandless, Yerger, & Malone, 2011; Muggli et al., 2002; Smith & Malone, 2003; Yerger & Malone, 2002).

THE PERSONAL BECOMES POLITICAL

I finally quit smoking for good after struggling for years. Going back to school helped build my confidence. In a postdoctoral fellowship, I began research on tobacco-control policy and I learned more about tobacco than I ever had in nursing school.

I learned that until the advent of the machine-rolled cigarette in the late 1800s, almost nobody ever died from lung cancer. It was once such a rare disease that most physicians never saw a case in their lifetimes. Those same entrepreneurs who introduced machine-rolled cigarettes also introduced aggressive, innovative advertising techniques that linked cigarettes with glamour, freedom, sexuality, and status (Kluger, 1997). I realized we were facing an industrially produced disease epidemic from tobacco.

More than 10 million internal tobacco company documents became publicly available as the result of multiple state attorneys general lawsuits in the late 1990s and are now accessible online at the Legacy Tobacco Documents Library. They offer an amazing window into this incredibly destructive industry. I developed a program of research drawing on these documents, and while doing this research, I stumbled upon the letters.

COMPELLING VOICES

"My father died last October at the age of 50 due to lung cancer," one read. "He purchased many of your items in your *Marlboro Country Store Catalog* with his cigarette coupons … Now myself and my 16 year old sister are left fatherless … smoking does cause cancer, does kill and destroy families. You don't need to be a scientist or conduct a study to figure that out, just visit my Dad's grave if you want proof." The words were in the fat, round script of a teenage girl, and the file I found contained many more such letters, written by every sort of human hand. Most were written on the backs of or in response to slick mailers from tobacco companies: catalogs, birthday cards, and offers of coupons for cigarette discounts. There were letters from grieving mothers, widows, sons, and daughters; letters from friends and family; and letters from dying smokers and those struggling to escape tobacco addiction. They were testimony: "I know that we all have to work to put food on the table and pay bills. But are there no other choices?"

The letters weren't asking for money, they wanted their human pain and loss to be acknowledged by those who had furthered it through promoting tobacco use. A woman, grieving over her mother's death at 57 from lung cancer, wrote, "My mother wanted to quit so badly … When I close my eyes at night, all I can see is my mother's face as she lay dying, and all the hell that she went through … that will haunt our family forever."

UNIT 5

As a nurse, I could easily fill in the terrible subtext accompanying every anguished word. Behind each letter were family members who had used every economic and emotional resource they had trying to cope with the suffering and loss of a loved one, orphaned children who would never have the guidance of a father or mother, and aging parents who helplessly watched their children die before them. I knew that the suffering from tobacco-related illnesses was often terrible to witness, and far worse to experience. And these stories were repeated more than 440,000 times every year, year after year, in the United States alone (HHS, 2013).

By the early 2000s, I knew the tobacco industry had tried to undermine the work of WHO and other public health bodies (Zeltner et al., 2000) and to interfere with tobacco-control efforts (WHO, 2009). I knew that the industry's political and philanthropic contributions bought silence from policymakers and groups that should have been protecting the public (Tesler & Malone, 2008; Yerger & Malone, 2002). But somehow, I had never once considered that these companies had been getting letters like these for decades and filing them away, year after deadly year. Although I tried to continue with my research projects the letters would not let me rest. It simply wasn't right for them to remain forever hidden in the tobacco industry's files.

Inspired by youth activists who had attended the Altria/Philip Morris shareholders' meeting to speak out about the industry's targeting of youth, I decided to buy one share of stock and go to the shareholders' meeting as a nurse, taking some of the letters with me to read aloud in protest. I recruited 11 other nurses from around the country who agreed to buy one share of Altria stock (only shareholders or their representatives could attend the meeting) and travel with me to the meeting in New Jersey. Other nurses paid for the airfares. We picked the Altria/Philip Morris meeting because Philip Morris is the largest U.S. tobacco company.

With our theme, nurses bearing witness, we sought to point out the contradictions in the company's claims to be changed and socially responsible while continuing the aggressive promotion of the most deadly consumer product ever made. Our key message: "A socially responsible company would not continue to promote products that it admits addict and kill." We were the first nursing group to confront Big Tobacco on its own turf (Schwarz, 2004, 2005).

STRATEGIC PLANNING

A nurse in New Jersey who was active with the American Lung Association scoped out the site for us. Other activists working with youth invited us to be part of a post-shareholder's meeting press conference. We assembled a selection of the letters into a 30-foot banner and made handouts about our efforts, including some of the letters and a press release (Box 80-1). We learned from other activists about the meeting format and how long we might have to speak. We wore white lab coats and black armbands, indicating solidarity with those who suffered from tobacco. That year, and every year since, the Nightingales Nurses have borne witness at tobacco company shareholder meetings.

KELLY'S STORY

When I first heard of the Nightingales, I searched the Internet to learn more and immediately joined. I had never heard of shareholder advocacy, but I had a long history of activism and advocacy for tobacco control. My own journey in tobacco policy had begun with my first cigarette puff in junior high school. I was nauseated and then embarrassed. The next year, while playing basketball, I realized that smoking and playing ball were in conflict, and I quit. I was one of the lucky ones, I escaped addiction.

In my first nursing position, I saw so many who did not escape. I once shut off the oxygen in an elderly man's room to allow him to smoke. I did not tell him about the dangers of smoking, but I found it ironic that he needed oxygen because of his smoking and yet he still desired to smoke. I now recognize this was a testament to nicotine's addictiveness.

Teaching smoking cessation classes in the late 1980s was moving, frustrating, and unsettling. Unfortunately, at the time, tobacco was considered a habit, and nicotine was not declared an addiction by the U.S. Surgeon General until 1988 (HHS, 1988). Midway through the program was quit day, but often less than a quarter of the participants

BOX 80-1 Nightingales' Press Release (Example)

PRESS RELEASE

NIGHTINGALES NURSES ACCUSE PHILIP MORRIS OF SOCIAL IRRESPONSIBILITY

DATE: Embargo release until 12:00 Noon Eastern Time Thursday April 29, 2010

CONTACT: Ruth Malone, RN, PhD, ruth.malone@ucsf .edu, (415) 123-4567

PRESS CONFERENCE: 12:00 Noon at Philip Morris entrance, 188 Rover Road, East Hanover, NJ

EAST HANOVER, NJ: Nurses from across America will attend the annual shareholders meeting of Philip Morris/ Altria tomorrow to call on the company to demonstrate genuine corporate social responsibility by voluntarily ending all active promotion and marketing of tobacco products. A press conference will be held immediately after the meeting, with the Nightingales Nurses reading and sharing letters sent to the company by its dying customers and their families.

"We're here to say that this can't go on," said Nightingales organizer Ruth Malone, RN, Professor of Nursing at the University of California, San Francisco, School of Nursing. "The tobacco industry spends more than $1 million an hour, 24/7, on making their deadly, addictive products look fun, cool, and glamorous—but these letters show the terrifying, painful reality of what cigarettes do."

As the largest group of health care providers, the nation's 3.1 million nurses are in a unique position at the bedside and in the community to witness firsthand the deadly effects of tobacco products. "A socially responsible company would not continue to promote a product that they themselves admit addicts and kills," said Diana Hackbarth, RN, Professor of Nursing at Loyola University in Chicago and a Fellow of the American Academy of Nursing.

Wearing black armbands to honor the memories of their patients who have suffered and died from cigarette-caused diseases, nurses are attending the meeting to tell their patients' stories, giving voice to those who can no longer speak because tobacco addiction has robbed them of breath and life.

The Nightingales is a group of nurses who use advocacy, activism, and education to focus public attention on the role of the tobacco industry in creating the epidemic of tobacco-caused suffering, disease, and death.

For more information or to join, visit the Nightingales Website at *www.nightingalesnurses.org.*

would remain quit for 48 hours, the disappointment and frustration showed clearly on their faces, if they came back to class at all. Seeing firsthand the power of addiction in people who strove so hard to quit was disturbing. Although smoking cessation success rates can be complex, currently 43% of all adults who tried to quit smoking succeeded for more than one day (Centers for Disease Control and Prevention [CDC], 2011). To increase success in cessation, best practices call for systems level changes to support individuals, increased coverage by insurance for cessation, and enhancements of state quit lines (CDC, 2014).

POLICY ADVOCACY

In 1992, I led a local public health tobacco prevention program in Minot, North Dakota. After developing a broad-based coalition, Stop Tobacco Access by Minors Program (STAMP), we successfully advocated for five local youth access laws. The policy and advocacy lessons learned through these efforts were invaluable for our later work on smoke-free environments that resulted in Minot being the first community in the state to pass a local smoke-free ordinance (Buettner-Schmidt, Muhlbrad & Brierley, 2003; Rosenbaum, Barnes & Glantz, 2012; Welle, Ibrahim & Glantz, 2004).

Our smoke-free environment efforts included public education events and billboard contests, collaborating with the American Cancer Society to encourage restaurants to be smoke-free the day of the Great American Smoke Out, and publicly recognizing restaurants that met public health standards and were smoke-free. In 2000, a new father and Minot city council member called me asking if the coalition would assist him in having restaurants become smoke-free. With a newborn, he was concerned about the exposure of his child and others to secondhand smoke. A partnership began and approximately 1 year later, after much political and media maneuvering, the city council passed the smoke-free ordinance. As we basked in our victory, however, opponents gathered enough signatures to put the new ordinance to a public vote. The battle-weary coalition began to meet weekly again to strategize how to defeat this referendum. Strategy for influencing city council members is vastly different from strategy to educate and influence an entire community. Thankfully, we were not alone in the fight. In conjunction with the Campaign for Tobacco Free Kids, Americans for Nonsmokers' Rights, the Robert Wood Johnson Foundation's Smokeless States program, the North Dakota Nurses Association, the North Dakota Medical Association, the American Lung Association, the American Cancer Society, the American Heart Association, and others, we defeated the referendum 55% to 45% on July 10, 2001. The new ordinance became effective January 1, 2002. With a chill, I later learned that the tobacco companies had also tracked STAMP's activities from at least 1996 (Nelson, 1996) through 2001 (Malito, 2001).

I later took a consulting position assisting other communities working on tobacco policy, helping pass several local ordinances and facilitating a statewide coalition that passed a bill banning tobacco use in certain public places and workplaces. I was involved in evaluating the effects of the local ordinance and the state law (Buettner-Schmidt, 2003, 2007; Buettner-Schmidt, Mangskau & Boots, 2007; Buettner-Schmidt & Moseley, 2003). In a university faculty role, I developed a project within my Community Health Nursing course wherein senior nursing students conducted an assessment of college-age smoking and smoking policies on university campuses. The students developed a smoke-free campus recommendation and presented it to the university president. After going through many committees, our campus became smoke-free in June 2006.

SHAREHOLDER ADVOCACY: "THE NURSES ARE COMING..."

After all this, when I heard about the Nightingales' call for more nurse volunteers to speak out at the shareholder meeting, I could not resist. I had seen the industry in action before. Locally, lobbyists of organizations who collaborated with the tobacco industry attempted to derail our city-level policy efforts. Statewide, the tobacco industry lobbyists themselves would roam the halls of the legislature, something I never would have believed in my pre-tobacco activist years.

Now I was on my way into the belly of the beast. After a long flight and a meeting with other nurse activists the night before, feeling the solidarity among colleagues working on tobacco control in many different roles, I was excited as we drove through luxurious acreage leading to the corporate offices. As we parked and entered the building, there were Men in Black everywhere speaking into hidden microphones and we could hear whispers: "The nurses are here...," "The nurses are coming..." It felt very James Bond–like, almost surreal.

Envision a cold-sounding CEO, a transfixing video presentation about cigarettes and other products, and an opulent environment; these are my memories of the shareholder meeting. After the video, CEO Louis Camilleri highlighted how successful the company had been in increasing cigarette sales worldwide and how profitable the stock was. Then it was time for the shareholder question-and-answer period. I told my family story and the stories of others whom I knew. Other nurses spoke of the suffering they had witnessed. A nurse practitioner spoke about the harm tobacco does to pregnant women, and a burn nurse spoke about caring for burn victims from cigarette-caused fires. Each time, the room fell silent as we spoke; I felt the symbolic power of our white lab coats and our nursing presence. Some of the protesting youths stood boldly to interrupt the meeting; the CEO repeatedly told them to sit down. Then the Men in Black forced the youths to the back of the room and out the door. I remember wondering if we had made an impact.

In our debriefing later and in self-reflection, I realized that although we cannot know whether our words on that one day will create change, it is essential for nurses to continue to speak out because we are nurses. People who profit from selling death should not be able to do so without, at the very least, hearing about the suffering and devastation that their product causes. As nurses, we have a responsibility to speak truth to power.

EXTENDING THE MESSAGE

Currently, we have Nightingales existing in more than half of the United States and in Canada. We annually attend both the Altria and Reynolds American tobacco company shareholders' meetings. We've challenged the company's claims of responsibility at Philip Morris public relations events. Our work is all voluntary.

Of course, tobacco companies are still promoting tobacco products but our efforts have borne fruit in several respects. First, we have sent a strong message to the tobacco industry that nurses are their opponents. Nurses such as Susan Priano and Elisabeth Gunderson, both from California, have found their voices after attending shareholder meetings. In 2011, cancer nurse Gunderson attracted international media attention when she told the story of her dying patient who said quitting smoking was harder than quitting heroin. The Philip Morris International CEO responded that "…it's not that hard to quit" and the story went viral (Daily Mail, 2011; USA Today, 2011, para 4), reminding the public of the tobacco industry's duplicity.

Nurses are trusted and respected by the public, and we owe it to our patients to speak out, tell the whole truth about Big Tobacco, and speak truth to power. Nurses need to promote public dialogue on how to end this industrially produced tobacco disease epidemic (Malone, 2010; Warner, 2013). From removing the profit from selling tobacco products (Borland, 2013) to decreasing cigarette nicotine levels until addiction does not occur (Benowitz & Henningfield, 2013) to setting a year where individuals born after that year are not allowed to possess tobacco products (Berrick, 2013) or phasing cigarettes off the market altogether (Proctor, 2013), many proposals are being discussed.

Whether our clients are starting to smoke or trying to quit, they receive constant messages from the tobacco industry, straight into their homes, and increasingly through more subtle marketing methods such as experiential programs, Internet marketing, and musical events. In 2003, Philip Morris had a database of more than 20 million smokers, which it uses to establish personalized relationships and targeted communications (Philip Morris USA, 2003). We need to help clients understand how the industry has studied their every psychological weakness, segmenting the market to reach everyone from starter replacement smokers,

as the industry calls youths, to worried older smokers whom they seek to reassure. We would not treat malaria victims without ever mentioning the mosquito that transmits the disease. As patient advocates, we must likewise name, discuss, and find ways to combat the industry vector of the tobacco disease epidemic.

Second, our efforts have inspired others. The youths we joined are still talking at meetings about the nurses and how we helped them feel part of something larger. Perhaps some of them will become nurses. We need their passion and political awareness in nursing. Finally, speaking out empowers us as nurses. As past shareholder meeting attendees have said: "This experience has changed the whole way I feel about being a nurse" and "Now I feel that I can say anything to anyone with confidence."

WHAT NURSES CAN DO

There is perhaps no other health issue on which nurses could have so much impact. Tobacco affects almost every body system and every demographic group across the lifespan. It affects individuals, families, and communities; there is no nurse for whom tobacco could not be relevant.

The tobacco industry has worried that nurses might take them on. Among the industry documents is a report on organizations the industry viewed as its opponents, with each one's strengths

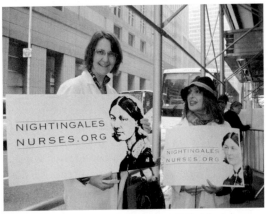

FIGURE 80-1 Nightingales at the 2013 Philip Morris International shareholders meeting.

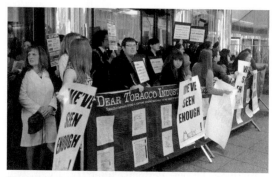

FIGURE 80-2 Nightingales participating in a press conference after the 2013 Phillip Morris International shareholders meeting in New York City.

appraised, including the American Nurses Association, the American Public Health Association, and others. "Nurses, as a group, feel strongly and negatively about tobacco use," the report reads. "As they become more active in politics … at all levels, they could easily become formidable opponents for the tobacco industry" (Osmon, 1990). Formidable opponents. We are not used to thinking of nurses in those terms. But when it comes to the tobacco industry, we need to be its formidable opponents in every possible way.

The Nightingales build on and inspire the great work of many nurses and nursing organizations. The newly formed Tobacco Control Nurses International's mission is to promote the visibility of nurses' involvement in tobacco control and facilitate professional collaboration and leadership to curb the tobacco epidemic (Global Bridges, 2013).

Tobacco Free Nurses, which aims to help nurses themselves quit smoking, is managed by Drs. Linda Sarna, Stella Bialous, and Erika Froelicher. Drs. Sarna and Bialous have been focusing on educating nurses on evidence-based tobacco dependence treatment interventions in the United States, China, the Czech Republic, and Poland. They recently collaborated with WHO on a monograph on enhancing nurses' role in addressing the non-communicable disease epidemic, in which tobacco plays a major role. At University College, Los Angeles (UCLA), Professor Sarna helped pass a policy against accepting tobacco industry research funding and more recently spearheaded the effort to make UCLA a tobacco-free campus.

Nightingales member and nursing professor Dr. Sophia S. Chan, PhD, RN, FAAN, is the first nurse in Hong Kong to be selected as a Fellow of the American Academy of Nursing. She conducted the first Asia Pacific Workshop on Tobacco Control and Nurses; in Hong Kong, developed the Women Against Tobacco Taskforce (WATT); launched the first Youth Quit line; and influenced the governmental funding of smoking cessation clinics.

The University of Kentucky's Tobacco Policy Research Program and the Kentucky Center for Smoke-free Policy are led by Ellen J. Hahn, PhD, RN, FAAN, and Carol A. Riker, MSN, RN. They are involved in community engagement, smoke-free and tobacco-free campus policy development, and research and have helped a total of 39 communities pass smoke-free laws or regulations since 2007.

In 2012, the Nightingales' founding member, Carol Southard, RN, MSN, won the American Lung Association and Koop Foundation Unsung Heroes in Tobacco Control award, making her the first woman and the first nurse to have ever received this honor. Since 2013, Carol has been involved with a Chicago Department of Public Health initiative, providing information at Town Hall meetings about the effects of flavored tobacco products and with the goal of recommending policies for curbing the use of these products and reducing health disparities.

Healthy Communities International currently at North Dakota State University and led by Buettner-Schmidt, was funded to conduct research and provide education and assistance to tobacco grantees throughout North Dakota. She assisted in a statewide ballot measure mandating tobacco settlement dollars be allocated to a fully funded, CDC Best Practices based, tobacco prevention program. North Dakota has the first tobacco prevention program in the country to be fully funded at the CDC recommended level.

Other nurse examples include Canadian Registered Nurse Joan O'Connor, who keeps statistics on every cigarette not smoked by members of her Tobacco Fighters and Survivors Club, a smoking reduction and cessation group for people living with mental illness. By 2011, more than 470,000 cigarettes were not smoked, equaling more than 23,000 packs not bought, 470,000 butts not in the environment, and approximately 30 pounds of tar not in human lungs. Nightingales founder Ruth Malone went on to become editor-in-chief of the leading international journal in the field, *Tobacco Control*, published by the British Medical Association.

Other nurses are organizing letter-writing campaigns, developing cessation services for special populations, conducting tobacco-related research, and working on a wide range of policy efforts to reduce tobacco's deadly toll. The Nightingales are always looking for more nurses to help; even writing a letter to the editor once a year can make a difference. Nurses play an active role as leaders of the global movement to end this preventable epidemic.

NURSING IS POLITICAL

Some nurses are afraid of being political, but health is political: resources, education, and care are unevenly distributed in our society. Tobacco is a social justice issue. Just caring about those beyond us and our immediate families is a deeply political act. Our most powerful nursing roots lie in our concern for those who feel voiceless and powerless, as exemplified by the early leaders in public health nursing.

As early as 1916, writings of Florence Nightingale referred to her knowledge of politics (Gourlay, 2004; Kopf, 1916; McDonald, 2006a, 2006b; Pfettscher, 2006). Nightingale emphasized having political will, using the media, and seeking the support of professionals and leaders (McDonald, 2006b). She encouraged others to lobby: "Agitate, agitate, agitate …" (McDonald, 2006b). Ms. Nightingale would surely support the Nightingales' tobacco-control policy efforts (Nightingale, 1946).

LESSONS LEARNED: NURSING ACTIVISM

The Power of a Few: The first lesson is that a few committed individuals can make a difference. It does not take a complex organization and big dollars to begin to become political on a local, state, or even national level. The Nightingales started with a few committed nurses and a loosely organized network and remain so, but now the group is also a member of the Framework Convention Alliance, a coalition of over 300 civil society organizations from more than 100 countries working on implementing the provisions of the world's first global public health treaty, the World Health Organization Framework Convention on Tobacco Control *(www.fctc.org)*.

Clarify Policy Goals: Second, determine your policy goals and objectives. Attempt to obtain a consensus, but also agree on a process for making decisions if there is disagreement.

Stakeholder Analysis: Third, educate yourself or your group. What are the arguments for and against the goals? Who are the opposition and how will you counter their arguments? Review the literature for the science behind your goals. Identify the personal stories that will allow policymakers, the media, and the public to connect to and support your cause. Determine how you will frame the issue. Identify a spokesperson or have all members prepared and ready to counter arguments.

Build Coalitions: Fourth, identify natural allies. Reach out to others to join forces. Build on common ground and share resources. For example, the Nightingales Nurses coordinated our press conferences with Essential Action, a youth-focused tobacco-control group.

Determine Leverage Points: Fifth, if you are seeking a policy change, determine who has the power to make that change. If it is a board or committee, try to identify amongst yourselves who on the board/committee strongly supports or opposes your goals. Identify those who influence the policymakers. Determine a strategy to educate those influential people and supportive policymakers and ask for their assistance and guidance, but maintain your organizational boundaries so you can attract support from people across the political spectrum. Seek an insider champion. Educate your group on the policy processes needed to change the policy. Develop a tentative and realistic timeframe, recognizing that this will need to be revisited as events change.

Engage Media: Sixth, develop a plan to engage the media. Media advocacy is a skill. For example, one of our group's aims was to get media coverage of our activism to change perspectives about the tobacco industry.

UNIT 5

Build on Your Strengths: Seventh, celebrate small successes to sustain energy. Build on the strengths of all members. With activism, realize that not everyone is comfortable with public speaking or confrontation; however, they may contribute in other ways, such as preparing press releases, managing logistics, or working on a website. Know that policy and politics is ongoing; once a policy passes, next is policy implementation and evaluation.

Use Your Power and Passion: Lastly, know that as an individual, it is easy to be a politically active nurse as many organizations use web-based advocacy opportunities. Find an entity focused on a health-related cause that stirs your passion, become a member, and express a willingness to become involved. Soon you may be emailing letters to your policymakers, meeting with editorial boards, and improving the health of your clients not only as individuals, but also at the policy level.

DISCUSSION QUESTIONS

1. Discuss a public problem that would benefit having nurses speak truth to power.
2. What health-related issue sparks your passion? Discuss existing organizations that advocate for this issue and the pros and cons of joining the organization or developing a new entity.
3. Do you think tobacco cessation is an important issue to nursing? Why or why not?

REFERENCES

Apollonio, D., & Malone, R. E. (2005). Marketing to the marginalized: Tobacco industry targeting of the homeless and mentally ill. *Tobacco Control, 14*(6), 409–415. doi:10.1136/tc.2005.011890.

Balbach, E. D., Gasior, R. J., & Barbeau, E. M. (2003). R.J. Reynolds' targeting of African Americans: 1988-2000. *American Journal of Public Health, 93*(5), 822–827.

Benowitz, N. L., & Henningfield, J. E. (2013). Reducing the nicotine content to make cigarettes less addictive. *Tobacco Control, 22*(S1), i14–i17. doi:10.1136/tobaccocontrol-2012-050860.

Bero, L. (2003). Implications of the tobacco industry documents for public health and policy. *Annual Review of Public Health, 24,* 267–288. doi:10.1146/annurev.publhealth.24.100901.140813.

Bero, L. A. (2005). Tobacco industry manipulation of research. *Public Health Reports, 120*(2), 200–208.

Berrick, A. J. (2013). The tobacco-free generation proposal. *Tobacco Control, 22*(S1), i22–i26. doi:10.1136/tobaccocontrol-2012-050865.

Borland, R. (2013). Minimising the harm from tobacco nicotine use: Finding the right regulatory framework. *Tobacco Control, 22*(S1), i6–i9. doi:10.1136/tobaccocontrol-2012-050843.

Brown and Williamson Tobacco Company. (1971). If you are worried about cigarettes—May we confuse you with some facts? (Advertisement). Retrieved from *legacy.library.ucsf.edu/tid/mgw93f00.*

Buettner-Schmidt, K. (2003). *Compliance of Minot restaurants with the Smoke-Free Restaurant Ordinance.* Minot, ND: Tobacco Education, Research and Policy Project, Minot State University, Department of Nursing.

Buettner-Schmidt, K. (2007). The economic impact of North Dakota's smoke-free law on restaurant and bar taxable sales. Minot, ND: Healthy Communities International, Minot State University, Department of Nursing. Retrieved from *www.ndhealth.gov/tobacco/Reports/Impact_Report _2007.pdf.*

Buettner-Schmidt, K., Mangskau, K., & Boots, C. (2007). An observational assessment of compliance with North Dakota smoke-free Law. Minot, ND: Healthy Communities International, Minot State University, Department of Nursing. Retrieved from *www.ndhealth.gov/tobacco/Reports/ Compliance_Report_2007.pdf.*

Buettner-Schmidt, K., & Moseley, F. (2003). *An economic analysis of a smoke-free restaurant ordinance in a Midwestern frontier state.* Minot, ND: Minot State University, Department of Nursing, North Dakota Center for Persons with Disabilities, & College of Business.

Buettner-Schmidt, K., Muhlbradt, M., & Brierley, L. (2003). *Why not Minot: The battle over North Dakota's first smoke-free ordinance.* Minot, ND: Minot State University, Department of Nursing.

Cataldo, J. K., & Malone, R. E. (2008). False promises: The tobacco industry, "low-tar" cigarettes, and older smokers. *Journal of the American Geriatrics Society, 56*(9), 1716–1723.

Centers for Disease Control and Prevention. (2011). Quitting smoking among adults—United States, 2001–2010. *Morbidity and Mortality Weekly Report, 60*(44), 1513–1519.

Centers for Disease Control and Prevention. (2014). *Best practices for comprehensive tobacco control programs—2014.* Retrieved from *www.cdc .gov/tobaccco/stateandcommunity/best-practices/index.htm.*

Cook, B. L., Wayne, G. F., Keithly, L., & Connolly, G. (2004). One size does not fit all: How the tobacco industry has altered cigarette design to target consumer groups with specific psychological and psychosocial needs. *Addiction (Abingdon, England), 99*(11), 1547–1561.

Daily Mail (2011). "It's not hard to quit": Tobacco boss sparks outrage after he's confronted by cancer nurse at AGM. Retrieved from *www .dailymail.co.uk/news/article-1386100/Tobacco-boss-Louis-C-Camilleri -tells-nurse-hard-quit-smoking.html#ixzz2ec8V2xxe.*

Federal Trade Commission. (2013). FTC releases reports on 2011 cigarette and smokeless tobacco advertising and promotion. Washington D.C. Retrieved from *www.ftc.gov/opa/2013/05/tobacco.shtm.*

Glantz, S., Slade, J., Bero, L., Hanauer, P., & Barnes, D. (1996). *The cigarette papers.* Berkeley: University of California Press.

Global Bridges. (2013). Global bridges: Healthcare alliance for tobacco dependence treatment. Nurses. Retrieved from *www.globalbridges.org/ Community/Nurses.*

Gourlay, J. (2004). Florence Nightingale: Still lighting the way for nurses. *Nurse Management, 11*(2), 14–15.

Halpin, P. (1994). Letter to Benson and Hedges in response to mailed survey. *Legacy Tobacco Documents Library.* Retrieved from *legacy .library.ucsf.edu/tid/usc62e00.*

Kluger, R. (1997). *Ashes to ashes: America's hundred-year cigarette war, the public health, and the unabashed triumph of Philip Morris.* New York: Vintage Books.

Kopf, E. W. (1916). Florence Nightingale as statistician. *Quarterly Publications of the American Statistical Association, 15*(116), 388–405.

Landrine, H., Klonoff, E. A., Fernandez, S., Hickman, N., Kashima, K., Parekh, B., et al. (2005). Cigarette advertising in Black, Latino, and White magazines, 1998-2002: An exploratory investigation. *Ethnicity and Disease, 15*(1), 63–67.

Malito, C. (2001). Newsedge—11/6/01. *Legacy Tobacco Documents Library*. Retrieved from *legacy.library.ucsf.edu/tid/xua17a00*.

Malone, R. E. (2009). The social and political context of the tobacco epidemic: Nursing research and scholarship on the tobacco industry. Invited [peer reviewed] review paper for Sarna, L. & Aguinaga-Bialous, S. (Eds.), Advancing nursing science and tobacco control. *Annual Review of Nursing Research, 27*, 63–90.

Malone, R. E. (2010). Imaging thinks otherwise: new endgame ideas for tobacco control. *Tobacco Control, 19*(5), 349–350. doi:10.1136/tc.2010.039727.

McCandless, P. M., Yerger, V. B., & Malone, R. E. (2011). Quid Pro Quo: Tobacco Companies and the Black Press. *American Journal of Public Health, 102*(4), 739–750. doi:10.2105/AJPH.2011.300180.

McDaniel, P. A., Intinarelli, G., & Malone, R. E. (2008). Tobacco industry issues management organizations: Creating a global corporate network to undermine public health. *Globalization and Health, 4*(2), doi:10.1186/1744-8603-4-2.

McDaniel, P. A., & Malone, R. E. (2009). The role of corporate credibility in legitimizing disease promotion. *American Journal of Public Health, 99*(3), 452–461. doi:10.2105/AJPH.2008.138115.

McDonald, L. (2006a). Florence Nightingale and public health policy: Theory, activism and public administration. Paper for Origins of Public Health Policy, CSAA Meetings, York University, 2006. Retrieved from *www.sociology.uoguelph.ca/fnightingale/Public%20Health%20Care/theory.htm*.

McDonald, L. (2006b). Florence Nightingale as a social reformer. *History Today, 56*(1), 9–15.

Muggli, M. E., Pollay, R. W., Lew, R., & Joseph, A. M. (2002). Targeting of Asian Americans and Pacific Islanders by the tobacco industry: Results from the Minnesota Tobacco Document Depository. *Tobacco Control, 11*(3), 201–209.

Nelson, B. (1996). Letter to Bob Fackler and others. Morning team notes 4/29. *Legacy Tobacco Documents Library*. Retrieved from *legacy.library.ucsf.edu/tid/poy72a00*.

Nightingale, F. (1946). Notes on nursing: What it is, and what it is not. In *Notes on nursing: What it is, and what it is not: Commemorative edition* (p. 8). Philadelphia: Lippincott.

Osmon, H. E. (1990). Letter to T. C. Harris and others: Attached is the updated overview of anti-smoking organizations. *Legacy Tobacco Documents Library*. Retrieved from *legacy.library.ucsf.edu/tid/dkf24d00*.

Pfettscher, S. A. (2006). Florence Nightingale, 1820-1910: Modern nursing. In A. M. Tomey & M. R. Alligood (Eds.), *Nursing theorists and their work* (6th ed., pp. 71–90). St. Louis: Mosby-Elsevier.

Philip Morris USA. (2003). PM USA adult smoker database marketing past, present and future. *Legacy Tobacco Documents Library*. Retrieved from *legacy.library.ucsf.edu/tid/msh95a00*.

Proctor, R. N. (2011). *Golden holocaust: Origins of the cigarette catastrophe and the case for abolition*. Berkeley: University of California Press.

Proctor, R. N. (2013). Why ban the sale of cigarettes? The case for abolition. *Tobacco Control, 22*(Supp1), i27–i30. doi:10.1136/tobaccocontrol-2012-050911.

Rosenbaum, D. J., Barnes, R. L., & Glantz, S. A. (2012). Tobacco control in North Dakota, 2004-2012; Reaching for higher ground. San Francisco: University of California, Center for Tobacco Control Research and Education. Retrieved from *escholarship.org/uc/item/2jk5n8p5*.

Schwarz, T. (2004). Nightingales vs. Big Tobacco: Nurses confront the nation's biggest public health threat. *American Journal of Nursing, 104*(6), 27.

Schwarz, T. (2005). Nightingales confront tobacco company, redux: Nurses from around the country gather to clear the smoke. *American Journal of Nursing, 105*(6), 35.

Smith, E. A. (2007). "It's interesting how few people die from smoking": Tobacco industry efforts to minimize risk and discredit health promotion. *European Journal of Public Health, 17*(2), 162–170.

Smith, E. A., & Malone, R. E. (2003). The outing of Philip Morris: Advertising tobacco to gay men. *American Journal of Public Health, 93*(6), 988–993.

Tesler, L., & Malone, R. E. (2008). Corporate philanthropy, lobbying and public health policy. *American Journal of Public Health, 98*(12), 2123–2133. doi:10.2105/AJPH.2007.128231.

USA Today. (2011). Philip Morris Int'l CEO: Tobacco not hard to quit. Retrieved from *usatoday30.usatoday.com/money/companies/management/2011-05-11-cigarettes-addictive-philip-morris_n.htm*.

U.S. Department of Health and Human Services [HHS]. (1988). The health consequences of smoking: Nicotine addiction. A report of the Surgeon General. Retrieved from *profiles.nlm.nih.gov/NN/B/B/Z/D/_/nnbbzd.pdf*.

U.S. Department of Health and Human Services [HHS]. (2013). *Tobacco control state highlights 2012*. Atlanta, GA: U.S. Department of Health and Human Services, Centers for Disease Control and Prevention, National Center for Chronic Disease Prevention and Health Promotion, Office on Smoking and Health.

U.S. Department of Health and Human Services [HHS]. (2014a). *Best practices for comprehensive tobacco control programs—2014*. Atlanta, GA: U.S. Department of Health and Human Services. Centers for Disease Control and Prevention, National Center for Chronic Disease Prevention and Health Promotion, Office on Smoking and Health.

Warner, K. E. (2013). An endgame for tobacco? *Tobacco Control, 22*(S1), i3–i5. doi:10.1136/tobaccocontrol-2013-050989.

Welle, J. R., Ibrahim, J. K., & Glantz, S. A. (2004). Tobacco control policy making in North Dakota: A tradition of activism. San Francisco: University of California, Center for Tobacco Control Research and Education. Retrieved from *repositories.cdlib.org/ctcre/tcpmus/ND2004*.

World Health Organization [WHO]. (2009). Tobacco industry interference with tobacco control. Retrieved from *www.who.int/tobacco/resources/publications /9789241597340.pdf*.

World Health Organization [WHO]. (2013). WHO report on the global tobacco epidemic, 2013. Enforcing bans on tobacco advertising, promotion and sponsorship. Executive summary. Retrieved from *apps.who.int/iris/bitstream/10665/85381/1/WHO_NMH_PND_13.2_eng.pdf*.

Yerger, V. B., & Malone, R. E. (2002). African American leadership groups: Smoking with the enemy. *Tobacco Control, 11*(4), 336–345. doi:10.1136/tc.11.4.336.

Zeltner, T., Kessler, D. A., Martiny, A., & Randera, F. (2000). Tobacco company strategies to undermine tobacco control activities at the World Health Organization. Geneva: World Health Organization. Retrieved from *www.who.int/tobacco/resources/publications/general/who_inquiry/en/*.

ONLINE RESOURCES

Legacy Foundation
www.legacyforhealth.org/our-issues
Legacy Tobacco Documents Library
legacy.library.ucsf.edu
Nightingale Nurses
www.nightingalesnurses.org
Tobacco Control Nurses International
www.globalnurses.org
Tobacco Free Nurses
www.tobaccofreenurses.org

UNIT 5

CHAPTER 81

Where Policy Hits the Pavement: Contemporary Issues in Communities

Katherine N. Bent

"I am of the opinion that my life belongs to the community, and as long as I live it is my privilege to do for it whatever I can."

George Bernard Shaw

Most people experience the effects of public policymaking in their communities. In daily life, people feel the outcomes of policy. In communities, nurses and other health professionals have immediate opportunities to advocate for policies that promote and protect health in multiple ways. This chapter explores the nature of communities, prospects for health in the community, the health-related conditions that shape and are shaped by policy, and how nurses, increasingly cross institutional boundaries to support improvements to those policies affecting health.

WHAT IS A COMMUNITY?

Although community is a part of our daily experience, the idea of community is elusive and can mean many things, particularly in a health care context (Bent, 2003). Attitudes about the role of community in health care and health policy differ when compared with attitudes regarding the role of community in other areas. For example, health care

entrepreneurs view health care communities as a market where they are likely to find a concentration of people to buy health care goods or services; however, public health professionals must be concerned about entire populations in a given area regardless of people's ability to buy, keeping in mind that where economic market potential is lower, health risks and needs may actually be higher (Geronimus, 2000). Although the concept of community has broad appeal, in a politically charged environment claims of community may serve to divide people more than to bring them together (Monroe, 1997). This effect has serious consequences for policies that support or define public health, such as those that mandate reporting of, or vaccination against, communicable diseases or policies that exclude certain health care treatments from government health insurance programs.

Milio (2002) noted that the basis for health lies in physical communities where homes, schools, recreation and entertainment centers, faith centers, businesses, and governmental and voluntary organizations, together with the means of communication and transportation, form a community's infrastructure. The quality, availability, and accessibility of the infrastructure make a difference to the health of the people who live there. Communities must share both spirit and a sense of place to build, achieve, and sustain health and well-being. Through attachment to place, communities share attachment to social responsibility for creating a healthy environment. Such an attachment does not exist among a dispersed population that may, however, share other interests such as targeted disease awareness or advocacy (Milio, 1996). As a nurse, Milio was an early advocate for what is now referred to as "place matters" in health: where people live, work, play, and learn (Bell & Rubin, 2007; Robert Wood Johnson Foundation [RWJF], 2014).

The health importance of physical and socioeconomic environments is well recognized. As noted by the Institute of Medicine (IOM), "the health risk conferred by place is above and beyond the risk that individuals carry with them" (IOM, 2003, p. 68). The Healthy People initiative, a federal effort to outline national public health objectives and which is now in its fifth edition, highlights how place, or the conditions in which people are born, live, work, and age, affects a wide range of health, functioning, and quality-of-life outcomes and risks, and how community resources can have a significant influence on population health outcomes (U.S. Department of Health and Human Services [HHS], 2010).

HEALTHY COMMUNITIES

In the late 1970s, the World Health Organization (WHO) challenged nations to provide a basic level of health for all citizens. The challenge remains relevant and open today with substantial social significance to health care and economic burden, awareness of lost opportunities, important health inequities, and again prompting widespread interest in reforming health systems. Many of today's leaders no longer limit their responsibility for health to survival and disease control, but undertake the building of systems that support health as a key resource and strength that people and societies value (WHO, 2013) (see Box 81-1).

The Robert Wood Johnson Foundation (RWJF) recently enacted new portfolios for Healthy Communities, Community Development and Health, and Violence Prevention, among others, thus leveraging their own funding with community funding and momentum to support the building of a culture of health. Signature initiatives, such as the Commission to Build a Healthier America, Roadmaps to Health Prize, and County Health Rankings, showcase how multiple sectors in the community can take action to address upstream determinants of health.

Today as national policies decentralize and commercialize, state policies localize, and individuals and communities are told they hold more responsibility than ever for their own health, we must not imply that the individual or the single community is responsible for the success (manifested through personal or population health measures) or failure (seen in ill health) of public health policy.

PARTNERSHIP FOR IMPROVING COMMUNITY HEALTH

Nurses have a tradition of actively creating and fostering partnerships for health promotion and community health, and their role remains vitally important today. Coalitions, as a particular type of partnership, are supported by evidence in the nursing, political, sociological, and organizational literature (Cary, 2012). Effective community collaborations are far more than nursing interventions; rather, they evolve through a dynamic process and with the philosophic underpinnings called for by true partnership. It is important to examine all partnerships critically so that they do not become a substitute for accountability in organizations or governments, as individuals and small coalitions are expected to assume the labor and costs associated with initiatives to improve health (see Box 81-2).

Roles for nurses in community initiatives focus on eliciting and supporting existing strengths within communities, community action, developing personal skills in community members, reorienting health care services, creating supportive environments, and participating actively in creating public policy to support health (see Box 81-3).

Efforts toward the making of public policy to support health rest on two explicit assumptions:
- Most people, most of the time, will make decisions and choices based on the options that are

UNIT 6

BOX 81-1 Evaluating a Healthy Community

Most communities have some processes in place for evaluating outcomes of health care at the community level, though the means by which they do so usually vary greatly. Variation in quality assessment strategies may allow the group asking the questions to capture issues of local importance (e.g., lead paint screening in communities with old housing stock, health career programs in schools, or enrollment assistance in public programs) but also complicates comparisons on issues of common concern across communities (e.g., how nonprofit

health care providers should be expected to benefit the communities they serve).

The CDC chart below is an example of evaluation data that track states, the District of Columbia, and New York City on whether they are recording vital events, including births, deaths, and fetal deaths, using the latest U.S. standard certificates, which are an important resource to generate standardized data for community health assessments.

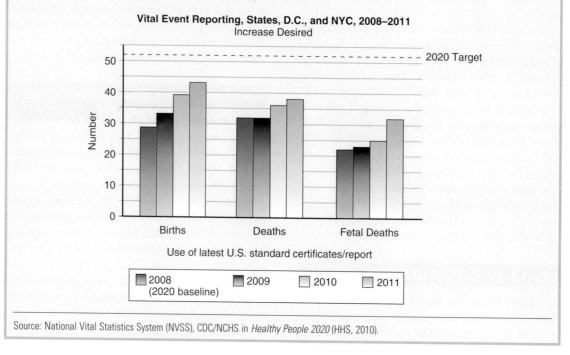

Vital Event Reporting, States, D.C., and NYC, 2008–2011
Increase Desired

Source: National Vital Statistics System (NVSS), CDC/NCHS in *Healthy People 2020* (HHS, 2010).

available. The results are not exclusively personal, nor are they the result of totally free choices about lifestyle made in isolation from social, economic, cultural, and political contexts.

• The options that are available, and from which people make choices, do not just happen, but rather are the result of prior policy choices that represent the scope of health-sustaining policy including energy, technology, pollution, employment, income maintenance, taxation, prices, food, agriculture, transportation, housing, health care, child care, and other services.

Within an emerging framework whereby public health is considered in all public policies (referred to as "health in all policies" [Rudolph et al., 2013]), policy can provide powerful disincentives to health-damaging conditions or actions. One example of the effect of such a framework can be seen in the body of laws and regulations that prohibit tobacco smoking in the workplace or other public areas. Along with tax measures, cessation measures, and education, policy supporting smoking bans is important in reducing smoking and promoting public health (WHO, 2004). Although smoking

BOX 81-2 Partnering with Veterans

With tens of thousands of veterans returning from service and looking to start new careers in a challenging economic environment, the nation is focused more than ever to help veterans transition into civilian careers.

Veterans face major hurdles as they transition into the civilian workforce. In 2012, 60% of veterans responding to a national survey said they had trouble translating military skills into civilian job experience (Prudential, Iraq and Afghanistan Veterans of America, 2012). Often veterans are required to repeat education to receive occupational credentials, even though their military training and experience overlaps with credential training requirements. In 2013, Maryland became the 13th state to enact legislation to facilitate the acceptance of military training and experience toward licensing requirements for more than 70 state licenses and certifications and to require public universities to translate military service into academic credit.

Nurses can highlight strategies to use talents and skills of veterans to both meet communities' most pressing needs and aid in community reintegration for veterans themselves. In states that have career-promoting provisions for veterans and their spouses, nurses can work with licensing boards and colleges to assure they are fully implemented. Nurses in other states that have not acted on these licensing and credentialing issues can urge policymakers to clear away unnecessary obstacles facing our veterans and their spouses.

BOX 81-3 Defining the Policy Focus

There are many examples of healthy public policy decisions that highlight both relationships and tensions in aspects of health and life. In August 2013, the California Supreme Court decided a case initiated 7 years earlier after the California Department of Education issued a directive allowing nonmedical school employees to administer insulin (Dolan, 2013). The directive was part of settling a federal class action lawsuit brought by 4 parents of students with diabetes, after a decade of proponents' failed efforts to pass state legislation that would have allowed unlicensed staff to administer insulin. The court case, brought by the American Nurses Association to block implementation of the directive and enforce state Nurse Practice Act law, pitted nurses, teachers, and other school employees against parents, disability advocates, the American Diabetes Association, and the Obama administration. The California Supreme Court decision, which overturned multiple lower courts' decisions, was the first time in the nation's history that state health care licensing law has been pre-empted by federal disability law (Daly & Davis-Aldritt, 2013). Is this case good for nursing? Is it good for communities?

laws vary widely, more than half of the states and the District of Columbia have enacted bans on smoking in all enclosed public places, including all bars and restaurants. When also considering local laws, according to the American Nonsmokers' Rights Foundation (2014), 82% of the U.S. population live under a ban on smoking in workplaces, restaurants, or bars. The rationale for smoke-free laws is to protect people from the effects of secondhand smoke, create incentives for smokers to quit, lower health care costs, improve work productivity, reduce fire risk, increase cleanliness, and reduce litter.

The increasing interest in smoke-free measures raises important questions for policymakers and offers opportunities for nurses to be active in providing accurate information that will have a meaningful effect on policy decisions. Most businesses and individuals willingly comply with the new laws, and the smoothest transitions occur in communities that make a significant effort to educate both the public and the affected business about the benefits of smoke-free establishments; nurses are ideal partners for these efforts (see Box 81-4).

The Affordable Care Act (ACA) includes support for public health and improving the health of communities. For example, the law requires that nonprofit community hospitals demonstrate their community benefit to retain their tax-exempt status by conducting a community health needs assessment, developing a plan for promoting the health of a community, and implementing the plan (Somerville, Nelson & Mueller, 2013). Nurses who work in such hospitals have an opportunity to lead these efforts and partner with community leaders to ensure that the hospital's efforts align with the needs, wants, and interests of a community.

BOX 81-4 Collaborative Processes for Information

Nurses working with the Red Cross in several locations have demonstrated the acceptability and success of engaging members of a local community to maintain a resource database to support community resilience and emergency response. Collaboratively gathering information raises awareness of risk and vulnerability within the community, can be economical, leads to an assessment of community strengths and resources, and mobilizes these resources and partnerships to support rapid assessment and response (Troy et al., 2008). This is one example of partnering to support the National Health Security Strategy (NHSS), and minimizes the negative health consequences of threats or incidents.

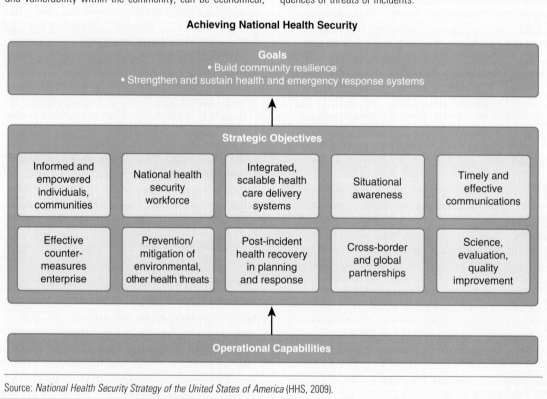

Achieving National Health Security

Source: *National Health Security Strategy of the United States of America* (HHS, 2009).

DETERMINANTS OF HEALTH

Within public policy arenas, views differ about what should be the main focus of health policy: Is the primary purpose of health policy to deliver health services to or to improve the health and well-being of populations? Researchers have increasingly documented that the portion of population health status attributable to health care services is modest when compared with the contributions of other factors, including the sociopolitical determinants of health. Indeed, Healthy People 2020 identified

access to health care as one of the leading indicators that, in addition to environmental quality and social indicators of health, could serve as measures for the health of the population (HHS, 2010).

Determinants of health are factors in the sociocultural and political environments that contribute to or detract from the health of individuals and communities. These factors include income, education, occupation, transportation, sanitation, housing, and access to services and resources linked to health, social support, and environmental hazards. Social forces are those that act at a collective level, such as a community decision to build sidewalks to promote safe walking opportunities, individual risk behaviors and health outcomes, and access to other resources that promote health.

For the first time in the history of this public health initiative, Healthy People 2020 used a framework of social determinants of health to establish and communicate goals and objectives for improving the nation's health and eliminating health disparities. The framework includes five areas, each reflecting a number of health critical issues and components: economic stability, education, social and community context, health and health care, and neighborhood and built environment. The framework has also been used to identify evidence-based resources and other tools or examples of how this approach may be implemented at a state as well as local level (HHS, 2010) (see Box 81-5).

SOCIOECONOMIC STATUS, HEALTH DISPARITIES, AND INEQUITIES

It is critical that nurses understand how determinants of health contribute to health inequities as well as how to advocate for policies to address the forces associated with poor health and quality of life outcomes. By working to establish policies that positively influence social and economic conditions and those that support healthy individual behaviors, we can improve health for large numbers of people in ways that can be sustained over time.

The link between the health status of a population and its socioeconomic status is well established in both the United States and other countries; many diseases are more common and life expectancy is shorter at the lower ends of the socioeconomic scale (WHO, 2003). Beyond a threshold of about $5,000 to $10,000 U.S. dollars per capita income, the gap between rich and poor, called income inequality, is a greater health hazard than absolute low income itself (Population Health Forum, 2009). This appears to be related to both access to resources for health, and relative social position among people with different levels of education, income, and types of jobs and among people who live in communities characterized by different levels of community wealth and infrastructure (Massey & Durrheim, 2007; Wilkinson & Marmot, 2003).

Because the United States compares poorly to other industrialized countries on the public health measure of teen birth rate, much research aims to describe the costs, outcomes, and consequences of early childbearing at individual, family, and societal levels and to identify interventions to promote deferred parenting. Rigorous studies in this field, which increasingly control for the background factors that predispose teens to become parents, are starting to show a vastly reduced link between early maternal age and what were previously believed to be negative outcomes of early maternal age, including: outcomes of mother's education, income, and welfare use; pregnancy complications; infant and child cognitive and behavioral outcomes; and public costs. The evidence now shows how early and enduring disadvantage, rather than age, shapes both short- and long-term maternal-child outcomes for teen mothers, their peers, and their sisters, regardless of age at first birth (SmithBattle, 2012). Thus there are gaps between scientific evidence on determinants and consequences of early childbearing and federal welfare policies in the United States that do not adequately account for the context in which behavior and choices are situated. For example, up to 60% of teen mothers dropped out of school before pregnancy; they were more likely to have undiagnosed learning problems or mental health conditions and were typically denied readmission to school after a prolonged absence; yet none of these barriers is addressed by Temporary Assistance for Needy Families (TANF), colloquially known as welfare (SmithBattle, 2012).

EDUCATION

Freudenberg and Ruglis (2007) identified a number of health interventions to reduce school dropout rates. The interventions, such as coordinated school health programs, violence prevention programs, and school-based health clinics, all show promising results in initial research. However, Freudenberg and Ruglis highlight a remaining need to coordinate, evaluate rigorously, and build theory around these interventions to better explain the mechanisms by which improving the health of students reduces dropout rates and to provide clearer paths to implementation in specific settings.

BOX 81-5 Healthy People 2020 and the Social Determinants of Health

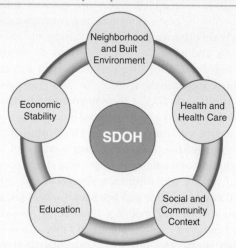

Each of these five determinant areas reflects a number of critical components/key issues that make up the underlying factors in the arena of social determinants of health.

- Economic stability, opportunity and mobility
  - Poverty
  - Employment status
  - Access to employment
  - Housing stability (e.g., homelessness, foreclosure)
- Education
  - High quality schools
  - High school graduation rates

- School policies that support health promotion
- School environments that are safe and conducive to learning
- Access to and enrollment in higher education
- Social and community context
  - Family structure
  - Social cohesion
  - Perceptions of discrimination and equity
  - Opportunities to participate in community life
  - Incarceration/institutionalization
- Health and health care
  - Access to health services, including clinical and preventive care
  - Access to primary care, including community-based health promotion and wellness programs
  - Health technology
- Neighborhood and build environment
  - Quality of housing, streets, sidewalks, and public spaces
  - Crime and violence
  - Environmental conditions
  - Access to healthy foods

In communities that have the resources, a sense of cohesion can bring about distribution of these resources to achieve sustainable health for the people who are part of those communities.

Source: *Healthy People 2020* (HHS, 2010).

Robust epidemiological evidence links educational achievement with quality and quantity of life, decreased health disparities, and improved personal health behaviors (National Poverty Center, 2007; RWJF, 2011). This intersection illuminates a path for nurses to apply an ecological perspective to developing and researching the broad scope of public policies that affect health.

ENVIRONMENTAL HEALTH

Environmental health is a rich public policy domain with considerable evidence linking local environment to health outcomes (Hawe & Shiell, 2000). Nurses in environmental health partnerships may address a wide range of topics, such as safety of fish consumption or of drinking water, bioterrorism, questions of environmental justice, or long-term health outcomes of community-wide exposures.

For example, Libby, Montana, is a rural community affected by generations of exposure to asbestos-contaminated mineral ores that were mined there for 78 years (Kuntz et al., 2009). Although mining operations provided jobs, roads, and economic development for the community, there were health consequences to residents. Libby was designated a federal Superfund site in 2002, after an analysis of mortality conducted by the Agency for Toxic Substances and Disease Registry

(ATSDR), in cooperation with the Montana Department of Public Health and Human Services (MDPHHS), found asbestosis mortality that was 40 to 80 times higher than expected when compared with Montana and the United States and found lung cancer mortality that was 20% to 30% higher than expected (Agency for Toxic Substances and Disease Registry [ATSDR], 2008, 2009).

There is a patchwork of federal agencies involved in public health management, policymaking, and regulation related to the health hazards associated with asbestos, but no single agency is responsible for coordination or oversight of these efforts. In addition, Libby is a highly uninsured/underinsured population in a Health Care Professional Shortage Area; thus, it is without sufficient access to health care services. Because community residents may or may not yet have disease, or may be in varying stages of disease, and because there is no umbrella agency taking leadership for comprehensive strategies and oversight to protect the health of residents, workers, and others affected by the contaminated ores, public health nurses and community members have been the most active partners in working collaboratively to identify the specific activities, strategies, and roles needed to address multiple, ambiguous health and policy issues such as community-level conflict, individual or community stigma, and generational health consequences in addition to long-term cleanup strategies (Kuntz et al., 2009).

Lessons learned from community health experiences and partnership processes in Libby may be equally applicable in communities in which hydraulic fracturing, known as fracking, is increasingly used to extract natural gas from the earth. These are often communities whose members face financial pressures that they may seek to relieve by allowing fracking operations on their land, and who thus become vulnerable to the effects of the known neurotoxins, carcinogens, and endocrine disruptors used in the process. Still undocumented health risks of fracking that may mirror those of other fossil fuel removal and combustion activities may also be present. In addition, there are known occupational hazards for community members doing the work (Rafferty & Limonik, 2013). The decisions individuals, families, and communities make about fracking are complex and nuanced. Community economic development and individual and family economic stability are important determinants of health, bringing quality housing, new roads and schools, healthier food options, access to clinical and preventive care, and other important health-supporting conditions. They may, however, come at a cost of environmental contamination and related health impacts, and communities face internal and external conflict and tension when attempting to balance these competing priorities.

Nurses can be actively involved in health monitoring and disease surveillance efforts, articulating individual and public health concerns in public venues when energy policies are discussed, keeping current on emerging scientific evidence about health outcomes associated with fracking practices, calling for full disclosure of chemicals used, identifying and advocating for alternative community development and economic opportunities, and being willing to take on roles on boards, commissions, and advisory councils for environmental and community health (McDermott-Levy, Kaktins & Sattler, 2013; Rafferty & Limonik, 2013).

DISCUSSION QUESTIONS

1. It is not easy to prove the effectiveness or value of community health prevention interventions or interventions to reduce health disparities; how can nurses use policy and policy analysis to strengthen the body of evidence available to community health nurses on a practical level?

2. For a community to improve its health, its members must often change aspects of the physical, social, organizational, and even political environments to eliminate or reduce factors that contribute to health problems or to introduce new elements that promote better health. What are the challenges of initiating and maintaining change in communities?

3. The Affordable Care Act (P.L. 111-148) contains several provisions that address systemic and structural gaps in access and care; have these policies had an effect on health disparities or other important community health indicators?

REFERENCES

Agency for Toxic Substances Disease Registry [ATSDR]. (2008). Summary report: Exposure to asbestos-containing vermiculite from Libby, Montana, at 28 processing sites in the United States. Retrieved from *www.atsdr.cdc.gov/asbestos/sites/national_map/index.html.*

Agency for Toxic Substances Disease Registry [ATSDR]. (2009). Mortality review: Mortality in Libby, Montana, 1979 to 1998. Retrieved from *www.atsdr.cdc.gov/asbestos/sites/libby_montant/mortality_review.html.*

American Nonsmokers' Rights Foundation. (2014). Overview list: How many smoke free laws? Retrieved from *http://www.no-smoke.org/pdf/mediaordlist.pdf.*

Bell, J., & Rubin, V. (2007). Why place matters: Building a movement for healthy communities. Retrieved from *www.policylink.org/sites/default/files/WHYPLACEMATTERS_FINAL.PDF.*

Bent, K. N. (2003). The people know what they want: An empowerment process of sustainable, ecological community health. *Advances in Nursing Science, 26*(3), 215–226.

Cary, A. H. (2012). The future of nursing depends on building coalitions. *Public Health Nursing, 29*(2), 97–98.

Daly, K. A., & Davis-Aldritt, L. (2013, May 28). California Supreme Court should forbid unlicensed school employees from administering insulin. *Mercurynews.com.* Retrieved from *www.mercurynews.com/opinionci_23338551.*

Dolan, L. (2013. August 12). Schools can administer insulin without licensed nurses, court says. *The Los Angeles Times.* Retrieved from *articles.latimes.com/2013/aug/12/local/la-me-school-nurses-20130813.*

Freudenberg, N., & Ruglis, J. (2007). Reframing school dropout as a public health issue. *Preventing Chronic Disease, 4*(4). Retrieved from *www.cdc.gov/pcd/issues/2007/oct/07_0063.htm.*

Geronimus, A. (2000). To mitigate, resist, or undo: Addressing structural influences on the health of urban populations. *American Journal of Public Health, 90*(5), 762–767.

Hawe, P., & Shiell, A. (2000). Social capital and health promotion: A review. *Social Science & Medicine, 51*(6), 871–875.

Institute of Medicine [IOM]. (2003). *The future of the public's health in the 21st century.* Washington, D.C.: The National Academies Press.

Kuntz, S. W., Winters, C. A., Hill, W. G., Weinert, C., Rowse, K., Hernandez, T., et al. (2009). Rural public health policy models to address an evolving environmental asbestos disaster. *Public Health Nursing, 26*(1), 70–78.

Massey, P., & Durrheim, D. (2007). Income inequality and health status: A nursing issue. *Australian Journal of Advanced Nursing, 25*(2), 84–88.

McDermott-Levy, R., Kaktins, N., & Sattler, B. (2013). Fracking, the environment, and health. *American Journal of Nursing, 113*(6), 45–51.

Milio, N. (1996). Linking health, communities, information technology and policy. In N. Milio (Ed.), *Engines of empowerment: Using information technology to create healthy communities and challenge public policy.* Chicago: Health Administration Press.

Milio, N. (2002). Where policy hits the pavement: Contemporary issues in communities. In D. J. Mason, J. K. Leavitt, & M. W. Chaffee (Eds.), *Policy & politics in nursing and health care* (4th ed., pp. 659–668). St. Louis: W.B. Saunders.

Monroe, J. A. (1997). Enemies of the people: The moral dimension to public health. *Journal of Health Politics, Policy and Law, 22*(4), 993–1020.

National Poverty Center. (2007). Policy brief #9: Education and health. Retrieved from *www.npc.umich.edu/publications/policy_briefs/brief9/policy_brief9.pdf.*

Population Health Forum, University of Washington. (2009). Advocating for action toward a healthier society. Retrieved from *depts.washington.edu/eqhlth/.*

Prudential, Iraq and Afghanistan Veterans of America. (2012). Veterans' employment challenges: Perceptions and experiences of transitioning from military to civilian life. Retrieved from *www.prudential.com/documents/public/VeteransEmploymentChallenges.pdf.*

Rafferty, M. A., & Limonik, E. (2013). Is shale gas drilling an energy solution or public health crisis? *Public Health Nursing, 30*(5), 454–462.

Rudolph, L., Caplan, J., Ben-Moshe, K., & Dillon, L. (2013). *Health in all policies: A guide for state and local governments.* Washington, DC and Oakland, CA: American Public Health Association and Public Health Institute. Retrieved from *www.apha.org/NR/rdonlyres/882690FE-8ADD-49E0-8270-94C0ACD14F91/0/HealthinAllPoliciesGuide169pages.PDF.*

Robert Wood Johnson Foundation [RWJF]. (2011). Education and health. Policy brief #5: Exploring the social determinants of health. Retrieved from *www.rwjf.org/content/dam/farm/reports/issue_briefs/2011/rwjf70447.*

Robert Wood Johnson Foundation [RWJF]. (2014). Place matters: Q&A with Brian Smedley, Joint Center for Political and Economic Studies. Retrieved from *www.rwjf.org/en/blogs/new-public-health/2014/04/place_matters_q_aw.html?cid=xtw_pubhealth.*

SmithBattle, L. (2012). Moving policies upstream to mitigate the social determinants of early childbearing. *Public Health Nursing, 29*(5), 444–454.

Somerville, M. H., Nelson, G. D., & Mueller, C. H. (2013). Hospital community benefits after the ACA: The state law landscape. Baltimore, MD: The Hilltop Institute. Retrieved from *www.hilltopinstitute.org/publications/HospitalCommunityBenefitsAfterTheACA-StateLawLandscapeIssueBrief6-March2013.pdf.*

Troy, D. A., Carson, A., Vanderbeek, J., & Hutton, A. (2008). Enhancing community-based disaster preparedness with information technology. *Disasters, 32*(1), 149–165.

U.S. Department of Health and Human Services [HHS]. (2009). National Health Security Strategy of the United States of America. Retrieved from *www.phe.gov/Preparedness/planning/authority/nhss/strategy/Documents/nhss-final.pdf.*

U.S. Department of Health and Human Services [HHS]. (2010). Healthy people 2020. Retrieved from *www.healthypeople.gov.*

Wilkinson, R., & Marmot, M. (Eds.), (2003). *Social determinants of health: The solid facts.* Copenhagen, Denmark: World Health Organization.

World Health Organization [WHO]. (2003). R. Wilkinson & M. Marmot (Eds.), *Social determinants of health: The solid facts* (2nd ed.). Retrieved from *www.euro.who.int/document/e81384.pdf.*

World Health Organization [WHO]. (2004). WHO Framework Convention on Tobacco Control. Retrieved from *www.who.int.fctc/en.*

World Health Organization [WHO]. (2013). *Alliance for Health Policy and Systems Research annual report 2012: Coming together as a community.* Geneva, Switzerland: World Health Organization.

ONLINE RESOURCES

Robert Wood Johnson Foundation, Healthy Communities Initiative
www.rwjf.org/en/topics/rwjf-topic-areas/healthy-communities.html
Robert Wood Johnson Foundation, Community Development and Health Initiative
www.rwjf.org/en/topics/rwjf-topic-areas/community-development-and-health.html
Healthy People 2020
www.healthypeople.gov
World Health Organization (WHO): Healthy People Initiative
www.who.int/topics/primary_health_care/en

CHAPTER 82

An Introduction to Community Activism

DeAnne K. Hilfinger Messias   Robin Dawson Estrada

"Never doubt that a small group of thoughtful, committed citizens can change the world. Indeed, it is the only thing that ever has."

Margaret Mead, anthropologist

Community activism is the means through which individuals, groups, and organizations work together to bring about specific, often radical, changes in social, economic, environmental, and cultural policies and practices. The broad goal of community activism is to enact social transformation that contributes directly to improving living conditions, enhancing community environments, and eliminating health and social disparities. Community activists engage in collaborative, sustained actions focused on changing underlying structures or removing barriers, be they political, social, economic, environmental, or cultural, with the ultimate aim of improving the lives of individuals or groups subjected to disparate, discriminatory, or oppressive conditions (Table 82-1). The primary focus on changing underlying or contributing structures, practices, or policies is what distinguishes community activism from community service, the provision of goods or services for underserved or underprivileged individuals or groups (Jennings et al., 2006; Jennings, Hardee, & Messias, 2010; Nam, 2012). It is further distinguished from community development, in which the primary focus is to enhance existing social and economic infrastructures through the creation of new service programs, leadership training, and innovative partnerships (Larsen, 2004; Dale & Newman, 2010). Another distinguishing characteristic of community activism is that the primary commitment and motivation for

change are generated from within the community of interest. In contrast, the motivation, expertise, and resources for community service and development often originate outside the local community.

KEY CONCEPTS

The concepts of social justice, community, consciousness-raising, critical reflection, praxis, and empowerment are integral to community activism (Figure 82-1).

Social justice is a philosophical, political, and public health concept rooted in the ideal of human rights and social equity (Reichert, 2007). The equitable distribution of resources and opportunities for a productive and fulfilling life is a human rights concern. Prerequisites for social justice include the establishment and assurance of equal treatment under the law, equal access to opportunities, and fair and equitable distribution of resources. Yet in many communities around the globe, availability and access to basic resources and opportunities such as clean air and water, adequate and nutritious food, appropriate housing, safe and secure neighborhoods, equitable educational opportunities, the means to a productive and fulfilling livelihood, culturally appropriate and affordable health services, and fair and equal treatment under the law are not equitably distributed among all individuals and groups (Braveman, 2006). Rather, factors such as social privilege or market forces determine the distribution of these key resources and opportunities, resulting in social injustices and inequities. Health inequities are avoidable differences in health status between groups, both within regions or countries and between countries (World Health

651

TABLE 82-1 Types and Definitions of Community Actions

Type of Community Action	Definition
Community Activism	Collaborative, sustained actions focused on changing structures or removing barriers with the ultimate aim of improving the lives of individuals or groups subjected to disparate, discriminatory, or oppressive social, economic, political, cultural, or environmental conditions.
Community Development	The creation of new programs and services to improve and enhance local social and economic infrastructures
Community Service	The provision of goods or services for underserved or underprivileged individuals or groups.

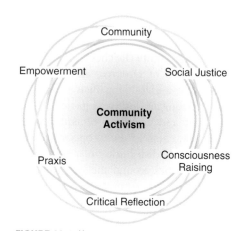

FIGURE 82-1 Key concepts of community activism.

Organization, n.d.). Overcoming health inequities and social injustice requires collective action and solutions on multiple fronts. One of the ways the ideal of social justice is translated into practice is through community activism.

Community is a dynamic and fluid concept, conceptualized and practiced in diverse ways. In relation to activism, community implies the actual involvement of individuals and groups directly impacted by the specific issues or conditions that are the focus of change. In a more traditional sense community, or grassroots, activism is considered to be locally generated and locally focused. Many community activists are located within and focused on creating change in a specific geographic location, such as the neighborhood, school district, or city where they live, study, or work. Neighborhood activists frequently mobilize around issues related to public safety, environmental health, education, land use, zoning, and economic development. The focus may be location-specific (e.g., getting traffic signs installed at busy intersections, organizing a neighborhood watch or clean-up effort, eliminating the presence of alcohol and tobacco advertising in low-income and minority neighborhoods) or may address broader structural issues such as economic development or environmental pollution.

In the United States, education is a common focus of activism involving students, parents, teachers, and the broader community. The implementation of bilingual education programs in southwest Chicago public schools came about in response to Mexican American community activism (Stovall, 2006). In 2013, education cuts to the North Carolina state budget led to demonstrations by students, parents, teachers, community and religious leaders, and members of national organizations including the National Education Association (NEA) and the National Association for the Advancement of Colored People (NAACP). The movement, which became known as Moral Mondays, included protests and rallies at the North Carolina Legislative Building, voter registration drives, and legal opposition to the proposed budget changes (Blythe, 2013).

Grassroots activists also mobilize across geographical and social communities. Historically, community activists have participated in broader social movements including the women's rights, civil rights, workers' rights, and environmental health movements. Much activism occurs within the context of communities formed through a shared sense of political responsibility or affiliation with a collective social identity (e.g., cultural or ethnic group, race, religion), exemplified by the effective mobilization of mothers and babies to rally against the use of bisphenol A (BPA) in baby bottles and other food and beverage containers (Smith & Lourie, 2009; Brewer & Ley, 2011). The increasingly widespread availability and decreased costs of devices that share written and visual information (such as cellular phones) allows activists to construct a new concept of community defined not by physical location but instead by connectedness with a common issue of concern (Tufekci & Wilson, 2012). Collective social identities related to specific health issues (e.g., HIV/AIDS, cancer, mental health, tuberculosis, women's reproductive health) have given rise to significant community activist movements. Over the past 25 years, what is now a global HIV/AIDS movement began as local activism within gay communities in the United States, Canada, Western Europe, and Australia. These early activists mobilized to educate their own communities around HIV prevention and, at the same time, demand responsive public action from governments, medical researchers, health care providers, pharmaceutical companies, and legal systems (Piot, 2006). Subsequent HIV/AIDS grassroots mobilizations have involved diverse communities, including persons living with AIDS in Brazil, Uganda, and South Africa, sex-workers in Thailand, religious and community leaders in Senegal, and impoverished mothers of childhood AIDS victims in Romania. Through relentless advocacy and demands for changes in public policy as well as local health care systems, HIV/AIDS community activists have provoked governmental and industry responses, resulting in more effective prevention and access to treatment and significantly impacting the global HIV/AIDS epidemic (Marcolongo, 2002; Piot, 2006; Gulaid & Kiragu, 2012).

Consciousness raising, critical reflection, and praxis are three interrelated components of community activism. Underlying liberatory approaches to community activism is the premise that empowerment emerges from engagement in focused dialogue, listening, critical reflection, and reflective action (Freire, 1970/1997, 1973/1993). One of the first steps to engaging participants in activist endeavors is to increase public awareness of specific issues and the associated root causes.

Consciousness-raising goes beyond simply presenting others with information, to actually engaging with others in critical reflection. Popular educator and community activist Paulo Freire originally defined and applied the concept of *conscientização* (Portuguese for conscientization) in his community-based work with illiterate Brazilian peasants. Conscientization is a reflective process in which individuals and groups examine their own particular situations and contexts to identify social, economic, cultural, political, and environmental forces contributing to those situations. Critical awareness arises through the reflective processes of problem-posing and interpretive decoding of lived experiences (Freire, 1970/1997).

Critical reflection is integral to understanding the linkages and connections between a local community's issues and problems and those of other communities across the globe. By engaging in critical dialogue and reflection, community activists begin to envision possibilities for collective action leading to transformation (Jennings, Hardee, & Messias, 2010). Critical reflection also involves attention to the political processes and actions necessary to challenge inequalities and effect change. Praxis is purposeful, reflective action arising out of individual and collective conscientization and theorizing, and grounded in a commitment to building a more just society through diverse means, including culture circles, critical pedagogies, action research, and community activism (Freire, 1970/1997, 1973/1993; Stovall, 2006; Hesse-Biber, 2007). Community activism is a form of critical social praxis, an iterative cycle of conscientization-reflection-reflective action in which relations of power and inequality are identified, challenged, and changed.

Empowerment is a multilevel construct that incorporates processes and outcomes of social action through which individuals, families, organizations, and communities gain control and mastery within the social, economic, and political contexts of their lives to attain greater equity and improve the quality of life (Jennings et al., 2006). At the individual level, empowerment may result from the generation of new knowledge and understanding of issues, and the development of new skills among community activists. This individual empowerment can then be linked to community organizing to support social action and political change, as well as to individual self-protective and other socially responsible behaviors (Wallerstein, Sanchez-Merki & Velarde, 2005). Collective empowerment occurs within families, organizations, and communities. It involves processes and structures that enhance members' skills, provides them with the mutual support necessary to effect change, improves their collective well-being, and strengthens intra- and inter-organizational networks and linkages to improve or maintain the quality of community life.

The process of making connections between personal experience and broader social issues is integral to personal and community empowerment and to effective action. In describing a youth empowerment program at an alternative high school for youth unable to succeed within the traditional educational system, Mitra (2008) reported an adult advisor's observation that "the kids involved are changing [from] delinquent into activists. [They can see] how they got sucked into being delinquent and the criminal justice system through their upbringing—not just their family, but the community and the policies" (p. 210). The purpose of empowerment education is to develop the requisite knowledge and skills for community activism, particularly among the youth. By participating in community action projects (peer teaching, the production of murals, cultural institutes, the creation of videos for use in educational efforts, or photo-voice projects) young people and other potential activists develop the requisite knowledge and skills for community activism as they engage in collective conscious-raising, critical reflection, and reflective action (Messias et al., 2008).

TAKING ACTION TO EFFECT CHANGE: CHARACTERISTICS OF COMMUNITY ACTIVISTS AND ACTIVISM

Activists not only recognize injustice but are willing to take action to correct it (Sherrod, 2006). Situated across the social, economic, and political spectrum,

activists share a desire to contribute to the collective welfare and create a more just and equitable society. Motivation and commitment of personal time and energy to social involvement, a willingness to take risks, and belief in the power and efficacy of groups to effect change are common characteristics among community activists. The motivation may be rooted in personal or professional experience, empathy, or solidarity (Lewis-Charp, Yu, & Soukamneuth, 2006; Montlake, 2009). Because of the risks embedded in social justice work, activists must individually and collectively assess the potential harm that may come from actions, help each other prepare if they choose to take calculated risks, and take steps to protect themselves and others as best as possible when they do (Cohen, de la Vega, & Watson, 2001).

Community activism grows out of the desire to change existing social, political, or environmental conditions. In their commitment to change and transform the way power is distributed or controlled, activists draw on the power of the people and the community (power within) and exert pressure on those who hold institutional power (power over). Characteristics of successful community activism include the ability to frame issues and envision a different reality, a clear commitment to change at various levels, the implementation of effective organizing practices and actions, and the ability to develop and sustain collaborative partnerships and relationships (Figure 82-2).

Envisioning change and possibilities for different realities: New ways of collective seeing, perceiving,

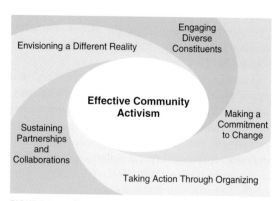

FIGURE 82-2 Characteristic processes of effective community activism.

and acting are essential for change (Jennings, Hardee & Messias, 2010). To create the momentum and sustain process toward social change, activists may need to refocus issues around commonalities rather than fuel polarization around differences. When working toward the goal of a new and different reality, the processes of consciousness-raising and critical reflection can result in collective redefinition and reframing of issues. For instance, in addressing problems such as educational inequality, activists may need to rethink commonly held wisdom and redirect the focus of their actions. Lightfoot (2008) provided an example of such rethinking and reframing, citing the case of local education activists changing the focus from replacing school segregation with integration to actively addressing the underlying racism that had fostered and perpetuated segregation in the first place. In the case of transnational activism to improve the lives of marginalized Filipino bar girls working in a country where prostitution is illegal, the commitment to change was informed by activists' understanding of the social and political context (Ralston & Keeble, 2009). Rather than framing the issue as eliminating prostitution, the activists focused on alleviating prostitutes' legal, financial, and social hardships, by changing the minds and practices of exploitative bar owners and clients, an unsympathetic community, and an insensitive court system.

Taking action: Beyond critical conceptualization and framing of issues, creating change requires action on multiple fronts and the participation of individuals with a wide range of skills, talents, and competencies. Activists work to create change in social norms, public policies, legislation, or environmental practices. Effecting change in policies, practices, and social structures entails integrated information, mobilization, relationship-building, and communication work. This requires extensive research and analysis of complex issues; monitoring of local power dynamics; and ongoing planning, implementation, and evaluation of the effectiveness of strategies and approaches.

Community activists organize and act to call attention to their issues, communicate and disseminate information, develop and maintain networks, and engage others in problem-solving and policy change strategies. Communication and information dissemination actions include door-to-door soliciting; writing letters to the editor; creating and distributing flyers, posters, and leaflets; and producing and disseminating print, radio, and television ads. Increasingly, activists employ Internet formats (e.g., websites, email, blogs, social networking sites) to communicate within their existing networks and to reach new audiences. In tailoring their messages for specific audiences, community activists use a range of media from art, storytelling, songs, theater, photography, videos, and multimedia presentations to expert panels, research reports, and policy briefs.

To engage community members and policymakers in problem solving and policy change, activists employ a variety of mobilization and organizing actions, such as conducting public meetings and forums; planning and carrying out mass demonstrations, rallies, and marches; supporting and participating in boycotts and strikes; collecting signatures on petitions and carrying out letter-writing campaigns; and conducting teach-ins, trainings, workshops, and community-based participatory research. The production of documentary films has been used as a strategy to expand the number of activists and to mobilize them for further action (Whiteman, 2009).

Creating and sustaining collaborations: Less visible but clearly as important is the behind-the-scenes work of networking, building relationships, and sustaining coalitions. Everyday social networks through home, school, and work provide potential connections and opportunities for activism (Martin, Hanson, & Fontaine, 2007). Collaboration is a key process within community activism and is necessary to develop and implement policies and practices to effect the desired changes. Collaboration requires considerable time, energy, skill, and the involvement of multiple stakeholders, but the power of collaboration is that by working together, concerned individuals and groups can create the synergy to produce a desired change that could not be generated by individual action alone.

Partnering with like-minded individuals and organizations strengthens activist movements, but to effect real change, activists often must build bridges and create collaborative relationships that cross differences in age, race, class, social position, location, or nationality and bring together groups with differing perspectives on the issues. Productive collaborations contribute to capacity-building among individuals, groups, and organizations, resulting in enhanced ability to achieve mutual goals. At its core, activism is relational work, as exemplified in the life and work of Ella Baker. Although not as well known or well recognized as Martin Luther King, Jr., Baker was an instrumental visionary and community organizer within the civil rights movements who dedicated her life to organizing and mentoring students and community members. Born and educated in the Jim Crow South, in 1927 Baker moved to New York City, which became the base for her activist career over the next 50 years. Ella Baker worked on social justice issues ranging from child welfare, youth services, school reform, and consumer education to police brutality, desegregation, and voting rights. Through her collaborative associations with other activists, educators, and policymakers in various organizations (including Parents in Action, NAACP, Southern Christian Leadership Conference, In Friendship, and the Student Nonviolent Coordinating Committee) Baker's activism was essential in developing the groundwork for legal and institutional changes of the civil rights movement and eventual de facto racial desegregation. Baker's approach to furthering human rights was to build "strong people" rather than to support a "strong leader" (Ransby, 2003).

CHALLENGES AND OPPORTUNITIES IN COMMUNITY ACTIVISM

Community activists in the 21st century face numerous challenges and opportunities, including making the choice between incremental or radical change, addressing local issues within the context of an increasingly globalized world, widening income gaps within and across countries, effectively harnessing the potential of new technologies, and

encouraging and empowering new activists. A major strategic challenge is the decision to pursue incremental or radical change, concomitantly balancing the potential costs with prospective gains of either strategy. Ralston and Keeble (2009) provided an example of this challenge in their assessment of transnational collaborative efforts to improve the lives of Filipino prostitutes. Although some of the partner activist organizations were steadfast in their commitment to the eradication of prostitution and an end to sexual exploitation, Ralston and Keeble recognized that to have begun with the explicit goal of "eliminating prostitution in such an exploitative context…would have prevented the germination of a project like ours, where the process of harm reduction to women in the sex trade began" (p. 161). Although making some headway in their collaborative effort to build the capacity of Filipino groups working directly with prostitutes, these activists also came to recognize the significance of actions and change at the individual level, arguing that transcending differences to work for social justice involved both standing with others and changing minds.

The forces of globalization and its concomitant movement of people, goods, services, technology, information, and ideas across geographical and political borders have impacted the form and focus of community activism. Today's community activists address local issues within the context of an increasingly globalized world. There are enormous opportunities for ongoing activism and engagement to overcome environmental, economic, and social inequalities and injustice on many fronts, and the ability to transcend local boundaries and become part of global movements is both a challenge and an opportunity. The growth of the activist movement against gender-based violence is an example of the opportunities for local activism to translate into global action and policy change. In communities across the globe, activists have worked to raise awareness about gender-based violence and to create and strengthen local resources to both support victims and prevent further violence against women and girls. The 16 Days of Activism campaign against gender violence is an example of a global network of community activists. This campaign originated with local activists who came together at the 1991 Women's Global Leadership Institute. An outcome of this event was the creation of the 16 Days Campaign, anchored by November 25, International Day Against Violence Against Women, and December 10, International Human Rights Day, and the symbolical linking of gender-based violence and the violation of human rights. As part of the early 16 Days Campaigns, local activists circulated petitions and collected signatures that were instrumental in shaping the agenda of the 1993 World Conference on Human Rights in Vienna. In recent years, 16 Days Campaign activists have focused on the intersections of HIV/AIDS and gender-based violence (Center for Women's Global Leadership, n.d.; The Joint United Nations Programme on HIV and AIDS [UNAIDS], 2006). Another example of transnational activism is the anti-sweatshop movement linking students, community residents, workers, and labor activists, in the United States and other countries. These activists work concomitantly to change the working conditions of workers, most of whom are women, and the creation of sweat-free business policies and practices in cities and campuses (Student Labor Action Coalition, n.d., United Students against Sweatshops, n.d.).

New technologies provide opportunities for activists to reach untapped audiences and disseminate interactive media. Components of online activism include public awareness and online advocacy, organization, and mobilization, and action and reaction (Vegh, 2003). Activists have used a variety of Internet-based media, from email and blogs to YouTube, Twitter, Facebook, and mobile-based apps (e.g., Vine, Instagram) that allow users to share and embed pictures and video on social networking sites. The use of social media subverts traditional means of activism by creating a space for protest that can be difficult for those in authority to control or suppress. In an increasingly globalized world, activists from these virtual communities use social media to provide real-time access to events of political significance and are able to rapidly mobilize protestors to action. The accessibility of Internet-based media, although democratizing, has the potential for negative outcomes.

Dissemination of information may have unintended consequences if that information is incorrect. Further, communities may coalesce around erroneous or inaccurate information. For nurses and health professionals, understanding the public health implications of social medial use is imperative. Consider, for example, the ramifications of increased infectious disease transmission associated with parents of young children basing the decision not to vaccinate their children on information gathered through social media (Salathé & Khandelwal, 2011).

Media literacy can be both the means and an end in community activism. Duncan-Andrade (2006) described how engaging youth in critical production of media texts can serve as a site for critique and analysis of urban social inequalities as well as a site of production for social change. A recent initiative of the Hesperian Foundation, the Community Action for Women's Health and Empowerment, combines the traditional print resource of a book with a web-based tool that will include examples of action strategies and community-based organizational tools from groups around the world with expertise in particular areas of women's health (Hesperian Foundation, 2009). Beyond employing information technology as a tool, another challenge global health activists face is to create access to appropriate technology, such as renewable energy sources (e.g., solar, wind) for remote rural health care clinics in developing countries. Of course, technology does not come without costs and challenges, which range from the investment costs, upkeep and maintenance, updates, and the costs of personnel and training. Ensuring intergenerational continuity of community work is another ongoing challenge among community activism movements (Naples, 1998). Thus, the work of successful community activists also includes encouraging, mentoring, and empowering new activists.

NURSES AS COMMUNITY ACTIVISTS

Nurses and other health professionals may be involved in activist endeavors as members of their local communities and in conjunction with their professional roles. The involvement of nurses in community activism is not surprising, given the shared ethics of care and social justice and the activism of early nursing leaders such as Florence Nightingale, Lillian Wald, and Lavinia Dock (Andrist, 2006; Drevdahl, 2006). In today's increasingly digital and global contexts, nurses around the world use a wide range of tools as they engage in grassroots to global activism to promote social, environmental, cultural, and health systems change (Beck, Dossey & Rushton, 2013). As environmental health activists, nurses have led efforts to implement smoke-free workplace policies, create physical-activity friendly neighborhood environments, establish and monitor standards for clean air and water, and mobilize communities impacted by environmental toxins and pollutants. Nurses have also joined in grassroots campaigns such as fire sprinkler mandates to promote public safety through legislation (Pertschuk et al., 2013). Within the women's health arena, examples of nurse-led activism include the establishment of community-based maternity care for underserved populations, implementation of hospital breastfeeding policies and practices, and advocacy and policy work in the areas of reproductive health and human trafficking. Nurse activists can be an important force for change within the health care system, as evidenced by recent efforts to implement policy and practice changes in the areas of patient safety, workplace injury prevention, and health care reform. The professional expectation that nurses be involved in policy development, implementation, and evaluation will require more nurses to develop an activist skill set in the future. As each new generation of nurses comes into practice, they must balance the need to sustain existing activist endeavors while addressing new challenges as they arise.

Opportunities for activism and social justice work exist across all types and configurations of communities. Every community faces the ongoing challenge of renewing the call to action, encouraging and empowering its members to actively participate in the processes and institutions that shape their social and economic lives, their health, and their well-being.

DISCUSSION QUESTIONS

1. What are the aims of community activism? Give some examples of social, economic, environmental, or cultural changes that have resulted from local community activism.

2. What are the key concepts underlying community activism? Give examples of how each of these concepts applies to a specific context.

3. What are the characteristics of successful community activist movements? Using a specific activist movement as an example, illustrate these various processes.

4. What are the challenges and opportunities community activists face in an increasingly globalized and technological world?

REFERENCES

Andrist, L. C. (2006). The history of the relationship between feminism and nursing. In L. C. Andrist, P. K. Nicholas, & K. A. Wolf (Eds.), *A history of nursing ideas* (pp. 5–22). Sudbury, MA: Jones and Bartlett.

Beck, D., Dossey, B. M., & Rushton, C. H. (2013). Building the Nightingale initiative for global health—NIGH: Can we engage and empower the public voices of nurses worldwide? *Nursing Science Quarterly, 26*(4), 336–371.

Blythe, A. (2013, July 23). Moral Monday demonstrators focus on voter rights, education cuts. *Raleigh News & Observer.* Retrieved from *www .newsobserver.com/2013/07/23/3049031_moral-monday-demonstrators -focus.html?rh=1.*

Braveman, P. (2006). Health disparities and health equity: Concepts and measurement. *Annual Review of Public Health, 27,* 167–194.

Brewer, P. R., & Ley, B. L. (2011). Multiple exposures: Scientific controversy, the media, and public responses to Bisphenol A. *Science Communication, 33*(1), 76–97.

Center for Women's Global Leadership. (n.d.). About the 16 Days: What is the 16 Days of Activism Against Gender Violence Campaign? Retrieved from *16dayscwgl.rutgers.edu/about/campaign-profile.*

Cohen, D., de la Vega, R., & Watson, G. (2001). *Advocacy for Social justice: A global action and reflection guide.* Bloomfield, Ct: Kumarian press.

Dale, A., & Newman, L. (2010). Social capital: A necessary and sufficient condition for sustainable community development? *Community Development Journal, 45*(1), 5–21.

Drevdahl, D. J. (2006). The concept of community in nursing history: Its narrative stream. In L. C. Andrist, P. K. Nicholas, & K. A. Wolf (Eds.), *A history of nursing ideas* (pp. 83–96). Sudbury, MA: Jones and Bartlett.

Duncan-Andrade, J. (2006). Urban youth, media literacy, and increased critical civic participation. In S. Ginwright, P. Noguera, & J. Cammarota (Eds.), *Beyond resistance! Youth activism and community change: New democratic possibilities for practice and policy for America's youth* (pp. 149–169). New York: Routledge.

Freire, P. (1970/1997). *Pedagogy of the oppressed* (20th-anniversary ed.). Trans. Myra Bergman Ramos. New York: Continuum.

Freire, P. (1973/1993). *Education for critical consciousness.* Trans. Myra Bergman Ramos. New York: Continuum.

Gulaid, L. A., & Kiragu, K. (2012). Lessons learnt from promising practices in community engagement for the elimination of new HIV infections in children by 2015 and keeping their mothers alive: summary of a desk review. *Journal of the International AIDS Society, 15*(Suppl. 2), 1–8.

Hesperian Foundation. (2009). Community action for women's health and empowerment. Retrieved from *www.hesperian.org/projects_inProgress _womensactionguide.php.*

Hesse-Biber, S. N. (2007). Feminist research: Exploring the interconnections of epistemology, methodology, and method. In S. N. Hesse-Biber (Ed.), *Handbook of feminist research: Theory and praxis* (pp. 1–26). Thousand Oaks: Sage.

Jennings, L., Hardee, S., & Messias, D. K. H. (2010). Addressing oppressive discourses and images of youth: Sites of possibility. In L. B. Jennings, P. C. Jewett, T. T. Laman, M. V. Souto-Manning, & J. L. Wilson (Eds.), *Sites of possibility: Critical dialogue across educational settings* (pp. 39–67). Cresskill NJ: Hampton Press.

Jennings, L. B., Parra-Medina, D., Messias, D. K. H., & McLoughlin, K. (2006). Toward a theory of critical social youth empowerment. *Journal of Community Practice, 14*(1/2), 29–54.

Larsen, S. C. (2004). Place, activism, and development politics in the Southwest Georgia United Empowerment Zone. *Journal of Cultural Geography, 22*(1), 27–49.

Lewis-Charp, H., Yu, H. C., & Soukamneuth, S. (2006). Civic activist approaches for engaging youth in social justice. In S. Ginwright, P. Noguera, & J. Cammarota (Eds.), *Beyond resistance! Youth activism and community change: New democratic possibilities for practice and policy for America's youth* (pp. 21–35). New York: Routledge.

Lightfoot, J. D. (2008). Separate is inherently unequal: Rethinking commonly held wisdom. In A. H. Normore (Ed.), *Leadership for social justice: Promoting equity and excellence through inquiry and reflective practice.* (pp. 37–59). Charlotte, NC: Information Age Publishing.

Marcolongo, M. (2002). The good mothers: Romania's HIV/AIDS activists are mostly poor mothers of thousands of children who contracted the disease due to poor medical practices under the Ceausescu regime. *Alternatives Journal, 28*(2), 23–25.

Martin, D. G., Hanson, S., & Fontaine, D. (2007). What counts as activism? The role of individuals in creating change. *Women's Studies Quarterly, 35*(3 & 4), 78–94.

Messias, D. K. H., McLoughlin, K., Fore, E., Jennings, L., & Parra-Medina, D. (2008). Images of youth: Representations and interpretations by youth actively engaged in their communities. *International Journal of Qualitative Issues in Education, 21*(2), 159–178.

Mitra, D. L. (2008). Student voice or empowerment? Examining the role of school-based youth-adult partnerships as an avenue toward focusing on social justice. In A. H. Normore (Ed.), *Leadership for social justice: Promoting equity and excellence through inquiry and reflective practice* (pp. 195–214). Charlotte, NC: Information Age Publishing.

Montlake, S. (2009). People making a difference: After her husband disappeared, housewife Angkhana Neelepaichit became a human rights activist. *Christian Science Monitor, 101*(86), 47.

Nam, C. (2012). Implications of community activism among urban minority young people for education for engaged and critical citizenship. *International Journal of Progressive Education, 8*(3), 62–76.

Naples, N. A. (1998). *Grassroots warriors: Activist mothering, community work, and the War on Poverty.* New York: Routledge.

Pertschuk, M., Hobart, R., Paloma, M., Larkin, M. A., & Balbach, E. D. (2013). Grassroots movement building and preemption in the campaign for residential fire sprinklers. *American Journal of Public Health, 103*(10), 1780–1787.

Piot, P. (2006). Diverse voices, common ground: Uniting the world against AIDS. Speech at Georgetown University, Washington D.C. March 7, 2006. Retrieved from *www.unaids.org/en/media/unaids/contentassets/ dataimport/pub/speechexd/2006/20060307_sp_piot_georgetown university_en.pdf.*

Ralston, M., & Keeble, E. (2009). *Reluctant bedfellows: Feminism, activism, and prostitution in the Philippines.* Sterling, VA: Kumarian Press.

Ransby, B. (2003). *Ella Baker and the Black freedom movement: A radical democratic vision.* Chapel Hill: University of North Carolina Press.

Reichert, E. (2007). *Challenges in human rights: A social work perspective.* New York: Columbia University.

Salathé, M., & Khandelwal, S. (2011). Assessing vaccination sentiments with online social media: Implications for infectious disease dynamics and control. *PLoS Computational Biology, 7*(10), e1002199.

Sherrod, L. R. (2006). Promoting citizenship and activism in today's youth. In S. Ginwright, P. Noguera, & J. Cammarota (Eds.), *Beyond resistance! Youth activism and community change: New democratic possibilities for practice and policy for America's youth* (pp. 287–299). New York: Routledge.

Smith, M., & Lourie, B. (2009). *Slow death by rubber duck.* Berkeley, CA: Counterpoint.

Stovall, D. (2006). From hunger strike to high school: Youth development, social justice, and school formation. In S. Ginwright, P. Noguera, & J. Cammarota (Eds.), *Beyond resistance! Youth activism and community change: New democratic possibilities for practice and policy for America's youth* (pp. 97–109). New York: Routledge.

Student Labor Action Coalition. (n.d.). Retrieved from *slacuw.com/.*

The Joint United Nations Programme on HIV and AIDS [UNAIDS]. (2006). Stop violence against women; stop HIV. Retrieved from *www.unaids.org/ en/KnowledgeCentre/Resources/FeatureStories/archive/2006/20061127 _Women_violence_en.asp.*

Tufekci, Z., & Wilson, C. (2012). Social media and the decision to participate in political protest: observations from Tahrir Square. *Journal of Communication, 62*(2), 363–379.

United Students Against Sweatshops. (n.d.). Whiteman, D. (2003). Reel impact: How nonprofits harness the power of documentary film. *Stanford Social Innovation Review, 1*(1), 60–63.

Vegh, S. (2003). Classifying forms of online activism: the case of cyberprotests against the World Bank. In M. McCaughey & M. D. Ayers (Eds.), *Cyberactivism: Online activism in theory and practice* (pp. 71–96). New York, NY: Routledge.

Wallerstein, N., Sanchez-Merki, V., & Verlade, L. (2005). Freirian praxis in health education and community organizing: A case study of an adolescent prevention program. In M. Minkler (Ed.), *Community organizing and community building for health* (2nd ed., pp. 218–239). New Brunswick, NJ: Rutgers University Press.

Whiteman, D. (2009). Documentary film as policy analysis: the impact of *Yes, In My Backyard* on activists, agendas, and policy. *Mass Communication and Society, 12*(4), 457–477.

World Health Organization (n.d.). Backgrounder 3: Key concepts: Health inequity. Retrieved from *www.who.int/social_determinants/final _report/key_concepts_en.pdf.*

ONLINE RESOURCES

The Body: HIV/AIDS Activist Central
www.thebody.com/index/govt/activist.html
GBV Prevention Network
www.preventgbvafrica.org
Race Forward
www.raceforward.org/?arc=1
Resilience—Building a World of Resilient Communities
www.resilience.org/about
16 Days of Activism
www.cwgl.rutgers.edu/16days/home.html
Soul of the City
www.ellabakercenter.org/index.php?p=sotc

UNIT 6

CHAPTER 83

TAKING ACTION:

The Canary Coalition for Clean Air in North Carolina's Smoky Mountains and Beyond

Jonathan Bentley   Jean Larson

> *"You cannot affirm the power plant and condemn the smokestack, or affirm the smoke and condemn the cough."*
>
> Wendell Berry, *The Gift of the Good Land,* 1981

I, Jonathan Bentley, moved to the Smoky Mountains of Western North Carolina in 1999, impressed by the region's lush mountains, kind people, and huge tracts of protected land. These blessings were marred, however, by some of the worst air quality in the nation. Pollution from motor vehicles and coal-fired power plants tended to accumulate in the mountains, and by the early years of the new millennium our air was compared to that of smoggy Los Angeles (Western North Carolina [WNC] Regional Air Quality, 2004).

Fortunately, people in our community were already working to clear the air. In 2000, I met Avram Friedman, Executive Director of the Canary Coalition. This grassroots organization took its name from canaries brought into coal mines, where the hapless birds served as early warning of poison gases or low oxygen levels. On behalf of modern-day canaries, such as asthma patients, Fraser firs, and human fetuses, Avram and supporters worked to organize everyday people and send a message to state lawmakers in Raleigh: "Clean air now!"

A prime example was the passage in 2002 of North Carolina's Clean Smokestacks Act, which promised to reduce nitrogen oxide and sulfur dioxide emissions from the state's 14 coal-fired power plants by approximately 75% within 10

years. To support passage of this legislation, the Canary Coalition organized a campaign to encourage people to write and call our state lawmakers to ask for their support. The next step was to visit these legislators in person. I had never considered being a lobbyist, and the same was probably true for eight other Canary Coalition members who boarded a van early one morning to go to the North Carolina General Assembly in Raleigh. With Avram's guidance, we visited lawmakers to highlight citizen support for the Clean Smokestacks Act, then just a bill. One representative showed us stacks of postcards and lists of e-mails and phone calls he had received on this issue, with a clear majority supporting the bill (Ross, 2009). Sitting across the desk from lawmakers, we helped put a face on the otherwise anonymous postcards and phone logs. Later that year, the North Carolina General Assembly signed the Clean Smokestacks Act into law with an overwhelming majority.

LESSONS IN COMMUNICATING

People felt empowered by this and joined our cause. In 2003, the Canary Coalition welcomed Jean Larson as a new member. Jean had worked as a nurse with neuropatients and later with high school students in a public health capacity. She brought new insights, energy, and dedication to our organization. She also helped me understand that citizens and legislators will usually listen to nurses, especially if we can maintain constructive interactions.

Nurses who talk with patients about health issues know that facts, force, and fear are not effective at changing behavior. We can motivate change by creating tension between current and desired states while imbuing a belief in the ability to change. Facts should be reinforced by persuasion that appeals to emotion rather than logic. To do this, we must listen to those who seem to have different views so we can understand their value drivers, match the problem to current concerns, and make the issue personal to them (Manns, 2008). The same is true in talking to people about climate and energy issues. If we listen openly and do not judge them, we may be surprised to find common ground such as maintaining our health, saving money, helping others, or providing for the future of our grandchildren. Discussing successes in other states or regions, telling hope-filled stories, and speaking from the heart can then move people to action.

PERSUASION: THE INTEGRATED RESOURCE PLAN EXAMPLE

Persuasive citizen testimony at Integrated Resource Plan (IRP) hearings is a powerful example of the Canary Coalition working with other environmental groups to improve citizens' effectiveness. Every 2 years utilities are required by the North Carolina Utilities Commission (NCUC) to submit an IRP explaining how power will be generated for the next 15 years. These public hearings had always been held in Raleigh and were seldom attended by anyone other than the utilities and the commission (North Carolina Utilities Commission [NCUC], 2012). But in 2011 a few environmental activists showed up, provided testimony, and started a groundswell. They inspired groups, such as NC Warn, Greenpeace, Beyond Coal, American Association of Retired Persons (AARP), Safe Carolinas, and the Canary Coalition, to encourage more everyday people to participate in subsequent hearings. NC Warn workshops helped people prepare personal, factual, heart-felt testimonies. The Canary Coalition's videotape of the Raleigh IRP testimony was helpful for aspiring speakers who had never attended a utilities commission hearing, and it allowed future testimony to cover points not already raised. Bowing to public pressure, the NCUC scheduled a second hearing in Charlotte, the first ever outside Raleigh.

SPEAKING TO POWER

Hundreds attended the IRP hearing in Charlotte as 91 people testified against NCUC approval of the new plan. Comments were not repetitious. Speakers quoted studies and detailed experiences in other states and countries. One child reported on her school science project in which she found arsenic in a puddle of water at her school. The school is next to a coal-burning power plant that, interestingly, was retired a few weeks later. As a result of persuasive public input, the commissioners made an unprecedented request for Duke Energy to respond to 18 points raised in the testimony (NCUC, 2013). Two of those selected points came from Canary Coalition members. Then, in a remarkable turn of events, the NCUC rejected Duke Energy's IRP, saying it lacked necessary information and should have incorporated more renewable energy options. This official recognition of citizen input gave us renewed hope that our air might continue to improve in years to come. To move forward, however, the Canary Coalition was being forced to reflect on our early years, when the air was dirtier and donations flowed more easily.

CLEAN AIR: A MIXED BLESSING

Ten years or more ago, people in the mountains could see, feel, and smell our smoggy air. First as a nursing student and later working in emergency departments, I observed that spikes in respiratory distress coincided with hazy days and high ground-level ozone. Frequent air quality alerts and ozone action days represented a clear and present danger, and people were motivated to support the Canary Coalition with their time, energy, and checkbooks. But as the promises of the 2002 Clean Smokestacks Act were fulfilled and local air quality improved, our relevance as an organization seemed less obvious. We had reached the end of an organizational cycle and needed to reforge our mission.

UNIT 6

Unlike smoggy vistas, the full picture of global climate change is hard to see. Clean air in the Smokies can be attributed to effective citizen activists, but our skies have also been scoured by changing weather patterns and record-breaking rainfall that move the pollution elsewhere (Daniel, 2013). Ironically, cleaner air in the Smokies may be an ominous sign of global climate change. The Canary Coalition has recognized this and has changed its focus accordingly.

THE CRUCIBLE OF FINANCIAL CHALLENGE

At a time when many donors are limited by effects of the Great Recession, we have moved beyond our established local support base into the climate change realm, which is already championed by well-organized entities such as Greenpeace and 350.org. The Canary Coalition has struggled financially in this new landscape and has been forced to adopt new fund-raising strategies. Although we retained our fundamental avoidance of donations from organizations and entities that might compromise our integrity, we did make some difficult changes. In our new plan, yearly membership dues are now required; board members assume a greater responsibility in fund-raising; and hiring a dedicated professional fund-raiser is being explored.

In drafting this new plan, we considered expert advice and evidence-based approaches. Fund-raising consultant Dan Hotchkiss suggests that people give to extend their own accomplishments. They want to help institutions "that have come to feel like an extension of themselves" (Hotchkiss, 2012). Avram and our board continue to look for ways to demonstrate that supporters' ideals and resources are leveraged by Canary Coalition activities. Videography has been one such tool. After a recent video release *(www.youtube.com/user/canarycoalition)* of testimony given by Avram at a 2013 rate-hike hearing, the organization received a significant inflow of funds. We saw bottom-line evidence that the video gave our donors renewed confidence in our plans and leadership.

Hotchkiss (2012) also writes that donors prefer giving to specific appeals and concrete projects

rather than general operations and staff salaries. Global climate change is a huge issue, but we do not know to what degree it motivates our potential membership base. A recent Yale study shows that "only one in three Americans say they discuss global warming at least occasionally with friends or family, down 8 points since November 2008" (Leiserowitz et al., 2013). With this in mind, we placed our primary focus on a new legislative movement, one that would provide immediate and concrete benefits locally while also addressing global climate change at its source.

EFFICIENT AND AFFORDABLE ENERGY RATES BILL

The 2002 Clean Smokestacks Act represented a crucial environmental success, but it did not address carbon dioxide, which has only recently been classified as pollution (Environmental Protection Agency, 2013). Starting in 2012, lobbying efforts by Canary Coalition members persuaded state legislators to introduce the Efficient and Affordable Energy Rates Bill, H401. Its key elements are: (1) to require the NCUC to establish tiered electricity rates for residential, commercial, public, and industrial customers to encourage energy conservation and energy efficiency; (2) to create the energy efficiency public benefit loan fund to be used for loans to customers for the costs of certain energy efficiency or renewable energy projects; and (3) to create an incentive for consumers to purchase Energy Star qualified household products (General Assembly of North Carolina, 2013).

Although our current rate structure subsidizes waste by decreasing the incremental cost of electricity as households and businesses use more energy, the new plan would reward efficiency. Efficient households and businesses would see even lower energy bills, while those who used more would pay higher rates. Less efficient customers could use special loan funds for efficiency upgrades, and their total bill including the loan payment would still be less than their power bills before the upgrade (General Assembly of North Carolina, 2013).

As an example, my family would be hard-pressed to pay several thousand dollars for a solar hot water

BOX 83-1 Efficient and Affordable Energy Rates Bill: H401 at a Glance

Economic Carrot and Stick for Investment in Efficiency and Independent Solar and Cogeneration Energy Systems	Efficiency Incentives	Tax the Wasters
Three separate rate structures: residential, commercial, and industrial. In each of these sectors is a set of tiered rate blocks of energy usage. The first block each month results in the lowest price per kilowatt/hour. As a rate-payer passes the threshold of each block into higher energy usage each month, the price per kilowatt/hour goes up dramatically.	Creation of an Energy Efficiency Bank that is administered through the monthly utility bill. Issues low-interest loans for energy efficiency, rooftop solar energy projects, and cogeneration systems that will result in lower monthly utility bills including monthly loan payments.	A 5% avoidable pollution fee paid at retail stores for the purchase of all non-Energy Star rated electrical appliances or equipment (e.g., incandescent light bulbs, washing machines, dryers, TVs, refrigerators). The money collected from this fee is earmarked as seed money for the Energy Efficiency Bank.

Designed by A. Freidman, executive director of the Canary Coalition. Retrieved from *www.canarycoalition.org*.

heating system, even with existing tax credits. But what if we could have such a system installed with no outlay of our own money, our monthly electric bills would become lower, and we could take hot showers even during a grid power outage? Even if we did not care about environmental stewardship or public health, the best choice would be clear (Box 83-1).

NURSES' ROLE IN ENVIRONMENTAL STEWARDSHIP

Like Florence Nightingale, the Canary Coalition believes that provision of fresh air is a key to health. The American Nurses Association (2007) calls for nurses to collaborate "with other professionals, policymakers, advocacy groups, and the public in promoting local, state, national, and international efforts to meet health needs." To do this, nurses can start by learning about environmental issues that affect public health in their own geographic areas. Will climate change bring new infectious diseases, displaced populations, or flooding and drought? Nurses can speak with facts and feeling to the decision makers. With our voices, time, and money, we can support advocacy groups that address these issues. We can be proactive by speaking clearly about our goal and persuading others to join us in promoting a healthy environment for current and future generations. In doing so, we may realize that we are all canaries.

REFERENCES

American Nurses Association. (2007). ANA's principles of environmental health for nursing practice with implementation strategies. Retrieved from *www.nursingworld.org/MainMenuCategories/WorkplaceSafety/Healthy-Nurse/ANAsPrinciplesofEnvironmentalHealthforNursingPractice.pdf*.

Daniel, M. (2013). U.S. Southeast experiencing extreme rainfall in 2013. *Earth.* Retrieved from *earthsky.org/earth/u-s-southeast-experiencing-extreme-rainfall-in-2013*.

Environmental Protection Agency. (2013). EPA fact sheet: Reducing carbon pollution from power plants, moving forward on the climate action plan. Retrieved from *www2.epa.gov/carbon-pollution-standards*.

General Assembly of North Carolina. (2013). Session 2013, House Bill 401: Efficient and affordable energy rates. Retrieved from *www.ncga.state.nc.us/Sessions/2013/Bills/House/HTML/H401v1.html*.

Hotchkiss, D. (2012). Unconventional wisdom: Fundraising beliefs. *Congregations Magazine, 3*(3).

Leiserowitz, A., Maibach, E., Roser-Renouf, C., & Feinberg, G. (2013). How Americans communicate about global warming in April 2013. New Haven, CT: Yale Project on Climate Change Communication, Yale University and George Mason University. Retrieved from *environment.yale.edu/climate-communication/article/how-americans-communicate-about-global-warming-april-2013/#sthash.Y4rNUpiX.dpuf*.

Manns, M. (2008, November). *The climate crisis: Transforming information into action.* Paper presented at University of North Carolina, Asheville, NC, Department of Management and Accountancy.

North Carolina Utilities Commission. (2012). Annual report regarding long range needs for expansion of electric generation facilities for service in North Carolina. Required pursuant to G.S. 62-110.1(C). Retrieved from *www.ncuc.commerce.state.nc.us/reports/2012ElectricReport.pdf*.

North Carolina Utilities Commission. (2013). Docket No. E-100, sub 137.

Ross, W. G., Jr. (2009). North Carolina's Clean Smokestacks Act. North Carolina Division of Air Quality. Retrieved from *daq.state.nc.us/news/leg/cleanstacks.shtml*.

Western North Carolina [WNC] Regional Air Quality. (2004). Do we really have air quality as bad as Los Angeles? Retrieved from *www.wncairquality.org/Documents/Asheville_air_quality.pdf*.

UNIT 6

How Community-Based Organizations Are Addressing Nursing's Role in Transforming Health Care

Mary Ann Christopher   Ann Campbell

"The day may soon dawn when we Americans can enjoy a measure of life and health that is consistent with our extraordinary resources and the intelligence of our people. The pioneers have begun their work; it is far from finished. New fields, new enterprises, are visible. The times call for the high spirit of the courageous pioneers among physicians, scientists, and nurses."

Lillian Wald

This is a time of rapid transformation in health care, one in which community health nursing has a critical role in advancing individual and public health. As the United States integrates the mandates of the Affordable Care Act (ACA), community health organizations have a pivotal role in affecting the health status of the nation, particularly for vulnerable populations. The Institute for Healthcare Improvement, through the construct of the Triple Aim, calls on all members of the health care team to improve the health of the population, improve the consumer experience and reduce the cost of care. The Institute of Medicine's (IOM) report on *The Future of Nursing* has charged nurses to become equal partners in the development of health policy and practice (IOM, 2011). The IOM report *Public Health and Primary Care* has challenged practitioners to coordinate efforts for the betterment of patients (IOM, 2012a).

Community-based organizations are strategically positioned to provide the leadership as well as the integration and coordination of services necessary to carry out these aims. Further, the community-based sector of the nursing profession is poised to influence the transformation of health care delivery by drawing on principles that are core to the discipline. By partnering with communities, creating innovative approaches to care as the system evolves, and engaging the communities they serve, community health nurses can deliver on the promise of quality health care for all. This chapter discusses the approaches of the Visiting Nurse Service of New York (VNSNY) to mobilize the strengths of the community to improve public health, establish cross-continuum interprofessional teams to affect the continuum of the patient care journey, and promote public policy to advance funding methodologies that more adequately consider risk factors of vulnerable populations.

COMMUNITY AS PARTNER AND THE COMMUNITY ANCHOR

Community Anchor is a concept that is being developed by the VNSNY as a way to build healthier communities. The Community Anchor is a term that suggests if nursing is going to exercise its responsibility for the individual as well as public health, the profession must recommit to its traditional focus on grassroots needs assessment and service provision, so brilliantly illustrated by the work of Lillian Wald, founder of the Henry Street Settlement House, the VNSNY, public health nursing, occupational health nursing, the first playground in New York City, and more. To best meet the health needs of individuals, nursing must work in partnership with the community. These partnerships act as bridges, connecting public health nursing both to individuals and to the wider community.

The Community Anchor works locally to build or support programs that address social determinants of health, offering reinforcement to communities as they work on revitalization efforts. The Community Anchor uses the community needs assessment to inform program development and create a foothold in the community's areas of vulnerability and strengths, and weaves solutions in tandem with the community. The Community Anchor teams comprise interprofessional members, who in most cases are members of the communities they serve. The following questions help the team to develop key organizing constructs that guide their interventions:

- What are the strengths and assets of the community?
- What are the needs and goals that the community identifies for itself?
- Who are the key stakeholders?
- What are the goals in care?
- What community initiatives are already underway upon which we can build?

Once these questions are answered, tools for the development of Community Anchor initiatives include:

- Mobilizing front-line public health visiting nurses to identify unmet needs and strategic directions of the community
- Mapping assets, or inventorying the assets and gaps in community resources and potential, across a broad spectrum of health, mental health, social service and housing providers, and faith-based coalitions
- Identifying existing community action groups and fostering collaboration
- Partnering with hospitals, ambulatory care networks, and other players to better address the health needs of the community

The Community Anchor strategy, by design, takes different forms based on unique characteristics of each community. In Washington Heights, a diverse, at-risk community in upper Manhattan, the anchor initiative has taken the form of a Health Village, aimed at impacting the self-care management of community residents 60 years of age and older diagnosed with diabetes mellitus. The VNSNY has partnered with supermarkets, housing providers, primary care providers, and an academic medical center to create a safety net of support around a low-income population struggling to follow through with treatment regimens. This patient-centered community network provides the access points for the residents to receive care and coaching in support of their self-management. In fact, residents can access any of the health or social services providers through this community network. It becomes the vehicle for their connection to a comprehensive system of health and social service providers.

In an area of the Rockaways on Long Island that was hit hard by Superstorm Sandy, the anchor initiative focuses on developing specialized registered nurses and licensed clinical social workers, called community wellness coaches (CWCs), with the goal of integrating medical and social services to achieve health promotion and disease prevention and to avert unnecessary emergency department visits. Funded by a New York State Social Services Block Grant, the CWCs direct teams of wellness navigators (WNs), who live in the neighborhoods they serve, centered around hot spots such as senior housing sites, pharmacies, churches, and community centers where health disparities are high and access to services is low. The VNSNY blends lessons learned from its experience in post-Superstorm Sandy recovery efforts with evidence-based elements from a number of coaching models that target at-risk populations, including the Geisinger ProvenHealth Navigator Model (Hospitals in Pursuit of Excellence, n.d.), the Kaiser Grace Model (Bielaszka-DuVernay, 2011), the Care Transitions Intervention (Coleman et al., 2006), and the Transitional Care Model (Naylor et al., 2011).

The objective of this Community Anchor initiative is to conduct outreach to 5000 community residents over a 24-month period through two programs: 1000 residents will be reached through a one-on-one intervention model, and 4000 will be impacted through a group-focused public health model. For the 1000 members in the CWC program who receive one-on-one coaching, community members are paired with the professional coaches for no less than 3 monthly visits. The community health nurses and social workers structure their interventions within the health coaching framework: self-management support, serving as a bridge between clinician and patients, navigation of the health care system, emotional support, and continuity (Bennett et al., 2010). To ensure that the intervention is culturally competent and relevant, WNs are recruited from the neighborhoods they serve to extend the intervention of the professional coaches. The role of the WNs involves fostering patient engagement, facilitating adherence to the plan of care, reinforcing health teaching, and assisting with negotiation of the health care system. The employment of local people likewise facilitates the economic development of the neighborhoods. Among those who serve as WNs are VNSNY home health aides who were promoted to this role and then immersed in a structured course of health navigation and coaching. With this enhanced competency, they now have advanced on the career ladder as well, fulfilling the charge of the IOM *Future of Nursing* report that each member of the interprofessional team function at their highest level of education and training (IOM, 2011). This commitment to the direct care workforce further supports the needs of economically disadvantaged communities.

Building on the assets of the community, the interprofessional teams promote public health by employing an aggregate approach to health intervention. Partnering with key community stakeholders, they design and implement Community Wellness Campaigns aimed at increasing awareness and linking community members to resources on weight management, age appropriate immunizations, health screenings, cardiovascular health, nutrition, and mental health.

ACCOUNTABLE CARE COMMUNITY

A longer-term initiative that will leverage these partnership approaches is the accountable care community (ACC). A concept developed in Akron, Ohio, the ACC focuses on integration within a specific geographic area to bring about improved health outcomes. The ACC encompasses the medical and public health systems, community stakeholders at the grassroots level, and community organizations whose work often encompasses the entire spectrum of the determinants of health (Janosky et al., 2013). Our goal is to obtain federal demonstration funding to test the model of care in collaboration with partners in Nassau County. Through this project, the VNSNY would extend its efforts through geographic morbidity and mortality mapping to at-risk neighborhoods. In a partnership with the community, a public hospital, local housing providers, and social services organizations, visiting nurses would function as population care coordinators to develop a population-based intervention model through which all partners, including community residents, have the opportunity to share in financial rewards that will result once improved health outcomes are achieved.

SUPERSTORM SANDY

This work expands on an approach that the VNSNY has been implementing in a community significantly devastated by Superstorm Sandy. Project Hope is a strengths-based model in which the VNSNY recruited members of the community who had effectively overcome the impact of the disaster to work as crisis counselors, fostering resiliency among survivors within the community. A survivor is defined as someone who is experiencing a "normal reaction to an abnormal situation," and the goal is to empower the survivor to draw upon his or her preexisting coping skills. The crisis counselors work with the survivor to problem solve, provide resources, and support the survivor in taking actions to recover, encompassing a range of behaviors, such as scheduling medical appointments, securing Federal Emergency Management Agency (FEMA) funding, negotiating home insurance coverage, and promoting optimal functioning within the family unit. The survivors regain a sense of control and accomplishment. Project Hope, funded through a public/private partnership, has resulted in the provision of over 20,000 community-based visits to those suffering posttraumatic stress from the impact of the storm. This strengths-based intervention model addresses the mental health impact of disaster and reaches out to those who have become isolated, toppling the disparities that arise when homes have been lost, communities leveled, and services destroyed.

This work has facilitated VNSNY's ability to highlight and institutionalize nursing's role in emergency and postemergency relief work. Through participation on city, state, and regional commissions, we have formalized the role of nursing in the standards for community response. Within the policy briefings that have been forthcoming from this event, community nursing stands embedded along with the environmental, health and human services, housing, communications, and transportation responses that impact societal resiliency.

Recognizing that the goals of the Triple Aim and the promise of the ACA depend on this commitment to community, the VNSNY made an intentional decision to transform the system of care in our market by enhancing the competency of our nurses to address both the individual and population health. Through a partnership with Duke University and New York University, the VNSNY has immersed cohorts of its nursing staff in a semester-long curriculum focused on population care coordination. Nurses gain enhanced exposure to the constructs of epidemiology, community assessment, predictive analytics, and social determinants of health. Armed with these competencies, nurses are assuming leadership roles in designing and implementing community anchor initiatives, accountable care organizations, and payer-based care coordination infrastructures. Nurses are demonstrating their roles as "...full partners, with physicians and other health care professionals, in redesigning health care ..." (IOM, 2010).

Nurses at the VNSNY are using these and other competencies to weave together a cross-continuum system of care that facilitates the safe and meaningful passage of patients. National statistics underscore the imperative for this cross-continuum coordination. In care for the chronically ill, studies have shown that only half of the recommended services are provided (IOM, 2010). If the quality of care were to improve in each state to match that in the highest performing states, an estimated 75,000 lives could be saved each year (IOM, 2012a, 2012b). Care quality, then, is critical to the path forward and partnerships are vital to this aim.

THE POPULATION CARE COORDINATOR

Shifting from a fee-for-service reimbursement environment to one that is value-based requires a change in practice among front-line community health nurses with regard to financial, quality, and population management concerns. In the past, reimbursement was based on the number of patients seen and the particular comorbidities of each patient. Under the value-based model, payment is based on a number of factors linked to care quality. Hospitals are penalized when their patients are readmitted within 30 days of being discharged, and patient satisfaction scores are measured and reported publicly, which influences consumer engagement and choice. Community health nurses must intentionally link discrete interventions to patient outcomes, most notably by preventing unnecessary rehospitalizations and by optimizing patient care experiences.

HOSPITAL PARTNERSHIPS AND TRANSITIONAL CARE

The VNSNY has collaborated with health system partners to establish transitional care programs that facilitate shorter lengths of stay, mitigate the need for subacute placement, and significantly reduce first 30-day all-cause readmissions. The critical components of these programs include: cross-continuum clinical pathways, interprofessional participation and endorsement, warm handoffs at the bedside between acute care and home care nurses, risk adjustment methodologies, and the leadership of advanced practice nurses.

Nurses in community-based settings are participating in convening tables with health system partners to redesign the models of care that are patient-focused and community-centric. In one initiative, hospital length of stay for postoperative patients recovering from hip and knee replacements was reduced by 1 day through an interprofessional team effort that included bedside handoffs, the more effective management and anticipation of uncontrolled diabetes, the advancement of a rehab home health aide coach, and the implementation of an intensive rehab program, which eliminated the need for a subacute stay. The readmission rate for these patients was under 2%.

In another case of patient postcardiothoracic surgery, warm handoffs at the bedside between the acute care and the home care nurse, including focused patient and caregiver engagement, resulted in avoidance of subacute placement, a reduction in substernal wound infections, reduction in length of stay, rehospitalization rates below 10%, and higher patient satisfaction and caregiver engagement.

Another opportunity for community nursing to transform the delivery system is to affect the system of care that results in avoidable emergency department visits with resultant admissions. By adding a community health nurse to the emergency department team, the perspectives of the home and community as assets in the plan of care result in an assess-and-release approach that is more conducive to patient outcome. Among 622 patients assessed in the emergency department of one hospital by VNSNY nurses over a 6-month period, 59% went home directly rather than being admitted to the hospital. The community health nurse in the emergency department interfaces with the home visiting nurse and the community-based nurse practitioner who stabilize the plan of care and create the bridge to the primary care provider. This program has been so effective that new start-up insurance companies on the New York State Health Exchange are contracting with the VNSNY so that home care nurses in the emergency department will be alerted via text when a member of their health plan arrives in the emergency room.

If nurses are truly to affect the system of care, they must also impact health insurance companies. Nurses at the VNSNY did just that by engaging a health insurance company as a partner. Using a modification of the Naylor transitions of care approach, the VNSNY nurses and nurse practitioners partnered with a major insurer and a community hospital to address the incidence of unnecessary hospitalizations among health plan members. Members of the interprofessional team included hospital physicians, nurses, and social workers; VNSNY nurses and nurse practitioners; and nurse practitioners from the health plan. Weekly case conferences, including staff from the hospital, VNSNY staff, and nurse practitioners from the health plan, are conducted virtually for the establishment of the plan of care. Members who were hospitalized received a bedside assessment by a VNSNY nurse to determine their risk of readmission. Among the variables that drive risk acuity are: multimorbidity, polypharmacy, cognitive disability, mental illness, substance abuse, and previous hospitalization or home care admission within the previous 6 months. For those who exhibit the highest risk, a VNSNY nurse practitioner enrolls the patient in a 30-day transitional care program with focused care coordination by an interprofessional team. The 24-hour access to a nurse practitioner, which addresses issues such as medication adjustment, anxiety, and the management of symptoms, many of which occur disproportionately after hours, has been a gold standard for this program. This cross-continuum model, designed by nurses, has effected a 49% reduction in first 30-day all-cause readmissions.

VULNERABLE PATIENT STUDY

Recognizing that the ultimate effectiveness of our work in impacting health care transformation rests on the degree to which it impacts reimbursement methodologies and policy considerations, the VNSNY has directed considerable effort to translating our knowledge of community-based health care to policy arenas. Through our care of vulnerable community-based populations, we have found that certain patient characteristics are predictive of the resource allocation that patients will ultimately require and that must influence reimbursement methodologies if these patients are to receive appropriate care. Through research conducted in partnership with the Visiting Nurse Associations of America, the VNSNY's Center for Home Care

Policy and Research and 23 Visiting Nurse Associations across the country identified patient characteristics that are not adequately considered in the Medicare home health methodology. Those characteristics include: presence of a caregiver, socioeconomic status, continence, clinical complexity, and uncontrolled chronic illness.

The results of this study have been shared with the Medicare Payment Advisory Commission, an independent organization established by the Balanced Budget Act of 1997, and the Centers for Medicare and Medicaid Services, which administers Medicare, Medicaid, and Children's Health Insurance Programs and coordinates with states to set up Health Insurance Marketplaces, expand Medicaid, and regulate private insurance (Centers for Medicare and Medicaid Services [CMS], 2013; Medicare Payment Advisory Commission [MedPAC], 2013). The goal of this advocacy has been to influence risk acuity of the Medicare system to more adequately address the needs of vulnerable populations. We are using similar predictive analytics and risk-adjusted methodologies to negotiate funding streams with private payers.

CONCLUSION

As the health care system continues to demand a commitment to the tenets of the Triple Aim, community health nurses have a central role to play in transforming the system of care. With a discipline anchored in an understanding of public health, with a practice that honors the assets of the community, and with a relationship-based competency that facilitates partnerships, community health nursing can and must execute on the IOM call for our profession to emerge as architects of a transformed health care system.

DISCUSSION QUESTIONS

1. What are the ways in which a population health focus might be applied in the transforming health care delivery system?

2. What are some of the new constructs that nurses are integrating in promoting the health of communities?

3. What are the key foundational elements of a successful transitional care program?

REFERENCES

Bennett, H., Coleman, E., Parry, C., Bodenheimer, T., & Chen, E. (2010). Health coaching for patients with chronic illness. *Family Practice Management, 17*(5), 24–29.

Bielaszka-DuVernay, C. (2011). The "GRACE" model: In-home assessments lead to better care for dual eligibles. *Health Affairs, 30*(3), 431–434.

Centers for Medicare and Medicaid Services [CMS]. (2013). CMS strategy: The road forward 2013-2017. Retrieved from *www.cms.gov/About -CMS/Agency-Information/CMS-Strategy/Downloads/CMS-Strategy .pdf.*

Coleman, E., Parry, C., Chalmers, S., & Min, S. (2006). The care transitions intervention: Results of a randomized controlled trial. *Archives of Internal Medicine, 166*(17), 1822–1828.

Hospitals in Pursuit of Excellence. (n.d.). Case study: Proven Health Navigation at Geisinger Health System. Retrieved from *www.hpoe.org/resources/ case-studies/1297.*

Institute of Medicine [IOM]. (2010). *The healthcare imperative: Lowering costs and improving outcomes.* Washington, DC: National Academies Press.

Institute of Medicine [IOM]. (2011). *The future of nursing: Leading change, advancing health.* Washington, DC: National Academies Press.

Institute of Medicine [IOM]. (2012a). *Public health and primary care: Exploring integration to improve population health.* Washington, DC: National Academies Press.

Institute of Medicine [IOM]. (2012b). *Best care at lower cost: The path to continuously learning health care in America.* Washington, DC: National Academies Press.

Janosky, J., Armoutliev, E., Benipal, A., Kingsbury, D., Teller, J., et al. (2013). Coalitions for impacting health of a community: The Summit County, Ohio, experience. *Population Health Management, 16*(4), 246–254.

Medicare Payment Advisory Commission [MedPAC]. (2013). About MedPAC. Retrieved from *www.medpac.gov/about.cfm.*

Naylor, M., Aiken, L., Kurtzman, E., Olds, D. M., & Hirschman, K. (2011). The importance of transitional care in achieving health reform. *Health Affairs, 30*(4), 746–754.

ONLINE RESOURCES

American Public Health Association
www.apha.org
Care Transitions Program (Eric Coleman's Model)
www.caretransitions.org
Institute for Healthcare Improvement
www.ihi.org/Pages/default.aspx
Transitional Care Model (Mary Naylor's Model)
www.transitionalcare.info
Visiting Nurse Associations of America
vnaa.org

UNIT 6

CHAPTER 85

TAKING ACTION:
From Sewage Problems to the Statehouse: Serving Communities

Mary L. Behrens

"All politics is local."

Thomas P. "Tip" O'Neill, former Speaker of the
U.S. House of Representatives

I have practiced as a family nurse practitioner, pediatric clinical specialist, and nurse educator. Running for political office was not one of my career goals. However, my father was a good role model, as he served on our local school board for 12 years. I attended college in the 1960s during a period of student activism and protests; that experience influenced me also. But it was a problem in my town that sparked my work in politics.

SEWAGE CHANGED MY LIFE

My leap into the political arena came because of a call from an upset friend who lived on property along the river that ran through our community. She told me there was raw sewage on her lawn that was washing up from the river. She had called the health department. They told her to call the state Department of Environmental Quality. That state department referred her to the health department. Out of frustration, she called me.

SEEING IS BELIEVING

I drove to my friend's neighborhood and saw the raw sewage on people's lawns. My friend told me that it appeared like clockwork when everyone flushed their toilets and used their dishwashers in the morning and evening. I decided to take action. I contacted local daycare centers and learned that they had noticed an increase in diarrhea in the children. I then called the two local TV stations and

three radio stations. I informed them of a serious problem on the river, and I gave them the time and location of a press conference I was planning.

At the press conference, I stated that I was a nurse and was concerned about the sewage being a serious health threat to citizens in our town. I discussed the increased diarrhea in children reported by local daycare centers. The news media representatives who attended my press conference could see the raw sewage and captured images with their cameras. The train was moving down the track! The city, the health department, and the state Department of Environmental Quality had to deal with the calls from the press and the citizens. Our local city government and the state had to provide funds to connect this housing development to city water and sewer to stop the pollution.

MY CAMPAIGNS

As I took action on the sewage problem, I attended several city council meetings. When I observed the city council in action, I thought to myself, "I can do this and bring a perspective to the council as a nurse, mother, and concerned citizen." At the next election, I ran for city council in my ward along with 13 other candidates. With the large field of candidates I knew I had to run a strategic campaign to win. I had a good neighbor who had been involved in other campaigns and was eager to help me. We ran a strong grassroots campaign. I walked door to door every free minute I had. I accepted every invitation to speak to various organizations, filled out questionnaires from interest groups, and looked for opportunities to meet with the press. I used a simple one-page flyer discussing my leadership skills. This helped keep expenses down. At Halloween we handed out balloons that said, "Vote for Mary."

I won! Since 1983, I have held three elected offices: city councilor and mayor, chair of the county commission, and representative in the state legislature.

Being involved in my professional associations was important to these successes. Professional membership allows you to meet other nurses around your state, encouraging leadership development, visibility, and confidence. Many nursing organizations encourage political involvement and mentoring. I have served as president of the Wyoming Nurses Association and as second vice president and first vice president of the American Nurses Association (ANA). I also served as chair of the ANA political action committee (PAC) and am the Wyoming representative for the American Association of Nurses Practitioners.

THE VALUE OF POLITICAL ACTIVITY IN YOUR COMMUNITY

At the local level, you have the opportunity to help address problems that affect people's lives. For example, a citizen came to a city council meeting one evening and said he wanted passing lanes on a street in the community. He had a persuasive personality and a reputation for getting what he wanted. His initial presentation was very convincing to other council members. But I lived in this neighborhood and was concerned about the safety implications of this proposal. Part of this street abutted a park where children played. Parents parked along the street to watch or pick up their children. If passing lanes were established in this area, speeds would increase, and the potential risk of a serious accident would rise. As a fellow council member, I asked every councilperson to visit the area, particularly in the late afternoon. All of the members voted against establishing passing lanes on the street.

AN OPPORTUNITY TO LEARN THE ROPES

The local community is an excellent starting place if you want to run for higher office. You can gain experience, confidence, name recognition, and respect. I had the chance to testify before the Federal Energy Regulatory Commission in Washington, DC about the high natural gas prices we were paying in our community. Because I was the only mayor to testify (the others providing testimony were senators, representatives, or governors), I was quoted and praised for bringing a refreshing perspective to the Commission.

NETWORKING

As mayor, I worked with citizens, state legislators, and our state's congressional delegation in Washington, DC. Richard B. (Dick) Cheney was our only representative in Congress when I served as mayor of Casper, Wyoming. I formed an important connection with him because of my mayoral service. This type of connection was an important part of my network when I decided to run for the state legislature and an international nursing endeavor.

Some of my work bridged both local and state-level work. I had joined the Seatbelt Coalition in Wyoming before running for the legislature. The coalition's mission was to educate Wyoming citizens about the need for seatbelt legislation and develop a model law for the Wyoming legislature to enact. As a freshman legislator, I cosponsored the first seatbelt legislation aimed at reducing fatalities on Wyoming highways. I also sponsored several pieces of legislation to help assist communities with high natural gas prices. My experience on the city council prepared me to hit the ground running with issues like this when I arrived at the Wyoming statehouse.

LEADERSHIP IN THE INTERNATIONAL COMMUNITY

I had traveled several times to do humanitarian work in Vietnam and had attended International Council of Nursing conferences. I was concerned about the nursing shortage, not just in the United States but also in the developing world. In 2006, I sent a one-page note to then-Vice President Cheney discussing how I might contribute to the World Health Assembly that meets annually in Geneva, Switzerland. I did not specify a year but rather how my experiences at the ANA and in Vietnam could add to the discussion for a future appointment.

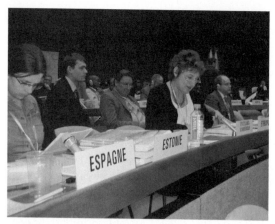

FIGURE 85-1 Mary Behrens testifying at the World Health Assembly in Geneva, Switzerland.

I was invited to meet with the vice president but had health issues that caused me to cancel (I could not believe I had to do that!). I was so disappointed to have missed out on this opportunity but was surprised a few weeks later when I answered the phone.

Someone said, "This is the White House." I grabbed my chair. My mind raced: "Am I dreaming this?" The vice president had recommended that I be part of the U.S. delegation to the World Health Assembly in 3 weeks. I notified the ANA and planned to work with Barbara Blakeney, then-ANA president, who would be attending also.

Soon I was involved in phone calls with staff on logistics and schedule. Before I knew it, I arrived in Geneva for the first meeting with the U.S. Secretary of Health and Human Services Michael Leavitt. I told staff I wanted to testify on behalf of the international nursing shortage (Figure 85-1).

Representatives of several countries had testified before me and had discussed their struggle to find nurses to provide basic services. When it was my turn, I shared my concern about the lack of nurses worldwide, especially in countries in Africa. Several nurses came up to me afterward to thank me for my remarks.

MENTORING OTHER NURSES FOR POLITICAL ADVOCACY

In 2009, the ANA launched the first American Nurses Advocacy Institute, an annual year-long

mentored program investing in growing nurses' competence in advocacy. Each year, state nurses' associations identify qualified candidates based upon previous grassroots experience and willingness to engage in either a project or series of activities designed to advance an initiative that pertains to the state nurses' association's legislative and regulatory agenda.

The program content resulted from dialogue by an ANA steering committee composed of members: nurse leaders/advocates. Face-to-face interactive sessions kick off the learning experience, followed by conference calls held every other month that permit continued engagement with ANA faculty and mentors. The calls provide member updates as well as an opportunity to delve more deeply into an advocacy tool or strategy. Examples of topics explored during the calls include: conducting a political environmental scan, bill analysis, preparing and delivering testimony, networking and coalition building, and communicating the value of a PAC.

Graduates of the program are also called upon to respond to federal initiatives, such as testimony delivered before the Senate Committee on Rural Health. Toni Decklever from the Wyoming Nurses Association graduated from the first ANA Institute and was invited to share the problems of access to primary care: 30 Million Patients and 11 Months to Go: Who Will Provide Their Primary Care? (Watch the hearing at *www.help.senate.gov/hearings/hearing/?id=dc487385-5056-a032-522c-082a29c4a406.*) Toni is also a lobbyist for the Wyoming Nurses Association in the capitol in Cheyenne. It is important to mentor new young nursing leaders if nursing is to continue to have a strong political voice.

RECOMMENDATIONS FOR BECOMING INVOLVED IN POLITICS

JOIN A POLITICAL PARTY

You do not have to agree with every part of a party's political platform, but joining a political party is an important step in learning the ropes. Organized political parties provide support and guidance on how to get started with a political campaign. They can provide you with the opportunity to gain experience by working on someone's campaign before actually running yourself. You can learn the steps for running a grassroots campaign; for example, how much money you need to raise; what forms are required; how to organize a campaign committee; and how to access mailing lists, voter registration, and past precinct results. The parties also raise money, which is used to support the total slate of offices in that particular party. The party can help you get your message out and reach all voters, especially those who might cross party lines.

CONNECT WITH OTHER NURSES

Nursing colleagues and associations can be extremely helpful in a political campaign. A group of nurses can send a powerful message of support when they back a candidate. Many state nurses associations have PACs to assist with endorsements and financial assistance.

LEARN FROM OTHERS IN YOUR COMMUNITY

Another helpful activity is to join the League of Women Voters. The name is derived from the women's suffrage movement, but today membership is open to women and men. Local leagues will often hold public forums on various issues such as health care. It is a wonderful opportunity to contribute to the dialogue and make connections. The League of Women Voters is also concerned about getting the vote out and what motivates people to go to the polls.

DEVELOP COST-EFFECTIVE CAMPAIGN STRATEGIES

When you are a candidate, you cannot be afraid to ask for money, and you need to take advantage of free and low-cost opportunities to get your message out. Flyers, mailing labels (usually the party you have joined will provide this at a bulk price),

newspaper and radio advertisements, yard signs, and billboards all cost money. Press releases, letters to the editor, speaking at meetings and forums, meetings at neighborhood cafes, and news coverage are free. My least expensive campaign was my first race for city council. We produced a one-page flyer and distributed it door-to-door. Whenever you choose a strategy like this, it is important to be aware of laws and regulations so you and your campaign staff do not run into problems. For example, you cannot leave flyers in a mailbox because it is a federal offense. If no one is at home, leaving a personal note stating "Sorry I missed you" can be an effective alternative. My husband made the political signs in our garage. It took a table saw, some nails, and stiff cardboard with my name and logo on it.

GET THE MESSAGE OUT

Getting out your message is critical to success. You must reach the voters. It does help to get some media training to help frame your messages. The press wants a good story and good sound bites, so your words should be carefully selected. Do not say anything you would not want to see in print or on TV. The press may not fully understand an issue, and you can help frame the story with your nursing knowledge. If you provide accurate information, members of the media will look forward to contacting you again. I have learned from my experience. Do not be afraid to tell the TV crew that you want a head and chest only shot of you because you did not have time to change your clothes.

Serving as an elected official can be a very rewarding experience and a great opportunity for advocating for community health improvements. We need nurses serving at all levels of government. We need nurses working for safe schools and safe drinking water at the local level, working for safe highways and seatbelt usage at the state level, and working for health care reform and funding for nursing education at the federal level.

UNIT 6

CHAPTER 86

Family and Sexual Violence: Nursing and U.S. Policy

Kathryn Laughon   Angela Frederick Amar

"If the numbers we see in domestic violence were applied to terrorism or gang violence, the entire country would be up in arms, and it would be the lead story on the news every night."

Rep. Mark Green, Wisconsin

Our society is steeped in violence. In the most recent national statistics, more than 26 per 1000 people aged 12 years or older will be the victims of a violent crime (Truman, Langton, & Planty, 2013). Most of our violence prevention strategies prepare potential victims to ward off violent attacks from strangers; yet, someone known to the victim perpetrates most violence against women, children, and older adults. The intimate nature of this violence, often perpetrated behind closed doors, has made these forms of violence less visible. However, the toll of violence on individuals and societies is substantial. The World Health Organization has framed violence as a significant public health problem (Truman, Langton, & Planty, 2013). A public health approach suggests an interdisciplinary, science-based approach with an emphasis on prevention. Effective strategies draw on resources in many fields, including nursing, medicine, criminal justice, epidemiology, and other social scientists.

The purpose of this chapter is to provide an overview of state, federal, and health sector policies regarding violence against women in the United States, briefly discuss policies related to violence against children and older adults, and outline the resulting implications for nurses and directions for future work.

INTIMATE PARTNER AND SEXUAL VIOLENCE AGAINST WOMEN

Intimate partner violence (IPV) is physical, sexual, or psychological harm inflicted by a current or former partner (same sex or not) or a current or former spouse (Black et al., 2011). Almost one third of American women experience being hit, slapped, or pushed by an intimate partner, and nearly a quarter will experience serious forms of IPV during their lifetimes. Additionally, nearly one in five women will experience a completed or attempted rape in their lifetimes. Men experience IPV and rape as well, although at far lower rates than do women. About a quarter of men will experience IPV (about 12% serious forms of violence) and nearly 1.5% a completed or attempted rape. Although more than half of women reporting rape report that the assailant was an intimate partner and 40% that the assailant was an acquaintance, men report that half of rapes were by acquaintances and 15% by strangers; the number raped by an intimate partner was too small to estimate.

The health effects of IPV and sexual violence are substantial and cost as much as $8.3 billion in health care and mental health services for victims (Max et al., 2004). Violence is associated with a wide range of health problems, including chronic pain recurring central nervous system symptoms, vaginal and sexually transmitted infections and other gynecological symptoms, and diagnosed gastrointestinal symptoms and disorders (Black et al., 2011). Mental health symptoms include depression, anxiety, posttraumatic stress disorder, and alcohol and drug use (Black et al., 2011; Campbell, 2002).

STATE LAWS REGARDING INTIMATE PARTNER AND SEXUAL VIOLENCE

State laws address a number of issues important for nurses to understand. Most often, crime of IPV and sexual violence are addressed through state laws. Most, although not all, states have laws specifically providing enhanced penalties for assault and battery that occurs between intimate partners. (It worth noting that most laws refer to domestic violence or family abuse rather than IPV.) For example, at least 23 states have some form of mandatory arrest for IPV (Hirschel, 2008). Research findings are mixed on whether mandatory arrest laws reduce reassault (Felson, Ackerman, & Gallagher, 2005; Hirschel et al., 2007), although findings from at least one study suggest that the overwhelming majority of victims support mandatory arrest laws (Barata & Schneider, 2004). Additionally, states may have enhanced penalties, such as escalating third offenses to felonies.

Until 1975, all states provided what is called the marital rape exemption under which it was legally impossible to commit rape against one's wife. Beginning in the mid-1970s, based in part on nursing research, these laws began to change (Campbell & Alford, 1989). Although all states now recognize marital rape as a crime, in some states it is still treated differently from rape by a nonspouse (Prachar, 2010).

Nonlethal strangulation of women is a significant but often overlooked threat to public safety. Most (80%) strangulations of women are committed by intimate partners (Shields et al., 2010). They can result in significant physical health problems for victims (Taliaferro et al., 2009) and substantially increase risk of later lethal violence (Glass et al., 2008). These cases can be difficult to charge and prosecute commensurate with the severity of the crime (Laughon, Glass, & Worrell, 2009); therefore, a growing number of states have strengthened laws related to strangulation.

All states provide for civil protective orders in cases where victims have a reasonable fear of violence from an assailant (Carroll, 2007). States vary widely, however, in who is eligible to obtain an order and how the orders are obtained. For example, in some states minors or dating partners may not be able to obtain orders of protection. Most states provide for civil protection orders against assailants who are accused of sexual assault, but the procedures may be different from those for protective orders against intimate partners. Studies of the effectiveness of these orders are mixed (Logan & Walker, 2009; Prachar, 2010).

In addition to these criminal justice remedies, state laws may address other issues related to IPV and sexual violence. As of 2010, 26 states had established intimate partner fatality review teams (Durborow et al., 2010). Fatality review teams use a multidisciplinary, public health approach to reviewing fatalities and identifying risk factors (Websdale, 1999). A handful of states require health care providers to report domestic violence against competent adults. It is important to understand that in most states, IPV and sexual assault are not mandatory reports unless there are other factors present.

FEDERAL LAWS RELATED TO INTIMATE PARTNER AND SEXUAL VIOLENCE

There are two significant federal laws that address violence against women. The Family Violence Prevention and Services Act was first authorized in 1984. It was most recently authorized through 2015 (Public Law [PL] 111-320 42 U.S.C. 10401, et seq.). It is the primary federal funding source for domestic violence shelters and service programs in the United States. It also funds the work of state coalitions on domestic violence, community-based violence prevention efforts, and a number of smaller training and assistance programs.

The Violence against Women Act (VAWA) was first authorized in 1994 (Title IV, sec. 40001-40703 of the Violent Crime Control and Law Enforcement Act of 1994, HR 3355, signed as PL 103-322). As states began creating the protective order and criminal statutes discussed earlier, the limitations of this patchwork of remedies became apparent.

UNIT 6

The VAWA was therefore created to address the gaps in state laws; create federal laws against domestic violence, including protection for immigrant women and enhanced gun control provisions; and fund a variety of violence-related training and other local programs (Valente et al., 2009). The law originally included a provision making crime motivated by gender a civil rights offense. This provision was, however, found unconstitutional in 2000 (*Brzonkala v. Morrison*, 2000).

The VAWA represented a significant turning point in public policy related to violence against women. Previously, women who received a protective order might find that violations that occurred in other states could not be enforced. The full faith and credit provision of the VAWA requires that protective orders be recognized and enforced across jurisdictional, state, and tribal boundaries within the United States. Likewise, by creating federal crimes of domestic violence and stalking, criminal acts that cross jurisdictional boundaries can now be more easily charged and prosecuted. Under the VAWA, it is illegal for individuals subject to certain types of protective orders or convicted of even misdemeanor domestic violence offenses to possess a firearm. Given that risk of intimate partner homicide increases dramatically when firearms are available to the assailant, this represents an important safeguard for women (Campbell et al., 2003). The VAWA addressed the significant hardships faced by both legal and illegal immigrant women experiencing abuse from their partners. The VAWA additionally funds a wide range of victim advocacy and training programs, with the goal of ensuring that victims of violence receive consistent, competent services in all communities.

Each subsequent renewal of the VAWA has strengthened these provisions. The latest renewal in 2013 expanded its definitions to explicitly include gay, lesbian, and transgender victims; expanded the safeguards available to women assaulted in tribal territories; expanded housing provisions to prohibit discrimination against victims of IPV in all forms of subsidized public housing; strengthened protections for immigrant women; and, for the first time, specifically addressed violence on college campuses (Violence against Women Act, 2013).

HEALTH POLICIES RELATED TO INTIMATE PARTNER AND SEXUAL VIOLENCE

As discussed earlier, the health consequences of violence are significant for women. Additionally, women who have experienced violence have significantly higher health care costs than women without a victimization history (Bonomi et al., 2009; National Center for Injury Prevention and Control, 2003). There is now a consensus that these health care settings offer a unique opportunity to identify and support women living with the effects of violence (Family Violence Prevention Fund, 2002; World Health Organization [WHO], 2013). The U.S. Preventative Services Taskforce recommends "clinicians screen women of childbearing age for IPV such as domestic violence, and provide or refer women who screen positive to intervention services." The Institute of Medicine identified screening and brief counseling for interpersonal violence as an essential and evidence-based practice necessary to ensure the well-being of women (National Research Council, 2011). A wide variety of medical and nursing professional organizations also recommend routine screening for violence (Amar et al., 2013). Significant evidence now exists for safety planning strategies to prevent homicide for women in abusive relationships. The Danger Assessment Instrument, for example, has been shown to have good predictive value and can assist women with making a realistic appraisal of their likelihood of experiencing lethal violence (Campbell, Webster, & Glass, 2008). Health care institutions should also have the appropriate capacity to provide care to women in the acute period after a physical or sexual assault (WHO, 2013).

Nurses and other health professionals have a role to play in community responses to violence. Many localities have created sexual assault response teams. These interdisciplinary teams work to ensure consistent, trauma-informed, and effective care for victims of sexual assault. Despite scant research on the effectiveness of these teams, they are a promising practice (Greeson & Campbell, 2013). Likewise, intimate partner/domestic violence fatality review teams review cases of intimate partner homicide with a public health approach. As with sexual assault response teams, there are little data on the effectiveness of these teams that have also been labeled a promising practice (Wilson & Websdale, 2006).

CHILD MALTREATMENT

Child maltreatment includes physical, sexual, and emotional abuse, as well as neglect. Actual prevalence of maltreatment is unknown, but there are more than 3 million referrals for more than 6 million children to child protective agencies annually, with nearly a quarter of these cases substantiated. An estimated 1570 children nationally died from abuse or neglect in 2011 (Administration on Children, Youth, and Families Children's Bureau, 2011; U.S. Government Accountability Office, 2011), a number that is believed to be undercounted. The estimated annual cost of child abuse and neglect in the United States for 2008 was $124 billion (Fang et al. 2012). Child maltreatment results in lifelong adverse physical and mental health consequences such as posttraumatic stress disorder, increased risk of chronic disease, lasting impacts or disability from physical injury, and reduced health-related quality of life (Corso et al. 2008).

STATE AND FEDERAL POLICIES RELATED TO CHILD MALTREATMENT

Because minors are considered to need additional protection as a result of their age, states not only have laws making the acts of abuse and neglect criminal offenses but also have laws requiring that certain adults must report suspected maltreatment to appropriate authorities. In some states, all adults are mandated reporters. In most states, specific professionals, teachers, health care professionals, social workers, law enforcement personnel, and others are mandated reporters (Child Welfare Information Gateway, 2011). At the federal level, the Child Abuse Prevention and Treatment Act (CAPTA) provides funding to states to support prevention, assessment, investigation, prosecution, and treatment activities related to child maltreatment and funding for research activities (Child Welfare Information Gateway, 2011, 2013).

HEALTH POLICIES RELATED TO CHILD MALTREATMENT

Children's Advocacy Centers coordinate investigation and intervention services for maltreated children by bringing together social work, legal, health care, and other professionals and agencies in a multidisciplinary team to create a child-focused approach to child abuse cases. Home visitation is another strategy that shows promise for improving child health and preventing child maltreatment (Avellar & Supplee, 2013).

OLDER ADULT MALTREATMENT

Best estimates indicate that 1 to 2 million Americans over the age of 65 years are abused, neglected, or exploited, most often by caregivers (National Center on Elder Abuse, 2005). Precise numbers are not available, attributable to differences in definitions of abuse, lack of a comprehensive national data system, and different state system reporting and data collection. Further, only a small fraction of abuse comes to the attention of Adult Protective Services (Dong & Simon, 2011). The U.S. aging population is rapidly increasing with projections for individuals 65 years and older to increase from 40.2 million in 2010 to 54.8 million in 2020 and to 72.1 million in 2030 (Dong & Simon, 2011). Legislation has been effective in bringing about reform.

STATE AND FEDERAL LEGISLATION RELATED TO OLDER ADULT MALTREATMENT

As with child maltreatment, state laws provide for criminal charges related to the abuse of older adults (the definition of which varies from state to state, but may be as young as 55 years of age). Most (but not all) states define certain individuals as mandated reporters of abuse of older adults as well. At the federal level, the Older American Act of 2006 developed and maintains the National Center on Elder Abuse, which provides funding for prevention activities, research, data collection, and long-term planning for elder justice. The Elder Justice Act (EJA) of 2010, which was part of the Patient

UNIT 6

Protection and Affordable Care Act (2010), is the first comprehensive strategy to address older adult abuse, neglect, and exploitation. It is important to note that the authorized funding has not been appropriated at this time and that the EJA is set to expire in 2014. Funding for older adult maltreatment is significantly less than for other types of violence and a national database has yet to be established.

HEALTH CARE POLICIES RELATED TO OLDER ADULT MALTREATMENT

Recent efforts have focused on using the primary care setting to identify and respond to older adult abuse (Perel-Levin, 2008). Case management strategies can be effective in providing consistency in monitoring of adult patient and caregiver behavior (Choi & Mayer, 2000). Research on effective intervention strategies in this area lags behind that of other areas of violence and is an area where nursing can make an impact.

OPPORTUNITY FOR NURSING

Nurses have the skills and education to take a leadership role in addressing violence and abuse on multiple levels, as providers, researchers, policy analysts, educators, and advocates. Efforts to address violence against children, women, and older adults have met with impressive successes over the past decades. These forms of violence, seen as largely justifiable and perhaps even necessary in the past, are now recognized as both crimes and important public health problems. The evidence base for interventions to prevent these forms of violence, end them when they start, and mitigate the related health consequences is growing. It is clear, however, that we still have important gaps in our understanding of both effective violence interventions and policies. Although we work to address these gaps in knowledge, we can continue to move forward on numerous fronts. Educators should ensure that curriculums at all levels include content on violence and abuse. Given the high rates and significant health effects of violence, all nurses

should have basic clinical knowledge of how to assess for, competently respond to, and appropriately refer all patients with a history of violence or abuse. Nurses can serve as powerful advocates for victims of violence, ensuring that state and federal laws meet the highest standards.

Violence and crime unite two powerful systems, health care and criminal justice, and involve multiple professionals including physicians, nurses, social services, police, lawyers, and judges. Prevention and intervention strategies require efforts at the individual, community, institutional, and public policy levels. Nurses can have a significant voice in ensuring the best possible prevention and advocacy services at the local, state, and federal levels. Nursing research and the testimony of nurses has been foundational for federal and state laws and resulting public policy related to violence.

DISCUSSION QUESTIONS

1. Consider the differences in the treatment of violence across states and what federal provisions might be advantageous to address the discrepancies.
2. How might nursing research help to fill the gaps in the knowledge?
3. It is apparent in the chapter that different strategies exist for violence against women, child maltreatment, and older adult abuse. Could the same strategies work across populations and abuse types? What might be the advantages/disadvantages to having similar strategies?

REFERENCES

Administration on Children, Youth, and Families Children's Bureau. (2011). *Child abuse and neglect fatalities 2011: Statistics and interventions*. Washington, DC: U.S. Department of Health and Human Services, Administration for Children and Families.

Amar, A., Laughon, K., Sharps, P., & Campbell, J. (2013). Screening and counseling for violence against women in primary care settings. *Nursing Outlook, 61*(3), 187–191.

Avellar, S. A., & Supplee, L. H. (2013). Effectiveness of home visiting in improving child health and reducing child maltreatment. *Pediatrics, 132*(10, Suppl. 2), S90–S99.

Barata, P. C., & Schneider, F. (2004). Battered women add their voices to the debate about the merits of mandatory arrest. *Women's Studies Quarterly, 32*(3–4), 148.

Black, M. C., Basile, K. C., Breiding, M. J., Smith, S. G., Walters, M. L., et al. (2011). *The national intimate partner and sexual violence survey (NISVS):*

2010 summary report. Atlanta, GA: National Center for Injury Prevention and Control, Centers for Disease Control and Prevention.

Bonomi, A. E., Anderson, M. L., Rivara, F. P., & Thompson, R. S. (2009). Health care utilization and costs associated with physical and nonphysical-only intimate partner violence. *Health Services Research, 44*(3), 1052–1067.

Brzonkala v. Morrison, 529 U.S. 598, 627 (2000).

Campbell, J. C. (2002). Health consequences of intimate partner violence. *Lancet, 359*(9314), 1331–1336.

Campbell, J. C., & Alford, P. (1989). The dark consequences of marital rape. *American Journal of Nursing, 89*(7), 946–949.

Campbell, J. C., Webster, D., Koziol-McLain, J., Block, C., Campbell, D., et al. (2003). Risk factors for femicide in abusive relationships: Results from a multisite case control study. *American Journal of Public Health, 93*(7), 1089–1097.

Campbell, J. C., Webster, D. W., & Glass, N. (2008). The danger assessment: Validation of a lethality risk assessment instrument for intimate partner femicide. *Journal of Interpersonal Violence, 24*(4), 653–674.

Carroll, C. A. (2007). *Sexual assault civil protection orders (CPOs) by state.* Washington, DC: American Bar Association Commission on Domestic and Sexual Violence.

Child Welfare Information Gateway. (2011). *About CAPTA: A legislative history.* Washington, DC: U.S. Department of Health and Human Services, Children's Bureau.

Child Welfare Information Gateway. (2013). *Long-term consequences of child abuse and neglect.* Washington, DC: U.S. Department of Health and Human Services. Retrieved from *www.childwelfare.gov/pubs/factsheets/long_term_consequences.cfm.*

Choi, N. G., & Mayer, J. (2000). Elder abuse, neglect, and exploitation: Risk factors and prevention strategies. *Journal of Gerontological Social Work, 33*(2), 5–25.

Corso, P. S., Edwards, V. J., Fang, X., & Mercy, J. A. (2008). Health-related quality of life among adults who experienced maltreatment during childhood. *American Journal of Public, 98*(6), 1094–1100.

Dong, X. Q., & Simon, M. A. (2011). Enhancing national policy and programs to address elder abuse. *JAMA: The Journal of the American Medical Association, 305*(23), 2460–2461.

Durborow, N., Lizdas, K. C., O'Flaherty, A., & Marjavi, A. (2010). *Compendium of state statutes and policies on domestic violence and health care.* San Francisco, CA: Family Violence Prevention Fund.

Family Violence Prevention Fund. (2002). *National consensus guidelines on identifying and responding to domestic violence victimization in health care settings.* San Francisco: Author.

Fang, X., Brown, D. S., Florence, C. S., & Mercy, J. A. (2012). The economic burden of child maltreatment in the United States and implications for prevention. *Child Abuse & Neglect, 36*(2), 156–165.

Felson, R. B., Ackerman, J. M., & Gallagher, C. A. (2005). Police intervention and the repeat of domestic assault. *Criminology, 43*(3), 563–588.

Glass, N., Laughon, K., Campbell, J., Block, C. R., Hanson, G., et al. (2008). Non-fatal strangulation is an important risk factor for homicide for women. *Journal of Emergency Medicine, 35*(3), 329–335.

Greeson, M. R., & Campbell, R. (2013). Sexual assault response teams (SARTs): An empirical review of their effectiveness and challenges to successful implementation. *Trauma, Violence and Abuse, 14*(2), 83–95.

Hirschel, D. (2008). *Domestic violence cases: What research shows about arrest and dual arrest rates.* Washington, DC: National Institute for Justice.

Hirschel, D., Buzawa, E., Pattavina, A., & Faggiani, D. (2007). Domestic violence and mandatory arrest laws: To what extent do they influence police arrest decisions? *Journal of Criminal Law & Criminology, 98*(1), 255–298.

Laughon, K., Glass, N., & Worrell, C. (2009). Review and analysis of laws related to strangulation in 50 states. *Evaluation Review, 33*(4), 358–369.

Logan, T., & Walker, R. (2009). Civil protective order outcomes: Violations and perceptions of effectiveness. *Journal of Interpersonal Violence, 24*(4), 675–692.

Max, W., Rice, D. P., Finkelstein, E., Bardwell, R. A., & Leadbetter, S. (2004). The economic toll of intimate partner violence against women in the United States. *Violence and Victims, 19*(3), 259–272.

National Center on Elder Abuse. (2005). *Fact sheet: Elder abuse prevalence and incidence.* Washington, DC: National Center on Elder Abuse.

National Center for Injury Prevention and Control. (2003). *Costs of intimate partner violence against women in the United States.* Atlanta: Centers for Disease Control and Prevention.

National Research Council. (2011). *Clinical preventive services for women: Closing the gaps.* Washington, DC: The National Academies Press.

Patient Protection and Affordable Care Act, 42 U.S.C. § 18001 (2010).

Perel-Levin, S. (2008). *Discussing screening for elder abuse at primary health care level.* Geneva: World Health Organization.

Prachar, M. (2010). The marital rape exemption: A violation of a woman's right of privacy. *Golden Gate University Law Review, 11,* 717.

Shields, L. B., Corey, T. S., Weakley-Jones, B., & Steward, D. (2010). Living victims of strangulation: A 10-year review of cases in a metropolitan community. *American Journal of Forensic Medicine and Pathology, 31,* 320–325.

Taliaferro, E., Hawley, D., McClane, G., & Strack, G. B. (2009). Strangulation in intimate partner violence. In C. Mitchell & D. Anglin (Eds.), *Intimate partner violence: A health-based perspective.* New York: Oxford University Press.

Truman, J., Langton, L., & Planty, M. (2013). *Criminal victimization, 2012 No. NCJ 243389.* Washington, DC: US Department of Justice, Office of Justice Programs, Bureau of Justice Statistics.

U.S. Government Accountability Office. (2011). *Child maltreatment: Strengthening national data on child fatalities could aid in prevention (GAO-11-599).* Washington, DC: U.S. Government Accountability Office.

Valente, R. L., Hart, B. J., Zeya, S., & Malefyt, M. (2009). The violence against women act of 1994: The federal commitment to ending domestic violence, sexual assault, stalking, and gender-based crimes of violence. In C. M. Renzetti, J. L. Edelson, & R. L. Bergen (Eds.), *Sourcebook on violence against women* (1st ed.). Thousand Oaks, CA: Sage.

Violence against Women Act, Public Law 113–4.

Violence Against Women Reauthorization Act of 2013. (2013).

Websdale, N. (1999). *Understanding domestic homicide.* Boston, MA: Northeastern University Press.

Wilson, J. S., & Websdale, N. (2006). Domestic violence fatality review teams: an interprofessional model to reduce deaths. *Journal of Interprofessional Care, 20*(5), 535–544.

World Health Organization [WHO]. (2013). *Responding to intimate partner violence and sexual violence against women: WHO clinical and policy guidelines.* Geneva: World Health Organization.

ONLINE RESOURCES

Child Welfare Information Gateway
www.childwelfare.gov
Futures without Violence
www.futureswithoutviolence.org
National Center of Elder Abuse
www.ncea.aoa.gov
Rape, Abuse, and Incest National Network
www.rainn.org

UNIT 6

CHAPTER 87

Human Trafficking: The Need for Nursing Advocacy

Barbara Glickstein

"I freed a thousand slaves. I could have freed a thousand more if only they knew they were slaves."

Harriet Ross Tubman, nurse abolitionist

Human trafficking is a serious crime of forced labor or enslavement. As defined under U.S. federal law, victims of human trafficking include children involved in the sex trade, adults age 18 years or over who are coerced or deceived into commercial sex acts, and anyone forced into different forms of labor or services, such as domestic workers held in a home or farm workers forced to labor against their will. A victim does not have to be physically transported from one location to another for the crime to fall under the definition of human trafficking (U.S. Department of State, 2013a).

Trafficking not only violates human rights but also contributes to harmful social, health, and economic conditions for the persons who are trafficked. Persons who are trafficked can experience intense psychological trauma, infectious disease (most notably HIV/AIDS), extensive physical injury, drug addiction, unwanted pregnancy, and malnutrition. Human trafficking also poses a significant public health problem.

Victim identification is the critical first step in stopping this crime. Nurses are well placed in every community to identify trafficking victims. They also bring a public health lens to this human rights issue, which contributes to their having a better understanding of the complexity of the issues a survivor faces. Nurses can focus on developing and implementing a victim-centered approach. The U.S. Department of Homeland Security Blue Campaign defines a victim-centered approach to combating human trafficking as one that places equal value on the identification and stabilization of victims, with the investigation and prosecution of traffickers (U.S. Department Homeland Security, 2013).

ENCOUNTERING THE VICTIMS OF HUMAN TRAFFICKING

Many nurses have treated victims of human trafficking without realizing it. Encountering modern-day slavery can provoke a strong visceral response, often followed by the urge to distance oneself. These feelings make it hard to imagine what you, one nurse, could possibly do to stop it. However, nurses are uniquely situated to make a difference.

Nurses should ask themselves one question: "What role can nurses have in stopping human trafficking?" (See Box 87-1.)

ADVANCING POLICY IN THE WORKPLACE

Does your place of employment have a policy on nursing's role in human trafficking? Does it have an action plan or protocol to follow when a person who is trafficked is identified? Networks of health care providers, law enforcement, lawyers, and nongovernmental organizations are developing evidence-based multisectored policies and protocols on how to proceed when a person has been identified as being trafficked. If your place of work does not have a policy, you can take the lead and get this process in motion to ensure that people who have been trafficked are given proper care, treated with respect, protected from harm, and

> **BOX 87-1 What Can You Do About Human Trafficking?**
>
> • Be well informed. Start with investigating what policy and protocols are in place at your health institution and if the issue of human trafficking is being addressed in the nursing curriculum in courses at your university or college.
>
> • If there are no policies in place, start an interdisciplinary task force to develop policies and pursue a plan to implement them.
>
> • Assess and educate community stakeholders, such as shelters, victim-assistance agencies, advocacy groups, and law enforcement agencies, and collaborate with them.
>
> • Become familiar with services and hotlines so that you can refer people who have been trafficked. Build a resource list, and keep it current. Access to reporting at the national level includes the National Human Trafficking Resource Center (NHTRC). The NHTRC is a national, toll-free hotline that operates 24 hours a day, 7 days a week, 365 days a year. The NHTRC can be reached by calling 1-888-3737-888 or text BeFree (233733).
>
> • Bring the issue of human trafficking to the public's attention in their local communities through public speaking in schools, places of worship, and social action groups. Use both traditional media and social media to launch campaigns and increase pressure on local authorities to act to stop human trafficking.

directed to social and legal services. Resources that can provide support to develop a protocol are the Polaris Project (2014), which offers training and technical assistance, and the International Organization for Migration handbook on Caring for Trafficked Persons (International Organization on Migration, 2009).

ROLE OF PROFESSIONAL NURSING ASSOCIATIONS

Historically, nursing organizations have played a critical role in developing and advancing policies on human rights issues. The International Council of Nurses' (ICN) Code of Ethics for Nurses position statement, Nurses and Human Rights, requires nurses to safeguard and promote human rights (ICN, 2006a, 2006b). This statement as well as other ICN advocacy and lobbying position statements cover a wide range of health issues where nurses must act to enforce human rights and to promote and protect health as a fundamental human right and a social goal (ICN, 2010).

In 2008, the New York State Nurses Association (NYSNA) invited me to deliver an address entitled *Nurses Working to Stop Human Trafficking* at their annual convention. The NYSNA board's response was immediate. They drafted and submitted an action proposal on human trafficking to the American Nurses Association (ANA), which was passed by the ANA House of Delegates in 2008. The resolution states that it will advocate legislation to reduce the incidence of human trafficking and will work to ensure that nurses know how to identify and assist victims. This is a commendable action by the ANA to educate nurses nationally and support stronger enforcement of the federal laws (American Nurses Association [ANA], 2008).

Investigate to see whether your state nurses' association and specialty nursing association has a position statement on nurses' role in human trafficking. You can be the person who takes the lead on this initiative if nothing exists to date. A good place to start would be to identify one or two state nurses' associations that have already developed a policy and ask for guidance from them on strategy and language for your state nurses' association.

ADVOCATING FOR STATE LEGISLATION AND POLICY ON HUMAN TRAFFICKING

Nurses can become part of a national network of health providers and advocacy groups challenging the lack of services available to victims of human trafficking by advocating for the allocation of resources on both the federal level and state level to address this void. They can also use their influence and leadership to advocate for better enforcement of existing antitrafficking laws in their state.

In 2000, the federal law Victims of Trafficking and Violence Protection Act (TVPA) was enacted, making human trafficking a federal crime. The TVPA includes a provision that each state could pass their own legislation to strengthen the work of the federal government and coordinate a partnership with local and federal law enforcement. The Federal Bureau of Investigation (FBI) and agents of Immigration and Customs Enforcement (ICE), a division under Homeland Security, are the main federal agencies involved in investigating human trafficking cases. Because states are enacting legislation and strengthening laws to prosecute traffickers and training law enforcement, we have an increase in investigating human trafficking. To date, not every one of the 50 states has done so. The website of the Center for Women Policy Studies (2014), an advocacy organization, provides an interactive map to learn about individual states and their statutes on human trafficking. If your state has legislation and an interagency antitrafficking task force working on a comprehensive plan to provide services for persons who have been trafficked, ask if there is a nurse on the task force. Once identified, ask how you can help. If there is no nurse on the task force, work toward getting a nurse appointed, or nominate yourself. If your state is one of the remaining states without antitrafficking laws, identify local and national advocacy organizations working toward this goal and work with them to pass this legislation. Contact and engage your state nurses' association to lobby to pass these comprehensive laws.

ADVANCING POLICY THROUGH MEDIA AND TECHNOLOGY

The media, both traditional media and digital media, is the single most powerful tool to educate, effect social change, and influence policies. Like most Americans, nurses' knowledge about human trafficking has been shaped by the media. A study by researchers Johnston, Friedman, and Scaefer (2012) evaluated print and broadcast media reports on human trafficking beginning in 2008 through 2012. They found that stories on the crime of sex trafficking dominated the coverage, while stories of survivors or the impact on public policy were less common. Dramatization of human trafficking appears more frequently in story lines on popular crime series on television and in movie plots in theaters. The news media have been the primary source of national policy and legislative issues about human trafficking.

Coverage of the issue about the health of the victims and the public health implications of human trafficking has been missing. A recent study on the dominant issues covered in the media on the issue of sex trafficking reported that only 1% of the news coverage addressed the issue of public health. When nurses become educated on the health implications of human trafficking they can become resources for the media's coverage on trafficking and shape the public's understanding of human trafficking beyond the issue that it is a crime. When the public is aware of the indicators of human trafficking and whom to contact if they see such indicators, victims can more readily be identified and helped.

Technologies are now being used for antitrafficking efforts. The Global Human Trafficking Hotline Network shares and analyzes data from hotlines to find and help victims and identify trafficking locations. One of them, the National Human Trafficking Resource Center (NHTRC) in the United States, answers calls from anywhere in the country and has started accepting text messages. Texting can be a safer form of connecting with victims and those seeking to report suspected human trafficking activities. When a text is received, a live, trained specialist receives the text and responds immediately. Texting provides secrecy that phone lines cannot provide if the person reporting feels threatened by others near them (Polaris Project, 2014).

TRAFFICKING AS A GLOBAL PUBLIC HEALTH ISSUE

There are more than 13 million nurses worldwide providing up to 80% of the health services in most countries (ICN, 2010). In every community where a nurse provides care, there are people who are vulnerable and could be targeted by traffickers. For nurses, trafficking in persons can be best understood as a very serious health risk, because trafficking, like other forms of violence, is associated with physical and psychological harm (International

Organization on Migration, 2009). It has serious public health implications related to the spread of infectious diseases such as tuberculosis, HIV, and other sexually transmitted infections. Victims of trafficking are highly prone to social, economic, and legal issues that further put them at risk for a variety of mental health issues, including substance abuse, addiction, posttraumatic stress disorder, anxiety, depression, and even suicide (Hynes & Raymond, 2002). Common abuses experienced by trafficked persons include rape, torture, and other forms of physical, sexual, and psychological violence (Zimmerman et al., 2008). Paradoxically, these victims who desperately require health services are less likely to have access as a result of discrimination, social stigma, fear of law enforcement, and other factors. Nurses can contribute their expertise by conducting research on human trafficking as a global public health issue.

Nurses are also at risk for being trafficked. As poorer nations prepare nurses for export to other countries, questionable recruiting practices have led some migrating nurses to be threatened with criminal charges and deportation when they object to exploitative working conditions. Raising nurses' awareness about human trafficking can lower their own risk.

THE WORLD OF THE VICTIMS

Without recruiters and criminals, human trafficking would not exist. Poverty, unemployment, economic collapse, war, natural disasters, and the lack of a promising future are compelling factors that facilitate the ease with which traffickers recruit people, but they are not the cause of trafficking. Traffickers take advantage of poverty, unemployment, and the desire to emigrate to recruit people and traffic them into dangerous situations. Tragically, recruiters often know their victims. A common way that many victims are recruited is through a friend or acquaintance (e.g., a cousin, neighbor, or boyfriend) or by an individual recommended to them by someone they trusted.

Finally, traffickers can be anyone. Traffickers brazenly operate in our neighborhoods. They advertise in our newspapers and on Craigslist. They are men and women of all ages. They run legal employment agencies. They are diplomats who often get diplomatic immunity when caught, and they work in all types of professions (General Accounting Office [GAO], 2008). They act alone or they may be members of international crime rings (Table 87-1).

INTERNATIONAL POLICY

The first international statement to use the term human rights was the Universal Declaration of Human Rights (UDHR), adopted by the United Nations General Assembly in Paris in 1948. The UDHR states that human rights are rights inherent to all human beings, whatever our nationality, place of residence, sex, national or ethnic origin, color, religion, language, or any other status. Among several protections covered by the UDHR, Article 4 of the UDHR states: "No one shall be held in slavery or servitude: slavery and the slave trade shall be prohibited in all their forms." The UDHR made history and is used by human rights activists globally (General Assembly of the United Nations, 1948).

The first international legal instrument to address human trafficking as a crime and to define trafficking was passed in 2000, when the United Nations Office on Drugs and Crime (2000) passed the Protocol to Prevent, Suppress, and Punish Trafficking in Persons. As of 2009, 136 Member States have signed the Protocol. It defines trafficking in persons as follows:

The recruitment, transportation, transfer, harboring or receipt of persons, by means of the threat or use of force or other forms of coercion, of abduction, of fraud, of deception, of the abuse of power or of a position of vulnerability or of the giving or receiving of payments or benefits to achieve the consent of a person having control over another person, for the purpose of exploitation. Exploitation shall include, at a minimum, the exploitation of the prostitution of others or other forms of sexual exploitation, forced labor or services, slavery or practices similar to slavery, servitude or the removal of organs. (United Nations, 2000)

UNIT 6

TABLE 87-1 Myths and Facts of Human Trafficking

The U.S. Department of Homeland Security's antitrafficking plan, called the Blue Campaign, provides a list of six myths and misconceptions about human trafficking:

Myth #1

Human trafficking does not occur in the United States. It only happens in other countries.

Fact

Human trafficking exists in every country, including the United States. It exists nationwide, in cities, suburbs, and rural towns, and possibly in your own community.

Myth #2

Human trafficking victims are only foreign-born individuals and those who are poor.

Fact

Human trafficking victims can be any age, race, gender, or nationality: young children, teenagers, women, men, runaways, U.S. citizens, and foreign-born individuals. They may come from all socioeconomic groups.

Myth #3

Human trafficking is only sex trafficking.

Fact

You may have heard about sex trafficking, but forced labor is also a significant and prevalent type of human trafficking. Victims are found in legitimate and illegitimate labor industries, including sweatshops, massage parlors, agriculture, restaurants, hotels, and domestic services. Note that sex trafficking and forced labor are both forms of human trafficking, involving exploitation of a person.

Myth #4

Individuals must be forced or coerced into commercial sex acts to be a victim of human trafficking.

Fact

According to U.S. federal law, any minor under the age of 18 years who is induced to perform commercial sex acts is a victim of human trafficking, regardless of whether he or she is forced or coerced.

Myth #5

Human trafficking and human smuggling are the same.

Fact

Human trafficking is not the same as smuggling. "Trafficking" is exploitation-based and does not require movement across borders. "Smuggling" is movement-based and involves moving a person across a country's border with that person's consent, in violation of immigration laws.

Although human smuggling is very different from human trafficking, human smuggling can turn into trafficking if the smuggler uses force, fraud, or coercion to hold people against their will for the purposes of labor or sexual exploitation. Under federal law, every minor induced to engage in commercial sex is a victim of human trafficking.

Myth #6

All human trafficking victims attempt to seek help when in public.

Fact

Human trafficking is often a hidden crime. Victims may be afraid to come forward and get help; they may be forced or coerced through threats or violence; they may fear retribution from traffickers, including danger to their families; and they may not be in possession or have control of their identification documents.

Retrieved from *www.dhs.gov/blue-campaign/myths-misconceptions.*

This International Protocol established the standard approach for governments developing policies on trafficking: the 3P Paradigm—prevention, prosecution, and protection of victims.

In 2007, the United Nations Global Initiative to Fight Human Trafficking (UN.GIFT) was established to coordinate global efforts to adopt the Protocol. In addition to working with governments, the UN.GIFT works with businesses, academia, civil society, and the media to develop effective tools to fight human trafficking (United Nations Office on Drugs and Crime [UNODC], 2009).

U.S. RESPONSE TO HUMAN TRAFFICKING

The U.S. Department of State began monitoring trafficking in persons in 1994, when the issue began to be covered in the Department's Annual Country Reports on Human Rights Practices. During the Clinton administration, the United States passed the TVPA of 2000. This Act established the standard for federal policy on trafficking, and responses to the Act were all based on the 3P Paradigm.

More recently, advocacy organizations globally are launching campaigns that focus on the demand side of slavery as a means of stopping this crime. These laws would take the focus off the women and children in prostitution and put it on the end user or customer. Another demand-reduction strategy is an education and awareness campaign that is aimed at boys and young men and focuses on the negative consequences of purchasing sex: from public and private health problems such as the spread of HIV and other sexually transmitted infections to the grim facts about who runs the sex trade and how customers are helping traffickers flourish and hurting those who have been trafficked.

The 2013 Trafficking in Persons (TIP) report (U.S. Department of State, 2013b) outlines major forms of human trafficking including forced labor, bonded labor, debt bondage among migrant laborers, involuntary domestic servitude, forced child labor, child soldiers, sex trafficking, and child sex trafficking and related abuses. The 2013 report focuses on victim identification as a top priority in the global movement to combat trafficking in persons. It details training and techniques that make identification efforts successful, and areas that need further focus such as culturally sensitive health services for all victims and better understanding in identifying boys, men, and lesbian, gay, bisexual, and transgender people who are trafficked. The 2013 TIP report stated that 47,000 victims of human trafficking were identified globally in 2013, a small percentage of the estimated 27 million women, men, and children being trafficked at any time. Global convictions of human traffickers increased by almost 20% from 2012 with 4746 convictions in 2013.

In January 2014, the White House released the 5-year federal strategic action plan Coordination, Collaboration, Capacity: Federal Strategic Action Plan on Services for Victims of Human Trafficking in the United States, 2013-2017. The Plan is a collaborative project involving 15 agencies across the federal government and nonprofits. This strategic plan includes significant input from survivors of trafficking. Development of the Plan was a collaborative, multiphase effort across a number of federal agencies, led by co-chairs from the U.S. Departments of Justice, Health and Human Services, and Homeland Security.

The Plan outlines a strategic coordinated effort with specific goals, objectives, and action items to better identify and provide services to victims of trafficking in the United States.

CONCLUSION

Although there is much work that needs to be done to understand and end human trafficking, great progress has been made since 2000. The international community has taken decisive action to end human trafficking. Greater research related to trafficking is a prerequisite for ending the abuse. Lack of data and failure to grasp the complexities that underlie human trafficking worldwide must be addressed. The media treatment of trafficking does not present the true dimensions of the problem, and we should work toward better reporting to help shatter the myths about human trafficking. Nongovernment agencies and advocacy groups dedicated to creating public awareness campaigns and developing victim services programs should be supported by volunteering your nursing expertise, time, and resources. Whether nurses are engaged in clinical care, advocacy, policy, or program activities, they can monitor human trafficking and have an impact on preventing it. Most activists agree that to stop human trafficking, global awareness of the problem must increase. Nurses can add their voices through advocacy and help build the global capacity needed to stop human trafficking.

DISCUSSION QUESTIONS

1. There is a clear need to develop, implement, and evaluate high-quality education and training programs that focus on human trafficking for nurses and other health care providers. How can you contribute to this unmet need?
2. What skills do you already have as a nurse when it comes to working with a patient who has experienced violence and trauma that can inform your work going forward advancing the health care needs of people who have been victims of human trafficking?
3. Consider researching a current news item on human trafficking and conduct a media analysis of how human trafficking is reported. Is this news item a blame narrative? Is the language sensitive to the victim or exploitive? Does it provide a health lens or public health lens? If not, consider a response pointing these issues out with a letter to the editor. Be sure to identify yourself as a registered nurse.

REFERENCES

American Nurses Association [ANA]. (2008). RN delegates to ANA biennial meeting take action to work toward greater nurse retention, address public health issues. Retrieved from *www.nursingworld.org/Functional MenuCategories/MediaResources/PressReleases/2010-PR/ANAs-Delegates -Take-Action.pdf.*

Center for Women Policy Studies. (2014). U.S. policy advocacy to combat trafficking (US PACT). Washington, DC: Center for Women Policy Studies. Retrieved from *www.centerwomenpolicy.org/programs/trafficking/ default.asp.*

General Accounting Office [GAO]. (2008). Human rights: U.S. government's efforts to address alleged abuse of household workers by foreign diplomats with immunity could be strengthened. Retrieved from *www.gao.gov/ new.items/d08892.pdf.*

General Assembly of the United Nations. (1948). Universal declaration of human rights. Retrieved from *www.un.org/en/documents/udhr.*

Hynes, P., & Raymond, J. G. (2002). Put in harm's way: The neglected health consequences of sex trafficking in the United States. In J. Stillman & A. Bhattacharjee (Eds.), *Policing the national body: Sex, race and criminalization.* Cambridge, MA: South End Press.

International Council of Nurses [ICN]. (2006a). ICN code of ethics for nurses. Retrieved from *www.icn.ch/images/stories/documents/about/icncode _english.pdf.*

International Council of Nurses [ICN]. (2006b). Nurses and human rights. Retrieved from *www.icn.ch/images/stories/documents/publications/ position_state ments/C06_Nurse_Retention_Migration.pdf.*

International Council of Nurses [ICN]. (2010). About ICN. Retrieved from *www.icn.ch/about-icn/about-icn.*

International Organization on Migration. (2009). Caring for trafficked persons. Geneva, Switzerland: International Organization for Migration. Retrieved from *http://publications.iom.int/bookstore/free/CT_Handbook.pdf.*

Johnston, A., Friedman, B., & Shafer, A. (2012). News framing of the problem of sex trafficking: Whose problem? What remedy? *Feminist Media Studies,* Retrieved from *dx.doi.org/10.1080/14680777.2012 .740492.*

Polaris Project. (2014). Tools for service providers and law enforcement. Retrieved from *www.polarisproject.org/resources/tools-for-service -providers-and-law-enforcement.*

United Nations [UN]. (2000). Protocol to prevent, suppress, and punish trafficking in persons, especially women and children, supplementing the United Nations Convention Against Transnational Organized Crime. Retrieved from *www.uncjin.org/Documents/Conventions/dcatoc/final _documents_ 2/convention_%20traff_eng.pdf.*

United Nations Office on Drugs and Crime [UNODC]. (2009). Global report on trafficking in persons. Retrieved from *www.unodc.org/documents/ human-trafficking/Global_Report_on_TIP.pdf.*

U.S. Department Homeland Security. (2013). Blue campaign. Retrieved from *www.dhs.gov/blue-campaign/about-blue-campaign.*

U.S. Department of State. (2013a). Trafficking in persons report. Retrieved from *www.state.gov/documents/organization/210737.pdf.*

U.S. Department of State. (2013b). Federal strategic action plan on services for victims of human trafficking in the United States 2013–2017. Retrieved from *www.state.gov/documents/organization/210737.pdf.*

Victims of Trafficking and Violence Protection Act [TVPA] of 2000, 22 U.S.C. § 7102(8).

Zimmerman, C., Hossain, M., Yun, K., Gajdadziev, V., & Guzun, N. (2008). The health of trafficked women: A survey of women entering post trafficking services in Europe. *American Journal of Public Health, 98*(1), 55–59.

ONLINE RESOURCES

General HEAL Trafficking Listserv
HEAL Trafficking
Health Professional Education, Advocacy, Linkage
Because Human Trafficking is a Health Issue
The purpose of the HEAL Trafficking Listserv is to discuss issues at the intersection of health and human trafficking. Although we recognize the value of learning about the breadth of antitrafficking efforts, please reserve nonhealth-related conversations for another forum. Please do not solicit funding on this Listserv and at no time discuss any protected health information, including identity, about any potential victim.
To post to this group, send an e-mail to: *human-trafficking-and-health -care@googlegroups.com*
Visit this group at: *groups.google.com/group/human-trafficking-and-health -care*
For more options, visit: *groups.google.com/d/optout*
ECPAT USA
www.ecpatusa.org/home
Polaris Project
www.polarisproject.org
U.S. Department of State Office to Monitor and Combat Human Trafficking
www.state.gov/j/tip

CHAPTER 88

TAKING ACTION:
A Champion of Change: For Want of a Hug

Cora Tomalinas

"From the earliest days of our founding, our nation has been shaped by ordinary people who have dared to dream and used their unique skills to do extraordinary things. Americans like you help carry this tradition forward by reaching for ideas that will help our country win the future. You and your fellow champions embody the change you want to see in the world. Together, we will out-innovate, out-educate, and out-build the rest of the world to keep our country strong."

President Obama in his letter to Cora Tomalinas

My name is Corazon Basa Cortes Tomalinas. I am a Pilipino American. I immigrated to the United States in 1961 and graduated from San Francisco State University with a bachelor's degree in nursing and a public health certificate in 1968. Soon after graduating I moved to San Jose to work. There I met and married my husband who is also a nurse and we started a family. We lived in a quiet neighborhood and were involved with our children, school, and church until our children became teenagers. What happened then plunged our family into the sad and painful experience of having to rescue our daughter from troubled peers and negative behavior.

WHAT HAPPENED?

When my daughter turned 13 years of age, our family spiraled into a type of hell. She became involved with party crews. Party crews have been called the junior varsity of street gangs. My daughter used drugs, ran away, and had many crises at school. She would attend school stoned. My husband and I were caught off guard; we clung to each other and our son for strength and hope. Finally, injured at a party she was arrested.

THE STRUGGLE TO FIND HELP

Although we were educated and articulate we struggled to find help for our daughter. We reached out to one organization that offered mental health services but not drug rehabilitation. Another organization provided rehabilitation but no mental health services. One organization would not admit patients on weekends. Once we found a program we believed would help her, another barrier arose: it cost us $18,000 for a 28-day stay in a rehabilitation center. We were forced to sell our rental property (our only savings) to pay for the treatment. We attended family therapy and she also received individual therapy at $97 an hour for 1 year. Most of this was not covered by insurance. Her high school objected to her leaving school for therapy sessions and the therapist had inflexible hours. I then had to take on the school to create an individual education plan for her.

During this time our son became a great support for his sister and for our family. My clergy also became a critical source of support. After 2 years of counseling and her rehabilitation program, we reclaimed each of our lives as a family. She attended a different high school and graduated with her class. Both of our children subsequently graduated from San Jose State University.

687

WE GOT HELP, BUT WHAT ABOUT OTHERS?

Gratitude for that grace inspired me to get more involved in our community and into community organizing to improve the quality of life for our children and families. I now serve with several community, faith-based, and government organizations and have done so for over 25 years. I wash dishes, fill food boxes, and distribute toys. I also serve as a commissioner and a board member when needed.

In 2012, I was nominated by the city of San Jose as one of President Barack Obama's Champions of Change and was invited to accept the award at the White House. The high point of that ceremony was the opportunity to address a global audience via telecast from the Indian Treaty Room. Here are parts of my address:

… The causes of the escalating youth violence and violence in general is as complex and varied as there are individuals. The solutions offered are as numerous as there are experts. My experience as a parent, as an engaged member of the community, and more importantly as a nurse, led me to believe that one of the root causes of violence is an absence and/or lack of meaningful bonding and close relationships which I label 'want of a hug.' While we cannot all start hugging everyone we meet literally, although we may start there; we can also give a hug in the form of policies and services that makes us a truly compassionate and just society …

We live in a world where the number and the quality of life between the rich and the poor grow ever wider. The high cost of living pulls us to a dizzying schedule of work to survive, to feed and shelter our families, and to keep them healthy and safe. Some of us labor at our jobs from dawn to dusk seven days a week. These demands leave us very little time to enjoy our families, to give and get hugs. The problem does not end there. Due to our budgeting and partisan wrangling our education system's much needed reform is slow to move ahead, leaving our workforce unprepared for existing jobs. Our health care reform is all but grinding to a halt due to differences of opinions by our elected representatives. The expansion and integration of much needed services are slow to

be implemented due to turf guarding. The fear of losing control over programs and resources grows, as departments, agencies, and organizations compete for the same and ever shrinking funding. Our jails are full despite the fact that incarceration is not the best way to rehabilitation, especially for our young offenders. Local services have yet to come to terms with the high price of prisons and to offer the more humane and sensible interventions of therapy, education, and support.

COMMITMENT IN MY COMMUNITY

There is hope! In my little corner of the world, we are fortunate to have individuals and elected officials who are working together: who believe in the value of hugs. We have residents who are engaged in community welfare and demand an equal voice as a stakeholder in moving toward a common goal: improving the quality of life for our families and maintaining a just and caring society. As a board member of the Silicon Valley Education Foundation, we continue to strongly support the STEM (science, technology, engineering, and mathematics) Initiative. Using technology and innovation, this program offers students, educators, and parents the opportunity to increase their skills to compete in these fields. It also encourages and supports their efforts in solving their own problems.

I have been a member of First 5 in Santa Clara County for over 12 years. Funded by Proposition 10, which is our state cigarette tax monies, this organization is a good example of partnerships that integrate services (First 5 Santa Clara County Annual Report, 2012). First 5 programming is based on the scientific evidence that the human brain develops most actively in the first 5 years of life and that learning is at its most efficient during this time. First 5 invests resources to support the healthy development of children from prenatal to 5 years old. Partnering with government and other community-based organizations, early developmental and behavioral screening is offered. Services start with prenatal care followed with coordination of referrals to appropriate therapy and medical care, thereby improving prognosis.

Other health issues such as obesity and diabetes are also addressed in our community by offering farmer's markets, water stations, and creative educational materials. Dental care is provided in more accessible locations and to more residents. Parenting, advocacy, and leadership development are offered at family resource centers and at houses of worship. All support and education materials as well as referrals are available at medical clinics and especially to pediatricians. Child-friendly materials, such as skits, videos, and books, have been developed to encourage children of all ages to read and are available to families, schools, museums, and community centers.

Educare is another important initiative I want to mention that is opening in San Jose. The first such Early Care and Education Program in the state of California comes through a partnership with the Buffett Foundation, school district, County Office of Education, Headstart, Silicon Valley Leadership Group, Hewlett Packard, and other private investment firms. Educare will be housed in a state-of-the-art building, in one of the neediest and most-challenged communities in the city. The program will have specially trained early care and education providers who will use innovative best practices of early learning in these classrooms and in the neighborhood. It will hug the pregnant mommies, the infants, the toddlers, and on up to 5 years old, to get them ready for school. Educare will provide support and hugs with all the necessary services at the ready to help when needed.

MEETING BASIC NEEDS

Many of our residents are laborers and have very little time or resources for their families. In San Jose, the heart of the community embraced the cause of those laborers. Community-based organizations such as PACT (People Acting in Community Together), Sacred Heart Community Services (of which I am a board member), along with San Jose State University students advocated and won a higher minimum wage rate. Hopefully, this will allow more time for families to be together, more people to be able to meet their basic needs, more opportunities to pursue their dreams; for more hugs.

We also have community- and faith-based organization partners who open their doors to provide timely emergency support for basic needs and guide clients toward a path to self-sufficiency with dignity and compassion. In turn, they become peer mentors to other families whose journey is toward their right to decide their own future, another form of hug. Hundreds of residents in all walks of life including myself advocated, marched, and financially support these organizations.

GANG VIOLENCE PREVENTION

Safety and feeling safe are key to a healthy community. Currently, I am a member of the police team of the San Jose Mayor's Gang Prevention Task Force. In addition to the Sheriff and Police Departments, San Jose and Santa Clara County have two unique programs working together to that end. San Jose Mayor's Gang Prevention Task Force (2011) with its continuum of prevention, intervention, suppression, and rehabilitation programs continues to evolve as we address violence and gang issues threatening our community's safety. Our faith community is also engaged as San Jose rolls out its Crisis Response Protocol in partnership with the Community Chaplains and Santa Clara Valley Medical Center. Legal and confidentiality concerns have been addressed and clergy can now be part of the response in the emergency room as well as aftercare, if requested by the patient following a violent incident. Community members not ready to volunteer for the intensity of a crisis response can contribute by joining on Beautiful Day. This day is spent helping with neighborhood clean ups including school and park upgrades annually.

The Santa Clara County Re-entry Network (I am also a member of the governing board) addresses the issue of returning ex-offenders into the neighborhood. The network with its partners and menu of services begin the work before release. The offenders' needs, weaknesses, and strengths are evaluated and individualized programs are developed. These individualized plans include physical and mental health, food, clothing, housing, and faith connections to prevent recidivism and hopefully increase our ex-offenders' strength to pick up the pieces of broken lives and families (Barnes, Irvine, & Ortega, 2012). Santa Clara County funded multiple points of access for these services in various areas of the community with one central center. The Re-entry Network Center is located near the court, police, and jail. It houses a registered nurse, a social worker, a peer mentor, clothing resources, housing referrals, and faith-based connections.

IT TAKES A VILLAGE

We all must work toward the goal of a just, compassionate, and violence-free society. We must be a people who value our children and safeguard the rights and dignity of individuals. We are making progress, albeit slow. The court's decision regarding Proposition 8 will go a long way to help the gay and lesbian community in their struggle for justice and dignity. California's AB 109 and the adjustment to the three-strikes law inches us closer to a more sensible approach to crime. Our federal government's Second Chance Act is helping cities with resources to decrease the rate of incarceration and recidivism. Sadly, when we see the news and look around us, we soon realize that we have much more work ahead to reach our goal. We will need government representatives who truly listen and act on the needs and priorities of their constituents. Programs, such as the aforementioned, need to be FUNDED, INTEGRATED, EVALUATED, REVISED, or EXPANDED as appropriate. This can only happen if the advocacy from our communities is articulated loudly, clearly, and consistently. Who will step up to lead that movement? We nurses certainly have practice in advocating for our patients. Are we strong enough and brave enough to continue the march so that all may have access to quality health care? A pastor I met from Chicago who lost his son to violence once said, "Do not waste the pain." Indeed, in that vulnerable moment a person is more likely to respond to a hug!

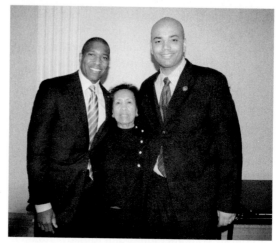

FIGURE 88-1 Author Cora Tomalinas with Associate Attorney General Tony West and National Director of Faith Based Services Eugene Sheenberger.

Will you help develop a crisis response plan in your place of work to make sure that violence victims and their families receive holistic care as early as possible, as well as the perpetrators? Will you join with your community and help beat the drums so that all who need these programs to improve their lives have access to them? Will you listen with your heart to the cry of our children and MOVE to become part of the solution? Will you take a chance and give our children a great big HUG?

REFERENCES

Barnes, M., Irvine, A., & Ortega, N. (2012). Santa Clara county adult re-entry strategic plan: Ready to change: Promoting safety and health for the whole community. National Council on Crime and Delinquency. Retrieved from www.nccdglobal.org/sites/default/files/publication_pdf/santa-clara-report.pdf.

First 5 Santa Clara County Annual Report. (2012). California Children and Families Commission. Retrieved from www.ccfc.ca.gov/pdf/annual_report_pdfs/Annual_Report_11-12.pdf.

Mayor's Gang Prevention Task Force—City of San Jose. (2011). Best evaluation report and summary. Retrieved from www.findyouthinfo.gov/youth-topics/preventing-youth-violence/forum-communities/san-jose/mayors-gang-prevention-task-force-city-san-josé.

CHAPTER 89

Lactivism: Breastfeeding Advocacy in the United States

Diane L. Spatz   Elizabeth B. Froh

"Formula feeding is the longest lasting uncontrolled experiment lacking informed consent in the history of medicine."

Frank Oski, MD

Lactivism is a term used to describe breastfeeding advocacy. Lactivists are those who support breastfeeding, advocate for the rights of breastfeeding mothers, ensure that breastfeeding mothers are not discriminated against, and aim to inform the public regarding the health benefits of breastfeeding. Lactivism occurs in many ways, and recently media attention has focused on human milk and breastfeeding. A woman breastfeeding her toddler was on the cover of *Time* magazine, adults in China are paying lactating women for their maternal breast milk, and the United States recently adapted federal legislation to protect the rights of breastfeeding women in the workplace. Additionally, American media continues to provide attention to stories surrounding wet nursing, informal milk sharing, and nurse-ins. At a nurse-in, mothers gather in public places to breastfeed their children.

WHY ADVOCATE FOR BREASTFEEDING?

Human milk is the preferred form of nutrition for all infants. The health benefits of human milk are so significant that virtually every professional organization including the American Academy of Pediatrics and the World Health Organization recommend exclusive breastfeeding for the first 6 months after birth followed by supplementary foods and continued breastfeeding for 1 to 2 years

or more as desirable by mother and child (American Academy of Pediatrics, 2012) (Figure 89-1). Although exclusive breastfeeding for the first 6 months is the recommended gold standard, few infants in the United States receive this dietary recommendation (16.4%). Why do suboptimal breastfeeding practices continue in the United States? What has led to the need for lactivism in the United States?

THE HISTORIC DECLINE IN BREASTFEEDING IN THE UNITED STATES

Until the mid-1800s, almost all infants in the United States were breastfed. In the 1890s and early 1900s, a shift began that transformed the culture to one in which bottle feeding became the norm. In the 1900s, infant formula manufacturers advertised their products in women's magazines and mothers had increasing doubts about being able to breastfeed successfully (meaning the woman reached her personal breastfeeding goal). As childbirth moved from the home into the hospital, medical practice began to interfere with establishment of lactation and breastfeeding. By 1948, only 38% of infants were receiving exclusive human milk feeds at 1 week of age, and by 1957, only 21% of infants were exclusively breastfed at the time of hospital discharge after birth (Apple, 1994).

The U.S. federal government has tracked breastfeeding trends only since 1999. Before this, the earliest, and now the longest, ongoing survey of breastfeeding initiation rates in the United States was produced by the baby formula industry (the Ross Mothers Survey). According to the Centers for

691

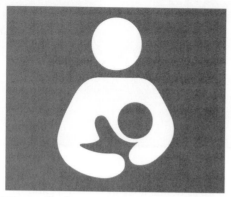

FIGURE 89-1 The International Breastfeeding Symbol. (Copyright © 2015 by breastfeedingsymbol.org.)

Disease Control and Prevention, breastfeeding initiation (defined as one instance of direct breastfeeding or pumping) and duration rates have risen since 1999; however, the increases have been modest. In 1999, approximately 68% of U.S. women initiated breastfeeding, and in 2011, 79.2% of women initiated breastfeeding, only an 11.2% increase. For infants born in 2011, only 18.8% of infants received human milk exclusively for 6 months, with any breastfeeding at 6 months increasing from 32.6% in 1999 to 44.3% in 2008 to 49.4% in 2011 (Centers for Disease Control and Prevention [CDC], 2009, 2011, 2014).

CULTURE OF BREASTFEEDING

The culture of breastfeeding in the United States has eroded over the past 100 years, and, despite the fact that more women now try breastfeeding, preference for both formula and bottle feeding persists. The United States remains a formula feeding society.

A sociocultural issue that appears to underlie resistance to breastfeeding is the dual roles female breasts have. Wolf (2008) wrote a commentary on why public breastfeeding remains so controversial in the United States. Wolf asserted that American culture focuses on female breasts for their sexual appeal, not for their primary function, which is to provide nourishment. The view that breastfeeding should be a private act, like sex, can make it challenging for some women to feel comfortable

breastfeeding or pumping outside their homes (Wolf, 2008). As an exemplar, in 2009 Berjuan Toys introduced the first breastfeeding toy for children, the Breast Milk Baby (The Breast Milk Baby, 2011). Children wear a vest over their chests that comes with a doll; the vest has two appliques of flowers located at the nipple line. When the doll is brought to a flower applique on the vest, it makes a soft sucking noise. After some time, the doll will stop and begin to cry, signaling the child to stop and burp the doll. Available in the United States this toy fostered strong negative media attention with many people seeing the doll as inappropriate for children (The Breast Milk Baby, 2011).

Because of these conflicting views, breastfeeding mothers have met with discrimination in public areas, stores, and restaurants. At a Toys "R" Us store in Times Square in New York, an employee asked a mother to move to a basement to breastfeed because there were children present. This resulted in a nurse-in at the Times Square location in 2006 (New York Civil Liberties Union, 2006). In 2004, Lori Charkoudian was asked by a Starbucks store employee in Silver Spring, Maryland, to cover up or use the women's restroom when she attempted to breastfeed her 15-month-old daughter. This also led to a nurse-in involving 30 mothers and their babies as well as family members and friends (Helderman, 2004). Similarly, a mother was ticketed for breastfeeding her son in Colorado at a beach, despite the fact that Colorado passed a law protecting breastfeeding in 2004 (The Denver Channel News, 2005). Table 89-1 provides a summary of breastfeeding incidents and lactivism events.

ACTION TO SUPPORT BREASTFEEDING

Efforts to improve breastfeeding rates have included federal and state legislation, changes in workplace policies, and individual activism to draw attention to discrimination against breastfeeding mothers.

FEDERAL EFFORTS

The U.S. federal government has attempted to address the need for changing breastfeeding outcomes in the United States. The U.S. national health

TABLE 89-1 Summary of U.S. Breastfeeding Incidents and Related Activities

Description of Breastfeeding Incident	Response	Source
Brooke Ryan was asked to cover the head of her infant while breastfeeding by a waitress and manager of an Applebee's restaurant in Lexington, Kentucky, in 2007. Both employees claimed that other customers were complaining about her breastfeeding in the restaurant.	A nurse-in was held on September 8, 2007. Jonathan R. Weatherby, Jr., Associate General Counsel for Applebee's attorney, wrote, "We regret that Ms. Ryan left without being served and would like the opportunity to personally invite her to return … we are also considering keeping blankets in the restaurants for use by breast-feeding mothers that may not have them readily available as a result of this incident."	www.mothering.com/discussions/showthread.php?t=739358
Danielle Glanvill was harassed twice by a female security guard for breastfeeding in the children's section of a New York library in 2009.	A written apology was granted, and the security guard was transferred to another branch.	www.nypost.com/seven/03242009/news/regionalnews/mom_wins_booby_prize_library_oks_breast__161094.htm
A mother was asked to cover up while breastfeeding at a Denny's restaurant in North Carolina.	A nurse-in was held in protest on February 22, 2009.	www.blogs.babiesonline.com/baby/nationwide-dennys-nurse-in-february-22/
Emily Gillette was asked to leave her Freedom Airlines flight if she would not cover her breasts while feeding her child.	News of the event spurred public nurse-ins at airports around the country, and Gillette filed a complaint with the Vermont Human Rights Commission.	www.msnbc.msn.com/id/16773617/wid/11915773/
A lifeguard told Laurie Waldherr to leave a public pool in Washington state when she was breastfeeding at the pool's edge for risk of bodily fluids getting into the pool.	Waldherr sued the city and reached a settlement out of court.	www.msnbc.msn.com/id/16773617/wid/11915773/
Julie Wheelan was asked to leave a shopping mall food court in Providence, Rhode Island, by a security guard when she was breastfeeding.	Wheelan suggested that the guard call the police, as she knew she was protected by law to breastfeed her child.	www.msnbc.msn.com/id/16773617/wid/11915773/
Dorian Ryan was ticketed for indecent exposure on July 14, 2005, at the Carter Lake Swimming beach in Larimer County, Colorado.	Ryan requested an apology, and Colorado lawmakers agreed. A law passed that gives women the right to breastfeed anywhere they are allowed to be in public.	www.thedenverchannel.com/news/4785183/detail.html
Lori Charkoudian was asked by a Silver Spring, Maryland, Starbucks store employee to cover up or use the women's restroom when she attempted to breastfeed her 15-month-old daughter in 2004.	A nurse-in was held in protest. A Starbucks spokesperson wrote, "We will instruct our Maryland store partners to inform any concerned customer that by Maryland law, mothers have the right to breastfeed in public and to suggest to the customer that they either avert their eyes or move to a different location within the store."	www.washingtonpost.com/wp-dyn/articles/A50610-2004Aug8.html

Continued

UNIT 6

TABLE 89-1 Summary of U.S. Breastfeeding Incidents and Related Activities—cont'd

Description of Breastfeeding Incident	Response	Source
Chelsi Meyerson was harassed for breastfeeding her infant at the Times Square, New York, Toys "R" Us store. An employee asked her to move to the basement to breastfeed. Chelsi refused. Four other female employees also pressed her to move to the basement.	A nurse-in was held at Toys "R" Us in Times Square on September 21, 2006. The New York Civil Liberties Union informed Toys "R" Us that it had violated civil rights law when employees told Meyerson she was not allowed to breastfeed in the store and that her breastfeeding was inappropriate because there were children around. Toys "R" Us has apologized to Meyerson and informed stores of its nursing policy, which specifies that nursing women may breastfeed their children in the place "of their choice" at Toys "R" Us stores.	*www.nyclu.org/news/mothers -gather-toys-r-us-nurse celebrating-right-breastfeed -public*
Cheryl Cruz was asked to cover up when breastfeeding at Universal Studios in Florida.	Cruz was permitted to breastfeed. A spokesman for the park said, "We're going to have the specific team members involved in this incident apologize to her, and we're going to make sure that our team members know how to proceed in these kinds of situations, moving forward."	*www.cbc.ca/canada/ newfoundland-labrador/story/ 2007/11/02/breastfeeding -orlando.html*
Lori Rueger asked if she could breastfeed her baby in a Victoria's Secret dressing room in Charleston, South Carolina. An employee told her no, it was against store policy, and suggested she go to the mall bathroom.	Anthony Hebron, spokesperson for The Limited Brands in Columbus, Ohio, said, "There was an unfortunate misunderstanding in the incident involving us, but you know what, if it's brought forth even greater things, that's fine."	*www.abcnews.go.com/US/ Health/story?id=1378087*
Heather Silvis was confronted in 2008 by a Walmart employee when she attempted to breastfeed. Her shopping cart and infant were taken from her and moved to a dressing room.	Two years earlier, Governor Mark Sanford signed an act protecting and promoting breastfeeding throughout the state. Walmart store management apologized to Silvis.	*www.midlandsconnect.com/news/ news_story.aspx?id=221405*

goals, Healthy People 2020, include objectives aimed at improving breastfeeding (CDC, 2009, 2011, 2014) (Table 89-2).

Workplace support for breastfeeding is critical. Breastfeeding mothers need support from supervisors and co-workers and need education regarding the benefits of continued breastfeeding. Co-workers can also benefit from education about the needs of breastfeeding employees. Mothers need time and a place to breastfeed or use a breast pump while at work. Unfortunately, without regulations and policies, it is unlikely that most employers will adopt these practices. For example, Heather Burgbacher, a school teacher from Colorado, was told her contract would not be renewed after she complained about the school's failure to accommodate her need to pump while at work (under the Colorado Nursing Mothers Act of 2008). The American Civil Liberties Union (ACLU) and the ACLU of Colorado reached a settlement in 2012 in which the

TABLE 89-2 Summary of Healthy People 2020 Goals

Healthy People 2020 Goals	Results
81.9% breastfeeding initiation	17 states have met this objective
60.6% breastfeeding at 6 months	7 states have met this objective
34.1% breastfeeding at 12 months	8 states have met this objective
46.2% exclusive breastfeeding through 3 months	14 states have met this objective
25.5% exclusive breastfeeding through 6 months	6 states have met this objective
To increase the percentage of employers who have worksite lactation programs to 38%	7%
To decrease the percentage of breastfed newborns who receive formula supplementation within the first 2 days of life to 14.2%	19.4%
To increase the percentage of live births that occur in facilities that provide recommended care for lactating mothers and their babies to 8.1%	7.79%

Source: www.cdc.gov/breastfeeding/pdf/2014breastfeedingreportcard.pdf.

school agreed to make policy changes for employees and provided monetary compensation to Burgbacher. This was the first public settlement brought under the Colorado Nursing Mothers Act (American Civil Liberties Union, 2012).

The Health Resources and Services Administration developed the Business Case for Breastfeeding program in 2008. It includes easy steps to support breastfeeding employees, an employee's guide to breastfeeding and working, an outreach marketing guide, and a tool kit. Representative Carolyn Maloney (D-NY) introduced the Breastfeeding Promotion Act of 2007 to amend the Civil Rights Act of 1964 to protect breastfeeding by new mothers, to provide performance standards for breast pumps, and to provide tax incentives for employers to encourage breastfeeding.

Legislation to protect the rights of working mothers was included in the passage of the U.S. Patient Protection and Affordable Care Act, Section 4207: Reasonable Break Time for Nursing Mothers, in March of 2010 under President Obama. This Act falls under Section 7 of the Fair Labor and Standard Act (FLSA) and requires employers to provide reasonable unpaid break time and a non-bathroom location (shielded from view and free from intrusion by co-workers and the public) for an employee to express milk for her child for up to 1 year after the child's birth. To be eligible one must be an employee covered by FLSA and employed by a business with 2 or more employees and (1) does

$500,000 in annual sales or business, or (2) is a hospital, care facility, school/preschool, or government agency. Employers with fewer than 50 employees are exempt if they claim undue hardship.

Increasing breastfeeding promotion among minorities is a national priority. The U.S. Department of Health and Human Services, Office on Women's Health sponsors the campaign It's Only Natural. This campaign is offers support to African-American women and families to better understand the benefits of breastfeeding for the family (U.S. Department of Health and Human Services, 2013).

STATE EFFORTS

Forty-nine states (West Virginia excluded) have enacted legislation to protect breastfeeding (CDC, 2014; National Conference of State Legislatures, 2011). However, the legislation varies significantly from state to state. In some states, breastfeeding is exempted from public indecency laws, and in others, breastfeeding is protected by allowing a mother to breastfeed in any private or public location (Chang & Spatz, 2006). Unfortunately, many women are not aware of their state laws and rights. Chang and Spatz (2006) advocate that nurses inform childbearing women of their rights and provide them with patient family education sheets (including both federal and state-specific legislation) before discharge from the birth hospital. These information sheets should also be available in primary care offices and urgent care facilities.

UNIT 6

BREASTFEEDING ADVOCACY ORGANIZATIONS

Much breastfeeding advocacy has occurred at the grassroots level led by organizations such as La Leche League. La Leche League was established in 1958 to provide mother-to-mother support and advocacy for breastfeeding. The National Alliance for Breastfeeding Advocacy was formed as the precursor to the U.S. Breastfeeding Committee (USBC). This committee is multidisciplinary and addresses the need for nationwide advocacy as it aims to move the breastfeeding agenda forward. The USBC was incorporated in Florida in 2000. Its mission is to improve the nation's health by working collaboratively to protect, promote, and support breastfeeding with a focus on collaboration, leadership, and advocacy (U.S. Breastfeeding Committee, 2003, 2005, 2008). USBC members consist of 46 nonprofit organizations, 8 regional breastfeeding coalitions and 7 governmental agencies that all have vested interests in breastfeeding advocacy.

HOSPITAL POLICIES

Few U.S. hospitals provide evidence-based lactation care. To change infant feeding practices, the World Health Organization and UNICEF sponsored the Baby-Friendly Hospital Initiative (BFHI), is a global program designed to support and encourage hospitals to enact the most beneficial infant feeding practices. The BFHI recognizes hospitals that have achieved optimal infant feeding goals (Baby-Friendly USA, 2013). Only 172 U.S. hospitals are designated as "baby-friendly," facilities, although there are more than 19,000 worldwide. Fewer than 7% of all U.S. births occur in baby-friendly facilities (Baby-Friendly USA, 2013). If hospital policies do not support, protect, and advocate for breastfeeding at all times, it is unlikely that women will be successful in their breastfeeding efforts. The BFHI is a designation available to birth hospitals only. Children and their mothers also may receive care at nonbirth hospitals (e.g., a children's hospital or an adult hospital where the mother is receiving care). These hospital personnel need to be aware of the need for breastfeeding education and advocacy. Spatz (2005a, 2005b) described the need for education of nurses and physicians, hospital-wide systems for managing breast milk, and the need for evidence-based standards of care.

THE NEED FOR BREASTFEEDING ADVOCACY EDUCATION

When the lack of hospital policies supporting breastfeeding and the lack of breastfeeding education received by health care providers is considered, the need for breastfeeding education becomes apparent. A model for integration of breastfeeding content into baccalaureate nursing curricula was developed that could be used for all health care disciplines (Spatz, Pugh, & American Academy of Nursing Expert Panel on Breastfeeding, 2007). A seminar course for undergraduate nursing students at the University of Pennsylvania serves as an example. Nursing students receive 28 hours of didactic and 14 hours of clinical experience related to current research topics in breastfeeding. In the CDC Guide to Strategies to Support Breastfeeding Mothers and Babies, step two on professional education features this course as an exemplary model for educating nurses (*www.cdc.gov/breastfeeding/pdf/BF-Guide-508.pdf*). A solid foundation in the science of breastfeeding makes nurses better prepared to serve as breastfeeding advocates.

One nurse can make a big difference in breastfeeding outcomes. In a hospital, nurses can provide education and support for new mothers and can also be effective in community advocacy efforts (Spatz & Sternberg, 2005). Since 1995, more than 300 students at the University of Pennsylvania have served as change agents in promoting breastfeeding. One student, who was motivated because her mother attempted breastfeeding her younger sibling born with spina bifida, wrote an article for the National Spina Bifida Association; this led to a second one published in a professional journal (Hurtekant & Spatz, 2007). Other students have targeted those not even planning to have children yet, such as presenting educational programs to their fraternity or sorority, athletic teams, and other organized groups (on and off campus). This type of advocacy work is vital because women make the decision on how they will feed their babies often before they are pregnant based on factors in their environment throughout their lifetime. Nurses are in ideal positions to influence breastfeeding in their clinical roles and as advocates in the workplace, community, and legislatures.

DISCUSSION QUESTIONS

1. Do you know your state's policies and legislation related to breastfeeding? Who would you contact on the state level if you had concerns regarding a violation of a person's rights related to breastfeeding?
2. Consider your school, college, or university. Are there any existing policies to promote and protect breastfeeding women and their families?
3. Working with your peers, brainstorm an advocacy project that you could implement in your community to promote or support breastfeeding.

REFERENCES

American Academy of Pediatrics. (2012). Breastfeeding and the use of human milk. *Pediatrics, 129*(3), 827–841.

American Civil Liberties Union [ACLU]. (2012). ACLU settles lawsuit vindicating the rights of Colorado mothers to pump breast milk in the workplace. Retrieved September 30, 2013, from *www.aclu.org/womens-rights/aclu-settles-lawsuit-vindicating-rights-colorado-mothers-pump-breast-milk-workplace.*

Apple, R. (1994). The medicalization of infant feeding in the United States and New Zealand: Two countries, one experience. *Journal of Human Lactation, 10*(1), 31–37.

Baby-Friendly USA. (2013). Find facilities. Retrieved from *www.babyfriendlyusa.org/find-facilities.*

The Breast Milk Baby. (2011). Berjuan Toys brings the breast milk baby doll to the U.S. retailers. Retrieved from *thebreastmilkbaby.com/2011/07/berjuan-toys-brings-the-breast-milk-baby-doll-to-the-u-s-retailers/.*

Centers for Disease Control and Prevention [CDC]. (2009). Healthy people 2020. Retrieved from *www.healthypeople.gov/hp2020/default.asp.*

Centers for Disease Control and Prevention [CDC]. (2011). Vital signs. Retrieved from *www.cdc.gov/vitalsigns/breastfeeding/.*

Centers for Disease Control and Prevention [CDC]. (2014). Breastfeeding report card—United States, 2012. Retrieved from *www.cdc.gov/breastfeeding/pdf/2014breastfeedingreportcard.pdf.*

Chang, K., & Spatz, D. L. (2006). The family & breastfeeding laws: What nurses need to know. *American Journal of Maternal Child Nursing, 31*(4), 224–230.

The Denver Channel News. (2005). Mother ticketed for breast-feeding son in public wants apology. *The Denver Channel News.* Retrieved from *www.thedenverchannel.com/news/4785183/detail.html.*

Helderman, R. S. (2004). Md. mom says no to coverup at Starbucks. *The Washington Post.* Retrieved from *www.washingtonpost.com/wp-dyn/articles/A50610-2004Aug8.html.*

Hurtekant, K. M., & Spatz, D. L. (2007). Special considerations for breastfeeding the infant with spina bifida. *Journal of Perinatal and Neonatal Nursing, 21*(1), 69–75.

National Conference of State Legislatures. (2011). Breastfeeding laws. Retrieved from *www.ncsl.org/issues-research/health/breastfeeding-state-laws.aspx.*

New York Civil Liberties Union. (2006). Mother's gather at Toys-R-Us for "nurse In" celebrating right to breastfeed in public. The New York Civil Liberties Union. Retrieved from *www.nyclu.org/news/mothers-gather-toys-r-us-nurse-celebrating-right-breastfeed-public.*

Spatz, D. L. (2005a). Breastfeeding education and training at a children's hospital. *Journal of Perinatal Education, 14*(1), 30–38.

Spatz, D. L. (2005b). The breastfeeding case study: A model for educating nursing students. *Journal of Nursing Education, 44*(9), 432–434.

Spatz, D. L., & Sternberg, A. (2005). Advocacy for breastfeeding: Making a difference one community at a time. *Journal of Human Lactation, 21*(2), 186–190.

Spatz, D. L., Pugh, L. C., & American Academy of Nursing Expert Panel on Breastfeeding. (2007). The integration of the use of human milk and breastfeeding in baccalaureate nursing curricula. *Nursing Outlook, 55*(5), 257–263.

U.S. Breastfeeding Committee. (2003). *State breastfeeding legislation* [issue paper]. Raleigh, NC: U.S. Breastfeeding Committee.

U.S. Breastfeeding Committee. (2005). *State legislation that protects, promotes, and supports breastfeeding: An inventory and analysis of state breastfeeding and maternity leave legislation.* Washington, DC: U.S. Breastfeeding Committee.

U.S. Breastfeeding Committee. (2008). Retrieved from *www.usbreastfeeding.org.*

U.S. Department of Health and Human Services. (2013). It's only natural. Retrieved from *womenshealth.gov/itsonlynatural/.*

Wolf, J. H. (2008). Got milk? Not in public! *International Breastfeeding Journal, 3*(11), 1–3.

ONLINE RESOURCES

Baby-Friendly USA
www.babyfriendlyusa.org
Centers for Disease Control and Prevention (CDC)
www.cdc.gov/breastfeeding
U.S. Breastfeeding
www.usbreastfeeding.org
Women's Health
womenshealth.gov/itsonlynatural

UNIT 6

CHAPTER 90

TAKING ACTION:

Reefer Madness: The Clash of Science, Politics, and Medical Marijuana

Mary Lynn Mathre   Bryan Krumm

"If you want to make enemies, try to change something."

Woodrow Wilson

A PLANT WITH AN IMAGE PROBLEM

It is a plant with an image problem, a botanical medicine that has been shown to help many patients but whose use is forbidden by federal law. We know it as marijuana, dope, pot, reefer, grass, weed, or ganja. In its clinical form, cannabis has been a valuable medicine used throughout the world. Cannabis (marijuana) and natural THC (the primary psychoactive substance in cannabis) remain in Schedule I, while dronabinol (Marinol), the synthetic form of THC, has since been reassigned from Schedule II to Schedule III (less controlled and more available) attributable to its safety and lack of diverted drug concerns (Box 90-1).

ONCE UPON A TIME, CANNABIS WAS LEGAL

Prior to the U.S. Congress passing the Marihuana Tax Act of 1937, cannabis was a medicine commonly used by physicians for a variety of ailments. *Cannabis sativa* and *Cannabis indica* were used to make cannabis tinctures (Figure 90-1), elixirs, salves, and even smokable products. Cannabis was listed in the U.S. Pharmacopoeia until 1942.

HOW AND WHY DID THE MARIJUANA PROHIBITION BEGIN?

A drug used by African-American jazz musicians in the American South and Mexicans in the Southwest was cannabis, but was called reefer by the African-American population and marijuana (or marihuana) by the Mexicans (Box 90-2). In 1936, the film *Reefer Madness* was released (a reefer being a marijuana cigarette) to warn the American population of the dangers of using marijuana. The film's plot involves tragic events that ensue when white high school students are lured by drug pushers into using marijuana. Few people realized at the time that this dangerous new drug was the same as the cannabis medicine that physicians prescribed. It was under this manufactured threat of marijuana that Congress ultimately passed the Marihuana Tax Act of 1937, despite opposition from the American Medical Association resulting from its recognition of cannabis as a safe and useful medicine (Bonnie & Whitebread, 1974).

MY INTRODUCTION TO THE PROBLEM OF MEDICAL CANNABIS USE

In the early 1980s, I, Mary Lynn Mathre, was working in a small hospital and encountered a cancer patient with experimental marijuana pills from the University of Washington. As this was

---

BOX 90-1 Schedule of Controlled Substances in the United States

21 U.S. Code §812(b) specifies the following classification system for drugs in the United States based on the purpose, safety, and effectiveness of the drug:

Schedule I Drugs

a. The drug or other substance has a high potential for abuse.
b. The drug or other substance has no currently accepted medical use in treatment in the United States.
c. There is a lack of accepted safety for use of the drug or other substance under medical supervision.

Schedule I drugs include marijuana (cannabis), heroin (diacetylmorphine), ecstasy (MDMA), psilocybin, GHB (gamma-hydroxybutyrate), LSD, mescaline, and peyote.

Schedule II Drugs

a. The drug or other substance has a high potential for abuse.
b. The drug or other substance has a currently accepted medical use in treatment in the United States or a currently accepted medical use with severe restrictions.
c. Abuse of the drug or other substance may lead to severe psychological or physical dependence.

Schedule II drugs are only available by prescription, and distribution is carefully controlled and monitored by the Drug Enforcement Administration. Schedule II drugs include cocaine, methylphenidate (Ritalin), most pure opioid agonists, meperidine, fentanyl, opium, oxycodone, morphine, and short-acting barbiturates, such as secobarbital, methamphetamine, and PCP.

Schedule III Drugs

a. The drug or other substance has a potential for abuse less than the drugs or other substances in Schedules I and II.
b. The drug or other substance has a currently accepted medical use in treatment in the United States.
c. Abuse of the drug or other substance may lead to moderate or low physical dependence or high psychological dependence.

Schedule III drugs are available only by prescription, although control of wholesale distribution is somewhat less stringent than for Schedule II drugs. Schedule III drugs include Marinol; anabolic steroids; intermediate-acting barbiturates, such as talbutal; preparations that combine codeine or hydrocodone with aspirin or acetaminophen; ketamine; and paregoric.

Schedule IV Drugs

a. The drug or other substance has a low potential for abuse relative to the drugs or other substances in Schedule III.
b. The drug or other substance has a currently accepted medical use in treatment in the United States.
c. Abuse of the drug or other substance may lead to limited physical dependence or psychological dependence relative to the drugs or other substances in Schedule III.

Schedule IV control measures are similar to those for Schedule III; drugs on this Schedule include benzodiazepines such as alprazolam (Xanax), chlordiazepoxide (Librium), and diazepam (Valium); long-acting barbiturates, such as phenobarbital; and some partial agonist opioid analgesics, such as propoxyphene (Darvon) and pentazocine (Talwin).

Schedule V Drugs

a. The drug or other substance has a low potential for abuse relative to the drugs or other substances in Schedule IV.
b. The drug or other substance has a currently accepted medical use in treatment in the United States.
c. Abuse of the drug or other substance may lead to limited physical dependence or psychological dependence relative to the drugs or other substances in Schedule IV.

Schedule V drugs are sometimes available without a prescription; drugs on this schedule include cough suppressants containing small amounts of codeine and preparations containing small amounts of opium, used to treat diarrhea.

From Title 21 U.S. Code (USC) Controlled Substances Act. Retrieved from *www.deadiversion.usdoj.gov/21cfr/21usc/802.htm#32a.*

---

a new experience for all nurses, we locked the prescribed marijuana pills in the narcotics cabinet. No problems were encountered, and I began researching these pills, Marinol (Figure 90-2), the synthetic marijuana pill. This led me to an organization called the Alliance for Cannabis Therapeutics (ACT), started by a glaucoma patient, Robert Randall, and his wife. In 1976, Randall had gained legal access to federally grown marijuana under the Compassionate Use Investigational New Drug (IND) program following a series of court battles because no other medicine could control his intraocular pressure. He formed ACT, a nonprofit organization, to let others know about the therapeutic benefits of cannabis and how patients could get a legal, federally approved supply of it. I was drawn to the issue; a patient was advocating for cannabis as medicine for glaucoma.

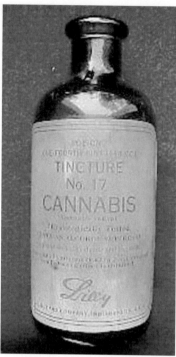

FIGURE 90-1 Historical photo. Tincture of cannabis no. 17 produced by Eli Lilly. (The Cannabis Museum, Elliston, VA, USA.)

AN OPPORTUNITY FOR EDUCATION

After earning my master's degree and conducting a survey on issues pertaining to medical marijuana, I accepted the volunteer position of Director of the NORML's Council on Marijuana and Health. NORML (National Organization for the Reform of Marijuana Laws) is a nonprofit organization committed to move public opinion to safely legalize marijuana. By 1990, there were five patients who had legal access to marijuana through the Compassionate Use IND program. At NORML's annual conference, a panel discussion comprising these 5 patients was aired on C-SPAN. This media exposure garnered national attention that resulted in numerous IND applications. Owing to the increased number of IND applications primarily from patients with HIV/AIDS, the Secretary of the U.S. Department of Health and Human Services, Dr. Louis Sullivan, responded by shutting down the

---

BOX 90-2 Cannabis Terms

Cannabis: A plant genus that is unique in the plant kingdom in that it contains a group of chemicals known as cannabinoids.

Cannabis indica: A species of the cannabis plant that has short, broad leaflets.

Cannabis sativa: A species of the cannabis plant that has long, narrow leaflets.

Cannabidiol (CBD): A nonpsychoactive cannabinoid with numerous therapeutic properties.

Cesamet—Nabilone: A synthetic derivative of THC that is available in Europe, Canada, and the United States.

Endocannabinoid system (ECS): A newly discovered molecular signaling system, present in all animals, which serves to keep us in balance and protect us from stressors.

Marijuana/marihuana: The obsolete pejorative Mexican name for cannabis, used by the U.S. federal government in their efforts to prohibit the use of the cannabis plant.

Marinol: A registered trademark of Unimed Pharmaceuticals. It is the commercial name for dronabinol (the synthetic form of delta-9-tetrahydrocannabinol), which is formulated with sesame oil and encapsulated in soft gelatin capsules. When first on the market, it was a Schedule II medication for use in the treatment of nausea and vomiting caused by chemotherapy, as well as appetite loss caused by AIDS.

Sativex: A cannabis extract oromucosal spray developed by GW Pharmaceuticals in the United Kingdom and first on the market in Canada in 2005 for use by patients with multiple sclerosis.

THC (Delta-9-tetrahydrocannabinol): The primary psychoactive ingredient in cannabis/marijuana; one of more than 60 cannabinoids.

IND access to marijuana in 1992. At that time, 15 patients were receiving marijuana; more than 30 patients had been approved and were waiting for their medication; and hundreds of applications were waiting for review (Randall & O'Leary, 1998). Only the 15 current patients would be allowed to continue in the program, closing the door to all others. Following the panel, we interviewed and videotaped each patient to create an 18-minute video called Marijuana as Medicine (Byrne &

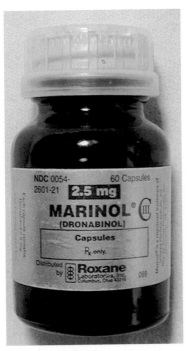

FIGURE 90-2 Marinol.

Mathre, 1992), which was designed to be a teaching aid.

These events helped me understand there was no justifiable reason for the marijuana prohibition. It has therapeutic value, it is safe, and patients benefit from it. I saw this as a problem that required patient advocacy and that had ethical implications. I believed it to be a professional responsibility to end the cannabis prohibition and make this medicine legally available to patients. This was not simply ignorance of the science but grounded in political ideology.

BARRIERS AND STRATEGIES

Over the years, I have encountered many barriers and tried various strategies; often the same strategies had been used under different circumstances. Barriers I have encountered include misinformation presented as facts, censorship of information, intimidation, laws and regulations that prevent research, federal promotion of an image based on racism and ideology rather than

science and reality, and pharmaceutical industry pressure to prevent potential competition.

I have used strategies such as finding a strong mentor; building a support system; mobilizing grassroots support; reframing the problem; partnering with patients; building a coalition; starting a nonprofit organization; providing continuing accredited education for health care professionals about cannabis; using the Internet; playing by the government's rules; teaching others; conducting research; disseminating research findings; educating the public through publications, the press, and the media; and helping to create a new nursing specialty organization, the American Cannabis Nurses Association. As you read about the barriers encountered and the strategies used, education and perseverance have been key to creating a massive grassroots movement to end the cannabis prohibition. Patients, family members, and their care providers are leading this grass-roots effort to end this costly, unfounded, unjust, and profit-motivated prohibition of cannabis.

PATIENTS OUT OF TIME

In 1995, following the deaths of a young couple with AIDS who were in the IND program, my husband and I felt the need to take legalizing medical marijuana more wholeheartedly. With the help of several IND patients and other health care professionals, we founded a national nonprofit organization, Patients Out of Time. We kept our mission simple: to educate health care professionals and the public about the therapeutic use of cannabis. Initially we focused on getting professional organizations, including the American Public Health Association, to issue resolutions in support of patient access to cannabis. We keep an updated list of supporting organizations on our website (*www.medical cannabis.com*). The American Nurses Association's resolution most clearly encompasses the issues of concern regarding the marijuana prohibition.

THE TIDE IS SHIFTING

In 2000, Patients Out of Time held the First National Clinical Conference on Cannabis Therapeutics with the University of Iowa's Colleges of Nursing and Medicine as cosponsors. We had an international conference faculty that included researchers, clinical experts, patients, and care providers. Since the first conference, we continue to hold biennial conferences, and the feedback is consistently positive.

The public's awareness and acceptance of therapeutic cannabis has increased over the years from 20% in the 1980s to 75% to 88% approval per recent public opinion polls (Medical Marijuana ProCon.org, 2013a; National Organization for the Reform of Marijuana Laws [NORML], 2013). Despite the federal prohibition, 23 states and Washington, DC now have laws allowing cannabis as medicine (Medical Marijuana ProCon.org, 2013b). Eric Holder, the U.S. Attorney General, issued a statement in 2009 clarifying that the U.S. federal government will no longer interfere with medical marijuana patients in states that have medical marijuana laws. President Obama made a statement in his inaugural address announcing that his administration would make policy changes based on science rather than ideology. These were viewed as positive steps toward ending the cannabis prohibition.

On July 22, 2010 the U.S. Department of Veterans Affairs issued a new directive (Medical Marijuana Directive 2011-004) in which it provides guidance on access to and the use of cannabis by veterans. This is a huge step forward by a U.S. federal agency. Veterans are allowed to use medicinal cannabis if they receive a recommendation from a civilian physician in one of the states permitting its use.

As states have been passing laws allowing for the medical use of cannabis, in the November 2012 elections both Colorado and Washington states passed initiatives legalizing marijuana for adult usage. In light of this bold step, the U.S. Department of Justice issued another memorandum on August 13, 2013 that states that the U.S. federal government will not challenge the state marijuana laws but will allow Colorado and Washington to regulate the growing and selling of cannabis in a regulated market. In 2010, I and a small group of nurses created a new specialty organization in nursing, the American Cannabis Nurses Association (www.cannabisnurse.org). The American Cannabis Nurses Association has experienced a growth spurt following this changing tide in the public acceptance of medicinal cannabis.

LOOKING AHEAD AT A PARADIGM SHIFT

The United States is in the midst of a seismic shift in the understanding of cannabis. The reefer madness myths are giving way to scientific discoveries and strong, positive public opinion and we as health care professionals need to embrace the science and role of cannabis for medicinal use. Medicinal cannabis products will likely in the future be removed from Schedule I and placed in the lowest restricted Schedule or removed from the controlled substances list all together. And ultimately, citizens should be allowed to grow this valuable plant in their own gardens.

REFERENCES

Bonnie, R. J., & Whitebread, C. H. (1974). *The marihuana conviction: A history of the marihuana prohibition in the United States.* Charlottesville, VA: University Press of Virginia.

Byrne, A., & Mathre, M. L. (1992). Marijuana as medicine (video). Retrieved from *www.medicalcannabis.com.*

The Marihuana Tax Act of 1937, Transcripts of Congressional hearings, additional statement of H. J. Anslinger, Commissioner of Narcotics. Retrieved from *druglibrary.org/schaffer/hemp/taxact/t10a.htm.*

Medical Marijuana. VHA Directive 2011-004. Washington, DC: Department of Veterans Affairs, Veterans Health Administration. Retrieved from *www1.va.gov/vhapublications/ViewPublication.asp?pub_ID=2276.*

Medical Marijuana ProCon.org. (2013a). Votes and polls, national. Retrieved from *medicalmarijuana.procon.org/view.additional-resource.php?resourceID=000151.*

Medical Marijuana ProCon.org. (2013b). 20 Legal medical marijuana states and DC laws, fees, and possession limits. Retrieved from *medical marijuana.procon.org/view.resource.php?resourceID=000881.*

National Organization for the Reform of Marijuana Laws (NORML). (2013). Surveys & polls. Retrieved from *norml.org/component/zoo/category/surveys-polls.*

Randall, R. C., & O'Leary, A. M. (1998). *Marijuana Rx: The patient's fight for medicinal pot.* New York: Thunder's Mouth Press.

CHAPTER 91

International Health and Nursing Policy and Politics Today: A Snapshot

Judith A. Oulton

"We cannot live for ourselves alone. Our lives are connected by a thousand invisible threads ... our actions run as causes and return to us as results."

Herman Melville

Nurses have a professional obligation to understand the world in its broader context and to base our decision making on an expanded understanding of ourselves, our patients, and our circumstances. By having a global view, we increase our capacity to synthesize a wider range of information to make more informed and thoughtful decisions. It begins with understanding the policies and politics of globalization and key international health and nursing issues.

GLOBALIZATION

Globalization, the growing interdependence of the world's people, means that national policy and action are increasingly shaped by international forces along with other aspects of our lives. For example, the increase in international travel means the ready spread of disease and threats to security as people move freely across borders and continents. Today, nations and health professionals must learn to care for new as well as reemerging illnesses, deal with the added risks of exposure, and handle acts of terrorism.

Globalization has increased the sharing of knowledge and technology and expanded gender and human rights advocacy. It has also meant that health services and the health professions are increasingly seen as commodities. Health tourism is gaining popularity as nations vie for patients interested in traveling to another country for high quality, lower cost health care. It is estimated that 7 million patients annually travel internationally for health care with India, the United States, and Thailand the favored destinations (Hodges, 2013; Lenhart, 2013).

The free movement of people and services has been aided by mutual recognition agreements (MRAs), legal instruments that accept the standards of another state or country as equal to their own, thus lowering barriers for people to work in other states within a country, or in other nations. For example, MRAs permit nurses to move freely within the European Union, 10 Southeast Asia nations, and 5 African countries. The MRAs aim to facilitate mobility of nursing professionals, exchange information and expertise on standards and qualifications, promote adoption of best practices, and provide opportunities for capacity building and training.

MRAs also occur within nations. The best known national MRA is in the United States where 24 states have signed the Nurse Licensure Compact. This agreement allows nurses to have one multistate license, with the ability to practice in both their home states and those of the other signatory states without dual licensure (National Council of State Boards of Nursing, 2013).

MIGRATION

Nurses are among the more than 230 million people moving to work, to study, to have fun, to receive health care or to escape violence, poverty, persecution, and famine in their native countries (United Nations [UN], 2013a). Migration brings with it problems of unemployment, racial tension, harmful cultural practices (e.g., female genital mutilation), and discrimination, and it is a United Nations (UN) priority. In 2013, the UN General Assembly held a high-level dialogue on International Migration and Development, which reaffirmed the need to protect all migrants' rights, no matter their status, with particular concern for women and children (UN, 2013b). Migration has been on the World Health Organization (WHO) agenda for several years. In 2010, the World Health Assembly (WHA), the annual meeting of Ministers of Health from Member States, created a nonbinding code of practice on the international recruitment of health personnel aimed at discouraging developed countries from recruiting from developing countries that have acute shortages of health professionals (WHO, 2013a).

The nursing community has been vocal nationally and internationally in addressing migration and workforce policy and practice. For example, the International Council of Nurses (ICN) has a policy on Ethical Nurse Recruitment and one on Nurse Retention and Migration (ICN, 2007a, 2007b). Both support the right of nurses to migrate (Box 91-1).

In line with the ICN, nurses' associations have condemned the practice of recruiting offshore rather than effectively addressing nursing workforce planning, including the problems that cause nurses to leave the profession. An excellent example of this is the work of the American Nurses Association (ANA), which takes a strong interest in ensuring positive employment conditions and support systems for foreign-educated nurses. The ANA participated along with representatives of business, labor, academia, and others in developing the 2008 voluntary Code of Ethical Conduct for the Recruitment of Foreign-Educated Nurses (ANA, 2008a, 2008b).

The ICN has created two centers addressing workforce issues, including migration. The International Centre on Nurse Migration (ICNM) serves as a global resource for the development, promotion, and dissemination of research, policy, and information on nurse migration (ICNM, 2013).

BOX 91-1 International Council of Nurses

The International Council of Nurses (ICN) is a federation of national nurses' associations representing nurses in more than 130 countries. Founded in 1899, the ICN is the world's first and widest-reaching international organization for health professionals. Operated by nurses for nurses, the ICN works to ensure high-quality nursing care for all, sound health policies globally, the advancement of nursing knowledge, and the presence worldwide of a respected nursing profession and a competent and satisfied nursing workforce.

The ICN advances nursing, nurses, and health through its policies, partnerships, advocacy, leadership development, networks, congresses, special projects, and work in the arenas of professional practice, regulation, and socioeconomic welfare. The ICN is particularly active in ethics, AIDS, advanced practice, research, leadership development, the international classification of nursing practice, women's health, regulation, human resources development, occupational health and safety, conditions of work, career development, and human rights.

The council works with agencies of the United Nations system, such as the World Health Organization (WHO), UNAIDS, UNICEF, UNESCO, United Nations Conference on Trade and Development (UNCTD), and International Labour Organization (ILO); other intergovernmental organizations such as the World Bank, World Trade Organization, and the International Organization on Migration; and international, regional, and national nongovernmental organizations.

For more information, visit: *www.icn.ch.*

The second center, the International Centre on Human Resources in Nursing, is an online resource for information and tools on nursing human resources (ICN, 2013).

Nurse migration affects policy, planning, and delivery of nursing education and patient care. It brings to the fore such issues as use of fraudulent credentials, ethical recruitment, and discriminatory workplace policy and practice, all of which affect safe care, safe practice, and a safe practice environment.

GLOBAL HEALTH

Globalization has also turned greater attention to global health. Today, university students from many developed nations are working side by side with their counterparts in Africa, Southeast Asia, and South America, learning firsthand about health care in resource-poor settings and connecting electronically to exchange views, experiences, and aspirations.

Along with universities, foundations (e.g., the Bill and Melinda Gates and the Clinton Foundations), industry (e.g., pharmaceutical and oil companies), nongovernmental organizations (NGOs), and new alliances (involving governmental, intergovernmental, and private sector groups) have entered the global health arena. The new players bring money, expertise, and influence that affect funding, services, and health policy. For example, the Bill and Melinda Gates Foundation (2014) has committed $1.5 billion to expand child immunization, and the Clinton Foundation's Health Access Initiative has been successful in lowering HIV/AIDS treatment costs in developing countries. NGOs, such as Médicins Sans Frontières (MSF, or Doctors Without Borders), have also gained influence, largely through delivery of humanitarian services in conflict, disaster, and poverty stricken countries and through their advocacy initiatives (Box 91-2).

The U.S. government, working with UN agencies and its own programs, makes major contributions to global health through the President's Emergency Plan for AIDS Relief (PEPFAR), USAID, and the Centers for Disease Control and Prevention (CDC). PEPFAR funding helps strengthen nursing and midwifery in several developing countries as a vehicle for addressing leadership in HIV/AIDS care. This takes the form of better regulation, leadership development, stronger nurses' associations, and expanded roles for nurses. Task-shifting for prescribing HIV medications and performing circumcisions (from physicians to nurses) is a current undertaking.

The CDC also plays an important role in global health and works in more than 60 countries (CDC, 2013a). As part of its 2012 to 2015 Global Health Strategy, the CDC is leading a consortium of national and international organizations to strengthen nursing and midwifery regulation in Sub-Saharan Africa (CDC, 2012, 2013b) (Box 91-3).

BOX 91-2 Médicins Sans Frontières

Médicins Sans Frontières (MSF) is a humanitarian nongovernmental organization created in 1971. Originally established in France, today its headquarters are in Geneva, Switzerland, not far from WHO. It has offices in 19 countries, including the United States. The organization is best known for its work in crisis countries, whether these are situations of conflict, war, or famine. Its 27,000 professionals (physicians, nurses, and others) currently work in 60 countries.

MSF prides itself on its neutrality and its independence from governments. More than 90% of its monies come from private sources. It pledged its 1999 Nobel Peace Prize money to the fight against neglected diseases that, along with HIV/AIDS, tuberculosis (TB), malnutrition, malaria, and vaccines, are the focus of its Access Campaign. It lobbies for lower costs of medicines and vaccines and against other restrictions on access, such as patents, as well as for better policies to fight malnutrition. Its record stands for itself, as the statistics from its 2012 report show (MSF, 2013):

- 8.3 million outpatient consultations
- 1.6 million patients treated for malaria
- 185,000 assisted births
- 284,000 patients with HIV on antiretroviral treatment
- 78,000 surgical procedures
- 276,000 children treated for malnutrition
  For more information, visit: *www.msf.org*.

THE POLICY ROLE OF THE WORLD HEALTH ORGANIZATION

WHO is a UN agency that leads on health, something it did successfully through its first half century. Both developed and developing countries refer to its leadership in areas such as primary health care, international health regulations, and counterfeit substances; however, its leadership in other areas is slipping.

Organizations such as the World Bank and influential NGOs have become increasingly frustrated by the inefficiency and ineffectiveness of WHO (Ng & Ruger, 2011). Ministries of health, although working with civil society and the private sector nationally, are reluctant to see other entities gain a policy voice, or greater influence, within WHO. Although the organization acknowledges that it cannot function effectively without engaging with

---

BOX 91-3 Centers for Disease Control and Prevention Global Health Goals, 2012 to 2015

Goal 1: Achieve health impact by improving the health and well-being of people around the world by focusing on:

- Preventing new HIV infections and serving the needs of individuals who are HIV-positive globally
- Reducing tuberculosis (TB)- and malaria-related deaths and disease
- Reducing morbidity and mortality among women and children
- Addressing specific neglected tropical diseases
- Controlling and ending vaccine-preventable diseases
- Decreasing the burden of noncommunicable diseases (NCDs)

Goal 2: Improve capabilities to prepare for and respond to infectious diseases, other emerging health threats, and public health emergencies by addressing:

- Increasing capacity to prepare for and detect infectious diseases and other emerging health threats
- Responding to international public health emergencies as well as helping improve country response capabilities

Goal 3: Build country public health capacity as a means to achieve lasting health improvements through focusing on helping counties to:

- Strengthen their public health institutions and infrastructure
- Improve their surveillance and use of strategic information
- Increase their workforce capacity
- Strengthen their laboratory systems and networks
- Improve their research capacity

Goal 4: Maximize the potential of the Centers for Disease Control and Prevention's (CDC) global programs to achieve impact by:

- Strengthening organizational and technical capacity to better support CDC's global health activities
- Enhancing communication to expand the impact of CDC's global health expertise (CDC, 2012)
  For more information, visit: *www.cdc.gov.*

---

nongovernmental players, it is unable to agree on how to move forward. Ng and Ruger (2011) note: "New actors bring new resources and ideas, but new actors and new forms of organization—e.g., networks and partnerships—also blur lines of responsibility" (Ng & Ruger, 2011, p. 2). Given that health policy is impacted by not only diverse players in the health arena but also indirectly by outside forces (trade, defense, migration, etc.), it is understandable that WHO's primacy in global health governance is threatened. Money is another key factor. Member nations fund less than a quarter of the annual budget; thus, WHO must rely on voluntary contributions from countries, intergovernmental agencies, and nongovernmental sources. Not surprisingly, a mammoth reform strategy is under way, reducing the budget, staff, and programs of WHO.

THE MILLENNIUM DEVELOPMENT GOALS

In 2000, the UN created a number of goals and targets to advance global welfare, several of which are of interest to nurses (UN, 2000) (Box 91-4). Nurses have been involved in promoting the millennium development goals (MDGs) and have benefited from work on the targets funded and/or carried out by countries, donors, and development agencies. Nurse and midwife numbers have grown in several countries; the profession has had access to more education and expanded roles; and educational institutions have been strengthened. Yet as we celebrate accomplishments, the data show that much remains to be done, with many opportunities for nurses to play a significant role, whether addressing poverty, HIV/AIDS, or other health issues.

The 2013 MDG report shows good, and sometimes remarkable, progress in many areas. However, the following situations persist (UN, 2013c; Volunteer Kenya, 2014; World Bank, 2013a,b; WHO, 2013a, 2013b):

- 1.2 billion people still live in extreme poverty, with women continuing to represent 70% of the absolute poor.
- Every day 1 in 8 people still go to bed hungry;
- 45 million children (mostly in Sub-Saharan Africa) are not in school.
- Fewer girls attend secondary school than boys overall, but the situation reverses in many regions when it comes to tertiary education.
- About 7% of children under age 5 years are overweight.

BOX 91-4 The Millennium Development Goals

(1) Eradicate extreme poverty and hunger
(2) Achieve universal primary education
(3) Promote gender equality and empower women
(4) Reduce child mortality
(5) Improve maternal health
(6) Combat HIV/AIDS, malaria, and other diseases
(7) Ensure environmental sustainability
(8) Develop a global partnership for development (United Nations [UN], 2000)

Along with the goals, 18 targets were set and 48 indicators, which evolved into 60 indicators as time progressed (UN, 2000, 2013c). Several of the targets are of particular interest to nurses. For example, between 1990 and 2015 the aim is to:

- Halve the proportion of people whose income is less than $1 a day.
- Halve the proportion of people who suffer from hunger.
- Ensure that all children everywhere will be able to complete primary school
- Eliminate gender disparity in primary and secondary education.
- Reduce by two thirds the under-five mortality rate.
- Reduce by three quarters the maternal mortality ratio.
- Achieve universal access to reproductive health.
- Halt and begin to reverse the spread of HIV/AIDS.
- Provide universal access to treatment for HIV/AIDS for all those who need it.
- Halt and begin to reverse the incidence of malaria and other major diseases.
- Halve the proportion of people without sustainable access to safe drinking water and basic sanitation.
- In cooperation with pharmaceutical companies, provide access to affordable essential drugs in developing countries (UN, 2013d).

For more information, visit: *www.un.org/millenniumgoals.*

- In Sub-Saharan Africa, 1 in 9 children die before age 5 years, more than 16 times the average for developed regions. Poverty, location, mother's education, conflict, political fragility, and violence all affect the mortality rate.
- Nearly 1 in 20 adults in Sub-Saharan Africa are HIV infected, accounting for 69% of the people living with HIV worldwide.

- Of the 17.3 million children who had lost at least one parent to HIV by 2011, 16 million (92.5%) live in Sub-Saharan Africa.
- In 2012, 8.6 million people contracted tuberculosis (TB), with Asia and Africa accounting for nearly 60% of new cases.

On the positive side, considerable progress has been made in some areas. For example:

- Bangladesh has shown remarkable falls in fertility and maternal mortality rates, which many attribute to women's increased literacy and education.
- According to the World Bank (2013b), enrolment of girls in Bangladesh's secondary schools has risen to over 6 million from 1.1 million in 1991.
- Of the 99 countries where malaria is prevalent, 50 are on track to meet the MDG target (UN, 2013c).
- The target for TB is on track, and WHO regions of the Americas and the West Pacific have already met the target. New diagnostic tests and new and repurposed TB drugs are being developed and vaccines for prevention are available and more are under way (WHO, 2013b).

BEYOND THE MILLENNIUM DEVELOPMENT GOALS

In 2013, the UN General Assembly agreed that the next set of goals, to be dealt with in September 2015, would be based on the principles of human rights, gender equality, and the rule of law. Women, young people, marginalized groups, and the environment were declared continuing concerns (Ford, L., 2013).

WHO and many countries are interested in seeing access to universal health coverage included among the next goals. WHO defines universal health coverage as ensuring that all people can use the preventive, curative, rehabilitative, and palliative health services they need, of sufficient quality to be effective, while also ensuring that the use of these services does not expose the user to financial hardship (WHO, 2013c). Every year 100 million people are pushed into poverty because they have to pay for health services directly (WHO, 2010a). To reduce these financial risks, countries such as

Thailand are moving away from a system funded largely by out-of-pocket payments to one funded by prepaid funds, a mix of taxes and insurance contributions (WHO, 2010a).

Clearly the new goals, being dubbed by many as the Sustainable Development Goals (SDGs), will need to include much of the unfinished worldwide agenda, such as poverty, women and children's health, and communicable disease, as well as environmental issues. They should also include noncommunicable diseases (NCDs), the leading cause of death globally. There is clear evidence of nurses' effectiveness in keeping patients with NCDs healthy and in keeping chronic care costs down.

HUMAN RESOURCES FOR HEALTH

Nearly a decade ago a worldwide shortage of health professionals, particularly nurses, midwives, and physicians, sparked a concentrated focus on human resources for health. Considerable funding led to a scale-up of training and employment in developing countries along with global and national advocacy for human resources for health (HRH). More recently, with funding restraints in developed countries, and WHO focused on internal reform, the focus on HRH has slipped.

Several developed countries have cut hospital nursing staff to save money, and in many countries new nurse graduates are not getting permanent jobs even though staffing is often known to be inadequate. The aging of the baby boomers, and their retirement, is adding pressure to overloaded systems. In the United States, expansion of Medicaid and changing health laws mean more demands on already stretched health care systems. For example, Illinois predicted that in 2014 it would have 32 million more insured persons and many more Medicare-aged baby boomers (Adorka, 2010).

Internationally, HRH growth has mainly been in the midwifery workforce and among community health workers, with donors embracing both as part of the push to decrease maternal and infant mortality. However, nurses continue to be in short supply. For example, England has a shortage of 20,000 nurses and is recruiting from abroad once again (Ford, S., 2013). India needs 2.4 million nurses to reach a nurse/patient ratio of 1 : 500 (WHO, 2010b), although the vacancy rate for nursing and midwifery positions in Malawi's public sector is 65% (Dwyer, 2012).

According to all predictions, the global situation will continue to worsen. For example, a 2009 WHO/ICN discussion paper estimated the shortfall of nurses will rise to 2.8 million by 2015 (Canadian Federation of Nurses Unions, 2012).

Although the West faces the issue of aging faculty, many developing countries have too few teachers, both in numbers and in academic preparation. Although technology is helping, many nursing institutions lack teaching-learning resources, classroom space, or the ability to provide clinical supervision of students.

Nurses everywhere share common workplace issues, although they vary in intensity. They feel stressed and understaffed. Overtime is common, although opportunities for continuing education and promotion are not. Nurses want more time with patients, a safe workplace, better compensation and benefits, a voice in policy, and supportive leaders. If nursing is to significantly contribute to patient care and population health, it is vital that nurses and nursing organizations work to improve workforce numbers and resolve workplace issues.

ADVANCED NURSING PRACTICE

Globalization, education, advocacy, disease burden, access to services, and resource issues have all played a part in the global growth of advanced practice. Although nurse midwives have been practicing for a century or more and nurse anesthetists for nearly as long, other advanced nursing practice nursing areas have been slower to develop. However, these have generally required a higher level of education than midwifery or anesthesia. Today, the education of nurse midwives ranges from certificate-level to master's-level preparation. Many countries in Africa and Asia continue to include midwifery as part of diploma-level programs, although there is increasing pressure for direct entry midwifery education.

Advanced practice continues to have two streams: the clinical nurse specialist (CNS) and the nurse practitioner (NP). The CNS role was the first to be taken up and remains the main advanced practice title and role in many countries, particularly in Southeast Asia. Although the United States has long promoted the CNS education level as a master's, in many nations it is less than this. The NP role development has been slower. Although it originated as a collaboration between a U.S. nurse and a physician, there has been considerable physician resistance to the role in many countries, but less so when the concept is introduced for rural and remote practice.

The United States has by far the largest number of advanced practice nurses (APNs), especially those who are master's prepared. In 2008, APNs represented 9% of all registered nurses (RNs) in the United States, 0.2% of RNs in Australia, and 1.5% in Canada; and in 2009, APNs made up 4% of nurses in Ireland (Lafortune, 2011). Numbers globally have been growing over the past 2 decades. In 1999, nurses' associations in 33 countries reported having some forms of advanced practice (Schober & Affara, 2006). By 2011, the ICN's International Nurse Practitioner/Advanced Nursing Practice Network (INP/APN) included nurses from 78 countries (Schober, 2013).

Korea has had nurse-midwives and nurse anesthetists since the 1950s and NPs since the 1980s (Schober & Affara, 2006). Thailand introduced NPs in the 1970s; today, NPs include those with 4 months post-basic training and others with master's-level education (Hanucharurnkul, 2007). Singapore has more than 100 master's-prepared NPs (Schober, 2012); although Japan launched its first program in 2009, it has had CNS programs for many years (Hindery, 2009).

Advanced practice is in various stages in Europe with little activity in Germany aside from nurse anesthetists and, according to a 2010 OECD study, is in its infancy in Belgium, the Czech Republic, France, and Poland (Delamaire & Lafortune, 2010), although France has more than 8500 nurse anesthetists (Frangou, 2007). NPs are well established in The Netherlands and Finland, as well as Sweden and the United Kingdom (Delamaire & Lafortune, 2010).

In Africa, Botswana has had a family nurse practitioner program since 1986 through both diploma and degree routes (Schober, 2013). The University of Addis Ababa is developing a pediatric NP program for Ethiopia (SickKids, 2012), and in 2012 the South African Nursing Council approved a position paper on advanced practice nursing that recognizes two levels of advanced practice: the nurse specialist, which requires a post-basic diploma, and the advanced nurse specialist, which requires master's preparation (South African Nursing Council, 2012).

Globally, advanced practice continues to face a number of hurdles. A 2012 survey by the ICN's INP/APN found wide variation in regulation, competencies, and autonomy (Heale & Rieck-Buckley, 2012). In addition, Schober (2012) identified variations in title, lack of recognition by others, varying scopes of practice and standards, and quality of programs as key global concerns. Despite these challenges, advanced nursing practice continues to move forward.

THE WORLD HEALTH ORGANIZATION AND NURSING

Nursing was once a visible, valued part of WHO. It had a senior nurse scientist, many country-based nursing staff, and a Global Advisory Group on Nursing and Midwifery (GAGNM) that provided policy advice to the Director General. The GAGNM has not met since 2010 and is not likely to meet again. In addition, the nurse scientist post has been vacant since 2010 and there are no plans to fill it as a result of reform and budget restrictions. Only three of the six WHO regions have a nurse who oversees nursing issues and most of them also carry other duties, such as human resources, women's issues, and so on.

An informal review of four WHO regions in 2012 by the author found that of the 120 countries comprising the four regions, only 11 (9%) had an official WHO nurse working in WHO offices. Fortunately, a few dedicated nursing staff within headquarters support and are supported by regional staff to keep nursing visible.

The one remaining potential voice having direct WHO and government involvement is the Triad meetings. Begun in 2006, by the ICN, WHO, and the International Confederation of Midwives (ICM), these strategic biennial meetings are held

BOX 91-5 World Health Organization

The World Health Organization (WHO), established in 1948, is governed by 194 member countries through the World Health Assembly. It has been in reform mode since 2010 and has downsized by approximately 1000 long-term and temporary staff. Latest available figures show total staff to be 7336 from more than 150 countries who work in WHO's 150 country offices, 6 regional offices, and its Geneva-based headquarters. The Director General heads the staff and is appointed by the Assembly (WHO, 2013c, 2013d).

WHO's objective is the attainment by all peoples of the highest possible level of health. It fulfills its mandate through its core functions as follows:

- Providing leadership on matters critical to health and engaging in partnerships where joint action is needed
- Shaping the research agenda and stimulating the generation, translation, and dissemination of valuable knowledge
- Setting norms and standards, and promoting and monitoring their implementation
- Articulating ethical and evidence-based policy options
- Providing technical support, catalyzing change, and building sustainable institutional capacity
- Monitoring the health situation and assessing health trends (WHO, 2013e)

WHO defines health as "a state of complete physical, mental, and social well-being and not merely the absence of disease or infirmity." The definition, adopted in 1948, has not changed, although attempts have been made to persuade WHO to add the concept of spiritual health to the definition (WHO, 2013f).

For more information, visit: *www.who.int*.

in advance of the WHA and attended by government chief nursing officers, nursing and midwifery regulators, and leaders of national nursing and midwifery organizations. They address key global issues, such as recruitment, retention, leadership, education, regulation, roles, and relationships, and their formal statements are used in policy and advocacy at national and regional levels (Box 91-5).

NURSING'S POLICY VOICE

Achieving nursing's policy potential is perhaps the greatest challenge facing the profession in the 21st century. The lack of a strong, united, nongovernmental nursing voice in many nations means that nursing continues to be disadvantaged in the policy arena.

Nursing's success in shaping policy varies depending on the country, the issue, and the group under consideration. By contrast, the limiting factors are fairly universal and include nursing's image, perceived value, and social status; educational requirements; gender issues; and numbers. The ratio of nurses to other health workers; the scope of practice, legislation, and cultural norms; and the presence of strong national nursing associations affect the influence of nurses. Equally important is the extent to which nurses are perceived to be interested in improving health for all versus being interested in only personal and professional gains.

Nursing's policy influence in the 21st century will require more nurse politicians, more unity of voice, and more strategic alliances, along with leadership development and added political and policy skills for all new graduates. Currently, a real danger in many countries is the potential split in the nursing voice as more specialty organizations develop, particularly outside the umbrella of the national nurses' associations. The United States has felt the impact of divided nursing interests for many years and has developed mechanisms, such as forums and issue-specific lobbies, to bring the nursing voice together on key issues. Such strategic alliances are part of today's socioeconomic and political fabric. Touted first by management gurus and then applied to industry, strategic alliances have come to the fore in global health.

GETTING INVOLVED

Any significant advancement toward realizing nursing's policy potential nationally, regionally, and internationally will require multiple strategies and joint efforts on many fronts. Ultimately, it means the commitment of individual nurses who share a vision and values and believe that nurses can make a difference for themselves and, most of all, for the people they serve. There are many ways to participate, as illustrated in Box 91-6.

If we are to achieve better health for all people, it will be through evidence that we are a strong profession that is committed to sound nursing and health policies and practices and skilled in policy, politics, and care. One of the key tenets of primary health care is that communities should participate in decisions affecting them. It follows, then, that nursing, as a community and as part of the global society, needs to engage in all aspects of health policy.

DISCUSSION QUESTIONS

1. Describe four aspects of globalization that are important for nursing to understand and why.
2. How can nurses help to address issues of MDGs and sustainable development?
3. How might you be more involved in positioning nursing locally? Nationally?

BOX 91-6 How to Get Involved

- Begin at home—think globally and act locally.
- Cultivate a worldview; be sensitive to the cultural aspects of policy and practice.
- Commit to learning more about trade agreements and how they affect your practice and your potential. Health services are now part of the World Trade Organization agenda.
- Through the association or your workplace, help colleagues in other countries as they work to strengthen nursing and health care.
- Undertake research to build evidence of nursing effectiveness.
- Advocate, initiate, and document nursing's role in policy.
- Know where your government stands on key international health and nursing matters, and lobby the government to support the initiative.
- Join others in ensuring that national and local structures are in place so that nursing's voice is heard in policy and practice.
- Ensure that new graduates know about policy and politics, how to analyze the environment, how to develop strategy, and how to work together.
- Get involved in international issues and team up with like-minded groups and individuals at home and internationally.
- Know the stance taken by regional and international organizations, such as the International Council of Nurses, on key nursing and health issues.
- Share your ideas and achievements through publications and the Internet and papers presented at international conferences.

REFERENCES

Adorka, C. (2010). Experts predict severe shortage of health care providers in 2014. Chicago, IL: Medill Reports. Retrieved from *newsarchive .medill.northwestern.edu/chicago/news.aspx?id=162934&terms =Experts%20predict%20severe%20shortage%20of%20health%20 care%20providers%20in%202014.*

American Nurses Association [ANA]. (2008a). The American Nurses Association advances the prevention of the unethical recruitment of foreign-educated nurses. Press release. Retrieved from *www.nursingworld.org/ FunctionalMenuCategories/MediaResources/PressReleases/2008PR/ ANAAdvancesthePreventionofUnethicalRecruitmentofForeigneducated Nurses.pdf.*

American Nurses Association [ANA]. (2008b). Voluntary code of ethical conduct for the recruitment of foreign-educated nurses to the United States. Retrieved from *www.nursingworld.org/MainMenuCategories/ ThePracticeofProfessionalNursing/workforce/ForeignNurses/Codeof ConductforRecruitmentofForeignEducatedNurses.pdf.*

Bill and Melinda Gates Foundation. (2014). Who we are. Foundation fact sheet. Retrieved from *www.gatesfoundation.org/Who-We-Are/General -Information/Foundation-Factsheet.*

Canadian Federation of Nurses Unions. (2012). The nursing workforce: Canadian Federation of Nurses Unions backgrounder. Retrieved from *nursesunions.ca/sites/default/files/2012.backgrounder.nursing_ workforce.e_0.pdf.*

Centers for Disease Control and Prevention [CDC]. (2012). Global health strategy 2012–2015. Retrieved from *www.cdc.gov/globalhealth/ strategy/pdf/cdc-globalhealthstrategy.pdf.*

Centers for Disease Control and Prevention [CDC]. (2013a). Global health, where we work. Retrieved from *www.cdc.gov/globalhealth/countries/ default.htm.*

Centers for Disease Control and Prevention [CDC]. (2013b). Strengthening the African health workforce. Retrieved from *www.cdc.gov/globalaids/ success-stories/arc.html.*

Delamaire, M.-L., & Lafortune, G. (2010). Nurses in advanced roles. A description and evaluation of experiences in 12 developed countries. OECD working paper #54. Directorate for Employment, Labour and Social Affairs Health Committee, OECD. Retrieved from *www.oecd -ilibrary.org/social-issues-migration-health/nurses-in-advanced-roles _5kmbrcfms5g7-en.*

Dwyer, S. (2012). Nurses needed: Partnering to scale up health worker education in Malawi. Voices #10. Retrieved from *www.capacityplus.org/ files/resources/Voices-10.pdf.*

Ford, L. (2013, September 25). New UN development goals must focus on rights and apply to all countries. *The Guardian.* Retrieved from *www*

.theguardian.com/global-development/2013/sep/25/new-development
-goals-un-general-assembly.

Ford, S. (2013, November 12). RCN warns of hidden crisis, as 20,000 nursing posts are unfilled. *Nursing Times.* Retrieved from *www.nursingtimes.net/ nursing-practice/clinical-zones/management/rcn-warns-of-hidden-crisis-as-20000-nursing-posts-are-unfilled/5065205.article.*

Frangou, C. (2007). Tensions rise in debate on role of Europe's CRNAs. *Anesthesiology News, 33,* 9.

Hanucharurnkul, S. (2007). Nurse practitioner practice in Thailand. Retrieved from *international.aanp.org/pdf/Nurse_practitioner_in_Thailand_ICN_ APNNP_rev.pdf.*

Heale, R., & Rieck-Buckley, C. (2012). Regulation of advanced nursing practice roles: A global update. INP/ANP Network Bulletin, Issue 18. Retrieved from *international.aanp.org/pdf/Nov2012.pdf.*

Hindery, R. (2009). UCSF serves as model for Japan's inaugural nurse practitioner program. *UCSF News.* Retrieved from *www.ucsf.edu/news/ 2009/04/8330/ucsf-guides-development-japanese-nursing-program.*

Hodges, J. (2013). Outsourcing health care: The global growth of medical tourism. *Humanosphere,* Retrieved from *www.humanosphere.org/2013/ 04/outsourcing-health-care-the-global-explosion-of-medical-tourism/.*

International Council of Nurses [ICN]. (2007a). Ethical nurse recruitment. ICN position statement. Geneva: International Council of Nurses. Retrieved from *www.icn.ch/images/stories/documents/publications/ position_statements/C03_Ethical_Nurse_Recruitment.pdf.*

International Council of Nurses [ICN]. (2007b). Nurse retention and migration. ICN position statement. Geneva: International Council of Nurses. Retrieved from *www.icn.ch/images/stories/documents/publications/ position_statements/C06_Nurse_Retention_Migration.pdf.*

International Council of Nurses [ICN]. (2013). *International Centre for Human Resources in Nursing.* Geneva: International Council of Nurses. Retrieved from *www.icn.ch/pillarsprograms/international-centre-for-human -resources-in-nursing-ichrn/.*

International Centre on Nurse Migration [ICNM]. (2013). International Centre on Nurse Migration: About us. Retrieved from *www.intlnursemigration .org/sections/about/aboutus.shtml.*

Lafortune, G. (2011, February 7). Development of advanced nursing roles in European and non-European countries. Presentation to the DG Sanco Working Group on Health Workforce, Brussels. Retrieved from *ec.europa.eu/health/workforce/docs/ev_20110207_co03_en.pdf.*

Lenhart, M. (2013). Survey sees robust growth for medical tourism. *Travel Market Report.* Retrieved from *www.travelmarketreport.com/articles/ Survey-Sees-Robust-Growth-for-Medical-Tourism.*

Médicins Sans Frontières [MSF]. (2013). Us. Retrieved from *www.msf.org/ about-msf.*

National Council of State Boards of Nursing. (2013). Nurse licensure compact. Retrieved from *www.ncsbn.org/nlc.htm.*

Ng, N. Y., & Ruger, J. P. (2011). Global health governance at a crossroads. *Global Health Governance, 3*(2), 1–37.

Schober, M. (2012, August 21). Globalisation of advanced practice: Global vision-global reality. Presentation to the 7th International ICN Nurse Practitioner/Advanced Practice Nursing Network Conference. Retrieved from *international.aanp.org/pdf/2012Pres1.pdf.*

Schober, M. (2013). Global perspectives on advanced nursing practice. In L. Joel (Ed.), *Advanced nursing practice: Essentials for role development* (3rd ed.). Philadelphia, PA: F.A. Davis Company.

Schober, M., & Affara, F. (2006). *Advanced nursing practice.* Oxford: Blackwell Publishing.

SickKids. (2012). Ethiopia-SickKids paediatric nurse practitioner training programme. Retrieved from *www.sickkids.ca/globalchildhealth/ Capacity%20Building%20Through%20Education/CIDA-SickKids/*
Ethiopia-SickKids/Ethiopia-SickKids-Paediatric-Nurse-Practitioner -Training-Programme.html.

South African Nursing Council. (2012). Advanced practice nursing. SANC's draft position paper/statement. Retrieved from *www.sanc.co.za/ position_advanced_practice_nursing.htm.*

United Nations [UN]. (2000). UN millennium summit. Retrieved from *www .un.org/en/events/pastevents/millennium_summit.shtml.*

United Nations [UN]. (2013a). 232 million international migrants living abroad worldwide–new UN global migration statistics reveal. Department of Social and Economic Affairs, Population Division. Press release, New York, September 11, 2013. Retrieved from *esa.un.org/unmigration/ wallchart2013.htm.*

United Nations [UN]. (2013b). Declaration of the high-level dialogue on international migration and development (draft). General Assembly, Sixty-eighth session. Agenda item 21(e) A/68/L.5l, October 2013. Retrieved from *www.un.org/ga/search/view_doc.asp?symbol=A/68 /L.5.*

United Nations [UN]. (2013c). The Millennium Develop Goals report 2013. Retrieved from *www.un.org/millenniumgoals/pdf/report-2013/mdg -report-2013-english.pdf.*

United Nations [UN]. (2013d). Official list of MDG indicators. The UN Statistics Division, Department of Economic and Social Affairs. Retrieved from *mdgs.un.org/unsd/mdg/host.aspx?Content=indicators/officiallist. htm.*

Volunteer Kenya. (2014). Microenterprise Development Program. The feminization of poverty in Western Kenya. Retrieved from *volunteerkenya.org/ index.php/programs/microenterprise.*

World Bank. (2013a). Poverty overview. Retrieved from *www.worldbank.org/ en/topic/poverty/overview.*

World Bank. (2013b). Girls education. overview. Retrieved from *web .worldbank.org/WBSITE/EXTERNAL/TOPICS/EXTEDUCATION/0,,content MDK:20298916~menuPK:617572~pagePK:148956~piPK:216618~theSit ePK:282386,00.html.*

World Health Organization [WHO]. (2010a). World health report 2010: Health systems financing the path to universal coverage. Geneva: World Health Organization. Retrieved from *www.who.int/whr/2010/en/.*

World Health Organization [WHO]. (2010b). Wanted: 2.4 million nurses, and that's just in India. *Bulletin of the World Health Organization, 88*(65), 321–400.

World Health Organization [WHO]. (2013a). Managing health workforce migration: The global code of practice. Geneva: World Health Organization. Retrieved from *www.who.int/hrh/migration/code/practice/en/.*

World Health Organization [WHO]. (2013b). Global tuberculosis report 2013. Geneva: World Health Organization. Retrieved from *apps.who.int/iris/ bitstream/10665/91355/1/9789241564656_eng.pdf.*

World Health Organization [WHO]. (2013c). Health financing for universal coverage: What is universal coverage? Geneva: World Health Organization. Retrieved from *www.who.int/health_financing/universal_coverage _definition/en/.*

World Health Organization [WHO]. (2013d). WHO: Its people and offices. Geneva: World Health Organization. Retrieved from *www.who.int/ about/structure/en/index.html.*

World Health Organization [WHO]. (2013e). Human resources: Annual report. Report by the Secretariat. Executive Board, 132nd Session, November 30, 2012. Provisional agenda item 14.3. Geneva: World Health Organization. Retrieved from *apps.who.int/gb/ebwha/pdf_files/EB132/B132 _38-en.pdf.*

World Health Organization [WHO]. (2013f). The role of WHO in public health. Geneva: World Health Organization. Retrieved from *www.who.int/ about/role/en/.*

CHAPTER 92

Infectious Disease: A Global Perspective

Catherine M. Dentinger   James Mark Simmerman

"Everything we do has microbial consequence."
Nicholas Ashbolt, PhD, School of Public Health,
University of Alberta, 2013

Not long ago, infectious diseases were thought to be well controlled by antibiotics, immunization, and hygiene measures. That perspective has changed as newly discovered pathogens and re-emerging diseases have increasingly garnered headlines around the world. Microbial evolution, driven by the interaction of factors, including population growth and urbanization, climate change, industrial food production and distribution, global travel and commerce, and the injudicious use of antimicrobials, have put communicable diseases back near the top of global health priorities (United Nations [UN], 2013). Limiting the impact of infectious diseases demands sustained attention, international cooperation, and considerable resources (Jones et al., 2008). Innovative approaches are needed to enhance detection, monitoring, and control of these diseases in the context of rapidly changing human-pathogen ecology. Nurses, the largest part of the global health care labor force, must participate in the development, implementation, and evaluation of these interventions (Bryar, Kendall, & Mogotlane, 2012).

BACKGROUND

By the 1960s, advances in public sanitation, immunization, and antibiotic therapy led to large declines in morbidity and mortality from infectious diseases and toward what was thought to be their eventual elimination as a human health concern (Burnet, 1962). Just 20 years later, the human immunodeficiency virus (HIV) pandemic and many other emerging pathogens demanded the attention of the medical and public health community. In 1992, Lederberg et al. coined the term emerging infectious disease (EID) to describe the introduction, transmission, and adaptation of pathogens in human populations, including those characterized by a resurgence or an extension of geographic range after a period of relative control (re-emergence). EID also referred to infections caused by newly discovered organisms, drug-resistant microbes, and intentionally released pathogens (Centers for Disease Control and Prevention [CDC], 1994; Lederberg, 1992).

It has been more than 30 years since the first acquired immunodeficiency syndrome (AIDS) cases were described, and HIV infection is now endemic in most countries. An estimated 32.2 to 38.8 million people are infected worldwide, and 1.9 to 2.7 million new infections occur each year (UNAIDS, 2013). More recently, coronaviruses causing severe acute respiratory syndrome (SARS) and Middle East respiratory syndrome (MERS) have emerged, while West Nile, monkeypox, and dengue viruses have become endemic or caused local transmission in areas where they had not previously circulated (CDC, 1999b, 2000, 2003, 2010b; Reed et al., 2004). Resurgences of disease caused by measles virus, poliovirus, and *Vibrio cholera* have occurred since 2010 following natural disasters, migration, political conflict, and declines in vaccination rates (CDC, 2013e; Cerda & Lee, 2013; MacDonald & Hebert, 2010). Drug-resistant pathogens have become increasingly common as antimicrobial use has increased both for human therapeutic interventions and as growth promoters in animal feed (Alexander et al., 2009; CDC, 2013a; van Panhuis et al., 2013). Influenza A viruses, which frequently mutate during replication and occasionally exchange entire genes, continue to cause substantial annual global mortality and intermittent pandemics (Dawood et al., 2009; Subbarao et al., 1998). Finally, the potential for intentional release of pathogens continues to require vigilance and resources (Kemp et al., 2012).

The introduction and transmission of pathogens in human populations originates from a complex interaction of host, agent, and environment and the adaption of microorganisms to pressures that are incompletely understood (Enright et al., 2002; Wolfe, Dunavan, & Diamond, 2007). Intervening in these complex relationships may inadvertently facilitate the emergence of new or more virulent infections or predispose the host to additional infections (CDC, 2012c; Specter, 2012). Multidrug resistant organisms, for example, are often identified in individuals requiring frequent antimicrobial treatment (CDC, 2013d). Factors often operate in concert to trigger emergence or re-emergence of infectious diseases (Plowright et al., 2008) (Figure 92-1). A traveler incubating *V. cholera* would not necessarily cause an outbreak in an area with adequate surveillance systems and public health infrastructure. When infected travelers from the Dominican Republic arrived in New York City (NYC) in 2011, no local transmission was detected (Baker, 2011). In contrast, large outbreaks of *V. cholera* occurred following the 2010 earthquake in Haiti (Patrick, 2013). Environmental changes alter ecosystems, which affect microorganisms and their vectors. The increasingly rapid movement of large numbers of people and goods via airplanes accelerates the rate of pathogen introduction and places all countries at risk (Arguin, Marano, & Freedman, 2009).

DETERMINANTS OF INFECTIOUS DISEASE INTRODUCTION AND TRANSMISSION

Complex multifactorial interactions promote pathogen emergence or re-emergence. In this chapter, we highlight four important drivers of this:

- Demographic and socioeconomic changes
- Industrialized food production and global commerce
- Climate change
- Antibiotic use and resistance

DEMOGRAPHICS AND SOCIOECONOMICS

Annawadi itself was nothing special in the context of the slums of Mumbai. Every house was off-kilter, so less off-kilter looked like straight. Sewage and sickness looked like life. (Katherine Boo, *Behind the Beautiful Forevers: Life, Death, and Hope in a Mumbai Undercity*)

The global population is more than 7.2 billion with a net average annual increase of about 80 million people (UN, 2012a). Since 1980, the world's population has increased by nearly 60%, although arable land, fresh water, and other natural resources have not (Tana, Lal, & Wiebe, 2005; Wyman, 2013). Although this rapid growth rate is thought to be slowing, the population will continue to increase and is projected to reach 9.3 billion by 2050 and 10.1 billion by 2100 (UN, 2012a). Most of the population growth through 2050 is predicted to occur in urban areas, and the number of megacities (cities with more than 10 million inhabitants) will increase (UN, 2012b). Urbanization and the expansion of human populations into new habitats following deforestation alter human-pathogen ecology (Wilcox, 2006).

The effect of urbanization on disease emergence and transmission may vary. In well-managed cities with planned growth, sufficient resources, and robust health systems, urbanization could lead to improved infection control. However, when urban areas expand rapidly and unplanned communities form haphazardly, with inadequate housing, sanitation, clean water, and health care, disease detection and control is difficult. As densely populated cities rapidly expand, animal husbandry and live animal markets often exist in close proximity to human populations, increasing the potential for zoonotic disease transmission (Finucane & Spencer, 2013; Yang, Utzinger, & Zhou, 2013). The movement of humans into new habitats is thought to have played a role in the introduction of pathogens including

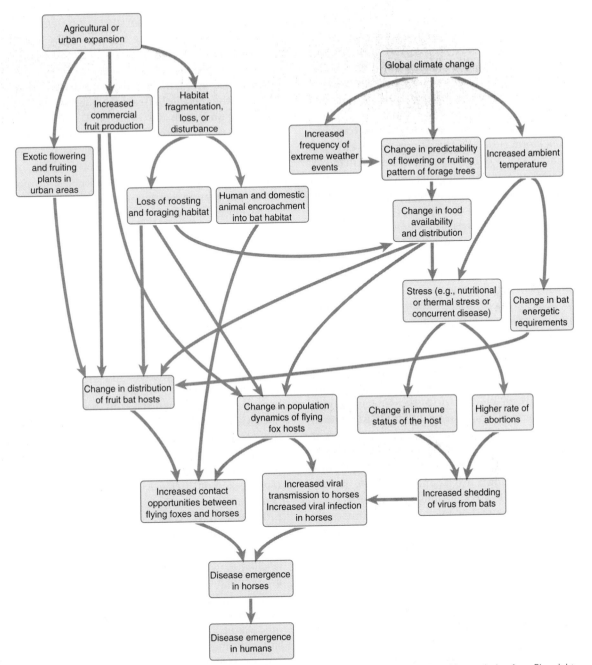

FIGURE 92-1 Causal diagram approach to examining Hendra virus emergence in Australia. (Used with permission from Plowright, R., Sokolow, S., Gorman, M., Daszak, P., & Foley, J. [2008]. Causal inference in disease ecology: Investigating ecological drivers of disease emergence. *Frontiers in Ecology and the Environment*, 6[8], 420–429.)

UNIT 6

HIV, Ebola virus, hantavirus, and tick-borne diseases such as ehrlichiosis and Lyme disease (Muehlenbein, 2012). Increases in arthropod-borne diseases including dengue and chikungunya are associated with increased population density in urban areas (Rogers, Suk, & Semenza, 2014; Weaver, 2013).

Poverty can also be a risk for disease transmission. World Health Organization (WHO) estimates indicate that 3 billion people live on less than U.S. $2 per day, an income that makes obtaining proper nutrition, hygienic living conditions, and preventive health care unlikely (WHO, 2012a). In megacities such as Dhaka, Lagos, or Mumbai, migration of rural populations in search of economic opportunity has resulted in the rapid growth of communities with minimal social or health services and inadequate housing and sanitation. These densely populated, impoverished urban areas pose enormous challenges for identifying and controlling infectious diseases (Afsana & Wahid, 2013).

Unanticipated displacement of large populations caused by natural disaster or conflict also results in the rapid growth of inadequately serviced communities. In June 2013, the United Nations High Commission on Refugees (UNHCR) reported that the number of global refugees under their mandate was 11.1 million, an increase of 600,000 persons in 6 months, representing one of the worst periods of human displacement in recent history (UNHCR, 2013). Populations fleeing conflict and disaster, either within their countries (internally displaced) or to bordering countries and beyond, often have poor baseline health and nutritional status and few resources. In settlements of displaced persons, communicable disease can spread rapidly (Gayer et al., 2007). For example, millions of Afghans displaced during years of war live in camps in Pakistan and experience a high burden of infectious disease (Rajabali et al., 2009). Natural disasters and conflict also disrupt public health programs for those who remain, and outbreaks of disease that were once eliminated or controlled can quickly resurface. The Syrian Arab Republic, which had been poliomyelitis-free since 1999, experienced outbreaks following the interruption of vaccination programs because of civil war (WHO, 2013).

Human population movement has increased with the expansion of air travel. In 2012 alone, nearly 3 billion people traveled by air for work, family obligation, to obtain health care services, or for leisure. These travelers may contribute importantly to the spread of disease (Hollingsworth, Ferguson, & Anderson, 2007) (Figure 92-2). The role of air travel in the spread of respiratory disease was well documented during the SARS outbreak in the spring of 2003 (Ruan, Wang, & Levin, 2006). In April 2009, NYC high school students returning from spring-break vacation in Mexico are thought to have been the source of the largest outbreak of influenza A (H1N1) in the United States at the time (France et al., 2010; Lessler et al., 2009).

INDUSTRIALIZED FOOD PRODUCTION AND GLOBAL COMMERCE

As the human population has grown exponentially, so too has the demand for food. Much of the global food supply is grown, processed, and distributed via a complex web of diverse businesses. Dominating this web are multinational companies seeking to maximize efficiency, increase profitability, and expand into new markets. This has resulted in cheaper food, especially animal protein, but the mass production of the food supply from livestock and farming to processing, packaging, and distribution creates opportunities for the introduction and rapid spread of diseases (Leibler et al., 2009). The complexity and massive volume of industrial food production, processing, and distribution makes detecting and containing pathogens in the global food supply exceptionally challenging. Food origin labeling is not mandated evenly across the globe, even though our food supply is global.

The transition to industrialized food production has occurred in parallel with urbanization. As food production became mechanized, populations shifted from rural to urban areas. In the early 20th century, farming was the livelihood for more than 50% of the U.S. population. Currently, approximately 1% to 2% of the U.S. population works on farms and about 85% live in cities. Rather than human labor, the modern food industry relies on machines, engineers, and technicians to rapidly grow and process huge volumes of food. A similar

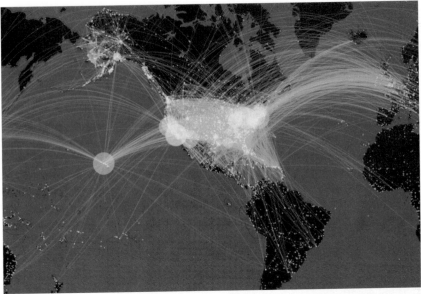

FIGURE 92-2 World map shows flight routes from the 40 largest U.S. airports. (Image from Christos Nicolaides, MIT. *cnicolaides.mit.edu.*)

technological and demographic shift is under way in many developing countries (Thornton, 2010; UN, 2012b).

LIVESTOCK PRODUCTION

Many zoonotic pathogens originate from domesticated animals raised for human consumption (Wolfe, Dunavan, & Diamond, 2007). Understanding the environment where food animals are raised is therefore critical for preventing disease introduction and interrupting transmission. Industrial food animal production is characterized by large numbers of animals raised in confinement with rapid turnover, forming ecosystems that can facilitate the evolution of pathogens (Leibler et al., 2009). Salmonella, often antibiotic-resistant strains, is commonly isolated from chicken, beef, turkey, and pork worldwide (Chaisatit et al., 2012; White et al., 2001). In industrial settings, food animals are bred and managed for rapid development and weight gain. To accomplish this, animals are housed in crowded pens to restrict movement, conditions that stress the animal and may adversely impact immune function, rendering them more susceptible to diseases (von Borell, 1995; Wells, 2013). The

concentration of large numbers of animals also complicates safe waste management and biocontainment (Figure 92-3).

Pathogens originating from food animal production facilities that spill into the surrounding environment pose health risks to communities downstream (Graham et al., 2008). For example, there is considerable evidence that the highly pathogenic avian influenza A (H5N1) virus originated in large-scale commercial poultry production systems and was transferred to wild birds and farmyard domesticated chickens, and from birds to humans, through occupational and environmental pathways across East and Southeast Asia (Graham et al., 2008).

Food processing plants are typically geographically concentrated to benefit from logistic and scale efficiencies. Products from diverse origins are shipped great distances to processing plants and then reshipped to distribution centers and retail outlets around the world. When meat and agriculture products are contaminated with microbial pathogens, they are often consumed far from their origin, resulting in widespread and difficult-to-trace outbreaks. In 1996, hepatitis A–contaminated

UNIT 6

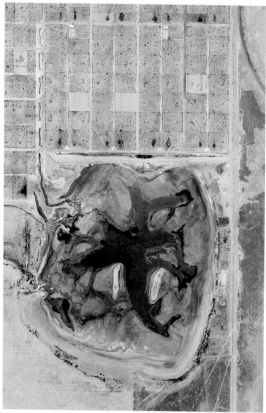

FIGURE 92-3 Satellite view of commercial cattle feedlot and waste pond. (Conorado Feeders, Dalhart, Texas. Mishka Henner, 2013. Courtesy of the artist. From *www.mishkahenner .com/Feedlots.*)

frozen strawberries were shipped from one California processing plant to school lunch programs across the United States, causing outbreaks among children in multiple states (Hutin et al., 1999). Furthermore, a single factory may process the same food item under different brand names, complicating investigations and recalls. In 2011, salmonella-contaminated peanut butter from a single processing plant sickened people in 20 U.S. states. Although only one brand of peanut butter was associated with illness, the plant produced peanut butter under different brand names (CDC, 2013g).

Advances in molecular techniques have improved our understanding of foodborne pathogens, our ability to link outbreaks, and our understanding of new vehicle-pathogen combinations. For example,

24 confirmed outbreaks of *Listeria monocytogenes* occurred in the United States from 1998 to 2004, many of them associated with ready-to-eat meats. However, foods, including sprouts, that had not previously been associated with this pathogen were also identified. In 2011, an outbreak of *L. monocytogenes* associated with cantaloupe from one U.S. farm sickened at least 147 individuals in 28 states, 33 of whom died (Cartwright et al., 2013; McCollum et al., 2013). In Europe, the same year, a novel strain of *Escherichia coli* that sickened nearly 4000 people and caused 53 deaths was eventually linked to seeds imported from Egypt, sprouted on a farm in Germany, and consumed throughout Europe (Buchholz et al., 2011; Griffin, 2010).

ANTIMICROBIAL USE IN AGRICULTURE

Enormous quantities of antibiotics and antivirals are fed to livestock and poultry every year, a practice that fuels the evolution of resistant organisms (Cyranoski, 2005; Mellon, Benbrook, & Benbrook, 2001). Subtherapeutic doses of antibiotics are used to prevent outbreaks in crowded cages and also for growth promotion in cattle, swine, and poultry (Hughes, 2011; Smith, Harris, Johnson, Silbergeld, & Morris, 2002). Low doses of certain antibiotics cause food animals to gain weight while consuming less feed, probably caused by disturbances of the intestinal microbiome in a direction that favors increased caloric absorption (Angelakis, Merhej, & Raoult, 2013; U.S. Food and Drug Administration [FDA], 2012). Use of antibiotics in food animals also destroys commensal (symbiotic) bacteria that are important for animal health and may accelerate the development of multidrug resistance (Hoogendoorn et al., 2013). Commensal bacteria, such as *Escherichia coli* and *Enterococcus* sp., may carry resistance genes that can be transmitted to people via the food supply or by direct exposure to infected animals (Aarestrup, Wegener, & Collignon, 2008; Heuer, Hammerum, Collignon, & Wegener, 2006). High rates of resistance to antibiotics have been documented among *E. coli*, *Campylobacter* and *Salmonella* isolated in food animals (Collignon, 2009; Johnson et al., 2009; Wang, Chen, & China Nosocomial Pathogens Resistance Surveillance Study Group, 2005).

The unregulated sale and indiscriminate use of antibiotics, limited quality controls on veterinary antibiotic production, and inadequate waste treatment systems facilitate the emergence and spread of resistant organisms. The contribution of foodborne transmission to antimicrobial resistant organisms in humans is not known, but is likely to be substantial. Studies suggest that most antibiotic-resistant *E. coli* in humans originates in livestock, especially chickens (Johnson et al., 2007). Mitigating the risks of antibiotic resistance to human health urgently requires development and enforcement of policies to reduce the use of antibiotics in food animals. After many years of consideration, in 2012 the U.S. Food and Drug Administration (FDA) issued voluntary guidelines to the food and pharmaceutical industries aimed at reducing the non-medical use of antibiotics in animal feeds (FDA, 2012; Kuehn, 2012). In sharp contrast to U.S. policy, the European Union finalized an involuntary ban on the use of antibiotics as growth promoters in animal feed beginning January 1, 2006 (European Commission, 2005).

CLIMATE CHANGE

Climate change refers to a significant and lasting difference in the statistical distribution of weather patterns. These include changes in average weather conditions, variability in patterns, and alterations in the frequency of extreme weather events (Intergovernmental Panel on Climate Change, 2007). Scientific consensus attributes these changes largely to human activity, primarily the release of greenhouse gases, carbon dioxide, and methane, and the changes are largely irreversible (Solomon et al., 2009; UN, 2012a). The effects of climate change have been observed over recent years and include increasing ocean and air temperatures, melting glaciers, rising sea levels, increased precipitation, decreased frequency of cold days, and extended droughts (National Research Council, 2012). Climate also influences the interaction of microbial pathogens, their hosts, and the environment. As environmental conditions change, the distribution of microorganisms and their vectors will change. Increased water temperatures in Katchemak Bay, Alaska in 2004 are thought to have contributed to the first outbreak of

Vibrio parahaemolyticus among individuals who ate oysters harvested from the bay (McLaughlin et al., 2005; Morin, Comrie, & Ernst, 2013). By 2004, WHO estimated that climate change was causing more than 140,000 excess all-cause deaths annually (McKinnon, 2012; WHO, 2009).

The poorest and most vulnerable populations are likely to suffer the greatest health consequences from climate change. In these communities, food insecurity will compromise overall health and host susceptibility; insufficient clean water will contribute to diarrheal diseases; and communicable disease incidence will likely increase (Haines et al., 2006; McMichael, Woodruff, & Hales, 2006). Governments and their partners made initial commitments to respond to climate change in the 2008 World Health Assembly resolution, Climate Change and Health (WHA61.19), urging member states to develop and integrate health adaptation measures (WHO, 2008). The resolution specifies that developing solutions to mitigate the impacts of climate change on health is a joint responsibility in which wealthy countries assist developing countries. Strengthening health systems to enable member countries to respond to anticipated changes in public health needs is a priority.

INCREASED INCIDENCE OF VECTOR-BORNE DISEASE

An increase in vector-borne infection is expected as climate patterns change. The observed increase in dengue virus infections is likely caused by climatic changes favoring wider distribution of the vector, *Aedes aegypti* and *Aedes albopictus* mosquitoes, combined with rapid urbanization (Morin et al., 2013). As the distribution of these mosquitoes has expanded, viral transmission is no longer limited to tropical and subtropical areas (WHO, 2012b). Vector expansion could expose populations with no underlying immunity to the virus, potentially resulting in high rates of disease. The magnitude of dengue virus outbreaks varies annually according to a number of determinants, but cases are seasonal and incidence is highly associated with rainfall and temperature (Viana & Ignotti, 2013). In Vietnam, a time-series study concluded that higher dengue incidence was associated with higher rainfall, humidity, and temperatures, and predicted that disease burden will increase following the impacts of climate change (Pham et al., 2011).

While the biologic rationale for climate change accelerating infectious disease incidence is strong, definitive evidence is currently lacking. A review of climate change impacts on mosquito-borne diseases in China (e.g., dengue, Japanese encephalitis and malaria) found that evidence was inconclusive and geographically inconsistent (Bai, Morton, & Liu, 2013). A review of studies in Asia indicates that although climatic changes are likely to impact the seasonal and geographic distribution of dengue, no clear evidence exists that such a change has occurred. Ultimately, the combination of pathogen, climatic, and socioeconomic determinants generates great complexity and uncertainty when estimating the health impact of climate change (Colon-Gonzalez et al., 2013).

ANTIBIOTIC USE AND RESISTANCE

The discovery and development of antibiotics has saved millions of lives and allowed for medical advancements including cancer treatments, joint replacement, and organ transplantation (McDermott & Rogers, 1982). The widespread use of antimicrobials has also accelerated the rate of microbial evolution and the development of resistance (Davies & Davies, 2010; Malhotra-Kumar et al., 2007). Infections with resistant organisms result in prolonged illness, poor patient outcomes, increased cost, and the need for more expensive and toxic medications (Roberts et al., 2009). New generations of antimicrobials to treat drug-resistant pathogens are difficult and costly to develop and often financially unattractive for industry to pursue (Infectious Diseases Society of America, 2010). Antibiotics are an essential and finite resource and must be used in a manner that preserves their effectiveness.

Like all living organisms, viruses, bacteria, parasites, and fungi must adapt to environmental pressures or succumb to them. Even as Alexander Fleming discovered that penicillin could kill bacteria, he expressed concerns that resistance could develop (Fleming, 1945). Pneumococci isolates that

were resistant to penicillin were described shortly after penicillin began to be used to treat pneumococcal infection; however, widespread resistance did not develop until the late 1970s (Campbell & Silberman, 1998). Antibiotic use can contribute to the development of resistance in part by reducing the population of susceptible pathogens and commensal species, leaving resistant variants to expand (Bronzwaer et al., 2002). Resistance genes can be transferred among organisms by a variety of mechanisms, both in the health care setting and in the community (Davies & Davies, 2010). Acquisition of antibiotic-resistant organisms has been described among hospitalized patients via contaminated surfaces, including hands of health care workers, and via person-to-person spread (Landelle et al., 2014).

Drug-resistant organisms are often initially detected in hospitals where compromised patients are treated for severe infections with multiple antibiotics. In the late 1980s, methicillin-resistant *Staphylococcus aureus* (MRSA) was primarily a hospital-acquired pathogen. However, in 1997, four previously healthy children with no medical facility exposures died from MRSA infection, an event that marked a transition to the era of community-acquired MRSA (CDC, 1999a). Initially, hospital-acquired and community-acquired MRSA infections were caused by different bacterial strains but, increasingly, that line is blurring (Stryjewski & Corey, 2014). Strains of several organisms, including *S. aureus*, *Mycobacterium tuberculosis*, and *Neisseria gonorrhea*, have developed resistance to multiple antibiotics (CDC, 2013a, 2013c, 2013f).

Antimicrobial use also affects the hosts' microbial balance, allowing organisms that might not normally cause illness to amplify. For example, diarrhea and yeast infections are well-described side effects of antimicrobial use (Tosh & McDonald, 2012). Antibiotics also reduce colonization resistance against *Clostridium difficile* bacteria (Theriot & Young, 2014). Colonized individuals are a source of outbreaks in health care and community settings (Jump et al., 2010; Khanna et al., 2012). In older adults and those with compromised immune systems, *C. difficile* infections can be fatal (Kenneley, 2014; Zilberberg, Shorr, & Kollef,

2008). Antibiotic-resistant pathogens, such as *Enterobacteriaceae* sp. resistant to the β-lactam class of antibiotics including carbapenems, can quickly spread around the world. This resistant strain was first identified in 2008 in a Swedish individual who had traveled to India, then in the United States in a patient who had been hospitalized in Greece (CDC, 2010a; Green et al., 2013; Henning, 2004), and has since spread worldwide (Hammerum et al., 2010).

Antibiotics are often prescribed empirically to treat illness in the absence of laboratory-confirmed infections or susceptibility testing, a practice that promotes the development and spread of resistance organisms (Barnett & Linder, 2014). In many countries, antibiotics can be purchased over-the-counter, which contributes to indiscriminate use and resistance (WHO, 2012c). A variety of strategies are being explored to slow the emergence of antibiotic-resistant organisms, including antimicrobial stewardship programs, information technology applications, educating clinicians and patients, development of rapid diagnostics to differentiate viral from bacterial infections, and effective incentives to develop new antimicrobials (Drew et al., 2009; Laxminarayan et al., 2013).

EBOLA VIRUS DISEASE OUTBREAK: WEST AFRICA, 2014

In early 2014, an outbreak of Ebola virus disease (EVD) occurred in a village of Guinea, West Africa, that bordered Sierra Leone and Liberia (Pannetier et al., 2014). EVD, one of several viral hemorrhagic diseases, has a high fatality rate and no known treatment or vaccine (CDC, 2014). Although this was the first identified EVD outbreak in West Africa (previous outbreaks had occurred in Central and Eastern African countries including the Democratic Republic of the Congo, Gabon, Uganda, and Sudan), it was thought that this cluster would be contained in the remote region where it began, as had occurred in previous outbreaks. Instead, for reasons that are not entirely understood but are thought to be partially related to human movement between the rural areas of Guinea, Sierra Leone, and Liberia and into the

urban areas of these countries, cases of EVD began to increase (Gatherer, 2014). The increase in cases quickly overwhelmed the fragile health infrastructure and limited public resources of these countries, some of the poorest on the globe. Resources to implement control measures that had been successful in previous outbreaks were inadequate. In July 2014, when EVD was diagnosed in a traveler from Liberia in Lagos, Nigeria (the most densely populated city in Africa) and subsequently in several of his contacts and care providers, the severity of the outbreak was understood by even those beyond the public health community (Shuaib et al., 2014). This was reinforced when an American physician and an aid worker became infected after caring for patients in Liberia and were transported to the United States for care (Binder & Grady, 2014). By the fall of 2014, disease modelers were estimating that many more individuals would become infected over the next few months while additional resources to control the epidemic were being put into place (Meltzer et al., 2014). In a world linked closely by air travel, diseases such as Ebola can move quickly to new populations and, in the absence of robust public health systems, can escalate rapidly.

Nurses have been, and will continue to be, critical to controlling EVD outbreaks globally. In 1976 in Zaire (now the Democratic Republic of the Congo), nurses cared for the first identified Ebola patients and became the first cases of health care–acquired EVD; nurses have been instrumental in caring for patients in all subsequent outbreaks (WHO, 1978) In September 2014, nurses at Emory University Hospital provided extraordinary care to the first cases of EVD treated in the United States (Ribner, 2014). Later in the fall, two of the nurses in Dallas, Texas, providing care to the first EVD case diagnosed inside the United States, became the first cases of health care–associated EVD in the United States, highlighting the risks of providing EVD care even in well-resourced settings (Chevalier et al., 2014). The collective experience of nurses providing care, preventing health care–associated infections, and designing public health measures to limit transmission must be captured and incorporated into plans to improve our ability to respond more effectively to future outbreaks.

UNIT 6

SURVEILLANCE AND REPORTING

Ongoing surveillance is essential for disease control. The goal of infectious disease surveillance is to monitor trends, respond to emergencies, identify risks, detect new pathogens, and target and evaluate interventions. Infectious disease surveillance relies on both formal and informal systems, may be syndrome-based or pathogen-specific, and is conducted on global and domestic platforms. Nurse epidemiologists and nurse clinicians are vital to these systems. It was a nurse in NYC who identified a large cluster of students presenting with influenza-like illness to her clinic and alerted public health authorities in the early stages of the 2009 influenza A (H1N1) pandemic (Balter et al., 2010; CDC, 2012b; Hartocollis, 2009).

GLOBAL DISEASE SURVEILLANCE

To monitor diseases across national borders, the World Health Assembly developed and periodically updates the International Health Regulations (IHR) and the 2005 revision is legally binding on WHO member states (WHO, 2007). The IHR include global surveillance for specific diseases as well as public health events of international concern. All members are required to develop, strengthen, and maintain core surveillance and response capacities, facilitate cross-border cooperation, and provide logistic and financial support to improve capacity for these activities (WHO, 2007). The IHR promote improved coordination with agricultural authorities such as the Food and Agriculture Organization (FAO) and the World Organization for Animal Health (OIE) to reduce the potential for outbreaks from food, livestock, and wild animal sources (Newell et al., 2010; Pavlin, Schloegel, & Daszak, 2009). WHO also conducts global and regional surveillance activities under the umbrella of Communicable Disease Surveillance and Response (CSR), including the Global Outbreak Alert and Response Network (GOARN), which monitors communicable diseases and food and water safety.

The U.S. CDC's Global Disease Detection (GDD) network is designed to detect and contain emerging global health threats (CDC, 2013b). The GDD operates regional centers in Thailand, Kenya, Guatemala, China, Egypt, India, South Africa, Bangladesh, Kazakhstan, and Georgia. In collaboration with the International Society of Travel Medicine, the CDC operates the Global Emerging Infections Sentinel (GeoSentinel) network. GeoSentinel consists of travel and tropical medicine clinics around the world that monitor trends in morbidity for 530 diagnoses among travelers according to region, date, and risk group (International Society of Travel Medicine and Centers for Disease Control and Prevention, 2013). The Global Public Health Intelligence Network (GHPIN) is managed by Canada's Public Health Agency and contributes to the WHO GOARN. GHPIN monitors Internet media, such as news wires and websites, in nine languages to help detect and report potential disease outbreaks or other health threats around the world (WHO, 2014).

DOMESTIC DISEASE SURVEILLANCE

In the United States, state and local health departments are responsible for disease surveillance. To monitor diseases of national concern, state organizations such as the Council for State and Territorial Epidemiologists (CSTE) work with the CDC to design national systems. The CDC's National Notifiable Disease Surveillance System (NNDSS) receives regular reports from state health departments to monitor diseases. The CDC also supports population-based sentinel surveillance systems that allow for more detailed information to be collected for specific diseases. For example, the Active Bacterial Core Surveillance (ABCs) system tracks bacterial diseases, such as invasive *Streptococcus pneumoniae* infections, in 10 sites representing approximately 42 million people across the United States (CDC, 2012a). Detailed clinical information is collected for each case of disease and bacterial isolates are submitted to the CDC for molecular characterization. To monitor antimicrobial resistance, the CDC works with the FDA and the U.S. Department of Agriculture to operate the National Antimicrobial Resistance Monitoring System (NARMS). Surveillance is also conducted for disease syndromes, such as influenza-like illness or diarrheal disease, rather than specific pathogens.

Disease surveillance systems designed to detect illness clusters earlier than traditional systems have been developed over the past several years. These systems take advantage of information such as pharmacy sales data or electronically transferred emergency department chief complaint data to identify early indicators of disease clusters. Data from such systems provide timely information and can be relatively inexpensive to operate because laboratory and case investigation data are not collected (Henning, 2004). Internet search–based systems developed by Yahoo and Google are being evaluated as tools for early indicators of influenza activity in communities. However, these systems can be less sensitive and specific than traditional public health surveillance systems (Ginsberg et al., 2009; Lazer et al., 2014). Data about diseases and outbreaks are disseminated online by government agencies and through informal channels, such as press reports, blogs, and chat rooms (Brownstein, Freifeld, & Madoff, 2009).

CONCLUSION

As the human population grows, as the climate changes, and as global commerce and travel increase, we can expect to encounter increasingly large and complex infectious disease outbreaks preventing and responding to these events will demand innovative approaches and global collaboration. Global health security will become a top policy priority in the United States and abroad to ensure the health of citizens in every country. Governments, nongovernmental organizations, academic institutions, health care professionals, private industry, and community representatives must leverage resources to develop effective policies and practices to improve public health infrastructure, mitigate the effects of climate change, and reduce the impact of infectious diseases. Research, education, and sustainable funding must be directed toward implementing and evaluating these policies and practices. Surveillance systems must be strengthened globally to detect outbreaks, identify risk factors for illness and death, and calibrate appropriate responses. For UN agencies and global donors, priority should be given to the lowest-income countries, displaced populations, and societies threatened by conflict and natural disasters. Ultimately, engagement in global health is not only a humanitarian concern but also a priority for our collective well-being, efficient use of limited resources, and protecting our future. Irrespective of national borders, nursing leadership at every level is needed to address these extraordinary challenges.

DISCUSSION QUESTIONS

1. How might nurses and nursing organizations improve policies to encourage the judicious use of antibiotics in humans?
2. How can nurses contribute to the policy discussions concerning human population growth and its impact on health?
3. How could nurses and nursing organizations respond to the health impacts of climate change?

REFERENCES

Aarestrup, F. M., Wegener, H. C., & Collignon, P. (2008). Resistance in bacteria of the food chain: Epidemiology and control strategies. *Expert Review of Anti-infective Therapy*, *6*(5), 733–750. doi:10.1586/14787210.6.5.733.

Afsana, K., & Wahid, S. S. (2013). Health care for poor people in the urban slums of Bangladesh. *Lancet*, *382*(9910), 2049–2051. doi:10.1016/S0140-6736(13)62295-3.

Alexander, T. W., Reuter, T., Sharma, R., Yanke, L. J., Topp, E., & McAllister, T. A. (2009). Longitudinal characterization of resistant *Escherichia coli* in fecal deposits from cattle fed subtherapeutic levels of antimicrobials. *Applied and Environmental Microbiology*, *75*(22), 7125–7134. doi:10.1128/AEM.00944-09.

Angelakis, E., Merhej, V., & Raoult, D. (2013). Related actions of probiotics and antibiotics on gut microbiota and weight modification. *The Lancet Infectious Diseases*, *13*(10), 889–899. doi:10.1016/S1473-3099(13)70179-8.

Arguin, P. M., Marano, N., & Freedman, D. O. (2009). Globally mobile populations and the spread of emerging pathogens. *Emerging Infectious Diseases*, *15*(11), 1713–1714. doi:10.3201/eid1511.091426.

Bai, L., Morton, L. C., & Liu, Q. (2013). Climate change and mosquito-borne diseases in China: A review. *Globalization and Health*, *9*, 10. doi:10.1186/1744-8603-9-10.

Baker, A. (2011). Three cases of cholera are confirmed by city officials. *New York Times*. Retrieved from *cityroom.blogs.nytimes.com/2011/02/05/city-confirms-three-cases-of-cholera/?_r=0*.

Balter, S., Gupta, L. S., Lim, S., Fu, J., & Perlman, S. E. (2010). Pandemic (H1N1) 2009 surveillance for severe illness and response, New York, NY, USA, April-July 2009. *Emerging Infectious Diseases*, *16*(8), 1259–1264. doi:10.3201/eid1608.091847.

Barnett, M. L., & Linder, J. A. (2014). Antibiotic prescribing to adults with sore throat in the United States, 1997–2010. *JAMA Internal Medicine*, *174*, 138–140.

Binder, A., & Grady, D. (2014). American doctor with ebola arrives in U.S. for Treatment. *New York Times*. Retrieved from *www.nytimes.com/2014/08/03/us/kent-brantley-nancy-writebol-ebola-treatment-atlanta.html?_r=0*.

Bronzwaer, S. L., Cars, O., Buchholz, U., Molstad, S., Goettsch, W., Veldhuijzen, I. K., et al. (2002). A European study on the relationship between antimicrobial use and antimicrobial resistance. *Emerging Infectious Diseases*, *8*(3), 278–282.

Brownstein, J. S., Freifeld, C. C., & Madoff, L. C. (2009). Digital disease detection–harnessing the Web for public health surveillance. *New England Journal of Medicine*, *360*(21), 2153–2155, 2157. doi:10.1056/NEJMp0900702.

Bryar, R., Kendall, S., & Mogotlane, S. M. (2012). *Reforming primary health care: A nursing perspective.* Geneva, Switzerland: International Council of Nurses, International Center for Human Resources in Nursing.

Buchholz, U., Bernard, H., Werber, D., Bohmer, M. M., Remschmidt, C., et al. (2011). German outbreak of *Escherichia coli* O104:H4 associated with sprouts. *New England Journal of Medicine*, *365*(19), 1763–1770. doi:10.1056/NEJMoa1106482.

Burnet, F. M. (1962). *Natural history of infectious disease* (3rd ed.). Cambridge, UK: Cambridge University Press.

Campbell, G. D., Jr., & Silberman, R. (1998). Drug-resistant *Streptococcus pneumoniae*. *Clinical Infectious Diseases*, *26*(5), 1188–1195.

Cartwright, E. J., Jackson, K. A., Johnson, S. D., Graves, L. M., Silk, B. J., & Mahon, B. E. (2013). Listeriosis outbreaks and associated food vehicles, United States, 1998–2008. *Emerging Infectious Diseases*, *19*(1), 1–9, quiz 184. doi:10.3201/eid1901.120393.

Centers for Disease Control and Prevention [CDC]. (1994). Addressing emerging infectious disease threats: A prevention strategy for the United States. Executive summary. *MMWR. Recommendations and Reports*, *43*(RR–5), 1–18.

Centers for Disease Control and Prevention [CDC]. (1999a). Four pediatric deaths from community-acquired methicillin-resistant *Staphylococcus aureus*—Minnesota and North Dakota, 1997–1999. *MMWR. Morbidity and Mortality Weekly Report*, *48*(32), 707–710.

Centers for Disease Control and Prevention [CDC]. (1999b). Update: Outbreak of Nipah virus—Malaysia and Singapore, 1999. *MMWR. Morbidity and Mortality Weekly Report*, *48*(16), 335–337.

Centers for Disease Control and Prevention [CDC]. (2000). West Nile virus activity—New York and New Jersey, 2000. *MMWR. Morbidity and Mortality Weekly Report*, *49*(28), 640–642.

Centers for Disease Control and Prevention [CDC]. (2003). Multistate outbreak of monkeypox—Illinois, Indiana, and Wisconsin, 2003. *MMWR. Morbidity and Mortality Weekly Report*, *52*(23), 537–540.

Centers for Disease Control and Prevention [CDC]. (2010a). Detection of Enterobacteriaceae isolates carrying metallo-beta-lactamase—United States, 2010. *MMWR. Morbidity and Mortality Weekly Report*, *59*(24), 750.

Centers for Disease Control and Prevention [CDC]. (2010b). Locally acquired Dengue—Key West, Florida, 2009-2010. *MMWR. Morbidity and Mortality Weekly Report*, *59*(19), 577–581.

Centers for Disease Control and Prevention [CDC]. (2012a). Active bacterial core surveillance (ABCs). Retrieved from *www.cdc.gov/abcs/index.html.*

Centers for Disease Control and Prevention [CDC]. (2012b). Centers for Disease Control and Prevention's vision for public health surveillance in the 21st century. *MMWR. Surveillance Summaries*, *61*(suppl.), 1–40.

Centers for Disease Control and Prevention [CDC]. (2012c). Vital signs: Preventing *Clostridium difficile* infections. *MMWR. Morbidity and Mortality Weekly Report*, *61*(9), 157–162.

Centers for Disease Control and Prevention [CDC]. (2013a). *Antibiotic resistance threats in the United States, 2013.* Atlanta, GA: Centers for Disease Control and Prevention.

Centers for Disease Control and Prevention [CDC]. (2013b). Centers for Disease Control and Prevention Global Disease Detection and Emergency Response. *Global Health*. Retrieved from *www.cdc.gov/globalhealth/gdder/.*

Centers for Disease Control and Prevention [CDC]. (2013c). Centers for Disease Control and Prevention grand rounds: The growing threat of multidrug-resistant gonorrhea. *MMWR. Morbidity and Mortality Weekly Report*, *62*(6), 103–106.

Centers for Disease Control and Prevention [CDC]. (2013d). *Clostridium difficile* infection. Healthcare-associated infections (HAIs). Retrieved from *www.cdc.gov/HAI/organisms/cdiff/Cdiff_infect.html.*

Centers for Disease Control and Prevention [CDC]. (2013e). Global control and regional elimination of measles, 2000–2011. *MMWR. Morbidity and Mortality Weekly Report*, *62*(2), 27–31.

Centers for Disease Control and Prevention [CDC]. (2013f). Multidrug-resistant *Bacteroides fragilis*—Seattle, Washington, 2013. *MMWR. Morbidity and Mortality Weekly Report*, *62*(34), 694–696.

Centers for Disease Control and Prevention [CDC]. (2013g). Notes from the field: *Salmonella* Bredeney infections linked to a brand of peanut butter—United States, 2012. *MMWR. Morbidity and Mortality Weekly Report*, *62*(6), 107.

Centers for Disease Control and Prevention [CDC]. (2014). Ebola virus disease. Retrieved from *www.cdc.gov/vhf/ebola/index.html.*

Cerda, R., & Lee, P. T. (2013). Modern cholera in the Americas: An opportunistic societal infection. *American Journal of Public Health*, *103*(11), 1934–1937. doi:10.2105/AJPH.2013.301567.

Chaisatit, C., Tribuddharat, C., Pulsrikarn, C., & Dejsirilert, S. (2012). Molecular characterization of antibiotic-resistant bacteria in contaminated chicken meat sold at supermarkets in Bangkok, Thailand. *Japanese Journal of Infectious Diseases*, *65*(6), 527–534.

Chevalier, M. S., Chung, W., Smith, J., Weil, L. M., Hughes, S. M., Joyner, S. N., et al. (2014). Ebola virus disease cluster in the United States—Dallas County, Texas, 2014. *MMWR*, *63*(46), 1087–1088.

Collignon, P. (2009). Resistant *Escherichia coli*—We are what we eat. *Clinical Infectious Diseases*, *49*(2), 202–204. doi:10.1086/599831.

Colon-Gonzalez, F. J., Fezzi, C., Lake, I. R., & Hunter, P. R. (2013). The effects of weather and climate change on dengue. *PLoS Neglected Tropical Diseases*, *7*(11), e2503. doi:10.1371/journal.pntd.0002503.

Cyranoski, D. (2005). China's chicken farmers under fire for antiviral abuse. *Nature*, *435*(7045), 1009. doi:10.1038/4351009a.

Davies, J., & Davies, D. (2010). Origins and evolution of antibiotic resistance. *Microbiology and Molecular Biology Reviews*, *74*(3), 417–433. doi:10.1128/MMBR.00016-10.

Dawood, F. S., Jain, S., Finelli, L., Shaw, M. W., Lindstrom, S., et al. (2009). Emergence of a novel swine-origin influenza A (H1N1) virus in humans. *New England Journal of Medicine*, *360*(25), 2605–2615. doi:10.1056/NEJMoa0903810.

Drew, R. H., White, R., MacDougall, C., Hermsen, E. D., & Owens, R. C., Jr. (2009). Insights from the Society of Infectious Diseases Pharmacists on antimicrobial stewardship guidelines from the Infectious Diseases Society of America and the Society for Healthcare Epidemiology of America. *Pharmacotherapy*, *29*(5), 593–607. doi:10.1592/phco.29.5.593.

Enright, M. C., Robinson, D. A., Randle, G., Feil, E. J., Grundmann, H., & Spratt, B. G. (2002). The evolutionary history of methicillin-resistant *Staphylococcus aureus* (MRSA). *Proceedings of National Academy of Sciences of the United States of America*, *99*(11), 7687–7692. doi:10.1073/pnas.122108599.

European Commission. (2005). Ban on antibiotics as growth promoters in animal feed enters into effect. (Regulation 1831/2003/EC on additives for use in animal nutrition, replacing Directive 70/524/EEC on additives in feeding-stuffs.) Retrieved from *europa.eu/rapid/press-release_IP-05-1687_en.htm.*

Finucane, M., & Spencer, J. H. (2013). *Rapid urbanization and infectious disease outbreaks: The case of avian influenza in Vietnam.* Recorded at the East-West Center Office in Washington, September 17, 2013. Honolulu, Hawaii: East-West Center.

Fleming, A. (1945). The assay of penicillin in the days before it was concentrated. *Health Organisation Bulletin, 12*(2), 250–252.

France, A. M., Jackson, M., Schrag, S., Lynch, M., & Zimmerman, C. (2010). Household transmission of 2009 influenza A (H1N1) virus after a school-based outbreak in New York City, April-May 2009. *Journal of Infectious Diseases, 201*(7), 984–992. doi:10.1086/651145.

Gatherer, D. (2014). The 2014 Ebola virus disease outbreak in West Africa. [Review]. *The Journal of General Virology, 95*(Pt. 8), 1619–1624. doi:10.1099/vir.0.067199-0.

Gayer, M., Legros, D., Formenty, P., & Connolly, M. A. (2007). Conflict and emerging infectious diseases. *Emerging Infectious Diseases, 13*(11), 1625–1631. doi:10.3201/eid1311.061093.

Ginsberg, J., Mohebbi, M. H., Patel, R. S., Brammer, L., Smolinski, M. S., & Brilliant, L. (2009). Detecting influenza epidemics using search engine query data. *Nature, 457*(7232), 1012–1014. doi:10.1038/nature07634.

Graham, J. P., Leibler, J. H., Price, L. B., Otte, J. M., & Pfeiffer, D. U. (2008). The animal-human interface and infectious disease in industrial food animal production: Rethinking biosecurity and biocontainment. *Public Health Reports, 123*(3), 282–299.

Green, D. A., Srinivas, N., Watz, N., Tenover, F. C., Amieva, M., & Banaei, N. (2013). A pediatric case of New Delhi metallo-beta-lactamase-1-producing *Enterobacteriaceae* in the United States. *The Pediatric Infectious Diseases Journal, 32*(11), 1291–1294. doi:10.1097/INF.0b013e31829eca34.

Griffin, D. E. (2010). Emergence and re-emergence of viral diseases of the central nervous system. *Progress in Neurobiology, 91*(2), 95–101. doi:10.1016/j.pneurobio.2009.12.003.

Haines, A., Kovats, R. S., Campbell-Lendrum, D., & Corvalan, C. (2006). Climate change and human health: impacts, vulnerability, and mitigation. *Lancet, 367*(9528), 2101–2109. doi:10.1016/S0140-6736(06)68933-2.

Hammerum, A. M., Toleman, M. A., Hansen, F., Kristensen, B., & Lester, C. H. (2010). Global spread of New Delhi metallo-beta-lactamase 1. *The Lancet Infectious Diseases, 10*(12), 829–830. doi:10.1016/S1473-3099(10)70276-0.

Hartocollis, A. (2009). Seeing warning signs of outbreak, school nurse set response in motion. *New York Times.* Retrieved from *www.nytimes.com/2009/04/27/nyregion/27response.html?pagewanted=all&_r=0.*

Henning, K. J. (2004). What is syndromic surveillance? *Morbidity and Mortality Weekly Report, 53*(Suppl.), 5–11.

Heuer, O. E., Hammerum, A. M., Collignon, P., & Wegener, H. C. (2006). Human health hazard from antimicrobial-resistant enterococci in animals and food. *Clinical Infectious Diseases, 43*(7), 911–916. doi:10.1086/507534.

Hollingsworth, T. D., Ferguson, N. M., & Anderson, R. M. (2007). Frequent travelers and rate of spread of epidemics. *Emerging Infectious Diseases, 13*(9), 1288–1294. doi:10.3201/eid1309.070081.

Hoogendoorn, M., Smalbrugge, M., Stobberingh, E. E., van Rossum, S. V., Vlaminckx, B. J., & Thijsen, S. F. (2013). Prevalence of antibiotic resistance of the commensal flora in Dutch nursing homes. *Journal of the American Medical Directors Association, 14*(5), 336–339. doi:10.1016/j.jamda.2012.11.001.

Hughes, J. M. (2011). Preserving the lifesaving power of antimicrobial agents. *JAMA: The Journal of the American Medical Association, 305*(10), 1027–1028. doi:10.1001/jama.2011.279.

Hutin, Y. J., Pool, V., Cramer, E. H., Nainan, O. V., Weth, J., et al. (1999). A multistate, foodborne outbreak of hepatitis A. National Hepatitis A Investigation Team. *New England Journal of Medicine, 340*(8), 595–602. doi:10.1056/NEJM199902253400802.

Infectious Diseases Society of America. (2010). The 10 ×'20 Initiative: Pursuing a global commitment to develop 10 new antibacterial drugs by 2020. *Clinical Infectious Diseases, 50*(8), 181–183.

Intergovernmental Panel on Climate Change [IPCC]. (2007). Fourth assessment report, Annex B: Glossary of terms. Retrieved from *http://www.ipcc.ch/pdf/assessment-report/ar4/wg3/ar4-wg3-annex1.pdf.*

International Society of Travel Medicine and Centers for Disease Control and Prevention. (2013). GeoSentinel: The Global Surveillance Network of the ISTM and CDC. Retrieved from *www.istm.org/geosentinel/main.html.*

Johnson, J. R., McCabe, J. S., White, D. G., Johnston, B., Kuskowski, M. A., & McDermott, P. (2009). Molecular analysis of *Escherichia coli* from retail meats (2002-2004) from the United States National Antimicrobial Resistance Monitoring System. *Clinical Infectious Diseases, 49*(2), 195–201.

Johnson, J. R., Sannes, M. R., Croy, C., Johnston, B., Clabots, C., et al. (2007). Antimicrobial drug-resistant *Escherichia coli* from humans and poultry products, Minnesota and Wisconsin, 2002-2004. *Emerging Infectious Diseases, 13*(6), 838–846. doi:10.3201/eid1306.061576.

Jones, K. E., Patel, N. G., Levy, M. A., Storeygard, A., & Balk, D. (2008). Global trends in emerging infectious diseases. *Nature, 451*(7181), 990–993. doi:10.1038/nature06536.

Jump, R. L., Riggs, M. M., Sethi, A. K., Pultz, M. J., Ellis-Reid, T., et al. (2010). Multihospital outbreak of *Clostridium difficile* infection, Cleveland, Ohio, USA. *Emerging Infectious Diseases, 16*(5), 827–829. doi:10.3201/eid1605.071606.

Kemp, M., Dargis, R., Andresen, K., & Christensen, J. J. (2012). A program against bacterial bioterrorism: Improved patient management and acquisition of new knowledge on infectious diseases. *Biosecurity and Bioterrorism, 10*(2), 203–207. doi:10.1089/bsp.2011.0055.

Kenneley, I. L. (2014). *Clostridium difficile* infection is on the rise. *American Journal of Nursing, 114*(3), 62–67. doi:10.1097/01.NAJ.0000444501.54723.5b.

Khanna, S., Pardi, D. S., Aronson, S. L., Kammer, P. P., Orenstein, R., et al. (2012). The epidemiology of community-acquired *Clostridium difficile* infection: A population-based study. *American Journal of Gastroenterology, 107*(1), 89–95. doi:10.1038/ajg.2011.398.

Kuehn, B. M. (2012). FDA aims to curb farm use of antibiotics. *JAMA: The Journal of the American Medical Association, 307*(21), 2244–2245. doi:10.1001/jama.2012.4560.

Landelle, C., Verachten, M., Legrand, P., Girou, E., Barbut, F., & Buisson, C. B. (2014). Contamination of healthcare workers' hands with *Clostridium difficile* spores after caring for patients with *C. difficile* infection. *Infection Control and Hospital Epidemiology, 35*(1), 10–15. doi:10.1086/674396.

Laxminarayan, R., Duse, A., Wattal, C., Zaidi, A. K., Wertheim, H. F., et al. (2013). Antibiotic resistance – the need for global solutions. *The Lancet Infectious Diseases, 13*(12), 1057–1098. doi:10.1016/S1473-3099(13)70318-9.

Lazer, D., Kennedy, R., King, G., & Vespignani, A. (2014). Big data. The parable of Google flu: Traps in big data analysis. *Science, 343*(6176), 1203–1205. doi:10.1126/science.1248506.

Lederberg, J. (1992). The interface of science and medicine. *The Mount Sinai Journal of Medicine, New York, 59*(5), 380–383.

Leibler, J. H., Otte, J., Roland-Holst, D., Pfeiffer, D. U., Soares Magalhaes, R., et al. (2009). Industrial food animal production and global health risks: Exploring the ecosystems and economics of avian influenza. *Ecohealth, 6*(1), 58–70. doi:10.1007/s10393-009-0226-0.

Lessler, J., Reich, N. G., Cummings, D. A., Nair, H. P., Jordan, H. T., & Thompson, N. (2009). Outbreak of 2009 pandemic influenza A (H1N1) at a New York City school. *New England Journal of Medicine, 361*(27), 2628–2636. doi:10.1056/NEJMoa0906089.

MacDonald, N., & Hebert, P. C. (2010). Polio outbreak in Tajikistan is cause for alarm. *Canadian Medical Association Journal, 182*(10), 1013. doi:10.1503/cmaj.100831.

Malhotra-Kumar, S., Lammens, C., Coenen, S., Van Herck, K., & Goossens, H. (2007). Effect of azithromycin and clarithromycin therapy on pharyngeal carriage of macrolide-resistant streptococci in healthy volunteers: A randomised, double-blind, placebo-controlled study. *Lancet, 369*(9560), 482–490. doi:10.1016/S0140-6736(07)60235-9.

McCollum, J. T., Cronquist, A. B., Silk, B. J., Jackson, K. A., O'Connor, K. A., et al. (2013). Multistate outbreak of listeriosis associated with cantaloupe. *New England Journal of Medicine, 369*(10), 944–953. doi:10.1056/NEJMoa1215837.

McDermott, W., & Rogers, D. E. (1982). Social ramifications of control of microbial disease. *The Johns Hopkins Medical Journal, 151*(6), 302–312.

McKinnon, M. (Ed..) (2012). *Climate vulnerability monitor: A guide to the cold calculus of a hot planet.* (2nd ed.). Madrid, Spain: Fundación DARA Internacional.

McLaughlin, J. B., DePaola, A., Bopp, C. A., Martinek, K. A., Napolilli, N. P., et al. (2005). Outbreak of *Vibrio parahaemolyticus* gastroenteritis associated with Alaskan oysters. *New England Journal of Medicine, 353*(14), 1463–1470. doi:10.1056/NEJMoa051594.

McMichael, A. J., Woodruff, R. E., & Hales, S. (2006). Climate change and human health: Present and future risks. *Lancet, 367*(9513), 859–869. doi:10.1016/S0140-6736(06)68079-3.

Mellon, M., Benbrook, C., & Benbrook, K. L. (2001). Hogging it: Estimates of antimicrobial abuse in livestock. *Union of Concerned Scientists,* (1), 23. Cambridge, MA: UCS Publications. Retrieved from *www.ucsusa.org/food_and_agriculture/our-failing-food-system/industrial-agriculture/hogging-it-estimates-of.html#.VliA4Vgo6L0.*

Meltzer, M. I., Atkins, C. Y., Santibanez, S., Knust, B., Petersen, B. W., Ervin, E. D., et al. (2014). Estimating the future number of cases in the ebola epidemic—Liberia and Sierra Leone, 2014-2015. *MMWR. Surveillance Summaries: Morbidity and Mortality Weekly Report. Surveillance Summaries, 63,* 1–14.

Morin, C. W., Comrie, A. C., & Ernst, K. (2013). Climate and dengue transmission: Evidence and implications. *Environmental Health Perspectives, 121*(11–12), 1264–1272. doi:10.1289/ehp.1306556.

Muehlenbein, M. (2012). Human-wildlife interactions and emerging infectious diseases. In E. Brondízio & E. Moran (Eds.), *Human-environment interactions: Current and future directions* (Vol. 1). London: Springer.

National Research Council. (2012). *Climate change. Evidence, impacts, choices. Answers to common questions about the science of climate change.* Washington, DC: National Academy of Sciences.

Newell, D. G., Koopmans, M., Verhoef, L., Duizer, E., Aidara-Kane, A., Sprong, H., et al. (2010). Food-borne diseases—The challenges of 20 years ago still persist while new ones continue to emerge. *International Journal of Food Microbiology, 139*(Suppl. 1), S3–S15.

Nicolaides, C., Cueto-Felgueroso, L., Gonzalez, M. C., & Juanes, R. (2012). A metric of influential spreading during contagion dynamics through the air transportation network. *PLoS ONE, 7*(7), e40961.

Nicolaides, C., Cueto-Felgueroso, L., & Juanes, R. (2012). The price of anarchy in mobility-driven contagion dynamics. *Journal of the Royal Society, Interface, 10*(87), 20130495.

Pannetier, D. B., Oestereich, L., Rieger, T., Koivogui, L., Magassouba, N., & Gunther, S. (2014). Emergence of Zaire Ebola virus disease in Guinea. [Research Support, Non-U.S. Government]. *The New England Journal of Medicine, 371*(15), 1418–1425. doi:10.1056/NEJMoa1404505.

Patrick, A. (2013). Cholera in Haiti takes a turn for the worse. *Lancet, 381*(9874), 1264.

Pavlin, B. I., Schloegel, L. M., & Daszak, P. (2009). Risk of importing zoonotic diseases through wildlife trade, United States. *Emerging Infectious Diseases, 15*(11), 1721–1726.

Pham, H. V., Doan, H. T., Phan, T. T., & Minh, N. N. (2011). Ecological factors associated with dengue fever in a Central Highlands province, Vietnam. *BMC Infectious Diseases, 11,* 172. doi:10.1186/1471-2334-11-172.

Plowright, R., Sokolow, S., Gorman, M., Daszak, P., & Foley, J. (2008). Causal inference in disease ecology: Investigating ecological drivers of disease emergence. *Frontiers in Ecology and the Environment, 6*(8), 420–429, doi. doi:10.1890/070086.

Rajabali, A., Moin, O., Ansari, A. S., Khanani, M. R., & Ali, S. H. (2009). Communicable disease among displaced Afghans: Refuge without shelter. *Nature Reviews. Microbiology, 7*(8), 609–614. doi:10.1038/nrmicro2176.

Reed, K. D., Melski, J. W., Graham, M. B., Regnery, R. L., Sotir, M. J., et al. (2004). The detection of monkeypox in humans in the Western Hemisphere. *New England Journal of Medicine, 350*(4), 342–350. doi:10.1056/NEJMoa032299.

Ribner, B. (2014). American health care workers who acquired disease while treating patients in West Africa. Infectious Disease Society of America Annual Conference, Philadelphia.

Roberts, R. R., Hota, B., Ahmad, I., Scott, R. D., 2nd, Foster, S. D., et al. (2009). Hospital and societal costs of antimicrobial-resistant infections in a Chicago teaching hospital: Implications for antibiotic stewardship. *Clinical Infectious Diseases, 49*(8), 1175–1184. doi:10.1086/605630.

Rogers, D. J., Suk, J., & Semenza, J. C. (2014). Using global maps to predict the risk of dengue in Europe. *Acta Tropica, 129,* 1–14. doi:10.1016/j.actatropica.2013.08.008.

Ruan, S., Wang, W., & Levin, S. A. (2006). The effect of global travel on the spread of SARS. *Mathematical Biosciences and Engineering, 3*(1), 2005–2018.

Shuaib, F., Gunnala, R., Musa, E. O., Mahoney, F. J., Oguntimehin, O., Nguku, P. M., et al. (2014). Ebola virus disease outbreak—Nigeria, July-September 2014. *MMWR, 63*(39), 867–872.

Smith, D. L., Harris, A. D., Johnson, J. A., Silbergeld, E. K., & Morris, J. G. (2002). Animal antibiotic use has an early but important impact on the emergence of antibiotic resistance in human commensal bacteria. *Proceedings of the National Academy of Sciences of the United States of America, 99*(9), 6434–6439.

Solomon, S., Plattner, G. K., Knutti, R., & Friedlingstein, P. (2009). Irreversible climate change due to carbon dioxide emissions. *Proceedings of National Academy of Sciences of the United States of America, 106*(6), 1704–1709. doi:10.1073/pnas.0812721105.

Specter, M. (2012). Germs are us. *The New Yorker.* Retrieved from *www.newyorker.tumblr.com/post/39657878414/germs-are-us.*

Stryjewski, M. E., & Corey, G. R. (2014). Methicillin-resistant *Staphylococcus aureus:* An evolving pathogen. *Clinical Infectious Diseases, 58*(Suppl. 1), S10–S19. doi:10.1093/cid/cit613.

Subbarao, K., Klimov, A., Katz, J., Regnery, H., Lim, W., et al. (1998). Characterization of an avian influenza A (H5N1) virus isolated from a child with a fatal respiratory illness. *Science, 279*(5349), 393–396.

Tana, Z. X., Lal, R., & Wiebe, K. D. (2005). Global soil nutrient depletion and yield reduction. *Journal of Sustainable Agriculture, 26*(1), 123–146.

Theriot, C. M., & Young, V. B. (2014). Microbial and metabolic interactions between the gastrointestinal tract and infection. *Gut Microbes, 5*(1), 86–95.

Thornton, P. K. (2010). Livestock production: Recent trends, future prospects. *Philosophical Transactions of the Royal Society. London B. Biological Sciences, 365*(1554), 2853–2867. doi:10.1098/rstb.2010.0134.

Tosh, P. K., & McDonald, L. C. (2012). Infection control in the multidrug-resistant era: Tending the human microbiome. *Clinical Infectious Diseases, 54*(5), 707–713. doi:10.1093/cid/cir899.

UNAIDS. (2013). *Global report: UNAIDS report on the global AIDS epidemic 2013.* New York: United Nations.

United Nations High Commission on Refugees [UNHCR]. (2013). UNHCR mid-year trends 2013. Retrieved from *www.unhcr.org/52af08d26.html.*

United Nations [UN]. (2012a). World population prospects: The 2012 revision. Retrieved December 17, 2013, from *esa.un.org/unpd/wpp/index.htm.*

United Nations [UN]. (2012b). World urbanization prospects, the 2011 revision. Retrieved from *www.un.org/en/development/desa/publications/world-urbanization-prospects-the-2011-revision.html*.

United Nations [UN]. (2013). *The millennium development goals report 2013*. New York: United Nations.

U.S. Food and Drug Administration [FDA]. (2012). The judicious use of medically important antimicrobial drugs in food-producing animals. Retrieved from *www.fda.gov/downloads/animalveterinary/guidancecomplianceenforcement/guidanceforindustry/ucm216936.pdf*.

van Panhuis, W. G., Grefenstette, J., Jung, S. Y., Chok, N. S., Cross, A., et al. (2013). Contagious diseases in the United States from 1888 to the present. *New England Journal of Medicine, 369*(22), 2152–2158. doi:10.1371/journal.pone.0040961.

von Borell, E. (1995). Neuroendocrine integration of stress and significance of stress for the performance of farm animals. *Applied Animal Behaviour Science, 44*(2–4), 219–227. doi:10.1001/jamainternmed.2013.11673.

Viana, D. V., & Ignotti, E. (2013). The occurrence of dengue and weather changes in Brazil: A systematic review. *Revista Brasileira de Epidemiologia, 16*(2), 240–256. doi:10.1590/S1415-790X2013000200002.

Wang, H., Chen, M., & China Nosocomial Pathogens Resistance Surveillance Study Group. (2005). Surveillance for antimicrobial resistance among clinical isolates of gram-negative bacteria from intensive care unit patients in China, 1996 to 2002. *Diagnostic Microbiology and Infectious Disease, 51*(3), 201–208. doi:10.1016/j.diagmicrobio.2004.09.001.

Weaver, S. C. (2013). Urbanization and geographic expansion of zoonotic arboviral diseases: Mechanisms and potential strategies for prevention. *Trends in Microbiology, 21*(8), 360–363. doi:10.1016/j.tim.2013.03.003.

Wells, K. D. (2013). Natural genotypes via genetic engineering. *Proceedings of National Academy of Sciences of the United States of America, 110*(41), 16295–16296. doi:10.1073/pnas.1315623110.

White, D. G., Zhao, S., Sudler, R., Ayers, S., Friedman, S., et al. (2001). The isolation of antibiotic-resistant *Salmonella* from retail ground meats. *New England Journal of Medicine, 345*(16), 1147–1154, doi. doi:10.1056/NEJMoa010315.

Wilcox, B. E. (2006). Forests and emerging infectious diseases of humans. Rome: Food and Agriculture Organization of the United Nations. Retrieved from *www.fao.org/docrep/009/a0789e/a0789e00.htm*.

Wolfe, N. D., Dunavan, C. P., & Diamond, J. (2007). Origins of major human infectious diseases. *Nature, 447*(7142), 279–283.

World Health Organization [WHO]. (1978). Ebola haemorrhagic fever in Zaire, 1976. *Bulletin of the World Health Organization, 56*(2), 271–293. Geneva: World Health Organization. Retrieved from *www.ncbi.nlm.nih.gov/pmc/articles/PMC2395567/*.

World Health Organization [WHO]. (2007). International health regulations 2005. Geneva: World Health Organization. Retrieved from *www.who.int/ihr/publications/9789241596664/en/index.html*.

World Health Organization [WHO]. (2008). *Climate change and health: Agenda item of the sixty first World Health Assembly*. Geneva: World Health Organization.

World Health Organization [WHO]. (2009). *Protecting health from climate change: Connecting science, policy and people*. Geneva: World Health Organization.

World Health Organization [WHO]. (2012a). *Global report for research on global diseases of poverty*. Geneva: World Health Organization.

World Health Organization [WHO]. (2012b). *Global strategy for dengue prevention and control 2012-2020*. Geneva: World Health Organization.

World Health Organization [WHO]. (2012c). Self-prescription of antibiotics boosts superbugs epidemic in the European region. Geneva: World Health Organization. Retrieved from *www.euro.who.int/en/media-centre/sections/latest-press-releases/self-prescription-of-antibiotics-boosts-superbugs-epidemic-in-the-european-region*.

World Health Organization [WHO]. (2013). Polio in the Syrian Arab Republic. Geneva: World Health Organization. Retrieved from *www.who.int/csr/don/2013_10_29/en/index.html*.

World Health Organization [WHO]. (2014). *Global Alert and Response (GAR)*. Geneva: World Health Organization. Retrieved from *www.who.int/csr/en/*.

Wyman, R. J. (2013). The effects of population on the depletion of fresh water. *Population and Development Review, 39*, 687–704. doi:10.1111/j.1728-4457.2013.00634.

Yang, G. J., Utzinger, J., & Zhou, X. N. (2013). Interplay between environment, agriculture and infectious diseases of poverty: Case studies in China. *Acta Tropica*. doi:10.1016/j.actatropica.2013.07.009.

Zilberberg, M. D., Shorr, A. F., & Kollef, M. H. (2008). Increase in adult *Clostridium difficile*-related hospitalizations and case-fatality rate, United States, 2000-2005. *Emerging Infectious Diseases, 14*(6), 929–931. doi:10.3201/eid1406.071447.

ONLINE RESOURCES

Careful Use of Antibiotics
www.cdc.gov/getsmart/index.html
Centers for Disease Control and Prevention (CDC)
www.cdc.org
Center for Infectious Disease Research and Policy (CIDRAP)
www.cidrap.unm.edu
One Health
www.onehealthinitiative.com
Promed
www.promedmail.org
World Health Organization (WHO)
www.who.int

Index

Page numbers followed by *b*, *t*, or *f* refer to boxes, tables, or figures, respectively.